Orthopedic Physical Assessment

Orthopedic Physical Assessment

THIRD EDITION

David J. Magee, Ph.D., B.P.T.

Professor
Department of Physical Therapy
Faculty of Rehabilitation Medicine
University of Alberta
Edmonton, Alberta, Canada

W.B. SAUNDERS COMPANY
A Division of Harcourt Brace & Company

Philadelphia   London   Toronto
Montreal   Sydney   Tokyo

W.B. SAUNDERS COMPANY

A Division of Harcourt Brace & Company

The Curtis Center
Independence Square West
Philadelphia, Pennsylvania 19106

Library of Congress Cataloging-in-Publication Data

Magee, David J.
Orthopedic physical assessment / David J. Magee.—3rd ed.

p.   cm.

Includes bibliographical references and index.

ISBN 0-7216-6290-0

1. Orthopedics—Diagnosis.   2. Physical diagnosis.   3. Physical
orthopedic tests.   I. Title.
[DNLM: 1. Bone Diseases—diagnosis. 2. Joint Diseases—
diagnosis.   3. Orthopedics—methods. 4. Physical
Examination—methods.   WE 168 M191o 1997]

RD734.M34 1997   617.3—dc20

DNLM/DLC   96-41121

ORTHOPEDIC PHYSICAL ASSESSMENT   ISBN 0-7216-6290-0

Printed in the United States of America.

Last digit is the print number: 9   8   7   6   5   4   3   2

To my parents,
who taught me to pick a goal
in life and to take it seriously

Preface to the First Edition

This manuscript was originally developed as part of a manual for physical therapy students at the University of Alberta. That original manual covered conditions and treatment as well as assessment.

The text is the result of my interpretation of the teachings of recognized experts in the field of orthopedic assessment: James Cyriax, Hans Debrunner, Stanley Hoppenfeld, Freddy Kaltenborn, Geoff Maitland, Robin McKenzie, John Mennell, and Alan Stoddard, to name a few. It is my belief that a book such as this will be of benefit to paramedical and medical students throughout their training and into their practice as well as to other health professionals.

The aim of the book is to provide the reader with a systematic approach to carry out an orthopedic assessment and an understanding of the reason for the various aspects of the assessment. Initially, in each chapter, pertinent arthrology is reviewed. The reader is then taken through history, observation, and examination of each joint of the body. The examination is organized in a consistent fashion beginning with active, passive, and resisted isometric movements. The movements are followed by tests designed by different individuals to evaluate specific structures, and a quick assessment of sensory distribution and reflexes to differentiate between peripheral nerves and nerve root problems. Palpation is discussed next to help the examiner pinpoint the problem. The assessment is concluded by a review of different roentgenographic views and the possible findings that the examiner might see in these views.

At the end of each chapter is a précis for quick review prior to beginning an assessment and a list of references should the examiner wish to do further in-depth reading.

The text is liberally provided with artistic renderings and photos to illustrate different points and to provide visual examples of the conditions and anatomic variations referred to in the manuscript.

This book is my first attempt at a project of this magnitude. Any feedback from readers with constructive ideas of how to improve the text would be greatly appreciated.

David J. Magee
1987

Preface to the Second Edition

The second edition of *Orthopedic Physical Assessment* is an update and rearrangement of information provided in the first edition. In most chapters, several different ways of testing structures are given. This is done not to confuse the reader but to give the reader a choice. The examiner should use the technique that he or she finds works the best and that gives the best results. By providing several tests for the same structures, the book acts as a reference source. I have added new sections dealing with functional assessment and new radiographic techniques to each chapter. Case studies included at the end of most chapters provide the reader with assessment exercises. Two new chapters, "Head and Face" and "Emergency Sports Assessment," have been added at the suggestion of some readers of the first edition.

I am grateful to all those who spoke to me or wrote offering suggestions and corrections to the first edition, especially the late Gail Gilewich. Their help was very much appreciated and many of their suggestions have been incorporated into the second edition. I hope readers will provide feedback to this edition as well.

David J. Magee
1992

Preface to the Third Edition

This third edition of *Orthopedic Physical Assessment* has been revised in response to comments from colleagues and students and to reflect the development of new knowledge in the field of neuromusculoskeletal assessment.

The aim of the book remains the same: to provide the reader with a systematic approach to perform a neuromusculoskeletal assessment and to understand the reason for the various aspects of the assessment. The principles and methods are the same, but new concepts and ideas have been added, as have many new references.

This edition has many new photographs and line drawings which will hopefully be clearer and make it easier to understand the concepts and methods of assessment. The different parts of the assessment are highlighted to a greater degree, as are important concepts and ideas. In response to my students' requests, in the special tests sections I have highlighted the more common tests performed at each joint. This does not mean the other tests are not useful or not important; they just are used less frequently. As well, I have gone into greater detail on peripheral nerve assessment so that one is able to differentiate between symptoms from radicular problems and symptoms from peripheral nerve problems in the context of neuromusculoskeletal assessment. I have included examples of differential diagnosis tables as examples of how the reader might decide what pathology is causing the problem. I have added a new chapter on Preparticipation Evaluation, as this information ties in very nicely with assessment of specific joints and is most commonly associated with neuromusculoskeletal assessment as well as assessment of other areas of the body.

I have been very fortunate in the acceptance of *Orthopedic Physical Assessment* by the health care professions. Its translation into French, Japanese, and Spanish is extremely gratifying and humbling. The feedback I have received has been very encouraging, and I appreciate very much the input from people in different health care professions who have taken the time to point out modifications and additions to the text that have made it better. Without the help of my students, my colleagues around the world—the people who did the research and developed the different concepts of assessment, and the individuals who have offered encouraging support, this book would not enjoy the success it does today.

David J. Magee

Acknowledgments

The writing of a book such as this, although a task undertaken by one person, is in reality the bringing together of ideas, concepts, and teachings developed and put forward by colleagues, friends, clinicians, and experts in the field of neuromusculoskeletal assessment.

In particular, I would like to thank the following people:

My family, for putting up with my moods and idiosyncrasies.

Bev Aindow, my irreplaceable secretary and the best developmental editor a person could ask for. Without her help, encouragement, and persistence, this edition would still be "on the drawing board"!

My undergraduate, graduate, and postgraduate students in Canada and the United States who provided me with many ideas for revisions and who collected many of the articles used as references.

The many authors and publishers who were kind enough to allow me to use their photographs, drawings, and tables in the text so that explanations could be clearer and more easily understood. Without these additions, the book would not be what I hoped.

My photographers, Paul Wodehouse and Gord Evjen, whose photographic talents along with those of Ted Huff, my artist, add immeasurably to the book.

My models, Alan Garard, Georgina Gray, Marney Dickey, Doug Gilroy, Martin Parfitt, Judy Chepeha, Doug Leong, Karen Fonteyne, Bev Aindow, Trent Brown, Ian Halworth, Dwayne Mandrusiak, Leslie Ann Marcuk, Kevin Wagner, Jim Meadows, and my family, Wendy, Shawn, and Bernice. Your patience and help is very much appreciated.

My colleagues who contributed ideas, suggestions, radiographs, and photographs and who typed and reviewed the manuscripts; in particular, Dr. David C. Reid, Dorothy Tomniuk, Dr. E. G. Parkinson, Ms. Kehoe, Martin Parfitt, and Donna Ford.

Margaret Biblis, Amy Norwitz, Shelley Hampton, Tracy Baldwin, Christa Fratantoro, and others at W.B. Saunders Company for their ideas, assistance, and patience in all three editions.

My teachers, colleagues, and mentors who encouraged me to pursue my chosen career.

To these people and many others—Thank you for your help and encouragement. Your support played a large part in the success and completion of this book.

David J. Magee

Contents

Orthopedic Physical Assessment

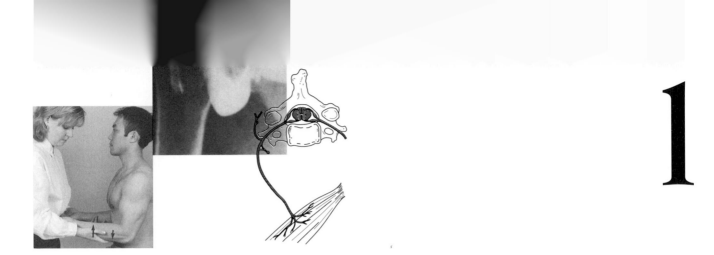

Principles and Concepts

To complete a musculoskeletal assessment of a patient, it is important to carry out a proper and thorough systematic examination. A correct diagnosis depends on a knowledge of functional anatomy, an accurate patient history, diligent observation, and a thorough examination. The differential diagnosis process can involve the use of clinical signs and symptoms, physical examination, knowledge of pathology and mechanisms of injury, provocative tests, and laboratory and diagnostic imaging techniques. It is only through a complete and systematic assessment that an accurate diagnosis can be made. The purpose of the assessment should be to fully and clearly understand the patient's problems, from the patient's perspective as well as the clinician's, and the physical basis for the symptoms that have caused the patient to complain. As James Cyriax stated, "Diagnosis is only a matter of applying one's anatomy."[1]

One of the more common assessment recording methods used is the problem-oriented medical records method, which uses "SOAP" notes.[2] SOAP stands for the four parts of the assessment: Subjective, Objective, Assessment, and Plan. This method is especially useful in helping the examiner to solve a problem. In this book, the subjective portion of the assessment is covered under Patient History, objective under Observation, and assessment under Examination.

Although the text deals primarily with orthopedic physical assessment on an outpatient basis, it can easily be adapted for the evaluation of inpatients. The primary difference is in adapting the assessment to the needs of a bedridden patient. Often, an inpatient's diagnosis has been made previously, and any continuing assessment is modified to determine how the patient's condition is responding to treatment. Likewise, the outpatient is continually assessed during treatment, and the assessment is modified to reflect the patient's response to treatment.

Regardless of which system is selected for assessment, the examiner should establish a **sequential method** to ensure that nothing is overlooked. The assessment must be organized, comprehensive, and reproducible. In general, the examiner compares one side of the body, which is assumed to be normal, with the other side of the body, which is abnormal or injured. For this reason, the examiner must come to understand and know the wide variability in what is considered normal. In addition, the examiner should focus attention on only one aspect of the assessment at a time.

Total Musculoskeletal Assessment

- Patient history
- Observation
- Examination of movement
- Special tests
- Reflexes and cutaneous distribution
- Joint play movements
- Palpation
- Diagnostic imaging

At the end of each chapter, the reader is provided with a summary, or précis, of the assessment procedures for that chapter. This section enables the examiner to quickly review the pertinent steps of assessment for the joint or structure being assessed. If further information is required, the examiner can refer to the more detailed sections of the chapter.

Patient History

A complete medical history should be taken and written to ensure reliability. Naturally, emphasis should be placed on that portion of the assessment having the greatest clinical relevance. Often, the examiner can make the diagnosis by simply **listening to the patient**. No subject areas should be skipped. Repetition helps the examiner to become familiar with the characteristic history of the patient's complaints, so that unusual deviation, which often indicates problems, can be noticed immediately. Even if the diagnosis is obvious, the history provides valuable information about the disorder, its prognosis, and the appropriate treatment. The history also enables the examiner to determine the type of person the patient is, the treatment the patient has received, and the behavior of the injury. In addition to the history of the present illness or injury, relevant past history, treatment, and results should be noted. Past medical history should include any major illnesses, surgery, accidents, or allergies. In some cases, it may be necessary to delve into the social and family histories of the patient if they appear relevant. Lifestyle habit patterns, including sleep patterns, stress, work load, and recreational pursuits, should also be noted.

It is important that the examiner keep the patient focused and discourage irrelevant information; this should be done politely but firmly. Questions and answers should provide practical information about the problem. At the same time, to obtain optimum results in the assessment, it is important to establish a good rapport with the patient. In addition, the examiner should listen for any potential "red flag" signs and symptoms (Table 1–1) that would indicate the need to involve a medical practitioner.[3]

The history is usually taken in an orderly sequence. It offers the patient an opportunity to describe the problem and the limitations caused by the problem as he or she perceives them. To achieve a good functional outcome, it is essential that the clinician pay heed to the patient's concerns and expectations for treatment. After all, the history is the patient's report of his or her own condition. The questions asked should be easy to understand and should not "lead" the patient. For example, the examiner should not say, "Does this increase your pain?" It would be better to say, "Does this alter your pain in any way?" The examiner should ask one question at a time and receive an answer to each question before proceeding with another question. Open-ended questions ask for narrative information; closed or direct questions ask for specific information. Direct questions are often used to fill in details of information given in open-ended questions, and they frequently require only a one-word answer, such as "yes" or "no." The examiner should seek answers to the following pertinent questions.

1. What is the patient's age? Many conditions occur within certain age ranges. For example, various growth disorders, such as Legg-Perthes disease or Scheuermann's disease, are seen in adolescents or teenagers. Degenerative conditions, such as osteoarthritis and osteoporosis, are more likely to be seen in an older population.

2. What is the patient's occupation? For example, a laborer probably has stronger muscles than a sedentary worker and may be less likely to suffer a muscle strain. However, laborers are more susceptible to injury because of the types of jobs they have. Because sedentary workers usually have no need for high levels of muscle strength, they may overstress their muscles or joints on weekends because of overactivity or participation in activity they are not used to. It is important to remember that habitual postures and repetitive strain caused by some occupations may indicate the location or source of the problem.

3. Why has the patient come for help? This is often referred to as the history of the present illness or chief

Table 1–1
"Red Flag" Findings in Patient History That Indicate Need for Referral to Physician

Cancer	Persistent pain at night
	Constant pain anywhere in the body
	Unexplained weight loss (e.g., 4.5 to 6.8 kg [10 to 15 lb] in 2 weeks or less)
	Loss of appetite
	Unusual lumps or growths
	Unwarranted fatigue
Cardiovascular	Shortness of breath
	Dizziness
	Pain or a feeling of heaviness in the chest
	Pulsating pain anywhere in the body
	Constant and severe pain in lower leg (calf) or arm
	Discolored or painful feet
	Swelling (no history of injury)
Gastrointestinal/ Genitourinary	Frequent or severe abdominal pain
	Frequent heartburn or indigestion
	Frequent nausea or vomiting
	Change in or problems with bladder function (e.g., urinary tract infection)
	Unusual menstrual irregularities
Miscellaneous	Fever or night sweats
	Recent severe emotional disturbances
	Swelling or redness in any joint with no history of injury
	Pregnancy
Neurological	Changes in hearing
	Frequent or severe headaches with no history of injury
	Problems with swallowing or changes in speech
	Changes in vision (e.g., blurriness or loss of sight)
	Problems with balance, coordination, or falling
	Fainting spells (drop attacks)
	Sudden weakness

Data from Stith, J.S., S.A. Sahrmann, K.K. Dixon, and B.J. Norton: Curriculum to prepare diagnosticians in physical therapy. J. Phys. Ther. Educ. 9:50, 1995.

complaint. This part of the history provides an opportunity for patients to describe in their own words what is bothering them and the extent to which it bothers them.

4. Was there any inciting trauma (macrotrauma) or repetitive activity (microtrauma)? In other words, what was the mechanism of injury, and were there any predisposing factors? If the patient was in a motor vehicle accident, for example, was the patient the driver or the passenger? Was he or she the cause of the accident? What part of the car was hit? How fast were the cars going? Was the patient wearing a seat belt? When asking questions about the mechanism(s) of injury, the examiner must try to determine the direction and magnitude of the injuring force and how the force was applied. By carefully listening to the patient, the examiner can often determine which structures were injured and how severely by knowing the force and mechanism of injury. For example, anterior dislocations of the shoulder usually occur when the arm is abducted and laterally rotated beyond the normal range of motion, and the "terrible triad" injury to the knee (medial collateral ligament, anterior cruciate ligament, and medial meniscus injury) usually occurs from a blow to the lateral side of the knee while the knee is flexed, the full weight of the patient is on the knee, and the foot is fixed. Likewise, the examiner should determine whether there were any predisposing, unusual, or new factors, such as sustained postures or repetitive activities, general health, or familial or genetic problems, that may have led to the problem.[4]

5. Was the onset of the problem slow or sudden? Did the condition start as an insidious, mild ache and then progress to continuous pain, or was there a specific episode in which the body part was injured? If inciting trauma has occurred, it is often relatively easy to determine the location of the problem. Does the pain get worse as the day progresses? Was the sudden onset caused by trauma, or was it sudden with locking? Is there anything that relieves the symptoms? Knowledge of these facts helps the examiner make a differential diagnosis.

6. Where are the symptoms that bother the patient? If possible, have the patient point to the area. Does the patient point to a specific structure, or is a more general area delineated? The latter may indicate a more severe condition or referral of symptoms. The way in which the patient describes the symptoms often helps delineate problems.

7. Where was the pain or other symptoms when the patient first had the complaint? Has the pain moved or spread? The patient should be asked to point to exactly where the pain was and where it is now. Are trigger points present? Trigger points are very localized areas of hyperirritability within the tissues; they are tender to compression, are often accompanied by tight bands of tissue, and, if sufficiently hypersensitive, may give rise to referred pain that is steady, deep, and aching. These

trigger points can lead to a diagnosis, because pressure on them reproduces the patient's symptoms. Trigger points are not found in normal muscles.[5]

In general, the area of pain enlarges or becomes more distal as the lesion worsens and becomes smaller or more localized as it improves. The more distal and superficial the problem, the more accurately the patient can determine the location of the pain. In the case of referred pain, the patient usually points out a general area; with a localized lesion, the patient points to a specific location. Referred pain tends to be felt deeply; its boundaries are indistinct, and it radiates segmentally without crossing the midline. The term **referred pain** means that the pain is felt at a site other than the injured tissue because the referred site is supplied by the same or adjacent neural segments. Pain also may shift as the lesion shifts. For example, with an internal derangement of the knee, pain may occur in flexion one time and in extension another time if it is caused by a loose body within the joint. The examiner must clearly understand where the patient feels the pain. For example, does the pain occur only at the end of the range of motion (ROM), in part of the range, or throughout the ROM?[4]

8. What are the exact movements or activities that cause pain? At this stage, the patient should not be asked to do the movements or activities; they will take place during the examination. However, the examiner should remember which movements the patient says are painful so that, when the examination is carried out, these movements can be done last to avoid overflow of painful symptoms. With cessation of the activity, does the pain stay the same, or how long does it take to return to normal? Are there any other factors that aggravate or help to relieve the pain? Is there any alteration in intensity of the pain with these activities? The answers to these questions give the examiner some idea of the irritability of the joint. Functionally, pain can be divided into seven levels, especially for repetitive stress conditions:

Level 1: Pain after specific activity
Level 2: Pain after specific activity resolving with
warm-up
Level 3: Pain during and after specific activity
which does not affect performance
Level 4: Pain during and after specific activity
which does affect performance
Level 5: Pain with activities of daily living (ADL)
Level 6: Constant dull aching pain at rest which
does not disturb sleep
Level 7: Dull aching pain which does disturb sleep

9. How long has the problem existed? What are the duration and frequency of the symptoms? Answers to these questions help the examiner to determine whether the condition is acute, subacute, chronic, or acute on chronic and to develop an idea of the patient's tolerance to pain. Generally, acute conditions are those that have

been present for 7 to 10 days. Subacute conditions have been present for 10 days to 7 weeks, and chronic conditions or symptoms have been present for longer than 7 weeks. In acute on chronic cases, the injured tissues usually have been reinjured. This knowledge is also beneficial in terms of how vigorously the patient can be examined. For example, the more acute the condition, the less stress the examiner is able to apply to the joints and tissues during the assessment. A full examination may not be possible in very acute conditions. In that case, the examiner must select those procedures of as-

sessment that will give the greatest amount of information with the least stress to the patient. Does the patient protect or support the injured part? If so, it is an indication of discomfort and fear of pain if the part moves.

10. Has the condition occurred before? If so, what was the onset like? Where was the site of the original condition, and has there been any radiation (spread) of the symptoms? If the patient is feeling better, how long did the recovery take? Did any treatment help to relieve symptoms? Does the current problem appear to be the same as the previous problem, or is it different? If it is

---

McGill-Melzack
PAIN QUESTIONNAIRE

Patient's name _____   Age _____
File No. _____   Date _____
Clinical category (e.g., cardiac, neurological, etc.):

Diagnosis : _____
_____
_____

Analgesic (if already administered):
   1. Type _____
   2. Dosage _____
   3. Time given in relation to this test _____
Patient's intelligence: circle number that represents best estimate

1 (low)   2   3   4   5(high)

****

This questionnaire has been designed to tell us more about your pain. Four major questions we ask are:
   1. Where is your pain?
   2. What does it feel like?
   3. How does it change with time?
   4. How strong is it?

It is important that you tell us how your pain feels now. Please follow the instructions at the beginning of each part.

© R. Melzack, Oct. 1970

Part 1.   Where Is Your Pain?

Please mark, on the drawings below, the areas where you feel pain. Put E if external, or I if internal, near the areas which you mark. Put EI if both external and internal.

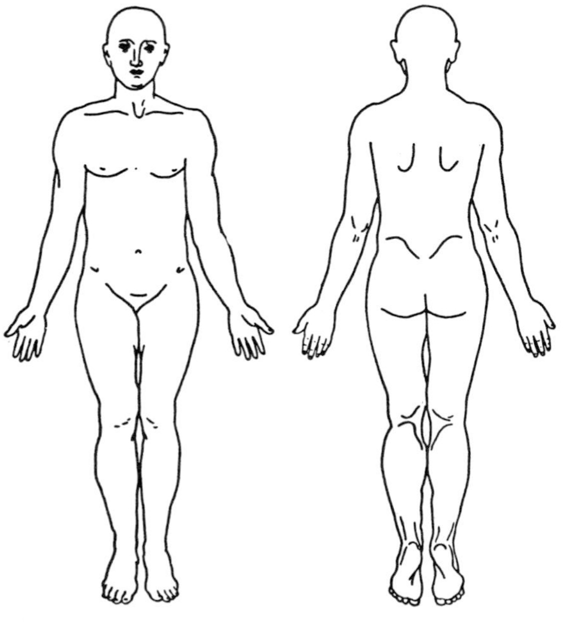

Part 2.   What Does Your Pain Feel Like?

Some of the words below describe your present pain. Circle ONLY those words that best describe it. Leave out any category that is not suitable. Use only a single word in each appropriate category—the one that applies best.

1	2	3	4
Flickering	Jumping	Pricking	Sharp
Quivering	Flashing	Boring	Cutting
Pulsing	Shooting	Drilling	Lacerating
Throbbing		Stabbing	
Beating		Lancinating	
Pounding			

5	6	7	8
Pinching	Tugging	Hot	Tingling
Pressing	Pulling	Burning	Itchy
Gnawing	Wrenching	Scalding	Smarting
Cramping		Searing	Stinging
Crushing			

9	10	11	12
Dull	Tender	Tiring	Sickening
Sore	Taut	Exhausting	Suffocating
Hurting	Rasping		
Aching	Splitting		
Heavy			

13	14	15	16
Fearful	Punishing	Wretched	Annoying
Frightful	Gruelling	Blinding	Troublesome
Terrifying	Cruel		Miserable
	Vicious		Intense
	Killing		Unbearable

17	18	19	20
Spreading	Tight	Cool	Nagging
Radiating	Numb	Cold	Nauseating
Penetrating	Drawing	Freezing	Agonizing
Piercing	Squeezing		Dreadful
	Tearing		Torturing

Part 3.   How Does Your Pain Change With Time?

1. Which word or words would you use to describe the pattern of your pain?

1	2	3
Continuous	Rhythmic	Brief
Steady	Periodic	Momentary
Constant	Intermittent	Transient

2. What kind of things relieve your pain?

3. What kind of things increase your pain?

Part 4.   How Strong Is Your Pain?

People agree that the following 5 words represent pain of increasing intensity. They are:

1	2	3	4	5
Mild	Discomforting	Distressing	Horrible	Excruciating

To answer each question below, write the number of the most appropriate word in the space beside the question.

1. Which word describes your pain right now?   _____
2. Which word describes it at its worst?   _____
3. Which word describes it when it is least?   _____
4. Which word describes the worst toothache you ever had?   _____
5. Which word describes the worst headache you ever had?   _____
6. Which word describes the worst stomach-ache you ever had?   _____

Figure 1–1

McGill-Melzack Pain Questionnaire. (From Melzack, R.: The McGill pain questionnaire: Major properties and scoring methods. Pain 1:280–281, 1975.)

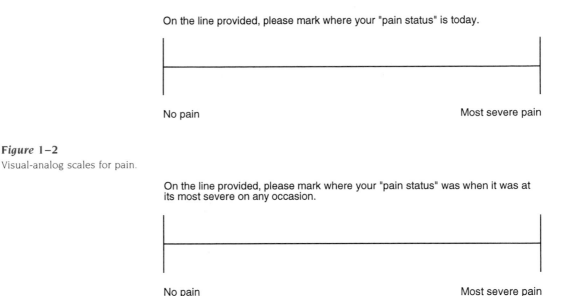

On the line provided, please mark where your "pain status" is today.

No pain   Most severe pain

Figure 1–2
Visual-analog scales for pain.

On the line provided, please mark where your "pain status" was when it was at its most severe on any occasion.

No pain   Most severe pain

different, how is it different? Answers to these questions help the examiner to determine the location and severity of the injury.

11. Are the intensity, duration, and/or frequency of pain or other symptoms increasing? These changes usually mean the condition is getting worse. A decrease in pain or other symptoms usually means the condition is improving. Is the pain static? If so, how long has it been that way? This question may help the examiner to determine the present state of the problem. These factors may become important in treatment and may help to determine whether a treatment is helping. Are pain or other symptoms associated with other physiological functions? For example, is the pain worse with menstruation? If so, when did the patient last have a pelvic examination? Questions such as these may give the examiner an indication of what is causing the problem or what factors affect the problem. It is often worthwhile to provide the patient with a pain questionnaire or a visual-analog scale (VAS) that can be completed while the patient is waiting to be assessed. In the McGill-Melzack pain questionnaire (Fig. 1–1),[6] three major classes of word descriptors—sensory, affective, and evaluative—are used by patients to describe their pain experience. Other pain-rating scales allow the patient to visually gauge the amount of pain along a solid 10-cm line (Fig. 1–2) or on a thermometer-type scale (Fig. 1–3).[7] It has been shown that an examiner should consistently use the same pain scales when assessing or reassessing patients to increase consistent results.[8–10] The examiner can use the completed questionnaire or scale as an indication of the pain as described or perceived by the patient.

12. Is the pain constant, periodic, episodic (occurring with certain activities), or occasional? Does the condition bother the patient at that exact moment? If the patient is not bothered at that exact moment, the pain is not constant. If the pain is periodic or occasional, the examiner should try to determine the activity, position, or posture that irritates or brings on the symptoms. At the same time, the examiner should be observing the patient. Does the patient appear to be in constant pain?

Pain Rating Scale

Instructions:
  Below is a thermometer with various grades of pain on it from "No pain at all" to "The pain is almost unbearable." Put an × by the words that describe your pain best. Mark how bad your pain is AT THIS MOMENT IN TIME.

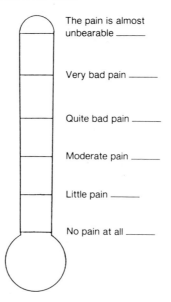

The pain is almost unbearable _____

Very bad pain _____

Quite bad pain _____

Moderate pain _____

Little pain _____

No pain at all _____

Figure 1–3
"Thermometer" pain rating scale. (From Brodie, D.J., J.V. Burnett, J.M. Walker, and D. Lydes-Reid: Evaluation of low back pain by patient questionnaires and therapist assessment. J. Orthop. Sports Phys. Ther. 11:528, 1990.)

Does the patient appear to be lacking sleep because of pain? Does the patient move around a great deal in an attempt to find a comfortable position?

13. Is the pain associated with rest? Activity? Certain postures? Visceral function? Time of day? Pain on activity that decreases with rest usually indicates a mechanical problem interfering with movement, such as adhesions. Morning pain with stiffness that improves with activity usually indicates chronic inflammation and edema. Pain or aching as the day progresses usually indicates increased congestion in a joint. Pain at rest and pain that is worse at the beginning of activity than at the end implies acute inflammation. Pain that is not affected by rest or activity usually indicates bone pain or could be related to organic or systemic disorders such as cancer or diseases of the viscera. Chronic pain is often associated with multiple factors such as fatigue or certain postures or activities. If the pain occurs at night, how does the patient lie in bed—supine, on the side, or prone? Does sleeping alter the pain, or does the patient wake when he or she changes position? Intractable pain at night may indicate serious pathology (e.g., a tumor). Symptoms of peripheral nerve entrapment (e.g., carpal tunnel syndrome) and thoracic outlet syndromes tend to be worse at night. Pain and cramping with prolonged walking may indicate lumbar spinal stenosis (neurogenic intermittent claudication) or vascular problems (circulatory intermittent claudication). Intervertebral disc pain is aggravated by sitting and bending forward. Facet joint pain is often relieved by sitting and bending forward. What types of mattress and pillow are used? Foam pillows often cause more problems for persons with cervical disorders because these pillows have more "bounce" to them than do feather pillows. Too many pillows, pillows improperly positioned, or too soft a mattress may also cause problems.

14. What type or quality of pain is exhibited? **Nerve pain** tends to be sharp, bright, and burning and also tends to run in the distribution of specific nerves. **Bone pain** tends to be deep, boring, and very localized. **Vascular pain** tends to be diffuse, aching, and poorly localized and may be referred to other areas of the body. **Muscle pain** is usually hard to localize, is dull and aching, is often aggravated by injury, and may be referred to other areas (Table 1–2).

15. What types of sensations does the patient feel, and where are there abnormal sensations? If the problem is in bone, there usually is very little radiation of pain. If pressure is applied to a nerve root, radicular pain results from pressure on the dura mater, which is the outermost covering of the spinal cord. If there is pressure on the nerve trunk, no pain occurs, but there is paresthesia or an abnormal sensation such as a "pins and needles" feeling or a tingling. If the nerve itself is affected, regardless of where the irritation occurs along the nerve, the pain is perceived by the brain as coming from the periphery. This is an example of referred pain. Muscular, ligamentous, and bursal types of pain are often indistinguishable.

16. Does a joint exhibit locking, unlocking, twinges, instability, or giving way? **Locking** may mean that the joint cannot be fully extended, as is the case with a meniscal tear, or it may mean that it does not extend one time and does not flex the next time (pseudolocking), as in the case of a loose body moving within the joint. Locking may mean that the joint cannot be put through a full ROM because of muscle spasm; this is sometimes referred to as spasm locking. **Giving way** is often caused by reflex inhibition of the muscles, so that the patient feels that the limb will buckle if weight is placed on it, or it may be caused by instability of the joint. Inhibition may be caused by anticipated pain or instability. There are two types of instability: mechanical and clinical.[11] **Mechanical (pathological) instability** refers to loss of control of the small joint movements (e.g., translation) that occur when the patient attempts to stabilize the joint during movement. **Clinical instability** refers to excessive gross movement in a joint and is sometimes referred to as **pathological hypermobility**; in nonpathological states, it is called **laxity** or **hypermobility**. Both types of instability can cause symptoms, and treatment centers on teaching the patient to develop muscular control of the joint and to improve reaction time and proprioceptive control. Both types of instability may be voluntary or involuntary. Voluntary instability is initiated by muscle contraction, and involuntary instability is the result of positioning.

17. Has the patient experienced any bilateral cord symptoms, fainting, or drop attacks? Is bladder function normal? Is there any "saddle" involvement or vertigo? Vertigo and dizziness are terms often used synonymously, although vertigo usually indicates more severe symptoms. The terms describe a swaying, spinning sensation accompanied by feelings of unsteadiness and loss of balance. These symptoms indicate severe neurological problems, such as cervical myelopathy, which must be dealt with carefully and can (e.g., in cases of altered bladder function) be emergency conditions potentially requiring surgery.

Table 1–2
Pain Descriptions and Related Structures

Type of Pain	Structure
Cramping, dull, aching	Muscle
Sharp, shooting	Nerve root
Sharp, bright, lightning-like	Nerve
Burning, pressure-like, stinging, aching	Sympathetic nerve
Deep, nagging, dull	Bone
Sharp, severe, intolerable	Fracture
Throbbing, diffuse	Vasculature

18. Are there any changes in color of the limb? Ischemic changes resulting from circulatory problems may include white, brittle skin; loss of hair; and abnormal nails on the foot or hand.

19. Has the patient been experiencing any life or economic stresses? Divorce, marital problems, financial problems, or job insecurity can contribute to increasing the pain or symptoms because of psychological stress.

20. Does the patient have any chronic or serious systemic illnesses that may influence the course of the pathology or the treatment?

21. Is there anything in the family history that may be related, such as tumors, arthritis, heart disease, diabetes, and allergies? Some disease processes and pathologies have a familial incidence.

22. Has the patient undergone an x-ray examination or other imaging techniques? If so, x-ray overexposure must be considered; if not, an x-ray examination may help yield a diagnosis.

23. Has the patient been receiving steroids or any other medication? If so, for how long? High dosages of steroids taken for long periods may lead to problems such as osteoporosis. Has the patient been taking any other medication that is pertinent? Patients may not regard over-the-counter formulations, birth control pills, and so on as "medications." If such medications have been taken for a long period, their use may not seem pertinent to the patient. How long has the patient been taking the medication? When did he or she last take the medication? Did the medication help?[12] It is also important to determine whether medication is being taken for the condition under review. If analgesics or anti-inflammatories were taken just before the patient's visit for the assessment, some symptoms may be masked.

24. Does the patient have a history of surgery? If so, when was the surgery performed, what was the site of operation, and what condition was being treated? Sometimes, the condition the examiner is asked to treat is the result of the surgery. Has the patient ever been hospitalized? If so, why?

It is evident that the taking of an accurate, detailed history is very important. With experience, the examiner is often able to make a **preliminary diagnosis** from the history alone. The observation and examination phases of the assessment are then used to confirm or refute the possible diagnoses.

Observation

In an assessment, observation is the "looking" or inspection phase. Its purpose is to gain information on visible defects, functional deficits, and abnormalities of alignment. Much of the observation phase involves assessment of normal standing posture (see Chapter 15). Normal posture covers a very wide range, and asymmetric findings are common. The key is to determine whether these findings are related to the pathology being presented. The examiner should note the patient's way of moving as well as the general posture, manner, attitude, and willingness to cooperate. Observation may begin in the waiting room or as the patient is being taken to the assessment area. Often the patient is unaware that observation is occurring at this stage and may present a different picture. The patient must be adequately undressed in a private assessment area to be observed properly. Male patients should wear only shorts, and female patients should wear a bra or halter top and shorts. Because the patient is in a state of undress, it is important for the examiner to explain to the patient that observation and detailed looking are an integral part of the assessment. This explanation may prevent a potentially embarrassing situation.

As the patient enters the assessment area, his or her gait should be observed (see Chapter 14). This initial gait assessment is only a cursory one; however, problems such as Trendelenburg sign or drop foot are easily noticed. If there apears to be an abnormality, the gait may be checked in greater detail after the patient has undressed.

The examiner should be positioned so that the dominant eye is used, and both sides of the patient should be compared simultaneously. During the observation stage, the examiner is only looking at the patient and does not ask the patient to move; the examiner usually does not palpate, except possibly to learn whether an area is warm or hot.

After the patient has undressed, the examiner should observe the posture and attempt to answer the following questions.

1. What is the normal body alignment? Anteriorly, the nose, xiphisternum, and umbilicus should be in a straight line. From the side, the tip of the ear, the tip of the acromion, the "high point" of the iliac crest, and the lateral malleolus (anterior aspect) should be in a straight line.

2. Is there any obvious deformity? Deformities may take the form of restricted ROM (e.g., flexion deformity), malalignment (e.g., genu varum), alteration in the shape of a bone (e.g., fracture), or alteration in the relaxation of two articulating structures (e.g., subluxation, dislocation). Structural deformities are present even at rest; examples include torticollis, fractures, scoliosis, and kyphosis. Dynamic deformities are caused by muscle action and therefore are not usually evident when the muscles are relaxed; these types of deformity are more likely to be seen during the examination phase.

3. Are the bony contours of the body normal and symmetric, or is there an obvious deviation? The body is not perfectly symmetric, and deviation may have no

clinical implications. For example, many people have a lower shoulder on the dominant side or demonstrate a slight scoliosis of the spine adjacent to the heart. However, any deviation should be noted, because it may contribute to a more accurate diagnosis.

4. Are the soft-tissue contours (e.g., muscle, skin, fat) normal and symmetric? Is there any obvious muscle wasting?

5. Are the limb positions equal and symmetric? The examiner should compare limb size, shape, any atrophy, color, and temperature.

6. Are the color and texture of the skin normal? Does the appearance of the skin differ in the area of pain or symptoms, compared with other areas of the body? Trophic changes in the skin resulting from peripheral nerve lesions include loss of skin elasticity, shiny skin, hair loss on the skin, and skin that breaks down easily and heals slowly. The nails may become brittle and ridged. Cyanosis, or a bluish color to the skin, is usually an indication of poor blood perfusion. Redness indicates increased blood flow or inflammation.

7. Are there any scars that indicate recent injury or surgery? Recent scars are red because they are still healing and contain capillaries; older scars are white and primarily avascular. Fibers of the dermis (skin) tend to run in one direction, along so-called cleavage or tension lines. Lacerations or surgical cuts along these lines produce less scarring. Cuts across joint flexion lines frequently produce excessive (hypertrophic) scarring. Some individuals are also prone to keloid (very excessive) scarring. Are there any callosities, blisters, or inflamed bursae, indicative of excessive pressure or friction to the skin? Are there any sinuses that may indicate infection? If so, are the sinuses draining or dry?

8. Is there any crepitus, snapping, or abnormal sound in the joints when the patient moves them? Crepitus may vary from a loud grinding noise to a squeaking noise. Snapping, especially if not painful, may be caused by a tendon moving over a bony protuberance. Clicking is sometimes heard in the temporomandibular joint and may be an indication of early nonsymptomatic pathology.

9. Is there any heat, swelling, or redness in the area being observed? All of these signs are indications of inflammation or an active inflammatory condition.

10. What attitude does the patient appear to have toward the condition or toward the examiner? Is the patient apprehensive, restless, resentful, or depressed? These questions give the examiner some indication of the patient's psychological state and how he or she will respond to treatment.

11. What is the patient's facial expression? Does the patient appear to be apprehensive, in discomfort, or lacking sleep?

12. Is the patient willing to move? Are patterns of movement normal? If not, how are they abnormal? Any

alteration should be noted and included in the observation portion of the assessment.

Examination
Principles

Because the examination portion of the assessment involves touching the patient and may, in some cases, cause the patient discomfort, the examiner must obtain a valid consent to perform the examination before it begins. A valid consent must be voluntary, must cover the procedures to be done (informed consent), and the patient must be legally competent to give the consent.[13]

The examination is used to confirm or refute the suspected diagnosis, which is based on the history and observation. The examination must be performed systematically, with the examiner looking for a consistent pattern of signs and symptoms that leads to a differential diagnosis. Special care must be taken if the condition of the joint is irritable or acute. This is especially true if the area is in severe spasm or if the patient complains of severe unremitting pain that is not affected by position or medication, severe night pain, severe pain with no history of injury, or nonmechanical behavior of the joint.

> ### "Red Flags" in Examination Indicating Need for Medical Consultation
>
> - Severe unremitting pain
> - Pain unaffected by medication or position
> - Severe night pain
> - Severe pain with no history of injury
> - Severe spasm
> - Psychologic overlay

In the examination portion of the assessment, a number of principles must be followed.

1. Unless bilateral movement is required, the normal side is tested first. Testing the normal side first allows the examiner to establish a baseline for normal movement and shows the patient what to expect, resulting in increased patient confidence and less patient apprehension.

2. Active movements are done before passive movements. Passive movements are followed by resisted isometric movements (see later discussion). In this way, the examiner has a better idea of what the patient thinks he or she can do before the structures are fully tested.

3. Any movements that are painful are done last, if possible, to prevent an overflow of painful symptoms to the next movement.

4. If active ROM is not full, overpressure is applied only with extreme care to prevent the exacerbation of symptoms.

5. During active movements, if the ROM is full, overpressure may be applied to determine the end feel of the joint. This often negates the need to do passive movements.

6. Each active, passive, or resisted isometric movement may be repeated several times or held (sustained) for a certain amount of time to see whether symptoms increase or decrease, whether a different pattern of movement results, whether there is increased weakness, and whether there is possible vascular insufficiency. This repetitive or sustained activity is especially important if the patient has complained that symptoms are altered by repetitive movement or sustained postures.

7. Resisted isometric movements are done with the joint in a neutral or resting position so that stress on the inert tissues is minimal. Any symptoms produced by the movement are then more likely to be caused by problems with contractile tissue.

8. For passive ROM or ligamentous tests, it is not only the degree (i.e., the amount) of the opening but also the quality (end feel) of the opening that is important.

9. When the examiner is testing the ligaments, the appropriate stress is applied gently and repeated several times; the stress is increased up to but not beyond the point of pain. In this way, maximum instability can be demonstrated without causing muscle spasm.

10. When testing **myotomes** (groups of muscles supplied by a single nerve root), each contraction is held for a minimum of **5 seconds** to see whether weakness becomes evident. Myotomal weakness takes time to develop.

Principles of Examination

- Test normal (uninvolved) side first
- Active movements first, then passive movements, then resisted isometric movements
- Painful movements are done last
- Apply overpressure with care
- Repeat or sustain movements if history indicates
- Do resisted isometric movements in a resting position
- With passive movements and ligamentous testing, both the degree and quality of opening are important
- With ligamentous testing, repeat with increasing stress
- With myotome testing, contractions must be held for 5 seconds
- Warn of possible exacerbations
- Refer if necessary

---

11. At the completion of an assessment, the examiner must warn the patient that he or she may experience exacerbation of symptoms as a result of the assessment.

12. If, at the conclusion of the examination, the examiner has found that the patient has presented with unusual signs and symptoms, or if the condition appears to be beyond his or her scope of practice, the examiner should not hesitate to refer the patient to another appropriate health care professional.

Scanning Examination

The examination described here emphasizes the joints of the body, their movement and stability. It is necessary to examine all appropriate tissues to delineate the affected area, which can then be examined in detail. Application of tension, stretch, or isometric contraction to specific tissues produces either a normal or an appropriate abnormal response. This action enables the examiner to determine the nature and site of the present symptoms and the patient's response to these symptoms. The examination shows whether certain activities provoke or change the patient's pain; in this way, the examiner can focus on the subjective response (the patient's feelings or opinions) as well as the test findings. The patient must be clear about his or her side of the examination. For instance, the patient must not confuse questions about movement-associated pain ("Does the movement make any difference to the pain?" "Does the movement bring on or change the pain?") with questions about already existing pain. In addition, the examiner attempts to see whether patient responses are measurably abnormal. Do the movements cause any abnormalities in function? A loss of movement or weakness in muscles can be measured and therefore is an objective response. Throughout the assessment, the examiner looks for two sets of data: (1) what the patient feels (subjective) and (2) responses that can be measured or are found by the examiner (objective).

The Scanning Examination Is Used When

- There is no history of trauma
- There are radicular signs
- There is trauma with radicular signs
- There is altered sensation in the limb
- There are spinal cord ("long track") signs
- The patient presents with abnormal patterns
- There is suspected psychogenic pain

To ensure that all possible sources of pathology are assessed, the examination must be extensive. This is especially true if there has been no history of trauma leading to symptoms. In this case, a scanning or screening examination is performed to rule out the possibility of referral of symptoms. Similarly, if there is any doubt about where the pathology is located, the scanning examination is essential to ensure a correct diagnosis.

In the upper part of the body, the scanning examination begins with the cervical spine and includes the temporomandibular joints, the entire scapular area, the shoulder region, and the upper limbs to the fingers. In the lower part of the body, the examination begins at the lumbar spine and continues to the toes. The goal of the scanning examination is to rule out potential problems in the upper or lower extremities that may have been referred from the spine to other areas; in addition, the examiner can identify areas needing more specific testing. The "scan" should add no more than 5 or 10 minutes to the assessment.

As with all assessments, the scanning examination begins with the history and observation. The scanning examination is a modification of the cervical or lumbar spinal assessment (Fig. 1–4). After the active, passive, and resisted isometric movements of the cervical or lumbar spine have been tested, the peripheral joints are "scanned," with the patient doing only a few movements at each joint. The movements should include those that may be expected to exacerbate symptoms. In reality, this quick look at the peripheral joints is the only part of the scanning examination that is different from the normal spine assessment. The examiner then tests the upper or lower limb myotomes. After these tests, the appropriate reflexes and cutaneous distributions can be checked or left until later. At this point, the examiner makes a decision or an educated guess as to whether the problem is in the cervical spine, lumbar spine, or a peripheral joint, based on the information gained so far. Once the decision is made, the examiner either continues with the spinal assessment or turns instead to a complete assessment of the appropriate peripheral joint (see Fig. 1–4).

The idea of the scanning examination was developed by Cyriax,[1] who also, more than any other author, originated the concepts of "contractile" and "inert" tissue, "end feel," and "capsular patterns" and contributed greatly to development of a comprehensive and systematic physical examination of the moving parts of the body.

Spinal Cord and Nerve Roots

To further comprehend and ensure the value of the scanning examination, the examiner must have a clear understanding of signs and symptoms arising from the spinal cord and nerve roots of the body and those arising from peripheral nerves. The scanning examination helps to determine whether the pathology is caused by tissues innervated by a nerve root that is referring symptoms distally.

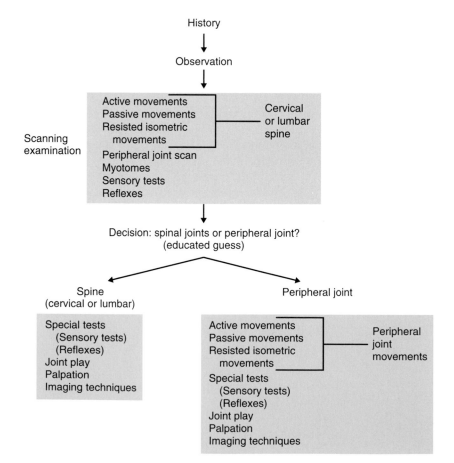

Figure 1–4
The scanning examination to rule out referral of symptoms from other tissues.

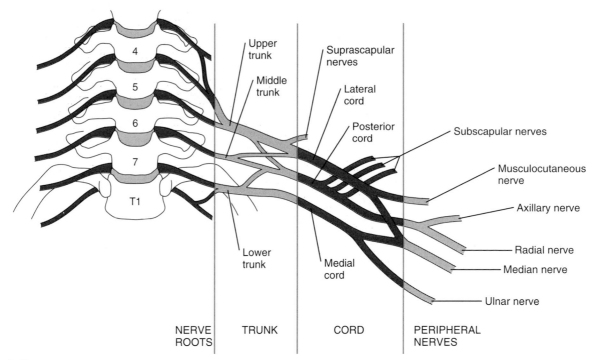

Figure 1–5

The inter-relationship of the spinal nerve roots, plexus, and peripheral nerves, using cervical spine and brachial plexus as an example.

The nerve root is that portion of a peripheral nerve that connects the nerve to the spinal cord. Nerve roots arise from each level of the spinal cord (e.g., C3, C4), and many, but not all, intermingle in a plexus (brachial, lumbar, or lumbosacral) to form different peripheral nerves (Fig. 1–5). This arrangement can result in a single nerve root supplying more than one peripheral nerve. For example, the median nerve is derived from the C6, C7, C8, and T1 nerve roots; the ulnar nerve is derived from the C7, C8, and T1 nerve roots; and the radial nerve is derived from the nerve roots of C5, C6, C7, C8, and T1. For this reason, if pressure is applied to the nerve root, the distribution of the sensation or motor function is often felt or exhibited in more than one peripheral nerve distribution (Table 1–3). Therefore, although the symptoms seen in a nerve root lesion (e.g., paresthesia, pain, muscle weakness) may be similar to those seen in peripheral nerves, the signs (e.g., area of paresthesia, where pain occurs, which muscles are weak) may be different. The examiner must be able to differentiate a dermatome (nerve root) from the sensory distribution of a peripheral nerve, and a myotome (nerve root) from muscles supplied by a specific peripheral nerve. In addition, neurological signs and symptoms such as paresthesia and pain may result from irritation of tissues such as facet joints and interspinous ligaments or other tissues supplied by the nerve roots, and they may be demonstrated in the dermatome, myotome, or sclerotome supplied by that nerve root. This irritation can contribute to the referred pain (see later discussion).

Nerve roots are made up of anterior (ventral) and posterior (dorsal) portions that unite near or in the intervertebral foramen to form a single **nerve root** or **spinal nerve** (Fig. 1–6). They are the most proximal parts of the peripheral nervous system.

Within the human body, there are 31 nerve root pairs: 8 cervical, 12 thoracic, 5 lumbar, 5 sacral, and 1 coccygeal. Each nerve root has two components: a **somatic** portion, which innervates the skeletal muscles and provides sensory input from the skin, fascia, muscles, and joints, and a **visceral** component, which is part of the autonomic nervous system.[14] The autonomic system

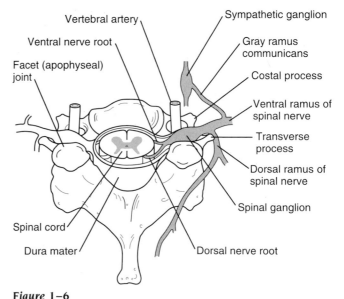

Figure 1–6

Spinal cord, nerve root portions, and spinal nerve in the cervical spine and their relation to the vertebra and vertebral artery.

Table 1–3
Nerve Root Dermatomes, Myotomes, Reflexes, and Paresthetic Areas

Nerve Root	Dermatome*	Muscle Weakness (Myotome)	Reflexes Affected	Paresthesias
C1	Vertex of skull	None	None	None
C2	Temple, forehead, occiput	Longus colli, sternocleidomastoid, rectus capitis	None	None
C3	Entire neck, posterior cheek, temporal area, prolongation forward under mandible	Trapezius, splenius capitis	None	Cheek, side of neck
C4	Shoulder area, clavicular area, upper scapular area	Trapezius, levator scapulae	None	Horizontal band along clavicle and upper scapula
C5	Deltoid area, anterior aspect of entire arm to base of thumb	Supraspinatus, infraspinatus, deltoid, biceps	Biceps, brachioradialis	None
C6	Anterior arm, radial side of hand to thumb and index finger	Biceps, supinator, wrist extensors	Biceps, brachioradialis	Thumb and index finger
C7	Lateral arm and forearm to index, long, and ring fingers	Triceps, wrist flexors (rarely, wrist extensors)	Triceps	Index, long, and ring fingers
C8	Medial arm and forearm to long, ring, and little fingers	Ulnar deviators, thumb extensors, thumb adductors (rarely, triceps)	Triceps	Little finger alone or with two adjacent fingers; *not* ring or long fingers, alone or together (C7)
T1 T2	Medial side of forearm to base of little finger Medial side of upper arm to medial elbow, pectoral and midscapular areas	Disc lesions at upper two thoracic levels do not appear to give rise to root weakness. Weakness of intrinsic muscles of the hand is due to other pathology (e.g., thoracic outlet pressure, neoplasm of lung, and ulnar nerve lesion). Dural and nerve root stress has T1 elbow flexion with arm horizontal. T1 and T2 scapulae forward and backward on chest wall. Neck flexion at any thoracic level.		
T3–T12	T3–T6, upper thorax; T5–T7, costal margin; T8–T12, abdomen and lumbar region	Articular and dural signs and root pain are common. Root signs (cutaneous analgesia) are rare and have such indefinite area that they have little localizing value. Weakness is not detectable.		
L1	Back, over trochanter and groin	None	None	Groin; after holding posture, which causes pain
L2	Back, front of thigh to knee	Psoas, hip adductors	None	Occasionally anterior thigh
L3	Back, upper buttock, anterior thigh and knee, medial lower leg	Psoas, quadriceps, thigh atrophy	Knee jerk sluggish, PKB positive, pain on full SLR	Medial knee, anterior lower leg
L4	Medial buttock, lateral thigh, medial leg, dorsum of foot, big toe	Tibialis anterior, extensor hallucis	SLR limited neck flexion pain, weak or absent knee jerk, side flexion limited	Medial aspect of calf and ankle
L5	Buttock, posterior and lateral thigh, lateral aspect of leg, dorsum of foot, medial half of sole, first, second, and third toes	Extensor hallucis, peroneals, gluteus medius, dorsiflexors, hamstring and calf atrophy	SLR limited one side, neck flexion painful, ankle decreased, crossed-leg raising—pain	Lateral aspect of leg, medial three toes
S1	Buttock, thigh, and leg posterior	Calf and hamstring, wasting of gluteals, peroneals, plantar flexors	SLR limited, Achilles reflex weak or absent	Lateral two toes, lateral foot, lateral leg to knee, plantar aspect of foot
S2	Same as S1	Same as S1 except peroneals	Same as S1	Lateral leg, knee, and heel
S3	Groin, medial thigh to knee	None	None	None
S4	Perineum, genitals, lower sacrum	Bladder, rectum	None	Saddle area, genitals, anus, impotence, massive posterior herniation

* In any part of which pain may be felt.

PKB = prone knee bending; SLR = straight leg raising.

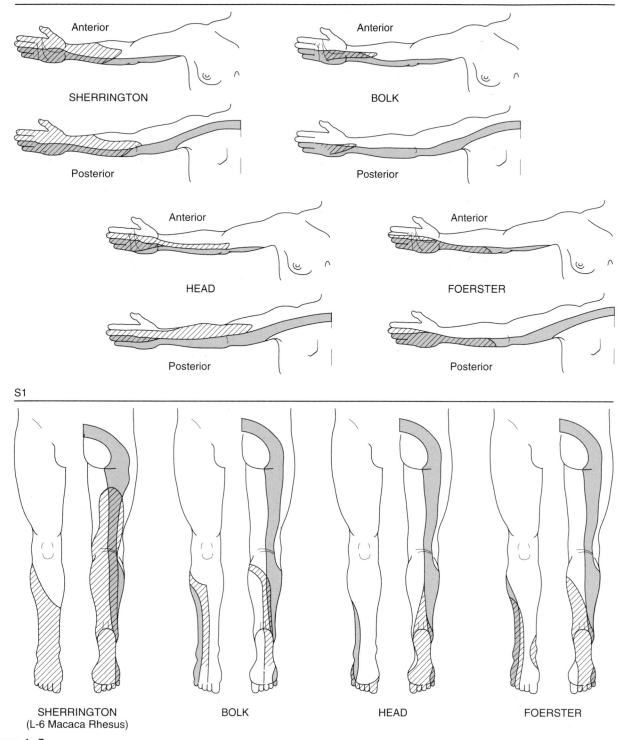

Figure 1–7

The variability of dermatomes at C8 and S1 as found by four researchers. Similar variability is demonstrated in most cervical, lumbar, and sacral vertebrae. (Redrawn from Keegan, J.J., and F.D. Garrett: The segmental distribution of the cutaneous nerves in the limbs of man. Anat. Rec. 101:430, 433, 1948. Copyright © 1948. Reprinted by permission of John Wiley & Sons, Inc.)

supplies the blood vessels, dura mater, periosteum, ligaments, and intervertebral discs, among many other structures.

The sensory distribution of each nerve root is called the **dermatome**. A dermatome is defined as the area of skin supplied by a single nerve root. The descriptions of dermatomes in the following chapters should be considered as examples only, because slight differences occur with each patient, and dermatomes also exhibit a great deal of overlap.[15] The variability in dermatomes was aptly demonstrated by Keegan and Garrett in 1948 (Fig. 1–7).[16] The overlap may be demonstrated by the fact that, in the thoracic spine, the loss of one dermatome is often not noticed because of the overlap of the adjacent dermatomes.

Spinal nerve roots have a poorly developed epineurium and lack a perineurium. This development makes the nerve root more susceptible to compressive forces, tensile deformation, chemical irritants (e.g., alcohol, lead, arsenic), and metabolic abnormalities. For example, compression of the nerve root could occur with a posterolateral intervertebral disc herniation, a "burner" or stretching of the nerve roots or the brachial plexus in a football player, alcoholic neuritis in an alcoholic, or metabolic peripheral neuropathy of one or more peripheral nerves in a diabetic. Pressure on nerve roots leads to loss of muscle tone and mass, but the loss is often not as obvious as when pressure is applied to a peripheral nerve. Because the peripheral nerve that innervates the muscle is usually supplied by more than one nerve root, more muscle fibers are likely to be affected if the peripheral nerve itself is damaged. In addition, the pattern of weakness (i.e., which muscles are affected) is different for an injury to a nerve root and to a peripheral nerve, because a nerve root supplies more than one peripheral nerve. Pressure on a peripheral nerve resulting in a neuropraxia leads to temporary nonfunction of the nerve. With this type of injury, there is primarily motor involvement, with little sensory or autonomic involvement, and although weakness may be demonstrated, muscle atrophy may not be evident. With more severe peripheral nerve lesions (e.g., axonotmesis and neurotmesis), atrophy is evident.

Myotomes are defined as groups of muscles supplied by a single nerve root. A lesion of a single nerve root is usually associated with paresis (incomplete paralysis) of the myotome (muscles) supplied by that nerve root. It therefore takes time for any weakness to become evident on resisted isometric or myotome testing, and for this reason, the isometric testing of myotomes is held **for at least 5 seconds.** On the other hand, a lesion of a peripheral nerve leads to complete paralysis of the muscles supplied by that nerve, especially if the injury results in axonotmesis or neurotmesis, and the weakness therefore is evident right away. Differences in the amount of resulting paralysis arise from the fact that more than one myotome contributes to the formation of a muscle embryologically.

A **sclerotome** is an area of bone or fascia supplied by a single nerve root (Fig. 1–8). As with dermatomes, sclerotomes can show a great deal of variability among individuals.

It is the complex nature of the dermatomes, myotomes, and sclerotomes supplied by the nerve root that can lead to **referred pain,** which is pain felt in a part of the body that is usually a considerable distance from the tissues that have caused it. Referred pain is explained as an error in perception on the part of the brain. Usually,

pain can be referred into the appropriate myotome, dermatome, or sclerotome from any somatic or visceral tissue innervated by a nerve root, but, confusingly, it sometimes is not referred according to a specific pattern.[17] It is not understood why this occurs, but clinically it has been found to be so.

Many theories of the mechanism of referred pain have been developed, but none has been proven conclusively. Generally, referred pain may involve one or more of the following mechanisms:

1. Misinterpretation by the brain as to the source of the painful impulses
2. Inability of the brain to interpret a summation of noxious stimuli from various sources
3. Disturbance of the internuncial pool by afferent nerve impulses.

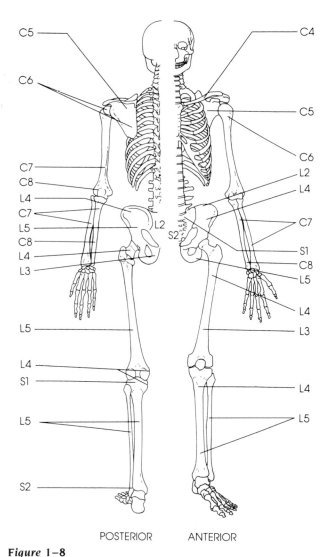

Figure 1–8

Sclerotomes of the body. Lines show areas of bone and fascia supplied by individual nerve roots.

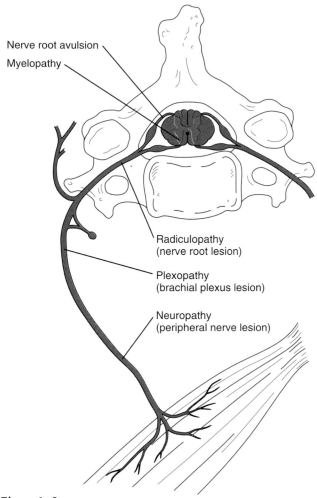

Figure 1–9
Path of neurological tissue from spinal cord to muscles, showing sites of neurological lesions.

Nerve root avulsion

Myelopathy

Radiculopathy
(nerve root lesion)

Plexopathy
(brachial plexus lesion)

Neuropathy
(peripheral nerve lesion)

segment that is at fault; it indicates that one of the structures innervated by a specific nerve root is causing signs and symptoms in other tissues supplied by that same nerve root. For example, pain in the L5 dermatome could arise from irritation around the L5 nerve root, from an L5 disc causing pressure on the L5 nerve root, from facet joint involvement at L4–L5 causing irritation of the L5 nerve root, from any muscle supplied by the L5 nerve root, or from any visceral structures having L5 innervation. Referred pain tends to be felt deeply; its boundaries are indistinct, and it radiates segmentally without crossing the midline. **Radicular** or **radiating pain,** a form of referred pain, is pain felt in a dermatome, myotome, or sclerotome because of direct involvement of a spinal nerve or nerve root.[12] It is sometimes referred to as a **radiculopathy.** A **myelopathy** is a neurogenic disorder involving the spinal cord or brain and resulting in an upper motor neuron lesion; the pattern of pain or symptoms is different from that of radicular pain, and often both upper and lower limbs are affected (Fig. 1–9).

Peripheral Nerves

Peripheral nerves are a unique type of "inert" tissue (see later discussion) in that they are not contractile tissue but they are necessary for the normal functioning of voluntary muscle. The examiner must be aware of potential injury to nervous tissue when examining both contractile and inert tissue. Table 1–4 shows some of the tissue changes that result when a peripheral nerve lesion occurs.

In peripheral nerves, the epineurium consists of a loose areolar connective tissue matrix surrounding the nerve fiber. It allows changes in growth length of the bundled nerve fibers (funiculi) without allowing the bundles to be strained. The perineurium protects the nerve bundles by acting as a diffusion barrier to irritants and provides tensile strength and elasticity to the nerve. Peripheral nerves therefore are most commonly affected by

Referral of pain is a common occurrence in problems associated with the musculoskeletal system. Pain is often felt at points remote from the site of the lesion. The site to which pain is referred is an **indicator** of the

Table 1–4
Signs and Symptoms of Mixed Peripheral Nerve (Lower Motor Neuron) Lesions*

Motor	Sensory	Sympathetic
Flaccid paralysis	Loss of or abnormal sensation	Loss of sweat glands (dryness)
Loss of reflexes	Loss of vasomotor tone: warm flushed (early); cold, white (later)	Loss of pilomotor response
Muscle wasting and atrophy		
Lost synergic action	Skin may be scaly (early); thin, smooth and shiny (later)	
Fibrosis, contractures, and adhesions	Shallower skin creases	
Joint weakness and instability		
Decreased range of motion and stiffness	Nail changes (striations, ridges, dry, brittle, abnormal curving, luster lost)	
Disuse osteoporosis of bone	Ulceration	
Growth affected		

* Primarily axonotmesis and neurotmesis.

pressure, traction, friction, anoxia, or cutting. Examples include pressure on the median nerve in the carpal tunnel, traction to the common peroneal nerve at the head of the fibula during a lateral ankle sprain, friction to the ulnar nerve in the cubital tunnel, anoxia of the anterior tibial nerve in a compartment syndrome, and cutting of the radial nerve with a fracture of the humeral shaft. Cooling, freezing, thermal or electrical injury may also affect peripheral nerves.

Nerve injuries are usually classified by the systems of Seddon[18] or Sunderland.[19] Seddon, whose system is most commonly used, classified nerve injuries into neuropraxia (most common), axonotmesis, and neurotmesis (Table 1–5). Sunderland followed a similar system but divided axonotmesis and neurotmesis into two levels each. Any examination of a joint must include a thorough peripheral nerve examination. The examiner must be able not only to differentiate inert tissue lesions from contractile tissue lesions but to determine whether a contractile tissue malfunction is the result of the contractile tissue itself or a peripheral nerve lesion or a nerve root lesion.

Sensory loss combined with motor loss should alert the examiner to lesions of nervous tissue.[20-22] Injury to a single peripheral nerve (e.g., the median nerve) is sometimes referred to as a **mononeuropathy**. Systemic diseases (e.g., diabetes) may affect more than one peripheral nerve. In this case, the pathology is referred to as a **polyneuropathy**. Careful mapping of the area of sensory loss and testing of the muscles affected by the motor loss allow the examiner to differentiate between a peripheral nerve lesion and a nerve root lesion. (An example is shown in Table 1–6.) If electromyographic studies are to be used to determine the grade of nerve injury, denervation cannot be evaluated for at least 3 weeks after injury to allow wallerian degeneration to occur and to allow regeneration (if any) to begin.[23-25] Muscle wasting usually becomes obvious after 4 to 6 weeks and progresses to reach its maximum by about 12 weeks following injury. Circulatory changes after nerve injury vary with time. In the initial or early stages, the skin is warm, but after about 3 weeks the skin becomes cooler as a result of decreased circulation. Because of the decreased circulation and disease, trophic changes occur to the skin and nails.

When assessing a patient, the examiner must also be aware of what has been called the double-crush syndrome or double-entrapment neuropathy.[26-29] The theory of this lesion (which has not yet been proved but has clinical supporting evidence) is that, whereas compression at one point along a peripheral nerve or nerve root may not be sufficient to cause signs and symptoms, compression at two or more points may lead to a cumulative effect that results in apparent signs and symptoms. Because of this cumulative effect, signs and symptoms may indicate one area of involvement (e.g., the carpal tunnel) while other areas (e.g., cervical spine, brachial plexus, thoracic outlet) may be contributing to the problem. Similarly, cervical lesions may be involved in tennis elbow syndromes. Upton and McComas[26] believed that compression proximally on the nerve trunk could increase the vulnerability of the peripheral nerves or nerve

Table 1–5
Classification of Nerve Injuries According to Seddon

Grade of Injury	Definition	Signs and Symptoms
Neuropraxia (Sunderland 1°)	A transient physiological block caused by ischemia from pressure or stretch of the nerve with no wallerian degeneration	Pain No or minimal muscle wasting Muscle weakness Numbness Proprioception affected Recovery time: minutes to days
Axonotmesis (Sunderland 2° and 3°)	Internal architecture of nerve preserved, but axons are so badly damaged that wallerian degeneration occurs	Pain Muscle wasting evident Complete motor, sensory and sympathetic functions lost (see Table 1–4) Recovery time: months (axon regenerates at rate of 1 inch/month, or 1 mm/day) Sensation is restored before motor function
Neurotmesis (Sunderland 4° and 5°)	Structure of nerve is destroyed by cutting, severe scarring, or prolonged severe compression	No pain (anesthesia) Muscle wasting Complete motor, sensory and sympathetic functions lost (see Table 1–4) Recovery time: months and only with surgery

Data from Seddon, H.J.: Three types of nerve injury. Brain 66:17–28, 1943.

Table 1–6
Comparison of Signs and Symptoms for C7 Nerve Root Lesion and Median Nerve Lesion at the Elbow

	C7 Nerve Root	Median Nerve
Sensory alteration	Lateral arm and forearm to index, long, and ring fingers on palmar and dorsal aspect	Palmar aspect of thumb, index, middle, and half of ring finger Dorsal aspect of index, middle, and possibly half of ring finger
Motor alteration	Triceps Wrist flexors Wrist extensors (rarely)	Pronator teres Wrist flexors (lateral half of flexor digitorum profundus) Palmaris longus Pronator quadratus Flexor pollicis longus and brevis Abductor pollicis brevis Opponens pollicis Lateral two lumbricals
Reflex alteration	Triceps	None*
Paresthesia	Index, long, and ring fingers on palmar and dorsal aspect	Same as sensory alteration

* No "common" reflexes are affected; if the examiner tested the tendon reflexes of the muscles listed, they would be affected.

roots at distal points along their paths because axonal transport would be disrupted. In addition, diseased nerves are more susceptible to injury; thus, the presence of systemic disease (e.g., diabetes, thyroid dysfunction) may make the nerve more susceptible to compression somewhere along its path.[21] Finally, the signs and symptoms could potentially be arising from both a nerve root lesion and a peripheral nerve lesion. Only with meticulous assessment can the clinician delineate where the true problems lie.

Similarly, the loss of extensibility at one site may produce increasing tensile loads when the peripheral nerve or nerve root is stretched, leading to mechanical dysfunction.[30] This is the principle behind the **neural tension** or **neurodynamic tests,** such as the straight leg raise, slump test, and upper limb tension test,[30–32] and may provide a partial explanation for lesions such as cervical spine lesions mimicking tennis elbow and carpal tunnel syndrome. These tests put neural tissue (e.g., neuraxis, meninges, nerve roots, peripheral nerves) under tension when they are performed and may duplicate symptoms that result during functional activity.[30, 32, 33] For example, sitting in a car is very closely mimicked by the action of the slump test and straight leg raising.

Neural tissue moves toward the joint at which elongation is initiated. Thus, if cervical flexion is initiated, the nerve roots, even those in the lumbar spine, move toward the cervical spine. Likewise, flexion of the whole spine causes movement toward the lumbar spine, and extension of the knee or dorsiflexion of the foot causes neural movement toward the knee or ankle.[30, 32, 33] These

"tension points" can potentially help determine where the restriction to movement is occurring. Normally, tension tests are not painful, although the patient is often aware of increased tension or discomfort in the spine and/or the limb. As tension tests give an indication of neural mobility and sensitivity to mechanical stresses, they are considered positive if they reproduce the patient's symptoms or if the patient's response is altered by movement of a body part distal to where the symptoms are felt (e.g., foot dorsiflexion causing symptoms in the lumbar spine), or if there is asymmetry in the response.[30] When doing tension tests, the examiner should note the angle or position at which the restriction occurs and what the resistance feels like. With irritable conditions, only those parts of the test that are needed to cause positive results should be performed. For example, in the slump test, if neck flexion and slumping cause positive signs, there is no need to cause further discomfort to the patient by doing knee extension and foot dorsiflexion.

Examination of Specific Joints

The examiner should use an unchanging, systematic approach to the examination that varies only slightly to elaborate certain clues given by the history or by asymmetric responses. For example, if the history is characteristic of a disc lesion, the examination should be a detailed one of all the tissues that may be affected by the disc and a brief one of all the other joints to exclude contradictory signs. If the history suggests arthritis of the hip, the examination should be a detailed one of the hip and a brief one of the other joints—again, to exclude contradictory signs. As the movements are tested, the examiner is looking sometimes for the patient's subjective responses and sometimes for clinical objective findings. For example, if examination of the cervical spine shows clear signs of a disc problem, as the examination is continued down the arm, the examiner looks more for muscle weakness (objective) rather than for elicitation of pain (subjective). In contrast, if the history suggests a muscle lesion, pain will probably be provoked when the arm is examined. In either case, the structures expected to be normal are not omitted from examination. There are only a few situations in which deviation from this systematic routine should occur: when there is uncertainty about where the pathology lies (in which case, a scanning examination must be performed, with combined assessment of the spine and one or more peripheral joints); when there is no history of trauma or indication of pathology in a specific joint yet the patient complains of pain in that joint (again, a scanning examination is performed); or when the joint to be assessed is too acutely injured to do the total systematic examination.

Active Movements

Active movements are "actively" performed by the patient's voluntary muscles and have their own special value in that they combine tests of joint range, control, muscle power, and the patient's willingness to perform the movement. These movements are sometimes referred to as physiological or anatomic movements. Contractile, nervous, and inert tissues are involved or moved during active movements. When active movements occur, one or more rigid structures (bones) move, and such movement results in movement of all structures that attach to or are in close proximity to that bone. Although active movements are usually the first movements done, they either are not performed at all or are performed with caution during fracture healing or if the movement could put stress on newly repaired soft tissues. The examiner should note which movements, if any, cause pain or other symptoms and the amount and quality of pain that results. For example, small, unguarded movements causing intense pain indicate an acute, irritable joint. If the condition is very irritable or acute, it may not be possible to elicit all the movements desired. In this case, only those movements that provide the most useful information should be performed. The examiner should note the rhythm of movement along with any pain, limitation, or trick movements that occur. Trick movements are modified movements that the patient consciously or unconsciously uses to accomplish what the examiner has asked the patient to do. For example, in the presence

of deltoid paralysis, if the examiner asks the patient to abduct the arm, the patient can accomplish this movement by laterally rotating the shoulder and using the biceps muscle to abduct the arm.

Contractile tissues may have tension placed on them by stretching or contraction.[1] These structures include the muscles, their tendons, and their attachments into the bone. **Nervous tissues** and their associated sheaths also have tension put on them by stretching and pinching, as do **inert tissues.** Inert tissues include all structures that would not be considered contractile or neurological, such as joint capsules, ligaments, bursae, blood vessels, cartilage, and dura mater. Table 1–7 demonstrates differential diagnosis of injuries to contractile tissue (strains and tendinitis) and inert tissue (sprains).

If there is an organic lesion, some movements will be abnormal or painful and others will not. Negative findings must balance positive ones, and the examination must be extensive enough to allow characteristic patterns to emerge. Determination of the problem is not made on the strength of the first positive finding; it is made only after it is clear that there are no other contradictory signs. Movements may be repeated several times quickly to rule out any problem such as vascular insufficiency or if the patient has indicated in the history that repetitive movements increase the symptoms. Likewise, sustained postures may be held for several seconds or combined movements may be performed if the history indicated increased symptoms with those postures or movements.

The active movement component of the examination is a functional test of the anatomic and dynamic aspects of the body and joints. When testing active movements, the examiner should note where in the arc of movement the symptoms occur. For example, pain occurs during abduction of the shoulder between 60° and 120° if there is impingement under the acromion process. Any increase in intensity and quality of pain should also be

---

On Active Movement, the Examiner Should Note

- When and where during each of the movements the onset of pain occurs
- Whether the movement increases the intensity and quality of the pain
- The reaction of the patient to pain
- The amount of observable restriction
- The pattern of movement
- The rhythm and quality of movement
- The movement of associated joints
- The willingness of the patient to move the part
- Any limitation and its nature

Table 1–7
Differential Diagnosis of Strains, Tendinitis, and Sprains

	1° Strain	2° Strain	3° Strain (rupture)	Tendinitis	1° Sprain	2° Sprain	3° Sprain
Definition	Few fibers of muscle torn	About half of muscle fibers torn	All muscle fibers torn (rupture)	Inflammation of tendon	Few fibers of ligament torn	About half of ligament torn	All fibers of ligament torn
Mechanism of injury	Overstretch Overload	Overstretch Overload Crushing	Overstretch Overload	Overuse Overstretch Overload	Overload Overstretch	Overload Overstretch	Overload Overstretch
Onset	Acute	Acute	Acute	Chronic Acute	Acute	Acute	Acute
Weakness	Minor	Moderate to major (reflex inhibition)	Moderate to major	Minor to moderate	Minor	Minor to moderate	Minor to moderate
Disability	Minor	Moderate	Major	Minor to major	Minor	Moderate	Moderate to major
Muscle spasm	Minor	Moderate to major	Moderate	Minor	Minor	Minor	Minor
Swelling	Minor	Moderate to major	Moderate to major	Minor to major (thickening)	Minor	Moderate	Moderate to major
Loss of function	Minor	Moderate to major	Major (reflex inhibition)	Minor to major	Minor	Moderate to major	Moderate to major (instability)
Pain on isometric contraction	Minor	Moderate to major	None to minor	Minor to major	None	None	None
Pain on stretch	Yes	Yes	No*	Yes	Yes	Yes	No*
Joint play	Normal	Normal	Normal	Normal	Normal	Normal	Normal to excessive
Palpable defect	No	No	Yes (if early)	No	No	No	Yes (if early)
Crepitus	No	No	No	Possible	No	No	No
Range of motion	Decreased	Decreased	May increase or decrease depending on swelling	Decreased	Decreased	Decreased	May increase or decrease depending on swelling Dislocation or subluxation possible

* Not if it is the only tissue injured; however, other structures may suffer 1° or 2° injuries and be painful.

noted. This information helps the examiner determine the particular tissue at fault. For example, bone pain, except in the case of a fracture or tumor, often is not altered with movement. By observing the patient's reaction to pain, the examiner can get some idea of how much the condition is affecting the patient and the patient's pain threshold. By noting the pattern of movement, the quality and rhythm of the movement, the movements in other joints, and the observable restriction, the examiner can tell if the patient is "cheating" (using accessory muscles) to do the movement and what tissues are affected. For example, "shoulder hiking" may indicate a capsular pattern of the shoulder.

Generally, active movements are performed once or twice in each desired direction while the examiner notes the pattern of movement and any discrepancies or "cheating" movements. If the patient has noted pain or difficulty with any particular movements, these movements should be done last to ensure no overflow of symptoms to other movements. If the patient has complained that certain repetitive movements or sustained postures are the problem, the examiner should ensure that the movements are repeated (5 to 10 times) or sustained (usually 5 to 20 seconds) until the symptoms are demonstrated.

There are standard movements for each joint and these movements tend to follow cardinal planes. However, if the patient complains of problems outside these standard movements, or if symptoms are more likely to be elicited by combined movements (i.e., movements in multiple planes or around combined axes), repeated movements, movements with speed, or movements under compression, then these should be performed.[34-36] In some cases, especially if the joints are not too reactive, overpressure may carefully be applied at the end of the active ROM. If the overpressure does not produce symptoms, the movement is considered normal and the examiner may decide that passive movements are unnecessary.

Passive Movements

With passive movement, the joint is put through its ROM by the examiner while the patient is relaxed. These movements may also be referred to as physiological or anatomic movements. The movement must proceed through as full a range as possible and should, if possible, involve the same motions as were performed actively. Differences in ROM between active and passive movements may be caused by muscle contraction or spasm, muscle deficiency, neurological deficit, contractures, or pain. ROM may be measured by goniometer, inclinometer, examiner estimation ("eyeballing"), or some similar measure.[37] With most of these methods, it is difficult to show consistent differences of less than 5°.[38] Goniometry is especially useful for measuring and recording joint or fracture deformities. Measurements at different times show progression or regression of the deformity. Although there are books that describe ROMs for various joints, the values given are averages and do not necessarily constitute the ROM needed to do specific activities or the ROM that is present in a specific patient. Normal

mobility is relative. For example, gymnasts tend to be classed as hypermobile in most joints, whereas elderly persons tend to be classed as hypomobile. For these individual populations, however, the available ROM may be considered normal. Certain pathological states may also affect ROM. For example, Ehlers-Danlos syndrome, a connective tissue disorder, results in hypermobility not only of joints but of the skin as well.

Each movement must be compared with the same movement in the opposite joint or, secondarily, with accepted norms. Although passive movement must be gentle, the examiner must determine whether there is any limitation of range (**hypomobility**) or excess of range (**hypermobility** or **laxity**) and, if so, whether it is painful. Hypermobile joints tend to be more susceptible to ligament sprains, joint effusion, chronic pain, recurrent injury, tendinitis resulting from lack of control (instability), and early osteoarthritis. Hypomobile joints are more susceptible to muscle strains, pinched nerve syndromes, and tendinitis resulting from overstress.[39, 40] Hypermobility is not the same as instability. Pathological instability involves loss of small joint movements such as translation, whereas pathological hypermobility refers to excessive gross anatomic movement. Although there are tests[41, 42] to demonstrate general hypermobility, these tests should be interpreted with caution because patients demonstrate a wide range of variability between joints. With careful assessment, one often finds that a joint may be hypermobile in one direction and hypomobile in another direction. It must also be remembered that evidence of hypomobility or hypermobility does not necessarily indicate a pathological state in the person being assessed. The examiner should attempt to determine the cause of the limitation (e.g., pain, spasm, adhesions, compression) and the quality of the movement (e.g., lead pipe, cogwheel).

End Feel[¹]

When assessing passive movement, the examiner should apply overpressure at the end of the ROM to determine the quality of end feel (the sensation the examiner "feels" in the joint as it reaches the end of the ROM) of each passive movement (Table 1–8). A proper evaluation of end feel can help the examiner to assess the type of pathology present, determine a prognosis for the condition, and learn the severity or stage of the problem.

There are three classic normal end feels.

Bone-to-Bone. This is a "hard," unyielding sensation that is painless. An example of normal bone-to-bone end feel is elbow extension.

Soft-Tissue Approximation. With this type of end feel, there is a yielding compression that stops further movement. Examples are elbow and knee flexion, in which movement is stopped by compression of the soft tissues, primarily the muscles. In a particularly slim person with

---

On Passive Movement, the Examiner Should Note

- When and where during each of the movements the pain begins
- Whether the movement increases the intensity and quality of pain
- The pattern of limitation of movement
- The end feel of movement
- The movement of associated joints
- The range of motion available

Table 1–8
Normal and Abnormal End Feel

End Feel	Example
Normal	
Bone-to-bone	Elbow extension
Soft tissue approximation	Knee flexion
Tissue stretch	Ankle dorsiflexion, shoulder lateral rotation, finger extension
Abnormal	
Early muscle spasm	Protective spasm after injury
Late muscle spasm	Spasm caused by instability
Hard capsular	Frozen shoulder
Soft capsular	Synovitis, soft tissue edema
Bone-to-bone	Osteophyte formation
Empty	Acute subacromial bursitis
Springy block	Meniscus tear

little muscle bulk, the end feel of elbow flexion may be bone-to-bone.

Tissue Stretch. There is a hard or firm (springy) type of movement with a slight give. Toward the end of ROM, there is a feeling of springy or elastic resistance. The normal tissue stretch end feel has a feeling of "rising tension." This feeling depends on the thickness of the tissue and may be very elastic, as in the Achilles tendon stretch, or slightly elastic, as in wrist flexion. Tissue stretch is the most common type of normal end feel; it is found when the capsule and ligaments are the primary restraints to movement. Examples are lateral rotation of the shoulder, and knee and metacarpophalangeal joint extension.

In addition to the three normal types of end feel, there are five classic abnormal end feels.[1]

Muscle Spasm. This end feel is invoked by movement, with a sudden dramatic arrest of movement often accompanied by pain. The end feel is sudden and hard. Cyriax calls this a "vibrant twang."[1] Some examiners divide muscle spasm into two parts. **Early muscle spasm** occurs early in the ROM, almost as soon as movement starts; this type of muscle spasm is associated with inflammation and is seen in more acute conditions. **Late muscle spasm** occurs at or near the end of the ROM. It is caused by instability and the resulting irritability caused by movement. An example is muscle spasm occurring during the apprehension test for anterior dislocation of the shoulder. Both types of muscle spasm are the result of the subconscious efforts of the body to protect the injured joint or structure.

Capsular. Although this end feel is very similar to tissue stretch, it does not occur where one would expect. ROM is obviously reduced, and the capsule can be postulated to be at fault. Muscle spasm usually does not occur

in conjunction with the capsular type of end feel. Some examiners divide this end feel into **hard capsular**, in which the end feel has a "thick" quality to it, and **soft capsular**, which is similar to normal but with a restricted ROM. The hard capsular end feel is seen in more chronic conditions or in full-blown capsular patterns. The limitation comes on rather abruptly after a smooth, friction-free movement. The soft capsular end feel is more often seen in acute conditions, with stiffness occurring early in the range and increasing until the end of range is reached. Maitland[43] calls this "resistance through range." Some authors[44] interpret this soft, boggy end feel as being the result of synovitis or soft-tissue edema. Major injury to ligaments often causes a softer end feel until the tension is taken up by other structures.[45]

Bone-to-Bone. This abnormal end feel is similar to the normal bone-to-bone type, but the restriction or sensation of restriction occurs before the end of ROM would normally occur or where a bone-to-bone end feel would not be expected. An example is a bone-to-bone end feel in the cervical spine resulting from osteophyte formation.

Empty. The empty end feel is detected when considerable pain is produced by movement. The movement cannot be performed because of the pain, although no real mechanical resistance is being detected. Examples include an acute subacromial bursitis or a tumor. Patients often have difficulty describing the empty end feel, and there is no muscle spasm involved.

Springy Block. Similar to a tissue stretch, this occurs where one would not expect it to occur; it tends to be found in joints with menisci. There is a rebound effect, and it usually indicates an internal derangement within the joint. A springy block end feel may be found with a torn meniscus of a knee when it is locked or unable to go into full extension.

Capsular Patterns[1]

With passive movement, a full ROM must be carried out in several directions. A short, too-soft movement in the midrange does not achieve the proper results or potential findings. In addition to evaluating the end feel, the examiner must look at the **pattern of limitation or restriction.** If the capsule of the joint is affected, the pattern of proportional limitation is the feature that indicates the presence of a **capsular pattern** in the joint. This pattern is the result of a total joint reaction, with muscle spasm, capsular contraction (the most common cause), and generalized osteophyte formation being possible mechanisms at fault. Each joint has a characteristic pattern of proportional limitation. The presence of this capsular pattern does not indicate the type of joint involvement; only an analysis of the end feel can do this. Only joints that are controlled by muscles have a capsular pattern; joints such as the sacroiliac and distal tibiofibular joints do not exhibit a capsular pattern. Table 1–9 illustrates some of the common capsular patterns seen in joints.

Noncapsular Patterns[1]

The examiner must also be aware of **noncapsular patterns,** for example, a limitation that exists but does not correspond to the classic capsular pattern for that joint. In the shoulder, abduction may be restricted but with very little rotational restriction (e.g., impingement syndrome). Although a total capsular reaction is absent, there are other possibilities, such as ligamentous adhesions, in which only part of a capsule or the accessory ligaments are involved. There may be a local restriction in one direction, often accompanied by pain, and full, pain-free ROM in all other directions. A second possibility is **internal derangement,** which commonly affects only certain joints, such as the knee and elbow. Intracapsular fragments may interfere with the normal sequence of motion. Movements causing impingement of the fragments will be limited, whereas other motions will be free. In the knee, for example, a torn meniscus may cause a blocking of extension, but flexion is usually free. Loose bodies cause limitation when they are caught between articular surfaces. A third possibility is **extra-articular lesions.** These lesions are revealed by disproportionate limitation, extra-articular adhesions, or an acutely inflamed structure limiting movement in a particular direction. For example, limited straight leg raising in the lumbar disc syndrome is referred to as a **constant length phenomenon.** This phenomenon results when the limitation of movement in one joint depends on the position in which another joint is held. The restricted tissue (in this case, the sciatic nerve) must lie outside the joint or joints (in this case, hip and knee) being tested. The constant length phenomenon may also result from muscle adhesions that cause restriction of motion.

Inert Tissue[1]

After the active and passive movements are completed, the examiner should be able to determine whether there are problems with any of the **inert tissues.** The examiner makes such a determination by judging the degree of pain and the limitation of movement within the joint. For lesions of inert tissue, the examiner may find that active and passive movements are painful in the same direction. Usually pain occurs as the limitation of motion approaches. Resisted isometric movements (discussed later) are not usually painful unless some compression is occurring.

Inert tissue refers to all tissue that is not considered contractile or neurological. Four classic patterns may be seen in lesions of inert issue, according to the ROM available and the amount of pain produced.

Table 1–9
Common Capsular Patterns of Joints

Joint	Restriction*
Temporomandibular	Limitation of mouth opening
Atlanto-occipital	Extension, side flexion equally limited
Cervical spine	Side flexion and rotation equally limited, extension
Glenohumeral	Lateral rotation, abduction, medial rotation
Sternoclavicular	Pain at extreme of range of movement
Acromioclavicular	Pain at extreme of range of movement
Humeroulnar	Flexion, extension
Radiohumeral	Flexion, extension supination, pronation
Proximal radioulnar	Supination, pronation
Distal radioulnar	Full range of movement, pain at extremes of rotation
Wrist	Flexion and extension equally limited
Trapeziometacarpal	Abduction, extension
Metacarpophalangeal and interphalangeal	Flexion, extension
Thoracic spine	Side flexion and rotation equally limited, extension
Lumbar spine	Side flexion and rotation equally limited, extension
Sacroiliac, symphysis pubis, and sacrococcygeal	Pain when joints are stressed
Hip†	Flexion, abduction, medial rotation (but in some cases medial rotation is most limited)
Knee	Flexion, extension
Tibiofibular	Pain when joint stressed
Talocrural	Plantar flexion, dorsiflexion
Talocalcaneal (subtalar)	Limitation of varus range of movement
Midtarsal	Dorsiflexion, plantar flexion, adduction, medial rotation
First metatarsophalangeal	Extension, flexion
Second to fifth metatarsophalangeal	Variable
Interphalangeal	Flexion, extension

* Movements are listed in order of restriction.

† For the hip, flexion, abduction, and medial rotation are always the movements most limited in a capsular pattern. However, the order of restriction may vary.

1. If the **range of movement is full and there is no pain,** there is no lesion of the inert tissues being tested by that passive movement; however, there may be lesions of inert tissue in other directions or around other joints.

2. The next pattern is one of **pain and limitation of movement in every direction.** In this pattern, the entire joint is affected, indicating arthritis or capsulitis. Each joint has its own capsular pattern (see Table 1–9), and the amount of limitation is not usually the same in each direction; however, although there is a set pattern for each joint, other directions may also be affected. All movements of the joint may be affected, but the motions described for the capsular pattern always occur in the particular order listed. For example, the capsular pattern of the shoulder is that lateral rotation is most limited, followed by abduction and medial rotation. In early capsular patterns, only one movement may be restricted; this movement is usually the one that has the potential for the greatest restriction. For example, in an early capsular pattern of the shoulder, only lateral rotation may be limited, and the limitation may be slight.

3. A patient with a lesion of inert tissue may experience **pain and limitation or excessive movement in some directions but not in others,** as in a ligament sprain or local capsular adhesion. In other words, a noncapsular pattern is presented. Movements that stretch, pinch, or move the affected structure cause the pain. Internal derangement that results in the blocking of a joint is another example of a lesion of inert tissue that produces a variable pattern. Extra-articular limitation occurs when a lesion outside the joint affects the movement of that joint. Because these movements pinch or stretch the involved structure (e.g., bursitis in the buttock, acute subacromial bursitis), pain and limitation of movement occur on stretch or compression of these structures. If a structure such as a ligament has been torn, the ROM may increase if swelling is minimal, indicating instability (pathological hypermobility) of the joint. Swelling often masks instability because it puts the tissues under tension. Pathological hypermobility, if present, results in greater than normal movement at the joint, causes pain, can put neurogenic structures at risk, and can result in progressive deformity and degeneration.[46] This clinical instability may be seen in the spine or peripheral joints.

4. There may be **limited movement that is pain free.** The end feel for this type of condition is often of the abnormal bone-to-bone type, and it usually indicates a symptomless osteoarthritis. That is, osteophytes are present and restricting movement, but they are not pinching or compressing any sensitive structures. If this situation is encountered, it should be left alone because it is not causing the patient any problem other than

restricted ROM and attempts at treatment could lead to further problems.

Patterns of Inert Tissue Lesions

- Pain-free, full range of motion
- Pain and limited range of motion in every direction
- Pain and excessive or limited range of motion in some directions
- Pain-free, limited range of motion

Resisted Isometric Movements

Resisted isometric movements are the movements tested last in the examination of the joints. This type of movement consists of a strong, static (isometric), voluntary muscle contraction, and it is used to determine whether the contractile tissue is the tissue at fault. If the muscle, its tendon, or the bone into which they insert is at fault, pain and weakness result; the amount of pain and weakness is related to the degree of injury and the patient's pain threshold. If movement is allowed to occur at the joint, inert tissue around the joint will also move, and it will not be clear whether any resulting pain arises from contractile or inert tissues. The joint, therefore, is put in a neutral or resting position so that minimal tension is placed on the inert tissue. The patient is asked to contract the muscle as strongly as possible while the examiner resists to prevent any movement from occurring and to ensure that the patient is using maximum effort. To keep movement to a minimum, it is best for the examiner to position the joint properly in the resting position and then to say to the patient, "Don't let me move you." In this way, the examiner can ensure that the contraction is isometric. Movement cannot be completely eliminated, but this method minimizes it. Some compression of the inert tissues (e.g., cartilage) occurs with the contraction, and there may be some joint shear as well, but it will be minimal if done as described.

On Resisted Isometric Movement, the Examiner Should Note

- Whether the contraction causes pain and, if it does, the pain's intensity and quality
- Strength of the contraction
- Type of contraction causing problem (concentric, isometric, eccentric)

If, as advocated, this isometric hold method is used, then movement against this resistance would require muscle strength of grade 3 to 5 on the muscle test grading scale (Table 1–10).[47] If the muscle strength is less than grade 3, then the methods advocated in muscle testing manuals[44, 48] must be used. If the examiner is having difficulty differentiating between grade 4 and grade 5 for the patient, an eccentric break method of muscle testing may be used. This method starts as an isometric contraction, but then the examiner applies sufficient force to cause an eccentric contraction or a "break" in the patient's isometric contraction. This method provides a more recognizable threshold for maximum isometric contraction.[47] It must be recognized, however, that all three methods are subjective for normal and good values. If, in the history, the patient has complained of symptoms in a different position than those commonly tested, the examiner may modify the isometric test to try to elicit the symptoms. If the patient has complained that a concentric, eccentric, or econcentric contraction has caused the problem, the examiner may include these movements, with or without load, in the examination, but only after the isometric tests have been completed. Econcentric contraction involves two-joint muscles in which the muscle is acting concentrically at one joint and eccentrically at the other joint, the result being minimal or no change in muscle length. In some cases, machines may be used to measure muscle strength, but care should be taken, because these tests are often not isometric, and they are not performed in functional positions or at functional speeds. They do, however, provide a comparison or ratio between right and left and between different movements.

Muscle weakness, if elicited, may be caused by an upper motor neuron lesion, injury to a peripheral nerve, pathology at the neuromuscular junction, a nerve root lesion, or a lesion of the muscle, its tendons, or the bony insertions themselves. For the first three of these causes, the system of muscle test grading may be used. For nerve root lesions, myotome testing is the method of choice. When testing for muscle lesions, it is more appropriate to test the resisted movements isometrically first, to determine which movements are painful, then perform individual muscle tests, as advocated in texts such as that of Daniels and Worthingham,[48] to determine exactly which muscle is at fault.

Causes of Muscle Weakness

- Muscle strain
- Pain/reflex inhibition
- Peripheral nerve injury
- Nerve root lesion (myotome)
- Upper motor neuron lesion
- Tendon pathology
- Avulsion
- Psychologic overlay

If the contraction appears weak, the examiner must make sure that the weakness is not caused by pain or by the patient's fear, unwillingness, or malingering. The examiner can often resolve such a finding by having the patient make a contraction on the good side first, which normally will not cause pain. Weakness that is not associated with pain or disuse is a positive neurological sign indicating that a nerve root, peripheral nerve, or upper motor neuron lesion is at least part of the problem.

Contractile Tissue[1]

With resisted isometric testing, the examiner is looking for problems of **contractile tissue,** which consists of muscles, tendons, their attachments (e.g., bone), and the nervous tissue supplying the contractile tissue. Both active movements and resisted isometric testing demonstrate symptoms if contractile tissue is affected. Usually, passive movements are normal; that is, passive movements are full and pain free, although pain may be exhibited at the end of the ROM when the contractile or nervous tissue is stretched. If contractile tissue has been injured, active movement is painful in one direction (contraction) and passive movement, if painful, is painful in the opposite direction (stretch). Resisted isometric testing is painful in the same direction as active movement. If the muscles are tested as previously described, not all movements will be found to be affected, except in patients with psychogenic pain and sometimes in patients with an acute joint lesion, in which even a small amount of tension on the muscles around the joint provokes pain. However, if the joint lesion is severe, passive movements, when tested, will be markedly affected, and there will be no confusion as to where the lesion lies.

Table 1–10
Muscle Test Grading

Grade	Value	Movement
5	Normal (100%)	Complete range of motion against gravity with maximal resistance
4	Good (75%)	Complete range of motion against gravity with some (moderate) resistance
3+	Fair +	Complete range of motion against gravity with minimal resistance
3	Fair (50%)	Complete range of motion against gravity
3−	Fair −	Some but not complete range of motion against gravity
2+	Poor +	Initiates motion against gravity
2	Poor (25%)	Complete range of motion with gravity eliminated
2−	Poor −	Initiates motion if gravity is eliminated
1	Trace	Evidence of slight contractility but no joint motion
0	Zero	No contraction palpated

As with inert tissue, there are four classic patterns that may be seen with lesions of contractile and nervous tissue.[1] (In this case, however, one is dealing with pain and strength rather than pain and limited or excessive ROM.)

1. Movement that is **strong and pain free** indicates that there is no lesion of the contractile unit being tested or the nervous tissue supplying that contractile unit, regardless of how tender the muscles may be when touched. The muscles and nerves function painlessly and are not the source of the patient's discomfort.

2. Movement that is **strong and painful** indicates a local lesion of the muscle or tendon. Such a lesion could be a first- or second-degree muscle strain. The amount of strength is usually determined by the amount of pain the patient feels on contraction, which results from reflex inhibition that leads to weakness or cogwheel contractions. A second-degree strain produces greater weakness and more pain than a first-degree strain. Similarly, tendinitis causes a strong (relative) and painful contraction, but one that is not usually as strong as on the good side, and the pain is in the tendon, not the muscle. If there is an avulsion fracture, again the movement will be strong and painful. However, if the avulsion is large, the movement will be weak and painful (see later discussion). Typically, there is no primary limitation of passive movement, except, for example, in the case of a gross muscle tear with hematoma where the muscle, which is often in spasm, is being stretched. In this case, the patient may develop joint stiffness secondary to disuse. This is often caused by protective muscle spasm of adjacent muscles that allows, for example, some joint contracture to be superimposed on the muscle lesion. This stiffness then takes precedence in the treatment. One should always remember that it is easier to maintain than it is to restore.

Patterns of Contractile Tissue and Nervous Tissue Lesions

- No pain, and movement is strong
- Pain, and movement is relatively strong
- Pain, and movement is weak
- No pain, and movement is weak

---

3. Movement that is **weak and painful** indicates a severe lesion around that joint, such as a fracture. The weakness that results is usually caused by reflex inhibition of the muscles around the joint, secondary to pain.

4. Movement that is **weak and pain free** indicates a rupture of a muscle (third-degree strain) or its tendon or involvement of the peripheral nerve or nerve root supplying that muscle. If the movement is weak and pain free, neurological involvement or a tendon rupture should be suspected first. With neurological involvement, the examiner must be able to differentiate between the muscle innervation of a nerve root (myotome) and the muscle innervation of a peripheral nerve (see Table 1–6 as an example). Also, the examiner should be able to differentiate between upper and lower motor neuron lesions (see Table 1–4; Table 1–11). Third-degree strains are sometimes masked, because if the force is great enough to cause a complete tear of a muscle, the surrounding muscles, which assisted the movement, may also be injured (first- or second-degree strain). The pain from these secondary muscles can mask the third-degree strain to the primary mover. The tested weakness, however, would be greater with the third-degree strain. Although significant pain can occur at the time of the third-degree injury, this pain usually quickly subsides to a dull ache, even when the muscle is contracting, because there is no tension on the muscle, which no longer has two attachment (origin and insertion) points. For this reason, a "gap" or hole in the muscle may be palpated. When the third-degree injured muscle does contract, the muscle may "bunch up," giving an obvious deformity.

If all movements around a joint appear painful, the pain is often a result of fatigue, emotional hypersensitivity, or emotional problems. Patients may equate effort with discomfort, and they must be told that they are not necessarily the same.

Janda[49] put forth an interesting concept by dividing muscles into two groups: postural and phasic. He believed that **postural** or **tonic muscles,** which are the muscles responsible for maintaining upright posture, have a tendency to become tight and hypertonic with pathology and to develop contractures but are less likely to atrophy, whereas **phasic muscles,** which include almost all other muscles, tend to become weak and inhibited with pathology. The examiner must be careful to note the type of muscle affected and the ROM available (active movements) as well as strength and production of pain (resisted isometric movements) when testing contractile tissue. Table 1–12 shows the muscles that are postural and prone to tightness and those that are phasic and prone to weakness. Table 1–13 shows the characteristics of postural and phasic muscles. If a muscle imbalance is present, the tight muscles must first be stretched to their normal length and tone before equalization of strength can be accomplished.[50, 51]

Table 1–11
Signs and Symptoms of Upper Motor Neuron Lesions

Spasticity

Hypertonicity

Hyperreflexia (deep tendon reflexes)

Positive pathological reflexes

Absent or reduced superficial reflexes

Extensor plantar response (bilateral)

Table 1–12
Functional Division of Muscle Groups*

Muscles Prone to Tightness (Postural Muscles)	Muscles Prone to Weakness (Phasic Muscles)
Gastrocnemius and soleus	Peronei
Tibialis posterior	Tibialis anterior
Short hip adductors	Vastus medialis and lateralis
Hamstrings	
Rectus femoris	Gluteus maximus, medius, and minimus
Iliopsoas	
Tensor fasciae latae	Rectus abdominis
Piriformis	Serratus anterior
	Rhomboids
Erector spinae (especially lumbar, thoracolumbar, and cervical portions)	Lower portion of trapezius
	Short cervical flexors
Quadratus lumborum	Extensors of upper limb
Pectoralis major	
Upper portion of trapezius	
Levator scapulae	
Sternocleidomastoid	
Scalenes	
Flexors of the upper limb	

* Janda considers all other muscles neutral.

Modified from Jull, G., and V. Janda: Muscles and motor control in low back pain. In Twomey, L.T., and J.R. Taylor (eds.): Physical Therapy for the Low Back: Clinics in Physical Therapy. New York, Churchill Livingstone, 1987, p. 258.

Other Findings

When carrying out the examination of the joints, the examiner must be aware of other findings that may become evident and may help to determine the nature and location of the problem. For example, it should be noted whether there is excessive ROM (hypermobility or laxity) within the joints. Comparison of the normal side with the involved side of the body gives some indication as to whether the findings on the affected side would be considered normal. For example, an apparently excessive range may just be the normal ROM for that patient. It must also be remembered that joints on the nondominant side tend to be more flexible than those on the dominant side.

It is also important to note whether a **painful arc** is present; this finding indicates that an internal structure is being squeezed. **Sounds** such as crepitus, clicking, or snapping should be noted. They may be caused by structures slipping over one another (e.g., tendons slipping over bone), loose bodies or arthritic changes in the joint, abnormal movement of structures (e.g., meniscus click on opening or closing of the temporomandibular joint), or a tear in a structure (e.g., a tear in the cartilage of the wrist). **Pain at the extreme of range of motion** may be caused by squeezing or stretching in which a particular joint is affected.

Table 1–13
Characteristics of Postural and Phasic Muscle Groups

Muscles Prone to Tightness (Postural Muscles)	Muscles Prone to Weakness (Phasic Muscles)
Predominantly postural function	Primarily phasic function
Associated with flexor reflexes	Associated with extensor reflexes
Primarily two-joint muscles	Primarily one-joint muscles
Readily activated with movement (shorter chronaxie)	Not readily activated with movement (longer chronaxie)
Tendency to tightness, hypertonia, shortening, or contractures	Tendency to hypotonia, inhibition, or weakness
Resistance to atrophy	Atrophy occurs easily

Adapted from Jull, G., and V. Janda: Muscles and motor control in low back pain. In Twomey, L.T., and J.R. Taylor (eds.): Physical Therapy for the Low Back: Clinics in Physical Therapy. New York, Churchill Livingstone, 1987.

Functional Assessment

Functional assessment plays a very important role in the evaluation of the patient. It is different from the analysis of specific movement patterns of active, passive, and resisted isometric movements to differentiate between inert, neurological, and contractile tissue. Functional assessment may involve task analysis or simply observation of certain patient activities. Determining what the patient hopes is an appropriate functional outcome and what the patient can and cannot do functionally can be extremely important in the choice of treatments that will be successful. Primarily, functional assessment helps the examiner establish what is important to the patient and the patient's expectations. It represents a measurement of a **whole-body task performance ability,** as opposed to isolated examination of a joint. Because it is part of each individual joint assessed, the functional testing should demonstrate whether an isolated impairment affects the patient's ability to perform everyday activities.

The examiner should attempt to establish what functional factors are important to the patient. For example, functional testing may include movements under different loads to determine the patient's ability to work or play. Likewise, repeated movements and sustained postures may be necessary for work, recreational, or social activities. In some cases, movements at different speeds or under different loads may be necessary to determine pathology.[36] Atraumatic shoulder instability, for example, may not be evident in a swimmer except when he or she is actually doing the activity at the speed and load at which the activity is done in the water.

Because functional testing relates to the effect of the injury on the patient's life, those activities that cause symptoms, those that are restricted by symptoms, and the factors (e.g., strength, power, flexibility) that are

Table 1-14
Examples of Functional and Clinical Outcomes

Clinical Outcomes	Functional Outcomes
Strength	Power
Range of motion	Agility
Proprioception	Kinesthetic awareness
Endurance (muscular)	Endurance (muscular and cardiovascular)
Swelling	
Pain	Speed
Psychological overlay	Activity specificity
	Pain
	Skill level required for activity
	Psychological preparedness
	Daily living skills

needed to perform the activities are considered. For example, if the patient is seated normally while a history is taken, the examiner knows the patient has the functional ROM (agility) for sitting with 90° of hip and knee flexion. Table 1-14 lists some functional outcome measures that should be considered. The activities should be simple, patient-oriented, and based on coordinated functional movement of the joints, and they should be activities the patient wants to do. Although most functional outcomes or tests are subjective, this does not make them any less effective.[52]

The functional assessment is important to determine the effect of the condition or injury on the patient's daily life, including his or her sex life. Functional impairment may be slightly annoying or completely disabling for the patient. Functional activities that should be tested, if appropriate, include self-care activities such as walking, dressing, daily hygiene (e.g., washing, bathing, shaving, combing hair), eating, and going to the bathroom; recreational activities such as reading, sewing, watching television, gardening, and playing a musical instrument; and activities such as driving, dialing a telephone, getting groceries, preparing meals, and hanging clothes. Goldstein[53] has nicely divided activities of human function into four broad areas, which are then broken down into more discrete levels (Table 1-15). The examiner should consider which of these are important to the patient and ensure that they are considered in the assessment. Figure 1-10 shows some of the daily living

Table 1-15
Goldstein's Divisions of Human Function

Function: Basic or Personal Activities of Daily Living (ADLs)

Activity	Examples	Activity	Examples
Bed activities	Moving in bed Managing pillows and blankets Reaching for objects Sitting up	Dressing activities	Putting on clothes Tying laces Putting on socks and shoes
Hygiene activities	Brushing teeth Bathing and showering Washing Toileting Combing hair Shaving Putting on makeup	Transfer activities	Bed to chair Sit to stand Getting into car
		Walking activities	Level and uneven surfaces Curbs and stairs Opening doors Walking and carrying items Distance and velocity Assistive devices Gait deviations
Eating activities	Using utensils Cutting meat Managing glass and cup		

Function: Instrumental (Advanced) Activities of Daily Living (IADLs)

Activity	Examples	Activity	Examples
Meal preparation	Cutting vegetables Turning on oven Measuring ingredients	Having sex	Manipulating clothing Changing positions
Light housework	Dusting Washing dishes Mopping floors	Driving car	Getting in and out Turning wheel Adjusting pedals, mirrors
Check writing	Manipulating pen Adding and subtracting	Gardening	Kneeling Raking Digging Watering
Shopping	Pushing cart Carrying groceries Reaching Getting money out of pocket	Communicating	Using writing tools Using telephone

Table continued on following page

Table 1–15
Goldstein's Divisions of Human Function (Continued)

Function: Work Activities

Activity	Examples	Activity	Examples
Lifting	From table and from floor	Kneeling	On all fours and just knees
Carrying	Small and large objects	Manipulating objects	Pen, salt shaker
Stooping	Wiping floor	Climbing	Stairs and ladder
Pushing	Broom	Standing	
Pulling	Drawer and door	Walking	Slow and fast
Reaching	Into cupboard		

Function: Sport and Recreational Activities

Activity	Example	Activity	Example
Walking	Forward and backward Sideways Level and uneven surfaces	Hitting	Baseball bat Tennis racquet Golf club
Jogging and sprinting	Different surfaces In water	Swimming	Different strokes Different kicks
Cutting	Circles Figure-eights Crossover and sidestep	Agility	Specific drills
		Open and closed kinetic chain	Throwing and pushing
Jumping and hopping	Vertical and distance Forward and backward Level and uneven surfaces	Speed and power	Moving different sized objects at different speeds
Throwing	Underhand and overhand Two-handed Different objects	Endurance	Aerobic and anaerobic Cardiovascular and muscle
Catching	One- and two-handed Different sizes and weights	Reaction time and proprioception	Blinking lights

Data from Goldstein, T.S.: Functional Rehabilitation in Orthopedics. Gaithersburg, Maryland, Aspen Pub. Inc., 1995, pp. 19–23.

Daily Living Skill and Mobility Questions for Functional Assessment

Daily Living Skills	**Mobility**

Daily Living Skills

Feeding
(7) Are you able to feed yourself from a tray or table using ordinary utensils? Can you cut meat? Can you pour liquids from open containers?
(4) If you use a spork or rocker knife or other helpful aid, are you able to feed yourself in a reasonable length of time?
(2) Are you able to feed yourself with some help from another person, for example, to help you raise a cup to your mouth or to cut meat?
(0) Do you depend on another person to feed you?

Dress Upper Body
(7) Are you able to get clothes out of your closets and drawers and put them on and remove them from your upper body by yourself, including bra, slip, pullovers, and front opening shirts and blouses, as well as managing zippers, buttons, and snaps?
(4) If someone lays your clothes out for you or hands them to you, are you able to dress your upper body by yourself even if it takes a little more time, or do you need some help with closures, such as buttons, zippers, snaps, or hooks? Do you use aids such as reachers, dressing hooks, button hooks, or zipper pulls?
(2) Does someone help you put on your blouse or shirt or sweater because you are limited by pain, lack of strength, or limited range of motion?
(0) Do you depend on another person to dress your upper body?

Mobility

Supine to Sit
(7) When you are lying on your back, can you sit up without using your arms or without rolling to the side? Can you do this smoothly and easily?
(4) Do you use your arms to help you sit up, or do you roll to the side before sitting up? Do you have to try several times before sitting up?
(2) Does someone help you to sit up?
(0) Are you unable to sit up?

Sitting to Standing
(7) Are you able to stand up from a regular chair without using your arms?
(4) Do you need to use your arms to help you stand up, or do you need to try several times?
(2) Does someone need to help you stand up out of a chair?
(0) Do you depend on someone else entirely to get you out of a chair?

Transfer—Toilet
(7) Are you able to get on and off the toilet easily and without using your hands?
(4) Do you need to use your arms to help you get on and off the toilet, or do you require assistive devices such as elevated toilet seats or grab bars?
(2) Does someone need to help you get on and off the toilet?
(0) Are you unable to use the toilet?

Figure 1–10

See legend on opposite page

Daily Living Skills	Mobility

Dress Lower Body

(7) Are you able to put on undergarments, slacks, socks, nylons, and shoes by yourself? Can you tie shoelaces?

(4) Are you able to put on undergarments, slacks, socks, nylons, and shoes by yourself if they are laid out for you or handed to you? Do you use dressing aids such as long handled reachers? Do you avoid shoes that have laces or buckles, or do you use elastic laces or velcro shoe closures by yourself?

(2) Does someone help you to put on undergarments, slacks, nylons, or shoes?

(0) Do you depend on another person to dress your lower body?

Grooming

(7) Are you able to comb and brush and shampoo your hair, shave, apply makeup, clean your teeth or dentures, and manage nail care by yourself without adaptations or modifications?

(4) Do you use assistive devices or adapted methods for grooming: If someone places what you need within reach, are you then able to complete grooming activities unaided? Do you use long-handled combs or brushes, suction brushes for cleaning nails or dentures, adapted shaving equipment or adapted key for rolling toothpaste tubes?

(2) Does someone actually help you shampoo or brush your hair, shave, apply makeup, clean your teeth or dentures, or manicure your nails?

(0) Do you depend on someone else entirely for your grooming needs?

Care of Perineum/Clothing at Toilet

(7) Are you able to go to the bathroom by yourself including managing your clothes, wiping yourself (and placing sanitary napkins or tampons)?

(4) Are you able to manage your clothing at the toilet and wipe yourself independently although it may be difficult, or do you use aids such as an extended reacher for wiping yourself or clothing aids?

(2) Does someone help you with your clothing at the toilet or assist you with wiping yourself (or in placement of sanitary napkins or tampons)?

(0) Do you depend on someone else to manage your clothes at the toilet for you or to wipe you (or to place sanitary napkins or tampons)?

Wash or Bathe

(7) Are you able to wash and dry your entire body by yourself, including your back and feet? Are you able to turn water faucets?

(4) Do you use bathing aids such as long handled bath brushes or sponges? Are you unable to reach some parts of your body for bathing or drying thoroughly but can still manage without help?

(2) Are you able to bathe and dry most parts of your body and have someone help you with the rest?

(0) Does someone else bathe you?

Vocational

(2) Are you employed full-time in your usual occupation? Are you a full-time homemaker and require no assistance? Are you retired for other than medical reasons?

(0) Not able to do the above

Transfer—Tub or Shower

(7) Are you able to get in and out of a tub or shower safely?

(4) Can you get in and out of a tub or shower using aids such as grab bars or special seat or lift?

(2) Does someone need to help you to get in and out of the tub or shower?

(0) Are you unable to get in and out of the tub or shower?

Transfer—Automobile

(7) Can you get in and out of a car easily, including opening and closing the door?

(4) Can you get in and out of a car by yourself if you use aids such as grab bars or if someone opens the door for you?

(2) Does someone help you get in and out of a car?

(0) Are you unable to get in and out of a car even with assistance?

Walk on Level

(7) Are you able to walk two blocks at an even pace without using a cane, crutches, walker, or adapted shoes?

(4) Do you need a cane, crutches, or walker to walk two blocks?

(2) Can you walk one block with assistance?

(0) Are you unable to walk one block even with assistance?

Walk Outdoors

(7) Are you able to walk outdoors at least two blocks without avoiding rough terrain such as grass, sand, gravel, curbs, ramps, or hills?

(4) Do you try to avoid uneven terrain? Do you use a crutch or cane for safety or balance purposes only when outside?

(2) Must you use a cane or crutches to walk at least two blocks on uneven terrain?

(0) Are you unable to walk on uneven terrain?

Up and Down Stairs

(7) Can you go up and down at least five steps safely, step over step without using the hand rail or other support?

(4) Are you able to go up and down at least five steps if you use a hand rail, cane, or crutches or if you go one step at a time?

(2) Do you need someone to help you go up and down at least five steps?

(0) Are you unable to go up and down at least five steps even with help?

Wheelchair/10 Yards

(7) Are you able to push your wheelchair without help for 10 yards? Can you turn corners and get close to bed, table, and toilet?

(4) Do you use a motorized wheelchair?

(2) Do you need someone to help you maneuver your wheelchair around corners or to help you position it?

(0) Are you unable to push your wheelchair 10 yards?

Figure 1–10 *Continued*

Daily living skill and mobility questions for function assessment. (Modified from Convery, F.R., M.A. Minteer, D. Amiel, and K.L. Connett: Polyarticular disability: A functional assessment. Arch. Phys. Med. Rehab. 58:498, 1977.)

skills and mobility questions that may be of concern to both the examiner and the patient. Other functional assessment tools that are available include the functional capacity evaluation (FCE),[53] the functional independence measure (FIM),[54] the physical performance test,[55] the functional status test,[56] the arthritis impact measurement scale (AIMS 2),[57] and the functional assessment tool (FAT).[58] The particular tool used depends on the needs of the patient and the presenting pathological problem.

Part of this functional assessment occurs during the history, when the examiner asks the patient which activities can be done easily, which with some difficulty, and which not at all. During the observation, the examiner notes what the patient can and cannot do within the confines of the assessment area. Finally, during the examination, functional testing or a work analysis may be performed. For example, when examining the hand, the examiner notes the power and dexterity exhibited during performance of fundamental maneuvers such as gripping and pinching. Similarly, Table 1–16 shows an example of a work activity analysis, which may be evaluated if the patient is hoping to return to that activity and to do it successfully.[59] Regardless of which functional test is used, it is important for the examiner to understand the purpose of the test. A functional test should not be done just because it is available. It should not be used in isolation but rather in conjunction with the overall assessment, so that a complete assessment picture of the patient can be developed.

Numerical scoring systems are often used as part of the functional assessment. These scoring systems are often more related to function as it applies to a specific joint rather than to the whole body (Fig. 1–11),[60] and for many, functional assessment plays only a small part. With these numerical systems, the clinician must ensure that the scoring systems really measure what they say

they measure. To be effective, a numerical scoring system must demonstrate universality, practicality, reliability, reproducibility, effectiveness, and inclusiveness, and it must have been validated.[61] The terminology and methods must be described precisely; the criteria should be related to functional outcome (what the patient desires) rather than clinical outcome (what the clinician desires), and the measures must be sensitive enough to show a difference.[62] Figure 1–12 shows a functional assessment involving the entire upper limb.[63] Table 1–17 demonstrates tests that could be used in an examination of simulated activities of daily living.[64] Similar charts can and have been developed for almost all joints of the body. However, many of these numerical scoring systems have been developed from the clinician's perspective rather than from what the patient thinks is important.

Functional tests may also be used as provocative tests to bring on the symptoms the patient has complained of or to determine how the patient is progressing or whether he or she is ready to return to activity. Examples of these tests include the hop test and disco test for the knee. These tests in reality could be used for all the weight-bearing (lower limb) joints. However, it must be remembered that many of these provocative or stress tests are designed for very active persons and are not suitable for all populations.

Special Tests

After the examiner has completed the history, observation, and evaluation of movement, special tests may be performed for the involved joint. Many special tests are available for each joint to determine whether a particular type of disease, condition, or injury is present. They are sometimes called clinical accessory, provocative, or structural tests. These tests, although strongly suggestive of a particular disease or condition when they yield positive results, do not necessarily rule out the disease or condition when they yield negative results. The findings of the tests depend primarily on the skill and ability of the examiner.

For each joint examination described in this book, specific tests are mentioned for specific conditions. Tests that the author has found to be particularly effective have been highlighted, but this does not rule out the use of other tests. Many of the tests are very similar and

Table 1–16
Example of an Analysis of Work Activity

Job title: *Packer*
Essential function: *Packing individual cobbler cups for shipping*
Steps:

1. Select a box
2. Place the box on the conveyor side rack
3. Pick up one cobbler cup in each hand
4. Place the cups into the packing box
5. Repeat steps 3 and 4 until 36 cups are in a box
6. Place the filled box on the "sealing table"
7. Fold the short flaps of the box lid
8. Fold the longer flaps of the box lid
9. Tape down the long flaps of the box using the manual taping machine
10. Place the sealed box on the pallet

From Ellexson, M.T.: Analyzing an industry: Job analysis for treatment, prevention, and placement. Orthop. Phys. Ther. Clin. 1:17, 1992.

Special Test Uses[35]

- To confirm a tentative diagnosis
- To make a differential diagnosis
- To differentiate between structures
- To understand unusual signs
- To unravel difficult signs and symptoms

Shoulder Evaluation Form

Diagnosis:
Aim of Procedure:
Operation:
Shoulder: right: left:
Arm Dominance: right: left:

The rating in each category can be adjusted
according to the AIM of the procedure

Patient's Name:
Hospital Unit #:
Date of Operation:
Date of Follow-up:
Surgeon:
Preoperative rating:
Postoperative rating:
Patient's Evaluation (circle):
Exc.   Good   Fair   Poor

Unit Rating
(circle one in
each category)

Unit Rating
(circle one in
each category)

I. PAIN (15)

1.	None	15
2.	Slight during activity	12
3.	Increased pain during activities	6
4.	Moderate/severe pain in activity	3
5.	Severe pain, dependent on medication	0 ___

II. STABILITY (25)

1.	Normal. Shoulder stable and strong in all positions	25
2.	Mild apprehension in normal use of arm. No subluxation or dislocation	20
3.	Avoids elevation and external rotation. Rare subluxation	10
4.	Recurrent subluxations ("Dead arm syndrome"). Positive apprehension test or recurrent dislocation	5
5.	Recurrent dislocation	0 ___

III. FUNCTION (25)

1.	Normal function. All activities of daily living. Performs all work, sport/recreation prior to injury. Lifting 30 + lb. Swimming, tennis, throwing. Combat	25
2.	Mild limitation in sports and work. Can throw, but limited in baseball. Strong in tennis, football, swimming, lifting (15–20 lb) and combat. Performs all personal care	20
3.	Moderate limitation in overhead work and lifting (10 lb) and athletics. Unable to throw or serve in tennis. Swims sidestroke. Difficulty with body care (perineal care, back pocket, combing hair, reaching back). Aid necessary at times	10
4.	Severe limitations. Unable to perform usual work or lifting. No athletics. Sedentary occupation. Unable to perform body care without aid. Can feed self and comb hair.	5
5.	Complete disability of extremity	0 ___

IV. MOTION (25)

Abduction and forward flexion

151 to 170°	15
121 to 150°	12
91 to 120°	10
61 to 90°	7
31 to 60°	5
Less than 30°	0 ___

IR   Thumb to scapula — 5
     Thumb to sacrum — 3
     Thumb to trochanter — 2
     Less than trochanter — 0 ___

ER   (with arm at side)
     80° — 5
     60° — 3
     30° — 2
     Less than 30° — 0 ___

V. STRENGTH (10) (compared to opposite shoulder)

(specify method = manual, spring gauge, Cybex)

Normal	10
Good	6
Fair	4
Poor	0 ___

TOTAL UNITS

Excellent   (100–85 units)   ___
Good   (84–70 units)
Fair   (69–50 units)
Poor   (49 units or less)

Figure 1–11

Shoulder evaluation form. (Modified from Rowe, C.R.: The Shoulder. Edinburgh, Churchill Livingstone, 1988, p. 632.)

show similar results; which ones to use depends on which give the best results for the individual examiner. For example, the **anterior drawer sign** was used for years to determine whether there was a problem with the anterior cruciate ligament of the knee. However, literature from the past few years has indicated that the **Lachman test** is much more effective.

Seldom are special tests taken in isolation to make a diagnosis. They should be considered as tests to confirm a tentative diagnosis, to make a differential diagnosis, to differentiate between structures, to understand unusual signs, or to unravel difficult signs and symptoms.[35] Often the examiner can design his or her own special tests or modify the described tests. Sometimes,

Upper Extremity Function Test

Basic Function	*Date* _____	
	Right	**Left**
Grasp		
1. Block 4 in. (Item 1)		
2. Block 3 in. (Item 2)		
3. Block 2 in. (Item 3)		
4. Block 1 in. (Item 4)		
Grip		
5. Pipe 1¾ in. (Item 5)		
6. Pipe ¾ in. (Item 6)		
Lateral Prehension		
7. Slate 1 × ⅝ × 4 in. (Item 7)		
Pinch		
8. Ball 3 in. (Item 8)		
Marble ⅝ in. (Item 9)		
9. Index finger and thumb		
10. Middle finger and thumb		
11. Ring finger and thumb		
12. Small finger and thumb		
Ball-bearing ⁷⁄₁₆ in. (Item 10)		
13. Index finger and thumb		
14. Middle finger and thumb		
15. Ring finger and thumb		
16. Small finger and thumb		
Ball-bearing ¼ in. (Item 11)		
17. Index finger and thumb		
18. Middle finger and thumb		
19. Ring finger and thumb		
20. Small finger and thumb		
Ball-bearing ⁵⁄₃₂ in. (Item 12)		
21. Index finger and thumb		
22. Middle finger and thumb		
23. Ring finger and thumb		
24. Small finger and thumb		
Placing		
25. Washer over nail (Item 13)		
26. Iron to shelf (Item 14)		
Supination and Pronation		
27. Pour water from pitcher to glass		
28. Pour water from glass to glass (pronation)		
29. Pour water back to first glass (supination)		
30. Place hand behind head		
31. Place hand on top of head		
32. Hand to mouth		
33. Write name _____		
	TOTAL _____	

Smedly Dynamometer Reading:
Does pain interfere with function?

Scoring:	3—Performs test normally
	2—Completes test, but takes abnormally long time or has great difficulty
	1—Performs test partially
	0—Can perform no part of test

Score:	0–25:	Trace
	26–50:	Very poor
	51–75:	Poor
	76–89:	Partial
	90–98:	Functional
	99–100:	Maximal (dominant hand) (96-nondominant hand)

Figure 1–12

Upper extremity function test. (Modified by permission of the publisher from Carroll, D.: A quantitative test of upper extremity function. J. Chron. Dis. 18:482, Copyright 1965 by Elsevier Science Inc.)

Table 1–17
Summary Description of Tests in Simulated Activities of Daily Living Examination (SADLE)

Test	Measure	Units	Instrumentation
Two leg standing, eyes open	Maximum time of three 30-second trials	Seconds	Stopwatch
One leg standing, eyes open	Maximum time of three 30-second trials	Seconds	Stopwatch
Two leg standing, eyes closed	Maximum time of three 30-second trials	Seconds	Stopwatch
One leg standing, eyes closed	Maximum time of three 30-second trials	Seconds	Stopwatch
Tandem walking with supports	Time to take 10 heel-to-toe steps	Steps/sec	Stopwatch and parallel bars
Tandem walking without supports	Time to take 10 heel-to-toe steps	Steps/sec	Stopwatch and parallel bars
Putting on a shirt	Average time of two trials	Seconds	Stopwatch and shirt
Managing three visible buttons	Average time of two trials	Seconds	Stopwatch and cloth with three buttons mounted on a board
Zipping a garment	Average time of two trials	Seconds	Stopwatch and cloth with zipper mounted on a board
Putting on gloves	Average time of two trials	Seconds	Stopwatch and two garden gloves
Dialing a telephone	Average time of two trials	Seconds	Stopwatch and telephone
Tying a bow	Average time of two trials	Seconds	Stopwatch and large shoelaces mounted on a board
Manipulating safety pins	Average time of two trials	Seconds	Stopwatch and two safety pins
Picking up coins	Average time of two trials	Seconds	Stopwatch and four coins placed on a plastic sheet
Threading a needle	Average time of two trials	Seconds	Stopwatch, thread, and large-eyed needle
Unwrapping a Band-Aid	Time for one trial	Seconds	Stopwatch and one Band-Aid
Squeezing toothpaste	Average time of two trials	Seconds	Stopwatch, tube of toothpaste, and a board
Cutting with a knife	Average time of two trials	Seconds	Stopwatch, plate, fork, knife, and permoplast
Using a fork	Average time of two trials	Seconds	Stopwatch, plate, fork, and permoplast

Modified from Potvin, A.R., W.W. Tourtellotte, J.S. Dailey, et al.: Simulated activities of daily living examination. Arch. Phys. Med. Rehab. 53:478, 1972.

the examiner can reproduce the same movement the patient described as the mechanism of injury, which may provoke the symptoms. However, the addition of too many special tests only makes the picture more confusing and the diagnosis more difficult. Also, care should be taken when performing these tests, because they are usually provocative tests and will provoke signs and symptoms, including pain and apprehension. Special tests should be done with caution and may be contraindicated in the presence of severe pain, acute and irritable conditions of the joints, instability, osteoporosis, pathological bone diseases, active disease processes, unusual signs and symptoms, major neurological signs, and patient apprehension.

In addition to the special tests, the examiner may also make use of **laboratory tests** for specific conditions. With osteomyelitis, for example, a positive blood culture is likely to be obtained, the white blood cell count will be elevated, and the erythrocyte sedimentation rate will be increased. The examiner, if a physician, may decide

Table 1–18
Normal Laboratory Values Used in Orthopedic Medicine*

Laboratory Test	Normal Range
White blood cell (WBC) count	$4–9 \times 10^9/L$
Red blood cell (RBC) count	$4.3–5.4 \times 10^{12}/L$ (male) $3.8–5.2 \times 10^{12}/L$ (female)
Hematocrit (HCT)	38–50% (male) 34–46% (female)
Hemoglobin (Hgb)	130–170 g/L (male) 115–160 g/L (female)
Erythrocyte sedimentation rate (ESR)	0–10 mm/hr (male) 0–15 mm/hr (female) 0–10 mm/hr (children)
Myoglobin (Mb)	30–90 ng/ml
Ferritin	25–465 μg/ml (male) 15–200 μg/ml (female)
Platelet count	140,000–350,000/mm³
Calcium	8.5–10.5 mg/dl
Ionized calcium	4.2–5.4 mg/dl
Alkaline phosphatase	25–92 U/L
Antinuclear antibodies screen	Negative
Uric acid	3.5–7.2 mg/dl (male) 2.6–6.0 mg/dl (female)
Rheumatoid arthritis factor	<1.20

* Values may vary slightly depending on equipment used.

to draw fluid out of a joint with a hypodermic needle to view the synovial fluid. Tables 1–18, 1–19, and 1–20 present normal laboratory values, laboratory findings in some bone diseases, and a classification of synovial fluid as examples of laboratory tests and values.

Reflexes and Cutaneous Distribution

After the special tests, the examiner can test the superficial, deep tendon, and/or pathological reflexes to obtain

Table 1–20
Classification of Synovial Fluid

Type	Appearance	Significance
Group 1	Clear yellow	Noninflammatory states, trauma
Group 2*	Cloudy	Inflammatory arthritis; excludes most patients with osteoarthritis
Group 3	Thick exudate, brownish	Septic arthritis; occasionally seen in gout
Group 4	Hemorrhagic	Trauma, bleeding disorders, tumors, fractures

* Inflammatory fluids will clot and should be collected in heparin-containing tubes. All group 2 or 3 fluids should be cultured if the diagnosis is uncertain.

From Curran, J.F., M.H. Ellman, and N.L. Brown: Rheumatologic aspects of painful conditions affecting the shoulder. Clin. Orthop. Relat. Res. 173:28, 1983.

an indication of the state of the nerve or nerve roots supplying the reflex. Most often, the deep tendon reflexes are tested with a reflex hammer. A deep tendon reflex can be elicited from almost any tendon with practice. The more common deep tendon reflexes tested are shown in Table 1–21. Tables 1–22 and 1–23 demonstrate superficial and pathological reflexes. Superficial reflexes are reflexes provoked by superficial stroking, usually with a sharp object. A pathological reflex is not normally present, and if it is present, it often serves as a sign of some pathological condition.

With a loss or abnormality of nerve conduction, there is a diminution (hyporeflexia) or loss (areflexia) of the stretch reflex. It should be remembered that there is a decreased response with aging. Upper motor neuron lesions (see Table 1–11) produce findings of spasticity, hyperreflexia, hypertonicity, extensor plantar responses, reduced or absent superficial reflexes, and weakness of muscles distal to the lesion. Lower motor neuron lesions involving nerve roots or peripheral nerves produce find-

Table 1–19
Laboratory Findings in Bone Disease

Condition	Calcium	Inorganic Phosphorus	Alkaline Phosphatase	Calcium	Phosphorus
Hyperparathyroidism, primary	↑	↓	↑	↑	↑
Hyperparathyroidism, secondary	N-↓	↑	R↑	↑	↑
Hyperthyroidism, marked	N	N	↑	↑	↑
Hypothyroidism	N	N	N	N	N
Senile osteoporosis	N	N-O↓	N	N	N
Rickets (child)	↓	↓	↑	N	N
Osteomalacia (adult)	N-↓	↓	↑	N	N
Paget's disease	R↑	R↓	↑	N	N
Multiple myeloma	↑	N-↑	R↑	↑	↑

N = normal; O = occasionally; R = rarely; ↑ = increased; ↓ = decreased.

Adapted from Quinn, J.: Introduction to the musculoskeletal system. In Meschan, I.: Synopsis of Analysis of Roentgen Signs in General Radiology. Philadelphia, W.B. Saunders Co., 1976, p. 27.

Table 1–21
Common Deep Tendon Reflexes

Reflex	Site of Stimulus	Normal Response	Pertinent Central Nervous System Segment
Jaw	Mandible	Mouth closes	Cranial nerve V
Biceps	Biceps tendon	Biceps contraction	C5–C6
Brachioradialis	Brachioradialis tendon or just distal to the musculotendinous junction	Flexion of elbow and/or pronation of forearm	C5–C6
Triceps	Distal triceps tendon above the olecranon process	Elbow extension	C7–C8
Patella	Patellar tendon	Leg extension	L3–L4
Medial hamstrings	Semimembranosus tendon	Knee flexion	L5, S1
Lateral hamstrings	Biceps femoris tendon	Knee flexion	S1–S2
Tibialis posterior	Tibialis posterior tendon behind medial malleolus	Plantar flexion of foot with inversion	L4–L5
Achilles	Achilles tendon	Plantar flexion of foot	S1–S2

Table 1–22
Superficial Reflexes

Reflex	Normal Response	Pertinent Central Nervous System Segment
Upper abdominal	Umbilicus moves up and toward area being stroked	T7–T9
Lower abdominal	Umbilicus moves down and toward area being stroked	T11–T12
Cremasteric	Scrotum elevates	T12, L1
Plantar	Flexion of toes	S1–S2
Gluteal	Skin tenses in gluteal area	L4–L5, S1–S3
Anal	Contraction of anal sphincter muscles	S2–S4

Table 1–23
Pathological Reflexes

Reflex	Elicitation	Positive Response	Pathology
Babinski's	Stroking of lateral aspect of side of foot	Extension of big toe and fanning of four small toes Normal reaction in newborns	Pyramidal tract lesion Organic hemiplegia
Chaddock's	Stroking of lateral side of foot beneath lateral malleolus	Same response as above	Pyramidal tract lesion
Oppenheim's	Stroking of anteromedial tibial surface	Same response as above	Pyramidal tract lesion
Gordon's	Squeezing of calf muscles firmly	Same response as above	Pyramidal tract lesion
Piotrowski's	Percussion of tibialis anterior muscle	Dorsiflexion and supination of foot	Organic disease of central nervous system
Brudzinski's	Passive flexion of one lower limb	Similar movement occurs in opposite limb	Meningitis
Hoffmann's (digital)	"Flicking" of terminal phalanx of index, middle, or ring finger	Reflex flexion of distal phalanx of thumb and of distal phalanx of index or middle finger (whichever one was not "flicked")	Increased irritability of sensory nerves in tetany Pyramidal tract lesion
Rossolimo's	Tapping of the plantar surface of toes	Plantar flexion of toes	Pyramidal tract lesion
Schaeffer's	Pinching of Achilles tendon in middle third	Flexion of foot and toes	Organic hemiplegia

ings of flaccidity, hyporeflexia or areflexia, hypotonicity, fasciculation, fibrillations, and weakness and atrophy of the involved muscles (see Table 1–4).[65]

To properly test the deep tendon reflexes, the patient must be relaxed and the examiner must ensure that the muscle of the tendon to be tested is relaxed. The tendon to be tested is put on slight stretch, and an adequate stimulus is applied by dropping the reflex hammer onto the tendon. The examiner should tap the tendon five or six times to uncover any fading reflex response, indicative of developing nerve root signs. If the deep tendon reflexes are difficult to elicit, the reflexes often can be enhanced by having the patient clench the teeth or squeeze the hands together (**Jendrassik maneuver**) when testing the lower limb or squeeze the legs together when testing the upper limb. These activities increase the facilitative activity of the spinal cord and thereby accentuate minimally active reflexes.[66]

Deep Tendon Reflex Grading

0—Absent

1—Diminished

2—Average (normal)

3—Exaggerated

4—Clonus, very brisk

Superficial reflexes are tested by stroking the skin with a moderately sharp object that does not break the skin. The expected responses are shown in Table 1–22. A great deal of practice is needed to become proficient in testing the superficial reflexes.

Pathological reflexes (see Table 1–23) may indicate upper motor neuron lesions if present on both sides or lower motor neuron lesions if present on only one side. Improper stimulation (e.g., too much pressure) may lead to voluntary withdrawal in normal subjects, and the examiner must take care not to confuse this reaction with the pathological response.

To be of clinical significance, findings must show asymmetry between bilateral reflexes unless there is a central lesion. The examiner should not be overly concerned if the reflexes are absent, diminished, or excessive on both sides, especially in young people, unless a central lesion is suspected. Exercise just before testing or patient anxiety or tenseness may lead to accentuated tendon reflexes.[32] Hyporeflexia or areflexia indicates a lesion of a peripheral nerve or spinal nerve root as a result of impingement, entrapment, or injury. Hyporeflexia or areflexia may be seen in the absence of muscle weakness or atrophy because of the involvement of the efferent loop of the reflex arc in the reflex. Hyperactive or exaggerated reflexes (hyperreflexia) indicate upper motor neuron lesions. In the cervical spine, if a disc herniation and compression occur above the cervical enlargement, the reflexes of the upper extremity are exaggerated. If the cervical enlargement is involved (which is more commonly the case), then some reflexes are exaggerated and some are decreased.[67]

At the same time, the examiner can perform a **sensory scanning examination** by checking the cutaneous distribution of the various peripheral nerves and the dermatomes around the joint being examined. The sensory examination is performed for several reasons. First, it is used to determine the extent of sensory loss, whether that loss is caused by nerve root lesions, peripheral nerve lesions, or compressive tunnel syndromes. Second, because function is often tied to sensation, it is used to determine the degree of functional impairment. Third, because sensory function returns before motor function, it can be used to determine nerve recovery after injury or repair as well as when re-education can commence. Finally, it is part of the total assessment and is often necessary for medicolegal reasons. Although the sensory distribution of peripheral nerves may vary from person to person, they tend to be much more consistent than dermatomes.[16, 68] The examiner must be able to differentiate between sensory loss involving a nerve root (dermatome) and that involving a peripheral nerve (see Table 1–6 for an example).

The sensory examination is begun with a quick "scan" of sensation. To do this, the examiner runs his or her relaxed hands relatively firmly over the skin to be tested and asks the patient whether there are any differences in sensation. The patient's eyes may be open. If the patient notes any differences in sensation between the affected and unaffected sides, then a more detailed sensory assessment is performed. The examiner should note the patient's ability to perceive the sensation being tested and the difference, if any, between the two sides of the body. In addition, distal and proximal sensitivities should be compared for each form of sensation tested. During the detailed sensory testing, the patient should keep the eyes closed so that the results will indicate the patient's perception and interpretation of the stimuli, not what the patient sees happening. With the detailed sensory testing, the examiner "marks out" the specific area of altered sensation and then correlates the area with the known dermatome and peripheral nerve distribution. However, the sensation felt does not necessarily come from the indicated nerve root or peripheral nerve; because of referred pain, it may come from any structure supplied by that nerve root. In some cases, the paresthesia may involve no specific pattern, or it may involve the entire circumference of a limb. This "opera glove" or "stocking" paresthesia or anesthesia may result from vascular insufficiency.

Superficial tactile sensation can be tested with a wisp of cotton or a soft hairbrush, and superficial pain can be tested with a flagged pin (holding a piece of tape attached to a pin), pinwheel, or other sharp object. Only light tapping should be used. About 2 seconds should elapse between each stimulus to avoid summation. It is the group II afferent fibers (Table 1–24) that are being tested. Perception to pin prick may range from absence of awareness, through pressure sensation, hyperanalgesia with or without radiation, localization, and sensation of sharpness, to normal perception.

If desired, the examiner may also test other sensations. Sensitivity to temperature (lateral spinothalamic tract and group III fibers) is tested by using two test tubes, one containing hot water and one containing cold water. A normal response to this test does not necessarily mean that the patient has normal temperature sensation. Rather, the patient can distinguish between hot and cold, each at one level in the range, but not necessarily between different degrees of hot and cold. Sensitivity to vibration (i.e., how long until vibration stops) may be tested by holding a tuning fork (usually 30- or 256-cps tuning forks are used) against bony prominences; this tests the integrity of group II fibers and the dorsal column and medial lemniscal systems. Deep pressure pain (group II Aβ fibers) can be tested by squeezing the Achilles tendon, the trapezius muscle, or the web space between the thumb and index finger or by applying a knuckle to the sternum. To test proprioception and motion (i.e., the skin and joint receptors, muscle spindles, dorsal column and medial lemniscal systems, and group I and II fibers), the patient's fingers or toes are passively moved, and the patient is asked to indicate the direction of movement and final position while keeping the eyes closed. To ensure that pressure on the patient's skin cannot be used as a clue to direction of movement, the test digit should be grasped between the thumb and index finger of the examiner.

Cortical and discriminatory sensations may be tested by two-point discrimination, point localization, texture discrimination, stereognostic function (i.e., identification of familiar objects held in the hand), and graphesthesia (i.e., recognition of letters or numbers written with a blunt object on the patient's palms or other body parts). These techniques also test the integrity of the dorsal column and lemniscal systems.

Joint Play Movements

All synovial and secondary cartilaginous joints, to some extent, are capable of an active ROM, termed voluntary movement. In addition, there is a small ROM that can be obtained only passively by the examiner; this movement is called **joint play** or **accessory movement**. These accessory movements are not under voluntary control; they are necessary, however, for full painless function of the joint and full ROM of the joint. **Joint dysfunction** signifies a loss of joint play movement.

The existence of joint play movement is necessary for full, pain-free voluntary movement to occur. An essential part of the detailed assessment of any joint includes an examination of its joint play movements. If any joint play movement is found to be absent, or decreased, this movement must be restored before functional voluntary movement can be fully accomplished. In most joints, this movement is normally less than 4 mm in any one direction.

Mennell's Rules for Joint Play Testing[69]

- The patient should be relaxed and fully supported
- The examiner should be relaxed and should use a firm but comfortable grasp
- One joint should be examined at a time
- One movement should be examined at a time
- The unaffected side should be tested first
- One articular surface is stabilized while the other surface is moved
- Movements must be normal and not forced
- Movements should not cause undue discomfort

Loose Packed (Resting) Position

To test joint play movement, the examiner places the joint in its resting position, which is the position in its ROM at which the joint is under the least amount of stress; it is also the position in which the joint capsule has its greatest capacity.[70] The resting position (sometimes called the loose packed position) is one of minimal congruency between the articular surfaces and the joint capsule, with the ligaments being in the position of greatest laxity and passive separation of the joint surfaces being the greatest. This position may be the anatomic resting position, which is usually considered in

Table 1–24
Nerve Fiber Classification

Sensory Axons	Axon Diameter (μm)	Conduction Velocity (m/sec)	Innervation
Ia (Aα)	12–22	65–130	Muscle spindles (annulospiral endings)
Ib (Aα)	12–22	65–130	Golgi tendon organs
II (Aβ)	5–15	20–90	Pressure, touch, vibration (flower spray endings)
III (Aδ)	2–10	6–45	Temperature, fast pain
IV (C)	0.2–1.5	0.2–2.0	Slow pain, visceral, temperature, crude touch

the midrange, or it may be just outside the range of pain and spasm. The advantage of the loose packed position is that the joint surface contact areas are reduced and are always changing to decrease friction and erosion in the joints. The position also provides proper joint lubrication and allows the movements of spin, slide, and roll. It is therefore the position for treatment using joint play mobilizations. Examples of resting positions are shown in Table 1–25.

Close Packed (Synarthrodial) Position

The close packed position should be avoided as much as possible during an assessment, because in this position the majority of joint structures are under maximum tension. In this position, the two joint surfaces fit together precisely; that is, they are fully congruent. The joint surfaces are tightly compressed; the ligaments and capsule of the joint are maximally tight; and the joint

Table 1–25
Resting (Loose Packed) Position of Joints

Joint	Position
Facet (spine)	Midway between flexion and extension
Temporomandibular	Mouth slightly open (freeway space)
Glenohumeral	55° abduction, 30° horizontal adduction
Acromioclavicular	Arm resting by side in normal physiological position
Sternoclavicular	Arm resting by side in normal physiological position
Ulnohumeral (elbow)	70° flexion, 10° supination
Radiohumeral	Full extension, full supination
Proximal radioulnar	70° flexion, 35° supination
Distal radioulnar	10° supination
Radiocarpal (wrist)	Neutral with slight ulnar deviation
Carpometacarpal	Midway between abduction-adduction and flexion-extension
Metacarpophalangeal	Slight flexion
Interphalangeal	Slight flexion
Hip	30° flexion, 30° abduction, slight lateral rotation
Knee	25° flexion
Talocrural (ankle)	10° plantar flexion, midway between maximum inversion and eversion
Subtalar	Midway between extremes of range of movement
Midtarsal	Midway between extremes of range of movement
Tarsometatarsal	Midway between extremes of range of movement
Metatarsophalangeal	Neutral
Interphalangeal	Slight flexion

Table 1–26
Close Packed Position of Joints

Joint	Position
Facet (spine)	Extension
Temporomandibular	Clenched teeth
Glenohumeral	Abduction and lateral rotation
Acromioclavicular	Arm abducted to 90°
Sternoclavicular	Maximum shoulder elevation
Ulnohumeral (elbow)	Extension
Radiohumeral	Elbow flexed 90°, forearm supinated 5°
Proximal radioulnar	5° supination
Distal radioulnar	5° supination
Radiocarpal (wrist)	Extension with radial deviation
Metacarpophalangeal (fingers)	Full flexion
Metacarpophalangeal (thumb)	Full opposition
Interphalangeal	Full extension
Hip	Full extension, medial rotation*
Knee	Full extension, lateral rotation of tibia
Talocrural (ankle)	Maximum dorsiflexion
Subtalar	Supination
Midtarsal	Supination
Tarsometatarsal	Supination
Metatarsophalangeal	Full extension
Interphalangeal	Full extension

* Some authors include abduction (e.g., Kaltenborn[70]).

surfaces cannot be separated by distractive forces. Ligaments, bone, or other joint structures, if injured, become more painful as the close packed position is approached. If a joint is swollen, the close packed position cannot be achieved.[45] In the close packed position, no accessory movement is possible. Examples of the close packed positions of most joints are shown in Table 1–26.

In some cases, joint play movements may be similar to or the same as movements tested during passive movements or ligamentous testing. This is most obvious in joints that have minimal movement and in joints that do not have muscles acting directly on them, such as the sacroiliac joints and superior tibiofibular joints.

Palpation

Initially, palpation for tenderness plays no part in the assessment, because referred tenderness is very real and can be misleading. Only after the tissue at fault has been identified is palpation for tenderness used to determine the exact extent of the lesion within that tissue, and then palpation is done only if the tissue lies superficially and within easy reach of the fingers. Palpation is an important assessment technique that must be practiced if it is to be used effectively.[71] Tenderness often does enable the examiner to name the affected ligament or the specific section or exact point of the tearing or bruising.

To palpate properly, the examiner must ensure that the area to be palpated is as relaxed as possible. For this to be done, the body part must be supported as much as possible. As the ability to perform palpation develops, the examiner should be able to accomplish the following.

1. Discriminate differences in tissue tension (e.g., effusion, spasm) and muscle tone (i.e., spasticity, rigidity, flaccidity). Spasticity refers to muscle tonus in which there may be a collapse of muscle tone during testing. Rigidity refers to involuntary resistance being maintained during passive movement and without collapse of the muscle. Flaccidity means there is no muscle tone.

2. Distinguish differences in tissue texture. For example, the examiner can, in some cases, palpate the direction of fibers or presence of fibrous bands.

3. Identify shapes, structures, and tissue type and thereby detect abnormalities. For example, bony deformity such as myositis ossificans may be palpated.

When Palpating, the Examiner Should Note

- Differences in tissue tension and texture
- Differences in tissue thickness
- Abnormalities
- Tenderness
- Temperature variation
- Pulses, tremors, and fasciculations
- Pathological state of tissues
- Dryness or excessive moisture
- Abnormal sensation

---

4. Determine tissue thickness and texture and determine whether it is pliable, soft, and resilient. Is there any obvious swelling? Edema is an abnormal accumulation of fluid in the intercellular spaces; swelling, on the other hand, is the abnormal enlargement of a body part. It may be the result of bone thickening, synovial membrane thickening, or fluid accumulation in and around the joint. It may be intracellular or extracellular (edema), intracapsular or extracapsular. Swelling may be localized (encapsulated), which may indicate intra-articular swelling, a cyst, or a swollen bursa. Swelling that develops immediately or in 2 to 4 hours after injury is probably caused by blood extravasation into the tissues or joint. Swelling that becomes evident after 8 to 24 hours is caused by inflammation and, in a joint, by synovial swelling. Bony or hard swelling may be caused by osteophytes or new bone formation (e.g., in myositis ossificans). Soft-tissue swelling such as edematous synovium produces a boggy, spongy feeling (like soft sponge rubber), whereas

fluid swelling is a softer and more mobile, fluctuating feeling. Blood swelling is usually a harder, thick, gel-like feeling, and the overlying skin is usually warmer. Pus is thick and less fluctuant; the overlying skin is warm, and the temperature is usually elevated. Older, long-standing soft-tissue swelling, such as a skin callus, feels like tough, dry leather. Synovial hypertrophy has a hard, thick feeling to it with little give. The more leathery the thickening feels, the more likely it is to be chronic and caused by local symptoms. Softer thickenings tend to be more acute and associated with recent symptoms.[43] Pitting edema is thick and slow moving, leaving an indentation after pressure is applied and removed. It is commonly caused by circulatory stasis. Long-lasting swelling may cause reflex inhibition of the muscles around the joint, leading to atrophy and weakness. Blood swelling within a joint is usually aspirated because of the irritating and damaging effect it has on the joint cartilage.

Swelling

- Comes on soon after injury → blood
- Comes on after 8 to 24 hours → synovial
- Boggy, spongy feeling → synovial
- Harder, tense feeling with warmth → blood
- Tough, dry → callus
- Leathery thickening → chronic
- Soft, fluctuating → acute
- Hard → bone
- Thick, slow-moving → pitting edema

---

5. Determine joint tenderness by applying firm pressure to the joint. The pressure should always be applied with care, especially in the acute phase.

Grading Tenderness on Palpation

Grade I: Patient complains of pain

Grade II: Patient complains of pain and winces

Grade III: Patient winces and withdraws the joint

Grade IV: Patient will not allow palpation of the joint

---

6. Feel variations in temperature. This determination is usually best done by using the back of the examiner's hand or fingers and comparing both sides. Joints tend to be warm in the acute phase, in the presence of infection, or with blood swelling.

7. Feel pulses, tremors, and fasciculations. Fasciculations result from contraction of a number of muscle cells innervated by a single motor axon. The contractions are very localized, are usually subconscious, and do not

involve the whole muscle. Tremors are involuntary movements in which agonist and antagonist muscle groups contract to cause rhythmic movements of a joint. Pulses are an indication of circulatory sufficiency and should be tested for rhythm and strength if circulatory problems are suspected. Table 1–27 indicates the more commonly palpated pulses that may be used to determine circulatory sufficiency and location.

8. Determine the pathological state of the tissues in and around the joint. The examiner should note any tenderness, tissue thickening, or other signs or symptoms that would indicate pathology.

9. Feel dryness or excessive moisture of the skin. For example, acute gouty joints tend to be dry, whereas septic joints tend to be moist. Nervous patients usually demonstrate increased moisture in the hands.

10. Note any abnormal sensation such as dysesthesia (diminished sensation), hyperesthesia (increased sensation), anesthesia (absence of sensation), or crepitus. Soft, fine crepitus may indicate roughening of the articular cartilage, whereas coarse grating may indicate badly damaged articular cartilage or bone. A creaking, leathery crepitus (snowball crepitation) is sometimes felt in tendons and indicates pathology. Tendons may "snap" over one another or over a bony prominence. Loud, snapping, pain-free noises in joints are usually caused by cavitation, in which gas bubbles form suddenly and transiently owing to negative pressure in the joint.

Palpation of a joint and surrounding area must be carried out in a systematic fashion to ensure that all structures are examined. This procedure involves having a starting point and working from that point to adjacent tissues to assess their normality or the possibility of pathological involvement. The examiner must work slowly and carefully, applying light pressure initially and working into a deeper pressure of palpation, "feeling" for pathological conditions or changes in tissue tension.[71] The uninvolved side should be palpated first so that the patient has some idea of what to expect. Any differences or abnormalities should be noted and contribute to the diagnosis.

Diagnostic Imaging

Plain Film Radiography

Conventional plain film radiography (also called x-rays) is the primary means of diagnostic imaging for musculoskeletal problems. It offers the advantages of being readily available, being relatively cheap, and providing good anatomic resolution. On the negative side, it does expose the patient to radiation, and it offers poor differentiation of soft-tissue structures. Although it is important, radiographic examination is usually used only to confirm a clinical opinion. Radiographs are not taken indiscriminately. Because x-rays have the potential for causing cell damage, there should be a clear indication of need before a radiograph is taken, and the process should not be considered routine.[72]

Normally, two projections at 90° orientation to each other are taken—most commonly, anteroposterior (AP) and lateral projections. Other views may be obtained, depending on clinical circumstances and specific needs.[72–75] In the lumbar spine, AP, lateral, and oblique views are commonly taken. Two views are necessary because x-rays take planar images, so that all structures in the path of the x-ray beam are superimposed on each other and abnormalities may be difficult to evaluate with only one view.

X-rays are part of the electromagnetic spectrum and have the ability to penetrate tissue to varying degrees. X-ray imaging is based on the principle that different tissues have different densities and produce images in different shades of gray.[76] The greater the density of the tissue, the less penetration of x-rays there is, and the whiter its image appears on the film. In order of descending degree of density are the following structures: metal, bone, soft tissue, water, fat, and air. These differences give the six basic densities on the x-ray plate. When viewing the x-rays, the examiner must identify the film, noting the name, age, date, and sex of the patient, and must identify the type of projection taken (e.g., AP, lateral, tunnel, skyline, weight-bearing, stress-type).

The x-ray plates that are developed after exposure to the roentgen rays enable the examiner to see any fractures, dislocations, foreign bodies, or radiopaque substances that may be present. The main function of plain x-ray examination is to rule out or exclude fractures or serious disease—such as infection (osteomyelitis), ankylosing spondylitis, or tumors—and structural body abnormalities such as developmental anomalies, arthri-

Table 1–27
Common Circulatory Pulse Locations

Artery	Location
Carotid	Anterior to sternocleidomastoid muscle
Brachial	Medial aspect of arm midway between shoulder and elbow
Radial	At wrist, lateral to flexor carpi radialis tendon
Ulnar	At wrist, between flexor digitorum superficialis and flexor carpi ulnaris tendons
Femoral	In femoral triangle (sartorius, adductor longus, and inguinal ligament)
Popliteal	Posterior aspect of knee (deep and hard to palpate)
Posterior tibial	Posterior aspect of medial malleolus
Dorsalis pedis	Between first and second metatarsal bones on superior aspect

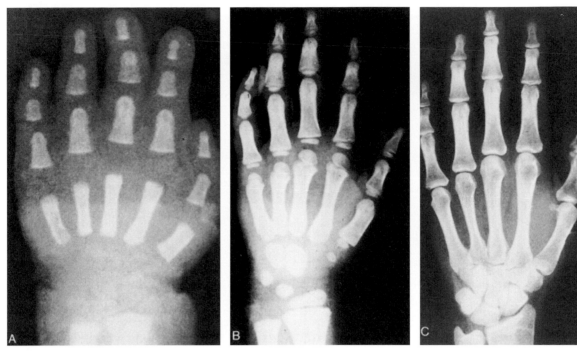

Figure 1–13
X-ray films showing skeletal maturity. (A) Male, newborn. (B) Male, 5 years old. (C) Female, 17 years old.

tis, and metabolic bone diseases. With soft-tissue injuries, clinical findings should take precedence over x-ray findings. It is desirable to know whether an x-ray has been taken so the examiner can obtain the films if necessary. The examiner should be aware of obvious and unusual x-ray findings that distract attention from other tissue that is actually the cause of the pain; such x-ray abnormalities are significant only if clinical examination bears out their relevance. With experience, the examiner becomes able to detect many important soft-tissue changes on x-ray examination, such as effusion in joints,

tendinous calcifications, ectopic bone in muscle, tissue displaced by tumor, and presence of air or foreign body material in the tissues. Radiographs may also be used to give an indication of bone loss. For osteoporosis to be evident on x-ray, approximately 30 to 35% of the bone must be lost.

The examiner should keep in mind the maturity of the patient when viewing films. Skeletal changes occur with age,[77] and the appearance and fusion of the epiphyses, for example, may be important in interpreting the pathology of the condition seen. Soft-tissue structures as well as bone can be seen, provided there is something to outline them. For example, the joint capsule may be silhouetted by the pericapsular fat, or a cardiac shadow may be silhouetted by air in the lungs. Anatomic variations and anomalies must be ruled out before pathology can be ruled in; for example, accessory navicular, bipartite patella, and os trigonum may be confused with fractures by the unsuspecting examiner. The fabella is often confused with a loose body in the knee in the AP projection x-ray film.

Radiographs may also be used to determine the maturity index of a patient. A special film of the wrist is taken to assess skeletal maturity (Fig. 1–13). These films can be compared with established films in a bone atlas such as that compiled by Gruelich and Pyle.[77] This is often done before epiphysiodesis and leg-lengthening procedures to ensure that the child is of a suitable skeletal age to do the procedure.

When Viewing an X-ray, the Examiner Should Note

- Overall size and shape of bone
- Local size and shape of bone
- Thickness of the cortex
- Trabecular pattern of the bone
- General density of the entire bone
- Local density change
- Margins of local lesions
- Any break in continuity of the bone
- Any periosteal change
- Any soft-tissue change
- Relation among bones
- Thickness of the cartilage (cartilage space within joints)

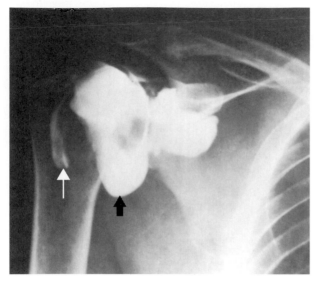

Figure 1–14

Normal arthrogram, shoulder in lateral rotation. Note the good dependent fold (*wide arrow*) and the outline of the bicipital tendon (*narrow arrow*). (From Neviaser, T.J.: Arthrography of the shoulder. Orthop. Clin. North Am. 11:209, 1980.)

Arthrography

Arthrography is an invasive technique in which air, a water-soluble contrast material containing iodine, or a combination of the two (double contrast) is injected into a joint space and a radiograph is taken of the joint. The air or contrast material outlines the structures within the joint or communicating with the joint (Fig. 1–14). It is especially useful in detecting abnormal joint and bursal communications. It is used primarily in the hip, knee, ankle, shoulder, elbow, and wrist.[72]

Computed Arthrography (CT-Arthrography)

This technique combines arthrography and computed tomography (CT). This method provides a three-dimensional definition of the joint, and the dye helps to delineate articular surfaces and joint margins. It is usually reserved for those cases in which conventional CT scanning has not provided adequate anatomic detail (e.g., shoulder instability).[11, 72, 75]

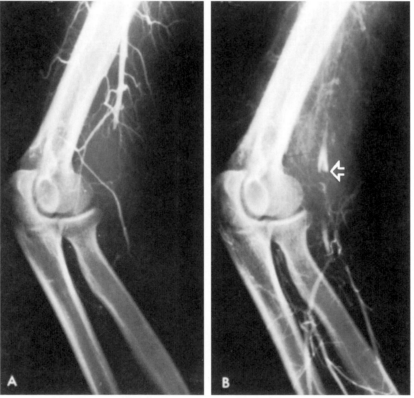

Figure 1–15

Occlusion of brachial artery. (A) Arteriogram of a young man with a previously reduced elbow dislocation and an ischemic hand shows an occluded brachial artery. (B) A later film shows fresh clot (*arrow*) in the brachial artery and reconstituted radial and ulnar arteries. Primary repair and thrombectomy treated the ischemic symptoms. (From McLean, G., and D.B. Frieman: Angiography of skeletal disease. Orthop. Clin. North Am. 14:267, 1983.)

Venogram and Arteriogram

With a venogram or an arteriogram, radiopaque dye is injected into specific vessels to outline abnormal conditions (Fig. 1–15). This technique may be used to diagnose arteriosclerosis, investigate tumors, and demonstrate blockage after traumatic injury.

Myelography

Myelography is an invasive imaging technique that is used to visualize the soft tissues within the spine. A water-soluble radiopaque dye is injected into the epidural space by spinal puncture and allowed to flow to different levels of the spinal cord, outlining the contour of the thecal sac, nerve roots, and spinal cord. A plain x-ray film is then taken of the spine (Figs. 1–16 and 1–17). In some cases, a CT scan may be taken in place of the x-ray.[72] This technique is used to detect disc disease, disc herniation, nerve root entrapment, spinal stenosis, and tumors of the spinal cord. The clinician should be aware that myelograms can have adverse side effects. Grainger[78] reported that 20 to 30% of patients receiving myelograms complained of headache, dizziness, nausea, vomiting, and seizures.[76]

Tomography and Computed Tomography

Tomography has become a common imaging technique for musculoskeletal disorders, especially when computer enhanced (CT scan). It produces cross-sectional images of the tissues. Conventional tomography, which is also called thin-section radiography or linear tomography, tends to show one small area or plane in focus with

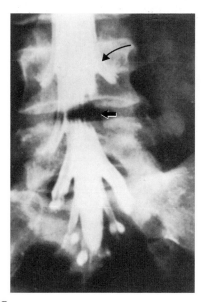

Figure 1–17

Myelogram of lumbar spine showing extrusion of nucleus pulposus of L4–L5 (*large arrow*). Note how radiopaque dye fills dural recesses (*small arrow*). (From Selby, D.K., A.J. Meril, K.J. Wagner, and R.R.G. Winans: Water-soluble myelography. Orthop. Clin. North Am. 8:82, 1977.)

other areas or planes appearing fuzzy or blurred. The conventional tomogram is seldom used today except when subtle bone density alterations are sought.

The CT scan involves the same thin cross sections or "slices" taken at specific levels (Fig. 1–18). CT scans produce cross-sectional images based on x-ray attenuation. Because of computer enhancement, CT produces superior tissue contrast resolution compared with conventional x-rays. CT provides excellent bony architecture detail and has good resolution of soft-tissue structures. Its disadvantages include limited scanning plane, cost, exposure to radiation (dosage similar to that of plain x-rays), alteration of the image by artifacts, and degradation of soft-tissue resolution in obese people.[11, 72] The CT scan, or CAT scan (computed axial tomography), is a radiological technique that may be used to assess for disc protrusions, facet disease, or spinal stenosis.[79] The technique may also be used to assess complex fractures and dislocations, especially those involving joints, patellofemoral alignment and tracking, osteonecrosis, tumors, and osteomyelitis. Because only a small cross-sectional area in one plane is viewed with each scan, multiple images or scans are taken to get a complete view of the area.[11]

Radionuclide Scanning

With bone scans (osteoscintigraphy), chemicals labeled with isotopes (radioactive tracers) such as technetium-

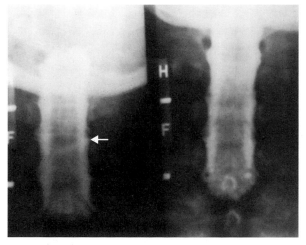

Figure 1–16

Myelogram of cervical spine. Note how radiopaque dye fills root sheaths (*arrow*).

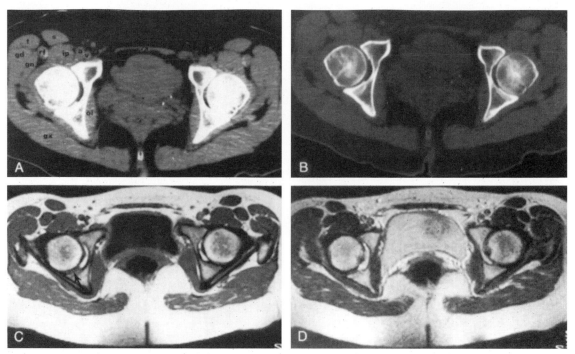

Figure 1–18
See legend on bottom of opposite page

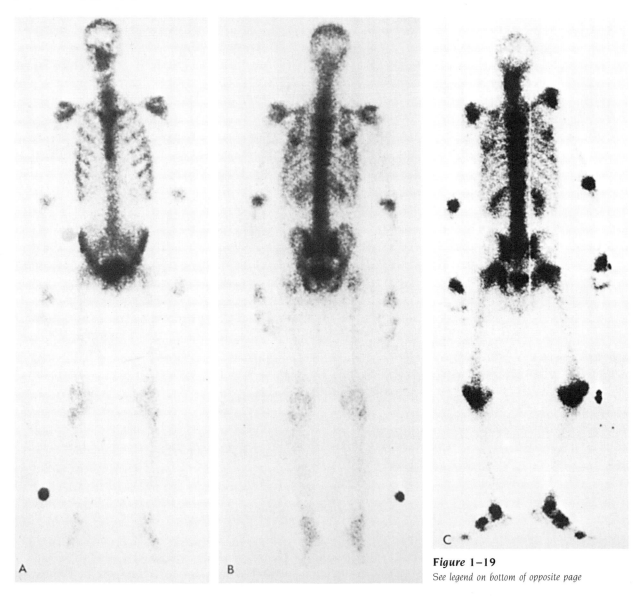

Figure 1–19
See legend on bottom of opposite page

99m–labeled methyl diphosphonate complexes are intravenously injected to localize specific organs that concentrate the particular chemical. The isotope is then localized where there is a high level of activity (bone turnover) relative to the rest of the bone. On the radiograph, a "hot spot" is seen (Fig. 1–19). Although plain film radiographs do not show bone disease or stress fractures until there is 30 to 50% bone loss, bone scans show bone disease or stress fractures with as little as 4 to 7% bone loss.[79] The bone scan images are usually taken 2 to 3 hours after the injection to allow uptake in the bone and clearance from the blood. Because the isotope is excreted by the kidneys, the kidneys and bladder are often visible in bone scans. Bone scans are used for lytic (bone-loss) diseases, infection, fractures, and tumors. They are highly sensitive to bone abnormalities but do not tell what the abnormality is. The whole body may be imaged, and the tracer is picked up by a gamma camera.[72]

Discography

The technique of discography involves injection of a small amount of radiopaque dye into the nucleus pulposus of an intervertebral disc (Fig. 1–20) under radiographic guidance. It is not a commonly used technique but may be used to determine disruptions in the nucleus pulposus or the annular fibrosus and is sometimes used as a provocative test to see whether injection into the disc brings on the patient's symptoms.[72]

Magnetic Resonance Imaging

Magnetic resonance imaging (MRI) is a noninvasive, painless imaging technique that uses exposure to magnetic fields, not ionizing radiation, to obtain an image of bone and soft tissue. MRI is based on the effect of a

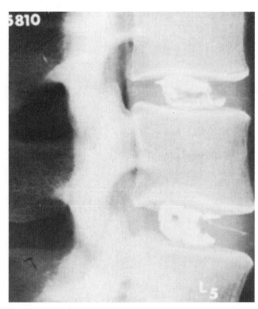

Figure 1–20

Normal discogram shown with barium paste. (From Farfan, H.F.: Mechanical Disorders of the Low Back. Philadelphia, Lea & Febiger, 1973, p. 96.)

strong magnetic field on hydrogen atoms. T1 images show very good anatomic detail (Fig. 1–21), whereas T2 images are used to demonstrate soft-tissue pathology that alters tissue water content.[11, 78] MRI offers excellent tissue contrast, is multiplanar (i.e., can image in any plane), and has no known adverse effects. In some patients, claustrophobia is a problem, and artifacts may result if the patient does not remain still.[78]

MRI is used to assess for spinal cord tumors, intracranial disease, and some types of central nervous system diseases (e.g., multiple sclerosis); it largely replaced myelography in the evaluation of disc pathology. It also aids in the diagnosis of meniscal and ligamentous tears,

Figure 1–18

(A) Normal computed tomographic (CT) image at the level of the midacetabulum obtained with soft-tissue window settings shows the homogenous, intermediate signal of musculature. a = common femoral artery; gd = gluteus medius; gn = gluteus minimus; gx = gluteus maximus; ip = iliopsoas; oi = obturator internus; ra = rectus abdominis; rf = rectus femoris; s = sartorius; t = tensor fascia lata; v = common femoral vein. (B) Axial CT at bone window settings reveals improved delineation of cortical and medullary osseous detail. Note anterior and posterior semilunar acetabular articular surfaces and the central nonarticular acetabular fossa. (C) Normal midacetabular T1-weighted axial 0.4-T magnetic resonance image (MRI) (TR, 600 msec; TE, 20 msec) of a different patient shows a normal, high-signal-intensity image of fatty marrow (adult pattern) and subcutaneous tissue, low-signal-intensity image of muscle, and absence of signal in the cortical bone. The thin articular hyaline cartilage is of intermediate signal intensity (*arrow*). (D) T2-weighted MRI (TR, 2,000 msec; TE, 80 msec) shows decreasing high signal intensity in fatty marrow and subcutaneous tissue with increased signal intensity in the fluid-filled urinary bladder. (From Pitt, M.J., P.J. Lund, and D.P. Speer: Imaging of the pelvis and hip. Orthop. Clin. North Am. 21:553, 1990.)

Figure 1–19

Whole body bone scans. (A) Normal adult anterior scan. (B) Normal adult posterior scan. (C) Posterior scan showing joint involvement of rheumatoid arthritis. (From Goldstein, H.A.: Bone scintigraphy. Orthop. Clin. North Am. 14:244, 250, 1983.)

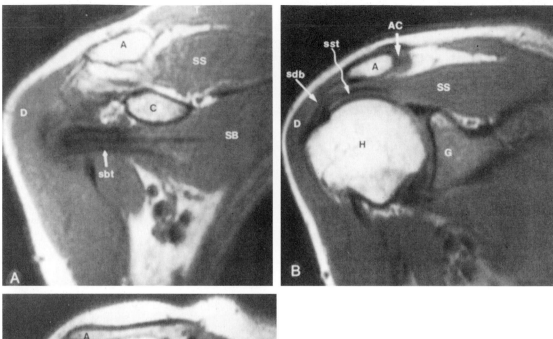

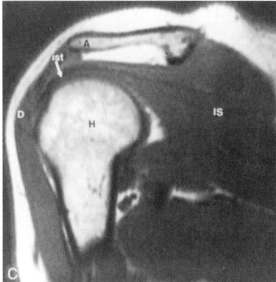

Figure 1-21
Magnetic resonance T1-weighted coronal oblique images from anterior (A) to posterior (C). T = trapezius muscle; A = acromion; SS = supraspinatus muscle; D = deltoid muscle; C = coracoid; SB = subscapularis muscle; sbt = subscapularis tendon; AC = acromioclavicular joint; sst = supraspinatus tendon; sdb = subdeltoid-subacromial bursa; H = humerus; G = glenoid of scapula; ist = infraspinatus tendon; IS = infraspinatus muscle. (From Mayer, S.J., and M.K. Dalinka: Magnetic resonance imaging of the shoulder. Orthop. Clin. North Am. 21:500, 1990.)

abnormal patellofemoral tracking, shoulder pathology, osteonecrosis, and osteochondral lesions.[11]

On the negative side, MRI is expensive, and specificity of pathology (e.g., tendon strain versus tendinitis) may not be possible with its use. Presence of some metallic objects such as cardiac pacemakers may make its use contraindicated because of the magnetic pull, especially if the objects are not solidly fixed to bone. It has been reported that MRI is safe with prosthetic joints and internal fixation devices.[72]

Fluoroscopy

Fluoroscopy is a technique that is used to show motion in joints through x-ray imaging; it also may be used as a guidance technique for injections (e.g., in discography). It is only rarely used because of the amount of radiation exposure. It is sometimes used to position fracture fragments and to demonstrate abnormal motion.

Diagnostic Ultrasound

Like therapeutic ultrasound, diagnostic ultrasound involves transmission of high-frequency sound waves (5 to 10 MHz) into the tissues by a transducer through a coupling agent, with calculation of the time it takes for the echo to return to the transducer from different interfaces. The depth of the structure is determined, and an image is formed. Each tissue has a unique echotexture that relates to its internal structure.[11]

In the hands of an experienced operator, ultrasound can provide good image detail and cross-sectional images in different planes. No radiation is used, and no harmful biological effects have been reported. It also has

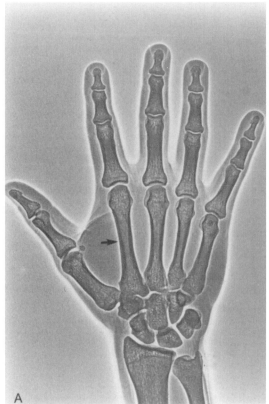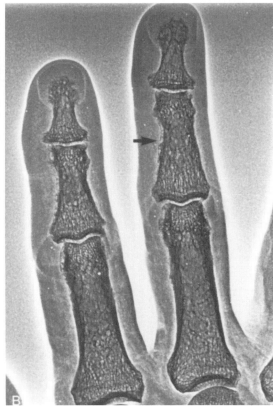

Figure 1–22

Xeroradiography. (A) Normal examination. Note the ability to demonstrate both soft tissues and bony structures on a single examination. The halo effect (*arrow*) around the bony cortices is an example of edge enhancement. (From Weissman, B.N.W., and C.B. Sledge: Orthopedic Radiology. Philadelphia, W.B. Saunders Co., 1986, p. 11.) (B) Hyperparathyroid bone changes shown on xeroradiography. The subperiosteal bone resorption (*arrow*) and distal tuft erosion are well seen. (From Seltzer, S.E., B.N. Weissman, H.J. Finberg, and J.A. Markisz: Improved diagnostic imaging in joint diseases. Semin. Arthritis Rheum. 11:315, 1982.)

the advantage of providing dynamic (moving) real-time images, so that tissues can be visualized as they move. It also allows localization of any tenderness or palpable mass[11] and therefore is used to assess soft-tissue injury such as tendon, ligament, or muscle pathology, soft-tissue masses (e.g., tumor, ganglion, cyst, inflamed bursa), effusion, and congenital dislocation of the hip.

The disadvantages of diagnostic ultrasound include limited contrast resolution, limited depth of penetration, small viewing field, and lack of penetration of bone.[11] The use of diagnostic ultrasound has a difficult learning curve, and the quality and interpretation of the images depend on the operator.

Xeroradiography

Xeroradiography is a technique in which a xeroradiographic plate replaces the normal x-ray film. On the plate, there is a thin layer of a photoconductor material which enhances the image (Fig. 1–22). This technique is used when the margins between areas of different densities need to be exaggerated.[75, 80]

Précis

At the end of each chapter, a précis of the assessment is presented as a quick reference. The précis does not follow the text description exactly but is laid out so that each assessment involves minimal movement of the patient, to decrease patient discomfort. For example, all aspects of the examination that are performed with the patient standing are done first, followed by those done with the patient sitting, and so on.

Case Studies

Case studies are provided as written exercises to help the examiner develop skills in assessment. Based on the presented case study, the reader should develop a list of appropriate questions to ask in the history, what things should especially be noted in observation, and what part of the examination is essential to make a definitive diagnosis. Where appropriate, example diagnoses are given in parentheses at the end of each question. At the end of the case study, the reader can develop a table showing the differential diagnosis for the case described. Tables 1–28 and 1–29 illustrate such differential diagnosis charts.

Conclusion

Having completed all parts of the assessment, the examiner can look at the pertinent objective and subjective facts, note the significant signs and symptoms to determine what is causing the patient's problems, and design a proper treatment regimen based on the findings. This is the normal and correct reasoning process. If the assessment is not followed through completely, the treatment regimen may not be implemented properly, and this may lead to unwarranted extended care of the patient and increased health care costs.

Occasionally, patients present with a mixture of signs and symptoms that indicates two or more possible problem areas. Only by adding the positive findings and subtracting the negative findings can the examiner determine the probable cause of the problem. In many cases, the decision may be an educated guess, because very few problems are "textbook perfect." Only the examiner's knowledge, clinical experience, and diagnosis, followed by trial treatment, can conclusively delineate the problem.

Finally, when the assessment has been completed, the clinician should not hesitate to refer the patient to another health care professional if the patient has presented with unusual signs and symptoms or if the condition appears to be beyond the scope of practice of the examiner.

Table 1–28
Differential Diagnosis of Claudication and Spinal Stenosis

Vascular Claudication	Neurogenic Claudication	Spinal Stenosis
Pain* is usually bilateral	Pain is usually bilateral but may be unilateral	Usually bilateral pain
Occurs in the calf (foot, thigh, hip, or buttocks)	Occurs in back, buttocks, thighs, calves, feet	Occurs in back, buttocks, thighs, calves, and feet
Pain consistent in all spinal positions	Pain decreased in spinal flexion	Pain decreased in spinal flexion
	Pain increased in spinal extension	Pain increased in spinal extension
Pain brought on by physical exertion (e.g., walking)	Pain increased with walking	Pain increased with walking
Pain relieved promptly by rest (1 to 5 minutes)	Pain decreased by recumbency	Pain relieved with prolonged rest (may persist hours after resting)
Pain increased by walking uphill		Pain decreased when walking uphill
No burning or dysesthesia	Burning and dysesthesia from the back to buttocks and leg or legs	Burning and numbness present in lower extremities
Decreased or absent pulses in lower extremities	Normal pulses	Normal pulses
Color and skin changes in feet—cold, numb, dry, or scaly skin, poor nail and hair growth	Good skin nutrition	Good skin nutrition
Affects ages from 40 to over 60	Affects ages from 40 to over 60	Peaks in seventh decade of life; affects men primarily

"Pain" associated with vascular claudication may also be described as an "aching," "cramping," or "tired" feeling.

Modified from Goodman, C.C., and T.E. Snyder: Differential Diagnosis in Physical Therapy, 2nd ed. Philadelphia, W.B. Saunders Co., 1995, p. 539.

Table 1–29
Differential Diagnosis of Contractile Tissue (Muscle) and Inert Tissue (Ligament) Pathology

	Muscle	Ligament
Mechanism of injury	Overstretching (overload) Crushing (pinching)	Overstretching (overload)
Contributing factors	Muscle fatigue Poor reciprocal muscle strength Inflexibility Inadequate warmup	Muscle fatigue Hypermobility
Active movement	Pain on contraction (1°, 2°) Pain on stretch (1°, 2°) No pain on contraction (3°) Weakness on contraction (1°, 2°, 3°)	Pain on stretch or compression (1°, 2°) No pain on stretch (3°) ROM decreased
Passive movement	Pain on stretch Pain on compression	Pain on stretch (1°, 2°) No pain on stretch (3°) ROM decreased
Resisted isometric movement	Pain on contraction (1°, 2°) No pain on contraction (3°) Weakness on contraction (1°, 2°, 3°)	No pain (1°, 2°, 3°)
Special tests	If test isolates muscle, weakness and pain on contraction (1°, 2°) or weakness and no pain on contraction (3°)	If test isolates ligament, ROM and pain affected
Reflexes	Normal unless 3°	Normal
Cutaneous distribution	Normal	Normal
Joint play movement (in resting position)	Normal	Increased ROM, unless restricted by swelling
Palpation	Point tenderness at site of injury Gap if palpated early Swelling (blood—ecchymosis late) Spasm	Point tenderness at site of injury Gap if palpated early Swelling (blood/synovial fluid)
Diagnostic imaging	MRI, arthrogram, and CT scan show lesion	MRI, arthrogram and CT scan show lesion Stress x-ray shows increased ROM

CT = computed tomography; MRI = magnetic resonance imaging; ROM = range of motion.

References

Cited References

1. Cyriax, J.: Textbook of Orthopaedic Medicine, vol. 1: Diagnosis of Soft Tissue Lesions, 8th ed. London, Balliere Tindall, 1982.
2. Weed, L.: Medical records that guide and teach: Part I. N. Engl. J. Med. 278:593–600, 1968.
3. Stith, J.S., S.A. Sahrmann, K.K. Dixon, and B.J. Norton. Curriculum to prepare diagnosticians in physical therapy. J. Phys. Ther. Educ. 9:46–53, 1995.
4. Maitland, G.D.: Neuro/musculo-skeletal Examination and Recording Guide. Glen Osmond, South Australia, Lauderdale Press, 1992.
5. Travell, J.G., and D.G. Simons: Myofascial Pain and Dysfunction: The Trigger Point Manual. Baltimore, Williams & Wilkins Co., 1983.
6. Melzack, R.: The McGill pain questionnaire: Major properties and scoring methods. Pain 1:277–299, 1975.
7. Brodie, D.J., J.V. Burnett, J.M. Walker, and D. Lydes-Reid: Evaluation of low back pain by patient questionnaires and therapist assessment. J. Orthop. Sports Phys. Ther. 11:519–529, 1990.
8. Scott, J., and E.C. Huskisson: Vertical or horizontal visual analogue scales. Ann. Rheum. Dis. 38:560, 1979.
9. Langley, G.B., and H. Sheppeard: The visual analogue scale: Its use in pain management. Rheumatol. Int. 5:145–148, 1985.
10. Carlsson, A.M.: Assessment of chronic pain. Aspects of the reliability and validity of the visual analogue scale. Pain 16:87–101, 1983.
11. Lee, M.: Biomechanics of joint movements. In Refshauge, K., and E. Gass (eds.): Musculoskeletal Physiotherapy. Oxford, England, Butterworth-Heinemann Ltd., 1995.
12. Goodman, C.C., and T.E. Snyder: Differential Diagnosis in Physical Therapy. Philadelphia, W.B. Saunders Co., 1995.
13. Refshauge, K.M., and J. Latimer: The physical examination. In Refshauge, K.M., and E. Gass (eds.): Musculoskeletal Physiotherapy. Oxford, England, Butterworth-Heinemann Ltd., 1995.

14. Williams, P., and R. Warwick (eds.): Gray's Anatomy, 36th British ed. Edinburgh, Churchill Livingstone, 1980.

15. Nitta, H., T. Tajima, H. Sugiyama, and A. Moriyama: Study on dermatomes by means of selective lumbar spinal nerve block. Spine 18:1782–1786, 1993.

16. Keegan, J.J., and E.D. Garrett: The segmental distribution of the cutaneous nerves in the limbs of man. Anat. Rec. 101:409–437, 1948.

17. Grieve, G.P.: Referred pain and other clinical features. In Boyling, J.D., and N. Palastanga (eds.): Grieve's Modern Manual Therapy: The Vertebral Column, 2nd ed. Edinburgh, Churchill Livingstone, 1994.

18. Seddon, H.J.: Three types of nerve injury. Brain 66:17–28, 1943.

19. Sunderland, S.: Nerve and Nerve Injuries. Edinburgh, Churchill Livingstone, 1978.

20. Wilgis, E.F.: Techniques for diagnosis of peripheral nerve loss. Clin. Orthop. 163:8–14, 1982.

21. Tardif, G.S.: Nerve injuries: Testing and treatment tactics. Phys. Sports Med. 23:61–72, 1995.

22. Omer, G.E.: Physical diagnosis of peripheral nerve injuries. Orthop. Clin. North Am. 12:207–228, 1981.

23. Harrelson, G.L.: Evaluation of brachial plexus injuries. Sports Med. Update 4:3–8, 1989.

24. Wilbourn, A.J.: Electrodiagnostic testing of neurologic injuries in athletes. Clin. Sports Med. 9:229–245, 1990.

25. Leffert, R.: Clinical diagnosis, testing, and electromyographic study in brachial plexus traction injuries. Clin. Orthop. 237:24–31, 1988.

26. Upton, A.R., and A.J. McComas: The double crush in nerve-entrapment syndromes. Lancet 2:359–362, 1973.

27. Mackinnon, S.E.: Double and multiple "crush" syndromes. Hand Clin. 8:369–390, 1992.

28. Lee Dellon, A., and S.E. Mackinnon: Chronic nerve compression model for the double crush hypothesis. Ann. Plast. Surg. 26:259–264, 1991.

29. Nemoto, K., N. Matsumoto, K. Tazaki, Y. Horiuchi, K. Uchinishi, and Y. Mori: An experimental study on the "double crush" hypothesis. J. Hand Surg. [Am] 12:552–559, 1987.

30. Butler, D.: Mobilisation of the Nervous System. Melbourne, Churchill Livingstone, 1991.

31. Elvey, R.L.: Treatment of arm pain associated with abnormal brachial plexus tension. Aust. J. Physiother. 32:225–230, 1986.

32. Shacklock, M.: Neurodynamics. Physiotherapy 81:9–16, 1995.

33. Shacklock, M., D. Butler, and H. Slater: The dynamic central nervous system: Structure and clinical neurobiomechanics. In Boyling, J.D., and N. Palastanga (eds.): Grieve's Modern Manual Therapy: The Vertebral Column, 2nd ed. Edinburgh, Churchill Livingstone, 1994.

34. Kaltenborn, F.M.: Manual Mobilization of the Extremity Joints. Oslo, Norway, Olaf Norlis Bokhandel, 1980.

35. Ombregt, L., P. Bisschop, H.J. ter Veer, and T. Van de Velde: A System of Orthopedic Medicine. London, W.B. Saunders Co., 1995.

36. Jull, G.A.: Examination of the articular system. In Boyling, J.D., and N. Palastanga (eds.): Grieve's Modern Manual Therapy: The Vertebral Column, 2nd ed. Edinburgh, Churchill Livingstone, 1994.

37. Lea, R.D., and J.J. Gerhardt: Range-of-motion measurements. J. Bone Joint Surg. Am. 77:784–798, 1995.

38. Bovens, A.M., M.A. van Baak, J.G. Vrencken, J.A. Wijnen, and F.T. Verstappen: Variability and reliability of joint measurements. Am. J. Sports Med. 18:58–63, 1990.

39. Beighton, P., R. Grahame, and H. Borde: Hypermobility of Joints. Berlin, Springer-Verlag, 1983.

40. Wynne-Davies, R.: Hypermobility. Proc. R. Soc. Med. 64:689–693, 1971.

41. Carter, C., and J. Wilkinson: Persistent joint laxity and congenital dislocation of the hip. J. Bone Joint Surg. Br. 46:40–45, 1969.

42. Nicholas, J.S., R.B. Grossman, and E.B. Hershman: The importance of a simplified classification of motion in sports in relation to performance. Orthop. Clin. North Am. 8:499–532, 1977.

43. Maitland, G.D.: Palpation examination of the posterior cervical spine: The ideal, average and abnormal. Aust. J. Physiother. 28:3–11, 1982.

44. Clarkson, H.M., and G.B. Gilewich: Musculoskeletal Assessment: Joint Range of Motion and Manual Muscle Strength. Baltimore, Williams & Wilkins, 1989.

45. Evans, P.: Ligaments, joint surfaces, conjunct rotation and close pack. Physiotherapy 74:105–114, 1988.

46. Pope, M.H., J.W. Frymoyer, and M.H. Krag: Diagnosing instability. Clin. Orthop. 279:60–67, 1992.

47. Sapega, A.A.: Muscle performance evaluation in orthopedic practice. J. Bone Joint Surg. Am. 72:1562–1574, 1990.

48. Hislop, H.J., and J. Montgomery: Daniels and Worthingham's Muscle Testing: Techniques of Manual Examination. Philadelphia, W.B. Saunders Co., 1995.

49. Janda, V.: On the concept of postural muscles and posture in man. Aust. J. Physiother. 29:83–85, 1983.

50. Jull, G.A., and V. Janda: Muscles and motor control in low back pain: Assessment and management. In Twomey, L.T., and J.R. Taylor (eds.): Physical Therapy of the Low Back. New York, Churchill Livingstone, 1987.

51. Schlink, M.B.: Muscle imbalance patterns associated with low back syndromes. In Watkins, R.G. (ed.): The Spine in Sports. St. Louis, C.V. Mosby Co., 1996.

52. Epstein, A.M.: The outcomes movement: Will it get us where we want to go? N. Engl. J. Med. 323:266–270, 1990.

53. Goldstein, T.S.: Functional Rehabilitation in Orthopedics. Gaithersburg, Maryland, Aspen Pub. Inc., 1995.

54. Research Foundation, State University of New York: Guide for Use of the Uniform Data Set for Medical Rehabilitation Including the Functional Independence Measure (FIM). Buffalo, New York, Research Foundation, State University of New York, 1990.

55. Rueben, D.B., and A.L. Siu: An objective measure of physical function of elderly outpatients. The physical performance test. J. Am. Geriatr. Soc. 38:1105–1112, 1990.

56. Jette, A.M.: Functional status index: Reliability of a chronic disease evaluation instrument. Arch. Phys. Med. Rehabil. 61:395–401, 1980.

57. Meenan, R.F., J.H. Mason, J.J. Anderson, et al.: AIMS 2: The content and properties of a revised and expanded arthritis impact measurement scales health status questionnaire. Arthritis Rheum. 25:1–10, 1990.

58. Brimer, M.A., G. Shuneman, and B.R. Allen: Guidelines for developing a functional assessment for an acute facility. Phys. Ther. Forum 12:22–25, 1993.

59. Ellexson, M.T.: Analyzing an industry: Job analysis for treatment, prevention, and placement. Orthop. Phys. Ther. Clin. 1:15–21, 1992.

60. Rowe, C.R.: The Shoulder. Edinburgh, Churchill Livingstone, 1988.

61. Lippitt, S.B., D.T. Harryman, and F.A. Matsen: A practical tool for evaluating function: The simple shoulder test. In Matsen, F.A., F.H. Fu, and R.J. Hawkins (eds.): The Shoulder: A Balance of Mobility and Stability. Rosemont, Illinois: American Academy of Orthopedic Surgeons, 1993.

62. Gerber, C.: Integrated scoring systems for the functional assessment of the shoulder. In Matsen, F.A., F.H. Fu, and R.J. Hawkins (eds.): The Shoulder: A Balance of Mobility and Stability. Rosemont, Illinois: American Academy of Orthopedic Surgeons, 1993.

63. Carroll, H.D.: A quantitative test of upper extremity function. J. Chron. Dis. 18:479–491, 1965.

64. Potvin, A.R., W.W. Tourtellotte, J.S. Dailey, et al.: Simulated activities of daily living examination. Arch. Phys. Med. Rehabil. 53:476–486, 1972.

65. Cervical Spine Research Society: The Cervical Spine. Philadelphia, J.B. Lippincott Co., 1989.

66. Hagbarth, K.E., G. Wallen, D. Burke, and L. Lofstedt: Effects of the Jendrassik manoeuvre on muscle spindle activity in man. J. Neurol. Neurosurg. Psych. 38:1143–1153, 1975.

67. Bland, J.H.: Disorders of the Cervical Spine. Philadelphia, W.B. Saunders Co., 1987.

68. Hockaday, J.M., and C.W.M. Whitty: Patterns of referred pain in the normal subject. Brain 90:481–495, 1967.

69. Mennell, J.McM.: Joint Pain. Boston, Little, Brown & Co., 1972.

70. Kaltenborn, F.M.: Mobilization of the Extremity Joints: Examination and Basic Treatment Techniques. Oslo, Norway, Olaf Norlis Bokhandel, 1980.

71. Lewit, K., and C. Liebenson: Palpation: Problems and implications. J. Manip. Physiol. Ther. 16:586–590, 1993.

72. Bigg-Wither, G., and P. Kelly: Diagnostic imaging in musculoskeletal physiotherapy. In Refshauge, K., and E. Gass (eds.): Musculoskeletal Physiotherapy. Oxford, England, Butterworth-Heinemann Ltd., 1995.

73. Jones, M.D.: Basic Diagnostic Radiology. St. Louis, C.V. Mosby Co., 1969.

74. Miller, W.T.: Introduction to Clinical Radiology. New York, MacMillan, 1982.

75. Gross, G.W.: Imaging. In Stanitski, C.L., J.C. DeLee, and D. Drez (eds.): Pediatric and Adolescent Sports Medicine. Philadelphia, W.B. Saunders Co., 1994.

76. Fischbach, F.: A Manual of Laboratory Diagnostic Tests, 3rd ed. Philadelphia, J.B. Lippincott Co., 1988.

77. Gruelich, W.W., and S.U. Pyle: Radiographic Atlas of Skeletal Development of the Wrist and Hand. Stanford, California, Stanford University Press, 1959.

78. Grainger, R.G.: The spinal canal. In Whitehouse, G.H., and B.S. Worthington (eds.): Techniques in Diagnostic Radiology. Oxford, England Blackwell Scientific Publications, 1983.

79. Evans, R.C.: Illustrated Essentials in Orthopedic Physical Assessment. St. Louis, Mosby–Year Book Inc., 1994.

80. Weissman, B.N.W., and C.B. Sledge: Orthopedic Radiology. Philadelphia, W.B. Saunders Co., 1986.

General References

Bassett, L.W., R.H. Gold, and L.L. Seeger: MRI of the Musculoskeletal System. London, Martin Dunitz Ltd., 1989.

Bombardier, D., and P. Tugwell: Measuring disability: Guidelines for rheumatology studies. J. Rheum. Suppl. 10:68–73, 1983.

Bonica, J.J.: The Management of Pain. Philadelphia, Lea & Febiger, 1953.

Chafetz, N., and H.K. Genant: Computed tomography of the lumbar spine. Orthop. Clin. North Am. 14:147–149, 1983.

Clark, C.R., and M. Bonfiglio: Orthopedics: Essentials of Diagnosis and Treatment. New York, Churchill Livingstone, 1994.

Cohen, J., M. Bonfiglio, and C.J. Campbell: Orthopedic Pathophysiology in Diagnosis and Treatment. Edinburgh, Churchill Livingstone, 1990.

Convery, F.R., M.A. Minteer, D. Amiel, and K.L. Connett: Polyarticular disability: A functional assessment. Arch. Phys. Med. Rehab. 58:494–499, 1977.

Cox, H.T.: The cleavage lines of the skin. J. Bone Joint Surg. Br. 29:234–240, 1942.

Curran, J.F., M.H. Ellman, and N.L. Brown: Rheumatologic aspects of painful conditions affecting the shoulder. Clin. Orthop. 173:27–37, 1983.

Currey, H.L.F.: Clinical Examination of the Joints: An Introduction to Clinical Rheumatology. Toronto, Pitman Medical, 1975.

Cyriax, J.: Examination of the spinal column. Physiotherapy 56:2–6, 1970.

Dahlin, L.B., and G. Lundberg: The neuron and its response to peripheral nerve compression. J. Hand Surg. 15B:5–10, 1990.

Farfan, H.F.: Mechanical Disorders of the Low Back. Philadelphia, Lea & Febiger, 1973.

Forrester, D.M., and J.C. Brown: The Radiology of Joint Disease. Philadelphia, W.B. Saunders Co., 1987.

French, S.: History taking in physiotherapy assessment. Physiotherapy 74:158–160, 1988.

Gartland, J.J.: Fundamentals of Orthopedics. Philadelphia, W.B. Saunders Co., 1979.

Goldstein, H.A.: Bone scintigraphy. Orthop. Clin. North Am. 14:243–256, 1983.

Goodman, C.C., and T.E. Snyder: Differential Diagnosis in Physical Therapy: Musculoskeletal and Systemic Conditions. Philadelphia, W.B. Saunders Co., 1990.

Grieve, G.P.: Common Vertebral Joint Problems. London, Churchill Livingstone, 1981.

Hammond, M.J.: Clinical examination and the physiotherapist. Aust. J. Physiother. 15:47–54, 1969.

Hawkins, R.J.: Musculoskeletal Examination. St. Louis, Mosby–Year Book Inc., 1995.

Health, J.R.: Problem oriented medical systems. Physiotherapy 64:269–270, 1978.

Hoppenfeld, S.: Physical Examination of the Spine and Extremities. New York, Appleton-Century-Crofts, 1976.

Jackson, R.: Headaches associated with disorders of the cervical spine. Headache 6:175–179, 1967.

Janda, V.: Muscle Function Testing. London, Butterworths, 1983.

Jones, M.A., and H.M. Jones: Principles of the physical examination. In Boyling, J.D., and N. Palastanga (eds.): Grieve's Modern Manual Therapy, 2nd ed. Edinburgh, Churchill Livingstone, 1994.

Judge, R.D., G.D. Zuidema, and F.T. Fitzgerald: Clinical Diagnosis: A Physiologic Approach. Boston, Little, Brown & Co., 1982.

Kaplan, R.M., J.W. Bush, and C.C. Berry: Health status: Types of validity and the index of well-being. Health Sci. Res. 11:478–507, 1976.

Lee, P., M.K. Jasani, W.C. Dick, and W.W. Buchanan: Evaluation of a functional index in rheumatoid arthritis. Scand. J. Rheum. 2:71–77, 1973.

Little, H.: The Rheumatological Physical Examination. Orlando, Grune & Stratton, Inc., 1986.

Loomis, J.: Rehabilitation outcomes: The clinician's perspective. Can. J. Rehab. 7:165–170, 1994.

MacConnaill, M.A., and J.V. Basmajian: Muscles and Movements: A Basis for Human Kinesiology. Baltimore, Williams & Wilkins, 1977.

Massey, E.W., T.L. Riley, and A.B. Pleet: Co-existent carpal tunnel syndrome and cervical radiculopathy (double crush syndrome). South. Med. J. 74:957–959, 1981.

Mayer, S.J., and M.K. Dalinka: Magnetic resonance imaging of the shoulder. Orthop. Clin. North Am. 21:497–513, 1990.

McLean, G., and D.B. Freiman: Angiography of skeletal disease. Orthop. Clin. North Am. 14:257–270, 1983.

Neviaser, T.J.: Arthrography of the shoulder. Orthop. Clin. North Am. 11:205–217, 1980.

Nilsson, N.: Measuring cervical muscle tenderness: A study of reliability. J. Manip. Physiol. Ther. 18: 88–90, 1995.

Novey, D.W.: Rapid Access Guide to the Physical Examination. Chicago, Year Book Medical Publishers, 1988.

Palmer, M.L., and M. Epler: Clinical Assessment Procedures in Physical Therapy. Philadelphia, J.B. Lippincott Co., 1990.

Pitt, M.J., P.J. Lund, and D.P. Speer: Imaging of the pelvis and hip. Orthop. Clin. North Am. 21:545–559, 1990.

Post, M.: Physical Examination of the Musculoskeletal System. Chicago, Year Book Medical Publishers, 1987.

Reading, A.E.: Testing pain mechanisms in persons in pain. In Wall, P.D., and R. Melzack (eds.): Textbook of Pain. Edinburgh, Churchill Livingstone, 1984.

Refshauge, K.M., and J. Latimer: The history. In Refshauge, K., and E. Gass (eds.): Musculoskeletal Physiotherapy. Oxford, England, Butterworth-Heinemann Ltd., 1995.

Saunders, H.D., and R. Saunders: Evaluation, Treatment and Prevention of Musculoskeletal Disorders, 3rd ed., vol. 1 and 2. Chaska, Minnesota, H.D. Saunders, 1993.

Saunders, H.D.: Evaluation of a musculoskeletal disorder. In Gould, J.A. (ed.): Orthopedics and Sports Physical Therapy. St. Louis, C.V. Mosby Co., 1990.

Schaible, H.G., and B.D. Grubb: Afferent and spinal mechanisms of joint pain. Pain 55:5–54, 1993.

Seidal, H.M., J.W. Ball, J.E. Dains, and G.W. Benedict: Mosby's Guide to Physical Examination. St. Louis, C.V. Mosby Co., 1987.

Selby, D.K., A.J. Meril, K.J. Wagner, and R.R.G. Winans: Water-soluble myelography. Orthop. Clin. North Am. 8:79–83, 1977.

Singer, K.P.: A new musculoskeletal assessment in a student
population. J. Orthop. Sports Phys. Ther. 8:34–41, 1986.

Smith, L.K.: Functional tests. Phys. Ther. Rev. 34:19–21, 1954.

Spengler, D.M.: Low Back Pain: Assessment and Management.
Orlando, Grune & Stratton, Inc., 1982.

Squire, L.F., W.M. Colaiace, and N. Strutynsky: Exercises in
Diagnostic Radiology, vol. 3: Bone. Philadelphia, W.B.
Saunders Co., 1972.

Starkey, C., and J. Ryan: Evaluation of Orthopedic and Athletic
Injuries. Philadelphia, F.A. Davis, 1996.

Wadsworth, C.T.: Manual Examination and Treatment of the Spine
and Extremities. Baltimore, Williams & Wilkins, 1988.

Warren, M.J.: Modern imaging of the spine: The use of computed
tomography and magnetic resonance. In Boyling, J.D., and N.
Palastanga (eds.): Grieve's Modern Manual Therapy, 2nd ed.
Edinburgh, Churchill Livingstone, 1994.

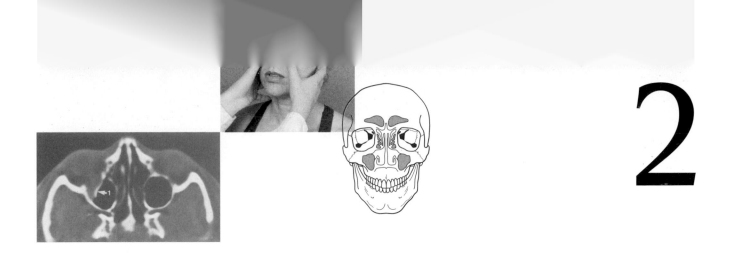

Head and Face

Assessment of the head and face is often performed by casualty officers and clinicians working in emergency care settings. In these settings, the assessment involves the bony aspects of the head and face as well as the soft tissues. The soft-tissue assessment involves primarily the sensory organs such as the skin, eyes, nose, and ears, whereas the muscles are tested only as they relate to injury to these structures. Joints and their integrity are not the main object of the assessment. Because the temporomandibular joints and cervical spine are discussed in Chapters 3 and 4, this chapter deals with only the head and face and associated structures.

Applied Anatomy

The head and face are made up of the cranial vault and facial bones. The **cranial vault,** or skull, is composed of several bones—one frontal, two sphenoid, two parietal, two temporal, and one occipital (Fig. 2–1). Of these, the strongest is the occipital bone, and the weakest are the temporal bones. The frontal bone forms the forehead, and the temporal and sphenoid bones form the antero-lateral walls of the skull, or the temples of the head. The parietal bones form the top and posterolateral portions of the skull, and the occipital bones form the posterior portion of the skull. The cranial vault reaches 90% of its ultimate size by age 5.

In addition to the cranial vault bones, there are 14 **facial bones.** These bones develop more slowly than the cranial bones, reaching only 60% of their ultimate size by age 6. The facial skeleton is composed of the mandible, which forms the lower jaw; the maxilla, which forms the upper jaw on each side; the nasal bones, which form the bridge of the nose; and the palatine, lacrimal, zygomatic, and ethmoid bones, which form the remainder of the face. It is the zygomatic bone that gives the cheek its prominence. The sphenoid bones also form

part of the orbital cavity. The facial skull has several cavities for the eyes (orbital), nose (nasal), and mouth (oral), as well as spaces for nerves and blood vessels to penetrate the bony structure. Weight is saved in the skull area by the addition of sinus cavities (Fig. 2–2).

The muscles of the head and face are controlled primarily by the 12 **cranial nerves.** The cranial nerves and their chief functions are shown in Table 2–1. The cranial nerves generally contain both sensory and motor fibers. However, some cranial nerves are strictly sensory (olfactory and optic), whereas others are strictly motor (oculomotor, trochlear, and hypoglossal).

The **external eye** is composed of the eyelids (upper and lower), conjunctiva (a transparent membrane covering the cornea, iris, pupil, lens, and sclera), lacrimal gland, eye muscles, and bony skull orbit (Fig. 2–3). Muscles of the eye, their actions, and their nerve supply are shown in Table 2–2. The muscles and movements of the eye are shown in Figure 2–4. To produce some of the actions, the various muscles of the eye must work in concert. The **eyelids** protect the eye from foreign bodies, distribute tears over the surface of the eye, and limit the amount of light entering the eye. The **conjunctiva** is a thin membrane covering the majority of the anterior surface of the eye. It helps to protect the eye from foreign bodies and desiccation (drying up). Tears (which keep the eye moist) are provided by the lacrimal gland (Fig. 2–5). The eye itself is made up of the sclera, cornea, and iris as well as the lens and retina (Fig. 2–6). The **sclera** is the dense white portion of the eye that physically supports the internal structures. The **cornea** is very sensitive to pain (e.g., the extreme pain that accompanies corneal abrasion) and separates the watery fluid of the anterior chamber of the eye from the external environment. It permits transmission of light through the lens to the retina. The **iris** is a circular, contractile muscular disc that controls the amount of light entering the eye and contains pigmented cells that give color to the eye. The **lens** is a crystalline structure located immediately

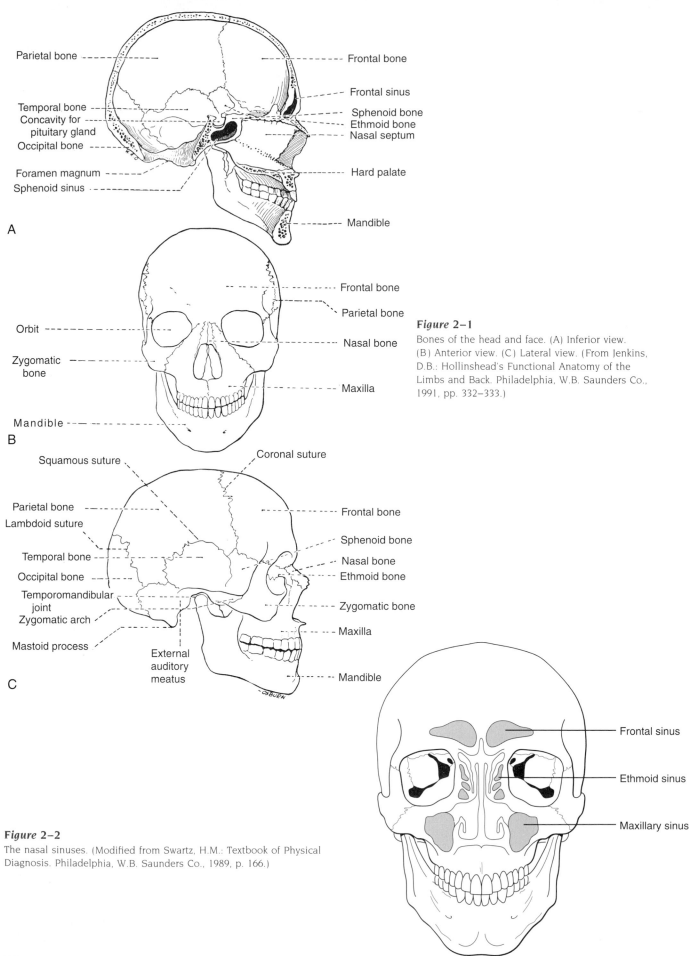

Parietal bone

Temporal bone
Concavity for
pituitary gland
Occipital bone

Foramen magnum
Sphenoid sinus

A

Frontal bone

Frontal sinus

Sphenoid bone
Ethmoid bone
Nasal septum

Hard palate

Mandible

Orbit

Zygomatic
bone

Mandible

B

Frontal bone

Parietal bone

Nasal bone

Maxilla

Figure 2–1

Bones of the head and face. (A) Inferior view.
(B) Anterior view. (C) Lateral view. (From Jenkins,
D.B.: Hollinshead's Functional Anatomy of the
Limbs and Back. Philadelphia, W.B. Saunders Co.,
1991, pp. 332–333.)

Squamous suture

Coronal suture

Parietal bone
Lambdoid suture

Temporal bone

Occipital bone

Temporomandibular
joint
Zygomatic arch

Mastoid process

C

External
auditory
meatus

Frontal bone

Sphenoid bone

Nasal bone
Ethmoid bone

Zygomatic bone

Maxilla

Mandible

Frontal sinus

Ethmoid sinus

Maxillary sinus

Figure 2–2

The nasal sinuses. (Modified from Swartz, H.M.: Textbook of Physical
Diagnosis. Philadelphia, W.B. Saunders Co., 1989, p. 166.)

Table 2–1
Cranial Nerves and Methods of Testing

Nerve	Afferent (Sensory)	Efferent (Motor)	Test
I. Olfactory	Smell: Nose	—	Identify familiar odors (e.g., chocolate, coffee)
II. Optic	Sight: Eye	—	Test visual fields
III. Oculomotor	—	Voluntary motor: Levator of eyelid; superior, medial, and inferior recti; inferior oblique muscle of eyeball Autonomic: Smooth muscle of eyeball	Upward, downward, and medial gaze Reaction to light
IV. Trochlear		Voluntary motor: Superior oblique muscle of eyeball	Downward and lateral gaze
V. Trigeminal	Touch, pain: Skin of face, mucous membranes of nose, sinuses, mouth, anterior tongue	Voluntary motor: Muscles of mastication	Corneal reflex Face sensation Clench teeth; push down on chin to separate jaws
VI. Abducens		Voluntary motor: Lateral rectus muscle of eyeball	Lateral gaze
VII. Facial	Taste: Anterior tongue	Voluntary motor: Facial muscles Autonomic: Lacrimal, submandibular, and sublingual glands	Close eyes tight Smile and show teeth Whistle and puff cheeks Identify familiar tastes (e.g., sweet, sour)
VIII. Vestibulocochlear (acoustic nerve)	Hearing: Ear Balance: Ear	—	Hear watch ticking Hearing tests Balance and coordination test
IX. Glossopharyngeal	Touch, pain: Posterior tongue, pharynx Taste: Posterior tongue	Voluntary motor: Unimportant muscle of pharynx Autonomic: Parotid gland	Gag reflex Ability to swallow
X. Vagus	Touch, pain: Pharynx, larynx, bronchi Taste: Tongue, epiglottis	Voluntary motor: Muscles of palate, pharynx, and larynx Autonomic: Thoracic and abdominal viscera	Gag reflex Ability to swallow Say "Ahhh"
XI. Accessory	—	Voluntary motor: Sternocleidomastoid and trapezius muscle	Resisted shoulder shrug
XII. Hypoglossal	—	Voluntary motor: Muscles of tongue	Tongue protrusion (if injured, tongue deviates toward injured side)

Adapted from Hollinshead, W.H., and D.B. Jenkins: Functional Anatomy of the Limbs and Back. Philadelphia, W.B. Saunders Co., 1981, p. 358; and Reid, D.C.: Sports Injury Assessment and Rehabilitation. New York, Churchill Livingstone, 1992, p. 860.

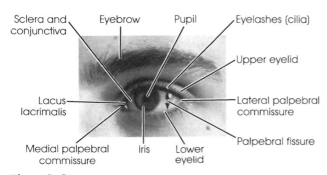

Sclera and conjunctiva · Eyebrow · Pupil · Eyelashes (cilia) · Upper eyelid · Lacus lacrimalis · Lateral palpebral commissure · Medial palpebral commissure · Iris · Lower eyelid · Palpebral fissure

Figure 2–3
External features of the eye.

behind the iris that permits images from varied distances to be focused on the retina. It is primarily the lens and its supporting ligaments that separate the eye into chambers—the anterior chamber (aqueous humor) and the posterior chamber (vitreous humor). Finally, the **retina** is the primary sensory structure of the eye that transforms light impulses into electrical impulses that are then transmitted by the optic nerve to the brain, which interprets the impulses as the objects seen.

The **external ear** consists of cartilage covered with skin. Its primary purpose is to direct sound and to protect the external auditory meatus, through which sound is

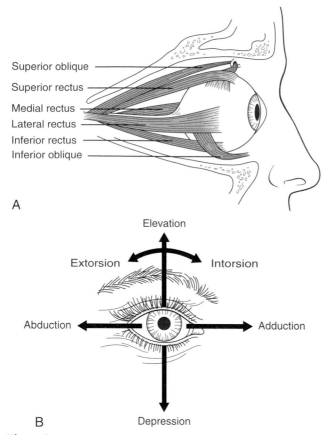

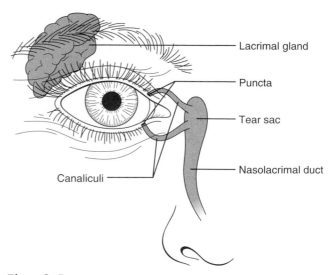

Figure 2–5

The lacrimal apparatus. (Modified from Swartz, H.M.: Textbook of Physical Diagnosis. Philadelphia, W.B. Saunders Co., 1989, p. 126.)

Figure 2–4

Muscles (A) and movements (B) of the eye. (Modified from Swartz, H.M.: Textbook of Physical Diagnosis. Philadelphia, W.B. Saunders Co., 1989, pp. 125–126.)

transmitted to the eardrum. The external ear, which is sometimes called the pinna, auricle, or trumpet, consists of the helix and lobule around the outside and the triangular fossa, antihelix, concha, tragus (cartilaginous projection anterior to external auditory meatus), and antitragus on the inside (Fig. 2–7). The **middle ear** structures consist of the tympanic membrane, or eardrum, which vibrates when sound hits it and sends vibrations through the ossicles—called the malleus (hammer), incus (anvil),

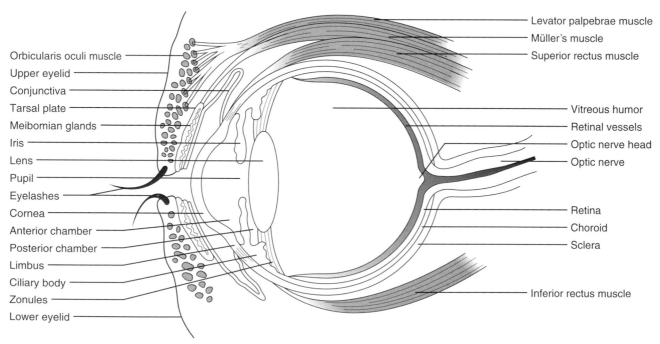

Figure 2–6

Cross section of the eye. (Modified from Swartz, H.M.: Textbook of Physical Diagnosis. Philadelphia, W.B. Saunders Co., 1989, p. 132.)

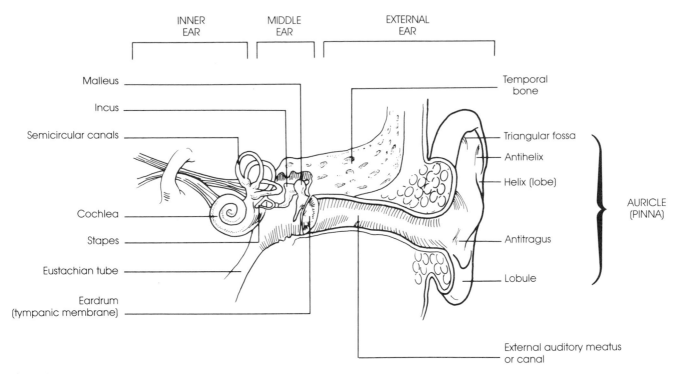

Figure 2–7
A cross-sectional view through the ear.

and stapes (stirrup)—to the cochlea. The cochlea, which is part of the **inner ear,** transmits the sound waves to the vestibulocochlear nerve (cranial nerve VIII), which transmits electrical impulses to the brain for interpretation. The semicircular canals, the other part of the inner ear, play a significant role in maintaining balance.

The **external nose,** like the external ear, consists primarily of cartilage covered with skin. However, its

proximal portion contains bone covered with skin. Figure 2–8 shows the bone and cartilage makeup of the nose. The floor of the nose consists of the hard and soft palates and forms the roof of the mouth (Fig. 2–9). The roof of

Table 2–2
Muscles of the Eye: Their Actions and Nerve Supply

Action	Muscles Acting	Nerve Supply
Moves pupil upward	Superior rectus	Oculomotor (CN III)
Moves pupil downward	Inferior rectus	Oculomotor (CN III)
Moves pupil medially	Medial rectus	Oculomotor (CN III)
Moves pupil laterally	Lateral rectus	Abducens (CN VI)
Moves pupil downward and laterally	Superior oblique	Trochlear (CN IV)
Moves pupil upward and laterally	Inferior oblique	Oculomotor (CN III)
Elevates upper eyelid	Levator palpebrae superioris	Oculomotor (CN III)

CN = cranial nerve.

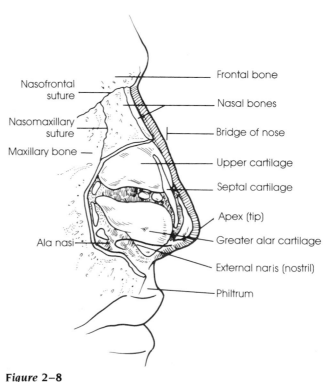

Figure 2–8
The bony and cartilaginous structures of the nose.

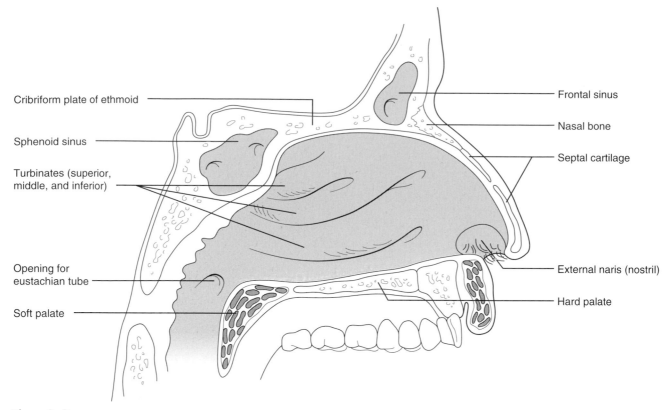

Figure 2-9
Cross section of the nose and nasopharynx.

Cribriform plate of ethmoid

Sphenoid sinus

Turbinates (superior, middle, and inferior)

Opening for eustachian tube

Soft palate

Frontal sinus

Nasal bone

Septal cartilage

External naris (nostril)

Hard palate

the nose is formed from cartilage and the nasal, frontal, ethmoid, and sphenoid bones. The frontal and maxillary bones form the nasal bridge. The lateral aspects of the nose are formed by three bony structures called turbinates (superior, middle, and inferior), which increase the surface area of the nose and thereby warm, humidify, and filter inspired air. The nose is divided into two chambers (vestibules) by a septum. These chambers are lined with a mucous membrane containing hairs that collect debris and other foreign substances from the inspired air. The cribriform plate of the ethmoid bone contains the sensory fibers of the olfactory nerve (cranial nerve I) for smell.

Patient History

In addition to the questions listed under Patient History in Chapter 1, the examiner should obtain the following information from the patient.

1. What happened? This question is asked to determine the mechanism of injury and, potentially, the area of the brain injured (Table 2–3). A forceful blow to a resting, moveable head usually produces maximum brain injury beneath the point of impact (Fig. 2–10). This type of injury, called a **coup injury,** is usually caused by linear or translational acceleration. It often causes focal ischemic lesions, especially in the cerebellum, leading to alterations in smooth, coordinated movements; equilibrium; and posture. If the head is moving and strikes an unyielding object such as the ground, maximum brain injury is usually sustained in an area opposite the site of impact. This **contrecoup injury** is the result of impact deceleration. The injury occurs on the side of the head

Table 2–3
Areas of the Brain and Their Function

Cerebrum	Cognitive aspects of motor control Memory Sensory awareness (e.g., pain, touch) Speech Special senses (e.g., taste, vision)
Cerebellum	Coordinate and integrate motor behavior Balance Motor learning Motor control (muscle contraction and force production)
Diencephalon (thalamus)	Regulation of body temperature and water balance Control of emotions Information processing to cerebrum
Brain stem	Control of respiratory and heart rates Peripheral blood flow control

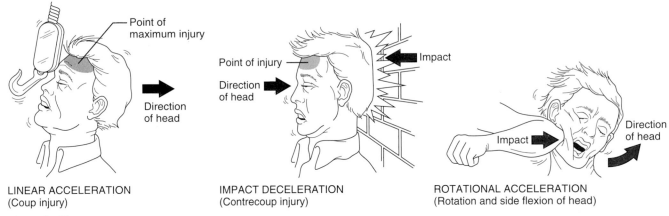

LINEAR ACCELERATION
(Coup injury)

IMPACT DECELERATION
(Contrecoup injury)

ROTATIONAL ACCELERATION
(Rotation and side flexion of head)

Figure 2–10
Mechanisms of injury to the brain.

opposite to that receiving the blow because the head is accelerating before impact, which squeezes the cerebrospinal fluid away from the trailing edge (the side away from the impact). The fluid is moved toward the impact side, thereby thickening the cerebrospinal fluid and offering a cushioning effect at the point of impact. Because of the lack of cushioning on the trailing edge, greater injury is likely to occur to the brain on the side opposite the impact. The brain may also experience a "shaking" caused by repeated reverberation within the brain after the head has been struck. This type of injury often results in the signs and symptoms of a concussion, with the degree of the concussion depending on the severity of the injury (Table 2–4). If the cervical spine is taken beyond its normal range of motion, especially into rotation or side flexion, there may be a twisting of the cerebral hemisphere, brain stem, carotid artery, or carotid sinus that results in injury to these structures or ischemia to the brain. Those areas of the brain that are most susceptible to damage include the temporal lobes, anterior frontal lobe, posterior occipital lobe, and upper portion of the midbrain.[1]

Table 2–4
Signs and Symptoms of Concussion (Torg Classification)

	Grade 1	Grade 2	Grade 3	Grade 4	Grade 5
Confusion	None or momentary	Slight	Moderate	Severe	Severe
Amnesia	No	Posttraumatic amnesia <30 min	Posttraumatic amnesia <30 min Retrograde amnesia	Posttraumatic amnesia >30 min Retrograde amnesia	Posttraumatic amnesia >24 hours Retrograde amnesia
Residual symptoms	No	Perhaps	Sometimes	Yes	Yes
Loss of consciousness	No	No	No	Yes (<5 min)	Yes (>5 min)
Tinnitus	No	Mild	Moderate	Severe	Often severe
Dizziness	No	Mild	Moderate	Severe	Usually severe
Headache	No	May be present (dull)	Often	Often	Often
Disorientation and unsteadiness	None or minimal	Some	Moderate	Severe (5–10 min)	Often severe (>10 min)
Blurred vision	No	No	No	Not usually	Possible
Postconcussion syndrome	No	Possible	Possible	Possible	Possible
Personality changes	No	No	No	Possible	Possible

Data from Vegso, J.J., and J.S. Torg: Field evaluation and management of intracranial injuries. In Torg, J.S. (ed.): Athletic Injuries to the Head, Neck and Face. St. Louis, Mosby–Year Book Inc., 1991, pp. 226–227.

2. Did the patient lose consciousness? If so, how long was the patient unconscious? Has the patient suffered a concussion before? These questions are often very difficult for the patient to answer or the examiner to know, because the patient may have been momentarily stunned and the time may have been so short that the patient believed there was no loss of consciousness. In other words, loss of consciousness may have been only momentary or, more traditionally, it may have lasted seconds to minutes. If the examiner is working with a sports team, accurate records are essential to record the severity (see later discussion) and number of concussions suffered by the athlete and to ensure that proper care is instituted and the athlete is not allowed to return to competition too soon. Concussions (which are examples of diffuse brain injuries) are the most common cause of loss of consciousness after trauma. **Concussions** can occur from a blow to the head or jaw or a fall on the buttocks from a height and can result in an inability to process information. There are many different grading systems for concussions, but the grades advocated by Torg[2] are described here. With each grade of concussion, the signs and symptoms worsen, and sequelae are more evident.

With a **grade I concussion,** the patient is slightly confused and may have a dazed look. The patient is completely lucid within 5 to 15 minutes; has no amnesia, sequelae, or residual symptoms; and has had no loss of consciousness. Some people refer to the grade I concussion as the patient's having his or her "bell rung."

With a **grade II concussion,** there is slight confusion, and posttraumatic amnesia becomes evident. Posttraumatic amnesia is the loss of memory for events occurring immediately after wakening or from the moment of injury. **Posttraumatic (anterograde) amnesia** is considered to be the length of time from injury until conscious memory returns. The patient who sustains a period of posttraumatic amnesia of less than 60 minutes is considered to have sustained a mild head injury. If the period of posttraumatic amnesia lasts from 1 to 24 hours, moderate head injury is considered to have occurred. If the posttraumatic amnesia lasts for more than 1 week, the patient is considered to have sustained a very serious head injury. If the duration of the posttraumatic amnesia is more than 7 days, full return to neurological function is highly unlikely.[3] With a grade II concussion, the patient may experience mild tinnitus (ringing in the ears), mild dizziness, and a dull headache with some disorientation. The patient who experienced a grade II concussion may also develop a postconcussion syndrome (i.e., have continual neurological problems after the concussion). The signs and symptoms of this syndrome include persistent headaches, especially with exertion; inability to concentrate; and irritability. The symptoms may last from several weeks to several years.

A patient with a **grade III concussion** has the same symptoms as someone with a grade II concussion and also experiences retrograde amnesia. **Retrograde amnesia** is loss of memory of events that occurred before the injury. It may take 5 to 10 minutes for retrograde amnesia to develop after the concussion, and amnesia may involve only a few minutes before the injury. For this reason, the patient should frequently be questioned about what happened before the injury occurred and how it occurred, to see if there is any change in the patient's memory pattern. There is always some degree of permanent retrograde amnesia with these patients.

Head Injury Severity Based on Length of Posttraumatic Amnesia

<60 *minutes*:	Mild
1–24 *hours*:	Moderate
>1 *week*:	Serious (full return of neurological function unlikely)

Levels of Consciousness

Coma	• No response to painful stimuli or any other stimuli
Stupor (semicoma)	• Responds to painful stimuli (withdrawal), shaking • Groans, mumbles • Reflex activity present
Obtundity	• Responds to loud voice or shake • Responds to painful stimulus (withdrawal) • Confused when aroused • Talks in monosyllables • Speech mumbled and incoherent • Needs constant stimulation to cooperate
Lethargy	• Sleeps when not stimulated • Drowsy, inattentive • Responds to name • Loses train of thought • Decreased spontaneous movement • Thinking is slow and fuzzy
Confusion	• Impaired memory • Confused and disoriented
Alertness	• Readily aroused, oriented and fully aware of surroundings

With a **grade IV concussion,** the patient loses consciousness for 5 minutes or less. The level of consciousness may vary; the patient may be comatose, stuporous, obtunded, lethargic, confused, or fully alert. The patient goes through the following stages of recovery: unconsciousness (also called paralytic coma), stupor, confusion (with or without delirium), near-lucidity with automatism, and finally full alertness. **Stupor** implies that the patient is only partially conscious and has reduced responsiveness. **Confusion** implies that the patient is disoriented in terms of time, place, or person. **Delirium** means that the patient may experience illusions, hallucinations, restlessness, or incoherence. **Lucidity with automatism** implies that the patient appears to be alert and fully recovered but acts only mechanically and is not really aware of what he or she is doing. With a grade IV concussion, there may be subtle changes in the patient's personality and memory function. Both retrograde and posttraumatic amnesia are evident, and the patient complains of mental confusion, tinnitus, and dizziness to a greater degree than is seen with a grade III concussion. The patient also has residual headaches and will be unsteady for 5 to 10 minutes after regaining consciousness.

With a **grade V concussion,** the patient has experienced a paralytic coma or unconsciousness for 5 minutes or longer. This grade of concussion involves bruising of the brain, and there is prolonged retrograde amnesia as well as posttraumatic amnesia. The patient complains of severe tinnitus, unsteadiness for longer than 10 minutes, blurred vision, poor light accommodation, and a headache that feels "different" from most headaches. Both the autonomic and the peripheral nervous systems are affected through their control by the brain. These patients may also experience nausea, vomiting, and sometimes convulsions. The recovery after a grade V concussion may be one of two types. In type A, the patient goes from a paralytic coma through stupor, confusion, lucidity, and full alertness, which is similar to a grade IV concussion but more severe. The individual with a type B grade V concussion experiences a paralytic coma that is associated with secondary cardiorespiratory collapse and is of much greater concern to the examiner, especially during the initial assessment, when the body's essential functions must be maintained.

More severe diffuse brain injuries are associated with more severe neurological dysfunction. With these injuries, loss of consciousness lasts for more than 24 hours and recovery is never complete, leading to deficits in intelligence, reasoning, and memory and to changes in personality. Shearing brain injuries tend to be more severe than diffuse brain injuries and lead to abnormal brain stem signs such as decerebrate rigidity.[2]

3. If the patient has had an injury to the head, are there any associated symptoms in the neck or problems with breathing, altered vision, discharge from the nose or ears, or urinary or fecal incontinence? These symptoms indicate severe brain or spinal cord injury, and the patient must be handled with extreme care.

Head Signs and Symptoms Requiring Specialist Care

- Presence of amnesia
- Prolonged residual symptoms
- Loss of consciousness
- Prolonged headache
- Postconcussion syndrome
- Personality changes
- More than one first- or second-degree concussion
- Prolonged disorientation, unsteadiness, or confusion (>2–3 min)
- Blurred vision
- Dizziness (>5 min)
- Tinnitus (>5 min)

---

4. What are the sites and boundaries of pain? This question can help the examiner determine what structures have been injured. It is important to keep in mind that the patient may be experiencing a referral of pain.

5. What type of pain is the patient experiencing? The type of pain will give an indication of the type of structure injured (see Table 1–2).

6. Is there any paresthesia, abnormal sensation, or lack of sensation? Are smell (cranial nerve I), vision (cranial nerve II), taste (cranial nerve VII), and hearing (cranial nerve VIII) normal? These questions give the examiner some idea of whether neurological structures have been injured and, if so, which ones.

7. What activities aggravate the particular problem?

8. What activities ease the particular problem?

9. Does the patient have a **headache** and, if so, where? (Tables 2–5 and 2–6) Is the headache tolerable? What type of headache is it? Is it a throbbing, pounding, boring, shocklike, dull, nagging, or constant-pressure type of headache? Is the pain of the headache aggravated by movement or by rest? What is the exact location of the headache? Is the headache affected by position or time of day? (Table 2–7) Does it cover the entire head, the sinus region, behind the eyes, the hat band distribution, the neck, or the occiput area? It is important for the examiner to record the location, character, duration, and frequency of the headache, as well as any factors that appear to either aggravate or relieve the pain, so that a diagnosis can be made and any changes can be noticed (Table 2–8).

10. Is the patient dizzy or unsteady or having problems with balance? The examiner should also note whether the dizziness is brought on by sudden standing up, turning, or bending or whether it occurs without

Table 2–5

Type of Headache Pain and Usual Causes

Type of Pain	Usual Causes
Acute	Trauma, acute infection, impending cerebrovascular accident, subarachnoid hemorrhage
Chronic, recurrent	Migraine (definite pattern of irregular interval); eyestrain; noise; excessive eating, drinking, or smoking; inadequate ventilation
Continuous, recurrent	Trauma
Severe, intense	Meningitis, aneurysm (ruptured), migraine, brain tumor
Intense, transient, shocklike	Neuralgia
Throbbing, pulsating (vascular)	Migraine, fever, hypertension, aortic insufficiency, neuralgia
Constant, tight (bandlike), bilateral	Muscle contraction

Table 2–7

Effect of Position or Time of Day on Headache

Position or Time of Day When Headache Is Worst	Usual Causes
Morning	Sinusitis, migraine, hypertension, alcoholism, sleeping position
Afternoon	Eyestrain, muscle tension
Night	Intracranial disease, osteomyelitis, nephritis
Bending	Sinusitis
Lying horizontal	Migraine

movement. It must be remembered that "dizziness" is a word sometimes used by patients to indicate unsteadiness in walking. Dizziness is usually associated with problems of the middle ear, vertebrobasilar insufficiency, or problems in the upper cervical spine. Vertigo implies a rotary component; the patient's environment seems to whirl around the patient, or the patient's body seems to rotate in relation to the environment. If the patient complains of dizziness or vertigo, the time of onset and duration of these attacks should be noted. A description of the type of motion that occurs and any other associated symptoms should be included. Balance may be affected by problems within the brain or the semicircular canals in the inner ear. The examiner should also note whether the patient is talking about unsteadiness, loss of balance, or actual falling.

11. Is the patient unduly irritated or having trouble concentrating? The patient's state will give an indication of the severity of the injury.

12. Does the patient know where he or she is, who he or she is, the day, and the time of day? Does the

Table 2–6

Location of Headache and Usual Causes

Location	Usual Causes
Forehead	Sinusitis, eye or nose disorder, muscle spasm of occipital or suboccipital region
Side of head	Migraine, eye or ear disorder, auriculotemporal neuralgia
Occipital	Myofascial problems, herniated disc, eyestrain, hypertension, occipital neuralgia
Parietal	Hysteria (viselike), meningitis, constipation, tumor
Face	Maxillary sinusitis, trigeminal neuralgia, dental problems, tumor

patient have some idea of what was happening when the injury occurred? These types of questions give an indication of the severity of the injury.

13. Does the patient have any memory of past events or what occurred before or after the injury? This type of question tests for retrograde amnesia, posttraumatic amnesia, and injury severity, which can be determined by asking the patient straightforward questions about events in the patient's own past, such as birthdate or year of graduation from high school or university. Questions about the injury, preceding events, and posttraumatic events may also be asked. The examiner must ensure that the answer to such questions is known by the examiner or someone present at the time of the examination. **Recent memory** can be tested by giving the patient two to five common objects or names, such as the color "red," the number "5," the name "Mr. Smith," and the word "pride" to remember and then asking the patient to name them 5 or 10 minutes later. The patient may be asked to repeat the words two or three times when the examiner initially says them to test immediate recall or to ensure that the patient can say and recall the words. **Immediate recall,** another form of memory, is best tested by saying a series of single digits and asking the patient to repeat them. Normally, a person can repeat at least six digits, and many people can repeat eight or nine. The patient may also be asked to repeat the months of the year backward in a similar type of test. Memory is generally thought to be formed and stored in certain regions of the temporal lobes. The parietal lobe of the brain is thought to enable one to have an appreciation of the environment, to interpret visual stimuli, and to communicate.

14. Can the patient solve simple problems? Because concussions reduce the ability to process information, it is important to determine the patient's **reasoning and processing abilty.** For example, does the patient know his or her home telephone number? Is the patient able to do the "minus 7" test (i.e., count backward from 100 by sevens)? This test gives the examiner some idea of the patient's calculating ability and concentration skills.

Table 2-8
Headaches: A Differential Diagnosis

Disorder	Sex/Age Predominance	Nature of Pain	Frequency	Location	Duration	Prodromal Events	Precipitating Factors	Cause	Familial Predisposition	Other Possible Symptoms
Migraine	Female/20 to 40 years	Builds to throbbing and intense	Usually not more than twice a week. May be nocturnal	Usually unilateral	Several hours to days	Visual disturbances can occur contralateral to pain site	Unknown, may be physical, emotional, hormonal, dietary	Vasomotor	Yes	Nausea, vomiting, pallor, photophobia, mood disturbances, fluid retention
Cluster (histamine) headache	Male/40 to 60 years	Excruciating, stabbing, burning, pulsating	1 to 4 episodes per 24 hours. Nocturnal manifestation	Unilateral, eye, temple, forehead	Minutes to hours	Sleep disturbances or personality changes can occur	Unknown, may be serotonin, histamine, hormonal, blood flow	Vasomotor	Minor	Ipsilateral sweating of face, lacrimation, nasal congestion or discharge
Hypertension headache	None	Dull, throbbing, nonlocalized	Variable	Entire cranium, especially occipital region	Variable	None	Activity that increases blood pressure	High blood pressure; diastolic >120 mm Hg	Only as related to hypertension	
Trigeminal neuralgia (tic douloureux)	Female/40 to 60 years	Excruciating, spontaneous, lancinating, lightning	Can occur many (12 or more) times per day	Unilateral along trigeminal nerve area	30 seconds to 1 minute	Disagreeable tingling	Touch (cold) to affected area	Neurological	None	Reddened conjunctiva, lacrimation
Glossopharyngeal neuralgia	Male/40 to 60 years	Excruciating, spontaneous, lancinating, lightning	Can occur many (12 or more) times per day	Unilateral retrolingual area to ear	30 seconds to 1 minute	None	Movement or contact of the pharynx	Neurological	None	
Cervical neuralgia	None	Dull pain or pressure in head	Variable	Bilateral, occipital, frontal, or facial	Variable	None	Posture or head movement	Neurological, pressure on roots of spinal nerves	None	Dizziness, auditory disturbances
Eye disorders	None	Generalized discomfort in or around the eyes	Intensify with sustained visual effort	Entire cranium	During and after visual effort	None	Impairment of eye function	Cornea, iris, or intraocular pain	Possible	Diminished vision, sensitivity to light, tearing
Sinus, ear, and nasal disorders	None	Dull, persistent	Variable	Frontal, temporal, ear, nose, occipital	Variable	None	Infection, allergy, chemical, bending, straining	Blockage, inflammation, infection	None	

Modified from Esposito, C.J., G.A. Grim, and T.K. Binkley: Headaches: A differential diagnosis. J. Craniomand. Pract. 4:320–321, 1986.

Mathematic ability (the ability to add, subtract, multiply, and divide) can also be evaluated to test processing ability. In addition, the patient can be asked to name several important people from the present in reverse chronological order (e.g., the last three presidents of the United States) or to give the names of some familiar capital cities. Finally, the patient should be tested on whether abstract relations can be comprehended. For example, one may quote a common proverb such as "a bird in the hand is worth two in the bush" and then ask the patient to explain what is meant. Patients with organic mental impairment and certain patients with schizophrenia may give a concrete answer, failing to recognize the abstract principle involved.[3] The ability to conceptualize, abstract, plan ahead, and formulate rational judgments of problems or events is largely a function of the frontal lobes.

15. Can the patient talk normally? Patients with lesions of the parietal lobe have great difficulty in communicating and understanding what is going on around them. **Dysarthria** indicates defects in articulation, enunciation, or rhythm of speech. It usually results from extraneural problems such as poor-fitting dentures, malformation of the oral structures, or impairment of the musculature of the tongue, palate, pharynx, or lips because of incoordination, weakness, or abnormal innervation. It is characterized by slurring, slowness of speech, indistinct speech, and breaks in normal speech rhythm. **Dysphonia** is a disorder of vocalization characterized by the abnormal production of sounds from the larynx. Dysphonia is usually caused by various abnormalities of the larynx itself or of its innervation. The principal complaint of dysphonia is hoarseness, ranging from mild roughness of the voice to inability to produce sound. **Dysphasia** denotes the inability to use and understand written and spoken words as a result of disorders involving cortical centers of speech or their interconnections in the dominant cerebral hemisphere. With all of these conditions, the peripheral mechanisms for speech remain intact.

16. Does the patient have any allergies, or is the patient receiving any medication? Allergies may affect the eyes and nose, as may medications. Medications themselves may mask some symptoms.

17. Is the patient having any problems with the eyes? Monocular **diplopia** (blurred vision when looking with one eye) may be due to hyphema, detached lens, or other trauma to the globe of the eye. Binocular diplopia (blurred vision when looking through both eyes) occurs in 10 to 40% of patients with a zygoma fracture. It may be caused by soft-tissue entrapment, neuromuscular injury (intraorbital or intramuscular), hemorrhage, or edema. It disappears when one eye is closed. Double vision, which occurs when the good eye is closed, indicates that some structure of the eye is injured. If it occurs with

both eyes open, there is something affecting the free movement of the eyes (Tables 2–9 and 2–10).

18. Does the patient wear glasses or contact lenses? If the patient wears glasses, are the lenses treated (hardened) or made of polycarbonate? If they are hardened, how long ago were they treated? If contact lenses were worn, are they hard, soft, or extended wear? Were eye protectors worn? If so, what type were they? Is there watering of the eyes? Is there any pain in the eyes? Small perforating injuries may be painless. If the patient complains of flashes of bright light, "a curtain falling in front of the eye," or floating black specks, these findings may be an indication of retinal detachment. These questions tell the examiner whether the eyewear or eyes need to be examined in greater detail.

19. Is the patient having any problem with hearing? Does the patient complain of an earache? If so, when was the onset and what is the duration of the earache?

Table 2–9
Common Visual Eye Symptoms and Disease States

Visual Symptom	Associated Causes
Loss of vision	Optic neuritis Detached retina Retinal hemorrhage Central retinal vascular occlusion
Spots	No pathological significance*
Flashes	Migraine Retinal detachment Posterior vitreous detachment
Loss of visual field or presence of shadows or curtains	Retinal detachment Retinal hemorrhage
Glare, photophobia	Iritis (inflammation of the iris) Meningitis (inflammation of the meninges)
Distortion of vision	Retinal detachment Macular edema
Difficulty seeing in dim light	Myopia Vitamin A deficiency Retinal degeneration
Colored haloes around lights	Acute narrow angle glaucoma Opacities in lens or cornea
Colored vision changes	Cataracts Drugs (digitalis increases yellow vision)
Double vision	Extraocular muscle paresis or paralysis

* May precede a retinal detachment or be associated with fertility drugs.

From Swartz, M.H.: Textbook of Physical Diagnosis. Philadelphia, W.B. Saunders Co., 1989, p. 132.

Table 2–10
Common Nonvisual Eye Symptoms and Disease States

Nonvisual Symptom	Associated Causes
Itching	Dry eyes Eye fatigue Allergies
Tearing	Emotional states Hypersecretion of tears Blockage of drainage
Dryness	Sjögren's syndrome Decreased secretion as a result of aging
Sandiness, grittiness	Conjunctivitis
Fullness of eyes	Proptosis (bulging of the eyeball) Aging changes in the lids
Twitching	Fibrillation of orbicularis oculi
Eyelid heaviness	Fatigue Lid edema
Dizziness	Refractive error Cerebellar disease
Blinking	Local irritation Facial tic
Lids sticking together	Inflammatory disease of lids or conjunctivae
Foreign body sensation	Foreign body Corneal abrasion
Burning	Uncorrected refractive error Conjunctivitis Sjögren's syndrome
Throbbing, aching	Acute iritis (inflammation of the iris) Sinusitis (inflammation of the sinuses)
Tenderness	Lid inflammations Conjunctivitis Iritis
Headache	Refractive errors Migraine Sinusitis
Drawing sensation	Uncorrected refractive errors

From Swartz, M.H.: Textbook of Physical Diagnosis. Philadelphia, W.B. Saunders Co., 1989, p. 133.

Does the patient complain of pain or a discharge from the ear? Is the earache associated with an upper respiratory tract infection, swimming, or trauma? The patient should also be questioned on the method of cleaning the ear. If there appears to be a hearing loss, the patient should be asked whether the hearing loss came on quickly or slowly, whether the patient hears best on the telephone (amplified sound) or in a quiet or noisy environment, and whether speech is heard soft or loud. Does the patient use a hearing aid?

20. Is the patient having any problems with the nose? Has the patient used nose drops or spray? If so, how much? How often? How long have these medica-tions been used? Does the patient have any nasal dis-charge, and if so, what is its character—watery, mucoid, purulent, crusty, or bloody? Does the discharge have any odor (indicative of infection), and is it unilateral or bilateral? Does the patient exhibit any associated nasal symptoms such as sneezing, nasal congestion, itching, or mouth breathing? Does the patient complain of a nosebleed, and has the patient had many nosebleeds? If so, how frequent are the nosebleeds, what is the amount of the bleeding, and what appears to be causing the bleeding? Positive responses to any of these ques-tions indicate that the nose must be examined in greater detail.

21. If the examiner is concerned about the mouth and teeth or the temporomandibular joints, questions related to these areas can be found in the chapter on temporomandibular joints (see Chapter 4). It is impor-tant, however, to ensure that the patient's dental occlu-sion and biting alignment have not been altered. Are all the teeth present, and are they symmetrical? Is there any swelling or bleeding around the teeth? Are the teeth mobile or is part of a tooth missing? Is the pulp exposed? Each of these questions helps determine whether the teeth have been injured. Teeth that have been avulsed, if intact, should be reimplanted as quickly as possible. If reimplanted after cleansing (rinsed in saline solution or water) within less than 30 minutes, the tooth has a 90% chance of being retained. If it is not possible to reimplant the tooth, it should be kept moist in saline, or the patient should keep it between the gum and cheek while dental care is sought.

22. Questions concerning the neck and cervical spine can be found in Chapter 3.

Observation

For proper observation[4-7] of the head and face, any hat, helmet, mouth guard, or face guard should be removed. If a neck injury is suspected or the patient presents an emergency situation, the examiner may take the time to remove only those items that are interfering with immediate emergency care. If a neck injury is suspected, extreme caution should be observed when removing the item. When assessing the head and face, the examiner must also observe and assess the posture of the cervical spine and the temporomandibular joints; see Chapters 3 and 4 for detailed descriptions of observation of these areas.

When observing the head and face, it is essential that the examiner look at the face to note the position and shape of the eyes, nose, mouth, teeth, and ears and look for deformity, asymmetry, facial imbalance, swell-ing, lacerations, foreign bodies, or bleeding during rest,

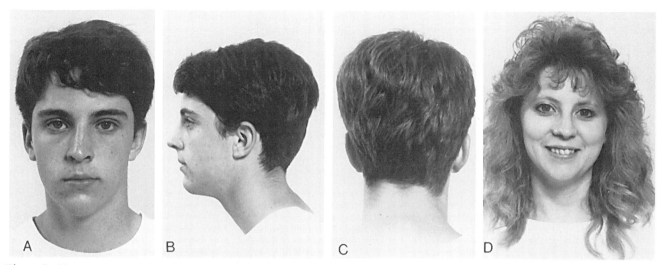

Figure 2-11
Views of the head and face. (A) Anterior. (B) Side. (C) Posterior. (D) Altered facial features with smile.

with movement, or with different facial expressions. One should also note, as much as possible, the individual's normal facial expression. The facial expression of the patient often reflects the patient's general feeling and well-being. A dazed or vacant look often indicates problems. While talking to the patient, the examiner should watch for any asymmetry of facial motion or change in facial expression when the patient answers; some slight facial asymmetry is common. In addition, small degrees or paralysis may not be obvious unless exaggerated expression is attempted. If some facial paralysis is suspected, the patient should be asked to make exaggerated facial expressions that will demonstrate the paralysis. If facial asymmetry is present, one should note whether all of the features on one side of the face are affected or only a portion of the face is affected. For example, with facial nerve (cranial nerve VII) paralysis, the entire side of the face is affected, although the most noticeable

differences will occur around the eye and one side of the mouth. If only one side of the mouth is involved, then a problem with the trigeminal nerve (cranial nerve V) should be suspected. Any changes in the shape of the face or unusual features such as masses, edema, puffiness, coarseness, prominent eyes, amount of facial hair, excessive perspiration, or skin color should be noted. Eye puffiness is often one of the earliest signs of edema in the face. Skin color may include cyanosis, pallor, jaundice, or pigmentation, and each may be indicative of different systemic problems.

The examiner should view the patient from the front, side, behind, and above, noting the area behind the ears, at the hairline, and around the crown of the head as well as on the face (Fig. 2–11). If one suspects a skull (cranial vault) injury, one should look behind the ears, at the hairline, and around the crown of the head for any deformity, bruising, or laceration.

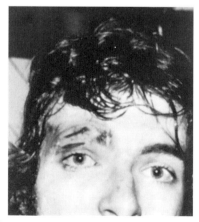

Figure 2-12
Lacerations to the upper eyelid and eyebrow.

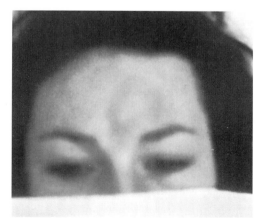

Figure 2-13
Contusion to the forehead caused by a racquetball ball.

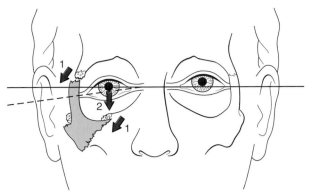

Figure 2-14

Inferior displacement of the zygoma (1) results in depression of the lateral canthus and pupil (2) because of depression of the suspensory ligaments that attach to the lateral orbital (Whitnall's) tubercle. (Modified from Ellis, E.: Fractures of the zygomatic complex and arch. *In* Fonseca, R.J., and R.V. Walker [eds.]: Oral and Maxillofacial Trauma. Philadelphia, W.B. Saunders Co., 1991, p. 446.)

Viewing from the front, the examiner should observe the patient's hairline, noting any abnormalities. The soft tissues such as the eyelids, eyebrows, cheeks, lips, nose, and chin should be inspected for lacerations, bruising, or hematoma (Figs. 2–12 and 2–13). The eyes should be level. For example, a zygoma fracture causes the eye on the affected side to drop (Fig. 2–14). The two eyes should be compared for prominence or retraction (Fig. 2–15).

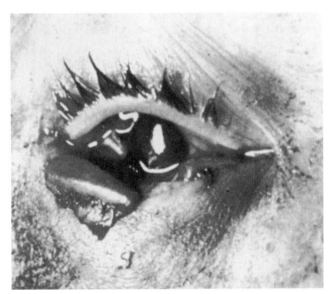

Figure 2-15

A severe glancing or direct blow to this right eye has resulted in a ruptured globe. Note the depressed eye. (From Pashby, T.J., and R.C. Pashby: Treatment of sports eye injuries. *In* Schneider, R.C., J.C. Kennedy, and M.L. Plant [eds.]: Sports Injuries—Mechanisms, Prevention and Treatment. Baltimore, Williams & Wilkins, 1985, p. 589.)

If there appears to be any bulging, especially unilaterally, the examiner should tilt the patient's head forward or back and, looking from above, compare each cornea with the lid below, noting whether one or both corneas bulge beyond the lid margins. If one or both eyes appear to bulge, the examiner can roughly measure the distance from the angle of the eye to the corneal apex with a pocket ruler.

Immediate referral for further examination by a specialist is required for an embedded corneal foreign body; haze or blood in the anterior chamber (hyphema); decreased or partial vision; irregular, asymmetric, or poor pupil action; diplopia or double vision; laceration of the eyelid or impaired lid function; perforation or laceration of the globe; broken contact lens or shattered eyeglass in the eye; unexplained eye pain that is stabbing or deep and throbbing; blurred vision that does not clear with blinking; loss of all or part of the visual field; protrusion

---

Eye Signs and Symptoms Requiring Specialist Care

- Foreign body that is not easily removed
- Eye does not move properly
- Altered pupil action
- Abnormal pupil size or shape
- Double vision
- Blurred vision
- Decreased or partial vision
- Loss of part or all of visual field
- Laceration of eye or eyelid
- Blood between cornea and iris (hyphema)
- Impaired eyelid function
- Penetration of eye or eyelid
- Eye pain
- Sharp or throbbing eye pain
- Protrusion or retraction of eye

---

of one eye relative to the other; an injured eye that does not move as fully as the uninjured eye; or abnormal pupil size or shape. A teardrop pupil usually indicates iris entrapment in a corneal or scleral laceration. In addition, the eyes should be observed from the lateral aspect. The normal distance from the cornea to the angle of the eye is 16 mm or less. The distances between the upper and lower lids should be the same for both eyes. When the eyes open, the superior eyelid should cover a portion of the iris but not the pupil itself. If it covers more of the iris than the other upper eyelid does, or if it extends over the iris or pupil, ptosis or drooping of that eyelid should be suspected. If the eyelid does not cover part of the iris, retraction of the eyelid should be suspected. Are the eyelids everted or inverted? Normally, they are

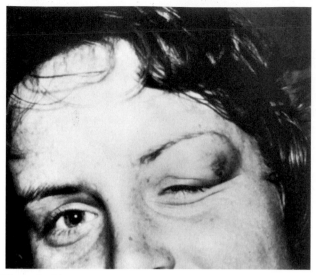

Figure 2–16
Black eye (periorbital ecchymosis).

to bring the eyelashes together. Any inflammation or masses, especially on the lid margin, should be noted. If present, a "black eye," or periorbital contusion, should also be noted (Fig. 2–16). The lashes should be viewed to see if there is even distribution along the lid margins. "Raccoon eyes," which are purple discolorations of the eyelids and orbital regions, may indicate orbital fractures, basilar skull fractures, or a fracture of the base of the anterior cranial fossa.[4] This sign takes several hours to develop.

The conjunctiva should be inspected for hemorrhage, laceration, and foreign bodies.[8] If the patient complains of "something in the eye," eversion of the upper eyelid usually reveals a foreign body that can often be easily brushed away. Displaced contact lenses are often found in this upper area of the eye. The conjunctival covering of the lower lid may be examined by having the patient look upward while the examiner draws the lower lid downward. The conjunctiva should be examined as being a continuous sheet of epithelium from the globe to the lids. The color of the sclera should also be noted. Posttraumatic conjunctival hemorrhage (Fig. 2–17) and possible scleral lacerations (Fig. 2–18) should be noted, if present. In dark-skinned patients, pigmented areas may show up as small dark spots or patches near the limbus. The shape and color of the cornea should be

neither. The examiner should also note whether the patient can close both eyes completely. If an eye injury is suspected, this action should be done very carefully, because closing the eyes can increase intraocular pressure. The lids should be pressed together only enough

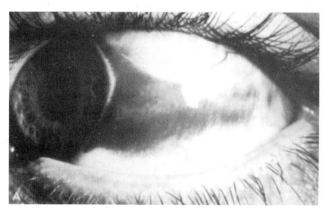

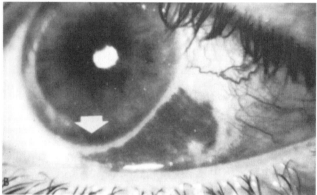

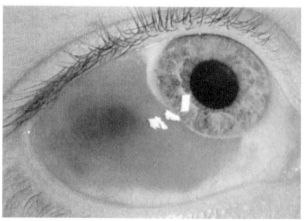

C

Figure 2–17
(A) Posttraumatic conjunctival hemorrhage without other ocular or orbital damage. (B) Posttraumatic conjunctival hemorrhage from blunt injury, with a small hyphema (*arrow*). In this case, the injury was significant because of the presence of blood in the anterior chamber. (From Paton, D., and M.F. Goldberg: Management of Ocular Injuries. Philadelphia, W.B. Saunders Co., 1976, p. 182.) (C) Subconjunctival ecchymosis with no lateral limit should suggest osseous orbital fractures. (From Lew, D., and D.P. Sinn: Diagnosis and treatment of midface fractures. In Fonseca, R.J., and R.V. Walker [eds.]: Oral and Maxillofacial Trauma. Philadelphia, W.B. Saunders Co., 1991, p. 250.)

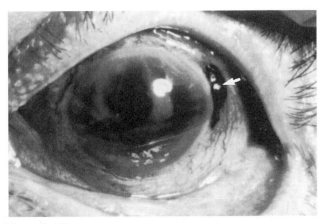

Figure 2–18

Scleral rupture (*arrow*) at the limbus after blunt trauma. The iris and ciliary body have prolapsed into the subconjunctival space. (From Paton, D., and M.F. Goldberg: Management of Ocular Injuries. Philadelphia, W.B. Saunders Co., 1976, p. 310.)

inspected. The anterior chambers of the eye should be inspected and compared for clarity and depth.[8] If present, hyphema in the form of haze or actual blood pooling (Fig. 2–19) in the anterior eye chamber should be noted. If there is any potential for or evidence of bleeding in the anterior chamber of the eye, the patient's activity should be curtailed, because increased activity increases the chances of secondary hemorrhage during the first week after injury. Examination of the cornea with a pen light shone obliquely on the eye should be carried out to look for foreign bodies, abrasions, or lacerations. Corneal injuries can lead to lacrimation (tearing), photophobia (intolerance to light), or blepharospasm (spasm of the

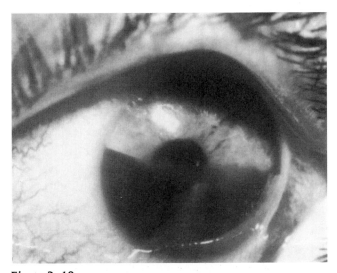

Figure 2–19

Hyphema in the anterior chamber of the eye. (From Easterbrook, M., and J. Cameron: Injuries in racquet sports. *In* Schneider, R.C., J.C. Kennedy, and M.L. Plant [eds.]: Sports Injuries—Mechanisms, Prevention and Treatment. Baltimore, Williams & Wilkins, 1985, p. 556.)

eyelid orbicular muscle) as well as extreme pain from exposure of sensory nerve endings. Abrasions are readily outlined by a fluorescein strip dipped into tears that have been exposed as the lower lid is pulled downward.

The pupillary size (diameter range, 2 to 6 mm; mean, 3.5 mm), shape (round), and symmetry should be compared with those of the other eye. Elliptical pupils often indicate a corneal laceration. The color of the irises of the eyes should be compared. When looking at the pupils, the examiner should note whether the pupils are equal. Are the pupils smaller or larger than normal? Are they round or irregularly shaped? The pupils are normally slightly unequal in 5% of the population, but inequality of pupil size should initially be viewed with suspicion. Pupils tend to be smaller in infants, the elderly, and persons with hyperopia (farsightedness), whereas they tend to be slightly dilated in persons with myopia (nearsightedness) or light-colored irises.

The nose should be inspected for any deviations in shape, size, or color. The skin should be smooth without swelling and should conform to the color of the face. The airways are usually oval and symmetrically proportioned. If a discharge is present, its character (i.e., color, smell, texture) should be noted and described. Bloody discharge occurs as a result of epistaxis or trauma such as a nasal fracture, zygoma fracture, or skull fracture. Mucoid discharge is typical of rhinitis. Bilateral purulent discharge can occur with upper respiratory tract infection. Unilateral purulent, thick, greenish, and often malodorous discharge usually indicates the presence of a foreign body.

Depression of the nasal bridge can result from a fracture of the nasal bone. Nasal flaring is associated with respiratory distress, whereas narrowing of the airways on inspiration may be indicative of chronic nasal obstruction and be associated with mouth breathing. The nasal mucosa should be deep pink and glistening. A film of clear discharge is often apparent on the nasal septum. The nasal septum should be close to midline and fairly straight, appearing thicker anteriorly than posteriorly. If present, a hematoma in the septal area should be noted. Asymmetric posterior nasal cavities may indicate a deviation of the nasal septum.

With the patient's mouth closed, the lips should be observed for symmetry, color, edema, and surface abnormalities. Lipstick should be removed before the assessment. The lips should be pink and have vertical and horizontal symmetry, both at rest and with movement. Dry, cracked lips may be caused by dehydration from wind or low humidity, whereas deep fissures at the corners of the mouth may indicate overclosure of the mouth or riboflavin deficiency.

Drooping of the mouth on one side, sagging of the lower eyelid, and flattening of the nasolabial fold suggest possible facial nerve (cranial nerve VII) involvement. The patient is also unable to pucker the lips to whistle.

The shape and position of the jaw and teeth should also be noted anteriorly and from the side. Asymmetry may indicate a fracture of the jaw (Fig. 2–20), whereas bleeding around the gums of the teeth may indicate fracture, avulsion, or loosening of the teeth (Fig. 2–21). If there are missing teeth, they must be accounted for. If they are not accounted for, an x-ray may be required to ensure that the teeth have not entered the abdominal or chest cavity. If pain occurs on percussion of the teeth, it often indicates damage to the periodontal ligament.

From the side, the examiner should look for any asymmetry or depression, which may indicate pathology. The examiner should inspect the auricles of the ears for size, shape, symmetry, landmarks, color, and position on the head. To determine the position of the auricle, the examiner can draw an imaginary line between the outer canthus of the eye and occipital protuberance (Fig. 2–22). The top of the auricle should touch or be above this line.[4] The examiner can then draw another imaginary line perpendicular to the previous line and just anterior to the auricle. The auricle's position should be almost vertical. If the angle is more than 10° posterior or anterior, it is considered abnormal. An auricle that is set low or is at an unusual angle may indicate chromosomal aberrations or renal disorders. In addition, the lateral and medial surfaces and surrounding tissues should be examined, noting any deformities, lesions, or nodules. The auricles should be the same color as the facial skin without moles, cysts, or other lesions or deformities.

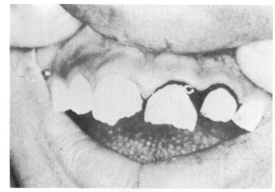

A

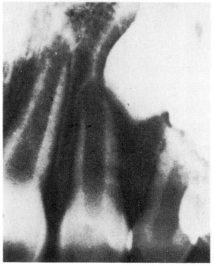

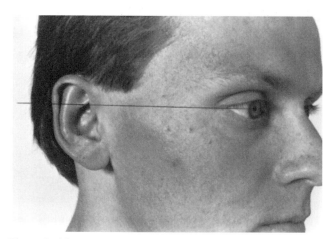

B

Figure 2–21

A 9-year-old boy was hit in the mouth with a ball while he was playing baseball. The right maxillary central and lateral incisors were chipped. (A) Avulsed teeth reimplanted with finger pressure. (B) Radiograph of root canal with wide-open apex. Reimplanted quickly, these teeth may not require root canal treatment. (From Torg, J.S.: Athletic Injuries to the Head, Neck and Face. Philadelphia, Lea & Febiger, 1982, p. 247.)

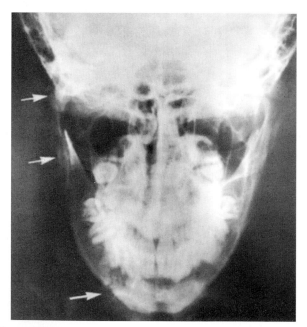

Figure 2–20

Fracture of the neck of the condyle on the right (*upper arrows*) with fracture through the mandible on the same side (*lower arrow*). When one fracture is shown in the mandible, search carefully for the second. (From O'Donoghue, D.H.: Treatment of Injuries to Athletes. Philadelphia, W.B. Saunders Co., 1984, p. 115.)

Figure 2–22

Auricle alignment. Normal position shown.

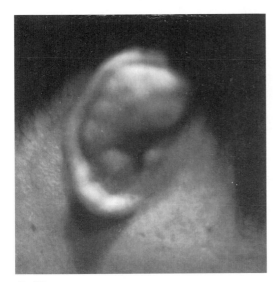

Figure 2–23
Hematoma auris seen in a wrestler.

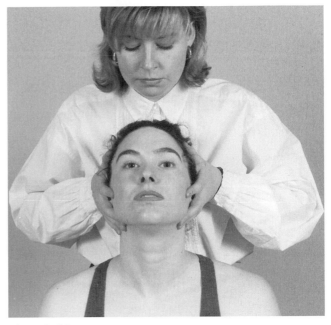

Figure 2–25
View of the patient from above to look for bilateral symmetry of the face.

Athletes, especially wrestlers, may exhibit a cauliflower ear (hematoma auris), which is a keloid scar forming in the auricle due to friction to or twisting of the ear (Fig. 2–23). Blueness may indicate some degree of cyanosis. Pallor or excessive redness may be the result of vasomotor instability or increased temperature. Frostbite can cause extreme pallor or blistering (Fig. 2–24).

The examiner should look posteriorly for any asymmetry or depression. The positions of the ears (height, protrusion) can be compared by observing from behind. A low hairline may indicate conditions such as Klippel-Feil syndrome. The examiner should also look for the presence of **Battle's sign**. This sign, which takes as long

as 24 hours to appear, is demonstrated by purple and blue discoloration of the skin in the mastoid area and may indicate a temporal bone or basilar skull fracture.

The examiner then views the patient from overhead (superior view) to note any asymmetry from above (Fig. 2–25). This method is especially useful when looking for a possible fracture of the zygoma (Fig. 2–26). The deformity is easier to detect if the examiner carefully places the index fingers below the infraorbital margins along the zygomatic bodies and then gently pushes into the edema to reduce the effect of the edema (Fig. 2–27).

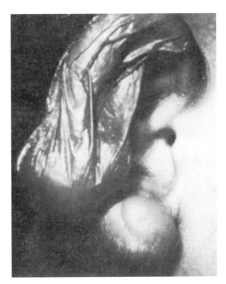

Figure 2–24
Auricular frostbite with development of massive vesicles that are beginning to resolve spontaneously. (From Schuller, D.E., and R.A. Bruce: Ear, nose, throat and eye. In Strauss, R.H. [ed.]: Sports Medicine, 2nd ed. Philadelphia, W.B. Saunders Co., 1991, p. 191.)

Signs and Symptoms of Maxillary and Zygomatic Fractures

- Facial asymmetry
- Loss of cheek prominence
- Palpable steps
  - Infraorbital rim (zygomaticomaxillary suture)
  - Lateral orbital rim (frontozygomatic suture)
  - Root of zygoma intraorally
  - Zygomatic arch between ear and eye (zygomaticotemporal suture)
- Hypoesthesia/anesthesia
  - Cheek, side of nose, upper lip, and teeth on the injured side
  - Compression of infraorbital nerve as it courses along floor of the orbit to exit into the face via the foramen beneath the orbital rim

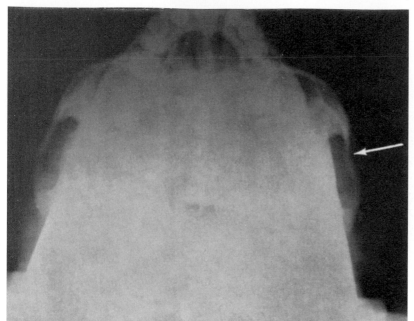

Figure 2–26

Typical fracture of zygomatic arch on the right (*arrow*). Note normal arch on the left. (From O'Donoghue, D.H.: Treatment of Injuries to Athletes. Philadelphia, W.B. Saunders Co., 1984, p. 114.)

Figure 2–27

Method of assessing posterior displacement of the zygomatic complex from behind the patient. The examiner should firmly but carefully depress the fingers into the edematous soft tissues while palpating along the infraorbital areas. (Modified from Ellis, E.: Fractures of the zygomatic complex and arch. *In* Fonseca, R.J., and R.V. Walker [eds.]: Oral and Maxillofacial Trauma. Philadelphia, W.B. Saunders Co., 1991, p. 443.)

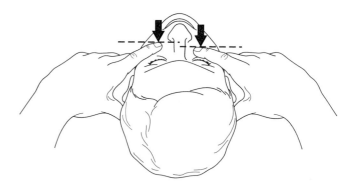

Table 2–11
Neural Watch Chart

Unit		Time 1 ( )	Time 2 ( )	Time 3 ( )	Unit		Time 1 ( )	Time 2 ( )	Time 3 ( )
I Vital signs	Blood pressure Pulse Respiration Temperature				VI Pupils	Size on right Size on left Reacts on right Reacts on left			
II Conscious and	Oriented Disoriented Restless Combative				VII Ability to move	Right arm Left arm Right leg Left leg			
III Speech	Clear Rambling Garbled None				VIII Sensation	Right side (normal/abnormal) Left side (normal/abnormal) Dermatome affected (specify) Peripheral nerve affected (specify)			
IV Will awaken to	Name Shaking Light pain Strong pain								
V Nonverbal reaction to pain	Appropriate Inappropriate "Decerebrate" None								

Modified from American Academy of Orthopedic Surgeons: Athletic Training and Sports Medicine. Park Ridge, IL, AAOS, 1984, p. 399.

Examination

The examination of the head and face differs from the orthopedic assessment of other areas of the body because the assessment does not involve articular joints. The only articular joints that could be included in the assessment are the temporomandibular joints, and these joints are discussed in Chapter 4.

Examination of the Head

Many problems in the head and face may be problems referred from the cervical spine, temporomandibular joint, or teeth. However, if one suspects a head injury, it is necessary to keep a close watch on the patient, noting any changes and when these changes occur. A **neural watch** should be implemented by the examiner so that any changes that occur over time can be determined easily (Table 2–11). The testing should occur at 15- or 30-minute intervals, depending on the severity of the injury and the changes recorded.

As the examination for a head injury is performed, the examiner should attempt to determine the degree of head injury, for example, the level of concussion suffered (see Table 2–4). This determination of degree of injury

---

Head Examination

- Concussion
- Headache
- Memory tests
- Neural watch (Glasgow Coma Scale)
- Expanding intracranial lesion
- Proprioception
- Coordination
- Head injury card

---

is important because it has an effect on when the patient will be allowed to return to activity (Table 2–12).[10, 11] The examiner should always be looking for the possibility of an expanding intracranial lesion resulting from a leaking or torn blood vessel. Normally, the brain has a fixed volume that is enclosed in a nonexpansile structure, namely, the skull and dura mater. These lesions may be caused by epidural hemorrhage (usually tearing of one of the meningeal arteries as a result of high-speed impact), subarachnoid hemorrhage (usually as a result of an aneurysm), or subdural hemorrhage (usually as a result of tearing of bridging veins between the brain and cavernous sinus). These injuries are emergency conditions that must be looked after immediately because of their high

---

Table 2–12
Timetable for Return to Competition After Concussion

Concussion Severity	First Concussion	Second Concussion	Third Concussion
1°	Return to activity after 10–30 minutes if asymptomatic*	Return in 1 week if asymptomatic	Return in 1 week if asymptomatic Must be cleared by specialist
2° (Posttraumatic [anterograde] amnesia)	Return to activity in 1 week if asymptomatic Must be cleared by specialist if some posttraumatic amnesia remains for ≤1 hour	Return in 2 weeks if asymptomatic after 1 week Must be cleared by specialist	No contact, collision, or high-risk activity for 3–6 months Must be cleared by specialist
3° (Retrograde amnesia)	Return to activity in 1 week if asymptomatic Must be cleared by specialist if some posttraumatic or retrograde amnesia remains for ≤1 hour	Return in 1 month if asymptomatic for final week Must be cleared by specialist	No contact, collision, or high-risk activity for 3–6 months Must be cleared by specialist
4° (Unconscious <5 min)	Return to activity in 1 month if asymptomatic for final week Must be cleared by specialist	No contact, collision, or high-risk activity for 3–6 months Must be cleared by specialist	No contact, collision, or high-risk activity for 3–6 months Must be cleared by specialist
5° (Unconscious >5 min)	Return to activity in 1–2 months if asymptomatic for final week Must be cleared by specialist	No contact, collision, or high-risk activity for 3–6 months Must be cleared by specialist	No contact, collision, or high-risk activity for 6–12 months Must be cleared by specialist

* Symptoms may include headache, dizziness, tinnitus, amnesia, disorientation, unsteadiness, blurred vision.

Data from Cantu, R.C.: Guidelines for return to contact sports after cerebral concussion. Phys. Sportsmed. 14:75–83, 1986; and Robert, W.O.: Who plays? Who sits? Managing concussions on the sidelines. Phys. Sportsmed. 20:66–72, 1992.

mortality rate (as much as 50%). An **expanding intracranial lesion** is indicated by an altered lucid state (state of consciousness), development of inequality of the pupils, unusual slowing of the heart rate that primarily occurs after a lucid interval, irregular eye movements, and eyes that no longer track properly. There is also a tendency for the patient to demonstrate increased body temperature and irregular respirations. Normal intracranial pressure measures from 4 to 15 mm Hg, and an intracranial pressure of more than 20 mm Hg is considered abnormal. Intracranial pressure of 40 mm Hg causes neurological dysfunction and impairment. Although in the emergency care setting there is no way of determining the intracra-

nial pressure, the signs and symptoms mentioned indicate that the pressure is increasing. Most patients who experience an increase in intracranial pressure complain of severe headache, and this symptom is often followed by vomiting (sometimes projectile vomiting). Finally, an expanding intracranial lesion causes increased weakness on one side of the body, the side opposite that on which the lesion has occurred.

Signs and symptoms that indicate a good possibility of recovery from a head injury, especially after the patient experiences unconsciousness, include response to noxious stimuli, eye opening, pupil activity, spontaneous eye movement, intact oculovestibular reflexes, and appropriate motor function responses. Neurological signs that indicate a poor prognosis after a head injury include nonreactive pupils, absence of oculovestibular reflexes, severe extension patterns or no motor function response at all, and increased intracranial pressure.[3]

It is important when examining the unconscious or conscious patient for a possible head injury to determine the level of consciousness of the individual, which may be done with the **Glasgow Coma Scale** (Table 2–13). The first test relates to eye opening. Eye opening may occur spontaneously, in response to speech, or in response to pain, or there may be no response at all. Each of these responses is given a numerical value: spontaneous eye opening, 4; response to speech, 3; response to pain, 2; and no response, 1. Spontaneous opening of the eyes indicates functioning of the ascending reticular activating system. This finding does not necessarily mean that the patient is aware of the surroundings or of what is happening, but it does imply that the patient is in a

---

Signs and Symptoms of an Expanding Intracranial Lesion

- Altered state of consciousness
- Nystagmus
- Pupil inequality
- Irregular eye movements
- Abnormal slowing of heart
- Irregular respiration
- Severe headache
- Intractable vomiting
- Positive expanding intracranial lesion tests (lateralizing)
- Positive coordination tests
- Decreasing muscle strength
- Seizure

Table 2–13
Glasgow Coma Scale

				Time 1 ( )	Time 2 ( )
Eyes	Open	Spontaneously	4		
		To verbal command	3		
		To pain	2		
		No response	1	_____	_____
Best motor response	To verbal command	Obeys	6		
	To painful stimulus*	Localizes pain	5		
		Flexion—withdrawal	4		
		Flexion—abnormal (decorticate rigidity)	3		
		Extension (decerebrate rigidity)	2		
		No response	1	_____	_____
Best verbal response†		Oriented and converses	5		
		Disoriented and converses	4		
		Inappropriate words	3		
		Incomprehensible sounds	2		
		No response	1	_____	_____
Total			3–15		

* Apply knuckles to sternum; observe arms.

† Arouse patient with painful stimulus if necessary.

state of arousal. A patient who opens his or her eyes in response to the examiner's voice is probably responding to the stimulus of sound, not necessarily to the command to open the eyes. If unsure, the examiner may try different sound-making objects (e.g., bell, horn) to elicit an appropriate response.

The second test involves motor response; the patient is given a grade of 6 if there is a response to a verbal command. Otherwise, the patient is graded on a five-point scale depending on the motor response to a painful stimulus (see Table 2–13). When scoring motor responses, it is the ease with which the motor responses are elicited that constitutes the criterion for the best response. Commands given to the patient should be simple, such as, "Move your arm." The patient should not be asked to squeeze the examiner's hand, nor should the examiner place something in the patient's hand and then ask the patient to grasp it. This action may cause a reflex grasp, not a response to a command.[3]

If the patient does not give a motor response to a verbal command, then the examiner should attempt to elicit a motor response to a painful stimulus. It is the type and quality of the patient's reaction to the painful stimulus that constitute the scoring criteria. The stimulus should not be applied to the face, because painful stimulus in the facial area may cause the eyes to close tightly as a protective reaction. The painful stimulus may consist of applying a knuckle to the sternum, squeezing the trapezius muscle, or squeezing the soft tissue between the thumb and index finger (Fig. 2–28). If the patient moves a limb when the painful stimulus is applied to more than one point or tries to remove the examiner's hand that is applying the painful stimulus, the patient is localizing, and a value of 5 is given. If the patient withdraws from the painful stimulus rapidly, a normal reflex withdrawal is being shown, and a value of 4 is given.

However, if application of a painful stimulus creates a decorticate or decerebrate posture (Fig. 2–29), an abnormal response is being demonstrated, and a value of 3 is given for the decorticate posture (injury above red nucleus) or a value of 2 is given for decerebrate posture (brain stem injury). **Decorticate posturing** results from lesions of the diencephalon area, whereas decerebrate posturing results from lesions of the midbrain. With decorticate posturing, the arms, wrists, and fingers are flexed, the upper limbs are adducted, and the legs are extended, medially rotated, and plantar flexed. **Decerebrate posturing,** which has a poorer prognosis, involves extension, adduction, and hyperpronation of the arms, whereas the lower limbs are the same as for decerebrate posturing.[12] Decerebrate rigidity is usually bilateral. If the patient exhibits no reaction to the painful stimulus, a value of 1 is given. It is important to be sure the "no" response is caused by a head injury and not a spinal cord injury leading to lack of feeling or sensation. Any

difference in reaction between limbs should be carefully noted; this finding may be indicative of a specific focal injury.[3]

In the third test, verbal response is graded on a five-point scale to measure the patient's speech in response to simple questions such as "Where are you?" or "Are you winning the game?" For verbal responses, the patient who converses appropriately shows proper orientation, being aware of oneself and the environment and is given a grade of 5. The patient who is confused is disoriented and unable to completely interact with the environment; this patient is able to converse using the appropriate words and is given a grade of 4. The patient exhibiting inappropriate speech is unable to sustain a conversation with the examiner; this person would be given a grade of 3. A vocalizing patient only groans or makes incomprehensible sounds; this finding leads to a grade of 2. Again, the examiner should make note of any possible mechanical reason for the inability to verbalize. If the patient makes no sounds and thus has no verbal response, a grade of 1 is assigned.

It is vital that the initial score on the Glasgow Coma Scale be obtained at the scene, as soon as possible after the onset of the injury. The scale can then be repeated at 15- or 30-minute intervals, especially in the early stages, if changes are noted. If the score is between 3 and 8, emergency care is required. With the Glasgow Coma Scale, the initial score is used as a basis for determining the severity of the patient's head injury. Patients who maintain a score of 8 or less on the Glasgow Coma Scale for 6 hours or longer are considered to have a serious head injury. A patient who scores between 9 and 11 is considered to be moderately head injured, and one who scores 12 or higher is considered to have a mild head injury.[3]

Head Injury Severity Based on Score Maintained on Glasgow Coma Scale (6 Hr+)

8 or less:	Severe head injury
9–11:	Moderate head injury
12+:	Mild head injury

The Rancho Los Amigos Scale of Cognitive Function may also be used to assess the patient's cognitive abilities. This scale is an eight-level progression from level I, in which the patient is nonresponsive, to level VIII, in which the patient's behavior is purposeful and appropriate (Table 2–14). The Rancho Los Amigos scale provides an assessment of cognitive function and behavior only, not of physical functioning.[3]

If a person receives a head injury such as a mild concussion and is not referred to the hospital, the examiner should ensure that someone accompanies the per-

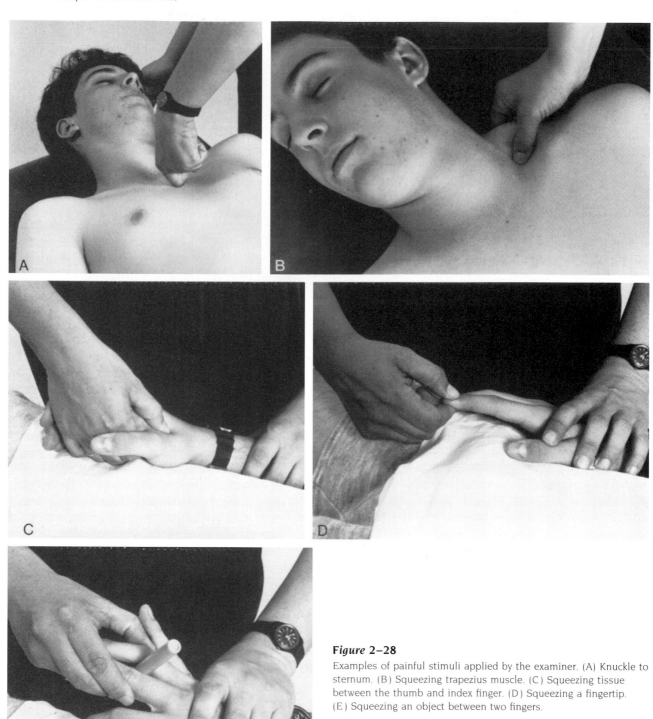

Figure 2–28
Examples of painful stimuli applied by the examiner. (A) Knuckle to sternum. (B) Squeezing trapezius muscle. (C) Squeezing tissue between the thumb and index finger. (D) Squeezing a fingertip. (E) Squeezing an object between two fingers.

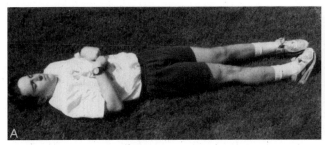 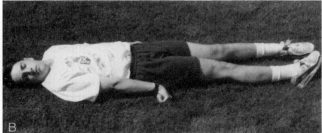

Figure 2–29
(A) Decorticate rigidity. (B) Decerebrate rigidity.

son home and that someone at home knows what has happened so he or she can monitor the patient in case the patient's condition worsens. Appropriate written instructions should be sent home concerning the individual. The **Head Injury Card** is such an example.

Levin and colleagues[13] reported the use of the Galveston Orientation and Amnesia Test (GOAT), which they believe measures orientation to person, place, and time and the memory of events preceding and following head trauma (Fig. 2–30). As the patient improves, the total GOAT score should increase.

The examiner may also wish to determine whether the patient has suffered an upper motor neuron lesion. Testing the deep tendon reflexes (see Table 1–21) or the pathological reflexes (see Table 1–23) or having the patient perform various balance and coordination tests may help to determine whether this type of lesion has occurred. However, the pathological reflexes may not be elicited owing to shock. Deep tendon reflexes are accentuated on the side of the body opposite that on which the brain injury has occurred. Balance can play an important role in the assessment of a head-injured patient. Balance involves the integration of several inputs (e.g., visual, proprioceptive, and vestibular systems), which are analyzed by the brain to allow a proper action. For example, in standing, the body is inherently unstable, and only the integration of input from various sources enables the patient to stand and to make appro-

Table 2–14
Rancho Los Amigos Scale of Cognitive Function

Level I	No response
Level II	Generalized response
Level III	Localized response
Level IV	Confused, agitated
Level V	Confused, inappropriate
Level VI	Confused, appropriate
Level VII	Automatic, appropriate
Level VIII	Purposeful, appropriate

From Hagen, C., D. Malkmus, and P. Durham: Levels of cognitive functioning. *In* Rehabilitation of the Brain Injured Adult—Comprehensive Management. Professional Staff Association of Rancho Los Amigos, Downey, California, 1980.

Head Injury Card
Please Read Carefully
(*Give one to an accompanying
person and one to the player*)

NAME _____ AGE _____

SUSTAINED A HEAD INJURY AT _____
                                                    (time)

ON _____
          (date)

Important Warning:
(S)He is to be taken to a hospital or a doctor immediately if (s)he:

• VOMITS
• DEVELOPS A HEADACHE
• BECOMES RESTLESS OR IRRITABLE
• BECOMES DIZZY OR DROWSY OR CANNOT BE ROUSED
• HAS A FIT (CONVULSION)
• EXPERIENCES ANYTHING ELSE UNUSUAL

For the **rest of today** (s)he should:

• REST QUIETLY
• NOT CONSUME ALCOHOL
• NOT DRIVE A VEHICLE

AND

(S)He should not train or play again without medical clearance by a doctor.

_____ PHONE _____
     (Doctor)

DATE _____

Queensland Health Department ● Division of Health Promotion

Galveston Orientation and Amnesia Test (GOAT)

Name _____ Date of test _____

Age _____   Sex   M   F   Day of the week   S   M   T   W   Th   F   S

Date of birth _____   Time   AM   PM

Diagnosis _____ Date of injury _____

	Error points

1. What is your name? (2) _____ When were you born? (4) _____ _____

   Where do you live? (4) _____

2. Where are you now? (city) (5) _____ Location (e.g., hospital) (5) _____ _____
   (unnecessary to state name of hospital)

3. On what date were you admitted to this hospital? (5) _____ _____

   How did you get here? (5) _____

4. What is the first event you can remember *after* the injury? (5) _____ _____
   Can you describe in detail (e.g., date, time, companions) the first event you can recall after injury?

   (5) _____

5. Can you describe the last event you recall *before* the accident? (5) _____ _____
   Can you describe in detail (e.g., date, time, companions) the first event you can recall before injury?

   (5) _____

6. What time is it now? _____ (1 for each 1/2 hour removed from correct time, to maximum of 5) _____

7. What day of the week is it? _____ (1 for each day removed from correct one) _____

8. What day of the month is it? _____ (1 for each day removed from correct date, to maximum _____
   of 5)

9. What is the month? _____ (5 for each month removed from correct one, to maximum of 5) _____

10. What is the year? _____ (10 for each year removed from correct one, to maximum of 30) _____

Total error points _____

Total GOAT score (100 minus total error points) _____

Figure 2–30
Galveston Orientation and Amnesia Test. Examiner adds up only error points, not positive responses.
For example, if patient remembers first name but not last name, he or she would get 1 error point.
(Modified from Levin, H.S., V.M. O'Donnell, and R.G. Grossman: The Galveston orientation and
amnesia test: A practical scale to assess cognition after head injury. J. Nerve Ment. Dis. 167:677, 1979.)

priate corrections to maintain proper standing posture. Balance and coordination can be tested in several ways. The patient can be asked to stand and walk a straight line with the eyes open and then with the eyes closed. The examiner should note any difference. The patient can be asked to bring the finger to the nose or the heel of the foot to the opposite knee with the eyes closed (Fig. 2–31). These tests, and others described under "Special Tests," assess balance and coordination.

Muscle tone and strength may also play a role in

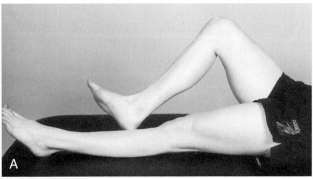

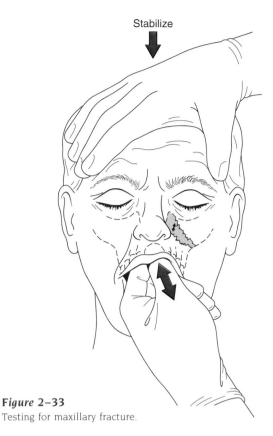

Figure 2–31
Performing coordination exercises. (A) Touching knee with opposite heel. (B) Touching nose with index finger with eyes closed.

Figure 2–33
Testing for maxillary fracture.

assessing the patient for head injury. Increased unilateral muscle tone usually implies contralateral cerebral peduncle compression. Flaccid muscle tone implies brain stem infarction, spinal cord transaction, or spinal shock. Unilateral effects such as hemiparesis may be seen with a stroke.

Examination of the Face[5–7, 14]

Once a head injury has been ruled out or if no head injury is suspected, the examiner can examine the face for injury. Major trauma and subsequent injury to the face should be assessed first. If major trauma has not occurred, only those areas of the face that have been

affected by the trauma (e.g., eyes, nose, ears) need be assessed. The patient may initially be tested for fractures with the use of a tongue depressor, if the patient can open the mouth. The patient is asked to bite down as hard as possible on the tongue depressor (Fig. 2–32A). The examiner should note whether the patient is able to bite down strongly and hold the contraction and where any pain is elicited.

To test for a maxillary fracture, the examiner grasps the anterior aspect of the maxilla with the fingers of one hand and places the fingers of the other hand over the bridge of the patient's nose or forehead. The examiner then gently pulls the maxilla forward (Fig. 2–33). If movement is felt by the fingers of the other hand at the nose

Figure 2–32
Testing for mandibular fracture. (A) Patient bites down on tongue depressor while examiner tries to pull it away. (B) Pressure at the angles of the mandible.

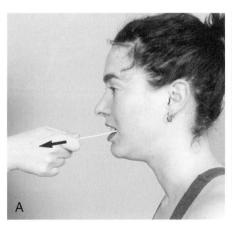

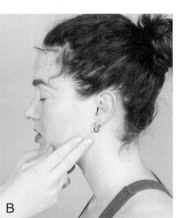

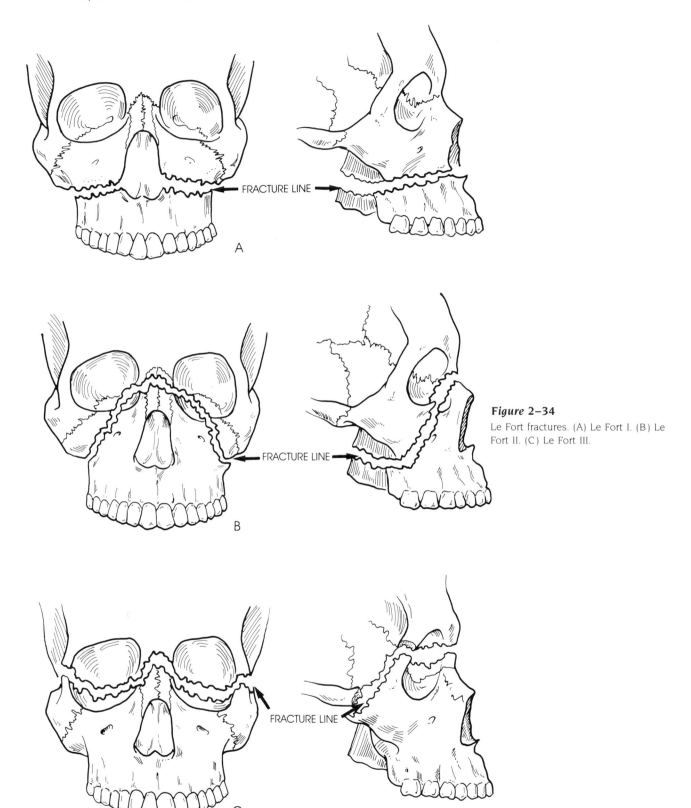

FRACTURE LINE

FRACTURE LINE

FRACTURE LINE

Figure 2-34
Le Fort fractures. (A) Le Fort I. (B) Le Fort II. (C) Le Fort III.

or the examiner feels the test hand moving forward, a Le Fort II or III fracture may be present (Fig. 2–34). If the maxilla moves without movement at the nose, either the maxilla is horizontally fractured or a Le Fort I fracture is present. With a Le Fort I fracture, the palate is separated from the superior portion of the maxilla, and the upper tooth-bearing segment of the face moves alone. The nasal bones, midportion of the face, and maxilla move if a Le Fort II fracture is present. With a Le Fort III fracture, the middle third of the face separates from the upper third of the face; this is often called a craniofacial separation. The patient may complain of lip or cheek anesthesia and double vision (diplopia) with any of these fractures.

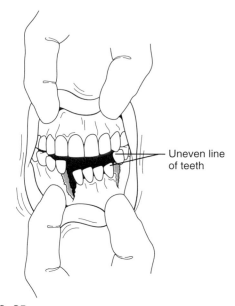

Figure 2–35

Malocclusion of teeth may be associated with fracture of mandible or maxilla.

Facial Examination

- Bone and soft tissue contours
- Fractures
  - Mandible
  - Maxilla
  - Zygoma
  - Skull
- Cranial nerves
- Facial muscles

The examiner then asks the patient to open the mouth slightly. The examiner carefully applies pressure bilaterally at the angles of the mandible (Fig. 2–32B). Localized pain, lower lip anesthesia, and intraoral laceration may indicate a fracture of the mandible.

Malocclusion of the teeth is often seen with fractures of the mandible or maxilla (Fig. 2–35). Alterations in smell (cranial nerve I) are often seen with frontobasal and nasoethmoid fractures. Skull fractures are often associated with clear nasal discharge (spinal fluid rhinorrhea), clear ear discharge (otorrhea), or a salty taste. If the fluid is accompanied by blood, the examiner can use a gauze pad to collect the fluid. If cerebrospinal fluid is mixed with the blood, a "halo" effect may be seen as the fluid collects on the gauze pad (Fig. 2–36). If the eardrum has not been perforated, blood may be seen behind it. Skull fractures may also result in blurred or double vision, loss of smell (anosmia), dizziness, tinnitus, and nausea and vomiting as well as signs and symptoms of concussion. Orbital floor fractures or dislocations are often accompanied by anesthesia of the skin in the midface or anesthesia of the cheek, lip, maxillary teeth, and gingiva.[15] Zygoma fractures are detected by observation (see Fig. 2–27). They may also cause unilateral epistaxis, double vision, and anesthesia and be asso-

ciated with eye injuries. Mouth opening may also be affected.

After major trauma has been ruled out, the examiner may test the muscles of the face (Table 2–15), especially if injury to these structures is suspected. The muscles of the face are different from most muscles in that they move the skin and soft tissues rather than joints, if one excludes the temporomandibular joint. For example, the frontalis muscle may be weak if the eyebrows do not raise symmetrically. The corrugator muscle draws the eyebrows medially and downward (frowning). The orbicularis oris muscle approximates and compresses the lips, whereas the zygomaticus muscles raise the lateral angle of the mouth (smiling).

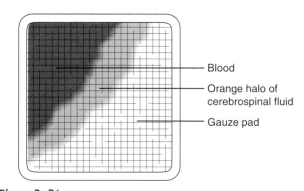

Figure 2–36

An orange halo will form around the blood on a gauze pad if cerebrospinal fluid is present.

Table 2–15
Muscles of the Face

	Action	Cranial Nerve
Muscles of the Mouth		
Orbicularis oris	Compresses lips against anterior teeth, closes mouth, protrudes lips	VII (Zygomatic, buccal, and mandibular branches)
Depressor anguli oris	Depresses angle of mouth	VII (Buccal and mandibular branches)
Levator anguli oris	Elevates angle of mouth	VII (Zygomatic and buccal branches)
Zygomaticus major	Draws angle of mouth upward and back	VII (Zygomatic and buccal branches)
Risorius	Draws angle of mouth laterally	VII (Zygomatic and buccal branches)
Muscle of the Lips		
Levator labii superioris	Elevates upper lip, flares nostril	VII (Zygomatic and buccal branches)
Muscle of the Cheek		
Buccinator	Compresses cheeks against molar teeth; sucking and blowing	VII (Buccal branches)
Muscle of the Chin		
Mentalis	Puckers skin of chin, protrudes lower lip	VII (Mandibular branches)
Muscle of the Nose		
Nasalis	Compresses nostrils Dilates or flares nostrils	VII (Zygomatic and buccal branches)
Muscle of the Eye		
Orbicularis oculi	Closes eye forcefully Closes eye gently Squeezes lubricating tears against eyeball	VII (Temporal and zygomatic branches)
Muscles of the Forehead		
Procerus	Transverse wrinkling of bridge of nose	VII (Temporal and zygomatic branches)
Corrugator	Vertical wrinkling of bridge of nose	VII (Temporal branches)
Frontalis	Pulls scalp upward and back	VII (Temporal branches)

Adapted from Liebgott, B.: The Anatomical Basis of Dentistry. St. Louis, C.V. Mosby, 1986, pp. 242–243.

Examination of the Eye[5-7]

If the eyelids are swollen shut, the examiner should assume that the globe has been ruptured. A penetrating wound of the eyelid should be assessed carefully, because it may be associated with a globe injury. The examiner should not force the eyelid open, because intraocular pressure can force extrusion of the ocular contents if the globe has been ruptured. The patient should also be instructed not to squeeze the eyelids tight, because this action increases the intraocular pressure from a normal value of 15 mm Hg up to approximately 70 mm Hg.

To examine the normal functioning of the eye muscles and several of the cranial nerves (II, III, IV, and VI), the examiner asks the patient to move through the six cardinal positions of gaze (Fig. 2–37). The examiner holds the patient's chin steady with one hand and asks the patient to follow the examiner's other hand while the examiner traces a large "H" in the air. The examiner should hold the index finger or pencil approximately 25 cm (10 inches) from the patient's nose. From the midline, the finger or pencil is moved approximately 30 cm (12 inches) to the patient's right and held. It is then moved up approximately 20 cm (8 inches) and held, moved down 40 cm (16 inches) (20 cm relative to midline) and held, and moved slowly back to midline. The same movement is repeated on the other side. The examiner

Eye Examination

- Six cardinal gaze positions
- Pupils (size, equality, reactivity)
- Nystagmus
- Visual field (peripheral vision)
- Visual acuity
- Symmetry of gaze
- Foreign objects/corneal abrasion
- Surrounding bone and soft tissue
- Hyphema

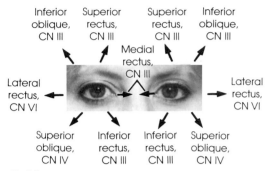

Figure 2–37

The six cardinal fields of gaze, showing eye muscles and cranial nerves (CN) involved in the movement.

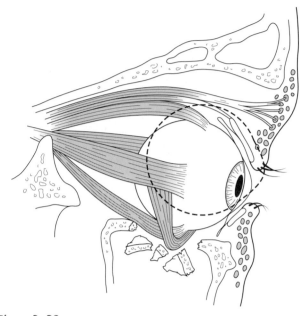

Figure 2–38

Blow-out fracture of the orbital floor. The dashed line indicates normal position of the globe. The inferior oblique and inferior rectus muscles are "caught" in the fracture site, preventing the eye from returning to its normal position. (Modified from Paton, D., and M.F. Goldberg: Management of Ocular Injuries. Philadelphia, W.B. Saunders Co., 1976, p. 63.)

should observe movement of both eyes, noting whether the eyes follow the finger or pencil smoothly. The examiner should also observe any parallel movement of the eyes in all directions. If the eyes do not move in unison or only one eye moves, there is something affecting the action of the muscles. One of the most common causes of one eye's not moving after trauma to the eye is a "blow-out" fracture of the orbital floor (Fig. 2–38). Because the inferior muscles become "caught" in the fracture site, the affected eye demonstrates limited movement (Fig. 2–39), especially upward. The patient with this type of fracture may also demonstrate depression of the eye globe, blurred vision, double vision, and conjunctival hemorrhage.

Occasionally, when looking to the extreme side, the eyes will develop a rhythmic motion called end-point nystagmus. **Nystagmus** is a rhythmic movement of the eyes with an abnormal slow drifting away from fixation and rapid return. With end-point nystagmus, there is a quick motion in the direction of the gaze followed by a slow return. This test differentiates end-point nystagmus from pathological nystagmus, in which there is a quick movement of the eyes in the same direction regardless of gaze. Pathological nystagmus exists in the region of full binocular vision, not just at the periphery. Cerebellar nystagmus is greater when the eyes are deviated toward the side of the lesion.

While testing the cardinal positions, the examiner should also watch for lid lag. Normally, the upper lid covers the top of the iris, rising when the patient looks up and quickly lowering as the eye lowers. With lid lag, the upper lid delays lowering as the eye lowers.

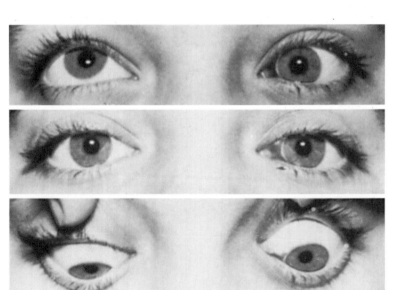

Figure 2–39

Fresh blow-out fracture of left orbit with limitation of upward (*top*) and downward (*bottom*) movements of the left eye. (From Paton, D., and M.F. Goldberg: Management of Ocular Injuries. Philadelphia, W.B. Saunders Co., 1976, p. 65.)

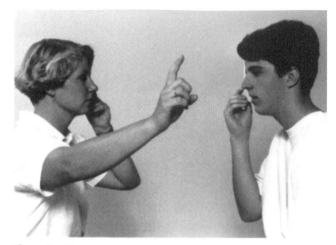

Figure 2–40
Confrontation eye test.

Peripheral vision or the visual field (peripheral limits of vision) can be tested with the **confrontation test** (Fig. 2–40). The patient is asked to cover the right eye while the examiner covers his or her own left eye, so that the open eyes of the examiner and of the patient are directly opposite each other. While the examiner and the patient look into each other's eye, the examiner fully extends his or her right arm, midway between the patient and the examiner, and then moves it toward them with the fingers waving. The patient tells the examiner when the moving fingers are first seen. The examiner then compares the patient's response with the time or distance at which the examiner first noted the fingers. The test is then repeated to the other side.

The nasal, temporal, superior, and inferior fields should all be tested in a similar fashion. The visual field should describe angles of 60° nasally, 90° temporally, 50° superiorly, and 70° inferiorly. Double simultaneous testing may also be performed. This method uses two stimuli (e.g., moving fingers) that are simultaneously presented in the right and left visual fields, and the patient is asked which finger is moving. Normally, the patient should say "both" without hesitation. With any loss of vision field (i.e., if the patient is unable to see in the same visual fields as before), the patient must be referred.

The eyelids should be everted to look at the underside of the eyelid and to give a clearer view of the globe, especially if the patient complains of a foreign body. The upper eyelid may be everted with the use of a special lid retractor or a cotton swab (Fig. 2–41). The patient is asked to look down and to the right and then down

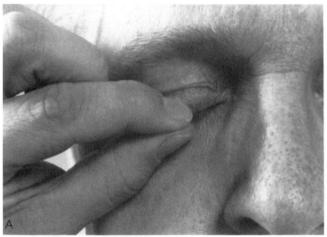

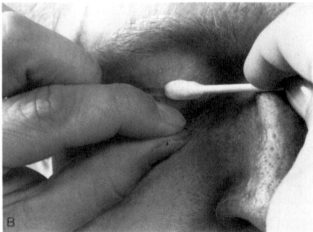

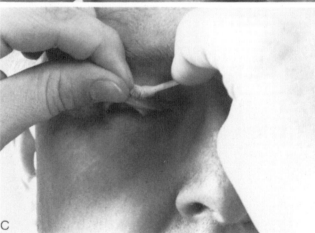

Figure 2–41
Eversion of the eyelid. (A) Grasping eyelash. (B) Putting moistened cotton-tipped applicator over eyelid. (C) Everting eyelid over the cotton-tipped applicator.

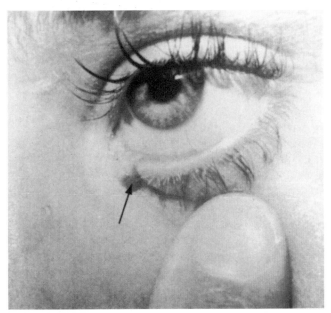

Figure 2–42
A lower lid laceration (*arrow*). (From Pashby, T.J., and R.C. Pashby: Treatment of sports eye injuries. *In* Schneider, R.C., J.C. Kennedy, and M.L. Plant [eds.]: Sports Injuries—Mechanisms, Prevention, and Treatment. Baltimore, Williams & Wilkins, 1985, p. 576.)

and to the left while the superior aspect of the eye is examined. The examiner can check the inferior aspect of the eye and its conjunctival lining by carefully pulling the lower eyelid downward and gently holding it against the bony orbit. Next, the patient is asked to look up and to the right and then up and to the left while the inferior aspect of the eye is examined. These two techniques may also be used to look for a contact lens that has migrated away from the cornea.

Both eyelids should be checked for laceration. Lacerations in the area of the lacrimal gland are especially important to detect because, if they are not looked after properly, the tearing function of the lacrimal gland may be lost (Fig. 2–42).

The reaction of the pupils to light should then be tested. First, the light in the room is dimmed. The pupils dilate in a dark environment or with a long focal distance and constrict in a light environment or with a short focal distance. The examiner shines a pen light directly into one of the patient's eyes for approximately 5 seconds (Fig. 2–43). Normally, constriction of the pupil occurs, followed by slight dilation. The pupillary reaction is classified as brisk (normal), sluggish, nonreactive, or fixed. An oval or slightly oval pupil or one that is fixed and dilated indicates increased intracranial pressure. The fixation and dilation of both pupils is a terminal sign of anoxia and ischemia to the brain. If the redilation is significant, an injury to the optic nerve may be suspected. If both pupils are midsize, midposition, and nonreactive, midbrain damage is usually indicated. In a fully conscious, alert patient who has sustained a blow near the eye, a dilated, fixed pupil usually implies injury to the ciliary nerves of the eye rather than brain injury. The other eye is tested similarly, and the results are compared.

Normally, both pupils constrict when a light is shined in one eye. The reaction of the eye being tested is called the **direct light reflex**; the reaction of the other pupil is called the **consensual light reflex**. This reaction is brisker in the young and people with blue eyes.[8] If the optic nerve is damaged, the affected pupil constricts in response to light in the opposite eye (consensual) and dilates in response to light shined into it (direct). If the oculomotor nerve is affected, the affected pupil is fixed and dilated and does not respond to light, either directly or consensually. If the pupils do not react, it is an indication of injury to the oculomotor nerve and its connections or of injury to the head. The eye also appears laterally displaced owing to paresis of the medial rectus muscle.

The pupil is then tested for "constriction to accommodation." The patient is asked to look at a distant object and then at a test object—a pencil or the examiner's finger held 10 cm (4 inches) from the bridge of the nose. The pupils dilate when the patient looks at a far object and constrict when the patient focuses on the near object. The eyes also adduct (go "cross-eyed") when the patient looks at the close object. These actions are called the **accommodation-convergence reflex**.[8] When

Figure 2–43
Testing the pupils for reaction to light. (A) Light shining in eye. (B) Light shining away from eye.

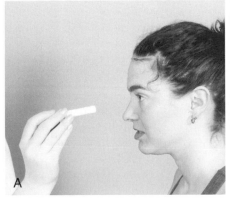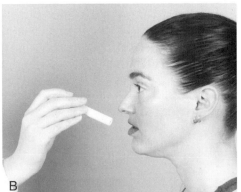

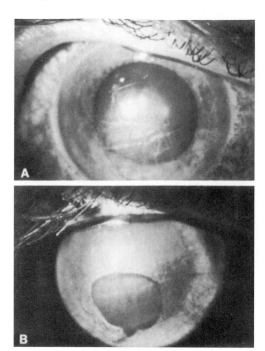

Figure 2–44
Corneal abrasion. (A) Without fluorescein. (B) With fluorescein. (From Torg, J.S.: Athletic Injuries to the Head, Neck and Face. Philadelphia, Lea & Febiger, 1982, p. 262.)

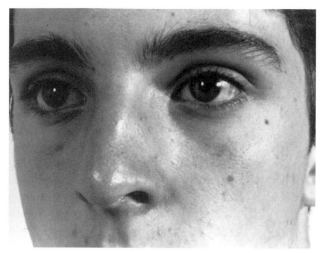

Figure 2–46
Symmetry of gaze. Note white "dots" of light on pupils.

looking at distant objects, the eyes should be parallel. Deviation or lack of parallelism is called **strabismus** and indicates weakness of one of the extraocular muscles or lack of neural coordination.[16]

When inspected under normal overhead light, the lens of the eye should be transparent. Shining a light on the lens may cause it to appear gray or yellow. The cornea should be smooth and clear. If the patient has extreme pain in the corneal area, a corneal abrasion

should be suspected (Fig. 2–44). An appropriate specialist may test for corneal abrasion by using a fluorescein strip and a slit lamp. The cornea should be crystal clear when it is viewed, and the iris details should match those of the other eye.

To check for depth of the anterior chamber of the eye or a narrow corneal angle, the examiner shines a light obliquely across each eye. Normally, it illuminates the entire iris. If the corneal angle is narrow because of a shallow anterior chamber, the examiner will be able to see a crescent-shaped shadow on the side of the iris away from the light (Fig. 2–45). This finding indicates an anatomic predisposition to narrow-angled glaucoma.

To test for **symmetry of gaze**, the examiner aims a light source approximately 60 cm (24 inches) from the patient while standing directly in front of the patient and

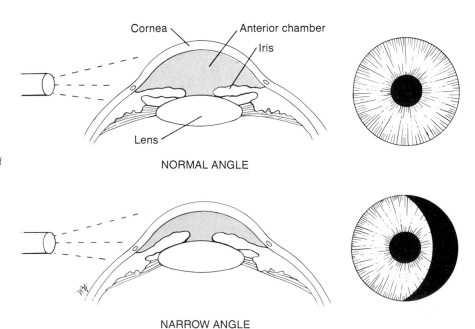

Figure 2–45
Normal and narrow corneal angle (depth of anterior chamber). (From Swartz, M.H.: Textbook of Physical Diagnosis. Philadelphia, W.B. Saunders Co., 1989, p. 144.)

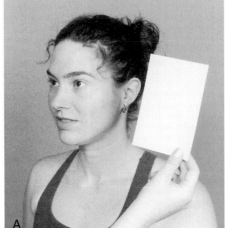
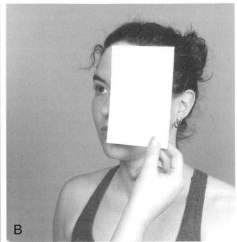

Figure 2–47
Cover-uncover test for mild ocular deviation. As patient gazes at a specific point (A), examiner covers one eye and looks for movement in uncovered eye (B).

holding the light distant enough to prevent convergence of the patient's gaze. The patient is asked to stare at the light. The dots of reflected light on the two corneas should be in the same relative location (Fig. 2–46). When one eye does not look directly at the light, the reflected dot of light moves to the side opposite the deviation. For example, if the eye deviates medially, the reflection appears more laterally placed than in the other eye. The examiner can approximate the angle of deviation by noting the position of the reflection. Each millimeter of displacement in the reflection represents approximately 7° of ocular deviation. To bring out a mild deviation, a **cover-uncover test** may be used (Fig. 2–47). The patient looks at a specific point, such as the bridge of the examiner's nose. One of the patient's eyes is then covered with a card. Normally, the uncovered eye will not move. If it moves, it was not straight before the other eye was covered. The other eye is then tested in a similar fashion.

Visual acuity is tested using a vision chart. Visual acuity is the ability of the eye to perceive fine detail, for example, when reading. If a standard eye wall chart is not available, a pocket visual acuity card may be used (Fig. 2–48). This pocket card is usually viewed at a distance of 35 to 36 cm (14 inches). As with the wall chart, the patient is asked to examine the smallest line possible. If neither eye chart is available, any printed material may be used. If glasses or contact lenses are worn, the patient should be tested both without and with the corrective lenses. The test is done quickly so the patient cannot memorize the chart. Visual acuity is recorded as a fraction in which the numerator indicates the distance of the patient from the chart (e.g., 20 ft) and the denominator indicates the distance at which the normal eye can read the line. Thus, 20/100 means the patient can read at 20 ft what the average person can read at 100 ft. The smaller the fraction, the worse the myopia (nearsightedness). Patients with corrected vision of less than 20/40 should be referred to the appropriate specialist.[8]

Intraocular examination with an ophthalmoscope, if available, may reveal lens, vitreous, or retinal damage.

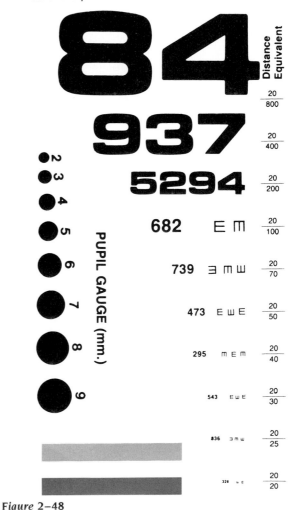

**CLARK'S CHARTS
EYE EXAM**

To test visual acuity: hold chart 14 inches from eyes in good light. Test each eye separately and then jointly, with and without corrective lenses. If bifocals are present have patient read with them.

Figure 2–48
Hand-held vision chart. (Top solid bar is red, and bottom solid bar is green.)

Examination of the Nose[5-7]

Patency of the nasal passages can be determined by occluding one of the patient's nostrils by pushing a finger against the side of it. The patient is then asked to breathe in and out of the opposite nostril with the mouth closed. The process is repeated on the other side. Normally, no sound is heard, and the patient can breathe easily through the open nostril.

If available, a nasal speculum and light may be used to inspect the nasal cavity. The nasal mucosa and turbinates can be inspected for color, foreign bodies, and abnormal masses (e.g., polyp). The nasal septum should be in midline and straight and is normally thicker anteriorly than posteriorly. If the nasal cavities are asymmetric, it may indicate a deviated septum. If the patient demonstrates a septal hematoma, it must be treated fairly quickly, because the hematoma may cause excessive pressure on the septum, making it avascular. This avascularity can result in a "saddle nose" deformity owing to necrosis and absorption of the underlying cartilage (Fig. 2–49).

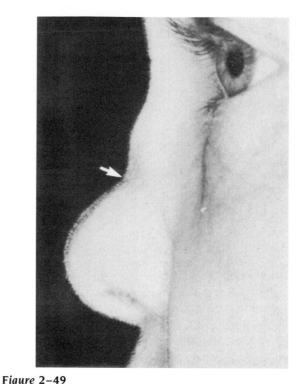

Figure 2–49
"Saddle nose" deformity (*arrow*) that occurred as a result of loss of septal cartilage support secondary to septal hematoma and abscess. (From Handler, S.D.: Diagnosis and management of maxillofacial injuries. In Torg, J.S. [ed.]: Athletic Injuries to the Head, Neck and Face. Philadelphia, Lea & Febiger, 1982, p. 232.)

Nasal Examination

• Patency
• Nasal cavities
• Sinuses
• Fracture
• Nasal discharge (bloody, straw-colored, clear)

Illumination of the frontal and maxillary sinuses may be performed if sinus tenderness is present or infection is suspected. The examination must be performed in a completely darkened room. To illuminate the maxillary sinuses, the examiner places the light source lateral to the patient's nose just beneath the medial aspect of the eye. The examiner then looks through the patient's open mouth for illumination of the hard palate. To illuminate the frontal sinuses, the examiner places the light source against the medial aspect of each supraorbital rim. The examiner looks for a dim red glow as light is transmitted just below the eyebrow. The sinuses usually show differing degrees of illumination. The absence of a glow indi-

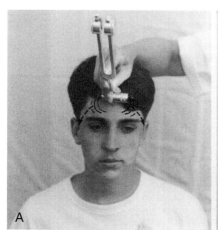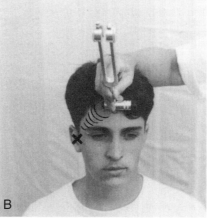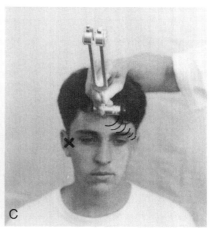

Figure 2–50
The Weber test. When a vibrating tuning fork is placed on the center of the forehead (A), the sound is heard in the center without lateralization to either side (normal response). (B) In the presence of a conductive hearing loss, the sound is heard on the side of the conductive loss. (C) In the presence of sensorineural loss, the sound is better heard on the opposite (unaffected) side.

cates either that the sinus is filled with secretions or that it has never developed.

Internal examination of the nose may be performed using a nasal illuminator or a light and nasal speculum, if available. In this case, the examiner observes the septum, nasal membrane, and turbinates for signs of pathology.

Examination of the Teeth[5-7]

The examiner should observe the teeth to see if they are in normal position and whether any teeth are missing, chipped, or depressed (see Fig. 2–21). Using the gloved index finger and thumb, the examiner can apply mild pressure to each tooth, pressing inward toward the tongue and outward toward the lips. Normally, a small amount of movement is seen. If a tooth is loose, a positive test is indicated by excessive movement or increased pain or numbness relative to other teeth. A tooth that has been avulsed may be cleansed with warm water and reinserted into the socket. The patient is then referred to the appropriate specialist.

Tooth Examination

- Number of teeth
- Position of teeth
- Movement of teeth
- Condition of teeth
- Condition of gums

Examination of the Ear[5-7]

Examination of the ear deals primarily with whether the patient is able to hear. There are several tests that may be used to test hearing.

Whispered Voice Test. The patient's response to the examiner's whispered voice can be used to determine hearing ability. The examiner masks the hearing in one of the patient's ears by placing a finger gently in the patient's ear canal. Standing approximately 30 to 60 cm (12 to 24 inches) away from the patient, the examiner whispers one- or two-syllable words very softly and asks the patient to repeat the words heard. If the patient has difficulty, the examiner gradually increases the loudness of the whisper until the patient responds appropriately. The procedure is repeated in the other ear. The patient should be able to hear softly whispered words in each ear at a distance of 30 to 60 cm (12 to 24 inches) and respond correctly at least 50% of the time.[4, 5]

Ticking Watch Test. The ticking watch test uses a non-electric ticking watch to test high-frequency hearing. The examiner positions the watch approximately 15 cm (6 inches) from the ear to be tested, slowly moving it toward the ear. The patient is asked to tell the examiner when the ticking is heard. The distance can be measured and

will give some idea of the patient's ability to hear high-frequency sound.[4, 5]

Weber Test. The examiner places the base of a vibrating tuning fork on the midline vertex of the patient's head. The patient is asked if the sound is heard equally well in both ears or is heard better in one ear (lateralization of sound). The patient should hear the sound equally well in both ears (Figs. 2–50 and 2–51). If the sound is

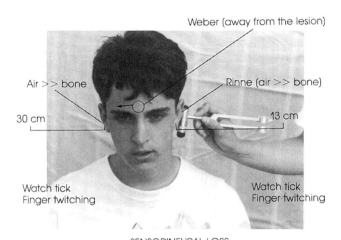

SENSORINEURAL LOSS

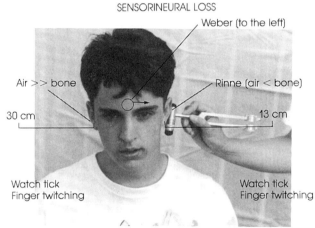

CONDUCTIVE LOSS

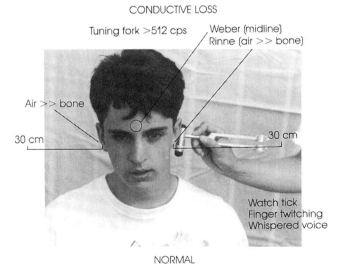

NORMAL

Figure 2–51
Bedside hearing tests and results with sensorineural or conductive loss in left ear and with normal hearing.

lateralized, the patient is asked to identify through which ear the sound is heard better. To test the reliability of the patient's response, the examiner repeats the procedure while occluding one ear with a finger and asks the patient through which ear the sound is heard better. It should be heard better in the occluded ear.[4, 5]

Rinne Test. The Rinne test is performed by placing the base of the vibrating tuning fork against the patient's mastoid bone. The examiner counts or times the interval with a watch. The patient is asked to tell the examiner when the sound is no longer heard, and the examiner notes the number of seconds. The examiner then quickly positions a still-vibrating tine 1 to 2 cm (0.5 to 0.8 inch) from the auditory canal, and the patient is asked to tell the examiner when the sound is no longer heard. The examiner then compares the number of seconds the sound was heard by bone conduction and by air conduction. The counting or timing of the interval between the two sounds determines the length of time that sound is heard by air conduction (see Fig. 2–51). Air-conducted sound should be heard twice as long as bone-conducted sound. For example, if bone conduction is heard for 15 seconds, the air conduction should be heard for 30 seconds.[4–6]

Schwabach Test. This test is a comparison of the patient's and examiner's hearing by bone conduction. The examiner alternately places the vibrating tuning fork against the patient's mastoid process and against the examiner's mastoid bone until one of them no longer hears a sound. The examiner and patient should hear the sound for equal amounts of time.[4, 5]

Conductive hearing loss implies that the patient experiences reduction of all sounds rather than difficulty in interpreting sounds. Sensorineural or perceptual hearing loss indicates that the patient has difficulty interpreting the sounds heard.

Internal examination of the ear may be accomplished with the use of an otoscope, if available. In this case, the examiner would observe the canal as well as the eardrum (tympanic membrane), noting any blockage, excessive wax, swelling, redness, transparency (usually pearly gray), bulging, retraction, or perforation of the eardrum.

Ear Examination

- Tenderness (exterior and interior)
- Ear discharge (bloody, straw-colored, clear)
- Hearing
- Balance

Special Tests

Only those special tests that the examiner thinks will have value are performed. For example, the tests for expanding intracranial lesions would not be performed with a facial injury unless an associated injury to the brain or other neurological tissues is suspected.

Tests for Expanding Intracranial Lesions

For each of these tests, the patient must be able to stand normally when the eyes are open.

Neurological Control Test—Upper Limb. The patient is asked to stand with the arms forward flexed 90° and the eyes closed. The patient is asked to hold this position for approximately 30 seconds. If the examiner notes that one arm tends to move or "drift" outward and downward, the test is considered positive for an expanding intracranial lesion on the side opposite the side with the drift.

Neurological Control Test—Lower Limb. The patient is asked to sit on the edge of a table or in a chair with the legs extended in front and not touching the ground. The patient is then asked to close the eyes for approximately 20 to 30 seconds. If the examiner notes that one leg tends to move or drift, the test is considered positive for an expanding intracranial lesion on the side opposite that with the drift.

Romberg Test. The patient is asked to stand with the feet together and arms by the sides with the eyes open. The examiner notes whether the patient has any problem with balance. The patient is then asked to close the eyes (for at least 20 seconds), and the examiner notes any differences. A positive Romberg test is elicited if the patient sways or falls to one side when the eyes are closed and is indicative of an expanding intracranial lesion.

Walk or Stand in Tandem. Patients with expanding intracranial lesions demonstrate increasing difficulty in walking in tandem ("walking the line") or standing in tandem (standing on 2 feet). Standing in tandem is more difficult to perform than walking in tandem.

Tests for Coordination

Finger-to-Nose Test. The patient stands or sits with the eyes open and is asked to bring the index finger to the nose. The test is repeated with the eyes closed. Both arms are tested several times with increasing speed. Normally, the tests should be accomplished easily, smoothly, and quickly with the eyes open and closed.

Finger-Thumb Test. The patient is asked to touch each finger with the thumb of the same hand. The normal or uninjured side is tested first, followed by the injured side. The examiner compares the two sides for coordination and timing.

Hand Flip Test. The patient is asked to touch the back of the opposite, stationary hand with the anterior aspect of the fingers, "flip" the test hand over, and touch the opposite hand with the posterior aspect of the fingers. The movement is repeated several times, with both sides being tested. The examiner compares the two sides for coordination and speed.

Finger Drumming Test. The patient is asked to "drum" the index and middle finger of one hand up and down as quickly as possible on the back of the other hand. The test is repeated with the opposite hand. The examiner compares the two sides for coordination and speed.

Hand-Thigh Test. The patient is asked to pat the thigh with the hand as quickly as possible. The uninjured side is tested first. The patient may be asked to supinate and pronate the hand between each hand-thigh contact to make the test more complex. The examiner watches for speed and coordination and compares the two sides.

Past Pointing Test. The patient and examiner face each other. The examiner holds up both index fingers approximately 15 cm (6 inches) apart. The patient is asked to lift the arms over the head and then bring the arms down to touch the patient's index fingers to the examiner's index fingers (Fig. 2–52). The test is repeated with the patient's eyes closed. Normally, the test can be performed without difficulty. Patients with vestibular disease have problems with past pointing. The test may also be used to test proprioception.

Heel-to-Knee Test. The patient, who is lying supine with the eyes open, is asked to take the heel of one foot and touch the opposite knee with the heel and then slide the heel down the shin. The test is repeated with the

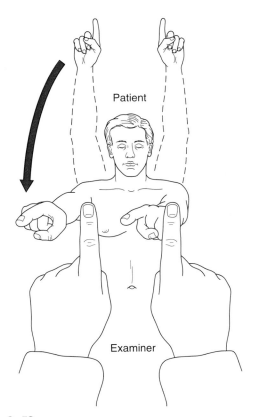

Figure 2–52
Past pointing. (Redrawn from Reilly, B.M.: Practical Strategies in Outpatient Medicine. Philadelphia, W.B. Saunders Co., 1991, p. 195.)

eyes closed, and both legs are tested. The test can be repeated several times with increasing speed, with the examiner noting any differences in coordination or the presence of tremor. Normally, the test should be accomplished easily, smoothly, and quickly with the eyes open and closed.

Tests for Proprioception

Proprioceptive Finger-Nose Test. The patient keeps the eyes closed. The examiner lightly touches one of the patient's fingers and asks the patient to touch the patient's nose with that finger. The examiner then touches another finger on the other hand, and the patient again touches the nose. Patients with proprioceptive loss have difficulty doing the test without visual input.

Proprioceptive Movement Test. The patient keeps the eyes closed. The examiner moves the patient's finger or toe up or down by grasping it on the sides to lessen clues given by pressure. The patient then tells the examiner which way the digit moved.

Proprioceptive Space Test. The patient keeps the eyes closed. The examiner places one of the patient's hands or feet in a selected position in space. The patient is then asked to imitate that position with the other limb or to find the hand or foot with the other limb. True proprioceptive loss causes the patient to be unable to properly position or to find the normal limb with the limb that has proprioceptive loss.

Past Pointing Test. The test is performed as described under Tests for Coordination.

Reflexes and Cutaneous Distribution

With a head injury patient, deep tendon reflexes (see Table 1–21) should be performed. Accentuation of one or more of the reflexes may indicate trauma to the brain on the opposite side. Pathological reflexes (see Table 1–23) may also be altered with a head injury.

The **corneal reflex** (trigeminal nerve, cranial nerve V) is used to test for damage or dysfunction to the pons. In some cases, the patient may look to one side to avoid involuntary blinking. The examiner touches the cornea (not the eyelashes or conjunctiva) with a small, fine point of cotton (Fig. 2–53). The normal response is a bilateral blink, because the reflex arc connects both facial nerve nuclei. If the reflex is absent, the test is considered positive.

The **gag reflex** may be tested using a tongue depressor that is inserted into the posterior pharynx and depressed toward the hypopharynx. The reflex tests cranial nerves IX and X, and its absence in a trauma setting may indicate caudal brain stem dysfunction.

Consensual light reflex may be tested by shining a light into one eye. This action causes the "lighted" pupil to constrict. If there is normal communication between

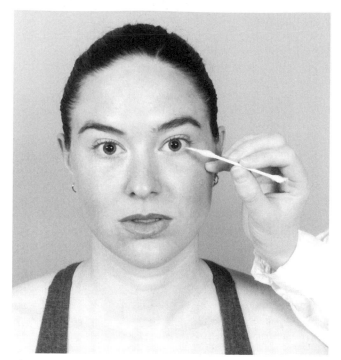

Figure 2–53
Test of corneal reflex.

the two oculomotor nerves, the "nonlighted" pupil also constricts.

The **jaw reflex** is usually tested only if the temporomandibular joint or cervical spine is being examined. The examiner should check the sensation of the head and face, keeping in mind the differences in dermatome and sensory nerve distributions (Fig. 2–54). Lip anesthesia or paresthesia is often seen in patients with mandibular fracture.

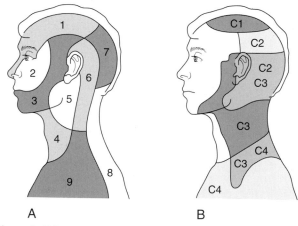

Figure 2–54
(A) Sensory nerve distribution of the head, neck and face. (1) Ophthalmic nerve. (2) Maxillary nerve. (3) Mandibular nerve. (4) Transverse cutaneous nerve of neck (C2–C3). (5) Greater auricular nerve (C2–C3). (6) Lesser auricular nerve (C2). (7) Greater occipital nerve (C2–C3). (8) Cervical dorsal rami (C3–C5). (9) Suprascapular nerve (C5–C6). (B) Dermatome pattern of the head, neck, and face. Note the overlap of C3.

Nerve Injuries of the Head and Face

Bell's palsy involves paralysis of the facial nerve (cranial nerve VII) and usually occurs where the nerve emerges from the stylomastoid foramen. Pressure in the foramen caused by inflammation or trauma affects the nerve and therefore the muscles of the face (occipitofrontalis, corrugator, orbicularis oculi, and the nose and mouth muscles) on one side. The inflammation may result from a middle ear infection, viral infection, chilling of the face, or tumor. The observable result is smoothing of the face on the affected side owing to loss of muscle action, the eye on the affected side remaining open and the lower eyelid sagging. The patient is unable to wink, whistle, purse the lips, or wrinkle the forehead. Speech sounds, especially those requiring pursing of the lips, are affected, resulting in slurred speech. The mouth droops, and it and the nose may deviate to the opposite side, especially in long-standing cases, of which there are remarkably few (90% of patients having complete recovery within 2 to 8 weeks). Facial sensation on the affected side is lost, and taste sensation is sometimes lost as well.

Joint Play Movements

Because no articular joints are involved in the assessment of the head and face, there are no joint play movements to test.

Palpation

During palpation of the head and face, the examiner should note any tenderness, deformity, crepitus, or other signs and symptoms that may indicate the source of pathology. The examiner should note the texture of the skin and surrounding bony and soft tissues. Normally, the patient is palpated in the sitting or supine position, beginning with the skull and moving from anterior to posterior, to the face, and finally to the lateral and posterior structures of the head.

The skull is palpated by a gentle rotary movement of the fingers, progressing systematically from front to back. Normally, the skin of the skull moves freely and has no tenderness, swelling, or depressions.

The temporal area and temporalis muscle should be laterally palpated for tenderness and deformity. The external ear or auricle and the periauricular area should also be palpated for tenderness or lacerations.

The occiput should be palpated posteriorly for tenderness. The presence of **Battle's sign** should be noted, if observed, because this sign is indicative of a basilar skull fracture.

The face is palpated beginning superiorly and working inferiorly in a systematic manner. Like the skull, the forehead is palpated by gentle rotary movements of the fingers, feeling the movement of the skin and the occipitofrontalis muscle underneath. Normally, the skin of the

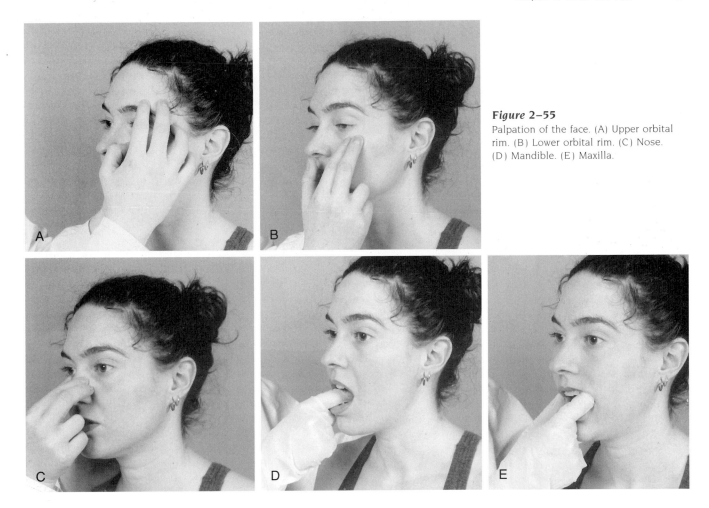

Figure 2–55
Palpation of the face. (A) Upper orbital rim. (B) Lower orbital rim. (C) Nose. (D) Mandible. (E) Maxilla.

forehead moves freely and is smooth and even with no tender areas. The examiner then palpates around the eye socket or orbital rim, moving over the eyebrow and supraorbital rims, around the lateral side of the eye, and along the zygomatic arch to the infraorbital rims, looking for deformity, crepitus, tenderness, and lacerations (Fig. 2–55A and B). The orbicularis oculi muscles surround the orbit, and the medial side of the orbital rim and nose are then palpated for tenderness, deformity, and fracture. The nasal bones, including the lateral and alar

cartilage, are palpated for any crepitus or deviation (Fig. 2–55C). The septum should be inspected to see if it has widened, which may indicate a septal hematoma, which often occurs with a fracture. It should also be determined whether the patient can breathe through the nose or smell.

The frontal and maxillary sinuses should be inspected for swelling. To palpate the frontal sinuses, the examiner uses the thumbs to press up under the bony brow on each side of the nose (Fig. 2–56A). The examiner then presses under the zygomatic processes using either

Figure 2–56
(A) Palpation of frontal sinuses.
(B) Palpation of maxillary sinuses.

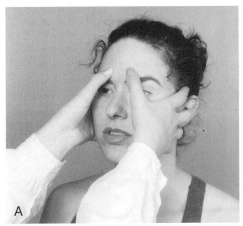
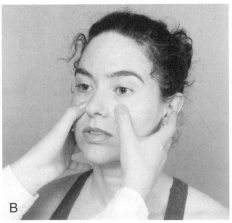

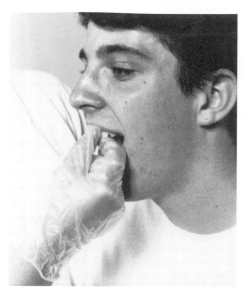

Figure 2–57

Palpation of maxillary fracture with anteroposterior "rocking" motion.

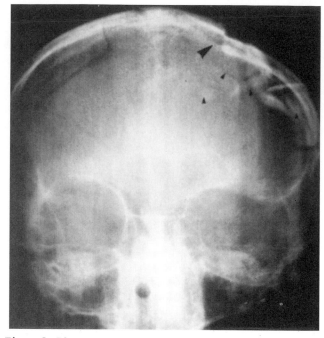

Figure 2–59

Anteroposterior skull radiograph showing a depressed parietal skull fracture (*large arrow*) with multiple bony fragments into the brain (*small arrows*). (From Albright, J.P., J. Van Gilder, G. El Khoury, E. Crowley, and D. Foster: Head and neck injuries in sports. *In* Scott, W.N., B. Nisonson, and J.A. Nicholas [eds.]: Principles of Sports Medicine. Baltimore, Williams & Wilkins, 1984, p. 53.)

the thumbs or index and middle fingers to palpate the maxillary sinuses (Fig. 2–56B). No tenderness or swelling over the soft tissue should be present. The sinus areas may also be percussed to detect tenderness. A light tap directly over each sinus with the index finger can be used to detect tenderness.

The examiner then moves inferiorly to palpate the jaw. The examiner palpates the mandible along its entire length, noting any tenderness, crepitus, or deformity. The examiner, using a rubber glove, may also palpate along the mandible interiorly, noting any tenderness or pain (Fig. 2–55D). The "outside" hand may be used to stabilize the jaw during this procedure. The mandible may also be tapped with a finger along its length to see if signs of tenderness are elicited. The muscles of the cheek (buccinator) and mouth (orbicularis oris) should be palpated at the same time.

The maxilla may be palpated in a similar fashion, both internally and externally, noting position of the teeth, tenderness, and any deformity (Fig. 2–55E). The examiner may grasp the teeth anteriorly to see if the teeth and mandible move in relation to the rest of the face, which may indicate a Le Fort fracture (Fig. 2–57).

The trachea should be palpated for midline position. The examiner places a thumb along each side of the trachea, comparing the spaces between the trachea and the sternocleidomastoid muscle, which should be symmetric. The hyoid bone and the thyroid and cricoid carti-

Figure 2–58

Incomplete fracture of angle of mandible on the left side (*arrows*). (A) Anteroposterior view. (B) Lateral view. (From O'Donoghue, D.H.: Treatment of Injuries to Athletes. Philadelphia, W.B. Saunders Co., 1984, p. 114.)

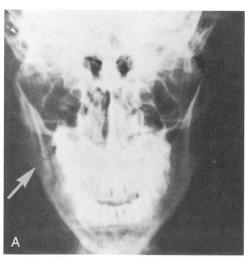

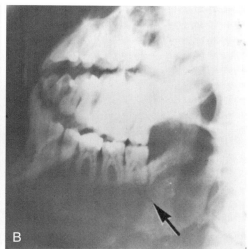

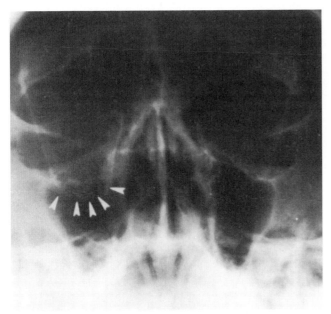

Figure 2–60

Plain posteroanterior view showing blow-out fracture of the orbit (*arrows*). (From Paton, D., and M.F. Goldberg: Management of Ocular Injuries. Philadelphia, W.B. Saunders Co., 1976, p. 70.)

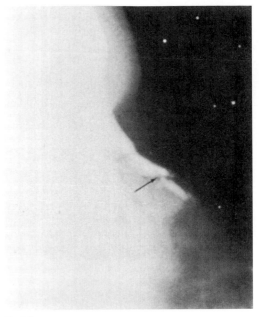

Figure 2–61

Lateral radiograph of the nasal bones demonstrating a nasal fracture (*arrow*). (From Torg, J.S.: Athletic Injuries to the Head, Neck and Face. Philadelphia, Lea & Febiger, 1982, p. 229.)

lages should be identified. Normally, they are smooth and nontender and move when the patient swallows.

Diagnostic Imaging

Plain Film Radiography

Anteroposterior View. The examiner should note the normal bone contours, looking for fractures of the various bones (Figs. 2–58 through 2–60).

Lateral View. The examiner should again note bony contours, looking for the possibility of fractures (Figs. 2–58 and 2–61).

Computed Tomography

Computed tomography scans help to differentiate between bone and soft tissue and give a more precise view of fractures (Figs. 2–62 and 2–63).

Magnetic Resonance Imaging

Magnetic resonance imaging is especially useful for demonstrating lesions of the soft tissues of the head and face and for differentiating between bone and soft tissue (Figs. 2–64 and 2–65).

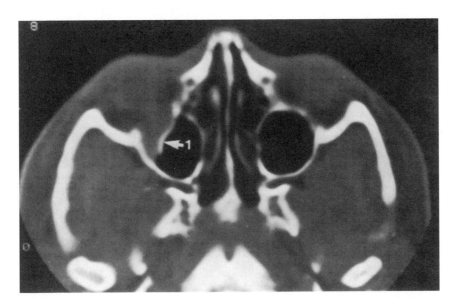

Figure 2–62

Axial computed tomogram of orbital blow-out fracture showing fracture of the orbit (1) with orbital contents herniated into the maxillary sinus. (From Sinn, D.P., and N.D. Karas: Radiographic evaluation of facial injuries. *In* Fonseca, R.J., and R.V. Walker [eds.]: Oral and Maxillofacial Trauma. Philadelphia, W.B. Saunders Co., 1991.)

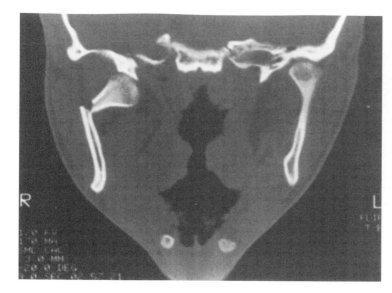

Figure 2–63
The computed tomographic scan is ideal for condylar fractures. (From Bruce, R., and R.J. Fonseca: Mandibular fractures. In Fonseca, R.J., and R.V. Walker [eds.]: Oral and Maxillofacial Trauma. Philadelphia, W.B. Saunders Co., 1991, p. 389.)

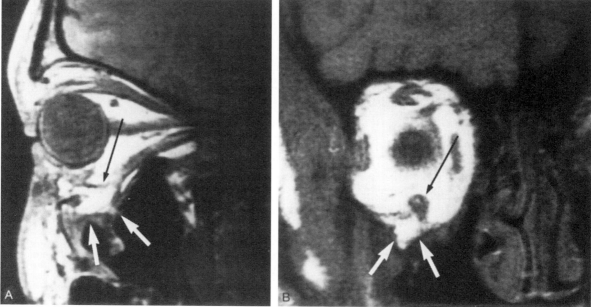

Figure 2–64
Magnetic resonance images showing blow-out fracture. Sagittal (A) and coronal (B) T1-weighted scans demonstrate a blow-out fracture of the right orbit with depression of the orbital floor (*white arrows*) into the superior maxillary sinus. The inferior rectus muscle (*long arrow*) is clearly identified and is not entrapped by the floor fracture. (From Harms, S.E.: The orbit. In Edelman, R.R., and J.R. Hesselink [eds.]: Clinical Magnetic Resonance Imaging. Philadelphia, W.B. Saunders Co., 1990, p. 619.)

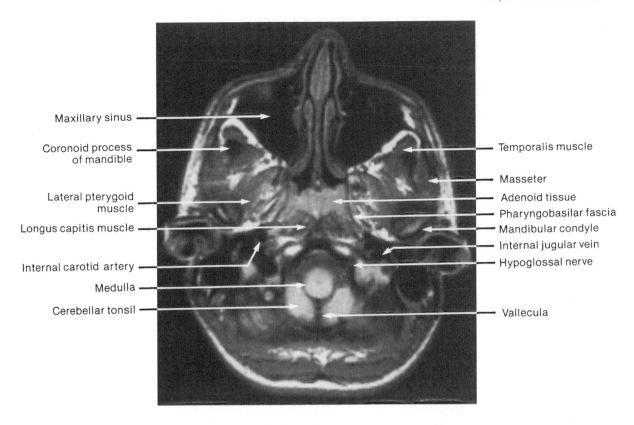

Maxillary sinus

Coronoid process
of mandible

Lateral pterygoid
muscle

Longus capitis muscle

Internal carotid artery

Medulla

Cerebellar tonsil

Temporalis muscle

Masseter

Adenoid tissue

Pharyngobasilar fascia

Mandibular condyle

Internal jugular vein

Hypoglossal nerve

Vallecula

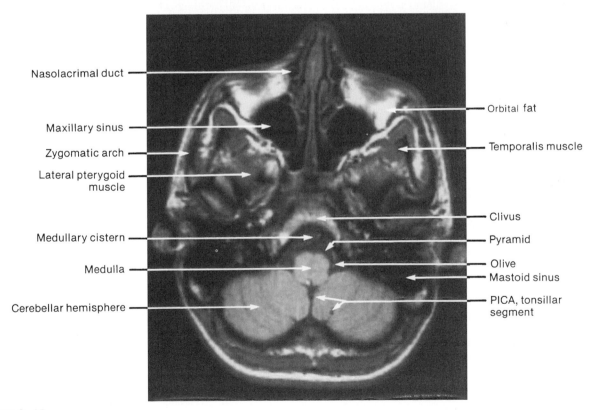

Nasolacrimal duct

Maxillary sinus

Zygomatic arch

Lateral pterygoid
muscle

Medullary cistern

Medulla

Cerebellar hemisphere

Orbital fat

Temporalis muscle

Clivus

Pyramid

Olive

Mastoid sinus

PICA, tonsillar
segment

Figure 2–65

T1-weighted axial magnetic resonance images of the head and brain at two levels. PICA, posterior
inferior cerebellar artery. (From Greenberg, J.J., et al: Brain: Indications, techniques, and atlas. In
Edelman, R.R., and J.R. Hesselink [eds.]: Clinical Magnetic Resonance Imaging. Philadelphia, W.B.
Saunders Co., 1990, p. 384.)

Précis of the Head and Face Assessment*

History (sitting)
Observation (sitting)
*Examination** (sitting)
    Head injury
        Neural watch
        Glasgow Coma Scale
        Concussion
        Memory tests
        Headache
        Expanding intracranial lesion
        Proprioception
        Coordination
        Head injury card
    Facial injury
        Bone and soft tissue contours
        Fractures
        Cranial nerves
        Facial muscles
    Eye injury
        Six cardinal gaze positions
        Pupils (size, equality, reactivity)
        Visual field (peripheral vision)
        Visual acuity
        Symmetry of gaze
        Hyphema
        Foreign objects, corneal abrasion
        Nystagmus
        Surrounding bone and soft tissue
    Nasal injury
        Patency
        Nasal cavities

        Sinuses
        Fracture
        Nose discharge (bloody, straw-colored, clear)
    Tooth injury
        Number of teeth
        Position of teeth
        Movement of teeth
        Condition of teeth
        Condition of gums
    Ear injury
        Tenderness or pain
        Ear discharge (bloody, straw-colored, clear)
        Hearing tests
        Balance
    Special tests
        Tests for expanding intracranial lesions
        Tests for coordination
        Tests for proprioception
    Reflexes and cutaneous distribution
    Palpation
    Diagnostic imaging

---

*When examining the head and face, if only one area has been injured (e.g., the nose), then only that area needs to be examined, provided the examiner is certain that adjacent structures have not also been injured.

After any examination, the patient should be warned of the possibility of exacerbation of symptoms as a result of the assessment.

Case Studies

When doing these case studies, the examiner should list the appropriate questions to be asked and why they are being asked, what to look for and why, and what things should be tested and why. Depending on the answers of the patient (and the examiner should consider different responses), several possible causes of the patient's problem may become evident (examples are given in parentheses). A differential diagnosis chart should be made up. (See Table 2–16 as an example.) The examiner can then decide how different diagnoses may affect the treatment plan.

1. A 27-year-old man was playing football. He received a "knee to the head," rendering him unconscious for approximately 3 minutes. How would you differentiate between a first-time, fourth-degree concussion and an expanding intracranial lesion?

2. A 13-year-old boy received "an elbow" in the nose and cheek while play-wrestling. The nose is crooked and painful and bled after the injury, and the cheek is sore. Describe your assessment plan for this patient (nasal fracture versus zygoma fracture).

3. A 23-year-old woman was in an automobile accident. She was a passenger in the front seat and was not wearing a seat belt. The car in which she was riding hit another car, which had run a red light. The woman's face hit the dashboard of the car, and she received a severe facial injury. Describe your assessment plan for this patient (Le Fort fracture versus mandibular fracture).

4. An 83-year-old man tripped in the bathroom and hit his chin against the bathtub, knocking himself unconscious. Describe your assessment plan for this patient (cervical spine lesion versus mandibular fracture).

5. An 18-year-old woman was playing squash. She was not wearing eye protectors and was hit in the eye with the ball. Describe your assessment plan for this patient (ruptured globe versus "blow-out" fracture).

6. A 15-year-old boy was playing field hockey. He was not wearing a mouth guard and was hit in the mouth and jaw by the ball. There was a large amount of blood. Describe your assessment plan for this patient (tooth fracture versus mandible fracture).

7. A 16-year-old male wrestler comes to you complaining of ear pain. He has just finished a match, which he lost. Describe your assessment plan for this patient (cauliflower ear versus external otitis).

8. A 17-year-old female basketball player comes to you complaining of eye pain. She says she received a "finger in the eye" when she went up to get the ball. Describe your assessment plan for this patient (hyphema versus corneal abrasion).

Table 2–16
Differential Diagnosis of 4° Concussion and Intracranial Lesion

	4° Concussion	Intracranial Lesion
Confusion	Yes, but should improve with time	Will have increased confusion with time
Amnesia	Posttraumatic, retrograde	Not usually
Loss of consciousness	Yes, but recovers	Lucid interval varies
Tinnitus	Severe	Not a factor
Dizziness	Severe, but improves	May get worse
Headache	Often	Severe
Nystagmus or irregular eye movements	Not usually	Possible
Pupil inequality	Not usually	Possible early; present later
Irregular respiration	No	Possible early; present later
Slowing of heart	No	Possible early; present later
Intractable vomiting	Not usually	Possible
Lateralization	No	Yes
Coordination affected	Yes, but improves	Yes, and gets worse
Seizure	Not usually	Possible early; probable late
Personality change	Possible	Possible

References

Cited References

1. Albright, J.P., J. Van Gilder, G. El Khoury, E. Crowley, and D. Foster: Head and neck injuries in sports. In Scott, W.N., B. Nisonson, and J.A. Nicholas (eds.): Principles of Sports Medicine. Baltimore, Williams & Wilkins, 1984.
2. Torg, J.S.: Athletic Injuries to the Head, Neck and Face. St. Louis, Mosby–Year Book Inc., 1991.
3. Manzi, D.B., and P.A. Weaver: Head Injury: The Acute Care Phase. Thorofare, New Jersey, Slack Inc., 1987.
4. Seidel, H.M., J.W. Ball, J.E. Dains, and G.W. Benedict: Mosby's Guide to Physical Examination. St. Louis, C.V. Mosby Co., 1987.
5. Swartz, M.H.: Textbook of Physical Diagnosis. Philadelphia, W.B. Saunders Co., 1989.
6. Reilly, B.M.: Practical Strategies in Outpatient Medicine. Philadelphia, W.B. Saunders Co., 1984.
7. Novey, D.W.: Rapid Access Guide to the Physical Examination. Chicago, Year Book Medical Publishers, 1988.
8. Pashby, T.J., and R.C. Pashby: Treatment of sports eye injuries. In Fu, F.H., and D.A. Stone (eds.): Sports Injuries—Mechanisms, Prevention, and Treatment. Baltimore, Williams & Wilkins, 1994.
9. Kelly, J.P.: Maxillofacial injuries. In Zachazewski, J.E., D.J. Magee, W.S. Quillen (eds.): Athletic Injuries and Rehabilitation. Philadelphia, W.B. Saunders Co., 1996.
10. Cantu, R.C.: Guidelines for return to contact sports after cerebral concussion. Phys. Sportsmed. 14:75–83, 1986.
11. Robert, W.O.: Who plays? Who sits? Managing concussions on the sidelines. Phys. Sportsmed. 20:66–72, 1992.
12. Topel, J.L.: Examination of the comatose patient. In Weiner, W.J., and C.G. Goetz (eds.): Neurology for the Non-Neurologist. Philadelphia, J.B. Lippincott, 1989.
13. Levin, H.S., V.M. O'Donnell, and R.G. Grossman: The Galveston orientation and amnesia test: A practical scale to assess cognition after head injury. J. Nerv. Ment. Dis. 167:675–684, 1979.
14. Fonseca, R.J., and R.V. Walker: Oral and Maxillofacial Trauma. Philadelphia, W.B. Saunders Co., 1991.
15. Pollock, R.A., and R.O. Dingman: Management and reconstruction of athletic injuries of the face, anterior neck, and upper respiratory tract. In Schneider, R.C., J.C. Kennedy, and M.L. Plant (eds.): Sports Injuries—Mechanisms, Treatment and Prevention. Baltimore, Williams & Wilkins, 1985.
16. Simpson, J.F., and K.R. Magee: Clinical Evaluation of the Nervous System. Boston, Little, Brown & Co., 1973.

General References

Ad Hoc Committee on Classification of Headache: Classification of headache. Arch. Neurol. 6:173–176, 1962.
American Academy of Orthopedic Surgeons: Athletic Training and Sports Medicine. Chicago, AAOS, 1991.
Booher, J.M., and G.A. Thibodeau: Athletic Injury Assessment. St. Louis, C.V. Mosby Co., 1989.
Boyd-Monk, H.: Examining the external eye. Nursing 80:58–63, 1980.
Bruce, R., and R.J. Fonseca: Mandibular fractures. In Fonseca, R.J., and R.V. Walker (eds.): Oral and Maxillofacial Trauma. Philadelphia, W.B. Saunders Co., 1991.
Brucker, A.J., D.M. Kozart, C.W. Nichols, and I.M. Raber: Diagnosis and management of injuries to the eye and orbit. In Torg, J.S. (ed.): Athletic Injuries to the Head, Neck and Face. St. Louis, Mosby–Year Book Inc., 1991.
Bruno, L.A., T.A. Gennarelli, and J.S. Torg: Head injuries in athletics. In Welsh, R.P., and R.J. Shephard (eds.): Current Therapy in Sports Medicine 1985–1986. St. Louis, C.V. Mosby Co., 1985.
Bruno, L.A., T.A. Gennarelli, and J.S. Torg: Management guidelines for head injuries in athletics. Clin. Sports Med. 6:17–29, 1987.
Burde, R.M.: Eye movements and vestibular system. In Pearlman, A.L., and R.C. Collins (eds.): Neurological Pathophysiology. New York, Oxford University Press, 1984.
Caillet, R.: Head and Face Pain Syndromes. Philadelphia, F.A. Davis Co., 1992.
Canter, R.C.: Guidelines for return to contact sports after a cerebral concussion. Phys. Sportsmed. 14:75–83, 1986.
Cox, M.S., C.L. Schepens, and H.M. MacKenzie Freeman: Retinal detachment due to ocular contusion. Arch. Ophthal. 76:678–685, 1966.
Crovitz, H.F., and W.F. Daniel: Length of retrograde amnesia after head injury: a revised formula. Cortex 23:695–698, 1987.

Diamond, G.R., G.E. Quinn, T.J. Pashby, and M. Easterbrook: Ophthalmologic injuries. Clin. Sports Med. 1:469–482, 1982.

Easterbrook, M., and J. Cameron: Injuries in racquet sports. In Schneider, R.C., J.C. Kennedy, and M.L. Plant (eds.): Sports Injuries—Mechanisms, Treatment and Prevention. Baltimore, Williams & Wilkins, 1985.

Edelman, R.R., and J.R. Hesselink: Clinical Magnetic Resonance Imaging. Philadelphia, W.B. Saunders Co., 1990.

Ellis, E.: Fractures of the zygomatic complex and arch. In Fonseca, R.J., and R.V. Walker (eds.): Oral and Maxillofacial Trauma. Philadelphia, W.B. Saunders Co., 1991.

Fahey, T.D.: Athletic Training—Principles and Practice. Palo Alto, California, Mayfield Pub. Co., 1986.

Foreman, S.M., and A.C. Croft: Whiplash Injuries—The Cervical Acceleration/Deceleration Syndrome. Baltimore, Williams & Wilkins, 1988.

Frost, D.E., and B.D. Kendall: Applied surgical anatomy of the head and neck. In Fonseca, R.J., and R.V. Walker (eds.): Oral and Maxillofacial Trauma. Philadelphia, W.B. Saunders Co., 1991.

Garrison, D.W.: Cranial Nerves—A Systems Approach. Springfield, Illinois, Charles C Thomas Pub., 1986.

Gorman, B.D.: Ophthalmology and sports medicine. In Scott, W.N., B. Nisonson, and J.A. Nicholas (eds.): Principles of Sports Medicine. Baltimore, Williams & Wilkins, 1984.

Greenberg, M.S., and P.S. Springer: Diagnosis and management of oral injuries. In Torg, J.S. (ed.): Athletic Injuries to the Head, Neck, and Face. St. Louis, Mosby–Year Book Inc., 1991.

Halling, A.H.: The importance of clinical signs and symptoms in the evaluation of facial fractures. Athletic Training 17:102–103, 1982.

Handler, S.D.: Diagnosis and management of maxillofacial injuries. In Torg, J.S. (ed.): Athletic Injuries to the Head, Neck and Face. Philadelphia, Lea & Febiger, 1982.

Havener, W.H., and T.A. Makley: Emergency management of ocular injuries. Ohio State Med. J. 71:776–779, 1975.

Hayward, R.: Management of Acute Head Injuries. Oxford, Blackwell Scientific Pub., 1980.

Hildebrandt, J.R.: Dental and maxillofacial injuries. Clin. Sports Med. 1:449–468, 1982.

Hollinshead, W.H., and D.B. Jenkins: Functional Anatomy of the Limbs and Back. Philadelphia, W.B. Saunders Co., 1981.

Hugenholtz, H., and M.T. Richard: Return to athletic competition following concussion. CMA J. 127:827–829, 1982.

Jenkins, D.B.: Hollinshead's Functional Anatomy of the Limbs and Back. Philadelphia, W.B. Saunders Co., 1991.

Jordan, B.D.: Head injury in sports. In Jordan, B.D., P. Tsairis, and R.F. Warren (eds.): Sports Neurology. Rockville, Maryland. Aspen Publishers Inc., 1989.

Kinderknecht, J.J.: Head injuries. In Zachazewski, J.E., D.J. Magee, W.S. Quillen (eds.): Athletic Injuries and Rehabilitation. Philadelphia, W.B. Saunders Co., 1996.

Kulund, D.N.: The Injured Athlete. Philadelphia, J.B. Lippincott Co., 1988.

Kumamoto, D.P., M. Jacob, and D. Nickelsen: Oral trauma: On field assessment. Phys. Sportsmed. 23:53–62, 1995.

Lampert, P.W., and J.M. Hardman: Morphological changes in brains of boxers. JAMA 251:2676–2679, 1984.

Lew, D., and D.P. Sinn: Diagnosis and treatment of midface fractures. In Fonseca, R.J., and R.V. Walker (eds.): Oral and Maxillofacial Trauma. Philadelphia, W.B. Saunders Co., 1991.

Liebgott, B.: The Anatomical Basis of Dentistry. St. Louis, C.V. Mosby, 1986.

Mueller, F.D.: Catastrophic head and neck injuries. Phys. Sportsmed. 7:710–714, 1979.

Nasher, L.M.: A Systems Approach to Understanding and Assessing Orientation and Balance Disorders. Clackamas, Oregon, NeuroCom International Inc., 1987.

O'Donoghue, D.H.: Treatment of Injuries to Athletes. Philadelphia, W.B. Saunders Co., 1984.

Pashby, R.C., and T.J. Pashby: Ocular injuries in sports. In Welsh, R.P., and R.J. Shephard (eds.): Current Therapy in Sports Medicine 1985–1986. St. Louis, C.V. Mosby Co., 1985.

Paton, D., and M.F. Goldberg: Management of Ocular Injuries. Philadelphia, W.B. Saunders Co., 1976.

Pavlov, H.: Radiographic evaluation of the skull and facial bones. In Torg, J.S. (ed.): Athletic Injuries to the Head, Neck, and Face. St. Louis, Mosby–Year Book Inc., 1991.

Powers, M.P.: Diagnosis and management of dentoalveolar injuries. In Fonseca, R.J., and R.V. Walker (eds.): Oral and Maxillofacial Trauma. Philadelphia, W.B. Saunders Co., 1991.

Reid, D.C.: Sports Injury Assessment and Rehabilitation. New York, Churchill Livingstone, 1992.

Rimel, R.W., B. Giordani, J.T. Barth, T.J. Boll, and J.J. Jane: Disability caused by minor head injury. Neurosurg. 9:221–228, 1981.

Root, J.D., B.D. Jordan, and R.D. Zimmerman: Delayed presentation of subdural hematoma. Phys. Sportsmed. 21:61–68, 1993.

Ross, R.J., I.R. Casson, O. Siegel, and M. Cole: Boxing injuries: Neurologic, radiologic and neuropsychologic evaluation. Clin. Sports Med. 6:41–51, 1987.

Rousseau, A.P.: Ocular trauma in sports. In MacKenzie Freeman, H.M. (ed.): Ocular Trauma in Sports. New York, Appleton-Century-Crofts, 1979.

Roy, S., and R. Irvin: Sports Medicine—Prevention, Evaluation, Management and Rehabilitation. Englewood Cliffs, New Jersey, Prentice-Hall Inc., 1983.

Sandusky, J.C.: Field evaluation of eye injuries. Athletic Training 16:254–258, 1981.

Schneider, R.C.: Head and Neck Injuries in Football—Mechanisms, Treatment and Prevention. Baltimore, Williams & Wilkins, 1973.

Schneider, R.C., T.R. Peterson, and R.E. Anderson: Football. In Schneider, R.C., J.C. Kennedy, and M.L. Plant (eds.): Sports Injuries—Mechanisms, Prevention and Treatment. Baltimore, Williams & Wilkins, 1985.

Schuller, D.E., and R.A. Bruce: Ear, nose, throat, and eye. In Strauss, R.H. (ed.): Sports Medicine, 2nd ed. Philadelphia, W.B. Saunders Co., 1991.

Schultz, R.C., and D.L. de Camara: Athletic facial injuries. JAMA 252:3395–3398, 1984.

Scott, W.N., B. Nisonson, and J.A. Nicholas (eds.): Principles of Sports Medicine. Baltimore, Williams & Wilkins, 1984.

Shell, D., G.A. Carico, and R.M. Patton: Can subdural hematoma result from repeated minor head injury? Phys. Sportsmed. 21:74–84, 1993.

Sinn, D.P., and N.D. Karas: Radiographic evaluation of facial injuries. In Fonseca, R.J., and V. Walker (eds.): Oral and Maxillofacial Trauma. Philadelphia, W.B. Saunders Co., 1991.

Sitler, M.: Nasal septal injuries. Athletic Training 21:10–12, 1986.

Solon, R.C.: Maxillofacial trauma. In Scott, W.N., B. Nisonson, and J.A. Nicholas (eds.): Principles of Sports Medicine. Baltimore, Williams & Wilkins, 1984.

Starkey, C., and J. Ryan: Evaluation of Orthopedic and Athletic Injuries. Philadelphia, F.A. Davis Co., 1996.

Untevharnscheidt, F.: Boxing injuries. In Schneider, R.C., J.C. Kennedy, and M.L. Plant (eds.): Sports Injuries—Mechanisms, Prevention and Treatment. Baltimore, Williams & Wilkins, 1985.

Vegso, J.J., and R.C. Lehman: Field evaluation and management of head and neck injuries. Clin. Sports Med. 6:1–15, 1987.

Vegso, J.J., and J.S. Torg: Field evaluation and management of intracranial injuries. In Torg, J.S. (ed.): Athletic Injuries to the Head, Neck and Face. Philadelphia, Lea & Febiger, 1982.

Vinger, P.F.: How I manage corneal abrasions and lacerations. Phys. Sportsmed. 14:170–179, 1986.

Wester, I.: Bell's palsy: the present status of electrodiagnosis and treatment. Physiother. Can. 23:218–221, 1971.

Zagelbaum, B.M., and M.A. Hochman: A close look at a 'red eye'—diagnosing vision-threatening causes. Phys. Sportsmed. 23:85–92, 1995.

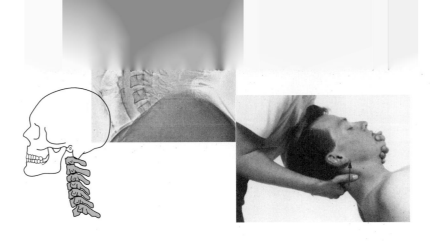

Cervical Spine

Examination of the cervical spine involves determining whether the injury or pathology occurs in the cervical spine or in a portion of the upper limb. Cyriax called this assessment the **scanning examination**.[1] In the initial assessment of a patient who complains of pain in the neck and/or upper limb, this procedure is always carried out unless the examiner is absolutely sure of the location of the lesion. If the injury is in the neck, the scanning examination is definitely called for. After the lesion site has been determined, a more detailed assessment of the affected area is performed if it is outside the cervical spine.

Because many conditions affecting the cervical spine can be manifested in other parts of the body, the cervical spine is a complicated area to assess properly, and adequate time must be allowed to ensure that as many causes or problems are examined as possible.

Applied Anatomy

The cervical spine consists of several joints. It is an area in which stability has been sacrificed for mobility, making the cervical spine particularly vulnerable to injury. The **atlanto-occipital joints** (C0–C1) are the two uppermost joints. The principal motion of these two joints is flexion-extension (15 to 20°), or nodding of the head. Side flexion is approximately 10°, whereas rotation is negligible. The **atlas** (C1) has no vertebral body as such. During development, the vertebral body of C1 evolves into the **odontoid process**, which is part of C2. The atlanto-occipital joints are ellipsoid and act in unison. Along with the atlanto-axial joints, these joints are the most complex articulations of the axial skeleton.

The **atlantoaxial joints** (C1–C2) constitute the most mobile articulations of the spine. Flexion-extension is approximately 10°, and side flexion is approximately 5°. Rotation, which is approximately 50°, is the primary movement of these joints. With rotation, there is a decrease in height of the cervical spine at this level as the vertebrae approximate because of the shape of the facet joints. The odontoid process of C2 acts as a pivot point for the rotation. This middle, or median, joint is classified as a **pivot (trochoidal) joint**. The lateral atlantoaxial, or facet, joints are classified as **plane joints**. Generally, if a person can talk and chew, there is probably some motion occurring at C1–C2.

It must be remembered that rotation past 50° in the cervical spine may lead to kinking of the contralateral vertebral artery; the ipsilateral vertebral artery may kink at 45° of rotation (Fig. 3–1). This kinking may lead to

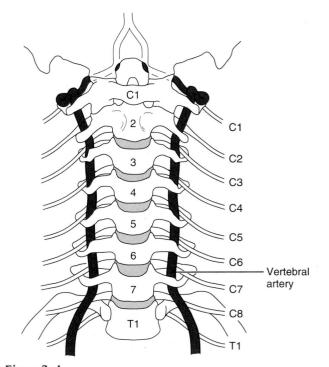

Figure 3–1
Course of vertebral artery in the cervical spine (anterior view). Note double turn at C1 as the artery wraps around the atlas.

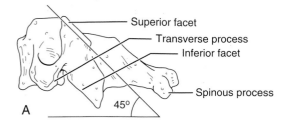

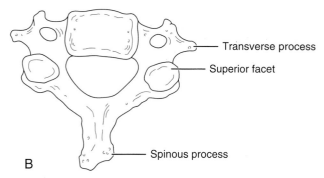

Figure 3–2

Cervical spine—plane of facet joints. (A) Lateral view. (B) Superior view.

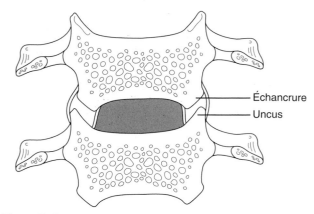

Figure 3–3

Joints of Luschka.

vertigo, nausea, tinnitus, "drop attacks" (fainting), visual disturbances, or in rare cases, stroke or death.

There are 14 **facet** (apophyseal) **joints** in the cervical spine. The upper four facet joints in the two upper thoracic vertebrae are often included in the examination of the cervical spine. The superior facets of the cervical spine face upward, backward, and medially; the inferior facets face downward, forward, and laterally (Fig. 3–2). This plane facilitates flexion and extension, but it prevents simple rotation or side flexion without both occurring to some degree together. These joints move primarily by gliding and are classified as **synovial (diarthrodial) joints**. The capsules are lax to allow for sufficient movement. At the same time, they provide support and a check-rein type of restriction. The greatest flexion-extension of the facet joints occurs between C5 and C6; however, there is almost as much movement at C4–C5 and C6–C7. Because of this mobility, degeneration is most likely to be seen at these levels. The neutral or resting position of the cervical spine is slightly extended. The close packed position of the facet joints is complete extension. The facet joints are highly innervated by the **recurrent meningeal or sinuvertebral nerve**.

Cervical Spine	
Resting position:	Slight extension
Close packed position:	Full extension
Capsular pattern:	Side flexion and rotation equally limited, extension

Some anatomists[2–5] refer to the costal or uncovertebral processes as **uncinate joints** or **joints of Luschka** (Fig. 3–3). These structures were described by von Luschka in 1858. The uncus gives a "saddle" form to the upper aspect of the cervical vertebra which is more pronounced posterolaterally; it has the effect of limiting side flexion. Extending from the uncus is a "joint" that appears to form because of a weakness in the annulus fibrosus. The portion of the vertebra above, which "articulates" or conforms to the uncus, is called the échancrure, or notch. Notches are found from C3 to T1, but according to most authors,[2–5] they are not seen until age 6 to 9 years and are not fully developed until 18 years of age. There is some controversy as to whether they should be classified as real joints, because some authors believe they are the result of degeneration of the intervertebral disc; degeneration tends to occur faster in the cervical spine than in any other part of the spine.

The **intervertebral discs** make up approximately 25% of the height of the cervical spine. No disc is found between the atlas and the occiput (C0–C1) or between the atlas and the axis (C1–C2). It is the discs rather than the vertebrae that give the cervical spine its lordotic shape (Fig. 3–4). The **nucleus pulposus** functions as a buffer to axial compression in distributing compressive forces, whereas the **annulus fibrosus** acts to withstand tension within the disc. Although it is generally believed that the intervertebral disc has no innervation, research indicates there may be some innervation on the periphery of the annulus fibrosus.[6, 7]

There are seven vertebrae in the cervical spine, with the body of each vertebra (except C1) supporting the weight of those above it. The facet joints may bear some of the weight of the vertebrae above, but this weight is minimal. However, even this slight amount of weight bearing can lead to spondylitic changes in these joints. The outer ring of the vertebral body is made of cortical bone, and the inner part is made of cancellous bone covered with the cartilaginous end plate. The vertebral arch protects the spinal cord; the spinous processes,

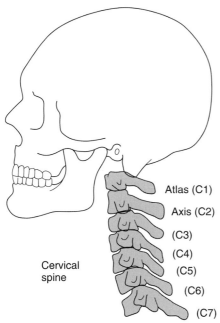

Figure 3–4
Lateral view of cervical spine and head.

most of which are bifid in the cervical spine, provide for attachment of muscles. The transverse processes have basically the same function. In the cervical spine, the spinous processes are at the level of the facet joints of the same vertebra. Generally, the spinous process is considered to be absent or at least rudimentary on C1. This is why the first palpable vertebra descending from

the external occiput protuberance is the spinous process of C2.

Although there are seven cervical vertebrae, there are eight **cervical nerve roots**. This difference occurs because there is a nerve root between the occiput and C1 that is designated the C1 nerve root. In the cervical spine, each nerve root is named for the vertebra below it. As an example, C5 nerve root exists between the C4 and C5 vertebrae (Fig. 3–5). In the rest of the spine, each nerve root is named for the vertebra above; the L4 nerve root, for example, exists between the L4 and L5 vertebrae. The switch in naming of the nerve roots from the one below to the one above is made between the C7 and T1 vertebrae. The nerve root between these two vertebrae is called C8, accounting for the fact that there are eight cervical nerve roots and only seven cervical vertebrae.

Patient History

In addition to the questions listed under Patient History in Chapter 1, the examiner should obtain the following information from the patient.

1. What is the patient's age? Spondylosis is often seen in persons 25 years of age or older, and it is present in 60% of those older than 45 years and 85% of those older than 65 years of age. Symptoms of osteoarthritis do not usually appear until a person is 60 years of age or older (Table 3–1).

2. How severe are the symptoms? Was the patient moving when the injury occurred? Watkins[8] provided a severity scale for neurological injury in football that can be used as a guideline for injury severity, especially if one is contemplating allowing the patient to return to activity (Fig. 3–6). A combined score (A+B) of 4 is considered a mild episode, 4 to 7 is a moderate episode, and 8 to 10 is a severe episode. This scale can be combined with radiologic information on canal size (score C) to give a general determination of the possibility of symptoms returning if the patient returns to activity. In this case, a score of 6 (A+B+C) indicates minimum risk, 6 to 10 is moderate risk, and 10 to 15 is severe risk. Watkins[8] also points out that extenuating factors such as age of patient, level of activity, and risk versus benefit also play a role and, although not included in the score, must be considered.

3. What was the mechanism of injury? Was trauma, stretching, or overuse involved? These questions help determine the type of injury. For example, trauma may cause a whiplash injury, stretching may lead to "burners," overuse or sustained postures may result in thoracic outlet symptoms, and a report of an insidious onset in someone older than 55 years of age may indicate cervical

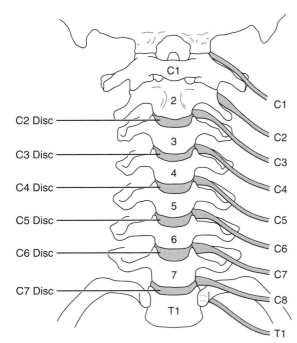

Figure 3–5
Anterior view of cervical spine showing nerve roots. Note how each cervical nerve root is numbered for the vertebra below it.

Table 3–1
Differential Diagnosis of Cervical Spondylosis, Spinal Stenosis, and Disc Herniation

	Cervical Spondylosis	Cervical Spinal Stenosis	Cervical Disc Herniation
Pain	Unilateral	May be unilateral or bilateral	May be unilateral (most common) or bilateral
Distribution of pain	Into affected dermatomes	Usually several dermatomes affected	Into affected dermatomes
Pain on extension	Increases	Increases	Increases
Pain on flexion	Decreases	Decreases	May increase or decrease (most common)
Pain relieved by rest	No	Yes	No
Age group affected	60% of those >45 yr 85% of those >60 yr	11–70 yr Most common: 30–60 yr	17–60 yr
Instability	Possible	No	No
Levels commonly affected	C5–C6, C6–C7	Varies	C5–C6
Onset	Slow	Slow (may be combined with spondylosis or disc herniation)	Sudden
Diagnostic imaging	Diagnostic	Diagnostic	Diagnostic

Watkins' Severity Scale for Neurological Deficit

Grade	Neurological Deficit
1	Unilateral arm numbness or dysesthesia; loss of strength
2	Bilateral upper extremity loss of motor and sensory function
3	Ipsilateral arm, leg, and trunk loss of motor and sensory function
4	Transient quadriparesis (temporary sensory loss in all 4 limbs)
5	Transient quadriplegia (temporary motor loss in all 4 limbs)

Score:_____ (A)

Grade	Time Symptoms Present
1	Less than 5 minutes
2	Less than 1 hour
3	less than 24 hours
4	Less than 1 week
5	Greater than 1 week

Score:_____ (B)

Severity Score: A + B = _____
(≤4: mild episode; 4–7: moderate episode; 8–10: severe episode)

Grade	Central Canal Diameter
1	>12 mm
2	Between 10–12
3	10 mm
4	8–10 mm
5	<8 mm

Score:_____ (C)

Return to Activity Score: A + B + C = _____
(≤6: minimum risk; 6–10: moderate risk; 10–15: severe risk)

Figure 3–6

Watkins' severity scale for neurological deficit. (Data from Watkins, R.G.: Neck injuries in football. In Watkins, R.G. [ed.]: The Spine in Sports. St. Louis, Mosby–Year Book Inc., 1996, p. 327.)

Table 3–2
Differential Diagnosis of Cervical Nerve Root and Brachial Plexus Lesions

	Cervical Nerve Root Lesion	**Brachial Plexus Lesion**
Cause	Disc herniation Stenosis Osteophytes Swelling with trauma Spondylosis	Stretching of cervical spine Compression of cervical spine Depression of shoulder
Contributing factors	Congenital defects	Thoracic outlet syndrome
Pain	Sharp, burning in affected dermatomes	Sharp, burning in all or most of arm dermatomes, pain in trapezius
Paresthesia	Numbness, pins and needles in affected dermatomes	Numbness, pins and needles in all or most arm dermatomes (more ambiguous distribution)
Tenderness	Over affected area of posterior cervical spine	Over affected area of brachial plexus or lateral to cervical spine
Range of motion	Decreased	Decreased but usually returns rather quickly
Weakness	Transient paralysis usually Myotome may be affected	Transient muscle weakness Myotomes affected
Deep tendon reflexes	Usually normal	May be depressed
Provocative test	Side flexion, rotation, and extension with compression increase symptoms Cervical traction decreases symptoms Upper limb tension tests positive	Side flexion with compression (same side) or stretch (opposite side) may increase symptoms Upper limb tension tests may be positive

spondylosis (Table 3–2). Was the patient hit from the side, front, or behind? Did the patient see the accident coming? "Burners" or "stingers" typically occur from a blow to part of the brachial plexus or from stretching or compression of the brachial plexus (Fig. 3–7). The answers to these questions help the examiner determine how the injury occurred, the tissues injured, and the severity of the injuries.

4. What is the patient's usual activity or pastime? Do any particular activities or postures bother the patient? What type of work does the patient do? Are there any positions that the patient holds for long periods (e.g., when sewing, typing, or working at a desk)? Does the patient wear glasses? If so, are they bifocals or trifocals?

Cervicothoracic joint problems are often painful when activities that require push-and-pull motion, such as lawnmowing, sawing, and cleaning windows, are performed.

5. Did the head strike anything, or did the patient lose consciousness? If the injury was caused by a motor vehicle accident, it is important to know whether the patient was wearing a seat belt, the type of seat belt (lap or shoulder), and whether the patient saw the accident coming. These questions give some idea of the severity and mechanisms of injury. If the patient was unconscious or unsteady, the character of each episode of altered consciousness should be noted (see Chapter 2).

6. Did the symptoms come on right away? Bone pain

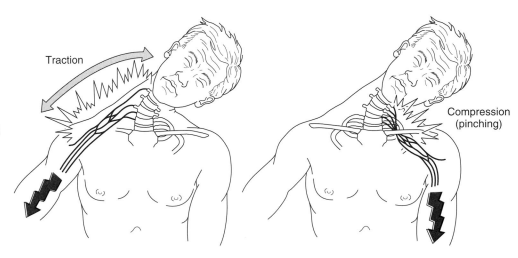

Figure 3–7
Mechanism of injury for brachial plexus (burner or stinger) pathology.

usually occurs immediately, but muscle or ligamentous pain can either come on immediately (e.g., a tear) or occur several hours or days later (e.g., stretching caused by a motor vehicle accident). How long have the symptoms been present? Myofascial pain syndromes demonstrate generalized aching and at least three trigger points, which have lasted for at least 3 months, with no history of trauma.[9]

7. What are the sites and boundaries of the pain? Have the patient point to the location or locations of the pain. Symptoms do not go down the arm for a C4

nerve root injury or for nerve roots above that level. **Cervical radiculopathy,** or injury to the nerve roots in the cervical spine, presents primarily with unilateral motor and sensory symptoms into the upper limb, with muscle weakness (myotome), sensory alteration (dermatome), reflex hypoactivity, and sometimes focal activity being the primary signs. **Cervical myelopathy,** or injury to the spinal cord itself, is more likely to present with spastic weakness, paresthesia, and possible incoordination in one or both lower limbs, as well as proprioceptive or sphincter dysfunction, or both (Table 3–3).[10]

Table 3–3
Differential Diagnosis of Neurological Disorders of the Cervical Spine and Upper Limb

Cervical Radiculopathy (Nerve Root Lesion)	Cervical Myelopathy	Brachial Plexus Lesion (Plexopathy)	Burner (Transient Brachial Plexus Lesion)	Peripheral Nerve (Upper Limb) Lesion
Arm pain in dermatome distribution	Hand numbness, head pain, hoarseness, vertigo, tinnitus, deafness	Pain more localized to shoulder and neck (sometimes face)	Temporary pain in dermatome	No pain
Pain increased by extension and rotation or side flexion	Extension, rotation, and side flexion may all cause pain	Pain on compression of brachial plexus	Pain on compression or stretch of brachial plexus	No pain early; if contracture occurs (late), pain on stretching
Pain may be relieved by putting hand on head	Arm positions have no effect on pain	Arm positions have no effect on pain*	Arm positions have no effect on pain*	Arm positions have no effect on pain*
Sensation (dermatome) affected	Sensation affected, abnormal pattern	Sensation (dermatome) affected	Sensation (dermatome) affected	Peripheral nerve sensation affected
Gait not affected	Wide-based gait, drop attacks, ataxia; proprioception affected	Gait not affected	Gait not affected	Gait not affected
Altered hand function	Loss of hand function	Loss of arm function	Loss of function temporary	Loss of function of muscles supplied by nerve
Bowel and bladder not affected	Possible loss of bowel and bladder control	Bowel and bladder not affected	Bowel and bladder not affected	Bowel and bladder not affected
Weakness in myotome but no spasticity	Spastic paresis (especially in lower limb early, upper limb affected later)	Weakness in myotome	Temporary weakness in myotome	Weakness of muscles supplied by nerve
Deep tendon reflexes (DTR) hyperactive Negative pathological reflex Negative superficial reflex	Lower limb DTR hyperactive Upper limb DTR hyperactive Positive pathological reflex Decreased superficial reflex	DTR hypoactive Negative pathological reflex Negative superficial reflex	DTR not affected Negative pathological reflex Negative superficial reflex	DTR may be decreased Negative pathological reflex Negative superficial reflex
Gait not affected	Gait affected	Gait not affected	Gait not affected	Gait not affected
Atrophy (late sign)	Atrophy	Atrophy	Atrophy	Atrophy (not usually with neuropraxia)

* Except in neurotension test positions.

8. Is there any radiation of pain? It is helpful to correlate this answer with dermatome and sensory peripheral nerve findings when performing sensation testing and palpation later in the examination. Is the pain deep? Superficial? Shooting? Burning? Aching? For example, when an athlete experiences a "burner," the sensation is a lightning-like, burning pain into the shoulder and arm, followed by a period of heaviness or loss of function in the arm.

9. Is the pain affected by laughing? Coughing? Sneezing? Straining? If so, an increase in intrathoracic or intra-abdominal pressure may be causing the problem.

10. Does the patient have any headaches? If so, where? How frequently do they occur? How intense are they? How long do they last? Are there any precipitating factors (e.g., food, stress, posture)? See Tables 2–5, 2–6, and 2–7 which indicate the influence of time of day, body position, headache location, and type of pain on diagnosis of the type of headache the patient may have. Table 2–8 outlines the salient features of some of the more common headaches. For example, C1 headaches occur at the base and top of the head, whereas C2 headaches are referred to the temporal area.

Signs of Headaches Having a Cervical Origin

- Occipital or suboccipital component to headache
- Neck movement alters headache
- Painful limitation of neck movements
- Abnormal head or neck posture
- Suboccipital or nuchal tenderness
- Abnormal mobility at C0–C1
- Sensory abnormalities in the occipital and suboccipital areas

11. Does a position change alter the headache or pain? If so, which positions increase or decrease the pain? Sometimes, the patient may state that the pain and referred symptoms are decreased or relieved by placing the hand or arm of the affected side on top of the head. This is called **Bakody's sign,** and it usually is indicative of problems in the C4 or C5 area.[11, 12]

12. Is paresthesia (a "pins and needles" feeling) present? This sensation occurs if pressure is applied to the nerve root. It may become evident if pressure is relieved from a nerve trunk. Numbness and/or paresthesia in the hands or legs and deteriorating hand function all may relate to cervical myelopathy.

13. Does the patient experience any tingling in the extremities? Are the symptoms bilateral? Bilateral symptoms usually indicate either systemic disorders (e.g., diabetes, alcohol abuse) that are causing neuropathies or central space-occupying lesions.

14. Are there any lower limb symptoms? This finding may indicate a severe problem affecting the spinal cord (myelopathy). These symptoms may include numbness, paresthesia, stumbling, difficulty walking, and lack of balance or agility. All of these symptoms could indicate cervical myelopathy. Likewise, signs of sphincter (bowel or bladder) or sexual dysfunction may be related to cervical myelopathy.

15. Does the patient have any difficulty walking? Does the patient have problems with balance? Does the patient stumble when walking, have trouble walking in the dark, or walk with feet wide apart? Positive responses may indicate a cervical myelopathy. Abnormality of the cranial nerves combined with gait alterations may indicate systemic neurological dysfunction.[13]

16. Does the patient experience dizziness, faintness, or seizures? What is the degree, frequency, and duration of the dizziness? Is it associated with certain head positions or body positions? Semicircular canal problems or vertebral artery problems can lead to dizziness. Complete passing out (fainting) is sometimes called a **drop attack.** Has the patient experienced any visual disturbances? Disturbances such as diplopia (double vision), **nystagmus** ("dancing eyes"), scotomas (depressed visual field), and loss of acuity may indicate severity of injury, neurological injury, and sometimes increased intracranial pressure (see Chapter 2).[11]

17. Does the patient exhibit or complain of any sympathetic symptoms? There may be injury to the cranial nerves or the sympathetic nervous system, which lies in the soft tissues of the neck anterior and lateral to the cervical vertebrae. The cranial nerves and their functions are shown in Table 2–1. Some of the sympathetic signs and symptoms the examiner may elicit are "ringing" in the ears, dizziness, blurred vision, photophobia, rhinorrhea, sweating, lacrimation, and hypothemia (loss of strength).

18. Is the condition improving? Worsening? Staying the same? The answers to these questions give the examiner some indication of the condition's progress.

19. Which activities aggravate the problem? Which activities ease the problem? Are there any head or neck positions that the patient finds particularly bothersome? These positions should be noted. For example, does reading (flexed cervical spine) bother the patient? If symptoms are not varied by a change in position, the problem is not likely to be mechanical in origin. Lesions of C3, C4, and C5 may affect the diaphragm and thereby affect breathing.

20. Does the patient complain of any restrictions when performing movements? If so, which movements are restricted? It is important that the patient not demonstrate the movements at this stage; the actual movements will be done during the examination.

21. Is the patient a mouth breather? Mouth breathing encourages forward head posture and increases activity of accessory respiratory muscles.

22. Is there any difficulty in swallowing (dysphagia), or have there been any voice changes? Such a change may be caused by neurological problems, mechanical pressure, or muscle incoordination. Pain on swallowing may be indicative of soft-tissue swelling in the throat, vertebral subluxation, osteophyte projection, or disc protrusion into the esophagus or pharynx. In addition, swallowing becomes more difficult and the voice becomes weaker as the neck is extended.

23. What can be learned about the patient's sleeping position? Is there any problem sleeping? How many pillows does the patient use, and what type are they (e.g., feather, foam)? Foam pillows tend to retain their shape and have more "bounce"; they do not offer as much support as a good feather pillow. What type of mattress does the patient use (e.g., hard, soft)? Does the patient "hug" the pillow or abduct the arms when sleeping? These positions can increase the stress on the lower cervical nerve roots.

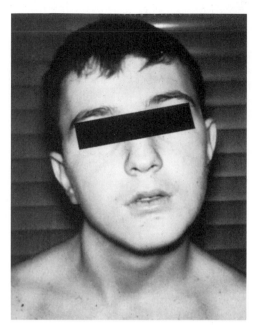

Figure 3–9

Example of torticollis showing prominent sternocleidomastoid muscle on the right. (From Gartland, J.J.: Fundamentals of Orthopedics. Philadelphia, W.B. Saunders Co., 1987, p. 279.)

Observation

For a proper observation, the patient must be suitably undressed. However, the examiner should also watch the patient as he or she enters the examination room, and before or while he or she undresses. The spontaneous movements of these activities can be very helpful in determining the patient's problems. For example, can the patient easily move the head when undressing? A male patient should wear only shorts, and a female patient should wear a bra and shorts for this part of the assessment. In some cases, the bra may have to be removed to determine whether there are any problems such as thoracic outlet syndrome, thoracic symptoms being referred to the cervical spine, or functional restriction of movement of the ribs. The examiner should note the willingness of the patient to move and the patterns of movement demonstrated. Facial expression of the patient can often give the examiner an indication of the amount of pain the patient is experiencing.

The patient may be seated or standing. Usually, a

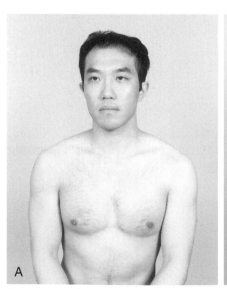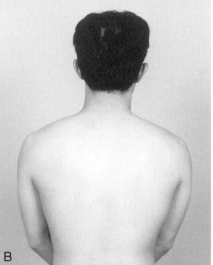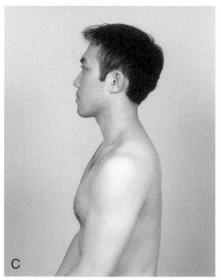

Figure 3–8

(A) through (C) Observation views of head and neck.

standing posture is best because the posture of the whole body can be observed (see Chapter 15). Abnormalities in one area frequently affect another area. For example, excessive lumbar lordosis may cause a "poking" chin to compensate for the lumbar deformity and to maintain the body's center of gravity. In the cervical spine region, the examiner should note the following.

Head and Neck Posture. Is the head in the midline (Fig. 3–8), or is there evidence of torticollis (Fig. 3–9), Klippel-Feil syndrome (Fig. 3–10), or other neck deformity? Does the patient exhibit a poking chin or a "military posture"? A habitual poking chin can result in adaptive shortening of the occipital muscles. Does the head sit in the middle of the shoulders? Is the head tilted or rotated to one side or the other, indicating possible torticollis? Does this posture appear to be habitual (in other words, does the patient always go back to this posture)? Habitual posture may result from postural compensation, weak muscles, hearing loss, temporomandibular joint problems, or wearing of bifocals or trifocals. The trapezius neck line should be equal on both sides. Head and neck posture should be checked with the patient sitting and then standing, and any differences should be noted.

Shoulder Levels. Usually the shoulder on the dominant side will be slightly lower than that on the nondominant side. With injury, the injured side may be elevated to provide protection. Rounded shoulders may be the result of or the cause of a poking chin. Rounding also causes the scapulae to protract, the humerus to medially rotate, and the anterior structures of the shoulder to tighten.

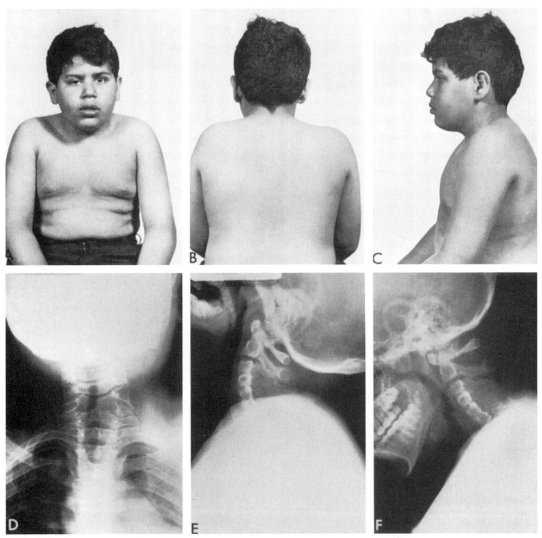

Figure 3–10
Klippel-Feil syndrome in a 12-year-old boy. (A) through (C) Clinical appearance of the patient. Note the short neck with the head appearing to sit directly on the thorax. (D) Anteroposterior and (E, F) lateral roentgenograms of the cervical spine. Note the failure of segmentation and the fusion into a homogeneous mass of bone of the four lower cervical vertebrae. (From Tachdjian, M.O.: Pediatric Orthopedics. Philadelphia, W.B. Saunders Co., 1972, p. 77.)

Muscle Spasm or Any Asymmetry. Is there any atrophy of the deltoid muscle (circumflex or axillary nerve palsy) or torticollis (spasm, prominence, or tightness of the sternocleidomastoid muscle)? (See Fig. 3–9.)

Facial Expression. The examiner should observe the patient's facial expression as the patient moves from position to position, makes different movements, and explains the problem. Such observation should give the examiner an idea of how much the patient is subjectively suffering.

Bony and Soft-Tissue Contours. If the cervical spine is injured, the head tends to be tilted and rotated away from the pain, and the face is tilted upward. If the patient is hysterical, the head tends to be tilted and rotated toward the pain, and the face is tilted down.

Evidence of Ischemia in Either Upper Limb. The examiner should note any altered coloration of the skin, ulcers, or vein distention as evidence of upper limb ischemia.

Normal Sitting Posture. The nose should be in line with the manubrium and xiphoid process of the sternum. From the side, the ear lobe should be in line with the acromion process and the high point on the iliac crest for proper postural alignment. The normal curve of the cervical spine is a lordotic type of curve. Referred pain from conditions such as spondylosis tends to occur in the shoulder and arm rather than the neck.

Examination

A complete examination of the cervical spine must be performed, including the neck and the upper limbs. Many of the symptoms that occur in an upper limb originate from the neck. Unless there is a history of definite trauma to a peripheral joint, a scanning examination must be done to rule out problems within the neck.

Active Movements

The first movements that are carried out are the active movements of the cervical spine, with the patient in the sitting position. The examiner is looking for differences in range of movement and in the patient's willingness to do the movement. The range of motion (ROM) taking place in this phase is the summation of all movements of the entire cervical spine, not just at one level. This combined movement allows for greater mobility in the cervical spine while still providing a firm support for the trunk and appendages. The ROM available in the cervical spine is the result of many factors, such as the flexibility of the intervertebral discs, the shape and inclination of the articular processes of the facet joints, and the slight laxity of the ligaments and joint capsules. Female patients tend to have a greater active range of motion than males, except in flexion, but the differences are not great.

The range available decreases with age, except rotation at C1–C2, which may increase.[14, 15]

The movements should be done in a particular order so that the most painful movements are done last and no residual pain is carried over from the previous movement.[1] If the patient has complained of pain on specific movements, these movements are done last. In the very acute cervical spine, only some movements—those that give the most information—are performed, to avoid undue exacerbation of symptoms.

While the patient performs the active movements, the examiner looks for limitation of movement and possible reasons for pain, spasm, stiffness, or blocking. As the patient reaches the full range of active movement, passive **overpressure** may be applied very carefully, but only if the movement appears to be full and pain free. The overpressure helps the examiner to test the end feel of the movement. The examiner must be careful when applying overpressure to rotation or any combination of rotation, side flexion, and extension.[16] In these positions, the vertebral artery is often compressed, which can lead to a decrease in blood supply to the brain. Should this occur, the patient may complain of dizziness or feel faint. If the patient exhibits these symptoms, the examiner must use extreme care during these movements, the rest of the assessment, and treatment.

The examiner can differentiate between movement in the upper and lower cervical spine. During flexion, **nodding** occurs in the upper cervical spine, whereas **flexion** occurs in the lower cervical spine. If the nodding movement does not occur, it indicates restriction of movement in the upper cervical spine; if flexion does not occur, it indicates restriction of motion in the lower cervical spine. Movement can occur between C1 and C2 without affecting the other vertebrae, but this is not true with other cervical vertebrae. In other words, for C2 to C7, if one vertebra moves, the ones adjacent to it will also move. The active movements that should be carried out in the cervical spine are as shown in Figure 3–11.

Flexion

For flexion, or forward bending, the maximum ROM is 80 to 90°. The extreme of ROM is normally found when the chin is able to reach the chest with the mouth closed; however, up to two finger widths between chin and chest

---

Active Movements of the Cervical Spine

- Flexion
- Extension
- Side flexion left and right
- Rotation left and right
- Combined movements (if necessary)
- Repetitive movements (if necessary)
- Sustained positions (if necessary)

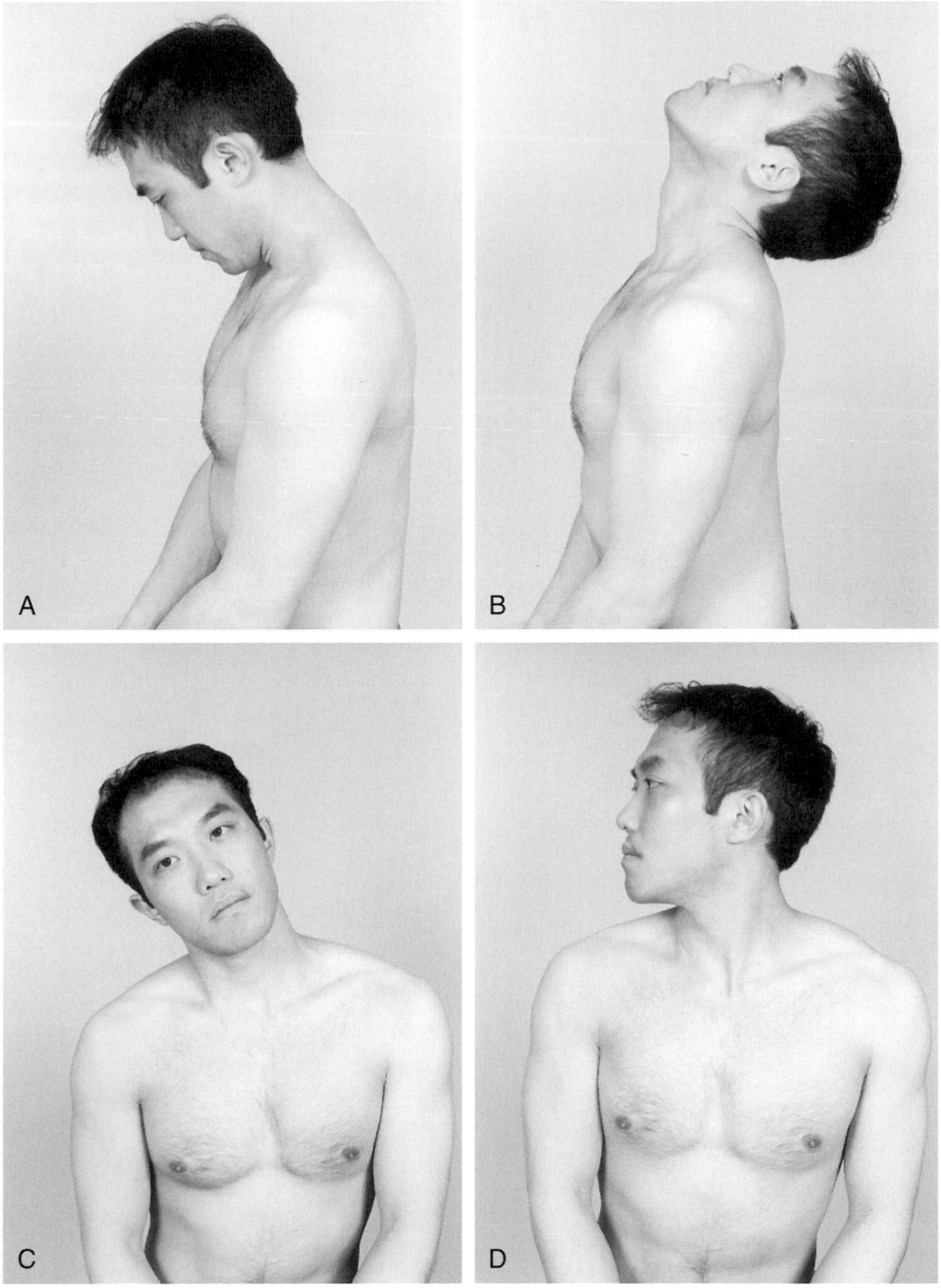

Figure 3–11

Active movements of the cervical spine. (A) Flexion. (B) Extension. (C) Side flexion. (D) Rotation.

is considered normal. In flexion, the intervertebral disc widens posteriorly and narrows anteriorly. The intervertebral foramen is 20 to 30% larger on flexion than on extension. The vertebrae shift forward in flexion and backward in extension. Also, the mastoid process moves away from the C1 transverse process on flexion and extension. As the patient forward flexes, the examiner should look for a posterior bulging of the spinous process of the axis. This bulging may result from forward subluxation of the atlas, which allows the spinous process of the axis to become more prominent. If this sign appears, the examiner should exercise **extreme caution** during the remainder of the cervical assessment. To verify the subluxation, the Sharp-Purser test (see under Special Tests) may be performed, but only with extreme care.

Extension

Extension, or backward bending, is normally limited to 70°. Because there is no anatomic block to stop movement going past this position, problems often result from whiplash or cervical strain. Normally, the plane of the nose and forehead is nearly horizontal. When the head is held in extension, the atlas tilts upward, resulting in posterior compression between the atlas and occiput.

Side Flexion

Side, or lateral, flexion is approximately 20 to 45° to the right and left. Most of the side flexion occurs between the occiput and C1 and between C1 and C2. When the patient does the movement, the examiner should ensure that the ear moves toward the shoulder and not the shoulder toward the ear.

Rotation

Normally, rotation is 70 to 90° right and left, and the chin does not quite reach the plane of the shoulder. Rotation and side flexion always occur together (coupled movement) in the cervical spine. This combined movement, which may or may not be visible in a given patient, occurs because of the shape of the articular surfaces of the facet joints; this shape is coronally oblique.

If, in the history, the patient has complained that **repetitive movements** or **sustained postures** have caused problems, not only should the specific movements be performed, but they should be either repeated several times or sustained to see if the symptoms are exacerbated. If a patient has complained in the history that a movement in other than a cardinal plane or a **combined movement** (e.g., side flexion, rotation, and extension combined) exacerbates the symptoms, then these movements should be performed as well. Figure 3–12 depicts active ROM of the cervical spine.

Passive Movements

If the patient does not have full ROM or the examiner has not applied overpressure to determine the end feel of the movement, the patient should be asked to lie in a supine position. The examiner then passively tests flexion, extension, side flexion, and rotation, as in the active movements. The passive ROM with the patient supine is normally greater than the active ROM with the patient sitting. For example, in sitting, active side flexion is about 45°, whereas in supine lying, passive side flexion is 75 to 80°, with the examiner often able to take the

---

> *Passive Movements of the*
> *Cervical Spine and Normal End Feel*
> _____
>
> - Flexion (tissue stretch)
> - Extension (tissue stretch)
> - Side flexion right and left (tissue stretch)
> - Rotation right and left (tissue stretch)

ear to the shoulder. This increased range in the supine position results from relaxation of the muscles that, in sitting, are trying to hold the head up against gravity. For the cervical spine, therefore, passive movements with overpressure should be performed along with active movements. Active movements with overpressure at end of range do not give a true impression of end feel for the cervical spine.

Passive movements are performed to determine the end feel of each movement. This may give the examiner an idea of the pathology involved. The normal **end feels** of the cervical spine motions are tissue stretch for all four movements. As with active movements, the most painful movements are done last. The examiner should also note whether a **capsular pattern** (i.e., side flexion and rotation equally limited; extension less limited) is present. Overpressure may be used to test the entire spine (Fig. 3–13A) by testing it at the end of the ROM, or proper positioning may be used to test different parts of the cervical spine.[17] For example, end feel for movement of the lower cervical spine into extension is tested with minimal extension and the head pushed directly posterior (Fig. 3–13C), whereas the upper cervical spine is tested by "nodding" the head into extension and pushing posteriorly at an approximate 45° angle (Fig. 3–13B).[18]

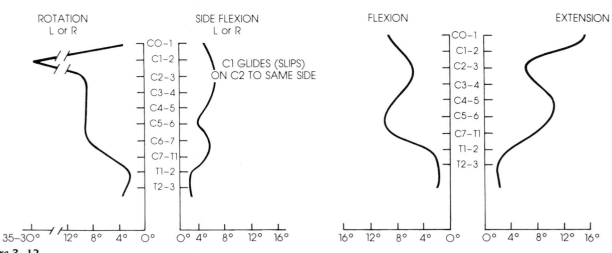

Figure 3–12

Average active range of motion in the cervical spine. Results for individual patients vary widely, depending on factors such as age and body type. (Adapted from Grieve, G.P.: Common Vertebral Joint Problems. Edinburgh, Churchill Livingstone, 1981, pp. 41, 42.)

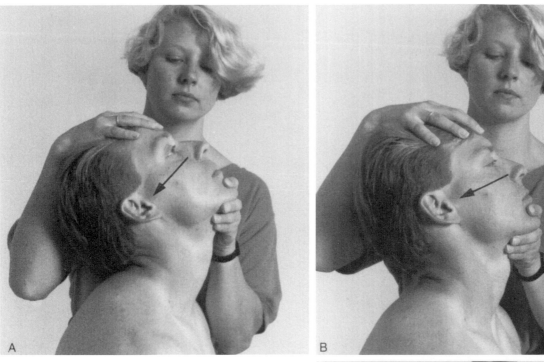

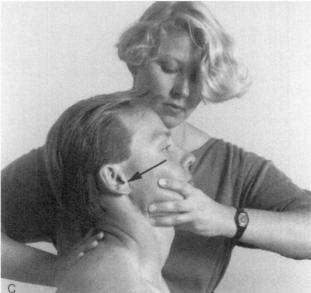

Figure 3–13

(A) Overpressure to the whole cervical spine. (B) Overpressure to the upper cervical spine. (C) Overpressure to the low cervical spine.

Resisted Isometric Movements

The same movements that were done actively (flexion, extension, side flexion, and rotation) are tested isometrically. It is better for the examiner to place the patient in the resting position and then say, "Don't let me move you," rather than to tell the patient, "Contract the muscle as hard as possible." In this way, the examiner ensures that the movement is as isometric as possible and that a minimal amount of movement occurs (Fig. 3–14). The examiner should ensure that these movements are done with the cervical spine in the neutral position and that painful movements are done last. Neck flexion tests cranial nerve XI and the C1 and C2 myotomes as well as

muscle strength or state. By using Table 3–4 and looking at the various combinations of muscles that cause the movement (Fig. 3–15), the examiner may be able to decide which muscle is at fault. If, in the history, the patient has complained that certain loaded or combined movements (those movements giving resistance other than gravity) are painful, the examiner should not hesitate to carefully test these movements isometrically to better ascertain the problem. If a neurological injury is suspected, the examiner must carefully assess for muscle weakness to determine the structures injured. If a severe neuropraxia or axonotmesis has occurred, there may be residual weakness even though muscle atrophy is not as evident.

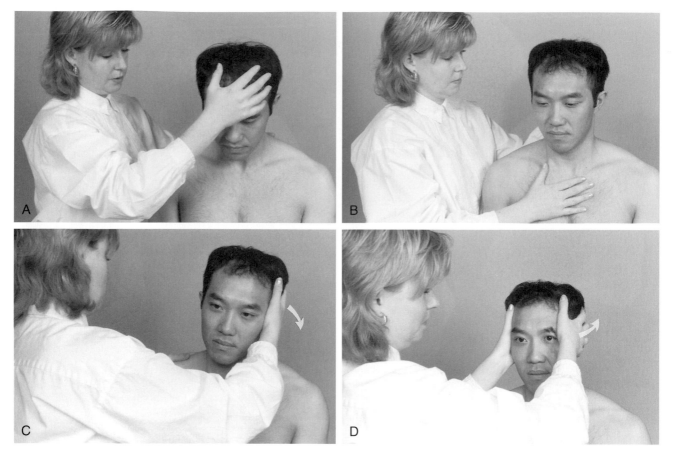

Figure 3–14

Positioning for resisted isometric movement. (A) Flexion. Note slight flexion of neck before giving resistance. (B) Extension. Note slight flexion of neck before giving resistance. (C) Side flexion (left side flexion shown). (D) Rotation (left rotation shown).

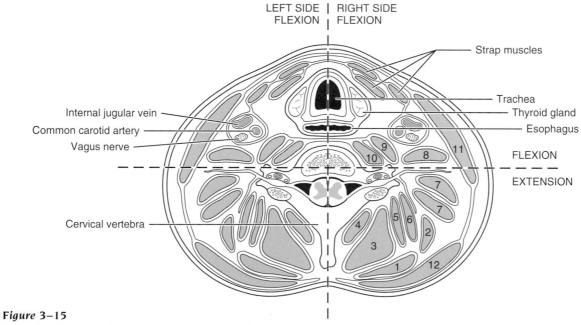

Figure 3–15

Anatomic relations of the lower cervical spine. (1) Splenius capitis. (2) Splenius cervicis. (3) Semispinalis cervicis and capitis. (4) Multifidus and rotatores. (5) Longissimus capitis. (6) Longissimus cervicis. (7) Levator scapulae. (8) Scalenus posterior. (9) Scalenus medius. (10) Scalenus anterior. (11) Sternocleidomastoid. (12) Trapezius.

Table 3–4
Muscles of the Cervical Spine: Their Actions and Nerve Supply

Action	Muscles Acting	Nerve Supply
Forward flexion of head	1. Rectus capitis anterior	C1–C2
	2. Rectus capitis lateralis	C1–C2
	3. Longus capitis	C1–C3
	4. Hyoid muscles	Inferior alveolar nerve
		Facial nerve
		Hypoglossal nerve
		Ansa cervicalis
	5. Obliquus capitis superior	C1
	6. Sternocleidomastoid (if head in neutral or flexion)	Accessory
		C2
Extension of head	1. Splenius capitis	C4–C6
	2. Semispinalis capitis	C1–C8
	3. Longissimus capitis	C6–C8
	4. Spinalis capitis	C6–C8
	5. Trapezius	Accessory
		C3–C4
	6. Rectus capitis posterior minor	C1
	7. Rectus capitis posterior major	C1
	8. Obliquus capitis superior	C1
	9. Obliquus capitis inferior	C1
	10. Sternocleidomastoid (if head in some extension)	Accessory
		C2
Rotation of head (muscles on one side contract)	1. Trapezius (face moves to opposite side)	Accessory
		C3, C4
	2. Splenius capitis (face moves to the same side)	C4–C6
	3. Longissimus capitis (face moves to same side)	C6–C8
	4. Semispinalis capitis (face moves to same side)	C1–C8
	5. Obliquus capitis inferior (face moves to same side)	C1
	6. Sternocleidomastoid (face moves to opposite side)	Accessory
		C2
Side flexion of head	1. Trapezius	Accessory
		C3–C4
	2. Splenius capitis	C4–C6
	3. Longissimus capitis	C6–C8
	4. Semispinalis capitis	C1–C8
	5. Obliquus capitis inferior	C1
	6. Rectus capitis lateralis	C1–C2
	7. Longus capitis	C1–C3
	8. Sternocleidomastoid	Accessory
		C2
Flexion of neck	1. Longus coli	C2–C6
	2. Scalenus anterior	C4–C6
	3. Scalenus medius	C3–C8
	4. Scalenus posterior	C6–C8
Extension of neck	1. Splenius cervicis	C6–C8
	2. Semispinalis cervicis	C1–C8
	3. Longissimus cervicis	C6–C8
	4. Levator scapulae	C3–C4
		Dorsal scapular
	5. Iliocostalis cervicis	C6–C8
	6. Spinalis cervicis	C6–C8
	7. Multifidus	C1–C8
	8. Interspinalis cervicis	C1–C8
	9. Trapezius	Accessory
		C3–C4
	10. Rectus capitus posterior major	C1
	11. Rotatores brevis	C1–C8
	12. Rotatores longi	C1–C8

Table continued on following page

Table 3-4
Muscles of the Cervical Spine: Their Actions and Nerve Supply (*Continued*)

Action	Muscles Acting	Nerve Supply
Side flexion of neck	1. Levator scapulae	C3–C4 Dorsal scapular
	2. Splenius cervicis	C4–C6
	3. Iliocostalis cervicis	C6–C8
	4. Longissimus cervicis	C6–C8
	5. Semispinalis cervicis	C1–C8
	6. Multifidus	C1–C8
	7. Intertransversarii	C1–C8
	8. Scaleni	C3–C8
	9. Sternocleidomastoid	Accessory C2
	10. Obliquus capitis inferior	C1
	11. Rotatores breves	C1–C8
	12. Rotatores longi	C1–C8
	13. Longus coli	C2–C6
Rotation* of neck (muscles on one side contract)	1. Levator scapulae (face moves to same side)	C3–C4 Dorsal scapular
	2. Splenius cervicis (face moves to same side)	C4–C6
	3. Iliocostalis cervicis (face moves to same side)	C6–C8
	4. Longissimus cervicis (face moves to same side)	C6–C8
	5. Semispinalis cervicis (face moves to same side)	C1–C8
	6. Multifidus (face moves to opposite side)	C1–C8
	7. Intertransversarii (face moves to same side)	C1–C8
	8. Scaleni (face moves to opposite side)	C3–C8
	9. Sternocleidomastoid (face moves to opposite side)	Accessory C2
	10. Obliquus capitis inferior (face moves to same side)	C1
	11. Rotatores brevis (face moves to same side)	C1–C8
	12. Rotatores longi (face moves to same side)	C1–C8

* Occurs in conjunction with side flexion owing to direction of facet joints.

Resisted Isometric Movements of the Cervical Spine

- Flexion
- Extension
- Side flexion right and left
- Rotation right and left

Peripheral Joint Scanning Examination

After the resisted isometric movements to the cervical spine have been completed, the peripheral joints should be quickly scanned to rule out obvious pathology in the extremities and to note areas that may need more detailed assessment.[1] The following joints are scanned bilaterally.

Temporomandibular Joints. The examiner checks the movement of the joints by placing the index or little fingers in the patient's ears (Fig. 3–16). The pulp aspect of the finger is placed forward to feel for equality of movement of the condyles of the temporomandibular joints and for clicking or grinding as well as to ensure that the ears are clear. Pain or tenderness, especially on closing the mandible, usually indicates posterior capsulitis. As the patient opens the mouth, the condyle moves forward. To open the mouth fully, the condyle must rotate and translate equally bilaterally. If this does not occur,

---

Peripheral Joint Scanning Examination

Temporomandibular joints	• Open mouth • Closed mouth
Shoulder joints	• Elevation through abduction • Elevation through forward flexion • Elevation through plane of scapula (SCAPTION) • Apley scratch test (right and left) • Rotation in 90° abduction
Elbow joints	• Flexion • Extension • Supination • Pronation
Wrist and hand joints	• Flexion • Extension • Abduction • Adduction • Opposition of thumb and little finger

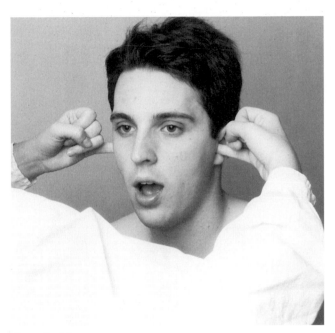

Figure 3–16
Testing temporomandibular joints.

each arm through abduction, followed by active elevation through forward flexion and elevation through the plane of the scapula (SCAPTION). In addition, the examiner quickly tests medial and lateral rotation of each shoulder with the arm at the side and with the arm abducted to 90°. Any pattern of restriction should be noted. If the patient is able to reach full abduction without difficulty or pain, the examiner may decide that there is no problem with the shoulder complex (see Chapter 5).

Elbow Joints. The elbow joints are actively moved through flexion, extension, supination, and pronation. Any restriction of movement or abnormal signs and symptoms should be noted, because they may be indicative of pathology (see Chapter 6).

Wrist and Hand. The patient actively performs flexion, extension, and radial and ulnar deviation of the wrist. Active movements (flexion, extension, abduction, adduction, and opposition) are performed for the fingers and thumb. These actions can be accomplished by having the patient make a fist and then spread the fingers and thumb wide. Again, any alteration in signs and symptoms or restriction of motion should be noted (see Chapter 7).

mouth opening will be limited or deviation of the mandible will occur, or both (see Chapter 4). The examiner should observe the patient as he or she opens and closes the mouth and should watch for any deviation during the movement.

Shoulder Girdle. The examiner quickly scans this complex of joints by asking the patient to actively elevate

Myotomes

Having completed the scanning examination of the peripheral joints, the examiner should then determine muscle power and possible neurological weakness originating from the nerve roots in the cervical spine by testing the myotomes (Table 3–5 and Fig. 3–17). Myotomes

Table 3–5
Myotomes of the Upper Limb

Nerve Root	Test Action	Muscles*
C1–C2	Neck flexion	Rectus lateralis, rectus capitis anterior, longus capitis, longus coli, longus cervicis, sternocleidomastoid
C3	Neck side flexion	Longus capitis, longus cervicis, trapezius, scalenus medius
C4	Shoulder elevation	Diaphragm, trapezius, levator scapulae, scalenus anterior, scalenus medius
C5	Shoulder abduction	Rhomboid major and minor, deltoid, supraspinatus, infraspinatus, teres minor, biceps, scalenus anterior and medius
C6	Elbow flexion and wrist extension	Serratus anterior, latissimus dorsi, subscapularis, teres major, pectoralis major (clavicular head), biceps, coracobrachialis, brachialis, brachioradialis, supinator, extensor carpi radialis longus, scalenus anterior, medius and posterior
C7	Elbow extension and wrist flexion	Serratus anterior, latissimus dorsi, pectoralis major (sternal head), pectoralis minor, triceps, pronator teres, flexor carpi radialis, flexor digitorum superficialis, extensor carpi radialis longus, extensor carpi radialis brevis, extensor digitorum, extensor digiti minimi, scalenus medius and posterior
C8	Thumb extension and ulnar deviation	Pectoralis major (sternal head), pectoralis minor, triceps, flexor digitorum superficialis, flexor digitorum profundus, flexor pollicis longus, pronator quadratus, flexor carpi ulnaris, abductor pollicis longus, extensor pollicis longus, extensor pollicis brevis, extensor indicis, abductor pollicis brevis, flexor pollicis brevis, opponens pollicis, scalenus medius and posterior
T1	Hand intrinsics	Flexor digitorum profundus, intrinsic muscles of the hand (except extensor pollicis brevis), flexor pollicis brevis, opponens pollicis

* Muscles listed may be supplied by additional nerve roots; only primary nerve root sources are listed.

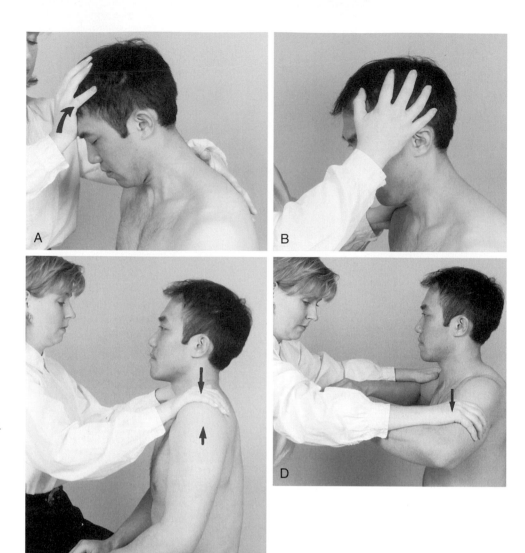

Figure 3–17
Positioning to test myotomes.
(A) Neck flexion (C1, C2).
(B) Neck side flexion to the left
(C3). (C) Shoulder elevation (C4).
(D) Shoulder abduction (C5).

are tested by resisted isometric contractions with the joint at or near the resting position. As with the resisted isometric movements previously mentioned, the examiner should position the seated patient and say, "Don't let me move you," so that an isometric contraction is obtained.

Cervical Myotomes

- Neck flexion: C1–C2
- Neck side flexion: C3
- Shoulder elevation: C4
- Shoulder abduction: C5
- Elbow flexion and/or wrist extension: C6
- Elbow extension and/or wrist flexion: C7
- Thumb extension and/or ulnar deviation: C8
- Abduction and/or adduction of hand intrinsics: T1

The contraction should be held for **at least 5 seconds** so that weakness, if any, can be noted. Where applicable, both sides are tested at the same time to provide a comparison. If possible, the examiner must not apply pressure over the joints, because this action may mask symptoms if the joints are tender.

To test neck flexion (C1–C2 myotome), the patient's head should be slightly flexed. The examiner applies pressure to the forehead while stabilizing the trunk with a hand between the scapulae (see Fig. 3–17A). To test neck side flexion (C3 myotome), the examiner places one hand above the patient's ear and applies a side flexion force while stabilizing the trunk with the other hand on the opposite shoulder (see Fig. 3–17B). Both right and left side flexion must be tested.

The examiner then asks the patient to elevate the shoulders (C4 myotome) to about one half of full elevation. The examiner applies a downward force on both of the patient's shoulders while the patient attempts to hold them in position (see Fig. 3–17C).

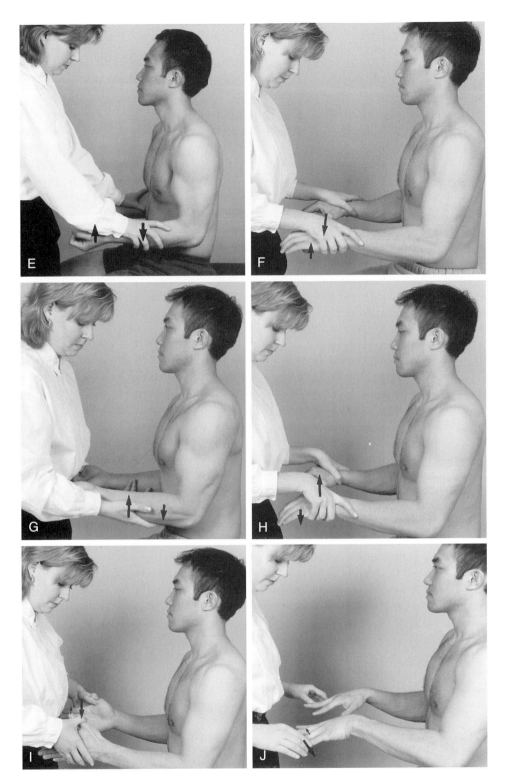

Figure 3–17 *Continued* (E) Elbow flexion (C6). (F) Wrist extension (C6). (G) Elbow extension (C7). (H) Wrist flexion (C7). (I) Thumb extension (C8). (J) Finger abduction (T1).

To test shoulder abduction (C5 myotome), the examiner asks the patient to abduct the arms about 75 to 80° with the elbows flexed to 90° and the forearms pronated or in neutral (see Fig. 3–17D). The examiner applies a downward force on the humerus while the patient attempts to hold the arms in position.

To test elbow flexion and extension, the examiner asks the patient to put the arms by the sides, with the elbows flexed to 90° and forearms in neutral. The examiner applies a downward isometric force (see Fig. 3–17E) to the forearms to test the elbow flexors (C6 myotome) and an upward isometric force (see Fig. 3–17G) to test the elbow extensors (C7 myotome).

For testing of wrist movements (extension, flexion, ulnar deviation) the patient's arms are by the side, elbows at 90°, forearms pronated, and wrists, hands, and fingers in neutral. The examiner applies a downward force (see Fig. 3–17F) to the hands to test wrist extension

(C6 myotome), an upward force (see Fig. 3–17H) to test wrist flexion (C7 myotome), and a lateral force (radially deviated) to test ulnar deviation (C8 myotome) while the patient maintains the position.

In the test for thumb extension (C8 myotome), the patient extends the thumb just short of full range of motion (see Fig. 3–17I). The examiner applies an isometric force to bring the thumbs into flexion. To test hand intrinsics (T1 myotome), the patient squeezes a piece of paper between the fingers while the examiner tries to pull it away; the patient may squeeze the examiner's fingers, or the patient may abduct the fingers slightly with the examiner isometrically adducting them (see Fig. 3–17J).

Functional Assessment

If, in the history, the patient has complained of functional difficulties or the examiner suspects some functional impairment, a series of functional tests or movements may be performed to determine the patient's functional capacity, keeping in mind the patient's age and health. These tests may include activities of daily living such as the following.

Functional Assessment of the Cervical Spine

- Activities of daily living
- Numerical scoring table (if desired)

Breathing. Normal, unlabored breathing should be seen with the mouth closed. There should be no gulping.

Swallowing. This is a complex movement involving muscles of the lips, tongue, jaw, soft palate, pharynx, and larynx as well as the suprahyoid and infrahyoid muscles.

Looking Up at the Ceiling. At least 40 to 50° of neck extension is necessary. If this range is not available, the patient will bend the back or the knees, or both, to obtain the desired range.

Looking Down at Belt Buckle or Shoe Laces. At least 60 to 70° of neck flexion is necessary. If this range is not available, the patient will flex the back to complete the task.

Shoulder Check. At least 60 to 70° of cervical rotation is necessary. If this range is not available, the patient will rotate the trunk to accomplish this task.

Tuck Chin In. This action produces upper cervical flexion with lower cervical extension.[18]

Poke Chin Out. This action produces upper cervical extension with lower cervical flexion.[18]

Neck Strength. In athletes, neck strength should be approximately 30% of body weight to decrease chance of injury.[19] Table 3–6 lists functional strength tests that can give the examiner some indication of the patient's functional strength capacity.

Paresthesia. Paresthesia may make cooking and handling utensils particularly difficult or even dangerous.

Vernon and Mior[20] have developed a numerical scoring functional test called the neck disability index (Fig. 3–18), which is a modification of the Oswestry low back pain index.

Table 3–6
Functional Strength Testing of the Cervical Spine

Starting Position	Action	Functional Test*
Supine lying	Lift head keeping chin tucked in (neck flexion)	6 to 8 repetitions: functional 3 to 5 repetitions: functionally fair 1 to 2 repetitions: functionally poor 0 repetitions: nonfunctional
Prone lying	Lift head backward (neck extension)	Hold 20 to 25 seconds: functional Hold 10 to 19 seconds: functionally fair Hold 1 to 9 seconds: functionally poor Hold 0 seconds: nonfunctional
Side lying (pillows under head so head is not side flexed)	Lift head sideways away from pillow (neck side flexion) (must be repeated for other side)	Hold 20 to 25 seconds: functional Hold 10 to 19 seconds: functionally fair Hold 1 to 9 seconds: functionally poor Hold 0 seconds: nonfunctional
Supine lying	Lift head off bed and rotate to one side keeping head off bed or pillow (neck rotation) (must be repeated both ways)	Hold 20 to 25 seconds: functional Hold 10 to 19 seconds: functionally fair Hold 1 to 9 seconds: functionally poor Hold 0 seconds: nonfunctional

* Younger patients should be able to do the most repetitions and for the longest time; with age, time and repetitions decrease.

Adapted from Palmer, M.L., and M. Epler: Clinical Assessment Procedures in Physical Therapy. Philadelphia, J.B. Lippincott, 1990, pp. 181–182.

Neck Disability Index

This questionnaire has been designed to give the doctor information as to how your neck pain has affected your ability to manage in everyday life. Please answer every section and mark in each section only the ONE box which applies to you. We realize you may consider that two of the statements in any one section relate to you, but please just mark the box which most closely describes your problem.

Section 1 — Pain Intensity

- ☐ I have no pain at the moment. (0)
- ☐ The pain is very mild at the moment. (1)
- ☐ The pain is moderate at the moment. (2)
- ☐ The pain is fairly severe at the moment. (3)
- ☐ The pain is very severe at the moment. (4)
- ☐ The pain is the worst imaginable at the moment. (5)

Section 2 — Personal Care (Washing, Dressing, etc.)

- ☐ I can look after myself normally without causing extra pain. (0)
- ☐ I can look after myself normally but it causes extra pain. (1)
- ☐ It is painful to look after myself and I am slow and careful. (2)
- ☐ I need some help but manage most of my personal care. (3)
- ☐ I need help every day in most aspects of self care. (4)
- ☐ I do not get dressed, I wash with difficulty and stay in bed. (5)

Section 3 — Lifting

- ☐ I can lift heavy weights without extra pain. (0)
- ☐ I can lift heavy weights but it gives extra pain. (1)
- ☐ Pain prevents me from lifting heavy weights off the floor, but I can manage if they are conveniently positioned, for example on a table. (2)
- ☐ Pain prevents me from lifting heavy weights, but I can manage light to medium weights if they are conveniently positioned. (3)
- ☐ I can lift very light weights. (4)
- ☐ I cannot lift or carry anything at all. (5)

Section 4 — Reading

- ☐ I can read as much as I want to with no pain in my neck. (0)
- ☐ I can read as much as I want to with slight pain in my neck. (1)
- ☐ I can read as much as I want with moderate pain in my neck. (2)
- ☐ I cannot read as much as I want because of moderate pain in my neck. (3)
- ☐ I can hardly read at all because of severe pain in my neck. (4)
- ☐ I cannot read at all. (5)

Section 5 — Headaches

- ☐ I have no headaches at all. (0)
- ☐ I have slight headaches that come infrequently. (1)
- ☐ I have moderate headaches which come infrequently. (2)
- ☐ I have moderate headaches which come frequently. (3)
- ☐ I have severe headaches which come frequently. (4)
- ☐ I have headaches almost all the time. (5)

Section 6 — Concentration

- ☐ I can concentrate fully when I want to with no difficulty. (0)
- ☐ I can concentrate fully when I want to with slight difficulty. (1)
- ☐ I have a fair degree of difficulty in concentrating when I want to. (2)
- ☐ I have a lot of difficulty in concentrating when I want to. (3)
- ☐ I have a great deal of difficulty in concentrating when I want to. (4)
- ☐ I cannot concentrate at all. (5)

Section 7 — Work

- ☐ I can do as much work as I want to. (0)
- ☐ I can do my usual work, but no more. (1)
- ☐ I can do most of my usual work, but no more. (2)
- ☐ I cannot do my usual work. (3)
- ☐ I can hardly do any work at all. (4)
- ☐ I cannot do any work at all. (5)

Section 8 — Driving

- ☐ I can drive my car without any neck pain. (0)
- ☐ I can drive my car as long as I want with slight pain in my neck. (1)
- ☐ I can drive my car as long as I want with moderate pain in my neck. (2)
- ☐ I cannot drive my car as long as I want because of moderate pain in my neck. (3)
- ☐ I can hardly drive at all because of severe pain in my neck. (4)
- ☐ I cannot drive my car at all. (5)

Section 9 — Sleeping

- ☐ I have no trouble sleeping. (0)
- ☐ My sleep is slightly disturbed (less than 1 hr. sleepless). (1)
- ☐ My sleep is mildly disturbed (1–2 hrs. sleepless). (2)
- ☐ My sleep is moderately disturbed (2–3 hrs. sleepless). (3)
- ☐ My sleep is greatly disturbed (3–5 hrs. sleepless). (4)
- ☐ My sleep is completely disturbed (5–7 hrs. sleepless). (5)

Section 10 — Recreation

- ☐ I am able to engage in all my recreation activities with no neck pain at all. (0)
- ☐ I am able to engage in all my recreation activities, with some pain in my neck. (1)
- ☐ I am able to engage in most, but not all, of my usual recreation activities because of pain in my neck. (2)
- ☐ I am able to engage in a few of my usual recreation activities because of pain in my neck. (3)
- ☐ I can hardly do any recreation activities because of pain in my neck. (4)
- ☐ I cannot do any recreation activities at all. (5)

Scores (out of 50):
- 0–4 No disability
- 5–14 Mild disability
- 15–24 Moderate disability
- 25–34 Severe disability
- >35 Complete disability

Figure 3–18

Neck disability index. (Modified from Vernon, H., and S. Mior: The neck disability index: A study of reliability and validity. J. Manip. Physiol. Ther. 14:411, 1991.)

Special Tests

There are several special tests that may be performed if the examiner believes they are relevant. Of these tests, some should always be done, and others should be done only if the examiner wants to use them as confirming tests.

Special Tests Commonly Performed on Cervical Spine

- Foraminal compression (Spurling's) test
- Distraction test
- Upper limb tension test
- Shoulder abduction test
- Vertebral artery (cervical quadrant) test

Tests for Neurological Symptoms

Foraminal Compression (Spurling's) Test.[21] The patient bends or side flexes the head (Fig. 3–19). The examiner carefully presses straight down on the head. Bradley and colleagues[13] advocate doing this test in three stages, each of which is increasingly provocative; if symptoms are produced, one does not proceed to the next stage. The first stage involves compression with the head in neutral. The second stage involves compression with the head in extension, and the final stage is with the head in extension and rotation to side of complaint, with compression. The third part of the test more closely follows the test as described by Spurling.[21] A test result is classified as positive if pain radiates into the arm toward which the head is side flexed during compression; this indicates pressure on a nerve root (cervical radiculitis). Radiculitis implies pain in the dermatomal distribution of the nerve root affected.[13] Neck pain with no radiation does not

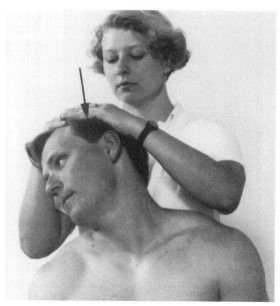

Figure 3–20
Maximum cervical compression test.

constitute a positive test. The dermatome distribution of the pain and altered sensation can give some indication as to which nerve root is involved. The test positions narrow the intervertebral foramen so that conditions such as stenosis, cervical spondylosis, osteophytes, trophic facet joints, or herniated disc, which also narrow the foramen, may lead to symptoms. If the pain is felt in the opposite side to which the head is taken, it is called a **reverse Spurling's sign** and is indicative of muscle spasm in conditions such as tension myalgia and whiplash syndromes.[22]

A very similar test is called the **maximum cervical compression test.** With this test, the patient side flexes the head and then rotates it to the same side. The test is repeated to the other side. A positive test is indicated if pain radiates into the arm.[7] If the head is taken into extension and compression is applied, the intervertebral foramina close maximally and symptoms are accentuated. Pain on the concave side indicates nerve root or facet joint pathology, whereas pain on the convex side indicates muscle strain (Fig. 3–20).[23] This second position may also compress the vertebral artery. If one is testing the vertebral artery, the position should be held for 20 to 30 seconds to elicit symptoms (e.g., dizziness, fainting feeling) that would indicate compression of the vertebral artery.

Distraction Test. To perform the distraction test, the examiner places one hand under the patient's chin and the other hand around the occiput, then slowly lifts the patient's head (Fig. 3–21). The test is classified as positive if the pain is relieved or decreased when the head is lifted or distracted, indicating pressure on nerve roots that has been relieved. This test may also be used to check the shoulder. If the patient abducts the arms while traction is applied, the symptoms are often further re-

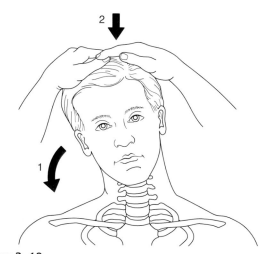

Figure 3–19
Foraminal compression test. Patient flexes head to one side (1), and examiner presses straight down on head (2).

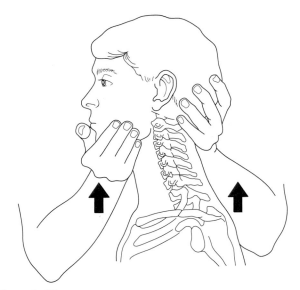

Figure 3–21
Distraction test.

Each phase is added until symptoms are produced. To further "sensitize" the test, side flexion of the cervical spine may be performed.[17, 23] Symptoms are more easily aggravated into the upper limb than the lower limb when doing tension tests,[24, 25] and if the neurological signs are worsening or in the acute phase, or if a cauda equina or spinal cord lesion is present, these stress tests are contraindicated.[24]

When positioning the shoulder, it is essential that a constant depression force be applied to the shoulder girdle so that, even with abduction, the shoulder girdle remains depressed. While the shoulder girdle is depressed, the glenohumeral joint is taken to the appropriate abduction position (110° or 10° depending on test), and the forearm, wrist, and fingers are taken to their appropriate end-of-range position; for example, in ULTT2 the wrist is in full extension (Fig. 3–22). Elbow extension stresses the radial and median nerves, whereas flexion stresses the ulnar nerve. Wrist and finger extension stress the median and ulnar nerve while releasing stress on the radial nerve.[24] If required (ULTT2, 3, and 4), the glenohumeral joint is appropriately rotated and held. The elbow position is often not done until last because the large elbow ROM is easiest to measure when recording available range to show improvement over time. As the elbow is taken toward its extreme (end-of-range) position, symptoms are usually felt.[25] Some of these symptoms are normal (Table 3–8), and some are pathological. If symptoms are minimal or no symptoms appear, the head and cervical spine are taken into contralateral side flexion. This final movement is sometimes referred to as a **sensitizing test**. This sensitizing test may be within or near the test limb (e.g., neck side flexion in ULTT), or it may be in another quadrant (e.g., right ULTT and right SLR).

The tests are designed to stress tissues. Although they stress the neurological tissues, they also stress some contractile and inert tissues. Differentiation among

lieved or lessened in the shoulder. In this case, the test would still be indicative of nerve root pressure in the cervical spine.

Upper Limb Tension Tests (Brachial Plexus Tension or Elvey Test). The upper limb tension tests (ULTT) are equivalent to the straight leg raise (SLR) test in the lumbar spine. They are tension tests designed to put stress on the neurological structures of the upper limb, although in truth stress is put on all the tissues of the upper limb. The neurological tissue is differentiated by what is defined as sensitizing tests (e.g., neck flexion with the SLR test). This test, first described by Elvey,[17] has since been divided into four tests (Table 3–7). Modification of the position of the shoulder, elbow, forearm, wrist, and fingers places greater stress on specific nerves (nerve bias).[24]

Each test begins by testing the good side first and positioning the shoulder, followed by the forearm, wrist, fingers, and last, because of its large ROM, the elbow.

Table 3–7
Upper Limb Tension Tests Showing Order of Joint Positioning and Nerve Bias

	ULTT1	ULTT2	ULTT3	ULTT4
Shoulder	Depression and abduction (110°)	Depression and abduction (10°)	Depression and abduction (10°)	Depression and abduction (10 to 90°), hand to ear
Elbow	Extension	Extension	Extension	Flexion
Forearm	Supination	Supination	Pronation	Supination
Wrist	Extension	Extension	Flexion and ulnar deviation	Extension and radial deviation
Fingers and thumb	Extension	Extension	Flexion	Extension
Shoulder	—	Lateral rotation	Medial rotation	Lateral rotation
Cervical spine	Contralateral side flexion	Contralateral side flexion	Contralateral side flexion	Contralateral side flexion
Nerve bias	Median nerve, anterior interosseous nerve, C5, C6, C7	Median nerve, musculocutaneous nerve, axillary nerve	Radial nerve	Ulnar nerve, C8 and T1 nerve roots

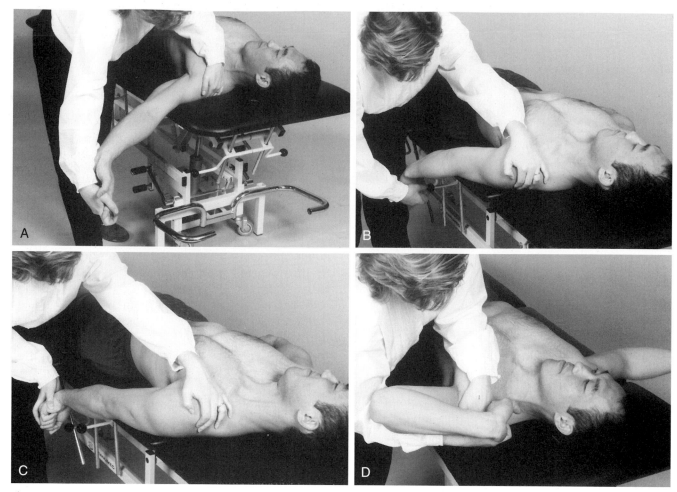

Figure 3–22
Upper limb tension tests (Elvey tests). (A) ULTT1. (B) ULTT2. (C) ULTT3. (D) ULTT4.

Table 3–8
Upper Limb Tension Test: Normal and Pathological Signs and Symptoms

Normal (Negative)	Pathological (Positive)
Deep ache or stretch in cubital fossa (99%)	Production of patient's symptoms (most important feature)
Deep ache or stretch into anterior and radial aspect of forearm and radial aspect of hand (80%)	A sensitizing test in the ipsilateral quadrant alters the symptoms
Tingling to the fingers supplied by appropriate nerve (nerve bias)	Different symptoms between right and left (contralateral quadrant)
Stretch in anterior shoulder area	
Above responses increased with contralateral cervical side flexion (90%)	
Above responses decreased with ipsilateral cervical side flexion (70%)	

Adapted from Butler, D.S.: Mobilisation of the Nervous System. Melbourne, Churchill Livingstone, 1991.

the types of tissues depends on the signs and symptoms presented (Table 3–9).

Finally, although specific ULTTs are described, if the patient describes neurological symptoms when doing functional movements (e.g., getting wallet out of back pocket) these movements should also be tested by positioning the limb and taking the joints toward their end range.

Evans[12] described a modification of the ULTT. The sitting patient abducts the arms with the elbows extended, stopping just short of the onset of symptoms. The patient laterally rotates the shoulder just short of symptoms, and the examiner then holds this position. Finally, the patient flexes the elbows so that the hands lie behind the head (Fig. 3–23). Reproduction of radicular symptoms with elbow flexion is considered a positive test. This test is similar to ULTT4 and stresses primarily the ulnar nerve and the C8 and T1 nerve roots.

Evans[12] outlined a second similar test. The seated patient abducts the arm to 90° with the elbow fully flexed. The arm is extended at the shoulder and then the elbow is extended (Fig. 3–24). If radicular pain results, the

Table 3–9
Differential Diagnosis of Contractile, Inert, and Nervous Tissue Based on Stretch or Tension

	Contractile Tissue	Inert Tissue (Ligament)	Neurogenic Tissue
Pain	Cramping, dull, ache	Dull → sharp	Burning, bright, lightning-like
Tingling	No	No	Yes
Constancy	Intermittent	Intermittent	Longer symptom duration
Dermatome pattern	No	No	Yes (if nerve root pathological)
Peripheral nerve sensory distribution	No	No	Yes (if peripheral nerve or nerve root is affected)
Resistance to stretch	Muscle spasm	Boggy, hard capsular	Soft capsular

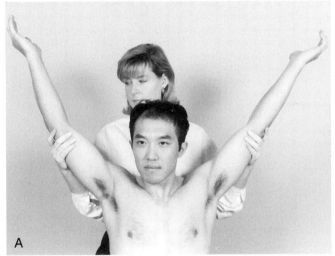
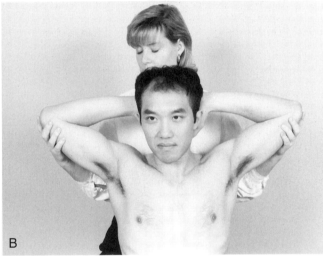

Figure 3–23
Brachial plexus tension test. (A) The patient abducts and then laterally rotates the arms until symptoms are felt; patient then lowers the arms until symptoms disappear and the examiner holds the patient's arms in the position. (B) While the shoulders are held in position, the patient flexes the elbows and places the hands behind the head. A positive test is indicated by return of symptoms.

Figure 3–24
Bikele's sign. (A) The arm is abducted to 90° with the elbow fully flexed. (B) The arm and then the elbow are extended.

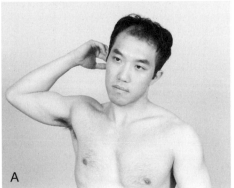
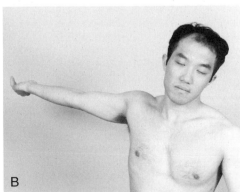

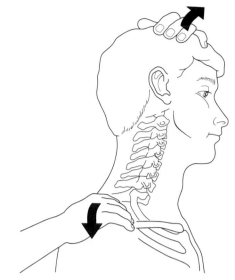

Figure 3–25
Shoulder depression test.

pain is positive (**Bikele's sign**). This test in reality is a modification of the ULTT done actively.

Shoulder Depression Test. The examiner side flexes the patient's head to one side while applying a downward pressure on the opposite shoulder (Fig. 3–25). If the pain is increased, it indicates irritation or compression of the nerve roots, foraminal encroachments such as osteophytes in the area, or adhesions around the dural sleeves of the nerve and adjacent joint capsule on the side being stretched. This test may also be used to evaluate for brachial plexus lesions (see Table 3–3) as this is the mechanism of injury for these lesions, plexopathies, and radiculopathies. With brachial plexus lesions, more than one nerve root is commonly affected.

Shoulder Abduction (Relief) Test. The patient is sitting or lying down, and the examiner passively or the patient actively elevates the arm through abduction, so that the hand or forearm rests on top of the head (Fig. 3–26).[11, 26] A decrease in or relief of symptoms indicates a cervical extradural compression problem such as a herniated disc, epidural vein compression, or nerve root compression, usually in the C4–C5 or C5–C6 area. Differentiation is by the dermatome distribution of the symptoms. This finding is also called **Bakody's sign**.[12] Abduction of the arm decreases the length of the neurological pathway and decreases the pressure on the lower nerve roots.[26, 27] If the pain increases with the positioning of the arm, it implies that pressure is increasing in the interscalene triangle.[12]

Lhermitte's Sign. The patient is in the long leg sitting position on the examining table. The examiner passively flexes the patient's head and one hip simultaneously, with the leg kept straight (Fig. 3–27). A positive test occurs if there is a sharp pain down the spine and into

the upper or lower limbs; it indicates dural or meningeal irritation in the spine or possible cervical myelopathy.[12] The test is similar to a combination of the Brudzinski test and the SLR test (see Chapter 9). If the patient can actively flex the head to the chest while in the supine lying position, the test is called the **Soto-Hall test**. If the hips are flexed to 135°, greater traction is placed on the spinal cord.[11]

Jackson's Compression Test. The patient rotates the head to one side. The examiner then carefully presses straight down on the head (Fig. 3–28). The test is repeated with the head rotated to the other side. The test is positive if, on testing, pain radiates into the arm, indicating pressure on a nerve root. The pain distribution (dermatome) can give some indication of which nerve root is affected.[11] This test is a modification of the foraminal compression test.

Scalene Cramp Test.[9] The patient sits and rotates the head to the affected side and pulls the chin down into the hollow above the clavicle by flexing the cervical spine. If pain increases, it is usually in the trigger points of the scalenes toward which the head rotates. Radicular signs may indicate plexopathy or thoracic outlet symptoms.

Valsalva Test. The examiner asks the patient to take a deep breath and hold it while bearing down, as if moving the bowels. A positive test is indicated by increased pain, which may be caused by increased intrathecal pressure. This increased pressure within the spinal cord usually results from a space-occupying lesion, such as a herniated disc, a tumor, or osteophytes. Test results are very subjective. The test should be done with care and caution, because the patient may become dizzy and pass out while performing the test or shortly afterward if the procedure blocks the blood supply to the brain.

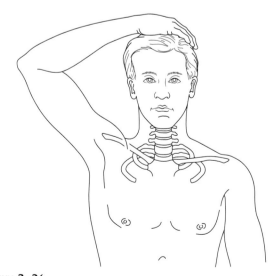

Figure 3–26
Shoulder abduction test.

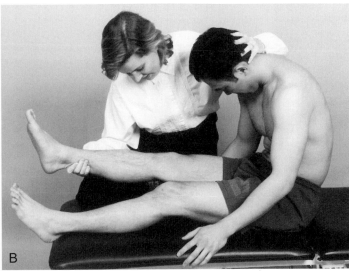

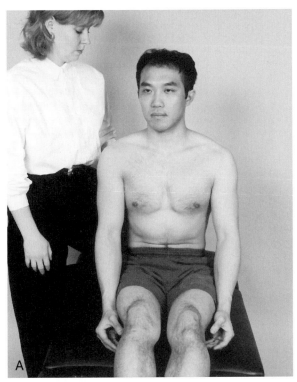

Figure 3–27
Lhermitte's sign. (A) Patient in long sitting. (B) Examiner flexes patient's head and hip simultaneously.

Tinel's Sign for Brachial Plexus Lesions.[28] The patient sits with the neck slightly side flexed. The examiner taps the area of the brachial plexus (Fig. 3–29) with a finger along the nerve trunks in such a way that the different nerve roots are tested. Pure local pain implies that there is an underlying cervical plexus lesion. A positive Tinel's sign (tingling sensation in the distribution of a nerve) means the lesion is anatomically intact and some recovery is occurring. If pain is elicited in the distribution of a peripheral nerve, the sign is positive for a neuroma and indicates a disruption of the continuity of the nerve.

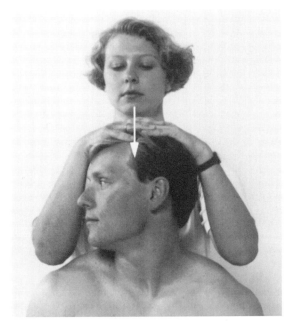

Figure 3–28
Jackson's compression test.

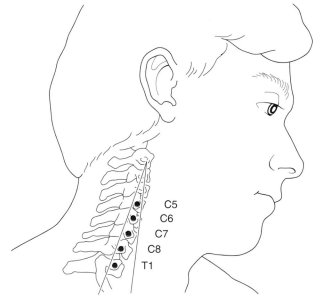

Figure 3–29
Tinel's sign for brachial plexus lesions. Dots indicate percussion points.

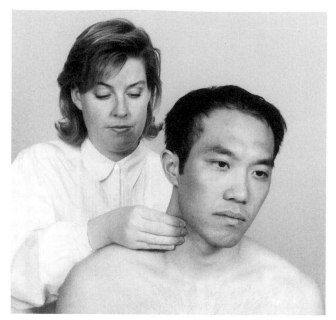

Figure 3–30
Maneuver to compress and squeeze the brachial plexus.

Brachial Plexus Compression Test.[29] The examiner applies firm compression to the brachial plexus by squeezing the plexus under the thumb or fingers (Fig. 3–30). Pain at the site is not diagnostic; the test is positive only if pain radiates into the shoulder or upper extremity. It is positive for mechanical cervical lesions having a mechanical component.

Tests for Upper Motor Neuron Lesions (Cervical Myelopathy)

Romberg's Test. For Romberg's test, the patient is standing and is asked to close the eyes. The position is held for 20 to 30 seconds. If the body begins to sway excessively or the patient loses balance, the test is considered positive for an upper motor neuron lesion.

Tests for Vascular Signs

Vertebral Artery (Cervical Quadrant) Test. With the patient supine, the examiner passively takes the patient's head and neck into extension and side flexion (Fig. 3–31).[30] After this movement is achieved, the examiner rotates the patient's neck to the same side and holds it for approximately 30 seconds. A positive test provokes referring symptoms if the side to which the head is taken is affected. This test must be done with care. If dizziness or nystagmus occurs, it is an indication that the vertebral arteries are being compressed. The **DeKleyn-Nieuwenhuyse test**[31] performs a similar function but involves extension and rotation instead of extension and side flexion. Both tests may also be used to assess nerve root compression in the lower cervical spine. To test the

upper cervical spine, the examiner "pokes" the patient's chin and follows with extension, side flexion, and rotation.

Static Vertebral Artery Tests. The examiner may test the following passive movements with the patient supine or sitting, as advocated by Grant,[32] watching for eye nystagmus and complaints by the patient of dizziness, lightheadedness, or visual disturbances. Each of these tests is increasingly provocative; if symptoms occur with the first test, there is no need to progress to the next test.

In *the sitting position*:

1. Sustained full neck and head extension
2. Sustained full neck and head rotation, right and left (if this movement causes symptoms, it is sometimes called a **Barre-Lieou sign**)[12]
3. Sustained full neck and head rotation with extension right and left (**DeKleyn's test**)[12]
4. Provocative movement position
5. Quick head movement into provocative position
6. Quick repeated head movement into provocative position
7. Head still, sustained trunk movement left and right
8. Head still, repeated trunk movement left and right

In *supine position*:

1. Sustained full neck and head extension
2. Sustained full neck and head rotation left and right
3. Sustained full neck and head rotation with extension left and right (if combined with side flexion, it is called the **Hallpike maneuver**[12])
4. Unilateral posteroanterior oscillation of C1–C2

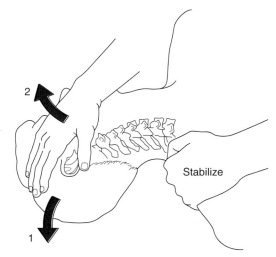

Figure 3–31
Vertebral artery (cervical quadrant) test. Examiner passively moves patient's head and neck into extension and side flexion (1), then rotation (2), holding for 30 seconds.

Table 3–10
Relationship of Head Position to Blood Flow to Head and Neurological Function

Head Position	Blood Flow	Neurological Space
Neutral	Normal	Normal
Flexion	Normal	Normal
Extension	Usually normal	Decreased
Side flexion	Slight decrease in ipsilateral artery Normal in contralateral artery	Decrease on ipsilateral side Increase on contralateral side
Rotation	Slight decrease in ipsilateral artery Significant decrease in contralateral artery	Decrease on ipsilateral side Increase on contralateral side
Extension and rotation	Bilateral decrease, greater in contralateral artery	Bilateral decrease, greater on ipsilateral side
Flexion and rotation	Bilateral decrease	Decrease on ipsilateral side Increase on contralateral side

facet joints (prone lying) with head rotated left and right

5. Simulated mobilization and manipulation position

Each position should be held for at least 10 to 30 seconds unless symptoms are evoked. Ten seconds should elapse between each test to ensure that there are no latent symptoms. Extension is more likely to test the patency of the intervertebral foramen, whereas rotation and side flexion are more likely to test the vertebral artery (Table 3–10). If symptoms are evoked, care should be taken concerning any treatment to follow. These tests are often more effective if done with the patient sitting, because the blood must flow against gravity and there is a restriction caused by the passive movement. However, the supine position allows greater passive range of movement.[33] Movements to the right tend to have more effect on the left vertebral artery, and movements to the left tend to have more effect on the right artery.

Aspinall[34] advocated the use of a progressive series of clinical tests to evaluate the vertebral artery. With these tests, the examiner progressively moves from the lower cervical spine and lower vertebral artery to the upper cervical spine and upper vertebral artery. Table 3–11 demonstrates Aspinall's progressive clinical tests for the vertebral arteries.

Table 3–11
Aspinall's Progressive Clinical Tests for Vertebral Artery Pathology

Vertebral Artery Area	Position Sitting	Position Lying	Test
Mid and lower cervical spine			
Area 1 (lower)	X		Active cervical rotation
Area 2 (middle)	X		Active cervical rotation
	X	X	Passive cervical rotation
	X		Active cervical extension
	X	X	Passive cervical extension
	X	X	Passive cervical extension with rotation
	X		Passive segmental extension with rotation
	X	X	Passive cervical flexion
	X	X	Cervical flexion with traction
		X	Accessory oscillatory anterior/posterior movement—transverse processes C2–C7 in combined extension and rotation
		X	Sustained manipulation position
Upper cervical spine			
Area 3 (upper)	X		Active cervical rotation
	X	X	Passive cervical rotation
	X		Active cervical extension
	X	X	Passive cervical extension
	X	X	Passive cervical rotation with extension
	X	X	Cervical rotation with extension and traction
	X		Cervical rotation with flexion
		X	Accessory oscillatory anterior/posterior movement—transverse processes C1–C2 in combined rotation and extension
		X	Sustained manipulation position

From Aspinall, W.: Clinical testing for the craniovertebral hypermobility syndrome. J. Orthop. Sports Phys. Ther. 12:180–181, 1989.

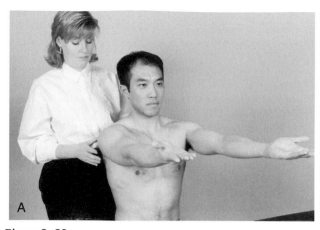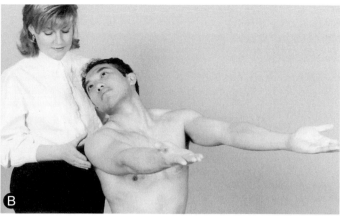

Figure 3–32
Positioning for Hautant's test. (A) Forward flexion of both arms to 90°. (B) Rotation and extension of neck with arms forward flexed to 90°.

Hautant's Test.[12, 35] This test has two parts and is used to differentiate dizziness or vertigo caused by articular problems from that caused by vascular problems. The patient sits and forward flexes both arms to 90° (Fig. 3–32). The eyes are then closed. The examiner watches for any loss of arm position. If the arms move, the cause is nonvascular. The patient is then asked to rotate or extend and rotate the neck and the eyes are again closed. If wavering of the arms occurs, the dysfunction is caused by vascular impairment to the brain.

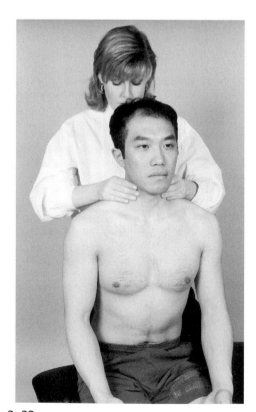

Figure 3–33
Naffziger's test (compression of jugular veins).

Barre's Test.[31] The patient stands with arms forward flexed to 90°, elbows straight and forearms supinated, palms up and eyes closed, holding the position for 10 to 20 seconds. The test is considered positive if one arm slowly falls with simultaneous forearm pronation. The cause is thought to be diminished blood flow to the brain stem. This test is identical to the first part of Hautant's test.

Underburg's Test.[12] The patient stands with the arms forward flexed to 90°, elbows straight and forearms supinated. The patient then closes the eyes and marches in place while holding the extended and rotated head to one side. The test is repeated with head movement to the opposite side. The test is considered positive if there is dropping of the arms, loss of balance, or pronation of the hands; a positive result indicates decreased blood supply to the brain.

Naffziger's Test.[12, 36] The patient is seated and the examiner stands behind the patient with his or her fingers over the patient's jugular veins (Fig. 3–33). The examiner compresses the veins for 30 seconds (Naffziger recommended 10 minutes!) and then asks the patient to cough. Pain may indicate a nerve root problem or space-occupying lesion (e.g., tumor). If lightheadedness or similar symptoms occur with compression of the jugular veins, the test should be terminated.

Tests for Vertigo and Dizziness

Temperature (Caloric) Test. The examiner alternately applies hot and cold test tubes just behind the patient's ears on the side of the head; each side is done in turn. A positive test is associated with the inducement of vertigo, which indicates inner ear problems.

Dizziness Test. The patient sits and the examiner grasps the patient's head. The examiner actively rotates the patient's head as far as possible to the right and then to the left, holding the head at the extreme of motion for a short time (10 to 30 seconds) while the shoulders remain stationary. The patient's shoulders are then actively rotated as far to the right as possible and then to the left as far as possible while keeping the head facing straight ahead. If the patient experiences dizziness in both cases, the problem lies in the vertebral arteries, because in both cases the vertebral artery may be "kinked," decreasing the blood flow. If the patient experiences dizziness only when the head is rotated, the problem lies within the semicircular canals of the inner ear.

Fitz-Ritson[37] advocates a modification of this test. For the first part of the test, he advocates that the examiner hold the shoulders still while the patient rapidly rotates the head left and right with the eyes closed. If vertigo results, the problem is in the vestibular nuclei or muscles and joints of the cervical spine. In addition, patients may lose their balance, veer to one side, or possibly vomit. The second stage is the same as previously mentioned, except that the eyes are closed. If vertigo is experienced this time, Fitz-Ritson believes that the problem is in the cervical spine because the vestibular apparatus is not being moved.

Tests for Instability

Sharp-Purser Test. This test should be performed **with extreme caution.** It is a test to determine subluxation of the atlas on the axis (Fig. 3–34). The examiner places one hand over the patient's forehead while the thumb of the other hand is placed over the spinous process of the axis to stabilize it (Fig. 3–35). The patient is asked to slowly flex the head; while this is occurring, the examiner presses backward with the palm. A positive test is indicated if the examiner feels the head slide backward dur-

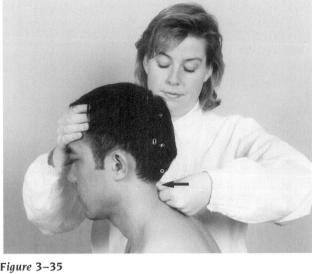

Figure 3–35
The Sharp-Purser test for subluxation of the atlas on the axis.

ing the movement. The slide backward indicates that the subluxation of the atlas has been reduced, and the slide may be accompanied by a "clunk."

Aspinall[38] advocates use of an additional test if the Sharp-Purser test is negative. The examiner stabilizes the occiput on the atlas in flexion and holds the occiput in this flexed position. The examiner then applies an anteriorly directed force to the posterior aspect of the atlas (Fig. 3–36). Normally, no movement or symptoms are perceived by the patient. For the test to be positive, the patient should feel a lump in the throat as the atlas moves toward the esophagus; this is indicative of hypermobility at the atlantoaxial articulation.

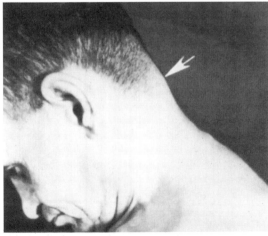

Figure 3–34
Subluxation of the atlas on neck flexion. Note the bulge in the posterior neck caused by the forward subluxation of the atlas, bringing the spinous process of the axis into prominence beneath the skin (*arrow*). (Courtesy of Harold S. Robinson, M.D., Vancouver, British Columbia.)

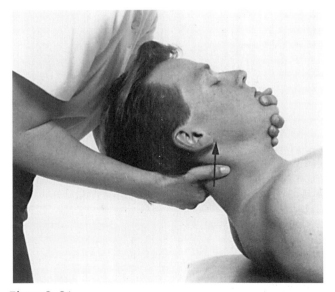

Figure 3–36
Aspinall's transverse ligament test.

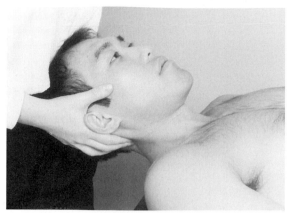

Figure 3–37
Testing the transverse ligament of C1. Examiner's hands support head and C1.

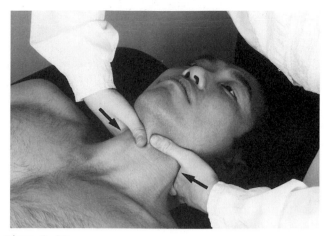

Figure 3–38
Atlantoaxial lateral shear test.

Transverse Ligament Stress Test.[35, 39] The patient lies supine with the examiner supporting the occiput with the palms and the third, fourth, and fifth fingers. The examiner places the index fingers in the space between the patient's occiput and C2 spinous process so that the fingertips are overlying the neural arch of C1. The head and C1 are then carefully lifted anteriorly together, allowing no flexion or extension (Fig. 3–37). This anterior shear is resisted by the transverse ligament. The position is held for 10 to 20 seconds to see whether symptoms occur, indicating a positive test. Positive symptoms include soft end feel, muscle spasm, dizziness, nausea, paresthesia of the lip, face, or limb, nystagmus, or a lump sensation in the throat. The test indicates hypermobility at the atlantoaxial articulation.

Lateral Shear Test.[35, 39] This test is used to determine instability of the atlantoaxial articulation caused by odontoid dysplasia. The patient lies supine with the head supported. The examiner places the radial side of one second metacarpophalangeal (MCP) joint against the transverse process of the atlas and the other MCP joint against the opposite transverse process of the axis. The examiner's hands are then carefully pushed together, causing a shear of one bone on the other (Fig. 3–38). Normally, minimal motion and no symptoms (cord or vascular) are produced.

Alar Ligament Stress Test.[35, 39] The patient lies supine while the examiner stabilizes the axis with a wide pinch grip around the spinous process and lamina (Fig. 3–39). The examiner then attempts to side flex the head and axis. Normally, if the ligament is intact, minimal side flexion occurs, with a strong capsular end feel.

Tests for First Rib Mobility

Although the first rib would normally be included with assessment of the thoracic spine, the examiner must always test for mobility of the first rib when examining the cervical spine, especially if side flexion is limited and there is pain or tenderness in the area of the first rib or T1.

For the first test, the patient lies supine while fully supported. The examiner palpates the first rib bilaterally lateral to T1 and places his or her fingers along the path of the patient's ribs to just posterior to the clavicles (Fig. 3–40). While palpating the ribs, the examiner notes the movement of both first ribs as the patient takes a deep breath in and out, and any asymmetry is noted. The examiner then palpates one first rib and side flexes the head to the opposite side until the rib is felt to move up. The range of neck side flexion is noted. The side flexion is then repeated to the opposite side, and results from the two sides are compared. Asymmetry may be caused by hypomobility of the first rib or tightness of the scalene muscles on the same side.

For the second test, the patient lies prone, and the examiner again palpates the first rib (Fig. 3–41). Using

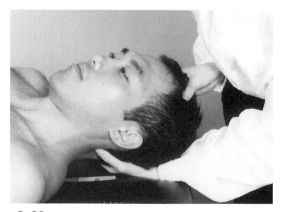

Figure 3–39
Alar ligament stress test. Examiner attempts to side flex the patient's head.

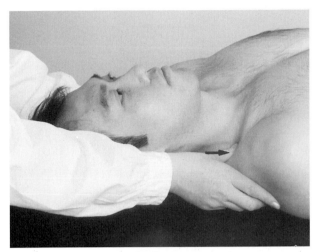

Figure 3–40
Testing mobility of the first rib (anterior aspect).

the thumb, reinforced by the other thumb, the examiner pushes the rib caudally, noting the amount of movement, end feel, and presence of pain. The other first rib is tested in a similar fashion, and the two sides are compared. Normally, a firm tissue stretch is felt with no pain, except possibly where the examiner's thumbs are pushing on the rib.

Tests for Thoracic Outlet Syndrome

See Special Tests in Chapter 5.

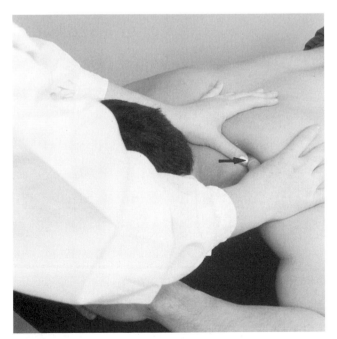

Figure 3–41
Testing mobility of the first rib (posterior aspect).

Reflexes and Cutaneous Distribution

The following reflexes should be checked for differences between the two sides, as shown in Figure 3–42: biceps (C5–C6), the brachioradialis (C5–C6), the triceps (C7–C8), and the jaw jerk (cranial nerve V). The reflexes are tested with a reflex hammer. The examiner tests the biceps and jaw jerk reflexes by placing his or her thumb over the patient's biceps tendon or at midpoint of the chin and then tapping the thumbnail with the reflex hammer to elicit the reflex. The jaw reflex may also be tested with a tongue depressor (see Fig. 3–42B). The examiner holds the tongue depressor firmly against the lower teeth and then strikes the tongue depressor with the reflex hammer. The brachioradialis and triceps reflexes are tested by directly tapping the tendon or muscle.

> ### Common Reflexes Checked in Cervical Spine Assessment
>
> - Biceps (C5, C6)
> - Triceps (C7, C8)
> - Hoffmann's sign (if upper motor neuron lesion suspected)

If an upper motor neuron lesion is suspected, the pathological reflexes (for example, **Babinski's reflex**) should be checked (see Table 1–23). **Hoffmann's sign** is the upper limb equivalent of the Babinski test. To test for Hoffmann's sign, the examiner holds the patient's middle finger and briskly flicks the distal phalanx. A positive sign is noted if the interphalangeal joint of the thumb of the same hand flexes. Denno and Meadows[40] advocated a dynamic Hoffmann's sign. The patient is asked to repeatedly flex and extend the head, and then the test is performed as described previously. Denno and Meadows believed that the dynamic test shows positive results earlier than the static or normal Hoffmann's sign. Because an upper motor neuron lesion affects both the upper and lower limb, initially unilaterally and at later stages bilaterally, Babinski's test may be performed if desired. Clonus, most easily seen by sudden dorsiflexion of the ankle resulting in four or five reflex twitches of the plantar flexors, is also a sign of an upper motor neuron lesion.[41]

The examiner then checks the **dermatome pattern** of the various nerve roots as well as the sensory distribution of the peripheral nerves (Figs. 3–43 and 3–44). Dermatomes vary from person to person and overlap a great deal, and the diagrams shown are estimations only. For example, in the thoracic spine, one dermatome may be completely absent with no loss of sensation. The examiner tests sensation by doing a **sensory scanning exami-**

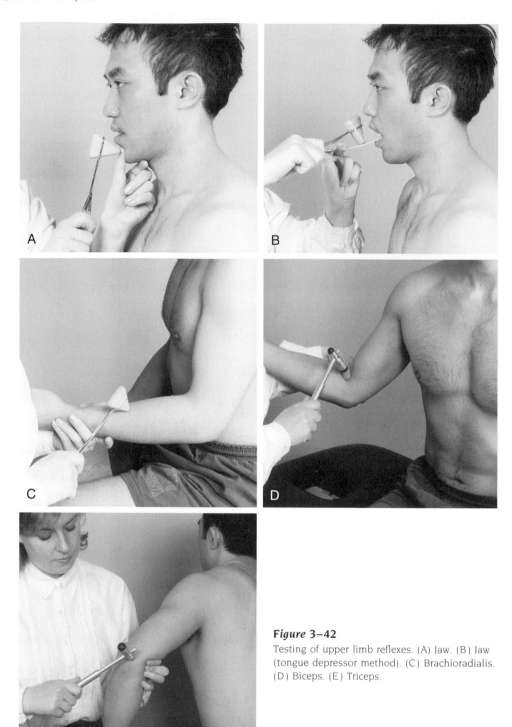

Figure 3–42

Testing of upper limb reflexes. (A) Jaw. (B) Jaw (tongue depressor method). (C) Brachioradialis. (D) Biceps. (E) Triceps.

nation. This is accomplished by running relaxed hands over the patient's head (sides and back); down over the shoulders, upper chest, and back; and down the arms, being sure to cover all aspects of the arm. If any difference is noted between the sides in this "sensation scan," the examiner may then use a pinwheel, pin, cotton batting, or brush, or a combination of these, to map out the exact area of sensory difference.

Because of the spinal cord and associated nerve roots and their relation to the other bony and soft tissues in the cervical spine, referred pain is a relatively common experience in lesions of the cervical spine. Within the cervical spine, the intervertebral discs, facet joints, and other bony and soft tissues may refer pain to other segments of the neck (dermatomes) or to the head, the shoulder, the scapular area, and the whole of the upper

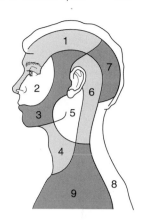

Figure 3–43

Sensory nerve distribution of the head, neck, and face. (1) Ophthalmic nerve. (2) Maxillary nerve.
(3) Mandibular nerve. (4) Transverse cutaneous nerve of neck (C2–C3). (5) Greater auricular nerve (C2–C3).
(6) Lesser auricular nerve (C2). (7) Greater occipital nerve (C2–C3). (8) Cervical dorsal rami (C3–C5).
(9) Suprascapular nerve (C5–C6).

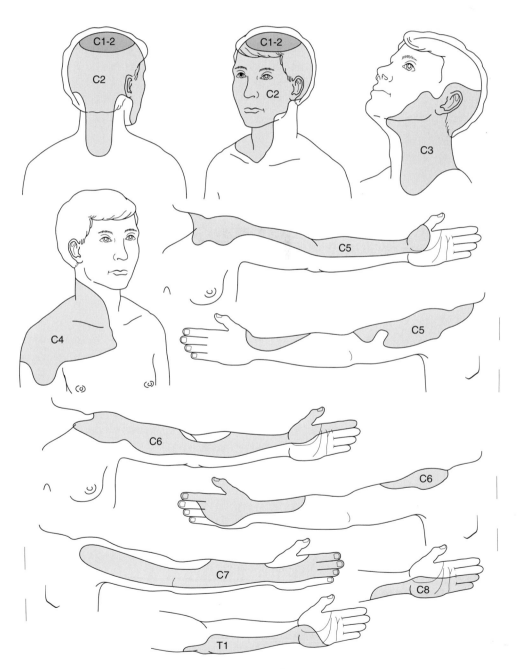

Figure 3–44

Dermatomes of the cervical spine.

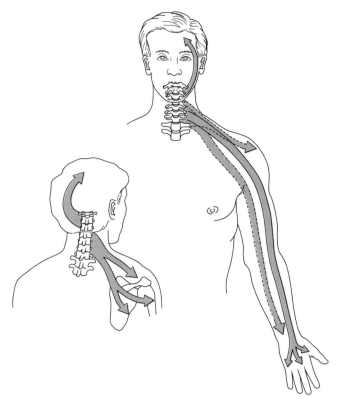

Figure 3–45
Referral of symptoms from the cervical spine to areas of the spine, head, shoulder girdle, and upper limb.

Table 3–12
Muscles of the Cervical Spine and Their Referral of Pain

Muscle	Referral Pattern
Trapezius	Right and left occiput, lateral aspect of head above ear to behind eye, tip of jaw
	Spinous processes to medial border of scapula and along spine of scapula; may also refer to lateral aspect of upper arm
Sternocleidomastoid	Back and top of head, front of ear over forehead to medial aspect of eye; cheek
	Behind ear, ear to forehead
Splenius capitis	Top of head
Splenius cervicis	Posterior neck and shoulder angle, side of head to eye
Semispinalis cervicis	Back of head
Semispinalis capitis	Band around head at level of forehead
Multifidus	Occiput to posterior neck and shoulder angle to base of spine of scapula
Suboccipital	Lateral aspect of head to eye
Scalene	Medial border of scapula and anterior chest down posterolateral aspect of arm to anterolateral and posterolateral aspect of hand

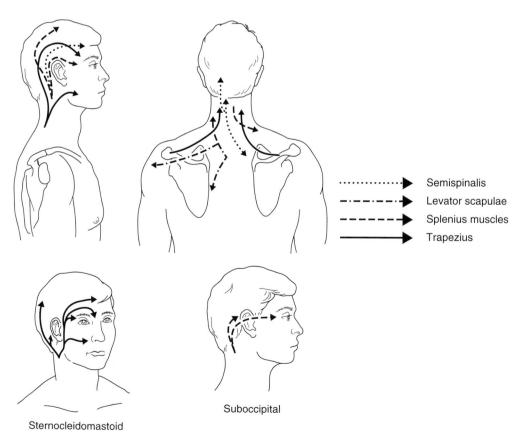

- · · · · · · · ▶ Semispinalis
- — · — · — ▶ Levator scapulae
- — — — — ▶ Splenius muscles
- ———— ▶ Trapezius

Sternocleidomastoid

Suboccipital

Figure 3–46
Muscles and their referred pain patterns. Diagram shows primarily one side.

limb (Fig. 3–45 and 3–46).[9, 14] Table 3–12 shows the muscles of the cervical spine and their referral of pain.

Brachial Plexus Injuries of the Cervical Spine

Erb-Duchenne Paralysis

This paralysis is an upper brachial plexus injury involving injury to the upper nerve roots (C5, C6) as a result of compression or stretching. The injury frequently occurs at Erb's point. With this injury, it is primarily the muscles of the shoulder region and elbow that are affected; the muscles of the hand (especially the intrinsic muscles) are not involved. However, sensation over the radial surfaces of the forearm and hand and the deltoid area are affected.

Klumpke (Dejerine-Klumpke) Paralysis

This injury involves the lower brachial plexus and results from compression or stretching of the lower nerve roots (C8, T1). Atrophy and weakness are evident in the muscles of the forearm and hand as well as in the triceps. The obvious changes are in the distal aspects of the upper limb. The resultant injury is a functionless hand. Sensory loss occurs primarily on the ulnar side of the forearm and hand.

Joint Play Movements

The joint play movements that are carried out in the cervical spine are, for the most part, general movements that involve the entire cervical spine and are not limited to one specific joint. As the joint play movements are performed, the examiner should note any decreased ROM, pain, or difference in end feel.

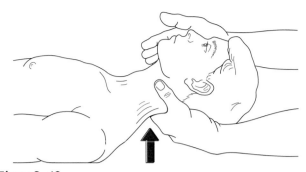

Figure 3–48
Anterior glide of the cervical spine.

Joint Play Movements of the Cervical Spine

- Side glide of the cervical spine (general)
- Anterior glide of the cervical spine (general)
- Posterior glide of the cervical spine (general)
- Traction glide of the cervical spine (general)
- Rotation of the occiput on C1 (specific)
- Posteroanterior central vertebral pressure (specific)
- Posteroanterior unilateral vertebral pressure (specific)
- Transverse vertebral pressure (specific)

Side Glide. The examiner holds the patient's head and moves it from side to side, keeping it in the same plane as the shoulder (Fig. 3–47).[42]

Anterior and Posterior Glide. The examiner holds the patient's head with one hand around the occiput and one hand around the chin, taking care to ensure that the patient is not choked.[18] The examiner then draws the head forward for anterior glide (Fig. 3–48) and posteriorly for posterior glide. While doing these movements, the examiner must prevent flexion and extension of the head.

Traction Glide. The examiner places one hand around the patient's chin and the other hand on the occiput.[19] Traction is the applied in a straight longitudinal direction, with the majority of the pull being through the occiput (Fig. 3–49).

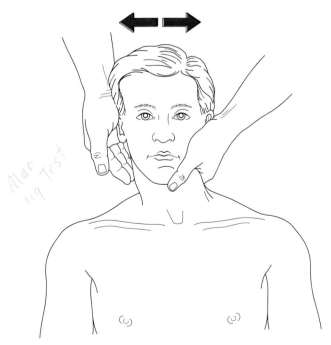

Figure 3–47
Side glide of the cervical spine. Glide to the right is illustrated.

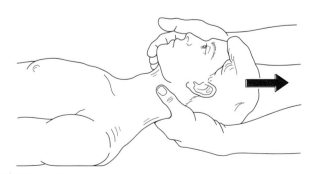

Figure 3–49
Traction glide of the cervical spine.

Rotation of the Occiput on C1. The examiner holds the patient's head in position and palpates the transverse processes of C1 (Fig. 3–50). The examiner must first find the mastoid process on each side and then move the fingers inferiorly and anteriorly until a hard bump (i.e., the transverse process of C1) is palpated on each side. Palpation in the area of the C1 transverse process is generally painful, so care must be taken. The examiner then rotates the patient's head while palpating the transverse processes; the transverse process on the side to which the head is rotated will seem to disappear in the normal case. If this disappearance does not occur, there is restriction of movement between C0 and C1 on that side.

Vertebral Pressures. For the last three joint play movements (Fig. 3–51), the patient lies prone with the forehead resting on the back of the hands.[16] These techniques are specific to each vertebra and are applied to each vertebra in turn or at least to the ones that the examination has indicated may be affected by pathology. The examiner palpates the spinous processes of the cervical spine, starting at the C2 spinous process and working

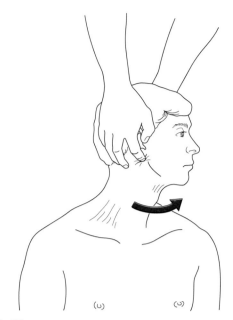

Figure 3–50
Left rotation of the occiput on C1. Note the index finger palpating the right transverse process of C1.

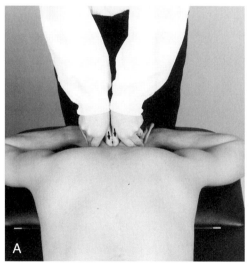

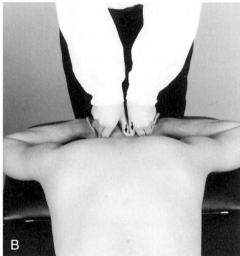

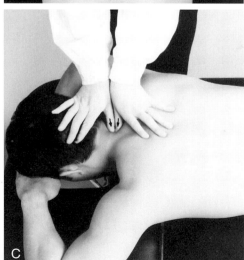

Figure 3–51
Vertebral pressures to the cervical spine.
(A) Posteroanterior central vertebral pressure.
(B) Posteroanterior unilateral vertebral pressure.
(C) Transverse vertebral pressure.

downward to the T2 spinous process. The positions of the examiner's hands, fingers, and thumbs in performing **posteroanterior central vertebral pressures** (PACVP) are shown in Figure 3–51A. Pressure is then applied through the examiner's thumbs, and the vertebra is pushed forward. The examiner must take care to apply pressure slowly, with carefully controlled movements, so as to "feel" the movement, which in reality is minimal. This "springing test" may be repeated several times to determine the quality of the movement and the end feel.

For **posteroanterior unilateral vertebral pressure** (PAUVP), the examiner's fingers move laterally away from the tip of the spinous process so that the thumbs rest on the lamina or transverse process, about 2 to 3 cm (1 to 1.5 inches) lateral to the spinous process of the cervical or thoracic vertebra (see Fig. 3–51B). Anterior springing pressure is applied as in the central pressure technique. This pressure causes a minimal rotation of the vertebral body. Both sides should be done and compared.

For **transverse vertebral pressure** (TVP), the examiner's thumbs are placed along the side of the spinous process of the cervical or thoracic spine (see Fig. 3–51C). The examiner then applies a transverse springing pressure to the side of the spinous process, feeling for the quality of movement. This pressure also causes rotation of the vertebral body.

Palpation

If, after completing the scanning examination of the cervical spine, the examiner decides the problem is in another joint, palpation should be delayed until that joint is completely examined. However, during palpation of the cervical spine, the examiner should note any tenderness, trigger points, muscle spasm, or other signs and symptoms that may indicate the source of the pathology.

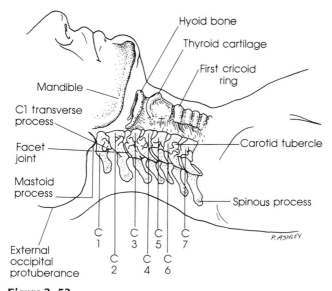

Figure 3–52
Palpation landmarks of the cervical spine.

As with any palpation, the examiner should note the texture of the skin and surrounding bony and soft tissues on the posterior, lateral, and anterior aspects of the neck. Usually, palpation is performed with the patient supine so that maximum relaxation of the neck muscles is possible. However, the examiner may palpate with the patient sitting (patient resting the head on forearms that are resting on something at shoulder height) or lying prone (on a table with a face hole) if it is more comfortable for the patient.

To palpate the posterior structures, the examiner stands behind the patient; the patient's head is "cupped" in the examiner's hand while the examiner palpates with the fingers of both hands. For the lateral and anterior structures, the examiner stands at the patient's side. If the examiner suspects that the problem is in the cervical spine, palpation is done on the following structures (Fig. 3–52).

Posterior Aspect

External Occipital Protuberance. The protuberance may be found in the posterior midline. The examiner palpates the posterior skull in midline and moves caudally until coming to a point where the fingers "dip" inward. The part of the bone just before the dip is the external occipital protuberance. The inion, or "bump of knowledge," is the most obvious point on the external occipital protuberance and lies in the midline of the occiput.

Spinous Processes and Facet Joints of Cervical Vertebrae. The spinous processes of C2, C6, and C7 are the most obvious. If the examiner palpates the occiput of the skull and descends in the midline, the C2 spinous process will be palpated as the first bump. The next spinous processes that are most obvious are C6 and C7, although C3, C4, and C5 can be differentiated with careful palpation. The examiner can differentiate between C6 and C7 by passively flexing and extending the patient's neck. With this movement, the C6 spinous process moves in and out and the C7 spinous process remains stationary. The movements between the spinous processes of C2 through C7 or T1 may be palpated by feeling between each set of spinous processes. While palpating between the spinous processes, the examiner's knees are flexed and extended, causing the cervical spine to flex and extend around the palpating finger. Relative movement between the cervical vertebrae can then be determined (i.e., hypomobility, normal movement, or hypermobility).[18] The facet joint may be palpated 1.3 to 2.5 cm (0.5 to 1 inch) lateral to the spinous process. Usually the facet joints are not felt as distinct structures but rather as a hard bony mass under the fingers. The muscles in the adjacent area may be palpated for tenderness, swelling, and other signs of pathology. Careful palpation should also include the suboccipital structures.

Mastoid Processes (Below and Behind Ear Lobe). If the examiner palpates the skull following the posterior aspect of the ear, there will be a point on the skull at which the finger again dips inward. The point just before the dip is the mastoid process.

Lateral Aspect

Transverse Processes of Cervical Vertebrae. The C1 transverse process is the easiest to palpate. The examiner first palpates the mastoid process and then moves inferiorly and slightly anteriorly until a hard bump is felt. If the examiner applies slight pressure to the bump, the patient should say it feels uncomfortable. These bumps are the transverse processes of C1. The other transverse process may be palpated if the musculature is sufficiently relaxed. After the C1 transverse process has been located, the examiner moves inferiorly, feeling for similar bumps. Normally, the bumps are not directly inferior but rather follow the lordotic path of the cervical vertebrae under the sternocleidomastoid muscle. These structures are situated more anteriorly than one might suspect (see Fig. 3–52). If the examiner rotates the patient's head while palpating the transverse processes of C1, the uppermost transverse process will protrude farther and the lower one will seem to disappear. During flexion, the space between the mastoid and the transverse processes increases. On extension, it decreases. On side flexion, the mastoid and transverse processes approach one another on the side to which the head is side flexed and separate on the other side.[18]

Lymph Nodes and Carotid Arteries. The lymph nodes are palpable only if they are swollen. The nodes lie along the line of the sternocleidomastoid muscle. The carotid pulse may be palpated in the midportion of the neck, between the sternocleidomastoid muscle and the trachea. The examiner should determine whether the pulse is normal and equal on both sides.

Temporomandibular Joints, Mandible, and Parotid Glands. The temporomandibular joints may be palpated anterior to the external ear. The examiner may either palpate directly over the joint or place the little or index finger (pulp forward) in the external ear to feel for movement in the joint. The examiner can then move the fingers along the length of the mandible, feeling for any abnormalities. The angle of the mandible is at the level of the C2 vertebra. Normally, the parotid gland is not palpable because it lies over the angle of the mandible. If it is swollen, however, it is palpable as a soft, boggy structure.

Anterior Aspect

Hyoid Bone, Thyroid Cartilage, and First Cricoid Ring. The hyoid bone may be palpated as part of the superior part of the trachea above the thyroid cartilage anterior to the C2–C3 vertebrae. The thyroid cartilage lies anterior to the C4–C5 vertebrae. With the neck in a neutral position, the thyroid cartilage can easily be moved. In extension, it is tight and crepitations may be felt. Adjacent to the cartilage is the thyroid gland, which the examiner should

palpate. If the gland is abnormal, it will be tender and enlarged. The cricoid ring is the first part of the trachea and lies above the site for an emergency tracheostomy. The ring moves when the patient swallows. Rough palpation of the ring may cause the patient to gag. While palpating the hyoid bone, the examiner should ask the patient to swallow; normally, the bone should move and cause no pain. The cricoid ring and thyroid cartilage also move when palpated as the patient swallows.

Paranasal Sinuses. Returning to the face, the examiner should palpate the paranasal sinuses (frontal and maxillary) for signs of tenderness and swelling (Fig. 3–53).

First Three Ribs. The examiner palpates the manubrium sternum and, moving the fingers laterally, follows the path of the first three ribs posteriorly. The examiner should palpate the ribs individually and with care, because it is difficult to palpate the ribs as they pass under the clavicle. The patient should be asked to breathe in and out deeply a few times so that the examiner can compare the movements of the ribs during breathing. Normally, there is equal mobility on both sides. The first

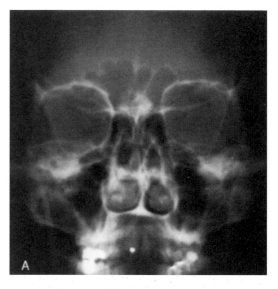

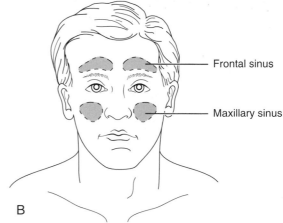

Figure 3–53

Paranasal sinuses. Radiograph (A) and illustration (B) of frontal and maxillary sinuses.

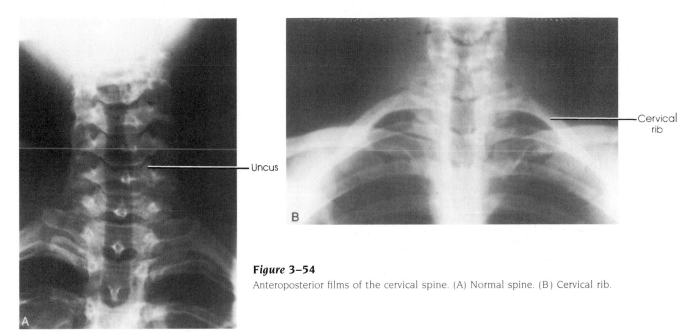

Uncus

Cervical rib

B

Figure 3–54
Anteroposterior films of the cervical spine. (A) Normal spine. (B) Cervical rib.

rib is more prone to pathology than the second and third ribs and can refer pain to the neck and/or shoulder.

Supraclavicular Fossa. The examiner can palpate the supraclavicular fossa, which is superior to the clavicle. Normally, the fossa is a smooth indentation. The examiner should palpate for swelling after trauma (possible fractured clavicle), abnormal soft tissue (possible swollen glands), and abnormal bony tissue (possible cervical rib). In addition, the examiner should palpate the sternocleidomastoid muscle along its length for signs of pathology, especially in cases of torticollis.

Diagnostic Imaging

Plain Film Radiography

Normally, a standard set of x-rays for the cervical spine is made up of an anteroposterior view, a lateral view, and an open or odontoid ("through-the-mouth") view. Other views are included if other pathologies are suspected.

Anteroposterior View. The examiner should look for or note the following (Figs. 3–54 and 3–55): the shape of

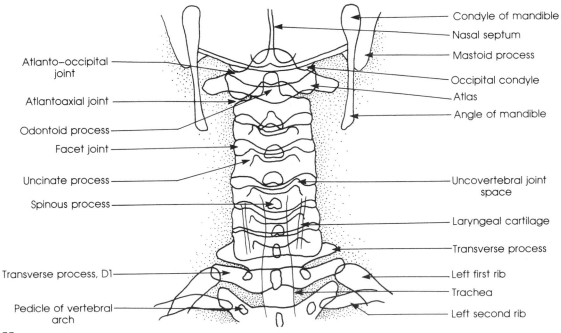

Atlanto-occipital joint
Atlantoaxial joint
Odontoid process
Facet joint
Uncinate process
Spinous process
Transverse process, D1
Pedicle of vertebral arch

Condyle of mandible
Nasal septum
Mastoid process
Occipital condyle
Atlas
Angle of mandible
Uncovertebral joint space
Laryngeal cartilage
Transverse process
Left first rib
Trachea
Left second rib

Figure 3–55
Diagram of structures seen on anteroposterior cervical spine film.

the vertebrae, the presence of any lateral wedging or osteophytes, the disc space, and the presence of a cervical rib. Frontal alignment should also be ascertained.

Lateral View. Lateral views of the cervical spine give the greatest amount of radiological information. The examiner should look for or note the following (Figs. 3–56, 3–57, and 3–58):

1. Normal or abnormal curvature. The curvature may be highly variable, because 20 to 40% of normal spines have a straight or slightly kyphotic curve in neutral.[43] Are the "lines" of the vertebrae normal? The line joining the anterior portion of the vertebral bodies (anterior

vertebral line) should form a smooth, unbroken arc from C2 to C7 (see Fig. 3–57). Similar lines should be seen for the posterior vertebral bodies (posterior vertebral line), which form the anterior aspect of the spinal canal, and the posterior aspect of the spinal canal (posterior canal line). Disruption of any of these lines would be an indication of instability possibly caused by ligamentous injury.

2. "Kinking" of the cervical spine. Kinking may be indicative of a subluxation or dislocation in the cervical spine.

3. General shape of the vertebrae. Is there any fusion, collapse, or wedging? The examiner should count

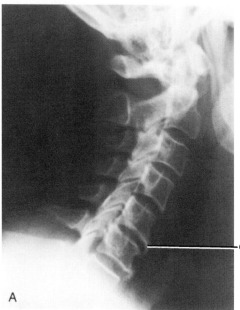

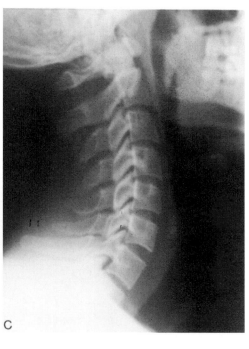

Figure 3–56
Lateral radiograph of the cervical spine.
(A) Normal curve showing osteophytic lipping.
(B) Cervical spine in flexion. (C) Cervical spine in extension.

Osteophyte

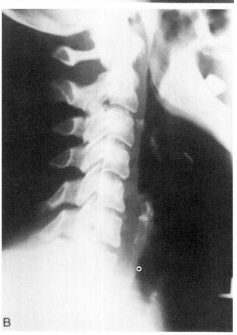

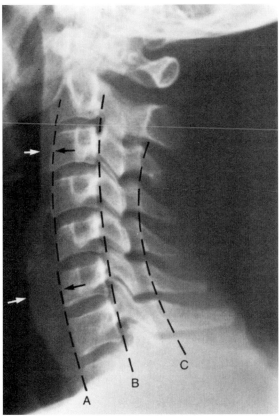

Figure 3–57

Normal cervical spine. Lateral projection. Note the alignment and appearance of the facet joints: A, anterior vertebral line; B, posterior vertebral line; C, posterior canal line. Retropharyngeal space (*between top arrows*) should not exceed 5 mm. Retrotracheal space (*between bottom arrows*) should not exceed 22 mm. (Modified from Forrester, D.M., and J.C. Brown: The Radiology of Joint Disease. Philadelphia: W.B. Saunders Co., 1987, p. 408.)

the vertebrae, because x-ray films do not always show C7 or T1, and it is essential that they be visualized for a proper radiological examination.

4. Displacement. Do the vertebrae sit in normal alignment with one another?

5. Disc space. Is it normal? Narrow? Narrowing may indicate cervical spondylosis.

6. Lipping (see Fig. 3–56A). Lipping indicates degeneration.

7. Osteophytes (see Fig. 3–56A). Osteophytes indicate degeneration or abnormal movement.

8. Normally, the ratio of the spinal canal diameter to the vertebral body diameter in the cervical spine is 1. If this ratio is less than 0.8, it is an indication of possible spinal stenosis.[10, 44, 45] This comparison is shown in Figure 3–57 (ratio AB:BC). Cantu[45] points out that this measurement is a static measurement and may not apply to stenosis that occurs during movement of the cervical spine.

9. Prevertebral soft-tissue width. Measured at the level of the anteroinferior border of the C3 vertebra, this width is normally 7 mm.[46] Edema or hemorrhage is suspected if the space is wider than 7 mm. The retropharyngeal space, lying between the anterior border of the vertebral body and the posterior border of the pharyngeal air shadow, should be from 2 to 5 mm in width at C3. From C4 to C7, the space is called the retrotracheal space and should be 18 to 22 mm in width (see Fig. 3–57).

10. Subluxation of the facets.

11. Abnormal soft-tissue shadows.

12. Forward shifting of C1 on C2. This finding indicates instability between C1 and C2. Normally, the joint space between the odontoid process and the anterior arch of the atlas (sometimes called the atlas dens index [ADI]) does not exceed 2.5 to 3 mm in the adult.

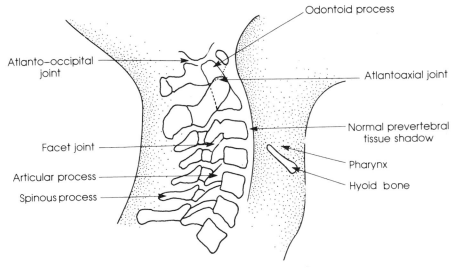

Figure 3–58

Diagram of structures seen on lateral film of the cervical spine.

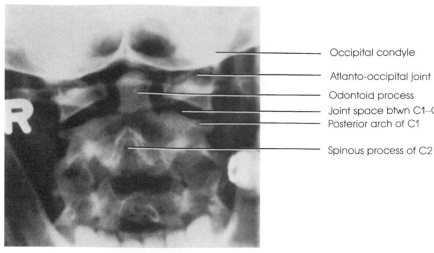

Occipital condyle
Atlanto-occipital joint
Odontoid process
Joint space btwn C1–C2
Posterior arch of C1
Spinous process of C2

Figure 3–59
Through-the-mouth radiograph.

13. Instability. Instability is present when more than 3.5 mm of horizontal displacement of one vertebra occurs in relation to the adjacent vertebra.

Open or Odontoid ("Through-the-Mouth") View. This anteroposterior view enables the examiner to determine the state of the odontoid process of C2 and its relation with C1 (Fig. 3–59). It may also show the atlanto-occipital and atlantoaxial joints.

Oblique View. This view provides information on the neural foramen and posterior elements of the cervical spine. The examiner should look for or note the following (Figs. 3–60 and 3–61):

1. Lipping of the joints of Luschka (osteophytes)
2. Overriding of the facet joints (subluxation, spondylosis)
3. Facet joints and intervertebral foramen (Fig. 3–61)

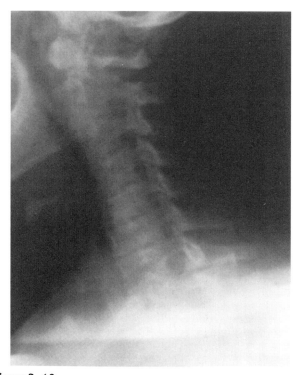

Figure 3–60
Abnormal x-ray findings on oblique view. Note loss of normal curve; narrowing at C4, C5, and C6; osteophytes and lipping of C4, C5, and C6; and encroachment on intervertebral foramen at C4–C5, C5–C6, and C6–C7.

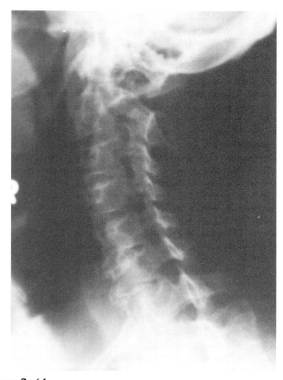

Figure 3–61
Oblique radiograph of the cervical spine showing intervertebral foramen and facet joints. Severe lipping in lower cervical spine and spondylosis are also evident.

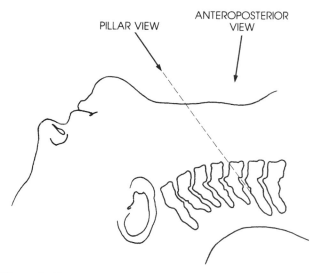

PILLAR VIEW   ANTEROPOSTERIOR VIEW

Figure 3–62
Diagram of pillar view showing orientation of facet joints.

Pillar View. This special view is used to evaluate the lateral masses of the cervical spine and especially the facet joints (Fig. 3–62). It is usually reserved for patients with suspected facet fractures.[47]

Computed Tomography

Computed tomography (CT) helps to delineate the bone and soft-tissue anatomy of the cervical spine in cross section and can show, for example, a disc prolapse. It also shows the true size and extent of osteophytes better than do plain x-rays (Fig. 3–63). CT scans are especially useful for showing bone fragments in the spinal canal

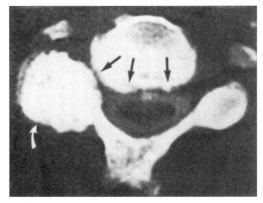

Figure 3–63
Foraminal stenosis caused by hypertrophic facet arthropathy and by spondylosis. Metrizamide-enhanced computed tomography scan through C5–C6 foramina details the markedly overgrown facet (*white arrow*) and the bony "bar," or spondylotic spurring (*black arrows*). The right foramen is almost occluded by abnormal bone. (From Dorwart, R.H., and D.L. LaMasters: Application of computed tomographic scanning of the cervical spine. Orthop. Clin. North Am. 16:386, 1985.)

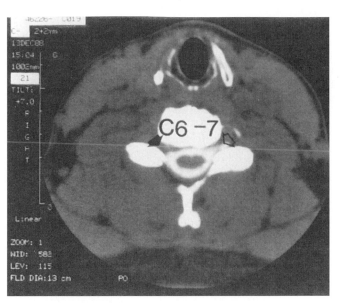

Figure 3–64
Postcontrast computed tomogram showing normally patent neural foramen at the C6–C7 level on the left side (*open arrow*). The nerve root sleeve fills with contrast medium and enters the neural foramen. On the right side (*closed arrow*), there is no evidence of filling of the nerve root sleeve within the neural foramen secondary to lateral C6–C7 disc herniation. (From Bell, G.R., and J.S. Ross: Diagnosis of nerve root compression: Myelography, computed tomography, and MRI. Orthop. Clin. North Am. 23:410, 1992.)

after a fracture and bony defects in the vertebral bodies and neural arches. CT scans may be combined with myelography to outline the spinal cord and nerve roots inside the thecal sac (Fig. 3–64). CT scans are used only after conventional radiographs have been taken and a need for them is shown.

Myelography

Myelograms are the modality of choice with brachial plexus avulsions, either Erb-Duchenne paralysis (C5 and C6) or Klumpke's paralysis (C7, C8, and T1). They may also be used to demonstrate narrowing in the intervertebral foramen and cervical spinal stenosis. They may be used to outline the contour of the thecal sac, nerve roots, and spinal cord (Fig. 3–65).

Magnetic Resonance Imaging

This noninvasive technique can differentiate between various soft tissues and bone (Fig. 3–66). Because it shows differences based on water content, magnetic resonance imaging (MRI) can differentiate between the nucleus pulposus and the annulus fibrosus. MRI may be used to reveal disc protrusions, but it has been reported that patients showing these lesions are often asymptomatic, highlighting the fact that radiographic abnormali-

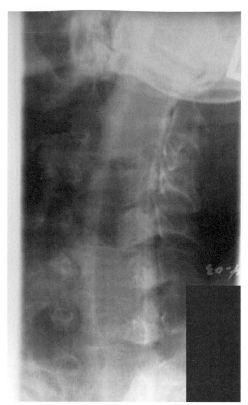

Figure 3–65
Myelogram of cervical spine.

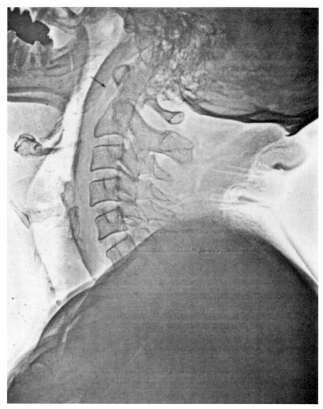

Figure 3–67
Xeroradiograph of cervical spine (lateral view). Arrow indicates calcified mass. (From Forrester, D.M., and J.C. Brown: The Radiology of Joint Disease. Philadelphia: W.B. Saunders Co., 1987, p. 420.)

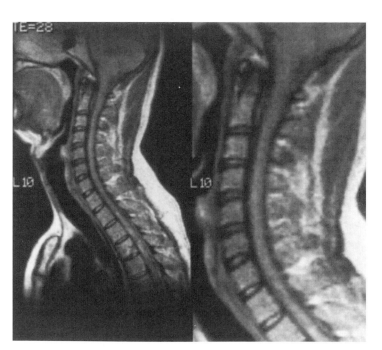

Figure 3–66
Magnetic resonance image of the cervical and upper thoracic spine. Sagittal view (*left*), with close-up of cervical spine (*right*). (From Foreman, S.M., and A.C. Croft: Whiplash Injuries: The Cervical Acceleration/Deceleration Syndrome. Baltimore: Williams & Wilkins Co., 1988, p. 126.)

ties should be considered only in relation to the history and examination.[48] An MRI allows visualization of the nerve roots, spinal cord, and thecal sac as well as the bone and bone marrow. It is also used to identify postoperative scarring and disc herniation.[49]

Xeroradiography

This technique also helps to delineate bone and soft tissue by enhancing the interfaces between tissues (Fig. 3–67).

Précis of the Cervical Spine Assessment*

History
Observation (standing or sitting)
Examination, sitting
  Active movements
    Flexion
    Extension
    Side flexion (right and left)
    Rotation (right and left)
    Combined movements (if necessary)
    Repetitive movements (if necessary)
    Sustained movements (if necessary)
  Resisted isometric movements (as in active movements)
  Peripheral joint scan
    Temporomandibular joints (open mouth and closed mouth)
    Shoulder girdle (elevation through abduction, elevation through forward flexion, elevation through plane of scapula, medial and lateral rotation with arm at side; medial and lateral rotation at 90° abduction)
    Elbow (flexion, extension, supination, pronation)
    Wrist (flexion, extension, radial and ulnar deviation)
    Fingers and thumb (flexion, extension, abduction, adduction, circumduction)
  Myotomes
    Neck flexion (C1–C2)
    Neck side flexion (C3)
    Shoulder elevation (C4)
    Shoulder abduction (C5)
    Elbow flexion (C6) and/or extension (C7)
    Wrist flexion (C7) and/or extension (C6)
    Thumb extension (C8) and/or ulnar deviation (C8)
    Hand intrinsics (abduction or adduction [T1])
  Special tests
    Foraminal compression (Spurling's) test
    Distraction test
    Shoulder abduction test
    Vertebral artery tests

  Reflexes and cutaneous distribution
    Biceps (C5–C6)
    Triceps (C7–C8)
    Hoffmann's sign
    Sensory scan
Examination, supine
  Passive movements
    Flexion
    Extension
    Side flexion
    Rotation
  Special tests
    Upper limb tension test
    Vertebral artery tests
  Joint play movements
    Side glide of cervical spine
    Anterior glide of cervical spine
    Posterior glide of cervical spine
    Traction glide of cervical spine
    Rotation of occiput on C1
  Palpation
Examination, prone
  Joint play movements
    Posteroanterior central vertebral pressure
    Posteroanterior unilateral vertebral pressure
    Transverse vertebral pressure
  Palpation
  Diagnostic imaging

---

* The précis is shown in an order that limits the amount of moving that the patient has to do but ensures that all necessary structures are tested.

After any examination, the patient should be warned of the possibility of exacerbation of symptoms as a result of the assessment.

Case Studies

When doing these case studies, the examiner should list the appropriate questions to be asked and why they are being asked, what to look for and why, and what things should be tested and why. Depending on the answers of the patient (and the examiner should consider different responses), several possible causes of the patient's problems may become evident (examples are given in parentheses). A differential diagnosis chart should be made up (see Table 3–13 as an example). The examiner can then decide how different diagnoses may affect the treatment plan.

1. A 2-month-old baby is brought to you by a concerned parent. The child does not move the head properly, and the sternocleidomastoid muscle on the left side is prominent. Describe your assessment plan before beginning treatment (congenital torticollis versus Klippel-Feil syndrome).

2. A 54-year-old man comes to you complaining of neck stiffness, especially on rising; sometimes he has numbness into his left arm. Describe your assessment plan (cervical spondylosis versus subacromial bursitis).

Table 3–13
Differential Diagnosis of Cervical Facet Syndrome, Cervical Nerve Root Lesion, and Thoracic Outlet Syndrome

Signs and Symptoms	Facet Syndrome	Cervical Nerve Root	Thoracic Outlet Syndrome
Pain referral	Possible	Yes	Possible
Pain on hyperextension and rotation	Yes (often without increased referral of symptoms)	Yes with increased symptoms	No
Spine stiffness	Yes	Possible	Possible
Paresthesia	No	Yes	Possible
Reflexes	Not affected	May be affected	May be affected
Muscle spasm	Yes	Yes	Yes
Tension tests	May or may not be positive	Positive	May be positive
Pallor and coolness	No	No	Possible
Muscle weakness	No	Possible	Not early (later small hand muscles)
Muscle fatigue and cramps	No	No	Possible

3. An 18-year-old male football player comes to you complaining of a "dead arm" after a tackle he made 2 days ago. Although he can now move the left arm, it still does not feel right. Describe your assessment plan (brachial plexus lesion versus acromioclavicular sprain).

4. A 23-year-old woman comes to you after a motor vehicle accident. Her car was hit from behind while stopped for a red light. She could tell the accident was going to occur because she could see in the rear-view mirror that the car behind her was not going to be able to stop. The car that hit her was going 50 kph (30 mph), and skid marks were visible for only 5 m from the location of her car. Describe your assessment plan (cervical sprain versus cervical facet syndrome).

5. A woman comes to you complaining of persistent headaches that last for days at a time. She is 35 years old and has recently lost her job. She complains that she sometimes sees flashing lights and cannot stand having anyone around her when the pain is very bad. Describe your assessment plan for this patient (migraine versus tension headache).

6. A 26-year-old man comes to you complaining of pain in his neck. The pain was evident yesterday when he got up and has not decreased significantly since then. He thinks that he may have "slept wrong." There is no previous history of trauma. Describe your assessment plan for this patient (acquired torticollis versus cervical disc lesion).

7. A 75-year-old woman comes to you complaining primarily of neck pain but also of stiffness. She exhibits a dowager's hump. There is no history of trauma. Describe your assessment plan for this patient (osteoporosis versus cervical spondylosis).

8. A 47-year-old man comes to you complaining of elbow and neck pain. There is no recent history of trauma, but he remembers being in a motor vehicle accident 19 years ago. He now works at a desk all day. Describe your assessment for this patient (cervical spondylosis versus tennis elbow versus double-crush injury).

9. A 16-year-old boy comes to you with a complaint of having hurt his neck. While "fooling" with some friends at the lake, he ran away from them and dove into the water to get away. The top of his head hit the bottom, and he felt a burning pain. The pain decreased as he came out of the water, but he still has a residual ache. Describe your plan for this patient (cervical fracture versus cervical sprain).

10. A 14-year-old girl comes to you complaining of neck pain. She has long hair. She states that when she "whipped" her hair out of her eyes, which she has done many times before, she felt a sudden pain in her neck. Although the pain intensity has decreased, it is still there, and she cannot fully move her neck. Describe your assessment plan for this patient (cervical sprain versus acquired torticollis).

References

Cited References

1. Cyriax, J.: Textbook of Orthopaedic Medicine, vol. 1: Diagnosis of Soft Tissue Lesions. London, Bailliere Tindall, 1982.
2. Boreades, A.G., and J. Gershon-Cohen: Luschka joints of the cervical spine. Radiology 66:181–187, 1956.
3. Hall, M.C.: Luschka's Joint. Springfield, Illinois, Charles C Thomas, 1965.
4. Silberstein, C.E.: The evolution of degenerative changes in the cervical spine and an investigation into the "joint of Luschka." Clin. Orthop. 40:184–204, 1965.
5. Willis, T.A.: Luschka's joints. Clin. Orthop. 46:121–125, 1966.
6. Ferlic, D.: The nerve supply of the cervical intervertebral disc in man. Johns Hopkins Hosp. Bull. 113:347, 1963.
7. Mednel, T., C.S. Wink, and M.L. Zimny: Neural elements in human cervical intervertebral discs. Spine 17:132–135, 1992.
8. Watkins, R.G.: Neck injuries in football. In Watkins, R.G. (ed.): The Spine in Sports. St. Louis, Mosby–Year Book Inc., 1996.
9. Travell, T.G., and D.G. Simons: Myofascial Pain and Dysfunction: The Trigger Point Manual, vol. 1. Baltimore, Williams & Wilkins, 1983.
10. Tsairis, P., and B. Jordan: Neurological evaluation of cervical spinal disorders. In Camins, M.B., and P.F. O'Leary (eds.): Disorders of the Cervical Spine. Baltimore, Williams & Wilkins, 1992.
11. Foreman, S.M., and A.C. Croft: Whiplash Injuries: The Cervical Acceleration/Deceleration Syndrome. Baltimore, Williams & Wilkins, 1988.

12. Evans, R.C.: Illustrated Essentials in Orthopedic Physical Assessment. St. Louis, Mosby–Year Book Inc., 1994.
13. Bradley, J.P., J.E. Tibone, and R.G. Watkins: History, physical examination, and diagnostic tests for neck and upper extremity problems. In Watkins, R.G. (ed.): The Spine in Sports. St. Louis, Mosby–Year Book Inc., 1996.
14. Youdas, J.W., T.R. Garrett, V.J. Suman, C.L. Bogard, H.O. Hallman, and J.R. Carey: Normal range of motion of the cervical spine: An initial goniometric study. Phys. Ther. 72:770–780, 1992.
15. Dvorak, J., J.A. Antinnes, M. Panjabi, D. Loustalot, and M. Bonomo: Age and gender related normal motion of the cervical spine. Spine 17:S393–S398, 1992.
16. Toole, J., and S.H. Tucker: Influence of head position upon cervical circulation. Arch. Neurol. 2:616–623, 1960.
17. Elvey, R.L.: The investigation of arm pain. In Boyling, J.D., and N. Palastanga (eds.): Grieve's Modern Manual Therapy: The Vertebral Column, 2nd ed. Edinburgh, Churchill Livingstone, 1994.
18. Magarey, M.E.: Examination of the cervical spine. In Grieve, G.P. (ed.): Modern Manual Therapy of the Vertebral Column. Edinburgh, Churchill Livingstone, 1986.
19. Schneider, R., H. Gosch, H. Norrell, M. Jerva, L. Combs, and R. Smith: Vascular insufficiency and differential distortion of brain and cord caused by cervicomedullary football injuries. J. Neurosurg. 33:363–375, 1970.
20. Vernon, H., and S. Mior: The neck disability index: A study of reliability and validity. J. Manip. Physiol. Ther. 14:409–415, 1991.
21. Spurling, R.G., and W.B. Scoville: Lateral rupture of the cervical intervertebral disc. Surg. Gynec. Obstet. 78:350–358, 1944.
22. Kelly, J.J.: Neurological problems in the athlete's shoulder. In Pettrone, F.A. (ed.): Athletic Injuries of the Shoulder. New York, McGraw-Hill, 1995.
23. Wells, P.: Cervical dysfunction and shoulder problems. Physiotherapy 68:66–73, 1982.
24. Butler, D.S.: Mobilisation of the Nervous System. Melbourne, Churchill Livingstone, 1991.
25. Slater, H., D.S. Butler, and M.O. Shacklock: The dynamic central nervous system: Examination and assessment using tension tests. In Boyling, J.D., and N. Palastanga (eds.): Grieve's Modern Manual Therapy: The Vertebral Column, 2nd ed. Edinburgh, Churchill Livingstone, 1994.
26. Davidson, R.I., E.J. Dunn, and J.N. Metzmaker: The shoulder abduction test in the diagnosis of radicular pain in cervical extradural compressive monoradiculopathies. Spine 6:441–446, 1981.
27. Farmer, J.C., and R.J. Wisneski: Cervical spine nerve root compression: An analysis of neuroforaminal pressure with varying head and arm positions. Spine 19:1850–1855, 1994.
28. Landi, A., and S. Copeland: Value of the Tinel sign in brachial plexus lesions. Ann. R. Coll. Surg. Engl. 61:470–471, 1979.
29. Uchihara, T., T. Furukawa, and H. Tsukagoshi: Compression of brachial plexus as a diagnostic test of a cervical cord lesion. Spine 19:2170–2173, 1994.
30. Maitland, G.D.: Vertebral Manipulation. London, Butterworths, 1973.
31. Ombregt, L., P. Bisschop, H.J. ter Veer, and T. Van de Velde: A System of Orthopedic Medicine. London, W.B. Saunders Co., 1995.
32. Grant, R.: Vertebral artery insufficiency: A clinical protocol for pre-manipulative testing of the cervical spine. In Boyling, J.D., and N. Palastanga (eds.): Grieve's Modern Manual Therapy: The Vertebral Column, 2nd ed. Edinburgh, Churchill Livingstone, 1994.
33. Wadsworth, C.T.: Manual Examination and Treatment of the Spine and Extremities. Baltimore, Williams & Wilkins, 1988.
34. Aspinall, W.: Clinical testing for cervical mechanical disorders which produce ischemic vertigo. J. Orthop. Sports Phys. Ther. 11:176–182, 1989.
35. Meadows, J.J., and D.J. Magee: An overview of dizziness and vertigo for the orthopedic manual therapist. In Boyling, J.D., and N. Palastanga (eds.): Grieve's Modern Manual Therapy: The Vertebral Column, 2nd ed. Edinburgh, Churchill Livingstone, 1994.
36. Gird, R.B., and H.C. Naffziger: Prolonged jugular compression:

A new diagnostic test of neurological value. Trans. Am. Neurol. Assoc. 66:45–49, 1940.
37. Fitz-Ritson, D.: Assessment of cervicogenic vertigo. J. Manip. Physiol. Ther. 14:193–198, 1991.
38. Aspinall, W.: Clinical testing for the craniovertebral hypermobility syndrome. J. Orthop. Sports Phys. Ther. 12:47–54, 1990.
39. Pettman, E.: Stress tests of the craniovertebral joints. In Boyling, J.D., and N. Palastanga (eds.): Grieve's Modern Manual Therapy: The Vertebral Column, 2nd ed. Edinburgh, Churchill Livingstone, 1994.
40. Denno, J.J., and G.R. Meadows: Early diagnosis of cervical spondylotic myelopathy: A useful clinical sign. Spine 16:1353–1355, 1991.
41. Refshauge, K., and E. Gass: The neurological examination. In Refshauge, K., and E. Gass (eds.): Musculoskeletal Physiotherapy. Oxford, Butterworth-Heinemann Ltd., 1995.
42. Mennell, J.M.: Joint Pain. Boston, Little, Brown & Co., 1964.
43. Helliwell, P.S., P.F. Evans, and V. Wright: The straight cervical spine: Does it indicate muscle spasm? J. Bone Joint Surg. Br. 76:103–106, 1994.
44. Pavlov, H., J.S. Torg, B. Robie, and C. Jahre: Cervical spine stenosis: Determination with vertebral body method. Radiology 164:771–775, 1987.
45. Cantu, R.C.: Functional cervical spinal stenosis: A contraindication to participation in contact sports. Med. Sci. Sports Exerc. 25:316–317, 1993.
46. Templeton, P.A., J.W. Young, S.E. Mirvis, et al.: The value of retropharyngeal soft tissue measurements in trauma of the adult cervical spine. Skeletal Radiol. 18:98–104, 1987.
47. Harris, J.H.: Radiographic evaluation of spinal trauma. Orthop. Clin. North Am. 17:75–86, 1986.
48. Reid, D.C.: Sports Injury Assessment and Rehabilitation. New York, Churchill Livingstone, 1992.
49. Bigg-Wither, G., and P. Kelly: Diagnostic imaging in musculoskeletal physiotherapy. In Refshauge, K., and E. Gass (eds.): Musculoskeletal Physiotherapy. Oxford, Butterworth-Heinemann Ltd., 1995.

General References

Aprill, C., A. Dwyer, and N. Bogduk: Cervical zygapophyseal joint pain patterns: A clinical evaluation. Spine 15:458–461, 1990.
Bassett, L.W., R.H. Gold, and L.L. Seeger: MRI Atlas of the Musculoskeletal System. London, Martin Dunitz Ltd., 1989.
Bateman, J.E.: The Shoulder and Neck. Philadelphia, W.B. Saunders Co., 1972.
Beatty, R.M., F.D. Fowler, and E.J. Hanson: The abducted arm as a sign of ruptured cervical disc. Neurosurgery 21:731–732, 1987.
Bell, G.R., and J.S. Ross: Diagnosis of nerve root compression: Myelography, computed tomography, and MRI. Orthop. Clin. North Am. 23:405–419, 1992.
Beggs, I.: Radiological assessment of degenerative diseases of the cervical spine. Semin. Orthop. 2:63–73, 1987.
Bland, J.H.: Disorders of the Cervical Spine. Philadelphia, W.B. Saunders Co., 1994.
Bogduk, N., and A. Marsland: The cervical zygapophyseal joints as a source of neck pain. Spine 13:610–617, 1988.
Bonica, J.J.: The Management of Pain. Philadelphia, Lea & Febiger, 1953.
Butler, D., and L. Gifford: The concept of adverse mechanical tension in the nervous system. Physiotherapy 75:622–636, 1989.
Cailliet, R.: Neck and Arm Pain. Philadelphia, F.A. Davis Co., 1964.
Campbell, A.M., and D.G. Phillips: Cervical disc lesions with neurological disorder. Br. Med. J. 2:480–485, 1960.
Cates, J.R., and M.M. Soriano: Cervical spondylotic myelopathy. J. Manip. Physiol. Ther. 18:471–475, 1995.
Cervical Spine Research Society: The Cervical Spine. Philadelphia, J.B. Lippincott, 1989.
Cibulka, M.T.: Evaluation and treatment of cervical spine injuries. Clin. Sports Med. 8:691–701, 1989.

Clark, C.R.: Examination of the neck. In Clark, C.R., and M. Bonfiglio (eds.): Orthopedics: Essentials of Diagnosis and Treatment. New York, Churchill Livingstone, 1994.

Clark, C.R., C.M. Igram, G.Y. El-Khoury, and S. Ehara: Radiologic evaluation of cervical spine injuries. Spine 13:742–747, 1988.

Collins, H.R.: An evaluation of cervical and lumbar discography. Clin. Orthop. 107:133–138, 1975.

Crouch, J.E.: Functional Human Anatomy. Philadelphia, Lea & Febiger, 1973.

Darnell, M.W.: A proposed chronology of events for forward head posture. J. Craniomand. Pract. 1:50–54, 1983.

Dorwart, R.H., and D.L. LaMasters: Application of computed tomographic scanning of the cervical spine. Orthop. Clin. North Am. 16:381–393, 1985.

Dvorak, J., and V. Dvorak: Manual Medicine: Diagnostics. New York, Thieme-Stratton Inc., 1984.

Edmeads, J.: Headaches and head pains associated with diseases of the cervical spine. Med. Clin. North Am. 62:533–544, 1978.

Edwards, B.C.: Combined movements in the cervical spine (C2–7): Their value in examination and technique choice. Aust. J. Physiother. 26:165–171, 1980.

Esposito, C.J., G.A. Crim, and T.K. Binkley: Headaches: A differential diagnosis. J. Craniomand. Pract. 4:318–322, 1986.

Ferlic, D.: The range of motion of the "normal" cervical spine. Johns Hopkins Hosp. Bull. 110:59, 1962.

Fielding, J.W.: Normal and selected abnormal motion of the cervical spine from the second cervical vertebra to the seventh cervical vertebra based on cineroentgenography. J. Bone Joint Surg. Am. 46:1779–1781, 1964.

Fielding, J.W., G.B. Cochran, J.F. Lawsing, and M. Hohl: Tears of the transverse ligament of the atlas: A clinical and biomechanical study. J. Bone Joint Surg. Am. 56:1683–1691, 1974.

Forrester, D.M., and J.C. Brown: The Radiology of Joint Disease. Philadelphia: W.B. Saunders Co., 1987.

Franco, J.L., and A. Herzog: A comparative assessment of neck muscle strength and vertebral stability. J. Orthop. Sports Phys. Ther. 8:351–356, 1987.

Frykholm, R.: Lower cervical vertebrae and intervertebral discs: Surgical anatomy and pathology. Acta Chir. Scand. 101–102:345–359, 1951–1952.

Gould, G.A.: The Spine. In Gould, G.A. (ed.): Orthopedic and Sports Physical Therapy. St. Louis, C.V. Mosby Co., 1990.

Grieve, G.P.: Mobilisation of the Spine, 3rd ed. New York, Churchill Livingstone, 1979.

Grieve, G.P.: Common Vertebral Joint Problems. New York, Churchill Livingstone, 1981.

Gundry, C.R., and K.B. Heithoff: Imaging evaluation of patients with spinal deformity. Orthop. Clin. North Am. 25:247–264, 1994.

Harrelson, G.L.: Evaluation of brachial plexus injuries. Sportsmed. Update 4:3–9, 1989.

Hensinger, R.N.: Congenital anomalies of the cervical spine. Clin. Orthop. 264:16–38, 1991.

Herrmann, D.B.: Validity study of head and neck flexion-extension motion comparing measurements of a pendulum goniometer and roentgenograms. J. Orthop. Sports Phys. Ther. 11:414–418, 1990.

Hershman, E.B.: Injuries to the brachial plexus. In Torg, J.S. (ed.): Athletic Injuries to the Head, Neck and Face. St. Louis, Mosby–Year Book, 1991.

Hohl, M.: Normal motions in the upper portion of the cervical spine. J. Bone Joint Surg. Am. 46:1777–1779, 1964.

Hohl, M., and H.R. Baker: The atlanto-axial joint: Roentgenographic and anatomic study of normal and abnormal motion. J. Bone Joint Surg. Am. 46:1739–1752, 1964.

Hohl, M.: Soft-tissue injuries of the neck. Clin. Orthop. 109:42–49, 1975.

Hollinshead, W.H., and D.B. Jenkins: Functional Anatomy of the Limbs and Back. Philadelphia, W.B. Saunders Co., 1981.

Hoppenfeld, S.: Physical Examination of the Spine and Extremities. New York, Appleton-Century-Crofts, 1976.

Hu, R., R. Burnham, D.C. Reid, M. Grace, and L. Saboe: Burners in contact sports. Clin. J. Sports Med. 1:236–242, 1991.

Jackson, R.: The Cervical Syndrome. Springfield, Illinois, Charles C Thomas, 1976.

Judge, R.D., G.D. Zuidema, and F.T. Fitzgerald: Clinical Diagnosis: A Physiological Approach. Boston, Little, Brown & Co., 1982.

Kapandji, I.A.: The Physiology of Joints, vol. 3: The Trunk and the Vertebral Column. New York, Churchill Livingstone, 1974.

Kaye, J.J., and E.P. Nance: Cervical spine trauma. Orthop. Clin. North Am. 21:449–462, 1990.

Kaye, S., and E. Mason: Clinical implications of the upper limb tension test. Physiotherapy 75:750–752, 1989.

Kettner, N.W.: The radiology of cervical spine injury. J. Manip. Physiol. Ther. 14:518–526, 1991.

Law, M.D., M. Bernhardt, and A.A. White: Evaluation and management of cervical spondylotic myelopathy. J. Bone Joint Surg. Am. 76:1420–1433, 1994.

Liebenson, C.S.: Thoracic outlet syndrome: Diagnosis and conservative management. J. Manip. Physiol. Ther. 11:493–499, 1988.

Liebgott, B.: The Anatomical Basis of Dentistry. Philadelphia, W.B. Saunders Co., 1982.

Lysell, E.: Motion in the cervical spine. Acta Orthop. Scand. Suppl. 123:1–61, 1969.

Macnab, I.: Cervical spondylosis. Clin. Orthop. 109:69–77, 1975.

Maigne, R.: Orthopaedic Medicine: A New Approach to Vertebral Manipulation. Springfield, Illinois, Charles C Thomas, 1972.

Maigne, R.: Diagnosis and Treatment of Pain of Vertebral Origin: A Manual Medicine Approach. Baltimore, Williams & Wilkins, 1996.

Mathews, J.A., and J. Pemberton: Radiologic anatomy of the neck. Physiotherapy 65:77–80, 1979.

Matsunaga, S., T. Sakou, E. Taketomi, M. Yamaguchi, and T. Okano: The natural course of myelopathy caused by ossification of the posterior longitudinal ligament in the cervical spine. Clin. Orthop. 305:1668–1677, 1994.

McRae, R.: Clinical Orthopaedic Examination. New York, Churchill Livingstone, 1976.

Meyer, S.A., K.R. Schulte, J.J. Callaghan, et al.: Cervical spinal stenosis and stingers in collegiate football players. Am. J. Sports Med. 22:158–166, 1994.

Palmer, M.L., and M. Epler: Clinical Assessment Procedures in Physical Therapy. Philadelphia, J.B. Lippincott Co., 1990.

Panjabi, M.M.: Cervical spine mechanics as a function of transection of components. J. Biomech. 8:327–336, 1975.

Patterson, R.H.: Cervical ribs and the scalenus muscle syndrome. Ann. Surg. 111:531–543, 1940.

Pavlov, H.: Radiographic evaluation of the cervical spine and related structures. In Torg, J.S. (ed.): Athletic Injuries to the Head, Neck and Face. St. Louis, Mosby–Year Book Inc., 1991.

Pavlov, H., J.S. Torg, B. Robie, and C. Jahre: Cervical spinal stenosis: Determination with vertebral body ratio method. Radiology 164:771–775, 1987.

Pedersen, H.E., C.F.J. Blunck, and E. Gardner: The anatomy of lumbosacral posterior rami and meningeal branches of spinal nerves (sinu-vertebral nerves). J. Bone Joint Surg. Am. 38:377–391, 1956.

Penning, L.: Functional pathology of the cervical spine. New York, Excerpta Medica Foundation, 1968.

Penning, L.: Normal movements of the cervical spine. Am. J. Roentgenol. 130:317–326, 1978.

Porterfield, J.A., and C. DeRosa: Mechanical Neck Pain. Philadelphia, W.B. Saunders Co., 1995.

Post, M.: Physical Examination of the Musculoskeletal System. Chicago, Year Book Medical Publishers, 1987.

Ratkovits, B.L.: Radiographic assessment. In Bland, J.H. (ed.): Disorders of the Lumbar Spine. Philadelphia, W.B. Saunders Co., 1994.

Refshauge, K.: Testing adequacy of cerebral blood flow (vertebral artery testing). In Refshauge, K., and E. Gass (eds.): Musculoskeletal Physiotherapy. Oxford, Butterworth-Heinemann Ltd., 1995.

Refshauge, K.M.: Rotation: A valid premanipulative dizziness test? Does it predict safe manipulation? J. Manip. Physiol. Ther. 17:15–19, 1994.

Rheault, W., B. Albright, C. Byers, et al.: Intertester reliability of the cervical range of motion device. J. Orthop. Sports Phys. Ther. 15:147–150, 1992.

Rockett, F.X.: Observations on the "burner": Traumatic cervical radiculopathy. Clin. Orthop. 164:18–19, 1982.

Rohim, K.A., and J.L. Stambough: Radiographic evaluation of the degenerative cervical spine. Orthop. Clin. North Am. 23:395–403, 1992.

Rorabech, C.H., and W.R. Harris: Factors affecting the prognosis of brachial plexus injuries. J. Bone Joint Surg. Br. 63:404–407, 1981.

Rothman, R.H.: The acute cervical disc. Clin. Orthop. 109:59–68, 1975.

Rothman, R.H., and F.A. Simeone: The Spine. Philadelphia, W.B. Saunders Co., 1982.

Saunders, H.D., and R. Saunders: Evaluation, Treatment and Prevention of Musculoskeletal Disorders. Chaska, Minnesota, Educational Opportunities, 1995.

Selvaratnam, P.J., T.A. Matyas, and E.F. Glasgow: Noninvasive discrimination of brachial plexus involvement in upper limb pain. Spine 19:26–33, 1994.

Sherk, H.H., W.C. Watters, and L. Zeiger: Evaluation and treatment of neck pain. Orthop. Clin. North Am. 13:439–452, 1982.

Southwick, W.O., and K. Keggi: The normal cervical spine. J. Bone Joint Surg. Am. 46:1767–1777, 1964.

Speer, K.P., and F.H. Bassett: The prolonged burner syndrome. Am. J. Sports Med. 18:591–594, 1990.

Stanwood, J.E., and G.H. Kraft: Diagnosis and assessment of brachial plexus injuries. Arch. Phys. Med. Rehabil. 52:52–60, 1971.

Stratton, S.A., and J.M. Bryon: Dysfunction, evaluation and treatment of the cervical spine and thoracic inlet. In Donatelli, R., and M.J. Wooden (eds.): Orthopedic Physical Therapy. New York, Churchill Livingstone, 1989.

Sunderland, S.: Meningeal-neural relations in the intervertebral foramen. J. Neurosurg. 40:756–763, 1974.

Tardiff, G.S.: Nerve injuries: Testing and treatment tactics. Phys. Sportsmed. 23:61–72, 1995.

Tatlow, W.F.T., and H.G. Bammer: Syndrome of vertebral artery compression. Neurology 7:331–340, 1957.

Templeton, P.A., J.W. Young, S.E. Mirvis, and E.U. Buddemeyer: The value of retrophalangeal soft tissue measurements in trauma of the adult cervical spine. Skeletal Radiol. 16:98–104, 1987.

Torg, J.S., H. Pavlov, and S.G. Glasgow: Radiographic evaluation of athletic injuries to the cervical spine. In Camins, M.B., and P.F. O'Leary (eds.): Disorders of the Cervical Spine. Baltimore, Williams & Wilkins, 1992.

Troost, B.T.: Dizziness and vertigo in vertebrobasilar disease. Stroke 11:413–415, 1980.

Vereschagin, K.S., J.J. Wiens, G.S. Fanton, and M.F. Dillingham: Burners: Don't overlook or underestimate them. Phys. Sportsmed. 19:96–106, 1991.

Waldron, R.L., and E.H. Wood: Cervical myelography. Clin. Orthop. 97:74–89, 1973.

Wasenko, J.J., and C.F. Lanzieri: Plain radiographic examination in cervical spine trauma. In Camins, M.B., and P.F. O'Leary (eds.): Disorders of the Cervical Spine. Baltimore, Williams & Wilkins, 1992.

Weir, D.C.: Roentgenographic signs of cervical injury. Clin. Orthop. 109:9–17, 1975.

White, A.A., R.M. Johnson, M.M. Panjabi, and W.O. Southwick: Biomechanical analysis of clinical stability in the cervical spine. Clin. Orthop. 109:85–96, 1975.

White, A.A., and M.M. Panjabi: The clinical biomechanics of the occipito-atlantoaxial complex. Orthop. Clin. North Am. 9:867–878, 1978.

White, A.A., and M.M. Panjabi: Clinical Biomechanics of the Spine. Philadelphia, J.B. Lippincott Co., 1978.

Williams, P., and R. Warwick (eds.): Gray's Anatomy, 36th British ed. Edinburgh, Churchill Livingstone, 1980.

Wong, A., and D.D. Nansel: Comparisons between active vs passive end-range assessments in subjects exhibiting cervical range of motion asymmetries. J. Manip. Physiol. Ther. 15:159–163, 1992.

Worth, D.R.: Movements of the head and neck. In Boyling, J.D., and N. Palastanga (eds.): Grieve's Modern Manual Therapy: The Vertebral Column, 2nd ed. Edinburgh, Churchill Livingstone, 1994.

Wyke, B.: Neurology of the cervical spine joints. Physiotherapy 65:72–76, 1979.

Yu, Y.L., E. Woo, and C.Y. Huang: Cervical spondylotic myelopathy and radiculopathy. Acta Neurol. Scand. 75:367–373, 1987.

Zatzkin, H.R., and F.W. Kveton: Evaluation of the cervical spine in whiplash injuries. Radiology 75:577–583, 1960.

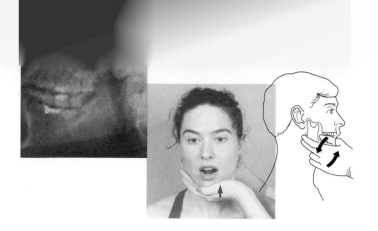

4

Temporomandibular Joint

The temporomandibular joints are two of the most frequently used joints in the body, but they probably receive the least amount of attention. Without these joints, we would be severely hindered when talking, eating, yawning, kissing, or sucking. In any examination of the head and neck, the temporomandibular joints should be included. Much of the work in this chapter has been developed from the teachings of Rocabado.[1]

Applied Anatomy

The temporomandibular joint is a synovial, condylar, and hinge-type joint with fibrocartilaginous surfaces rather than hyaline cartilage and an articular disc; this disc completely divides each joint into two cavities (Fig. 4–1). Both joints, one on each side of the jaw, must be considered together in any examination. Along with the teeth, these joints are considered to be a "trijoint complex."

Gliding, translation, or sliding movement occurs in the upper cavity of the temporomandibular joint, whereas rotation or hinge movement occurs in the lower cavity. Rotation occurs from the beginning to the midrange of movement. The upper head of the lateral pterygoid muscle draws the disc, or meniscus, anteriorly and prepares for condylar rotation during movement. The rotation occurs through the two condylar heads between the articular disc and the condyle. In addition, the disc provides congruent contours and lubrication for the joint. Gliding, which occurs as a second movement, is a translatory movement of the condyle and disc along the slope of the articular eminence. Both gliding and rotation are essential for full opening and closing of the mouth (Fig. 4–2). The capsule of the temporomandibular joints is thin and loose. In the resting position, the mouth is slightly open, the lips are together, and the teeth are not in contact but slightly apart. In the close packed position, the teeth are tightly clenched, and the heads of the condyles are in the posterior aspect of the joint.

Centric occlusion is the relation of the jaws and teeth when there is maximum contact of the teeth, and it is the position assumed by the jaw in swallowing.

> ### Temporomandibular Joints
>
> - Resting position: Mouth slightly open, lips together, teeth not in contact
> - Close packed position: Teeth tightly clenched
> - Capsular pattern: Limitation of mouth opening

The temporomandibular joints actively displace only anteriorly and slightly laterally. When the mouth is opening, the condyles of the joint rest on the disc in the articular eminences, and any sudden movement, such as a yawn, may displace one or both condyles forward. As the mandible moves forward on opening, the disc moves medially and posteriorly until the collateral ligaments and lateral pterygoid stop its movement. The disc is then "seated" on the head of the mandible, and both disc and mandible move forward to full opening. If this "seating" of the disc does not occur, full range of motion at the temporomandibular joint is limited. In the first phase, mainly rotation occurs, primarily in the inferior joint space. In the second phase, in which the mandible and disc move together, mainly translation occurs in the superior joint space.[2]

The temporomandibular joints are innervated by branches of the auriculotemporal and masseteric branches of the mandibular nerve. The disc is innervated along its periphery but is aneural and avascular in its intermediate (force-bearing) zone.

The temporomandibular, or lateral, ligament restrains movement of the lower jaw and prevents compression of the tissues behind the condyle. In reality, this collateral ligament is a thickening in the joint capsule. The sphenomandibular and stylomandibular ligaments act as "guiding" restraints to keep the condyle,

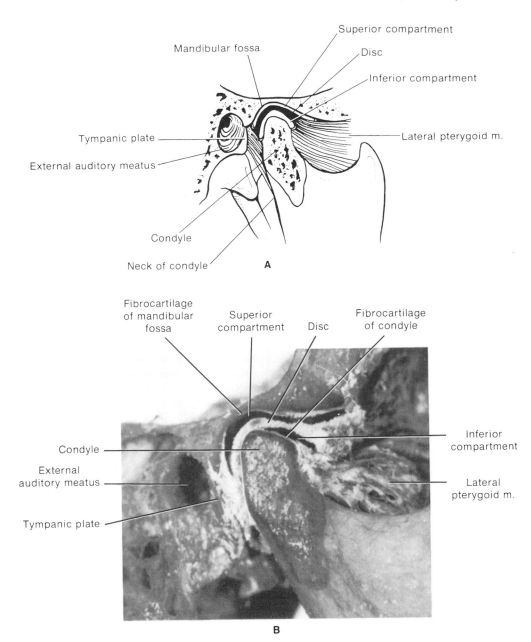

Figure 4–1
The temporomandibular joint. (A) Diagram of the sagittal section. (B) Sagittal section. (From Liebgott, B.: The Anatomical Basis of Dentistry. St. Louis, C.V. Mosby Co., 1986.)

disc, and temporal bone firmly opposed. The stylomandibular ligament is a specialized band of deep cerebral fascia with thickening of the parotid fascia.

In the human, there are 20 deciduous, or temporary ("baby"), teeth and 32 permanent teeth (Fig. 4–3). The temporary teeth are shed between the ages of 6 and 13 years. In the adult, the incisors are the front teeth (four maxillary and four mandibular), with the maxillary incisors being larger than the mandibular incisors. The incisors are designed to cut food. The canine teeth (two maxillary and two mandibular) are the longest permanent teeth and are designed to cut and tear food. The premolars crush and break down the food for digestion; usually they have two cusps. There are eight premolars in all, two on each side, top and bottom. The final set of teeth are the molars, which crush and grind food for digestion. They have four or five cusps, and there are two or three on each side, top and bottom (total 8 to 12). The third molars are called wisdom teeth. Missing teeth, abnormal eruption, malocclusion, or dental caries (decay) may lead to problems of the temporomandibular joint. By convention, the teeth are divided into four quadrants—the upper left, the upper right, the lower left, and the lower right quadrants (Fig. 4–4).

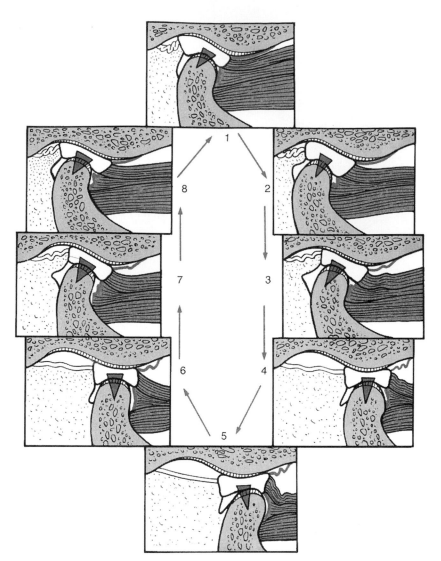

Figure 4–2

Normal functional movement of the condyle and disc during the full range of opening and closing. Note that the disc is rotated posteriorly on the condyle as the condyle is translated out of the fossa. The closing movement is the exact opposite of the opening movement. (From Myers, R. [ed.]: Saunders Manual of Physical Therapy Practice. Philadelphia, W.B. Saunders Co., 1995, p. 680.)

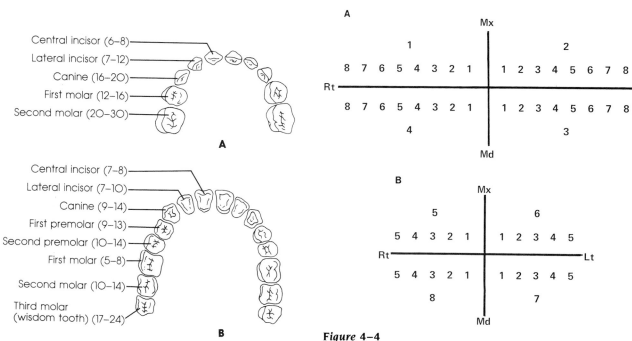

Central incisor (6–8)
Lateral incisor (7–12)
Canine (16–20)
First molar (12–16)
Second molar (20–30)

A

Central incisor (7–8)
Lateral incisor (7–10)
Canine (9–14)
First premolar (9–13)
Second premolar (10–14)
First molar (5–8)
Second molar (10–14)
Third molar (wisdom tooth) (17–24)

B

Figure 4–3

Teeth in a child (A) and in an adult (B). Numbers indicate age (in months for a child, in years for an adult) at which teeth erupt.

A

Mx

1   2
8 7 6 5 4 3 2 1   1 2 3 4 5 6 7 8
Rt ─────────────────────────── Lt
8 7 6 5 4 3 2 1   1 2 3 4 5 6 7 8
4   3

Md

B

Mx

5   6
5 4 3 2 1   1 2 3 4 5
Rt ─────────────────── Lt
5 4 3 2 1   1 2 3 4 5
8   7

Md

Figure 4–4

Numeric symbols for dentition in an adult (A) and in a child (B). (From Liebgott, B.: The Anatomical Basis of Dentistry. St. Louis, C.V. Mosby Co., 1986.)

Patient History

In addition to the questions listed under Patient History in Chapter 1, the examiner should obtain the following information from the patient.

1. Is there pain on opening or closing of the mouth? Pain in the fully opened position (e.g., pain associated with opening to bite an apple, yawning) is probably caused by an extra-articular problem, whereas pain associated with biting firm objects is probably caused by an intra-articular problem.[3]

2. Is there pain on eating? Does the patient chew on the right? Left? Both sides equally? Loss of molars or worn dentures can lead to loss of vertical dimension, which can make chewing painful. Often, chewing on one side is the result of malocclusion.[3]

3. What movements of the jaw cause pain? A history of stiffness on waking with pain on function that disappears as the day goes on suggests osteoarthritis.[4]

4. Do any of these actions cause pain or discomfort: Yawning? Biting? Chewing? Swallowing? Speaking? Shouting? If so, where?

5. Does the patient breathe through the nose or the mouth? Normal breathing is through the nose with the lips closed and no "air gulping." If the patient is a "mouth breather," the tongue does not sit in the proper position against the palate. In the young, if the tongue does not push against the palate, developmental abnormalities may occur, because the tongue provides internal pressure to shape the mouth. The buccinator and orbicularis oris muscle complex provides external pressure to counterbalance the internal pressure of the tongue. Loss of normal neck balance often results in the individual's becoming a mouth breather and an upper respiratory breather, using the accessory muscles of respiration. Conditions such as adenoids, tonsils, and upper respiratory tract infections may cause the same problem.

6. Has the patient complained of any **clicking?** Normally, the condyles of the temporomandibular joint slide out of the concavity and onto the rim of the disc. Clicking may occur when the condyle slides back off the rim into the center (Fig. 4–5).[5] Clicking is the result of abnormal

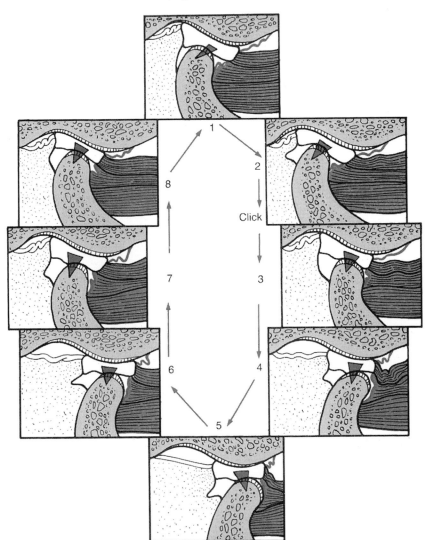

Figure 4–5

Single click. Between positions 2 and 3, a click is felt as the condyle moves across the posterior border into the intermediate zone of the disc. Normal condyle-disc function occurs during the remaining opening and closing movement. In the closed joint position (1), the disc is again displaced forward (and medially) by activity of the superior lateral pterygoid muscle. (From Myers, R. [ed.]: Saunders Manual of Physical Therapy Practice. Philadelphia, W.B. Saunders Co., 1995, p. 692.)

motion of the disc and mandible. If the disc sticks or is bunched slightly, opening causes the condyle to abruptly move over the disc and into its normal position, resulting in a single click (see Fig. 4–5).[6] There may be a partial anterior displacement (subluxation) or dislocation of the disc, which the condyle must override to reach its normal position when the mouth is fully open (Fig. 4–6). This override may also cause a click. Similarly, a click may occur if the disc is displaced anteriorly and/or medially and the condyle, finally and later than normal in the movement, overrides the posterior rim of the disc during mouth opening. This is referred to as disc displacement with reduction. If clicking occurs in both directions, it is called **reciprocal clicking** (Fig. 4–7). The opening click occurs somewhere during the opening or protrusive path, and the click indicates the condyle is slipping over the thicker posterior border of the disc to its position in the thinner middle or intermediate zone. The closing (reciprocal) click occurs near the end of the closing or retrusive path as the pull of the superior lateral pterygoid muscle causes the disc to slip more anteriorly and the condyle to move over its posterior border.

Clicks may also be caused by adhesions (Fig. 4–8), especially in people who clench their teeth (bruxism). These "adhesive" clicks occur only once, after the period of clenching.[7] If adhesions occur in the superior or inferior joint space, translation or rotation will be limited. This presents as a temporary closed lock, which then opens with a click.

If the articular eminence is abnormally developed (i.e., short, steep posterior slope or long, flat anterior slope), the maximum anterior movement of the disc may be reached before maximum translation of the condyle has occurred. As the condyle overrides the disc, a loud crack is heard, and the condyle-disc leaps (subluxes) forward.[7]

"Soft" or "popping" clicks that are sometimes heard in normal joints are caused by ligament movement, articular surface separation, or sucking of loose tissue behind the condyle as it moves forward. These clicks usually result from muscle incoordination. "Hard" or "cracking" clicks are more likely to indicate joint pathology or joint surface defects. Soft crepitus (like rubbing knuckles together) is a sound that sometimes occurs in symptom-

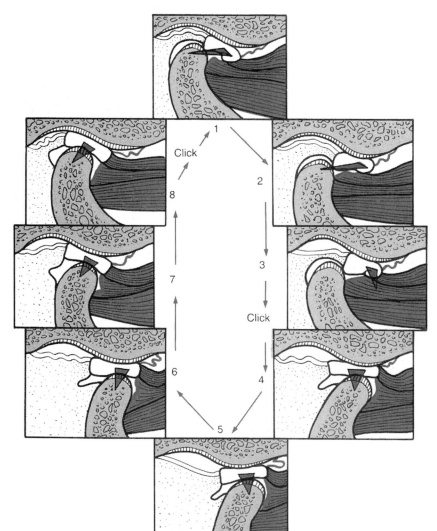

Figure 4–6

Functional dislocation of the disc with reduction. During opening, the condyle passes over the posterior border of the disc into the intermediate area of the disc, thus reducing the dislocated disc. (From Myers, R. [ed.]: Saunders Manual of Physical Therapy Practice. Philadelphia, W.B. Saunders Co., 1995, p. 694.)

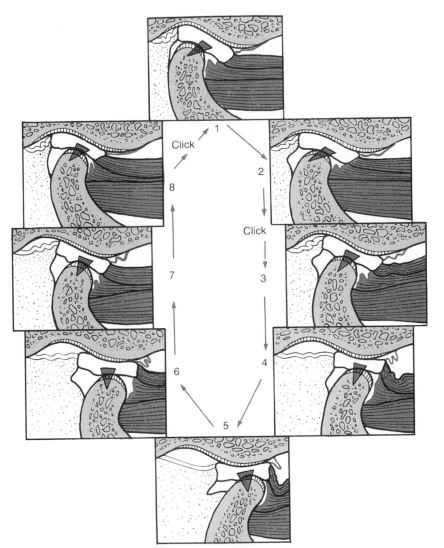

Figure 4–7

Reciprocal click. Between positions 2 and 3, a click is felt as the condyle moves across the posterior border of the disc. Normal condyle-disc function occurs during the remaining opening and closing movement until the closed joint position is approached. A second click is heard as the condyle once again moves from the intermediate zone to the posterior border of the disc between positions 8 and 1. (From Myers, R. [ed.]: Saunders Manual of Physical Therapy Practice. Philadelphia, W.B. Saunders Co., 1995, p. 693.)

less joints and is not necessarily an indication of pathology. Hard crepitus (like a footstep on gravel) is indicative of arthritic changes in the joints. The clicking may be caused by uncoordinated muscle action of the lateral pterygoid muscles, a tear or perforation in the disc, osteoarthrosis, or occlusal imbalance. Normally, the upper head of the lateral pterygoid muscle pulls the disc forward. If the disc does not move first, the condyle clicks over the disc as it is pulled forward by the lower head of the lateral pterygoid muscle. Iglarsh and Snyder-Mackler[2] have divided disc displacement into four stages (Table 4–1).

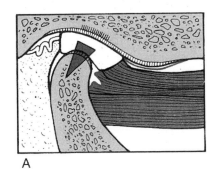
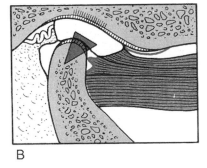
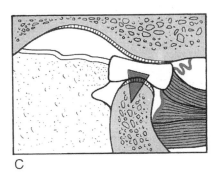

A   B   C

Figure 4–8

(A) Adhesion in the superior joint space. (B) The presence of the adhesion limits the joint to rotation only. (C) If the adhesion is freed, normal translation can occur. (From Myers, R. [ed.]: Saunders Manual of Physical Therapy Practice. Philadelphia, W.B. Saunders Co., 1995, p. 704.)

Table 4–1
Temporomandibular Disc Dysfunction

Stage	Characteristics
Stage 1	Disc slightly anterior and medial on mandibular condyle Inconsistent click (may or may not be present) Mild or no pain
Stage 2	Disc anterior and medial Reciprocal click present (early on opening, late on closing) Severe consistent pain
Stage 3	Reciprocal consistent click present (later on opening, earlier on closing) Most painful stage
Stage 4	Click rare (disc no longer relocates) No pain

7. Has the mouth or jaw ever locked? If the jaw has locked in the closed position, the locking is probably caused by a disc, with the condyle being posterior or anteromedial to the disc. If locking occurs in the open position, it is probably caused by subluxation of the joint or possibly by posterior disc displacement (Fig. 4–9). Even if translation is blocked (e.g., "locked" disc), the mandible can still open 30 mm by rotation. Locking is usually preceded by reciprocal clicking. Locking may imply that the mouth does not fully open or it does not fully close. If there is functional dislocation of the disc with reduction (see Fig. 4–6), the disc is usually positioned anteromedially, and opening is limited. The patient complains that the jaw "catches" sometimes, so the locking occurs only occasionally and, at those times, opening is limited. If there is functional anterior dislocation of the disc without reduction, a **closed lock** occurs. Closed lock implies there has been anterior and/or medial displacement of the disc, so that the disc does not return to its normal position during the entire movement of the condyle. In this case, opening is limited to about 25 mm, the mandible deviates to the affected side (see Fig. 4–9), and lateral movement to the uninvolved side is reduced.[7] With an **open lock,** there are two clicks on opening, when the condyle moves over the posterior rim of the disc and then the anterior rim of the disc, and

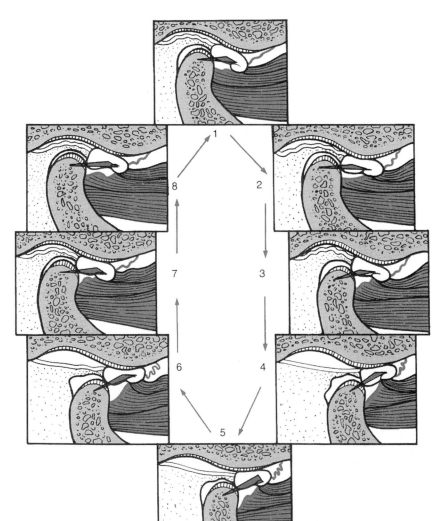

Figure 4–9
Closed lock. The condyle never assumes a normal relation to the disc but instead causes the disc to move forward ahead of it. This condition limits the distance it can translate forward. (From Myers, R. [ed.]: Saunders Manual of Physical Therapy Practice. Philadelphia, W.B. Saunders Co., 1995, p. 695.)

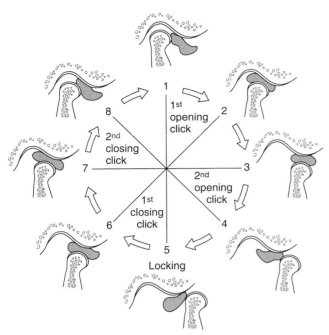

Figure 4–10

Open lock (disc incoordination). (1) The disc always stays in anterior position with the jaw closed. (1–4) Disc is displaced posterior to the head with one or two opening clicks. (5–6) The disc disturbs jaw closing after maximum opening. (6–1) The disc is again displaced to anterior position from the posterior with one or two clicks.

two clicks on closing. If, after the second click occurs on opening, the disc lies posterior to the condyle, it may not allow the condyle to slide back (Fig. 4–10).[8] If the condyle dislocates outside the fossa, it is a true dislocation with open lock; the patient cannot close the mouth, and the dislocation must be reduced.[8]

8. Does the patient have any habits such as pipe smoking, using a cigarette holder, leaning on the chin, chewing gum, biting the nails, chewing hair, pursing and chewing lips, continually moving the mouth, or any other nervous habits? All these activities place additional stress on the temporomandibular joints.

9. Does the patient grind the teeth or hold them tightly? **Bruxism** is the forced clenching and grinding of the teeth, especially during sleep. If the front teeth are in contact and the back ones are not, facial and temporomandibular pain may develop as a result of malocclusion.

10. Are any teeth missing? If so, which ones and how many? The presence or absence of teeth and their relation to one another must be noted on a table similar to the one shown in Figure 4–4. Their presence or absence can have an effect on the temporomandibular joints and their muscles. If some teeth are missing, others may deviate to fill in the space, altering the occlusion. The examiner should watch the patient's jaw movement while the patient is talking.

11. Are any teeth painful or sensitive? This finding may be indicative of dental caries or abscess. Tooth pain may lead to incorrect biting when chewing, which puts abnormal stresses on the temporomandibular joints.

12. Does the patient have any difficulty swallowing? Does the patient swallow normally or gulp? What happens to the tongue when the patient swallows? Does it move normally, anteriorly, or laterally? Is there any evidence of tongue thrust or thumb sucking? For example, the facial nerve (cranial nerve VII) and the trigeminal nerve (cranial nerve V), which control facial expression and mastication and contribute to speech, also control anterior lip seal. If lip seal is weakened, the teeth may move anteriorly, an action which would be accentuated in "tongue thrusters." The normal resting position of the tongue is against the anterior palate (Fig. 4–11). It is the position in which one would place the tongue to make a "clicking" sound.

13. Are there any ear problems such as hearing loss, ringing in the ears, blocking of the ears, earache, or dizziness? Symptoms such as these may be caused by inner ear, cervical spine, or temporomandibular joint problems.

14. Does the patient have any habitual head postures? For example, holding the telephone between the

Figure 4–11

(A) Normal resting position of the tongue. Tongue position cannot be seen because of teeth. Upper and lower teeth are not in contact. (B) Mouth opened to show tongue against upper anterior palate. This would not be considered the normal resting position because the mouth is open too much.

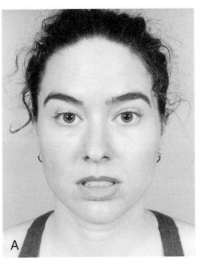

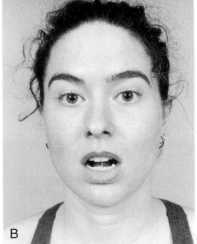

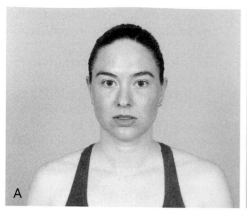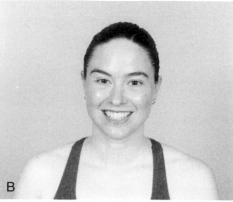

Figure 4–12
Facial symmetry. Look for symmetry both vertically and horizontally. Also note the changes in symmetry occurring with no smile (A) and smile (B).

ear and the shoulder compacts the temporomandibular joint on that side. Reading or listening to someone while leaning one hand against the jaw has the same effect.

15. Has the patient noticed any voice changes? Changes may be caused by muscle spasm.

16. Does the patient have headaches? If so, where? Temporomandibular joint problems can refer pain to the head. Is there any history of infection or swollen glands?

17. Does the patient ever feel dizzy or faint?

18. Has the patient ever worn a dental splint? If so, when? For how long?

19. Has the patient ever been seen by a dentist? A periodontist (a dentist who specializes in the study of tissues around the teeth and diseases of these tissues)? An orthodontist (a dentist who specializes in correction and prevention of irregularities of the teeth)? An endodontist (a dentist who specializes in the treatment of diseases of the tooth pulp, root canal, and periapical areas)? If so, why did the patient see the specialist, and what was done?

Observation

When assessing the temporomandibular joints, the examiner must also assess the posture of the cervical spine and head. For example, it is necessary that the head be "balanced" on the cervical spine.

1. Is the face symmetrical horizontally and vertically, and are facial proportions normal (Fig. 4–12)? The examiner should check the eyebrows, eyes, nose, ears, and corners of the mouth for symmetry on both horizontal and vertical planes. Horizontally, the face of an adult is divided into thirds (Fig. 4–13); this demonstrates normal vertical dimension. Vertical dimension is the distance between any two arbitrary points on the face, one of these points being above and the other below the mouth, usually in midline. Usually the upper and lower teeth are used to measure vertical dimension. The horizontal bipupital, otic, and occlusive lines should be parallel to each other (Fig. 4–14). A quick way to measure the vertical dimension is to measure from the lateral edge of the eye to the corner of the mouth and from the nose to the chin (Fig. 4–15). Normally, the two measurements are equal. If the second measurement is smaller than the first by 1 mm or more, there has been a loss of vertical dimension, which may have resulted from loss of teeth, overbite, or temporomandibular joint dysfunction. In children, elderly persons, and those with massive tooth loss, the lower third of the face is not well developed (lack of teeth) or has recessed (Fig. 4–16). As the teeth grow, the lower third develops into its normal proportion. The examiner should notice whether there is any paralysis, which could be indicated by **ptosis** (drooping of

Figure 4–13
Divisions of the face (vertical dimension).

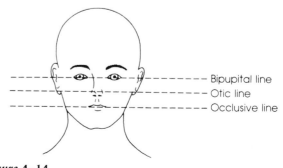

Figure 4–14
Normally, bipupital, otic, and occlusive lines are parallel.

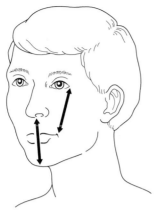

Figure 4–15

A quick measurement of vertical dimension. Normally, the distance from lateral edge of eye to corner of mouth (A–B) equals the distance from nose to point of chin (C–D).

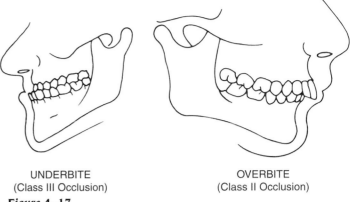

UNDERBITE
(Class III Occlusion)

OVERBITE
(Class II Occlusion)

Figure 4–17

Illustrations of underbite and overbite.

an eyelid) or by drooping of the mouth on one side (Bell's palsy).

2. The examiner should note whether there is any crossbite, underbite, or overbite (Fig. 4–17). With **crossbite,** the teeth of the mandible are lateral to the upper (maxillary) teeth on one side and medial on the opposite side. There is abnormal interdigitation of the teeth. With anterior crossbite, the lower incisors are ahead of the upper incisors. With posterior crossbite, there is a transverse abnormal relation of the teeth. In **underbite,** the mandibular teeth are unilaterally, bilaterally, or in pairs in **buccoversion** (i.e., they lie anterior to the maxillary teeth). In **overbite,** the anterior maxillary incisors extend below the anterior mandibular incisors when the jaw is in centric occlusion. A small amount of overbite (2 to 3 mm) anteriorly is the most common position of the teeth. This is because the maxillary arch is slightly longer than the mandibular arch. **Overjet** (Fig. 4–18) is the distance that the maxillary incisors close over the mandibular incisors. This distance is normally 2 to 3 mm. **Occlusal interference** refers to premature teeth contact, which tends to deflect the jaw laterally and/or anteriorly.[9]

Any orthodontic appliances or false teeth present should also be evaluated for fit and possible sore spots.

3. The examiner should note whether there is any **malocclusion** that may result in a faulty bite. Malocclusion may be a major factor in the development of disc problems of the temporomandibular joints. Occlusion occurs when the teeth are in contact and the mouth is closed. Malocclusion is defined as any deviation from

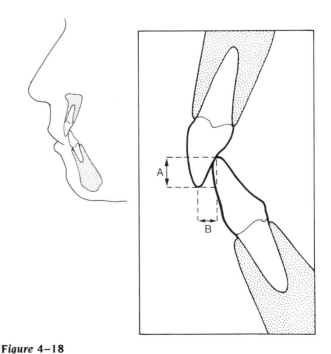

Figure 4–18

Overlap of maxillary anterior teeth. (A) Vertical overlap (overbite). (B) Horizontal overlap (overjet). (From Friedman, M.H., and J. Weisberg: The temporomandibular joint. *In* Gould, J.A. [ed.]: Orthopedics and Sports Physical Therapy. St. Louis, C.V. Mosby Co., 1990, p. 578.)

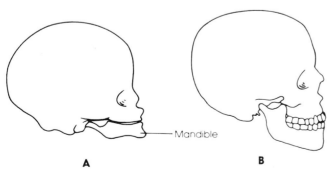

A   B

Figure 4–16

Human skull at birth (A) and in the adult (B). Note the difference brought about by development of the teeth and lower jaw in the adult.

normal occlusion. Class I occlusion refers to the normal anteroposterior relation of the maxillary teeth to mandibular teeth. A slight modification with only the incisors affected and overjet slightly larger is sometimes classed as a Class I occlusion or malocclusion. Class II malocclusion (overbite) occurs when the mandibular teeth are positioned posterior to their normal position relative to the maxillary teeth. This malocclusion deformity involves all the teeth, including the molars. The designation Class II Division 1 malocclusion (also called large overjet or **horizontal overlap**) indicates that the maxillary incisors demonstrate significant overjet. Class II Division 2 malocclusion (also called deep overbite or **vertical overlap**) implies that overjet is not significant but there is overbite and lateral flaring of the lateral maxillary incisors.[10] Class III malocclusion (e.g., underbite) occurs when the mandibular teeth are positioned anterior to their normal position relative to the maxillary teeth. If maxillary and mandibular teeth are on the same vertical plane, a Class III malocclusion would be present.

4. What is the facial profile? The orthognathic profile is the normal, "straight-jawed" form. With this facial profile, a vertical line dropped perpendicular to the bipupital line would touch the upper and lower lips and the tip of the chin. In a person with a retrognathic profile, the chin would lie behind the vertical line, and the person would be said to have a "receding chin." With the prognathic profile, the chin would be in front of the vertical line, and the person would have a protruded or "strong" chin (Fig. 4–19).[10]

5. The examiner should note whether the patient demonstrates normal bony and soft-tissue contours. When the patient bites down, do the masseter muscles bulge as they normally should? Hypertrophy caused by overuse may lead to abnormal wear of the teeth. When looking at the soft tissues, it is important to note symmetry. The upper lip should normally cover two thirds of the maxillary teeth at rest. If it does not, the lip is said to be short.[2] If the lip can be drawn over the upper teeth, however, the upper lip is said to be functional and no treatment is necessary. The lower lip normally covers the mandibular teeth and, when the mouth is closed, part of the maxillary teeth.

6. Is the patient able to move the tongue properly? Can the patient move the tongue up to and against the palate? Can the tongue be protruded? Is the patient able to "click" the tongue? **Tongue thrusting** refers to forward movement of the tongue, usually to push against the lower teeth; it also occurs when the tongue is pushed against the upper teeth and the lower teeth are closed firmly against it, creating an oral seal.[11] Tongue thrusters find it easier to thrust the tongue if the head is protruded. Therefore, to test for tongue thrusting, the patient's head posture is corrected and the patient is asked to swallow. In the tongue thruster, swallowing causes the tongue to move forward resulting in protrusion of the head.

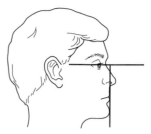

Orthognathic

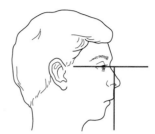

Retrognathic

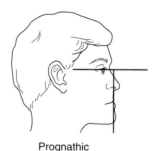

Prognathic

Figure 4–19
Facial profiles.

7. Where does the tongue rest? Is the tongue bitten frequently? Does the tongue have any scalloping or ridges? Does the patient swallow normally? Do the lips part when swallowing? What is the tongue position when swallowing? Do the facial muscles tighten on swallowing? All of these factors give the examiner some idea of the mobility of the structures of the mouth and jaw and their neurological mechanisms.

Examination

The examiner must remember that many problems of the temporomandibular joints may be the result of or related to problems in the cervical spine or teeth. Therefore, the cervical spine is at least partially included in a temporomandibular assessment.

Active Movements

With the patient in the sitting position, the examiner watches the active movements, noting whether they deviate from what would be considered normal range of motion and whether the patient is willing to do the movement. The patient is first asked to carry out active movements of the cervical spine. The most painful movements, if any, should be done last.

During flexion of the neck, the mandible moves up and forward, and the posterior structures of the neck become tight. During extension, the mandible moves down and back and the anterior structures of the neck become tight. The examiner should note whether the patient can flex and extend the neck while keeping the mouth closed or whether the patient must open the mouth to do these movements. The patient should be asked to place a fist under the chin and then open the mouth while keeping the fist in place and the lower jaw against it. If the mouth opens in this way, movement of the neck into extension is occurring. This test movement would be especially important if the patient subjectively feels that there is a loss of neck extension. With side flexion of the neck to the right, maximum occlusion occurs on the right. Side flexion and rotation of the neck occur to the same side, so that if these movements are carried out to the right, maximum occlusion also occurs to the right.

Having observed the neck movements, the examiner goes on to note the active movements of the temporomandibular joints. The movements of the mandible can be measured with a millimeter ruler, depth gauge, or Vernier calipers. When using the ruler, the examiner

should pick a midline point from which to measure opening and lateral deviation. This same ruler can be used to measure protrusion and retrusion.

Opening and Closing of the Mouth

With opening and closing of the mouth, the normal arc of movement of the jaw is smooth and unbroken; that is, both temporomandibular joints are working in unison with no asymmetry or sideways movement, and both joints are bilaterally rotating and translating equally. Any alteration may cause or indicate potential problems in the temporomandibular joints. The first phase of opening is rotation, which can be tested by having the patient open the mouth as widely as possible while maintaining the tongue against the roof (hard palate) of the mouth. Usually this movement causes minimal pain and occurs even in the presence of acute temporomandibular dysfunction. The second phase of opening is translation and rotation as the condyles move along the slope of the eminence. This phase begins when the tongue loses contact with the roof of the mouth.[2] Most of the clicking sensations occur during this phase.

Normally, the mandible should open and close in a straight line (Fig. 4–20). If deviation occurs to the left on opening (Fig. 4–21), the left temporomandibular joint is said to be hypomobile or the right temporomandibular joint hypermobile. If, on opening of the mouth, the deviation is a C-type curve, hypomobility is evident toward the side of the deviation; if the deviation is an S-type curve, the problem is probably muscular imbalance or

Figure 4–20
Mandibular motion.

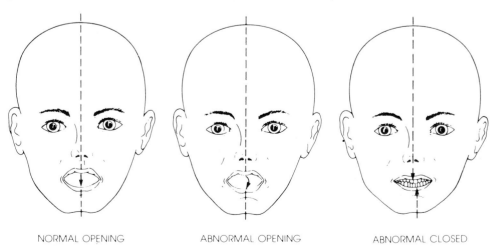

NORMAL OPENING   ABNORMAL OPENING   ABNORMAL CLOSED

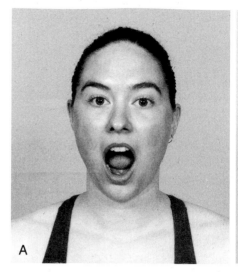

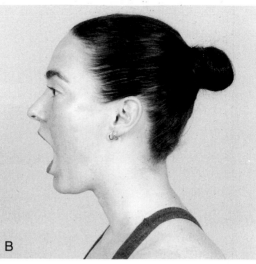

Figure 4–21
Active opening of mouth.
(A) Anteroposterior view. (B) Side
view.

medial displacement as the condyle "walks around" the disc. The chin deviates toward the affected side, usually because of spasm of the pterygoid or masseter muscles or an obstruction in the joint. Early deviation on opening is usually caused by muscle spasm, whereas late deviation on opening is usually a result of capsulitis. Pain or tenderness, especially on closing, indicates posterior capsulitis.

The examiner should then determine whether the patient's mouth can functionally be opened. The **functional opening** is determined by having the patient try to place two or three flexed proximal interphalangeal joints within the mouth opening (Fig. 4–22). This opening should be approximately 35 to 50 mm. Normally, only about 25 to 35 mm of opening is needed for everyday activity. If the space is less than this, the temporomandibular joints are said to be hypomobile.

As the mouth opens, the examiner should palpate the external auditory meatus with the finger (fleshy part anterior). The patient is then asked to close the mouth. When the examiner first feels the condyle touch the

finger, the temporomandibular joints are in the resting position. This resting position of the temporomandibular joints is called the **freeway space**, or **interocclusal space**. The freeway space is the potential space or vertical distance that is found between the teeth when the mandible is in the resting position. To determine the freeway space, the examiner marks a point on the chin and a point vertically above on the upper lip below the nose. The patient closes the mouth into centric occlusion, and the distance between the two points is measured. Then the patient is asked to say three simple words (e.g., "boy, boy, boy") and then maintain this position of the jaw without moving. The distance between the two points is measured again. The difference between the two measurements is the freeway space.[9] Normally, the space between the front teeth at this point is 2 to 4 mm.

If rotation does not occur at the temporomandibular joint, the mouth cannot open fully. There may be gliding at the temporomandibular joint, but rotation has not occurred. If translation (gliding) does not occur, the mandible may still open up to 30 mm as a result of rotation. Normally, when the mouth opens, the disc moves forward approximately 7 mm, and the condyle moves forward approximately 14 mm.[12]

Protrusion of the Mandible

The examiner asks the patient to protrude or jut the lower jaw out past the upper teeth. The patient should be able to do this without difficulty. The normal movement is 3 to 6 mm, measured from the resting position to the protruded position. The normal values vary depending on the degree of overbite (greater movement) or underbite (less movement).

Retrusion of the Mandible

The examiner asks the patient to retrude or pull the lower jaw in or back as far as possible. In full retention

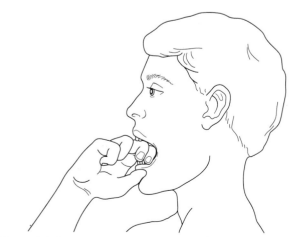

Figure 4–22
Functional opening "knuckle" test.

or centric relation, the temporomandibular joint is in a close packed position. The normal movement is 3 to 4 mm.[3]

Lateral Deviation or Excursion of Mandible

For lateral deviation, the teeth are slightly disoccluded and the patient moves the mandible laterally, first to one side and then to the other. With the joints in resting position, two points are picked on the upper and lower teeth that are at the same level. When the mandible is laterally deviated, the two points, which have moved apart, are measured, giving the amount of lateral deviation. The normal lateral deviation is 10 to 15 mm. During lateral deviation, the opposite condyle moves forward, down, and toward the motion side. The condyle on the motion side (e.g., left condyle on left lateral deviation) remains relatively stationary and becomes more prominent.[3] When charting any changes, the examiner should note the opening deviation as well as the functional opening and any lateral deviation (Fig. 4–23). Any lateral deviation from the normal opening position or abnormal protrusion to one side indicates that the lateral pterygoid, masseter, or temporalis muscle, the disc, or the lateral ligament on the opposite side is affected.

Mandibular Measurement

Next, the examiner should measure the mandible from the posterior aspect of the temporomandibular joint to the notch of the chin (Fig. 4–24). Both sides are measured and compared for equality (the normal distance is 10 to 12 cm). Any difference indicates a developmental problem or structural change; the patient may not be able to obtain balancing in the midline.

Swallowing and Tongue Position

The patient is asked to relax and then swallow. The patient is asked to leave the tongue in the position it assumed when swallowing occurred. The examiner, wearing rubber gloves, then separates the lips and notes the position of the tongue (between teeth? at upper anterior palate?).[9]

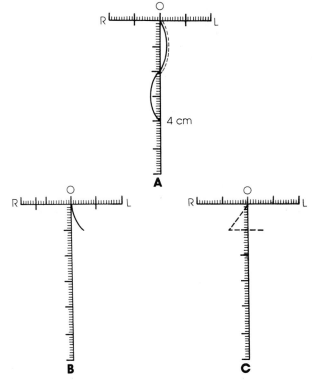

Figure 4–23
Charting temporomandibular motion. (A) Deviation to both right (R) and left (L) on opening; maximum opening, 4 cm; lateral deviation equal (1 cm each direction); protrusion on functional opening (*dashed lines*). (B) Capsule-ligamentous pattern; opening limited to 1 cm; lateral deviation greater to R than L; deviation to L on opening. (C) Protrusion is 1 cm; lateral deviation to R on protrusion (indicates weak lateral pterygoid on opposite side).

Cranial Nerve Testing

If injury to the cranial nerves is suspected, the cranial nerves should be tested (Table 4–2).

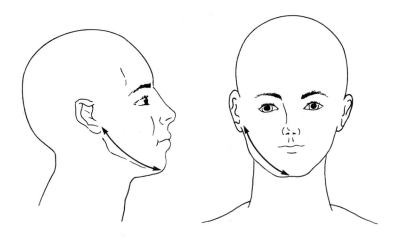

Figure 4–24
Measurement of the mandible.

Table 4–2
Muscles of the Temporomandibular Joint: Their Actions and Nerve Supply

Action	Muscles Acting	Nerve Supply
Opening of mouth (depression of mandible)	1. Lateral (external) pterygoid 2. Mylohyoid* 3. Geniohyoid* 4. Digastric*	Mandibular (CN V) Inferior alveolar (CN V) Hypoglossal (CN XII) Inferior alveolar (CN V) Facial (CN VII)
Closing of mouth (elevation of mandible or occlusion)	1. Masseter 2. Temporalis 3. Medial (internal) pterygoid	Mandibular (CN V) Mandibular (CN V) Mandibular (CN V)
Protrusion of mandible	1. Lateral (external) pterygoid 2. Medial (internal) pterygoid 3. Masseter* 4. Mylohyoid* 5. Geniohyoid* 6. Digastric* 7. Stylohyoid* 8. Temporalis (anterior fibers)*	Mandibular (CN V) Mandibular (CN V) Mandibular (CN V) Inferior alveolar (CN V) Hypoglossal (CN XII) Inferior alveolar (CN V) Facial (CN VII) Facial (CN VII) Mandibular (CN V)
Retraction of mandible	1. Temporalis (posterior fibers) 2. Masseter* 3. Digastric* 4. Stylohyoid* 5. Mylohyoid* 6. Geniohyoid*	Mandibular (CN V) Mandibular (CN V) Inferior alveolar (CN V) Facial (CN VII) Inferior alveolar (CN VII) Inferior alveolar (CN V) Hypoglossal (CN XII)
Lateral deviation of mandible	1. Lateral (external) pterygoid (ipsilateral muscle) 2. Medial (internal) pterygoid (contralateral muscle) 3. Temporalis* 4. Masseter*	Mandibular (CN V) Mandibular (CN V) Mandibular (CN V) Mandibular (CN V)

* Act only when assistance is required.
CN = cranial nerve.

Cranial Nerve Testing

CN I:	Smell coffee or some similar substance with eyes closed	eye on one side, the symptoms may be indicative of Bell's palsy (paralysis of the facial nerve).
CN II (*optic nerve*):	Read something with one eye closed	
CN III, IV, VI:	Eye movements; note any ptosis	CN VIII (*auditory nerve*): Eyes closed; talk to patient and have him or her repeat what was said
CN V (*trigeminal nerve*):	Contract muscles of mastication (masseter and temporalis)	CN IX: Have patient swallow
CN VII (*facial nerve*):	Move eyebrows up and down, purse lips, show teeth. This cranial nerve is the most commonly injured one. If the patient is unable to whistle or wink or close an	CN X (*vagus nerve*): Have patient swallow CN XI (*spinal accessory*): Have patient contract sternomastoid CN XII: Have patient stick out tongue, move it to right and left

Passive Movements

Very seldom are passive movements carried out for the temporomandibular joints except when the examiner is attempting to determine the end feel of the joints. The normal end feel of these joints is tissue stretch on opening and teeth contact ("bone to bone") on closing. When the teeth are in maximum contact, the horizontal overjet is sometimes measured. The overjet is the horizontal distance from the edge of the upper central incisors to the lower central incisors (see Fig. 4–18). If the lower teeth extend over the upper teeth, this malocclusion condition is called an underbite. Overbite is the vertical overlap of the teeth.

Normal End Feel at the Temporomandibular Joints

- Opening: Tissue stretch
- Closing: Bone to bone

Resisted Isometric Movements

Resisted isometric movements of the temporomandibular joints are relatively difficult to test. The jaw should be in the resting position. The examiner applies firm but gentle resistance to the joints and asks the patient to hold the position, saying "Don't let me move you."

Resisted Isometric Movements of the Temporomandibular Joints

- Depression (opening)
- Occlusion (closing)
- Lateral deviation left and right

---

1. Opening of the mouth (depression). This movement may be tested by applying resistance at the chin or, using a rubber glove, over the teeth with one hand while the other hand rests behind the head or neck or over the forehead to stabilize the head (Fig. 4–25A).

2. Closing of the mouth (elevation or occlusion). One hand is placed over the back of the head or neck to stabilize the head while the other hand is placed under the chin of the patient's slightly open mouth to resist the movement (Fig. 4–25B). In a second method, the examiner uses a rubber glove and places two fingers over the patient's lower teeth (mandible) to resist the movement (Fig. 4–25C).

3. Lateral deviation of the jaw. One of the examiner's hands is placed over the side of the head above the

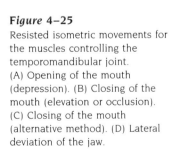

Figure 4–25
Resisted isometric movements for the muscles controlling the temporomandibular joint. (A) Opening of the mouth (depression). (B) Closing of the mouth (elevation or occlusion). (C) Closing of the mouth (alternative method). (D) Lateral deviation of the jaw.

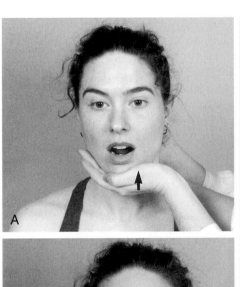
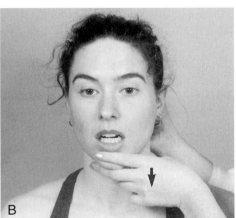
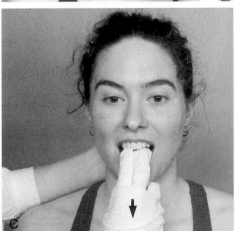
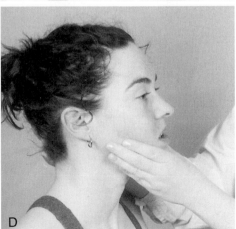

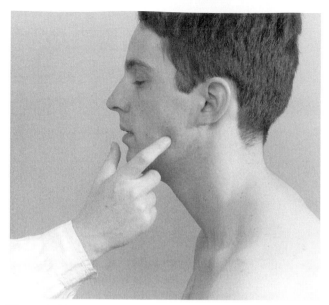

Figure 4–26
Chvostek test.

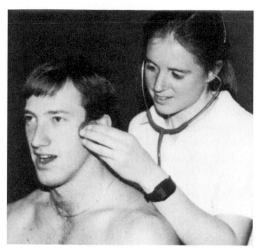

Figure 4–27
Auscultation of the left temporomandibular joint.

temporomandibular joint to stabilize the head. The other hand is placed along the jaw of the patient's slightly open mouth, and the patient pushes out against it (Fig. 4–25D). Both sides are tested individually.

Functional Assessment

After the basic movements of the temporomandibular joints have been tested, the examiner should test functional activities or activities of daily living involving the use of the temporomandibular joints. These activities include chewing, swallowing, coughing, talking, and blowing.

Special Tests

There are no routine special tests for the temporomandibular joints. The **Chvostek test** is used to determine whether there is pathology involving the seventh cranial (facial) nerve (Fig. 4–26). The examiner taps the parotid gland overlying the masseter muscle. If the facial muscles twitch, the result is positive.

The examiner can listen to (auscultate) the temporomandibular joints during movement (Fig. 4–27). The movements "listened to" include opening and closing of the mouth, lateral deviation of the mandible to the right and left, and mandibular protrusion. Normally, only on occlusion would a sound be heard. This is a single, solid sound, not a "slipping" sound. A slipping sound could occur if the teeth are not "hitting" simultaneously. The most common joint noise is reciprocal clicking (see

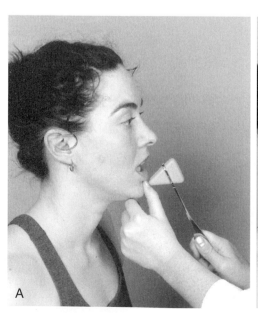

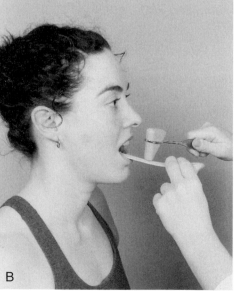

Figure 4–28
Testing of the jaw reflex.
(A) Hitting examiner's thumb.
(B) Hitting tongue depressor.

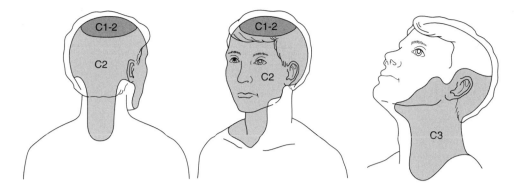

Figure 4–29
Dermatomes of the head.

Fig. 4–7), which occurs when the mouth opens and when it closes. It is clinical evidence that the disc is self-reducing. The opening click results when the condyle slips under the posterior aspect of the disc (reduces) or slips anterior to the disc (subluxes) on opening. The second click, which is quieter, occurs when the condyle slips posterior to the disc (subluxes) or into its proper position and reduces. A single click may occur if the condyle gets caught behind the disc on opening (see Fig. 4–5) or if the condyle slips behind the disc on closing. On opening, the later the click occurs, the more anterior lies the disc. The later the opening click, the more the disc is displaced anteriorly and the more likely it is to lock. A closing click is usually caused by loosening of the structures attaching the disc to the condyle. Clicking is more likely to occur in hypermobile joints.[13, 14]

Grating noise (crepitus) is usually indicative of degenerative joint disease or a perforation in the disc. Painful crepitus usually means that the disc has eroded, the condyle bone and temporal bone are rubbing together, and much of the fibrocartilage has been lost. While the examiner is listening, each movement should be done four or five times to ensure a correct diagnosis.

Reflexes and Cutaneous Distribution

The reflex of the temporomandibular joints is called the **jaw reflex.** The examiner's thumb is placed on the chin of the patient with the patient's mouth relaxed and open in the resting position. The examiner then taps the thumbnail with a neurological hammer (Fig. 4–28A). The jaw reflex may also be tested by using a tongue depressor (Fig. 4–28B). The examiner holds the tongue depressor firmly against the bottom teeth; while the patient relaxes the jaw muscles, the examiner taps the tongue depressor with the reflex hammer. The reflex closes the mouth and is a test of cranial nerve V.

The examiner must be aware of the dermatome patterns for the head and neck (Fig. 4–29) as well as the sensory nerve distribution of the peripheral nerves (see Fig. 3–43). Pain may be referred from the temporomandibular joint to the teeth, neck, or head, and vice versa (Fig. 4–30). Table 4–3 shows the muscles of the temporomandibular joint and their referral of pain.

Joint Play Movements

The joint play movements of the temporomandibular joints are then tested. Wearing rubber gloves, the examiner places both thumbs on the patient's lower teeth inside the mouth and both index fingers on the mandible outside the mouth. The mandible is then distracted by

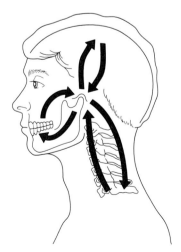

Figure 4–30
Referred pain patterns to and from the temporomandibular joint in the teeth, head, and neck.

Table 4–3
Temporomandibular Muscles and Referral of Pain

Muscle	Referral Pattern
Masseter	Cheek, mandible to forehead or ear
Temporalis	Maxilla to forehead and side of head above ear
Medial pterygoid	Posterior mandible to temporomandibular joint
Lateral pterygoid	Cheek to temporomandibular joint
Digastric	Lateral cervical spine to posterolateral skull
Occipitofrontal	Above eye, over eyelid, and up over lateral aspect of skull

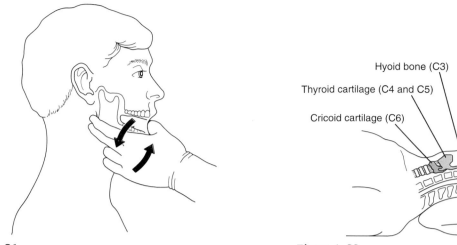

Figure 4–31

Joint play of the temporomandibular joints when each side is tested individually.

Figure 4–32

Position of hyoid bone, thyroid cartilage, and cricoid cartilage.

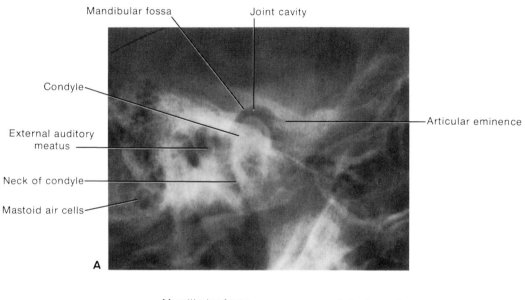

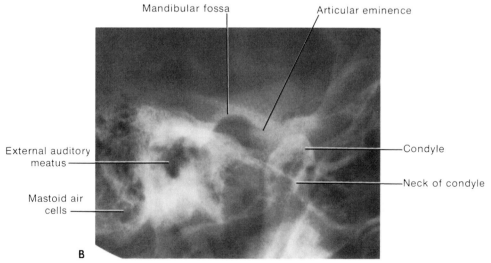

Figure 4–33

Radiographs of the right temporomandibular joint. (A) Mouth closed. (B) Mouth open. (From Liebgott, B.: The Anatomical Basis of Dentistry. St. Louis, C.V. Mosby Co., 1986, p. 295. Courtesy of Dr. Friedman.)

pushing down with the thumbs and pulling down and forward with the index fingers while the other fingers push against the chin, acting as a pivot point. The examiner should feel the tissue stretch of the joint. Each joint may also be done individually while the other hand and arm stabilize the head. This individual technique is the one more commonly used (Fig. 4–31). Lateral movements may also be accomplished by pushing on the side of first one mandible and then the other.

Palpation

To palpate the temporomandibular joints, the examiner places the fingers (padded part anteriorly) in the patient's external auditory canals and asks the patient to actively open and close the mouth. As this is being done, the examiner determines whether both sides are moving simultaneously and whether the movement is smooth. If the patient feels pain on closing, the posterior capsule is usually involved.

The examiner then places the index fingers over the mandibular condyles and feels for elicited pain or tenderness on opening and closing of the mouth. The examiner may also palpate the medial pterygoid, the medial and lower border of the inferior head of the lateral pterygoid, the temporalis and its tendon, and the masseter muscles and any other soft tissues for tenderness or indications of pathology. This procedure is followed by palpation of the following structures.

Mandible. The examiner palpates the mandible along its entire length, feeling for any differences between the left and right sides. As the examiner moves along the superior aspect of the angle of the mandible, the fingers pass over the parotid gland. Normally, the gland is not palpable, but with pathology (e.g., mumps), the site feels "boggy" rather than having the normal hard and bony feel.

Teeth. The examiner should note the position, absence, or tenderness of the teeth. The examiner wears a rubber glove and palpates inside the patient's mouth. At the same time, the interior cheek region and gums may be palpated for pathology.

Hyoid Bone (Anterior to C2–C3 Vertebrae). While palpating the hyoid bone (Fig. 4–32), the examiner asks the patient to swallow. Normally, the bone moves and causes no pain. The hyoid bone is part of the superior trachea.

Thyroid Cartilage (Anterior to C4–C5 Vertebrae). While the neck is in the neutral position, the thyroid cartilage can be easily moved; while in extension, it is tight and the examiner may feel crepitations. The thyroid gland, which is adjacent to the cartilage, may be palpated at the same time. If abnormal or inflamed, it will be tender and enlarged.

Mastoid Processes. The examiner should palpate the skull, following the posterior aspect of the ear. The examiner will come to a point on the skull where the finger

dips inward (see Fig. 3–52). The point just before the dip is the mastoid process.

Cervical Spine. Beginning on the posterior aspect at the occiput, the examiner systematically palpates the posterior structures of the neck (spinous processes, facet joints, and muscles of the suboccipital region), working from the head toward the shoulders. On the lateral aspect, the transverse processes of the vertebrae, the lymph nodes (palpable only if swollen), and the muscles should be palpated for tenderness. A more detailed description of the palpation of these structures is given in Chapter 3.

Diagnostic Imaging

Plain Film Radiography

On the anteroposterior view, the examiner should look for condylar shape and normal contours. On the lateral view, the examiner should look for condylar shape and contours, position of condylar heads in the opened and closed positions (Fig. 4–33), amount of condylar movement (closed versus open), and relation of temporomandibular joint to other bony structures of the skull and cervical spine (Fig. 4–34).

Magnetic Resonance Imaging

This technique is used to differentiate the soft tissue of the joint, mainly the disc, from the bony structures. It has the advantage of using nonionizing radiation (Fig. 4–35).

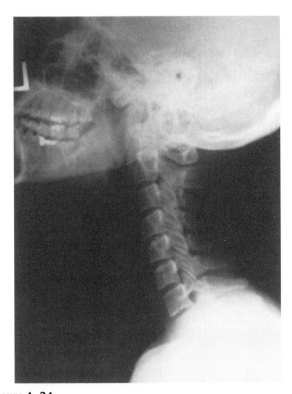

Figure 4–34
Lateral radiograph of the skull, left temporomandibular joint, and cervical spine.

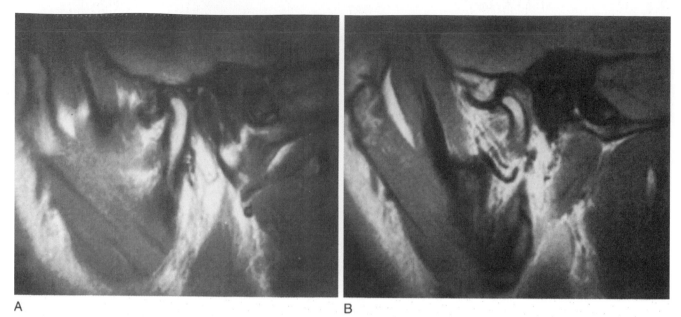

A   B

Figure 4–35

Magnetic resonance images of anterior disc displacement with reduction. (A) The T1-weighted image (SE 250/25) demonstrates anterior displacement of the articular disc in the closed-mouth position. The posterior band lies at approximately 9 o'clock with respect to the condyle. (B) The T1-weighted image (SE 250/25) shows reduction of the disc in the open-mouth positon. (Adapted from Bassett, L.W., R.H. Gold, and L.L. Seeger: MRI Atlas of the Musculoskeletal System. London, Martin Dunitz Ltd., 1989, p. 67.)

Précis of the Temporomandibular Joint Assessment*

History
Observation
Examination
    Active movements
      Neck flexion
      Neck extension
      Neck side flexion (left and right)
      Neck rotation (left and right)
      Extend neck by opening mouth
      Assess functional opening
      Assess freeway space
      Open mouth
      Closed mouth (occlusion)
      Measure protrusion of mandible
      Measure retrusion of mandible
      Measure lateral deviation of mandible (left and right)
      Measure mandibular length
      Swallowing and tongue position
      Cranial nerve testing (if necessary)

Passive movements (as in active movements, if necessary)
Resisted isometric movements
    Open mouth
    Closed mouth (occlusion)
    Lateral deviation of jaw
Special tests
Reflexes and cutaneous distribution
Joint play movements
Palpation
Diagnostic imaging

---

* Usually the entire assessment is done with the patient sitting.

After any examination, the patient should be warned of the possibility of exacerbation of symptoms as a result of the assessment.

Case Studies

When doing these case studies, the examiner should list the appropriate questions to be asked and why they are being asked, what to look for and why, and what things should be tested and why. Depending on the answers of the patient (and the examiner should consider different responses), several possible causes of the patient's problem may become evident (examples are given in parentheses). A differential diagnosis chart should be made up (see Table 4–4 as an example). The examiner can then decide how different diagnoses may affect the treatment plan.

1. A 49-year-old woman comes to you complaining of neck and left temporomandibular joint pain. The pain is

Table 4–4
Differential Diagnosis of Cervical Spondylosis and Temporomandibular Joint (TMJ) Dysfunction

	Cervical Spondylosis	TMJ Dysfunction
History	Insidious onset May complain of referred pain into arm or head Stiff neck	Insidious onset May be related to biting something hard Pain may be referred to neck or head
Observation	Muscle guarding of neck muscles	Minimal or no muscle guarding
Active movements	Cervical spine movements limited TMJ movements normal	Cervical movements may be limited if they compress or stress TMJ TMJ movements may or may not be painful but range of motion is altered
Passive movements	Restricted May have altered end feel: muscle spasm or bone-to-bone	Restricted
Resisted isometric movements	Relatively normal Myotomes may be affected	Normal
Special tests	Spurling's test may be positive Distraction test may be positive	None
Reflexes and cutaneous distribution	Deep tendon reflexes may be hyporeflexic See history for referred pain	No effect See history for referred pain

worse when she eats, especially if she chews on the left. Describe your assessment plan for this patient (cervical spondylosis versus temporomandibular dysfunction; see Table 4–4).

2. A 33-year-old woman comes to you complaining of pain and clicking when opening her mouth, especially when the mouth is open wide. She states that there is a small click on closing but minimal pain. Describe your assessment plan for this patient (temporomandibular joint arthritis versus temporomandibular disc dysfunction).

3. An 18-year-old male hockey player comes to you stating that he was hit in the jaw while playing. He is in severe pain and has difficulty speaking. Describe your assessment plan for this patient (cervical sprain versus temporomandibular joint dysfunction).

4. A 35-year-old man comes to you with his jaw locked open. Describe your assessment plan for this patient (temporomandibular disc dysfunction versus temporomandibular arthritis).

5. A 42-year-old woman comes to you complaining of jaw pain and headaches. She slipped on some wet stairs 3 days ago and fell, hitting her chin on the stairs. Describe your assessment plan for this patient (temporomandibular joint dysfunction versus head injury).

6. A 27-year-old nervous woman with long hair comes to you complaining of jaw pain. She has recently had a new dental plate installed. Describe your assessment plan for this patient (cervical sprain versus temporomandibular joint dysfunction).

References

Cited References

1. Rocabado, M.: Course notes. Course on temporomandibular joints. Edmonton, Canada, 1979.
2. Iglarsh, Z.A., and L. Snyder-Mackler: Temporomandibular joint and the cervical spine. In Richardson, J.K., and Z.A. Iglarsh (eds.): Clinical Orthopedic Physical Therapy. Philadelphia, W.B. Saunders Co., 1994.
3. Trott, P.H.: Examination of the temporomandibular joint. In Grieve, G. (ed.): Modern Manual Therapy of the Vertebral Column. Edinburgh, Churchill Livingstone, 1986.
4. Day, L.D.: History taking. In Morgan, D.H., L.R. House, W.P. Hall, and S.J. Vamvas (eds.): Diseases of the Temporomandibular Apparatus. St. Louis, C.V. Mosby Co., 1982.
5. Isberg-Holm, A.M., and P.L. Westesson: Movement of the disc and condyle in temporomandibular joints with clicking. Acta Odontol. Scand. 40:151–164, 1982.
6. Bush, F.M., J.H. Butler, and D.M. Abbott: The relationship of TMJ clicking to palpable facial pain. J. Craniomand. Pract. 1:44–48, 1983.
7. Bourbon, B.: Craniomandibular examination and treatment. In Myers, R. (ed.): Saunders Manual of Physical Therapy Practice. Philadelphia, W.B. Saunders Co., 1995.
8. Hondo, T., T. Shimoda, J.J. Moses, and H. Harada: Traumatically induced posterior disc displacement without reduction of the TMJ. J. Craniomand. Pract. 12:128–132, 1994.
9. Curnette, D.C.: The role of occlusion in diagnoses and treatment planning. In Morgan, D.H., L.R. House, W.P. Hall, and S.J. Vamvas (eds.): Diseases of the Temporomandibular Apparatus. St. Louis, C.V. Mosby Co., 1982.
10. Enlow, D.H.: Handbook of Facial Growth. Philadelphia, W.B. Saunders Co., 1975.
11. Mew, J.: Tongue posture. Br. J. Orthod. 8:203–211, 1981.
12. Friedman, M.H., and J. Weisberg: The temporomandibular joint. In Gould, J.A. (ed.): Orthopedic and Sports Physical Therapy. St. Louis, C.V. Mosby Co., 1990.
13. Friedman, M.H., and J. Weisberg: Application of orthopedic principles in evaluation of the temporomandibular joint. Phys. Ther. 62:597–603, 1982.
14. Rocabado, M.: Arthrokinematics of the temporomandibular joint. Dent. Clin. North Am. 27:573–594, 1983.

General References

Anthony, C.P., and N.J. Kotthoff: Textbook of Anatomy and Physiology. St. Louis, C.V. Mosby Co., 1971.

Atkinson, T.A., S. Vossler, and D.L. Hart: The evaluation of facial, head, neck and temporomandibular joint pain patients. J. Orthop. Sports Phys. Ther. 3:193–199, 1982.

Bassett, L.W., R.H. Gold, and L.L. Seeger: MRI Atlas of the Musculoskeletal System. London: Martin Dunitz Ltd., 1989.

Bell, W.E.: Understanding temporomandibular biomechanics. J. Craniomand. Pract. 1:28–33, 1983.

Clarke, G.T.: Examining temporomandibular disorder patients for cranio-cervical dysfunction. J. Craniomand. Pract. 2:56–63, 1984.

Crawford, W.A.: Centric relation reappraised. J. Craniomand. Pract. 2:40–45, 1984.

Crouch, J.E.: Functional Human Anatomy. Philadelphia, Lea & Febiger, 1973.

Curl, D.D.: The visual range of motion scale: Analysis of mandibular gait in a chiropractic setting. J. Manipulative Physiol. Ther. 15:115–122, 1992.

Dawson, P.E.: Evaluation, Diagnosis, and Treatment of Occlusal Problems. St. Louis, C.V. Mosby Co., 1984.

de Leuw, R., G. Boering, B. Stegenga, and L.G. de Bont: Symptoms of temporomandibular joint osteoarthrosis and internal derangement 30 years after nonsurgical treatment. J. Craniomand. Pract. 13:81–88, 1995.

Dworkin, S.F., K.H. Huggins, L. LeResche, et al.: Epidemiology of signs and symptoms in temporomandibular disorders: Clinical signs in cases and controls. J. Am. Dent. Assoc. 120:273–281, 1990.

Eriksson, L., P.L. Westesson, and H. Sjoberg: Observer performance in describing temporomandibular joint sounds. J. Craniomand. Pract. 5:33–35, 1987.

Eversaul, G.A.: Dental Kinesiology. Las Vegas, Nevada, G.A. Eversaul, 1977.

Fain, W.D., and J.M. McKinney: The TMJ examination form. J. Craniomand. Pract. 3:138–144, 1985.

Farrar, W.B., and W.L. McCarty: Inferior joint space arthrography and characteristics of condylar paths in internal derangements of the TMJ. J. Prosthet. Dent. 41:548–555, 1979.

Farrar, W.B., and W.L. McCarty: The TMJ dilemma. J. Alabama Dent. Assoc. 63:19–26, 1979.

Friedman, M.H., and J. Weisberg: Joint play movements of the temporomandibular joint: Clinical considerations. Arch. Phys. Med. Rehabil. 65:413–417, 1984.

Frumker, S.C.: Determining masticatory muscle spasm and TMJ capsulitis. J. Craniomand. Pract. 1:52–58, 1983.

Gelb, H.: Clinical Management of Head, Neck and TMJ Pain and Dysfunction. Philadelphia, W.B. Saunders Co., 1977.

Gelb, H.: An orthopaedic approach to occlusal imbalance and temporomandibular joint dysfunction. Dent. Clin. North Am. 23:181–197, 1979.

Gelb, H., and J. Tarte: A two-year clinical dental evaluation of 200 cases of chronic headache: The craniocervical-mandibular syndrome. J. Am. Dent. Assoc. 91:1230–1236, 1975.

Graber, T.M.: Overbite: The dentist's challenge. J. Am. Dent. Assoc. 79:1135–1145, 1969.

Helland, M.M.: Anatomy and function of the temporomandibular joint. J. Orthop. Sports Phys. Ther. 1:145–152, 1980.

Helland, M.M.: Anatomy and function of the temporomandibular joint. In Grieve, G. (ed.): Modern Manual Therapy of the Vertebral Column. Edinburgh, Churchill Livingstone, 1986.

Hollinshead, W.H., and D.B. Jenkins: Functional Anatomy of the Limbs and Back. Philadelphia, W.B. Saunders Co., 1981.

Hoppenfeld, S.: Physical Examination of the Spine and Extremities. New York, Appleton-Century-Crofts, 1976.

Humberger, H.C., and N.W. Humberger: Physical therapy evaluation of the craniomandibular pain and dysfunction patient. J. Craniomand. Pract. 10:138–143, 1992.

Klineberg, I.: Structure and function of temporomandibular joint innervation. Ann. R. Coll. Surg. Engl. 49:268–288, 1971.

Liebgott, B.: The Anatomical Basis of Dentistry, 2nd ed. St. Louis, C.V. Mosby Co., 1986.

Maitland, G.D.: The Peripheral Joints: Examination and Recording Guide. Adelaide, Australia, Virgo Press, 1973.

Ombregt, L., P. Bisschop, H.J. ter Veer, and T. Van de Velde: A System of Orthopedic Medicine. London, W.B. Saunders Co., 1995.

Paesani, D., P.L. Westesson, M. Hatala, R.H. Tallents, and K. Kurita: Prevalence of temporomandibular joint internal derangement in patients with craniomandibular disorders. Am. J. Orthod. Dentofac. Orthop. 101:41–47, 1992.

Palmer, M.L., and M. Epler: Clinical Assessment Procedures in Physical Therapy. Philadelphia, J.B. Lippincott Co., 1990.

Pollmann, L.: Sounds produced by the mandibular joint in young men. J. Max. Fac. Surg. 8:155–157, 1980.

Raustia, A.M., O. Tervonen, and J. Pyhtinen: Temporomandibular joint findings obtained by brain MRI. J. Craniomand. Pract. 12:28–32, 1994.

Sherriff, J.: Tongue posture. Br. J. Orthod. 8:203–211, 1981.

Silver, C.M., S.D. Simon, and A.A. Savastano: Meniscus injuries of the temporomandibular joint. J. Bone Joint Surg. Am. 38:541–552, 1956.

Snow, D.F.: Initial examination. In Morgan, D.H., L.R. House, W.P. Hall, and S.J. Vamvas (eds.): Diseases of the Temporomandibular Apparatus. St. Louis, C.V. Mosby Co., 1982,

Stein, J.L.: The temporomandibular joint. In Little, H. (ed.): Rheumatological Physical Examination. Orlando, Grune & Stratton, 1986.

Talley, R.L., G.J. Murphy, S.D. Smith, M.A. Baylin, and J.L. Hadon: Standards for the history, examination, diagnosis and treatment of temporomandibular disorders: A position paper. J. Craniomand. Pract. 8:60–77, 1990.

Thilander, B.: Innervation of the temporomandibular joint capsule in man. Transactions of the Royal Schools of Dentistry No. 7, 1961.

Travell, J.: Temporomandibular joint pain referred muscles of the head and neck. J. Prosthet. Dent. 10:745–763, 1960.

Travell, J.G., and D.G. Simons: Myofacial Pain and Dysfunction: The Trigger Point Manual. Baltimore, Williams & Wilkins, 1983.

Watt, D.M.: Temporomandibular joint sounds. J. Dent. 8:119–127, 1980.

Weinberg, L.A.: Temporomandibular joint injuries. In Foreman, S.M., and A.C. Croft (eds.): Whiplash Injuries. Baltimore, Williams & Wilkins, 1988.

Williams, P., and R. Warwick (eds.): Gray's Anatomy, 36th British ed. Edinburgh, Churchill Livingstone, 1980.

Wright, E.F.: A simple questionnaire and clinical examination to help identify possible non-craniomandibular disorders that may influence a patient's CMD symptoms. J. Craniomand. Pract. 10:228–234, 1992.

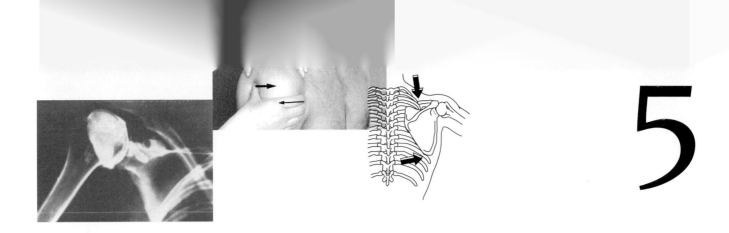

Shoulder

5

The prerequisite to any treatment of a patient with pain in the shoulder region is a precise and comprehensive picture of the signs and symptoms as they present during the assessment and as they existed until that time. This knowledge ensures that the techniques used will be suited to the condition and that the degree of success will be estimated against this background. Shoulder pain can be caused by intrinsic disease of the shoulder joints or pathology in the periarticular structures, or it may originate from the cervical spine, chest, or visceral structures. The shoulder complex is difficult to assess because of its many structures (most of which are located in a small area), its many movements, and the many lesions that can occur either inside or outside the joints. Influences such as referred pain from the cervical spine and the possibility of more than one lesion at one time, as well as the difficulty in deciding what weight to give to each response, make the examination even more difficult to understand. Assessment of the shoulder region often necessitates an evaluation of the cervical spine (see Chapter 3) to rule out referred symptoms, and the examiner must be prepared to include the cervical spine and its scanning examination in any shoulder assessment.

Applied Anatomy

The **glenohumeral joint** is a multiaxial, ball-and-socket, synovial joint that depends on muscles rather than bones or ligaments for its support, stability, and integrity. The **labrum,** which is the ring of fibrocartilage, surrounds and slightly deepens the glenoid cavity of the scapula. Only part of the humeral head is in contact with the glenoid at any one time. This joint has three axes and three degrees of freedom. The resting position of the glenohumeral joint is 55° of abduction and 30° of horizontal adduction. The close packed position of the joint is full abduction and lateral rotation. When relaxed, the humerus sits in the upper part of the glenoid cavity; with contraction of the rotator cuff muscles, it is pulled down into the lower, wider part of the glenoid cavity. If this "dropping down" does not occur, full abduction is impossible. The glenoid in the resting position has a 5° superior tilt or inclination and a 7° retroversion (slight internal rotation). The angle between the humeral neck and shaft is about 130°, and the humeral head is retroverted 30 to 40° relative to the line joining the epicondyle.[1] The rotator cuff muscles play an integral role in

Glenohumeral Joint

Resting position:	55° abduction, 30° horizontal adduction (scapular plane)
Close packed position:	Full abduction, lateral rotation
Capsular pattern:	Lateral rotation, abduction, medial rotation

shoulder movement. Their positioning on the humerus may be visualized by "cupping" the shoulder with the thumb anteriorly, as shown in Figure 5–1. The biceps tendon runs between the thumb and index finger just anterior to the index finger. The primary ligaments of the glenohumeral joint—the superior, middle, and inferior glenohumeral ligaments—play an important role in stabilizing the shoulder.[1] The capsular pattern of the glenohumeral joint is lateral rotation most limited, followed by abduction and medial rotation. Branches of the posterior cord of the brachial plexus and the suprascapular, axillary, and lateral pectoral nerves innervate the joint.

The **acromioclavicular joint** is a plane synovial joint that augments the range of motion (ROM) in the hu-

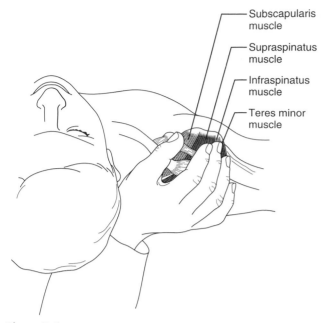

Subscapularis muscle

Supraspinatus muscle

Infraspinatus muscle

Teres minor muscle

Figure 5–1

Positioning of the rotator cuff with thumb over subscapularis, index finger over supraspinatus, middle finger over infraspinatus, and ring finger over teres minor.

merus. The bones making up this joint are the acromion process of the scapula and the lateral end of the clavicle. The joint has three degrees of freedom. The capsule, which is fibrous, surrounds the joint. An articular disc may be found within the joint. Rarely does the disc separate the acromion and clavicular articular surfaces. This joint depends on ligaments (primarily the acromiocla-

Acromioclavicular Joint

Resting position:	Arm by side
Close packed position:	90° abduction
Capsular pattern:	Pain at extremes of range of motion, especially horizontal adduction and full elevation

vicular and coracoclavicular) for its strength. In the resting position of the joint, the arm rests by the side in the normal standing position. In the close packed position of the acromioclavicular joint, the arm is abducted to 90°. The indication of a capsular pattern in the joint is pain at the extreme ROM, especially in horizontal adduction (cross-flexion) and full elevation. This joint is innervated by branches of the suprascapular and lateral pectoral nerve.

The **sternoclavicular joint,** along with the acromioclavicular joint, enables the humerus to move through a full 180° of abduction. It is a saddle-shaped synovial joint with three degrees of freedom and is made up of

the medial end of the clavicle, the manubrium sternum, and the cartilage of the first rib. There is a substantial disc between the two bony joint surfaces, and the capsule is thicker anteriorly than posteriorly. The disc separates the articular surfaces of the clavicle and sternum and adds significant strength to the joint because of attachments, thereby preventing medial displacement of the clavicle. Like the acromioclavicular joint, it depends

Sternoclavicular Joint

Resting position:	Arm at side
Close packed position:	Full elevation
Capsular pattern:	Pain at extremes of range of motion, especially horizontal adduction and full elevation

on ligaments for its strength. The movements possible at this joint and at the acromioclavicular joint are elevation, depression, protrusion, retraction, and rotation. The close packed position of the sternoclavicular joint is full or maximum rotation of the clavicle, which occurs when the upper arm is in full elevation. The resting position and capsular pattern are the same as with the acromioclavicular joint. The joint is innervated by branches of the anterior supraclavicular nerve and the nerve to the subclavius muscle.

Although the **scapulothoracic joint** is not a true joint, it functions as an integral part of the shoulder complex and must be considered in any assessment. Some texts call this structure the scapulocostal joint. This joint consists of the body of the scapula and the muscles covering the posterior chest wall. The medial border of the scapula is not parallel with the spinous processes but is angled about 3° away (top to bottom), and the scapula lies 20 to 30° forward relative to the sagittal plane.[1] Because it is not a true joint, it does not have a capsular pattern or a close packed position. The resting position of this joint is the same as for the acromioclavicular joint. The scapula extends from the level of T2 spinous process to T7 or T9 spinous process, depending on the size of the scapula.

Patient History

In addition to the questions listed under Patient History in Chapter 1, the examiner should obtain the following information from the patient.

1. What is the patient's age? Many problems of the shoulder can be age related. For example, rotator cuff degeneration usually occurs in patients who are between

40 and 60 years of age. Calcium deposits may occur between the ages of 20 and 40. Chondrosarcomas may be seen in those older than 30 years of age, whereas frozen shoulder is seen in persons between the ages of 45 and 60 years if it results from causes other than trauma (Table 5–1).

2. Does the patient support the upper limb in a protected position (Fig. 5–2) or hesitate to move it? This action could mean that one of the joints of the shoulder complex is unstable or that there is an acute problem in the shoulder.

3. If there was an injury, what exactly was the mechanism of injury? Did the patient fall on an outstretched hand ("FOOSH" injury), which could indicate a fracture or dislocation of the glenohumeral joint? Did the patient fall on or receive a blow to the tip of the shoulder, or

Table 5–1
Differential Diagnosis of Rotator Cuff Degeneration, Frozen Shoulder, Atraumatic Instability, and Cervical Spondylosis

	Rotator Cuff Lesion	Frozen Shoulder	Atraumatic Instability	Cervical Spondylosis
History	Age 30–50 years Pain and weakness after eccentric load	Age 45+ (insidious type) Insidious onset or after trauma or surgery Functional restriction of lateral rotation, abduction, and medial rotation	Age 10–35 years Pain and instability with activity No history of trauma	Age 50+ years Acute or chronic
Observation	Normal bone and soft tissue outlines Protective shoulder hike may be seen	Normal bone and soft-tissue outlines	Normal bone and soft-tissue outlines	Minimal or no cervical spine movement Torticollis may be present
Active movement	Weakness of abduction or rotation, or both Crepitus may be present	Restricted ROM Shoulder hiking	Full or excessive ROM	Limited ROM with pain
Passive movement	Pain if impingement occurs	Limited ROM, especially in lateral rotation, abduction, and medial rotation (capsular pattern)	Normal or excessive ROM	Limited ROM (symptoms may be exacerbated)
Resisted isometric movement	Pain and weakness on abduction and lateral rotation	Normal, when arm by side	Normal	Normal, except if nerve root compressed Myotome may be affected
Special tests	Drop-arm test positive Empty can test positive	None	Load and shift test positive Apprehension test positive Relocation test positive Augmentation tests positive	Spurling's test positive Distraction test positive ULTT positive Shoulder abduction test positive
Sensory function and reflexes	Not affected	Not affected		Dermatomes affected Reflexes affected
Palpation	Tender over rotator cuff	Not painful unless capsule is stretched	Anterior or posterior pain	Tender over appropriate vertebra or facet
Diagnostic imaging	Radiography: upward displacement of humeral head; acromial spurring MRI diagnostic	Radiography: negative Arthrography: decreased capsular size	Negative	Radiography: narrowing; osteophytes

MRI = magnetic resonance imaging; ROM = range of motion; ULTT = upper limb tension test.

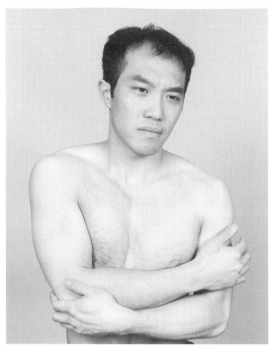

Figure 5–2
Patient supports the upper limb in protected position.

did the patient land on the elbow, driving the humerus up against the acromion? This finding may indicate an acromioclavicular dislocation or subluxation. Did the shoulder feel unstable or feel like it was "coming out" during movement? This may indicate gross instability, as in recurrent shoulder dislocation, or subtle translation instability. The spectrum of instability varies from the TUBS type (**T**raumatic onset, **U**nidirectional anterior with a **B**ankart lesion responding to **S**urgery) to the AMBRI type (**A**traumatic cause, **M**ultidirectional with **B**ilateral shoulder findings with **R**ehabilitation as appropriate treatment and, rarely, **I**nferior capsular shift surgery). AMBRI is referred to by some as AMBRII. The second "I" refers to surgery that also includes reconstruction of the rotator interval lesion.[2]

4. Are there any movements that cause the patient pain or problems? If so, which ones? The examiner must keep in mind that cervical spine movements may cause pain in the shoulder. Persons who have had recurrent dislocations of the shoulder may find that any movement involving lateral rotation bothers them, because this movement is involved in anterior dislocations of the shoulder. Excessive abduction and lateral rotation may lead to "dead-arm" syndrome in which the patient feels a sudden "paralyzing" pain and weakness in the shoulder. This finding is often an indication of anterior shoulder instability. If the patient complains of pain during specific phases of pitching (for example, during the late

cocking and acceleration phases), anterior instability should be considered even in the presence of minimal clinical signs.[3] Commonly, instability and impingement occur together. Night pain and resting pain are often related to rotator cuff tears and, on occasion, to tumors; activity-related pain usually signifies tendinitis. Acromioclavicular pain is especially evident at greater than 90° of abduction and tends to be localized to the joint.

5. What is the extent and behavior of the patient's pain? For example, deep, boring, toothache-like pain in the neck or shoulder region, or both, may indicate **thoracic outlet syndrome** (Fig. 5–3) or acute brachial plexus neuropathy. Strains of the rotator cuff usually cause dull, toothache-like pain that is worse at night, whereas acute calcific tendinitis usually causes a hot, burning type of pain.

6. Are there any activities that cause or increase the pain? For example, bicipital tendinitis is often seen in skiers and may be the result of holding on to a ski tow; in cross-country skiing, it may be the result of poling (using the pole for propulsion). Elite swimmers may train for more than 15,000 m daily, which can lead to stress overload (repetitive microtrauma) of the structures of the shoulder. Does throwing or reaching alter the pain? If so, what positions cause pain or discomfort? These questions may give an indication of the structures that are injured.

7. Do any positions relieve the pain? Patients with nerve root pain may find that elevation of the arm over the head gives relief of symptoms. Lifting the arm over the head by a patient with instability or inflammatory conditions usually exacerbates shoulder problems.

8. What is the patient unable to do functionally? Is the patient able to talk or swallow? Is the patient hoarse? These signs could indicate an injury to the sternoclavicular joint if there is swelling, or a posterior dislocation.

9. How long has the problem bothered the patient? For example, idiopathic frozen shoulder goes through three stages: the condition becomes progressively worse, plateaus, and then progressively improves, with each stage lasting 3 to 5 months.[4]

10. Is there any indication of muscle spasm, deformity, bruising, wasting, paresthesia, or numbness?

11. Does the patient complain of a feeling of weakness and heaviness in the limb after activity? Does the limb tire easily? Are there any other venous symptoms, such as swelling or stiffness, which may extend all the way to the fingers? Are there any arterial symptoms, such as coolness or pallor in the upper limb? These complaints may be the result of pressure on an artery, a vein, or both. An example is thoracic outlet syndrome (see Fig. 5–3), in which pressure may be applied to the vascular and/or neurological structures as they enter the

upper limb in three locations: at the scalene triangle, at the costoclavicular space, and under the pectoralis minor and the coracoid process.[5, 6] Excessive repetitive demands placed on the shoulder, such as those seen in pitching, may lead to thoracic outlet syndrome, axillary artery occlusion, effort thrombosis, or pressure in the quadrilateral space. (The quadrilateral space has as its boundaries the medial border of the humerus laterally, the lateral border of the long head of triceps medially, the inferior border of teres minor, and the superior border of teres major.)[7]

12. Is there any indication of nerve injury? The examiner should evaluate the nerves and the muscles supplied by the nerves to determine possible nerve injury. Any history of weakness, numbness, or paresthesia may indicate nerve injury (Table 5–2). For example, the suprascapular nerve may be injured as it passes through the suprascapular notch under the transverse scapular ligament, leading to atrophy and paralysis of the supraspinatus and infraspinatus muscles. The examiner should listen to the history carefully, because this condition could mimic a third-degree (rupture) strain of the supra-

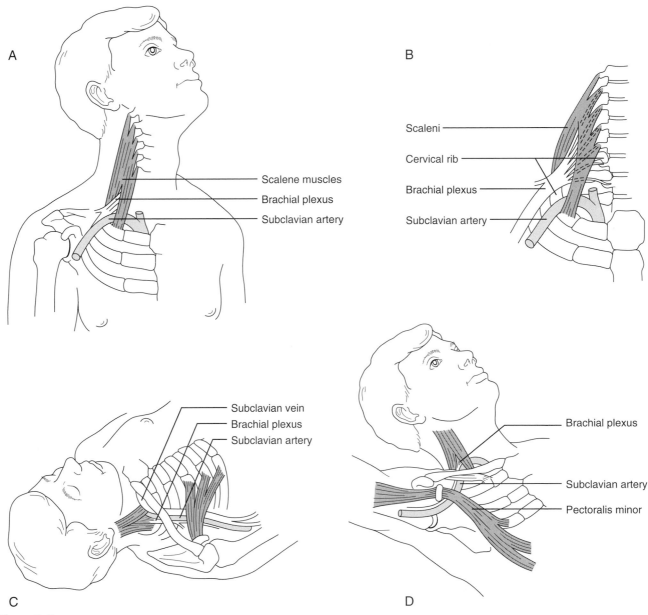

Figure 5–3

Location and causes of thoracic outlet syndrome. (A) Scalenus anterior syndrome. (B) Cervical rib syndrome. (C) Costoclavicular space syndrome. (D) Hyperabduction syndrome.

Table 5–2
Peripheral Nerve Injuries (Neuropathy) About the Shoulder

Affected Nerve (Root)	Muscle Weakness	Sensory Alteration	Reflexes Affected	Mechanism of Injury
Suprascapular nerve (C5–C6)	Supraspinatus, infraspinatus (arm lateral rotation)	Top of shoulder from clavicle to spine of scapula Pain in posterior shoulder radiating into arm	None	Compression in suprascapular notch Stretch into scapular protraction plus horizontal adduction Compression in spinoglenoid notch Direct blow Space occupying lesion (e.g., ganglion)
Axillary (circumflex) nerve (posterior cord; C5–C6)	Deltoid, teres minor (arm abduction)	Deltoid area Anterior shoulder pain	None	Anterior glenohumeral dislocation or fracture of surgical neck of humerus Forced abduction Surgery for instability
Radial nerve (C5–C8, T1)	Triceps, wrist extensors, finger extensors (shoulder, wrist, and hand extension)	Dorsum of hand	Triceps	Fracture humeral shaft Pressure (e.g., crutch palsy)
Long thoracic nerve (C5–C6, [C7])	Serratus anterior (scapular control)			Direct blow Traction Compression against internal chest wall (backpack injury) Heavy effort above shoulder height Repetitive strain
Musculocutaneous nerve (C5–C7)	Coracobrachialis, biceps, brachialis (elbow flexion)	Lateral aspect of forearm	Biceps	Compression Muscle hypertrophy Direct blow Fracture (clavicle and humerus) Dislocation (anterior) Surgery (Putti-Platt, Bankart)
Spinal accessory nerve (cranial nerve XI; C3–C4)	Trapezius (shoulder elevation)	Brachial plexus symptoms possible because of drooping of shoulder Shoulder aching	None	Direct blow Traction (shoulder depression and neck rotation to opposite side) Biopsy
Subscapular nerve (posterior cord; C5–C6)	Subscapularis, teres major (medial rotation)	None	None	Direct blow Traction
Dorsal scapular nerve (C5)	Levator scapulae, rhomboid major, rhomboid minor (scapular retraction and elevation)	None	None	Direct blow Compression
Lateral pectoral nerve (C5–C6)	Pectoralis major, pectoralis minor	None	None	Direct blow
Thoracodorsal nerve (C6–C7, [C8])	Latissimus dorsi	None	None	Direct blow Compression
Supraclavicular nerve	—	Mild clavicular pain Sensory loss over anterior shoulder		Compression

spinatus tendon. Another potential nerve injury is one to the axillary (circumflex) nerve (Fig. 5–4) or musculocutaneous nerve (Fig. 5–5) after dislocation of the glenohumeral joint. With an axillary nerve injury, the deltoid muscle and the teres minor muscle are atrophied and weak or paralyzed. The radial nerve (see Fig. 5–4) is sometimes injured as it winds around the posterior aspect of the shaft of the humerus. The injury frequently occurs when the humeral shaft is fractured. If the nerve is damaged in this location, the extensors of the elbow,

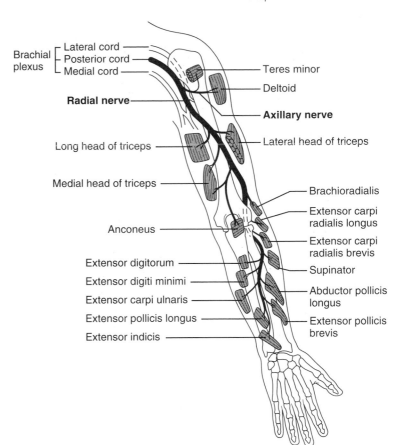

Figure 5–4
Motor distribution of the radial and axillary nerves.

wrist, and fingers are affected and an altered sensation occurs in the radial nerve sensory distribution.

13. Which hand is dominant? Often the dominant shoulder is lower than the nondominant shoulder and the ROM may not be the same for both. Usually, the dominant shoulder shows greater muscularity and often less ROM.

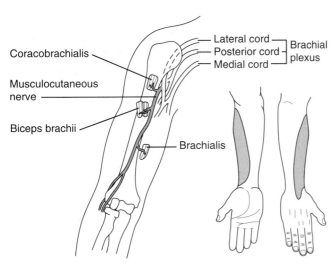

Figure 5–5
Motor and sensory distribution of musculocutaneous nerve.

Observation

The patient must be suitably undressed so that the examiner can observe the bony and soft-tissue contours of both shoulders and determine whether they are normal and symmetric. When observing the shoulder, the examiner looks at the head, the cervical spine, the thorax (especially the posterior aspect), and the entire upper limb. The hand, for example, may show some vasomotor changes that result from problems in the shoulder, including shiny skin, loss of hair, swelling, and muscle atrophy.

It is important to observe the patient as he or she removes clothes from the upper body and later replaces them. For example, is the affected arm undressed last or dressed first? The patient's actions give some indication of functional restriction, pain, and/or weakness in the upper limb.

Anterior View

When looking at the patient from the anterior view (Fig. 5–6A), the examiner should begin by ensuring that the head and neck are in the midline of the body and observing their relation to the shoulders. While observing the shoulder, the examiner should look for the possibility

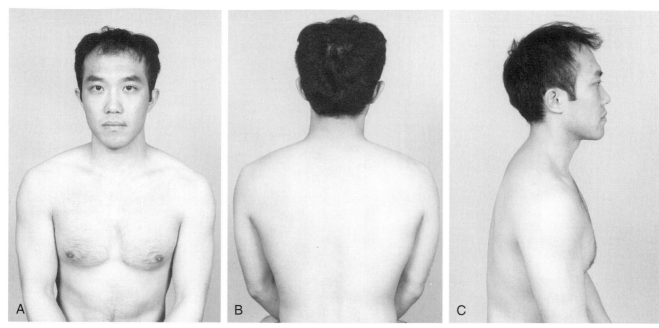

Figure 5–6
Anterior (A), posterior (B), and side (C) views of the shoulder.

of a **step deformity** (Fig. 5–7). Such a deformity may be caused by an acromioclavicular dislocation, with the distal end of the clavicle lying superior to the acromion process. If a deformity appears when traction is applied to the arm, it may be caused by multidirectional instability, leading to inferior subluxation of the glenohumeral joint. This sign is referred to as a **sulcus sign** because of the appearance of a sulcus below the acromion process. Flattening of the normally round deltoid muscle area may indicate an anterior dislocation of the glenohumeral joint or paralysis of the deltoid muscle (Fig. 5–8). The examiner should note any abnormal bumps or malalign-

ment in the bones that may indicate past injury, such as a fracture of the clavicle.

In most people, the dominant side is lower than the nondominant side. This difference may be caused by the extra use of the dominant side, which results in stretching of the ligaments, joint capsules, and muscles, allowing the arm to "sag" slightly. Tennis players[8] and others who stretch their upper limbs in a reaching action show even greater differences along with gross hypertrophy of the muscles on the dominant side (Fig. 5–9). If the patient is very protective of the shoulder, however, it may appear that the injured shoulder, whether dominant or

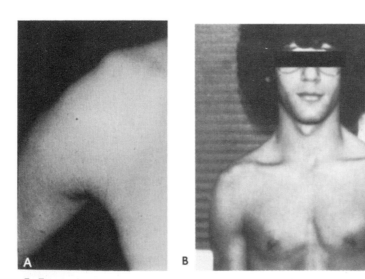
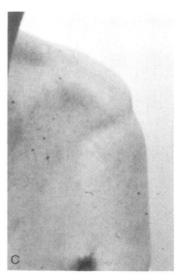

Figure 5–7
(A) Step deformity resulting from acromioclavicular dislocation. (B) Sulcus sign for shoulder instability. (From Warren, R.F.: Subluxation of the shoulder in athletes. Clin. Sports Med. 2:339, 1983). (C) Subluxation of glenohumeral joint following a stroke (paralysis of deltoid muscle).

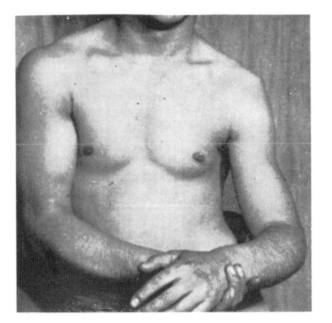

Figure 5–8

Subcoracoid dislocation of the shoulder. Note the prominent acromion, the arm held away from the side, and the flat deltoid. (From McLaughlin, H.L.: Trauma. Philadelphia, W.B. Saunders Co., 1959, p. 246.)

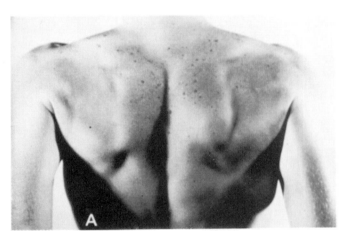

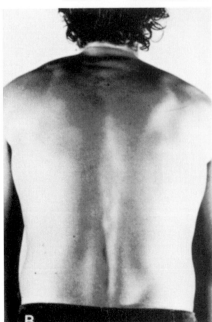

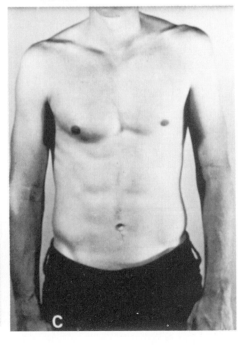

Figure 5–9

Depressed right shoulder in a right-dominant individual—in this case, a tennis player. (A) Hypertrophy of playing shoulder muscles. (B) With muscles relaxed, the distance between spinous processes and medial border of scapula is widened on the right. (C) Depressed shoulder. (From Priest, J.D., and D.A. Nagel: Tennis shoulder. Am. J. Sports Med. 4:33, 1976.)

nondominant, is higher than the normal side (see Fig. 5–2).

The examiner notes whether the patient is able to assume the normal functional position for the shoulder, which is in the scapular plane with 60° of abduction and the arm in neutral or no rotation. The examiner should be aware that if the patient's arm is medially rotated from this position to bring the hand into midline, the biceps tendon is forced against the lesser tuberosity of the medial wall of the bicipital (intertubercular) groove. If this position is maintained for long periods, there may be increased wear of the biceps tendon, which can lead to bicipital tendinitis. The bicipital groove may vary in width and depth (Fig. 5–10), possibly leading to problems if the shoulder is overused. Especially wide or deep grooves lead to the greatest problems. The wide grooves tend to allow the tendon too much lateral movement, leading to inflammation; the deep grooves tend to be too narrow, compressing the tendon.[9]

Posterior View

When viewing the patient from behind (Fig. 5–6B), the examiner again notes bony and soft-tissue contours and body alignment. For example, atrophy of the upper trapezius may indicate spinal accessory nerve palsy, whereas atrophy of supraspinatus and/or infraspinatus may indicate supraspinous nerve palsy.[10] The spines of the scapulae, which begin medially at the level of the third (T3) thoracic vertebra, should be at the same angle. The scapula itself should extend from the T2 spinous process to the T7 spinous process of the thoracic vertebrae. If the scapula is sitting lower than normal against the chest wall, the superior medial border of the scapula may "washboard" over the ribs, causing a snapping or clunking sound (snapping scapula) during abduction and adduction.[11] The inferior angles of the scapulae should be equidistant from the spine. The examiner should note the possible presence of **winging** of the scapula, a condition in which the medial border moves away from the posterior chest wall (Fig. 5–11), or **rotary winging,** in which the inferior angle of one scapula is rotated farther from the spine than the inferior angle of the other scapula. **Dynamic winging** (i.e., winging with movement) may be caused by a lesion of the long thoracic nerve affecting serratus anterior, trapezius palsy (spinal accessory nerve), rhomboid weakness, multidirectional instability, voluntary action, or a painful shoulder resulting in splinting of the glenohumeral joint, which in turn causes reverse scapulohumeral rhythm.[12] The two most common causes of dynamic winging—long thoracic nerve palsy and spinal accessory nerve palsy—cause different positioning of the scapula. Spinal accessory nerve palsy causes the scapula to depress and move laterally, with the inferior angle rotated laterally. Long thoracic nerve

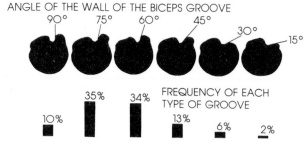

ANGLE OF THE WALL OF THE BICEPS GROOVE

Figure 5–10

Different shapes of the bicipital groove. (Adapted from Hitchcock, H.H., and C.O. Bechtol: Painful shoulder: Observation on the role of the tendon of the long head of the biceps brachii in its causation. J. Bone Joint Surg. Am. 30:267, 1948.)

palsy causes the scapula to elevate and move medially, with the inferior angle rotating medially[13] (Fig. 5–12). Radiculopathies at C3, C4 (trapezius), C5 (rhomboids), and C7 (serratus anterior, rhomboids) can also cause winging.[14, 15] **Static winging** (i.e., winging occurring at rest) is usually caused by a structural deformity of the scapula, clavicle, spine, or ribs.[16] **Scapular tilt** (superior or inferior border tilt, away from the chest wall) may also occur with weakness or instability. **Sprengel's deformity,** which

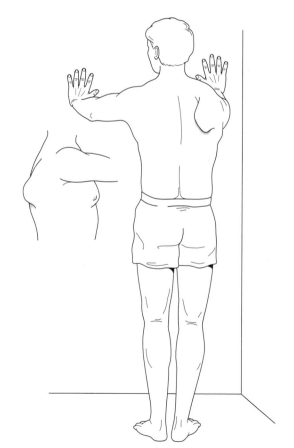

Figure 5–11

Winging of the scapula.

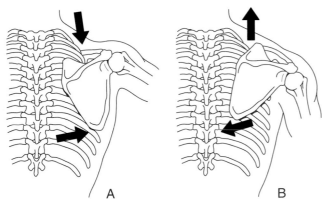

Figure 5–12
Scapular movement resulting in scapular winging caused by trapezius palsy (A) and serratus anterior palsy (B).

is a congenitally high or undescended scapula (Fig. 5–13), may also be seen.[17, 18] With this deformity, the scapular muscles are poorly developed or are replaced by a fibrous band. The condition may be unilateral or bilateral, and the range of the shoulder abduction is decreased, although functional disability may be slight. Usually, the scapula is smaller than normal and is medially rotated.

The shoulder muscles may be accentuated by having the patient place the hands on the hips and contract the muscles. The examiner should check closely for wasting in the supraspinatus and infraspinatus muscles (suprascapular nerve palsy), in the serratus anterior muscle (long thoracic nerve palsy), and in the trapezius muscle

(spinal accessory nerve palsy), all of which can lead to winging of the scapula.

Examination

Because assessment of the shoulder may include an assessment of the cervical spine, the examination can be an extensive one. If there is any doubt in the examiner's mind as to the location of the lesion, a cervical spine assessment (see Chapter 3) should be performed. In addition, the examiner must remember that the arm, of which the shoulder is an integral part, may act as an open kinetic chain when the hand is free to move or as a closed kinetic chain when the hand is fixed to some relatively immovable object. These **kinetic chains** and the intricate and complex interplay of the components of the kinetic chain have different effects on the shoulder. Eating, reaching, and dressing are considered open kinetic chain activities, whereas crutch walking and pushing up from a chair are considered closed kinetic chain movements.

As with any assessment, the examiner is comparing one side of the body with the other. This comparison is necessary because of the individual differences among normal people.

Active Movements

The first movements to be examined are the active movements. These movements are usually done in such a way that the painful movements are performed last.

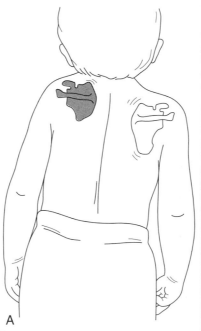
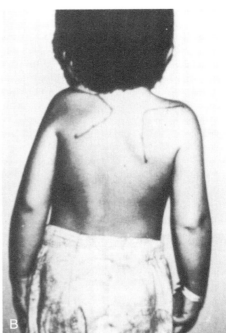

Figure 5–13
Diagram (A) and photograph (B) of child with Sprengel's deformity. Note elevated shoulder and poorly developed scapula on the left (A, modified from Gartland J.J.: Fundamentals of Orthopaedics. Philadelphia, W.B. Saunders Co., 1979, p. 73. B, courtesy of Dr. Roshen Irani.)

Active Movements of the Shoulder Complex

- Elevation through abduction (170 to 180°)
- Elevation through forward flexion (160 to 180°)
- Elevation through the plane of the scapula (170 to 180°)
- Lateral (external) rotation (80 to 90°)
- Medial (internal) rotation (60 to 100°)
- Extension (50 to 60°)
- Adduction (50 to 75°)
- Horizontal adduction/abduction (cross-flexion/cross-extension; 130°)
- Circumduction (200°)
- Combined movements (if necessary)
- Repetitive movements (if necessary)
- Sustained positions (if necessary)

Active elevation through abduction is normally 170 to 180°. The extreme of the ROM is found when the arm is abducted and lies against the head on the same side (Fig. 5–14). Active elevation through forward flexion is normally 160 to 180°, and at the extreme of the ROM the arm is in the same position as for active elevation through abduction. Active elevation (170 to 180°) through the plane of the scapula (30 to 45° of forward flexion), termed **scaption,** is the most natural and func-

tional position of abduction (see Fig. 5–14). Elevation in this position is sometimes called neutral elevation. The exact angle is determined by the contour of the chest wall on which the scapula rests. Often, movement into elevation is less painful in this position than elevation through abduction in which the glenohumeral joint is actually in extension. Movement in the plane of the scapula puts less stress on the capsule and surrounding musculature and is the position in which most of the functions of daily activity are performed. Strength testing in this plane also gives higher values. Patients with weakness spontaneously choose this plane when elevating the arm.[19, 20]

Active lateral rotation is normally 80 to 90° but may be greater in some athletes such as gymnasts and pitchers. Care must be taken when applying overpressure with this movement, because it could lead to anterior dislocation of the glenohumeral joint, especially in those with recurrent dislocation problems. Active medial rotation is normally 60 to 100°. This is usually assessed by measuring the height of "hitchhiking" thumb (thumb in extension) reaching up the person's back. Common reference points include the greater trochanter, buttock, waist, and spinous processes, with T5 to T10 representing the normal degree of medial rotation.[21]

Active extension is normally 50 to 60°. The examiner must ensure that the movement is in the shoulder and not in the spine, because some patients may flex the spine or bend forward, giving the appearance of increased shoulder extension.

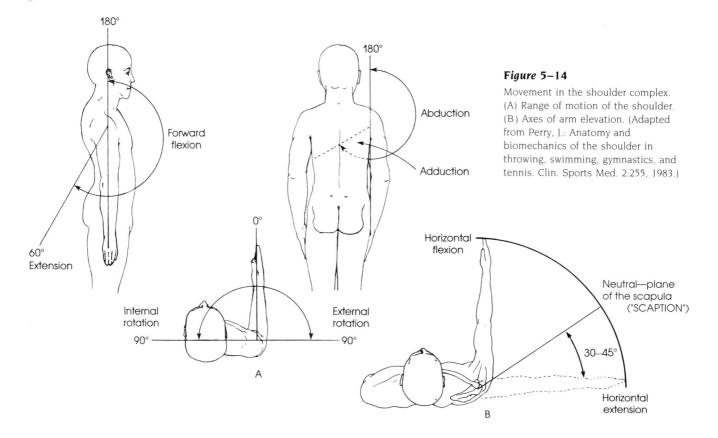

Figure 5–14

Movement in the shoulder complex. (A) Range of motion of the shoulder. (B) Axes of arm elevation. (Adapted from Perry, J.: Anatomy and biomechanics of the shoulder in throwing, swimming, gymnastics, and tennis. Clin. Sports Med. 2:255, 1983.)

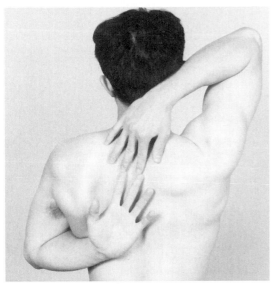

Figure 5–15

Apley's scratch test. The right arm is in lateral rotation and abduction, and the left arm is in medial rotation and adduction.

Adduction is normally 50 to 75° if the arm is brought in front of the body. Horizontal adduction, or cross-flexion, is normally 130°. To accomplish this movement, the patient first abducts the arm to 90° and then moves the arm across the front of the body. Horizontal abduction, or cross-extension, is approximately 45°. After abducting the arm to 90°, the patient moves the straight arm in a backward direction. Circumduction is normally approximately 200° and involves taking the arm in a circle on the vertical plane.

When observing these movements, the examiner may ask the patient to perform them in combination, especially if the history has indicated that combined movements are bothersome. For example, **Apley's scratch test** combines medial rotation with adduction and lateral rotation with abduction (Fig. 5–15). This method may decrease the time required to do the assessment. In addition, by having the patient do the combined movements, the examiner is given some idea of the functional capacity of the patient. For example, abduction combined with lateral rotation or adduction combined with medial rotation is needed to comb the hair, to zip a back zipper, or to reach for a wallet in a back pocket. However, the examiner must take care to notice which movements are restricted and which ones are not, because several movements are performed at the same time. Often, the dominant shoulder shows greater restriction than the nondominant shoulder, even in normal persons. If, in the history, the patient has complained that shoulder movements in certain postures are painful or that sustained or repetitive movements increase symptoms, the examiner should consider having the patient hold a sustained arm position (10 to 60 seconds) or do the movements repetitively (10 to 20 repetitions).

As the patient elevates the upper extremity by abducting the shoulder, the examiner should note whether a **painful arc** is present[22] (Fig. 5–16). A painful arc may

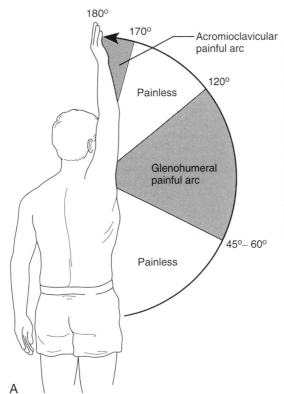

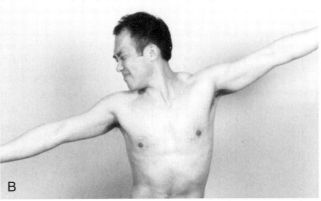

Figure 5–16

Painful arc in the shoulder. (A) Painful arc of the glenohumeral joint. In the case of acromioclavicular joint problems only, the range of 170° to 180° would elicit pain. (Modified from Hawkins, R.J., and P.E. Hobeika: Impingement syndrome in the athletic shoulder. Clin. Sports Med. 2:391, 1983.) (B) Note the impingement causing pain on the right at approximately 85°.

Table 5–3
Classification of Glenohumeral Painful Arcs

	Anterior	Posterior	Superior
Night pain	Yes	Yes	Maybe
Age	50+	50+	40+
Sex ratio	F > M	F > M	M > F
Aggravated by	Lateral rotation and abduction	Medial rotation and abduction	Abduction
Tenderness	Lesser tuberosity	Posterior aspect of greater tuberosity	Greater tuberosity
Acromioclavicular joint involvement	No	No	Often
Calcification (if present)	Supraspinatus, infraspinatus, and/or subscapularis	Supraspinatus and/or infraspinatus	Supraspinatus and/or subscapularis
Third-degree strain biceps brachii (long head)	No	No	Occasional
Prognosis	Good	Very good	Poor (without surgery)

From Kessel, L., and M. Watson: The painful arc syndrome. J. Bone Joint Surg. Br. 59:166, 1977.

be caused by subacromial bursitis, calcium deposits, or a tendinitis of the rotator cuff muscles. The pain is the result of pinching of inflamed or tender structures under the acromion process and the coracoacromial ligament. Initially, the structures are not pinched under the acromion process, so the patient is able to abduct the arm 45 to 60° with little difficulty. As the patient abducts further (60 to 120°), the structures become pinched and the patient is often unable to abduct fully because of pain. If full abduction is possible, however, the pain diminishes after approximately 120° because the pinched soft tissues have passed under the acromion process and are no longer being pinched. Often, the pain is greater going up (against gravity) than coming down, and there is more pain on active abduction than on passive abduction. If the movement is very painful, the patient often elevates the arm through forward flexion or "hikes" the shoulder in an attempt to decrease the pain. If the pain is greater as the patient reaches full elevation, the examiner should consider the possibility of an acromioclavicular joint problem. Table 5–3 presents the signs and symptoms of three types of painful arc in the shoulder, with the superior type being the most common. The arc of pain may be present also during elevation through forward flexion and scaption, although the pain is usually less severe on these movements. The interconnection of the subacromial, subcoracoid, and subscapularis bursae with each other and with the glenohumeral joint capsule often produces a broad area of signs and symptoms.

A second painful arc may be seen during the same abduction movement. This painful arc (see Fig. 5–16) occurs toward the end of abduction, in the last 10 to 20° of elevation, and is caused by pathology in the acromioclavicular joint or by a positive impingement test. In the case of the acromioclavicular joint lesion, the pain tends to be localized to the joint. With the impingement syndrome, the pain is usually found in the anterior shoulder region.

When examining the movement of elevation through abduction, the examiner must take time to observe **scapulohumeral rhythm** of the shoulder complex (Fig. 5–17), both anteriorly and posteriorly.[23, 24] That is, during 180° of abduction, there is roughly a 2:1 ratio of movement of the humerus to the scapula, with 120° of movement occurring at the glenohumeral joint and 60° at the scapulothoracic joint. During this total movement, there are three phases:

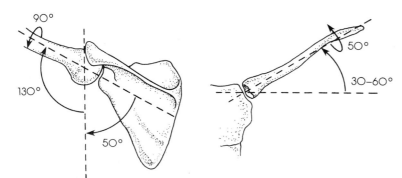

Figure 5–17
Movement of the scapula, humerus, and clavicle during scapulohumeral rhythm.

Scapulohumeral Rhythm

Phase 1:	Humerus	30° abduction
	Scapula	minimal movement
	Clavicle	0–15° elevation
Phase 2:	Humerus	40° abduction
	Scapula	20° rotation
	Clavicle	30–36° elevation
Phase 3:	Humerus	60° abduction
		90° lateral rotation
	Scapula	30° rotation
	Clavicle	30–50° posterior rotation
		up to 30° elevation

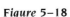

1. In the first phase of 30° of elevation through abduction, the outer end of the clavicle may elevate from 0 to 15° while the scapula is said to be "setting." This setting phase means that the scapula may rotate in, rotate out, or not move at all. Thus, there is no 2:1 ratio of movement during this phase. The angle between the scapular spine and the clavicle also increases by 10°, but there is no rotation of the clavicle.

2. During the next 60° of elevation (second phase), the scapula rotates 30° and the clavicle elevates 30 to 36°. There is a 2:1 ratio of scapulohumeral movement. There still is no rotation of the clavicle at this stage.

3. During the final 90° of motion (third phase), there continues to be a 2:1 ratio of scapulohumeral movement,

and the angle between the scapular spine and the clavicle increases an additional 10°. It is in this stage that the clavicle rotates posteriorly 30 to 50° on a long axis and elevates up to a further 30°. Also during this final stage, the humerus laterally rotates 90°, so that the greater tuberosity of the humerus avoids the acromion process.

It should be pointed out that some authors do not agree with the 2:1 ratio. Although they concede that there is more movement in the glenohumeral joint than in the scapulothoracic joint, Davies and colleagues[25] believe the ratio is greater, at least to 120° of abduction, whereas Poppen and associates[26] believe the ratio is less (5:4) after 30° of abduction. Therefore, it is more important to look for asymmetry between the injured and the good sides than to be concerned with the actual degree of movement.

If the clavicle does not rotate and elevate, elevation through abduction at the glenohumeral joint is limited to 120°. If the glenohumeral joint does not move, elevation through abduction is limited to 60°, which occurs totally in the scapulothoracic joint. If there is no lateral rotation of the humerus during abduction, the total movement available is 120°, 60° of which occurs at the glenohumeral joint and 60° of which occurs at the scapulothoracic articulation. The normal end of ROM is reached when there is contact of a surgical neck of humerus with the acromion process. **Reverse scapulohumeral rhythm** (Fig. 5–18) means that the scapula moves more than the humerus. This is seen in conditions such as frozen

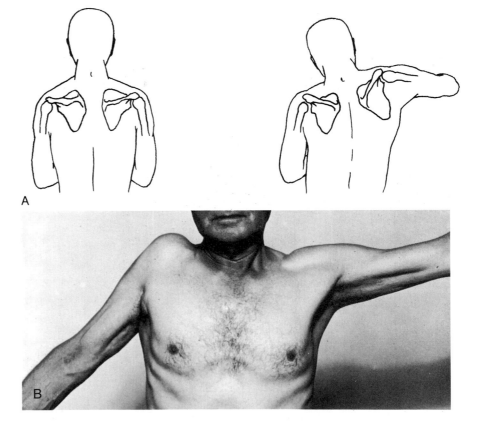

Figure 5–18
Reverse scapulohumeral rhythm (notice shoulder hiking). Examples include frozen shoulder (A) or tear of rotator cuff (B). (B, from Beetham, W.P., H.F. Polley, C.H. Slocum, and W.F. Weaver: Physical Examination of the Joints. Philadelphia, W.B. Saunders Co., 1965, p. 41.)

shoulder. The patient appears to "hike" the entire shoulder complex rather than produce a smooth coordinated abduction movement.

It must be remembered that the biceps tendon does not move in the bicipital groove during movement; rather, the humerus moves over the fixed tendon. From adduction to full elevation of abduction, a given point in the groove moves along the tendon at least 4 cm. If the examiner wants to keep excursion of the biceps tendon to a minimum, the arm should be elevated with the humerus in medial rotation; elevation of the arm with the humerus laterally rotated causes maximum excursion of the biceps tendon. This laterally rotated position is sometimes used by patients who have deltoid or supraspinatus pathology, because lateral rotation allows the biceps tendon to be used as a shoulder abductor in a "cheating" movement.

As the patient does the various movements, the examiner watches to see whether the components of the shoulder complex move in normal, coordinated sequence and whether the patient exhibits any apprehension when doing a movement. With **anterior instability** of the shoulder, the shoulder girdle often droops, and excessive scapulothoracic movement may be seen on abduction. With **posterior instability,** horizontal adduction (cross-flexion) may cause excessive scapulothoracic movement. Any apprehension suggests the possibility of instability. The examiner should also watch for **winging of the scapula.** Winging of the medial border of the scapula is indicative of injury to the serratus anterior muscle or the long thoracic nerve; rotary winging of the scapula or scapular tilt is indicative of upper trapezius pathology or injury to the spinal accessory nerve (cranial nerve XI; Table 5–4).[10, 21, 27] In some cases, it may be necessary to load the appropriate muscle isometrically or to hold the contraction for 10 to 15 seconds to demonstrate the winging. It has been reported that application of a resistance to adduction at 30° and at 60° of shoulder abduction is the best way to show scapular winging.[21] Eccentric loading of the shoulder in different positions may also demonstrate winging.

If the scapula appears to wing, the examiner asks the patient to forward flex the shoulder to 90°. The examiner then pushes the straight arm toward the patient's body

Table 5–4
Winging of the Scapula: Dynamic Causes and Effects

Cause	Effect
Trapezius or spinal accessory nerve lesion	Inability to shrug shoulder
Serratus anterior or long thoracic nerve lesion	Difficulty elevating arm above 120°
Strain of rhomboids	Difficulty pushing elbow back against resistance (with hand on hip)
Muscle imbalance or contractures	Winging of upper margin of scapula on adduction and lateral rotation

Table 5–5
Peripheral Nerve Tests

Spinal accessory nerve	Inability to abduct arm beyond 90°
	Pain in shoulder on abduction
Long thoracic nerve	Pain on flexing fully extended arm
	Inability to flex fully extended arm
	Winging starts at 90° forward flexion
Suprascapular nerve	Increased pain on forward shoulder flexion
	Shoulder weakness (partial loss of humeral control)
	Pain increases with scapular abduction
	Pain increases with cervical rotation to opposite side
Axillary (circumflex) nerve	Inability to abduct arm with neutral rotation
Musculocutaneous nerve	Weak elbow flexion with forearm supinated

while the patient resists. If there is weakness of the upper trapezius muscle, the serratus anterior muscle, or the nerves supplying these muscles, their inability to contract will cause the scapula to wing. Winging of the scapula may also be tested by having the patient stand and lean against the wall. The patient is then asked to do a "push-up" away from the wall while the examiner watches for winging (see Figs. 5–11 and 5–12).

Injury to other nerves in the shoulder region must not be overlooked (Table 5–5). As previously mentioned, damage to the suprascapular nerve affects the supraspinatus and infraspinatus muscles, whereas injury to the musculocutaneous nerve can lead to paralysis of the coracobrachialis, biceps, and brachialis muscles. These changes affect elbow flexion and supination and forward flexion of the shoulder. There is also a loss of the biceps reflex. Injury to the axillary (circumflex) nerve leads to paralysis of the deltoid and teres minor muscles, affecting abduction and lateral rotation of the shoulder. There is also a sensory loss over the deltoid insertion area. Damage to the radial nerve affects all of the extensor muscles of the upper limb, including the triceps. Triceps paralysis may be overlooked unless arm extension is attempted along with elbow extension against gravity. Both of these movements are affected in high radial nerve palsy, although some triceps function may remain (e.g., in radial nerve palsy after a humeral shaft fracture).

Passive Movements

If the ROM is not full during the active movements and the examiner is unable to test the end feel, all passive movements of the shoulder should be performed to determine the end feel and passive ROM, and any restriction should be noted.

Passive Movements of the Shoulder Complex and Normal End Feel

- Elevation through forward flexion of the arm (tissue stretch)
- Elevation through abduction of the arm (bone-to-bone or tissue stretch)
- Elevation through abduction of the glenohumeral joint only (bone-to-bone or tissue stretch)
- Lateral rotation of the arm (tissue stretch)
- Medial rotation of the arm (tissue stretch)
- Extension of the arm (tissue stretch)
- Adduction of the arm (tissue approximation)
- Horizontal adduction (tissue stretch or approximation) and abduction of the arm (tissue stretch)
- Quadrant test

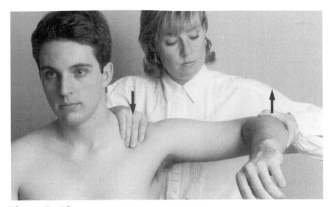

Figure 5–19

Passive abduction of the glenohumeral joint.

Particular attention must be paid to passive medial and lateral rotation if the examiner suspects a problem with the glenohumeral joint capsule. **Subcoracoid bursitis** may limit full lateral rotation and **subacromial bursitis** may limit full abduction because of compression or pinching of these structures. If lateral rotation of the shoulder is limited, the examiner should check forearm supination with the arm forward flexed to 90°. Patients who have a posterior dislocation at the glenohumeral joint exhibit restricted lateral rotation of the shoulder and limited supination in forward flexion (**Rowe sign**).[28] Even if overpressure has been applied on active movement, it is still necessary for the examiner to perform elevation through abduction of the glenohumeral joint only (Fig. 5–19) and the quadrant test.

Passive elevation through abduction of the glenohumeral joint with the clavicle and scapula fixed is performed by the examiner to determine the amount of abduction in the glenohumeral joint alone. Normally, this movement should be 120°.

To test the **quadrant position,**[29] the examiner stabilizes the scapula and clavicle by placing the forearm under the patient's scapula on the side to be tested and extending the hand over the shoulder to hold the trapezius muscle and prevent shoulder shrugging (Fig. 5–20). To test the position, the upper limb is elevated to rest alongside the patient's head with the shoulder externally rotated. The patient's shoulder is then adducted. Because adduction occurs on the coronal plane, a point (the quadrant position) is reached at which the arm will move forward slightly from the coronal plane. At approximately 60° of adduction (from the arm beside the head), this position of maximum forward movement occurs even if a backward pressure is applied. As the shoulder is further adducted, the arm falls back to the previous coronal plane. The quadrant position indicates the position at which the arm has medially rotated during its descent to the patient's side.

The rotation of the humerus in the quadrant position demonstrates Codman's "pivotal paradox"[20, 30] and MacConaill's[31] conjunct rotation in diadochal movement. For

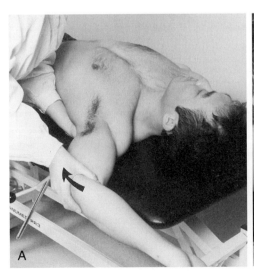
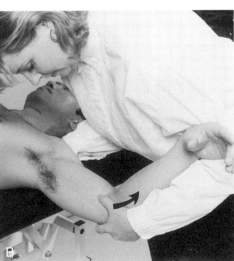

Figure 5–20

Quadrant position. (A) Adduction test. (B) Abduction test (locked quadrant).

example, if the arm, with the elbow flexed, is laterally rotated when the arm is at the side and then abducted in the coronal plane to 180°, the shoulder will be in 90° of medial rotation even though no apparent rotation has occurred. The path traced by the humerus during the quadrant test, in which the humerus moves forward at approximately 120° of abduction, is the unconscious rotation occurring at the glenohumeral joint. The examiner should not only feel the movement but also determine the quality of the movement and the amount of anterior humeral movement. This test and the following locked quadrant test assess one area or quadrant of the 200° of circumduction. It is the quadrant of the circumduction movement in which the humerus must rotate to allow full pain-free movement. Although both of these tests should normally be pain free, the examiner should be aware that they place a high level of stress on the soft tissues of the glenohumeral joint, and discomfort should not be misinterpreted as pathological pain. If movement is painful and restricted, the tests indicate early stages of shoulder pathology.[32]

The quadrant position also may be found by abducting the medially rotated shoulder while maintaining extension. In this case, the quadrant position is reached (at approximately 120° of abduction) when the shoulder no longer abducts because it is prevented from laterally rotating by the catching of the greater tuberosity in the subacromial space. This position is referred to as the **locked quadrant position.** If the arm is allowed to move forward, lateral rotation occurs and full abduction can be achieved.

The capsular pattern of the shoulder is lateral rotation showing the greatest restriction, followed by abduction and medial rotation. Each of these movements normally has a tissue-stretch end feel. Other movements may be limited, but not in the same order and not with as much restriction. Finding of limitation, but not in the order described, is indicative of a noncapsular pattern.

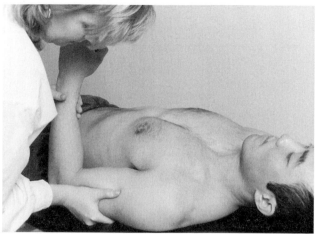

Figure 5–21
Positioning of the patient for resisted isometric movements.

Resisted Isometric Movements

Having completed the active and passive movements, which are done while the patient is standing, sitting, or lying supine (in the case of quadrant test), the patient lies supine to do the resisted isometric movements (Fig. 5–21). It has been advocated that the muscles should be tested in more than one position to determine the mechanical effect of the contraction in different situations. If pain is found in the initial position, other positions (e.g., position of injury, position of mechanical advantage) may be tried to further differentiate the specific contractile tissue that is injured. During the active movements, the examiner should have noted which movements caused discomfort or pain so that this information can be correlated with that obtained from resisted isometric movements. By carefully noting which movements cause pain on isometric testing, the examiner should be able to determine which muscle or muscles are at fault (Table 5–6). For example, if the patient

Table 5–6
Muscles About the Shoulder: Their Actions, Nerve Supply, and Nerve Root Derivation

Action	Muscles Acting	Nerve Supply	Nerve Root Derivation
Forward flexion	1. Deltoid (anterior fibers)	Axillary (circumflex)	C5–C6 (posterior cord)
	2. Pectoralis major (clavicular fibers)	Lateral pectoral	C5–C6 (lateral cord)
	3. Coracobrachialis	Musculocutaneous	C5–C7 (lateral cord)
	4. Biceps (when strong contraction required)	Musculocutaneous	C5–C7 (lateral cord)
Extension	1. Deltoid (posterior fibers)	Axillary (circumflex)	C5–C6 (posterior cord)
	2. Teres major	Subscapular	C5–C6 (posterior cord)
	3. Teres minor	Axillary (circumflex)	C5–C6 (posterior cord)
	4. Latissimus dorsi	Thoracodorsal	C6–C8 (posterior cord)
	5. Pectoralis major (sternocostal fibers)	Lateral pectoral	C5–C6 (lateral cord)
		Medial pectoral	C8, T1 (medial cord)
	6. Triceps (long head)	Radial	C5–C8, T1 (posterior cord)
Horizontal adduction	1. Pectoralis major	Lateral pectoral	C5–C6 (lateral cord)
	2. Deltoid (anterior fibers)	Axillary (circumflex)	C5–C6 (posterior cord)

Table 5–6
Muscles About the Shoulder: Their Actions, Nerve Supply, and Nerve Root Derivation (Continued)

Action	Muscles Acting	Nerve Supply	Nerve Root Derivation
Horizontal abduction	1. Deltoid (posterior fibers)	Axillary (circumflex)	C5–C6 (posterior cord)
	2. Teres major	Subscapular	C5–C6 (posterior cord)
	3. Teres minor	Axillary (circumflex)	C5–C6 (brachial plexus trunk)
	4. Infraspinatus	Suprascapular	C5–C6 (brachial plexus trunk)
Abduction	1. Deltoid	Axillary (circumflex)	C5–C6 (posterior cord)
	2. Supraspinatus	Suprascapular	C5–C6 (brachial plexus trunk)
	3. Infraspinatus	Suprascapular	C5–C6 (brachial plexus trunk)
	4. Subscapularis	Subscapular	C5–C6 (posterior cord)
	5. Teres minor	Axillary (circumflex)	C5–C6 (posterior cord)
	6. Long head of biceps (if arm laterally rotated first, trick movement)	Musculocutaneous	C5–C7 (lateral cord)
Adduction	1. Pectoralis major	Lateral pectoral	C5–C6 (lateral cord)
	2. Latissimus dorsi	Thoracodorsal	C6–C8 (posterior cord)
	3. Teres major	Subscapular	C5–C6 (posterior cord)
	4. Subscapularis	Subscapular	C5–C6 (posterior cord)
Medial rotation	1. Pectoralis major	Lateral pectoral	C5–C6 (lateral cord)
	2. Deltoid (anterior fibers)	Axillary (circumflex)	C5–C6 (posterior cord)
	3. Latissimus dorsi	Thoracodorsal	C6–C8 (posterior cord)
	4. Teres major	Subscapular	C5–C6 (posterior cord)
	5. Subscapularis (when arm is by side)	Subscapular	C5–C6 (posterior cord)
Lateral rotation	1. Infraspinatus	Suprascapular	C5–C6 (brachial plexus trunk)
	2. Deltoid (posterior fibers)	Axillary (circumflex)	C5–C6 (posterior cord)
	3. Teres minor	Axillary (circumflex)	C5–C6 (posterior cord)
Elevation of scapula	1. Trapezius (upper fibers)	Accessory C3–C4 nerve roots	Cranial nerve XI C3–C4
	2. Levator scapulae	C3–C4 nerve roots Dorsal scapular	C3–C4 C5
	3. Rhomboid major	Dorsal scapular	(C4), C5
	4. Rhomboid minor	Dorsal scapular	(C4), C5
Depression of scapula	1. Serratus anterior	Long thoracic	C5–C6, (C7)
	2. Pectoralis major	Lateral pectoral	C5–C6 (lateral cord)
	3. Pectoralis minor	Medial pectoral	C8, T1 (medial cord)
	4. Latissimus dorsi	Thoracodorsal	C6–C8 (posterior cord)
	5. Trapezius (lower fibers)	Accessory C3–C4 nerve roots	Cranial nerve XI C3–C4
Protraction (forward movement) of scapula	1. Serratus anterior	Long thoracic	C5–C6, (C7)
	2. Pectoralis major	Lateral pectoral	C5–C6 (lateral cord)
	3. Pectoralis minor	Medial pectoral	C8, T1 (medial cord)
	4. Latissimus dorsi	Thoracodorsal	C6–C8 (posterior cord)
Retraction (backward movement) of scapula	1. Trapezius	Accessory	Cranial nerve XI
	2. Rhomboid major	Dorsal scapular	(C4), C5
	3. Rhomboid minor	Dorsal scapular	(C4), C5
Lateral (upward) rotation of inferior angle of scapula	1. Trapezius (upper and lower fibers)	Accessory C3–C4 nerve roots	Cranial nerve XI C3–C4
	2. Serratus anterior	Long thoracic	C5–C6, (C7)
Medial (downward) rotation of inferior angle of scapula	1. Levator scapulae	C3–C4 nerve roots Dorsal scapular	C3–C4 C5
	2. Rhomboid major	Dorsal scapular	(C4), C5
	3. Rhomboid minor	Dorsal scapular	(C4), C5
	4. Pectoralis minor	Medial pectoral	C8, T1 (medial cord)
Flexion of elbow	1. Brachialis	Musculocutaneous	C5–C6, (C7)
	2. Biceps brachii	Musculocutaneous	C5–C6
	3. Brachioradialis	Radial	C5–C6, (C7)
	4. Pronator teres	Median	C6–C7
	5. Flexor carpi ulnaris	Ulnar	C7–C8
Extension of elbow	1. Triceps	Radial	C6–C8
	2. Anconeus	Radial	C7–C8, (T1)

experiences pain primarily on medial rotation but also on abduction and adduction, a problem would be suspected in the subscapularis muscle, because the other muscles involved in these actions were found to be pain free in other movements. To do the initial resisted isometric tests, the examiner positions the patient's arm at the side with the elbow flexed to 90°. The muscles of the shoulder are then tested isometrically with the examiner positioning the patient and saying, "Don't let me move you."

Resisted Isometric Movements of the Shoulder Complex

- Forward flexion of the shoulder
- Extension of the shoulder
- Adduction of the shoulder
- Abduction of the shoulder
- Medial rotation of the shoulder
- Lateral rotation of the shoulder
- Flexion of the elbow
- Extension of the elbow

Resisted isometric elbow flexion and extension must be performed, because some of the muscles (e.g., biceps, triceps) act over the elbow as well as the shoulder. The examiner should watch for the possibility of a third-degree strain (rupture) of the long head of biceps tendon ("Popeye muscle") when testing isometric elbow flexion (Fig. 5–22).

During the testing, the examiner will find differences in the relative strengths of the various muscle groups around the shoulder. The relative percentages for isometric testing will be altered for tests at faster speeds and tests in different planes. If, in the history, the patient complained that concentric, eccentric, or econcentric movements were painful or caused symptoms, these movements should also be tested, with loading or no loading, as required.

Relative Isometric Muscle Strengths

- Abduction should be 50 to 70% of adduction
- Forward flexion should be 50 to 60% of adduction
- Medial rotation should be 45 to 50% of adduction
- Lateral rotation should be 65 to 70% of medial rotation
- Forward flexion should be 50 to 60% of extension
- Horizontal adduction should be 70 to 80% of horizontal abduction

---

Functional Assessment

The shoulder complex plays an integral role in the activities of daily living, sometimes acting as part of an open kinetic chain and sometimes acting as part of a closed kinetic chain. Assessment of function plays an important part of the shoulder assessment. Limitation of function can greatly affect the patient. For example, placing the hand behind the head (e.g., to comb the hair) requires full lateral rotation, whereas placing the hand in the small of the back (e.g., to get a wallet out of a back pocket or undo a bra) requires full medial rotation. Matsen and colleagues[11] have listed the functional ROM necessary to do some of the functional activities of daily living (Table 5–7).

The functional assessment may be based on activities of daily living, work, or recreation, because these activities are of most concern to the patient, or it may be based on numerical scoring charts (Figs. 5–23, 5–24, 5–25), which are derived from clinical measures as well

Text continued on page 197

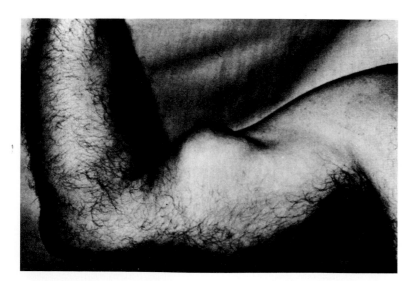

Figure 5–22

Rupture of the long head of the biceps brachii caused by the patient's awkward catch of partner in gymnastics. Bunching of muscle is attended by complete loss of function of the long head. (From O'Donoghue, D.H.: Treatment of Injuries to Athletes, 4th ed. Philadelphia, W.B. Saunders Co., 1984, p. 53.)

Athletic Shoulder Outcome Rating Scale

Name _____ Age _____ Sex _____

Dominant Hand (R) _____ (L) _____ (Ambidextrous) _____

Date of Examination _____ Position Played _____

Surgeon _____ Years Played _____

Type of Sport _____ Prior Injury _____

Activity Level

1) Professional (major league)
2) Professional (minor league)
3) College
4) High school
5) Recreational (full time)
6) Recreational (occasionally)

Diagnosis

1) Anterior instability
2) Posterior instability
3) Multidirectional instability
4) Recurrent dislocations
5) Impingement syndrome
6) Acromioclavicular separation
7) Acromioclavicular arthrosis
8) Rotator cuff repair (partial)
9) Rotator cuff tear (complete)
10) Biceps tendon rupture
11) Calcific tendinitis
12) Fracture

Subjective (90 Points)

I. Pain

	Points
No pain with competition	10
Pain after competing only	8
Pain while competing	6
Pain preventing competing	4
Pain with ADLs	2
Pain at rest	0

II. Strength/Endurance

No weakness, normal competition fatigue	10
Weakness after competition, early competition fatigue	8
Weakness during competition, abnormal competition fatigue	6
Weakness or fatigue preventing competition	4
Weakness or fatigue with ADLs	2
Weakness or fatigue preventing ADLs	0

III. Stability

No looseness during competition	10
Recurrent subluxations while competing	8
Dead-arm syndrome while competing	6
Recurrent subluxations prevent competition	4
Recurrent subluxations during ADLs	2
Dislocation	0

IV. Intensity

	Points
Preinjury versus postinjury hours of competition (100%)	10
Preinjury versus postinjury hours of competition (less than 75%)	8
Preinjury versus postinjury hours of competition (less than 50%)	6
Preinjury versus postinjury hours of competition (less than 25%)	4
Preinjury and postinjury hours of ADLs (100%)	2
Preinjury and postinjury hours of ADLs (less than 50%)	0

V. Performance

At the same level, same proficiency	50
At the same level, decreased proficiency	40
At the same level, decreased proficiency, not acceptable to athlete	30
Decreased level with acceptable proficiency at that level	20
Decreased level, unacceptable proficiency	10
Cannot compete, had to switch sport	0

Objective (10 Points)

Range of Motion

	Points
Normal external rotation at 90°–90° position; normal elevation	10
Less than 5° loss of external rotation; normal elevation	8
Less than 10° loss of external rotation; normal elevation	6
Less than 15° loss of external rotation; normal elevation	4
Less than 20° loss of external rotation; normal elevation	2
Greater than 20° loss of external rotation, or any loss of elevation	0

Overall Results

Excellent:	90–100 points
Good:	70–89 points
Fair:	50–69 points
Poor:	Less than 50 points

Figure 5–23

Athletic shoulder outcome rating scale. (From Tibone, J.E., and J.P. Bradley: Evaluation of treatment outcomes for the athlete's shoulder. *In* Matsen, F.A., F.H. Fu, and R.J. Hawkins [eds.]: The Shoulder: A Balance of Mobility and Stability. Rosemont, Illinois, American Academy of Orthopedic Surgeons, 1993, pp. 526–527.)

Table 5-7

Range of Motion Necessary at the Shoulder to Do Certain Activities of Daily Living

Activity	Range of Motion	Activity	Range of Motion
Eating	70–100° horizontal adduction* 45–60° abduction	Hand behind head	10–15° horizontal adduction* 110–125° forward flexion 90° lateral rotation
Combing hair	30–70° horizontal adduction* 105–120° abduction 90° lateral rotation	Put something on shelf	70–80° horizontal adduction* 70–80° forward flexion 45° lateral rotation
Reach perineum	75–90° horizontal abduction 30–45° abduction 90°+ medial rotation	Wash opposite shoulder	60–90° forward flexion 60–120° horizontal adduction*
Tuck in shirt	50–60° horizontal abduction 55–65° abduction 90° medial rotation		

* Horizontal adduction is from 0 to 90° of abduction.

Adapted from Matsen, F.A., S.B. Lippitt, J.A. Sidles, and D.T. Harryman: Practical Evaluation and Management of the Shoulder. Philadelphia, W.B. Saunders Co., 1994, pp. 20, 24.

Walch-Duplay Rating Sheet for Anterior Instability of the Shoulder

Family Name: _____ First name: _____ Date: _____

Sport

(1) Type of Sport Practiced

C = competition
L = leisure (spare time)
N = not practicing a sport

(2) Type of Sport

0 = no sport

1 = risk free   athletics, rowing, fencing, swimming, breaststroke, underwater diving, voluntary gymnastics, cross-country skiing, shooting, sailing.

2 = with contact   martial arts, cycling, motorcycling or biking, scrambling, soccer, rugby, waterskiing, downhill skiing, parachute jumping, horse riding.

3 = with cocking of the arm   climbing, weight lifting, shot-putting, swimming overarm and butterfly, pole vaulting, figure skating, canoeing, golf, hockey, tennis, baseball.

4 = with blocked cocking or "high risk"   basketball, handball, volleyball, hang gliding, kayaking, water polo, javelin throwing, judo, karate, wrestling, sky diving, wind surfing, diving, ice hockey, acrobatics, gymnastics (floor, using apparatus).

(3) Side

D = dominant
d = nondominant

(4) Functional Score of the Shoulder (100 points) with respect to

resuming sport	25 points
stability	25 points
pain	25 points
mobility	25 points

Figure 5-24

Walch-Duplay rating sheet for anterior instability of the shoulder. (From Walch, G.: Directions for the use of the quotation of anterior instabilities of the shoulder. Abstracts of the First Open Congress of the European Society of Surgery of the Shoulder and Elbow. Paris, 1987, pp. 51–55.)

Walch-Duplay Rating Sheet for Anterior Instability of the Shoulder (*Continued*)

Daily Activity

Return to the same level in the same sport * No discomfort	+25 points
Decrease of level in the same sport practiced * Slight discomfort in forceful movements	+15 points
Change in sport * Slight discomfort during simple movements	+10 points
Decrease of level and change, or stop sport * Severe discomfort	0 points

Stability

No apprehension	+25 points
Persistent apprehension	+15 points
Feeling of instability	0 points
True recurrence	−25 points

Pain

No pain or pain during certain climatic conditions	+25 points
Pain during forceful movements or when tired	+15 points
Pain during daily life	0 points

Mobility

Pure frontal abduction against a wall: symmetric Internal rotation (IR) limited to less than three vertebrae External rotation (ER) at 90° abduction limited to less than 10% of the opposite side	+25 points
Pure frontal abduction against a wall <150° IR: limited to less than three vertebrae ER: limited to less than 30% of the opposite side	+15 points
Pure frontal abduction against a wall <120° IR: limited to less than six vertebrae ER: limited to less than 50% of the opposite side	+5 points
Pure frontal abduction against a wall <90° IR: limited to more than six vertebrae ER: limited to more than 50% of the opposite side	0 points

Total points _____

Overall Functional Result

Excellent:	**91 to 100 points**
Good:	**76 to 90 points**
Medium:	**51 to 75 points**
Poor:	**50 points or less**

* Criterion if the patient did not participate in sports before the operation

Figure 5–24 *Continued*

as functional measures. Some numerical evaluation scales are designed for specific populations, such as athletes (see Fig. 5–23), or specific injuries, such as anterior instability (see Fig. 5–24). Other shoulder rating scales are also available.[33–37] When using numerical scoring charts, the examiner should not place too much reliance on the form, because most of these charts are based primarily on the examiner's clinical measures and not the patient's subjective functional, hoped-for outcome, which is the primary concern of the patient. Proba-

American Shoulder and Elbow Surgeons' Shoulder Evaluation Form

Name _____ Hosp # _____ Date _____ Shoulder: R / L

I. Pain: (5 = none, 4 = slight, 3 = after unusual activity, 2 = moderate, 1 = marked, 0 = complete disability, NA = not available) _____

II. Motion:

A. Patient Sitting
1. Active total elevation of arm: _____ degrees*
2. Passive internal rotation:
   (Circle segment of posterior anatomy reached by thumb)
   (Note if reach restricted by limited elbow flexion)

1 = Less than trochanter	5 = L5	9 = L1	13 = T9	17 = T5
2 = Trochanter	6 = L4	10 = T12	14 = T8	18 = T4
3 = Gluteal	7 = L3	11 = T11	15 = T7	19 = T3
4 = Sacrum	8 = L2	12 = T10	16 = T6	20 = T2
				21 = T1

3. Active external rotation with arm at side: _____ degrees

4. Active external rotation at 90° abduction: _____ degrees
   (Enter "NA" if cannot achieve 90° of abduction)

B. Patient Supine

1. Passive total elevation of arm: _____ degrees*

2. Passive external rotation with arm at side: _____ degrees

* Total elevation of arm measured by viewing patient from side and using goniometer to determine angle between *arm* and *thorax.*

III. Strength: (5 = normal, 4 = good, 3 = fair, 2 = poor, 1 = trace, 0 = paralysis)

A. Anterior deltoid _____   C. External rotation _____

B. Middle deltoid _____   D. Internal rotation _____

IV. Stability: (5 = normal, 4 = apprehension, 3 = rare subluxation, 2 = recurrent subluxation, 1 = recurrent dislocation, 0 = fixed dislocation, NA = not available)

A. Anterior _____   B. Posterior _____   C. Inferior _____

V. Function: (4 = normal, 3 = mild compromise, 2 = difficulty, 1 = with aid, 0 = unable, NA = not available)

A. Use back pocket	_____	I. Sleep on affected side	_____
B. Perineal care	_____	J. Pulling	_____
C. Wash opposite axilla	_____	K. Use hand overhead	_____
D. Eat with utensil	_____	L. Throwing	_____
E. Comb hair	_____	M. Lifting	_____
F. Use hand with arm at shoulder level	_____	N. Do usual work (specify _____)	_____
G. Carry 10–15 lb with arm at side	_____	O. Do usual sport (specify _____)	_____
H. Dress	_____		

VI. Patient Response: (3 = much better, 2 = better, 1 = same, 0 = worse, NA = not available/applicable) _____

Figure 5–25

American Shoulder and Elbow Surgeons' shoulder evaluation form. (Courtesy of the American Shoulder and Elbow Surgeons.)

Name: _____ Date: __/__/__ Age: _____
     Last   First   M.I.

Address: _____ Occupation: _____
     Street/Apt #   City   State Zip Code

Phone: (___) ___ - _____   (___) ___ - _____   (___) ___ - _____
        Home   Business   Relative

Circle one	Circle one
Dominant Hand: Right / Left / Ambidextrous	Shoulder Evaluated: Right / Left

Answer Each Question Below by Checking "Yes" or "No"   **Response**

Yes No

1. Is your shoulder comfortable with your arm at rest by your side?   ☐ ☐ 1

2. Does your shoulder allow you to sleep comfortably?   ☐ ☐ 2

3. Can you reach the small of your back to tuck in your shirt with your hand?   ☐ ☐ 3

4. Can you place your hand behind your head with the elbow straight out to the side? ☐ ☐ 4

5. Can you place a coin on a shelf at the level of your shoulder without bending your elbow? ☐ ☐ 5

6. Can you lift one pound (a full pint container) to the level of your shoulder without bending your elbow? ☐ ☐ 6

7. Can you lift eight pounds (a full gallon container) to the level of your shoulder without bending your elbow? ☐ ☐ 7

8. Can you carry twenty pounds at your side with the affected extremity?   ☐ ☐ 8

9. Do you think you can toss a softball underhand ten yards with the affected extremity? ☐ ☐ 9

10. Do you think you can toss a softball overhand twenty yards with the affected extremity? ☐ ☐ 10

11. Can you wash the back of your opposite shoulder with the affected extremity?   ☐ ☐ 11

12. Would your shoulder allow you to work full-time at your regular job?   ☐ ☐ 12

Office Use Only

Diagnosis: DJD RA AVN IMP RCT FS TUBS AMBRII Other: _____

Dx Confirmed? _____ Pt# _____ Physician _____

SST: Initial / Pre-op / Follow-up: 6 mon 1 yr 18 mon 2 yr 3 yr 4 yr 5 yr Other: _____

Initial SST Date: ___/___/___ Rx: _____ Surgery Date: ___/___/___

Figure 5–26
Simple shoulder test questionnaire form. (From Lippitt, S.B., D.T. Harryman, and F.A. Matsen: A
practical tool for evaluating function: The simple shoulder test. *In* Matsen, F.A., F.H. Fu, and R.J.
Hawkins [eds.]: The Shoulder: A Balance of Mobility and Stability. Rosemont, Illinois, American
Academy of Orthopedic Surgeons, 1993, p. 514.)

bly the most functional numerical shoulder test from a patient's perspective is the **simple shoulder test** (Fig. 5–26) developed by Lippitt and associates.[11, 38] Table 5–8 provides the examiner with a method of determining the patient's functional shoulder strength and endurance. This table is based on the general population and would not indicate a true functional reading of athletes or persons who do heavy work involving the shoulders.

Table 5-8
Functional Testing of the Shoulder

Starting Position	Action	Functional Test*
Sitting	Forward flex arm to 90°	Lift 4 to 5 lb weight: Functional Lift 1 to 3 lb weight: Functionally fair Lift arm weight: Functionally poor Cannot lift arm: Nonfunctional
Sitting	Shoulder extension	Lift 4 to 5 lb weight: Functional Lift 1 to 3 lb weight: Functionally fair Lift arm weight: Functionally poor Cannot lift arm: Nonfunctional
Side lying (may be done in sitting with pulley)	Shoulder medial rotation	Lift 4 to 5 lb weight: Functional Lift 1 to 3 lb weight: Functionally fair Lift arm weight: Functionally poor Cannot lift arm: Nonfunctional
Side lying (may be done in sitting with pulley)	Shoulder lateral rotation	Lift 4 to 5 lb weight: Functional Lift 1 to 3 lb weight: Functionally fair Lift arm weight: Functionally poor Cannot lift arm: Nonfunctional
Sitting	Shoulder abduction	Lift 4 to 5 lb weight: Functional Lift 1 to 3 lb weight: Functionally fair Lift arm weight: Functionally poor Cannot lift arm: Nonfunctional
Sitting	Shoulder adduction (using wall pulley)	Lift 4 to 5 lb weight: Functional Lift 1 to 3 lb weight: Functionally fair Lift arm weight: Functionally poor Cannot lift arm: Nonfunctional
Sitting	Shoulder elevation (shoulder shrug)	5 to 6 Repetitions: Functional 3 to 4 Repetitions: Functionally fair 1 to 2 Repetitions: Functionally poor 0 Repetitions: Nonfunctional
Sitting	Sitting push-up (shoulder dysfunction)	5 to 6 Repetitions: Functional 3 to 4 Repetitions: Functionally fair 1 to 2 Repetitions: Functionally poor 0 Repetitions: Nonfunctional

* Younger, more fit patients should easily be able to do more than the values given for these tests. A comparison between the good side and the injured side gives the examiner some idea about the patient's functional strength capacity.

Data from Palmer, M.L., and M. Epler: Clinical Assessment Procedures in Physical Therapy. Philadelphia, J.B. Lippincott, 1990, pp. 68–73.

Special Tests

In the examination of the shoulder, special tests are often done to confirm findings or a tentative diagnosis. The examiner must be proficient in those tests that he or she decides to use. Proficiency increases the reliability of the findings. Depending on the history, some tests are compulsory, and others may be used as confirming or excluding tests. If the history indicates instability, then at least one test each for anterior, posterior, and multidirectional instability should be performed. Also, because of the interrelation of impingement and instability, tests for both should be applied if the history indicates that either condition may be present.[39] Jobe and colleagues[40] believed that impingement and instability often went together in throwing athletes and, based on that assumption, developed the following classification:

Grade I: Pure impingement (often seen in older patients)

Grade II: Secondary impingement and instability caused by capsular and labral trauma

Grade III: Secondary impingement and instability caused by hypermobility

Grade IV: Primary instability

It is important when looking at shoulder instability to differentiate between gross laxity or hypermobility, seen with the TUBS lesion, and instability (excessive translation), seen with AMBRI lesions[11] (Table 5–9). With the instability tests, the examiner is trying to duplicate the patient's symptoms as well as feel for abnormal movement. Therefore, a response of "That's what my shoulder feels like when it bothers me" is much more significant than the degree of laxity or translation found.[11]

Table 5–9
Differential Diagnosis of Shoulder Instability (AMBRI) Versus Traumatic Anterior Dislocation (TUBS)

	Shoulder Instability	Traumatic Anterior Dislocation
History	Feeling of shoulder slippage with pain Feeling of insecurity when doing specific activities No history of injury	Arm elevated and laterally rotated relative to body Feeling of insecurity when in specific position (of dislocation) Recurrent episodes of apprehension
Observation	Normal	Normal (if reduced) (if not, loss of rounding of deltoid caused by anterior dislocation)
Active movement	Normal ROM May be abnormal or painful at activity speed	Apprehension and decreased ROM in abduction and lateral rotation
Passive movement	Normal ROM Pain at extreme of ROM possible	Muscle guarding and decreased ROM in apprehension position
Resisted isometric movement	Normal in test position May be weak in provocative position	Pain into abduction and lateral rotation
Special tests	Load and shift test is positive	Apprehension positive Augmentation positive Relocation positive
Reflexes and cutaneous distribution	Normal reflexes and sensation	Reflexes normal Sensation normal, unless axillary or musculocutaneous nerve is injured
Palpation	Normal	Anterior shoulder is tender
Diagnostic imaging	Normal	Normal, unless still dislocated; defect possible

ROM = range of motion.

Special Tests Commonly Performed on the Shoulder

Instability, anterior:	Load and shift test Crank (apprehension) and relocation tests
Instability, posterior:	Load and shift test Posterior apprehension test
Instability, inferior:	Sulcus sign
Labral lesions:	Clunk test Anterior slide test
Scapular stability tests:	Lateral scapular slide tests
Muscle tendon pathology:	Speed's test Yergason's test Empty can test Lift-off sign
Impingement tests:	Neer test Hawkins-Kennedy test
Neurological involvement:	Upper limb tension test
Thoracic outlet syndromes:	Roos test (EAST)

Tests for Anterior Shoulder Instability

Load and Shift Test.[21, 41] The patient sits with no back support and with the hand of the test arm resting on the thigh. The examiner stands or sits slightly behind the patient and stabilizes the shoulder with one hand over the clavicle and scapula (Fig. 5–27A). With the other hand, the examiner grasps the head of the humerus with the thumb over the posterior humeral head and the fingers over the anterior humeral head (Fig. 5–27B). The humerus is then gently pushed into the glenoid to seat it properly in the glenoid fossa. This is the "load" portion of the test, and this "seating" of the humerus allows true translation to occur. If the load is not applied (anterior drawer test), movement will be greater and the "feel" will be altered. The examiner then pushes the humeral head anteriorly (anterior instability) or posteriorly (posterior instability), noting the amount of translation. This is the "shift" portion of the test.

Translation of 25% of the humeral head diameter or less anteriorly is considered normal. Hawkins and Mohtadi[41] advocate a three-grade system for anterior translation (Fig. 5–28). Normally, the head translates 0 to 25% of the diameter of the humeral head. Up to 50% of humeral head translation, with the head riding up to the glenoid rim and spontaneous reduction, is considered grade I. For grade II, the humeral head has more

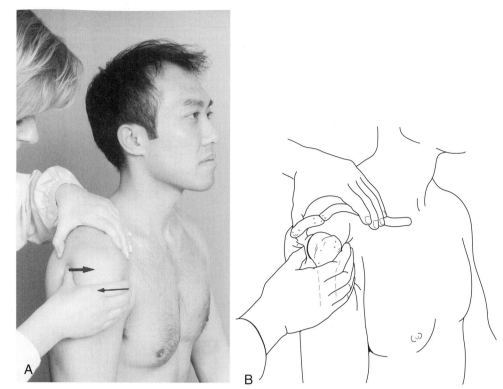

Figure 5–27

(A) Load and shift test. Anterior shift shown. (B) Line drawing showing position of examiner's hands in relation to bones of patient's shoulder. Notice that examiner's left thumb holds the spine of the scapula for stability.

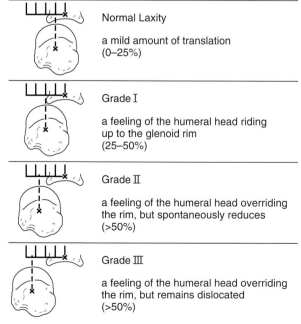

Figure 5–28

Grades of anterior glenohumeral translation.

than 50% translation; the head feels as though it is riding over the glenoid rim but spontaneously reduces. Grade III implies that the humeral head rides over the glenoid rim and does not spontaneously reduce. For posterior translation, translation of 50% of the diameter of the humeral head is considered normal. Thus, normally, one would expect greater posterior translation than anterior translation when doing the test. Differences between affected and normal sides should be compared in terms of the amount of translation and the ease with which it occurs. This comparison, along with reproduction of the patient's symptoms, is often considered more important than the amount of movement obtained. If the patient has multidirectional instability, both anterior and posterior translation may be excessive on the affected side compared with the normal side. The test may also be done with the patient in supine lying position.

Apprehension (Crank) Test for Anterior Shoulder Dislocation. The examiner abducts the arm to 90° and laterally rotates the patient's shoulder slowly (Fig. 5–29). A positive test is indicated by a look or feeling of apprehension

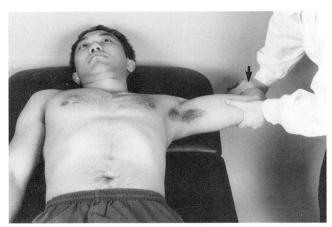

Figure 5–29
Anterior apprehension (crank) test.

apprehension, the pain decreases, and further lateral rotation is possible before the apprehension returns (Fig. 5–30). This relocation is sometimes referred to as the **Fowler sign** or **Fowler test** or the **Jobe relocation test**. The test is considered positive if pain decreases during the maneuver, even if there was no apprehension.[41] If the arm is released (**release test**) in the newly acquired range, pain and forward translation of the head are noted in positive tests.[39] The resulting pain from this release procedure may be caused by anterior shoulder instability, labral lesion (Bankart lesion or SLAP lesion—superior labrum, anterior posterior), or bicipital tendinitis. It has also been reported to cause pain in older patients with rotator cuff pathology and no instability.[43] This release maneuver should be done with care because it often causes apprehension and distrust on the part of the patient and it could cause a dislocation, especially in patients who have had recurrent dislocations. For most patients, therefore, lateral rotation should be released before the posterior stress is released.

or alarm on the patient's face and the patient's resistance to further motion. The patient may also state that the feeling experienced is what it felt like when the shoulder was previously dislocated. It is imperative that this test be done slowly. If the test is done too quickly, the humerus may become dislocated. Hawkins and Bokor[42] noted that the examiner should observe the amount of lateral rotation that exists when the patient becomes apprehensive. If the examiner then applies a posterior stress to the arm (**relocation test**), the patient loses the

The crank test may be modified to test lateral rotation at different degrees of abduction, depending on the history and mechanism of injury. The Rockwood test described next is simply a modification of the crank test.

Rockwood Test for Anterior Instability.[44] The examiner stands behind the seated patient. With the arm at the patient's side, the examiner laterally rotates the shoul-

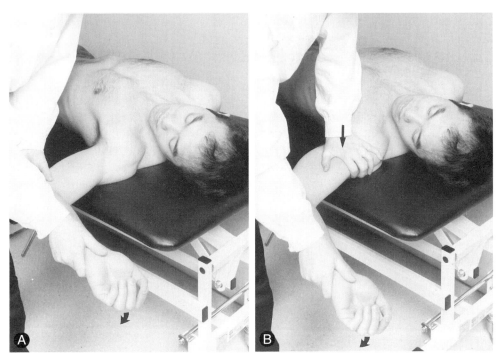

Figure 5–30
Relocation test. (A) Abduction and lateral rotation (crank test). (B) Abduction and lateral rotation combined with posterior translation of the humerus (relocation test).

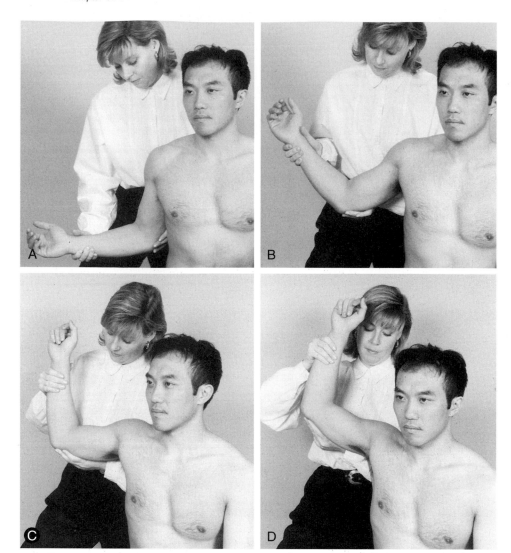

Figure 5–31
Rockwood test for anterior instability. (A) Arm at side. (B) Arm at 45°. (C) Arm at 90°. (D) Arm at 120°.

der. The arm is abducted to 45°, and passive lateral rotation is repeated. The same procedure is repeated at 90° and 120° (Fig. 5–31). These different positions are performed because the stabilizers of the shoulder vary as the angle of abduction changes. For the test to be positive, the patient must show marked apprehension with posterior pain when the arm is tested at 90°. At 45° and 120°, the patient shows some uneasiness and some pain; at 0°, there is rarely apprehension.

Similarly, the Rowe and fulcrum tests stress the anterior shoulder structures. They are more likely to bring on apprehension sooner, because they stress the anterior structures sooner (i.e., the head of the humerus is pushed forward). In effect, they are the opposite to the relocation test; they are therefore called **augmentation tests**.

Rowe Test for Anterior Instability.[45] The patient lies supine and places the hand behind the head. The examiner places one hand (clenched fist) against the posterior humeral head and pushes up while extending the arm slightly (Fig. 5–32). A look of apprehension or pain is indicative of a positive test for anterior instability.

Fulcrum Test.[46] The patient lies supine with the arm abducted to 90°. The examiner places one hand under the glenohumeral joint to act as a fulcrum. The examiner then extends and laterally rotates the arm gently over the fulcrum (Fig. 5–33). A positive test for anterior instability is a look of apprehension by the patient.

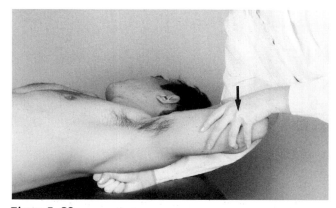

Figure 5–32
Rowe test for anterior instability.

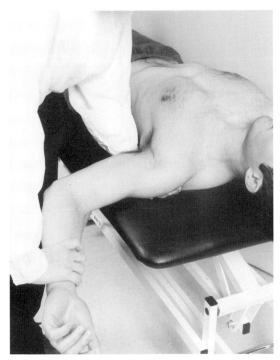

Figure 5–33
Fulcrum test.

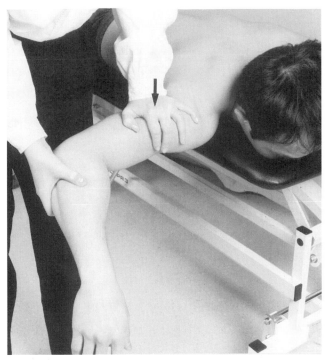

Figure 5–34
Prone anterior instability test. Examiner stabilizes the arm in 90° abduction and lateral rotation and then pushes anteriorly on the humerus.

The following anterior instability tests are modifications of the anterior load and shift test in that they are designed to cause anterior translation of the head of the humerus in the glenoid. As with the load and shift test, the examiner can determine or grade the amount of anterior translation. Therefore, these tests can be used as substitutes for the load and shift test.

Prone Anterior Instability Test.[47] The patient lies prone. The examiner abducts the patient's arm to 90° and laterally rotates it 90°. While holding this position with one hand at the elbow, the examiner places the other hand over the humeral head and pushes it forward (Fig. 5–34). A positive test for anterior instability is indicated by reproduction of the patient's symptoms.

Andrews' Anterior Instability Test.[47] The patient lies supine with the shoulder abducted 130° and laterally rotated 90°. The examiner stabilizes the elbow and distal humerus with one hand and uses the other hand to grasp the humeral head and lift it forward (Fig. 5–35). Reproduction of the patient's symptoms gives a positive test for anterior instability. If an anterior labral tear is present, a clunk may be heard.

Anterior Drawer Test of the Shoulder.[48] The patient lies supine. The examiner places the hand of the affected shoulder in the examiner's axilla, holding the patient's hand with the arm so that the patient remains relaxed. The shoulder to be tested is abducted between 80° and 120°, forward flexed up to 20°, and laterally rotated up to 30°. The examiner then stabilizes the patient's scapula with the opposite hand, pushing the spine of the scapula

forward with the index and middle fingers. The examiner's thumb exerts counterpressure on the patient's coracoid process. Using the arm that is holding the patient's hand, the examiner places his or her hand around the patient's relaxed upper arm and draws the humerus forward. The movement may be accompanied by a click or by patient apprehension or both. The amount of movement available is compared with that of the normal side. A positive test is indicative of anterior instability (Fig. 5–36), depending on the amount of anterior translation. The click may indicate a labral tear or slippage of the humeral head over the glenoid rim.

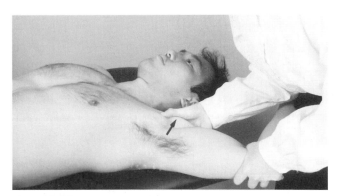

Figure 5–35
Andrews' anterior instability test.

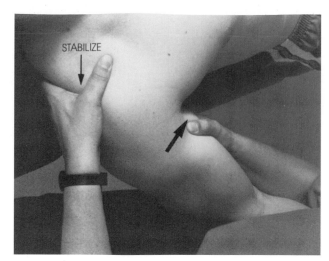

Figure 5–36
Anterior drawer test of the shoulder.

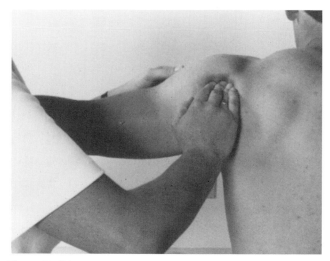

Figure 5–37
Protzman test for anterior instability (posterior view).

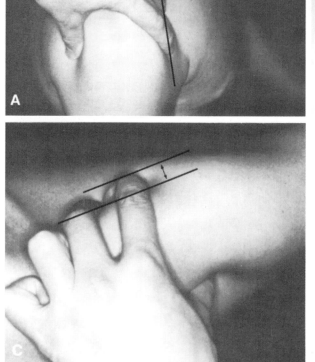

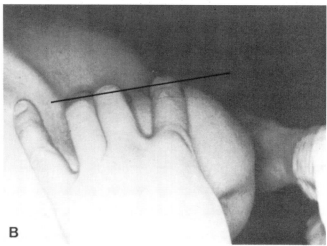

Figure 5–38
Anterior instability test. (A) Side view and (B) superior view. With the patient's arm by the side, the examiner's fingers are in the same plane. (C) With a positive test, on abduction and lateral rotation, the index and middle fingers are no longer in the same plane. (Adapted from Leffert, R.D., and G. Gumbery: The relationship between dead arm syndrome and thoracic outlet syndrome. Clin. Orthop. 223:22–23, 1987.)

Protzman Test for Anterior Instability.[49] The patient is sitting. The examiner abducts the patient's arm to 90° and supports the arm against the examiner's hip so that the patient's shoulder muscles are relaxed. The examiner palpates the anterior aspect of the head of the humerus with the fingers of one hand deep in the patient's axilla while the fingers of the other hand are placed over the posterior aspect of the humeral head. The examiner then pushes the humeral head anteriorly and inferiorly (Fig. 5–37). If this movement causes pain and if palpation indicates abnormal anteroinferior movement, the test is positive for anterior instability. Normally, anterior translation should be no more than 25% of the diameter of the humeral head.[50] A click may sometimes be palpated as the humeral head slides over the glenoid rim. The test may also be done with the patient in the supine lying position with the elbow supported on a pillow.

Anterior Instability Test.[51] The examiner stands behind the shoulder being examined while the patient sits. The examiner places his or her near hand over the shoulder so that the index finger is over the head of the humerus anteriorly and the middle finger is over the coracoid process. The thumb is placed over the posterior humeral head. The examiner's other hand grasps the patient's wrist and carefully abducts and laterally rotates the arm (Fig. 5–38). If, on movement of the arm, the finger palpating the anterior humeral head moves forward, the test is said to be positive for anterior instability. Normally, the two fingers remain in the same plane. With a positive test, when the arm is returned to the starting position, the index finger returns to the starting position as the humeral head glides backward.

Dugas' Test.[52] This test is used if an unreduced anterior shoulder dislocation is suspected. The patient is asked to place the hand on the opposite shoulder and then attempt to lower the elbow to the chest. With an anterior dislocation, this is not possible, and pain in the shoulder results. If the pain is only over the acromioclavicular joint, problems in that joint should be suspected.

Tests for Posterior Shoulder Instability

Load and Shift Test. This test is described under anterior shoulder instability.

Posterior Apprehension or Stress Test.[53] The examiner forward flexes the patient's shoulder in the plane of the scapula to 90° (Fig. 5–39). The examiner then applies a posterior force on the patient's elbow. While applying the axial load, the examiner horizontally adducts and medially rotates the arm. A positive result is indicated by a look of apprehension or alarm on the patient's face and the patient's resistance to further motion or the reproduction of the patient's symptoms. Pagnani and Warren[54] reported that pain production is more likely than apprehension in a positive test. They reported that

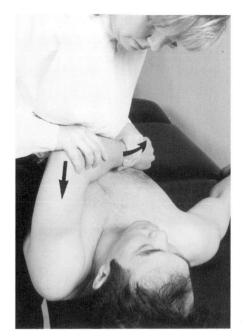

Figure 5–39
Posterior apprehension test.

with atraumatic multidirectional (inferior) instability, the test is negative. If the test is done with the patient in the sitting position, the scapula must be stabilized. The test is indicative of a posterior instability or dislocation of the humerus. The test should also be performed with the arm in 90° of abduction. The examiner palpates the head of the humerus with one hand while the other hand pushes the head of the humerus posteriorly. In either case, if the humeral head moves posteriorly more than 50% of its diameter (Fig. 5–40), posterior instability is evident.[50] The movement may be accompanied by a clunk as the humeral head passes over the glenoid rim.

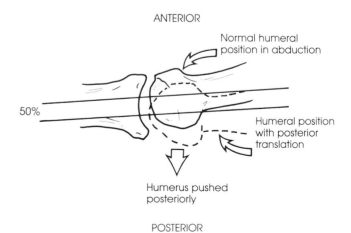

Figure 5–40
The posterior stress examination should normally produce no translation beyond 50% of the diameter of the humeral head in the glenoid.

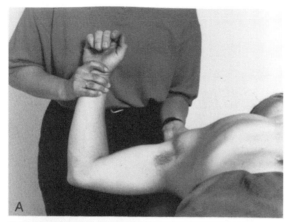

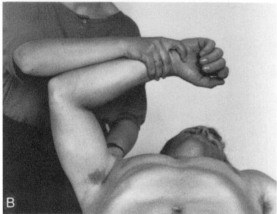

Figure 5–41

Norwood stress test for posterior shoulder instability. (A) Arm abducted 90°. (B) Arm forward flexed.

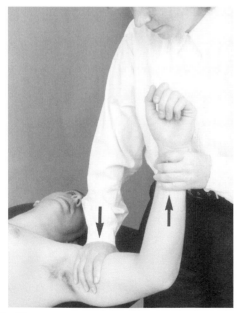

Figure 5–42

Push-pull test.

Norwood Stress Test for Posterior Instability.[55] The patient lies supine with the shoulder abducted 60 to 100° and laterally rotated 90° and with the elbow flexed to 90° so that the arm is horizontal. The examiner stabilizes the scapula with one hand, palpating the posterior humeral head with the fingers, and stabilizes the upper limb by holding the forearm and elbow at the elbow. The examiner then brings the arm into forward flexion (Fig. 5–41). Cofield and Irving[56] recommend medially rotating the forearm approximately 20° after the forward flexion, then pushing the elbow posteriorly to enhance the effect of the test. A positive test is indicated by the humeral head's slipping posteriorly relative to the glenoid. Care must be taken because the test does not cause apprehension but may cause subluxation or dislocation. The patient confirms that the sensation felt is the same as that felt during activities. The arm is returned to the starting position, and the humeral head is felt to reduce. A clicking caused by the passage of the head over the glenoid rim may accompany either subluxation or reduction.

Push-Pull Test.[46] The patient lies supine. The examiner holds the patient's arm at the wrist, abducts the arm 90°, and forward flexes it 30°. The examiner places the other hand over the humerus close to the humeral head. The examiner then pulls up on the arm at the wrist while pushing down on the humerus with the other hand (Fig. 5–42). Normally, 50% posterior translation can be accomplished. If more than 50% posterior translation occurs or if the patient becomes apprehensive or pain results, the examiner should suspect posterior instability.

Posterior Drawer Test of the Shoulder.[48] The patient lies supine. The examiner stands at the level of the shoulder and grasps the patient's proximal forearm with one hand, flexing the patient's elbow to 120° and the shoulder to between 80° and 120° of abduction and between 20° and 30° of forward flexion. With the other hand, the examiner stabilizes the scapula by placing the index and middle fingers on the spine of the scapula and the thumb on the coracoid process. The examiner then rotates the forearm medially and forward flexes the shoulder to between 60° and 80° while at the same time taking the thumb of the other hand off the coracoid process and pushing the head of the humerus posteriorly. The head of the humerus can be felt by the index finger of the same hand (Fig. 5–43). The test is usually pain free, but the patient may exhibit apprehension. A positive test is indicative of posterior instability and demonstrates significant posterior translation (>50% humeral head diameter).

Jerk Test.[46] The patient sits with the arm medially rotated and forward flexed to 90°. The examiner grasps the patient's elbow and axially loads the humerus in a proximal direction. While maintaining the axial loading, the examiner moves the arm horizontally (cross-flexion)

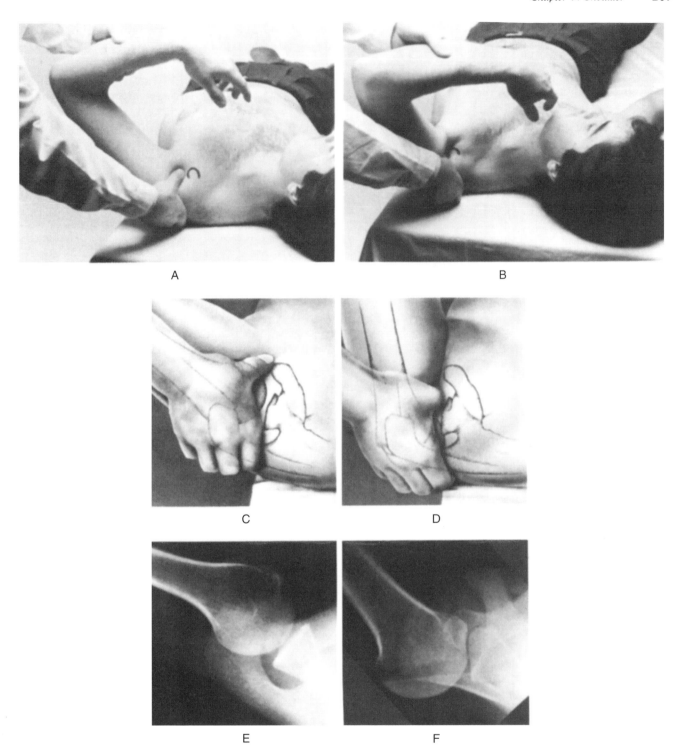

Figure 5–43

Posterior drawer test of the shoulder. (A) and (B) The test. (C) and (D) Superimposed view of bones involved in test. (E) and (F) Radiographic images of test. (From Gerber, C., and R. Ganz: Clinical assessment of instability of the shoulder. J. Bone Joint Surg. Br. 66:554, 1984.)

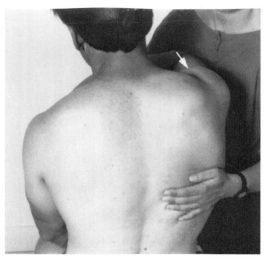

Figure 5–44
Jerk test.

across the body (Fig. 5–44). A positive test for recurrent posterior instability is the production of a sudden jerk or clunk as the humeral head slides off (subluxes) the back of the glenoid (Fig. 5–45). When the arm is returned

to the original 90° abduction position, a second jerk may be felt as the head reduces.

Tests for Inferior and Multidirectional Shoulder Instability

It is believed that if a patient demonstrates inferior instability, multidirectional instability is also present. Therefore, the patient with inferior instability will also demonstrate anterior and/or posterior instability.

Test for Inferior Shoulder Instability (Sulcus Sign).[46, 48] The patient stands with the arm by the side and shoulder muscles relaxed. The examiner grasps the patient's forearm below the elbow and pulls the arm distally (Fig. 5–46). The presence of a **sulcus sign** (Fig. 5–47; see Fig. 5–7B) is indicative of inferior instability. The sulcus sign may be graded by measuring from the inferior margin of the acromion to the humeral head. A +1 sulcus implies a distance of less than 1 cm; +2 sulcus, 1 to 2 cm; and +3 sulcus, more than 2 cm.

It has been reported that the best position to test for inferior instability is at 20 to 50° of abduction with neutral rotation. Thus, more than one position should

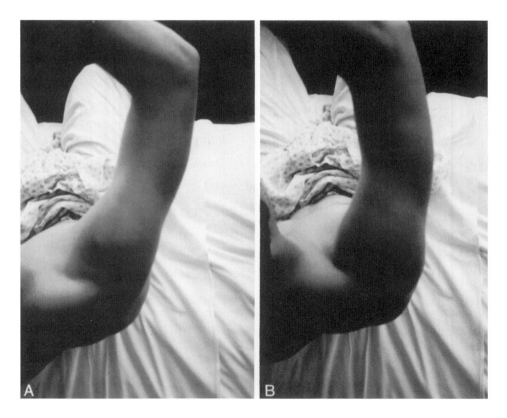

Figure 5–45
Positive jerk test. (A) Normal appearance of the shoulder before the patient performs a jerk test. (B) With axial loading and movement of the arm horizontally across the body, the humeral head slides off the back of the glenoid, as demonstrated by the prominence in the anterior aspect of the patient's shoulder. This maneuver resulted in a sudden jerk and some discomfort. (From Matsen, F.A., S.C. Thomas, and C.A. Rockwood: Glenohumeral instability. In Rockwood, C.A., and F.A. Matsen [eds.]: The Shoulder. Philadelphia, W.B. Saunders Co., 1990, p. 551.)

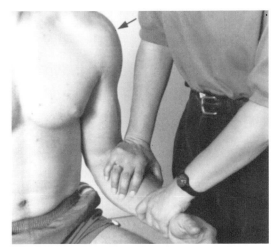

Figure 5–46

Test for inferior shoulder instability (sulcus test). Arrow indicates where to look for sulcus, which is not evident in this patient.

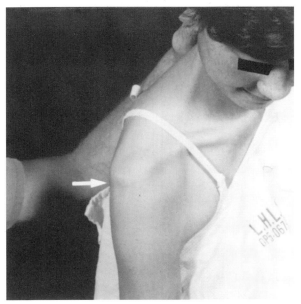

Figure 5–47

Positive suclus sign. (Adapted from Hawkins, R.J., and D.J. Boker: Clinical evaluations of shoulder problems. In Rockwood, C.A., and R.A. Matsen [eds.]: The Shoulder. Philadelphia, W.B. Saunders Co., 1990, p. 169.)

be tested.[13, 54, 57] Depending on the history, the examiner should test the patient in the position in which the sensation of instability is reported.

Feagin Test.[44] The Feagin test is a modification of the sulcus sign test with the arm abducted to 90° instead of being at the side. The patient stands with the arm abducted to 90° and the elbow extended and resting on the top of the examiner's shoulder. The examiner's hands are clasped together over the patient's humerus, between the upper and middle thirds. The examiner pushes the humerus down and forward (Fig. 5–48). A look of apprehension on the patient's face indicates a positive test

and the presence of anteroinferior instability (Fig. 5–49). This test position also places more stress on the inferior glenohumeral ligament.

Rowe Test for Multidirectional Instability.[45] The patient stands forward flexed 45° at the waist with the arms relaxed and pointing at the floor. The examiner places one hand over the shoulder so that the index and middle fingers sit over the anterior aspect of the humeral head and the thumb sits over the posterior aspect of the hu-

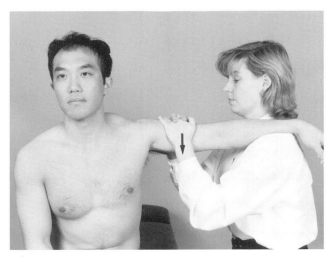

Figure 5–48

Feagin test.

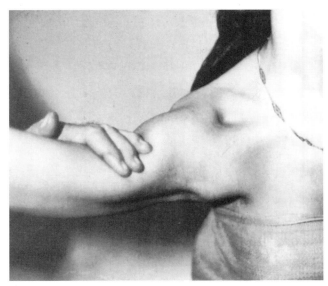

Figure 5–49

A 21-year-old woman whose shoulder could be dislocated inferiorly and anteriorly and subluxated posteriorly. She was unable to carry books, reach overhead, or use the arm for activities such as tennis or swimming. There were associated episodes of numbness and weakness of the entire upper extremity that at times lasted for 1 or 2 days. (Neer, C.S., and C.R. Foster: Inferior capsular shift for involuntary inferior and multidirectional instability of the shoulder. J. Bone Joint Surg. Am. 62:900, 1980.)

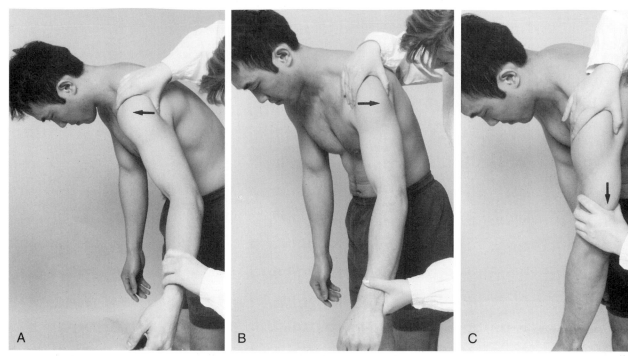

Figure 5–50
Rowe test for multidirectional instability. (A) Testing for anterior instability. (B) Testing for posterior instability. (C) Testing for inferior instability.

meral head. The examiner then pulls the arm down slightly (Fig. 5–50). To test for anterior instability, the humeral head is pushed anteriorly with the thumb while the arm is extended 20 to 30° from the vertical position. To test for posterior instability, the humeral head is pushed posteriorly with the index and middle fingers while the arm is flexed 20 to 30° from the vertical position. For inferior instability, more traction is applied to the arm, and the sulcus sign is evident.

Tests for Labral Tears

Injuries to the labrum are relatively common, especially in throwing athletes. The tear may be a Bankart lesion, in which the anteroinferior labrum is torn, or the superior labrum may have been injured, causing a **SLAP lesion** (superior labrum, anterior and posterior). Snyder and colleagues[58] have divided these SLAP lesions into four types:

Type I: Superior labrum markedly frayed but attachments intact
Type II: Superior labrum has small tear and there is instability of the labral-biceps complex (most common)
Type III: Bucket-handle tear of labrum that may displace into joint; labral biceps attachment intact
Type IV: Bucket-handle tear of labrum that extends to biceps tendon, allowing tendon to sublux into joint

Clunk Test. The patient lies supine. The examiner places one hand on the posterior aspect of the shoulder over the humeral head. The examiner's other hand holds the humerus above the elbow. The examiner fully abducts the arm over the patient's head. The examiner then pushes anteriorly with the hand over the humeral head while the other hand rotates the humerus into lateral rotation (Fig. 5–51). A clunk or grinding sound indicates a positive test and is indicative of a tear of the labrum.[59] The test may also cause apprehension if anterior instability is present. Walsh[60] indicated that if the examiner

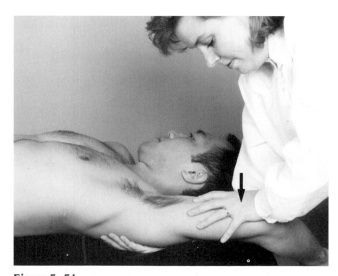

Figure 5–51
Clunk test.

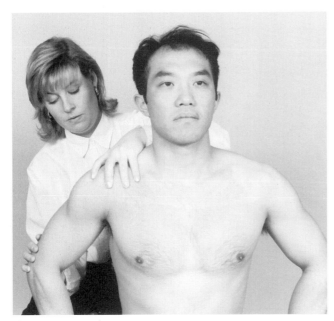

Figure 5–52

Anterior slide testing. Note position of examiner's hands and patient's arms.

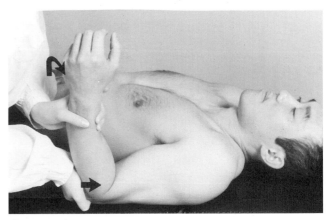

Figure 5–53

Compression-rotation test.

follows these maneuvers with horizontal adduction that relocates the humerus, a clunk or click may also be heard, indicating a tear of the labrum.

Anterior Slide Test.[61, 62] The patient is sitting with the hands on the waist, thumbs posterior. The examiner stands behind the patient and stabilizes the scapula and clavicle with one hand. With the other hand, the examiner applies an anterosuperior force at the elbow (Fig. 5–52). If the labrum is torn (SLAP lesion), the humeral head slides over the labrum with a pop or crack and the patient complains of anterosuperior pain.

Compression Rotation Test.[63] The patient lies relaxed in supine position. The examiner grasps the arm and flexes the elbow with the arm abducted to about 20°. The examiner then pushes or compresses the humerus in the glenoid by pushing up on the elbow while the examiner's other hand rotates the humerus medially and laterally

(Fig. 5–53). If a snapping or catching sensation is felt when the humeral head is felt, the test is positive for a labral tear (Bankart or SLAP lesion).

Posterior Inferior Ligament Test.[61] The patient sits while the examiner forward flexes the arm to between 80° and 90° and then horizontally adducts the arm 40° with medial rotation (Fig. 5–54). While doing the movement, the examiner palpates the posteroinferior region of the glenoid. If the humerus protrudes or pain is felt in the area, the test is considered positive and indicates a lesion of the posterior portion of the inferior glenohumeral ligament.

Tests for Scapular Stability

In order for the muscles of the glenohumeral joint to work in a normal coordinated fashion, the scapula must be stabilized by its muscles. Thus, when doing the tests the examiner is watching for movement patterns of the scapula as well as winging of the scapula.

Lateral Scapular Slide Test.[25, 64] This test is used to determine the stability of the scapula during glenohumeral movements. The patient sits with the arm resting at the side. The examiner measures the distance from the base of the spine of the scapula to the spinous process of

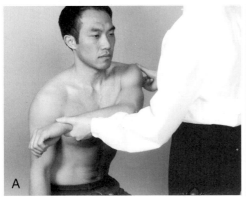
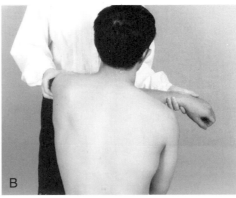

Figure 5–54

Posterior inferior ligament test. (A) Anterior view. (B) Posterior view.

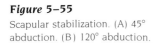

Figure 5–55
Scapular stabilization. (A) 45° abduction. (B) 120° abduction.

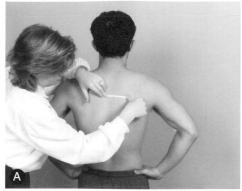

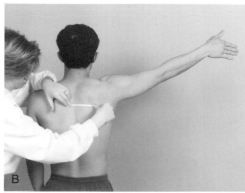

T2–T3, from the inferior angle of the scapula to the spinous process of T7–T9, or from T2 to the superior angle of the scapula. The patient is then tested holding two[64] (Fig. 5–55) or four[25] other positions: 45° abduction (hands on waist, thumbs posteriorly),[25, 64] 90° abduction with medial rotation,[25, 64] 120° abduction,[25] and 150° abduction.[25] Davies and Dickoff-Hoffman[25] and Kibler[64] state that in each position the distance measured should not vary more than 1 to 1.5 cm (0.5 to 0.75 inch) from the original measure. However, there may be increased distances above 90° as the scapula rotates during scapulohumeral rhythm. It therefore is important to look for asymmetry of movement between left and right sides, as well as the amount of movement, when determining scapular stability. In the different positions, the examiner may test for scapular and humeral stability by performing an eccentric movement at the shoulder by pushing the arm forward. One arm is tested at a time. As the arm is pushed forward eccentrically, the examiner should watch the relative movement at the scapulothoracic joint and the glenohumeral joint. Normally, more movement (relatively) will occur at the glenohumeral joint. If instability exists at either joint, excessive movement will be seen at that joint relative to the other joint. In addition, the examiner should watch for winging of the scapula, which indicates scapular instability. The test may also be performed by loading the arm (providing resistance) at 45° and greater abduction (scapular load test). Again, the scapula should not move more than 1.5 cm (0.75 inch).

Tests for Other Shoulder Joints

Acromioclavicular Shear Test.[50] With the patient in the sitting position, the examiner cups his or her hands over the deltoid muscle, with one hand on the clavicle and one hand on the spine of the scapula. The examiner then squeezes the heels of the hands together (Fig. 5–56). A positive test is indicated by pain or abnormal movement at the acromioclavicular joint and is indicative of acromioclavicular joint pathology.

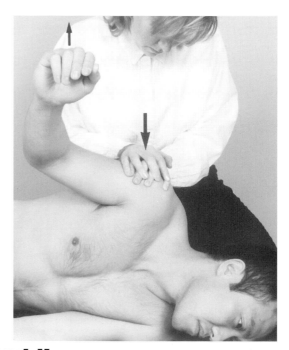

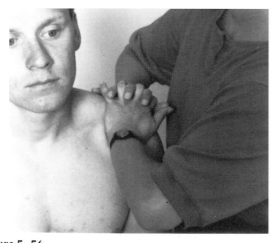

Figure 5–56
Acromioclavicular shear test.

Figure 5–57
Ellman's compression-rotation test for glenohumeral arthritis.

The integrity of the conoid portion of the coracoacromial ligament may be tested by placing the patient in side lying on the unaffected side. The examiner stabilizes the clavicle while pulling the inferior angle of the scapula away from the chest wall. The trapezoid portion of the ligament may be tested from the same position. The examiner stabilizes the clavicle and pulls the medial border of the scapula away from the chest wall. Pain in either case in the area of the ligament constitutes a positive test.

Ellman's Compression Rotation Test.[65, 66] The patient lies on the unaffected side. The examiner compresses the humeral head into the glenoid while the patient rotates the shoulder medially and laterally. If the patient's symptoms are reproduced, glenohumeral arthritis is suspected (Fig. 5–57).

Tests for Muscle or Tendon Pathology

Common Muscle and Tendon Pathology Tests

- Speed's test (biceps)
- Yergason's test (biceps)
- Empty can test (supraspinatus)
- Lift-off test (subscapularis)

Speed's Test (Biceps or Straight-Arm Test). The examiner resists shoulder forward flexion by the patient while the patient's forearm is first supinated, then pronated, and the elbow is completely extended. The test may also be performed by forward flexing the patient's arm to 90° and then asking the patient to resist an eccentric movement into extension (Fig. 5–58). A positive test elicits increased tenderness in the bicipital groove and is indicative of bicipital tendinitis. Speed's test is more effective than Yergason's test because the bone moves over the tendon during the test. It has been reported[63] that this

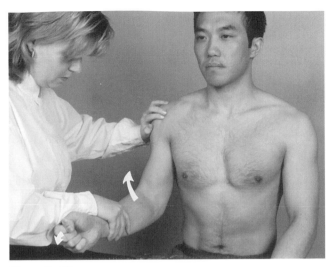

Figure 5–59
Yergason's test.

test may cause pain and will therefore be positive if a SLAP lesion is present. If profound weakness is found on resisted supination, a severe second- or third-degree (rupture) strain of the distal biceps should be suspected.[67]

Yergason's Test. With the patient's elbow flexed to 90° and stabilized against the thorax and with the forearm pronated, the examiner resists supination while the patient also laterally rotates the arm against resistance[68] (Fig. 5–59). A positive result is tenderness in the bicipital groove (or the tendon may pop out of the groove) and is indicative of bicipital tendinitis. This test is not as effective as Speed's test, because the tendon moves only a small amount in the bicipital groove during the test and because biceps tendon pain tends to occur with motion or palpation rather than with tension.

Ludington's Test.[69] The patient clasps both hands on top of or behind the head, allowing the interlocking fingers to support the weight of the upper limbs (Fig. 5–60). This action allows maximum relaxation of the biceps

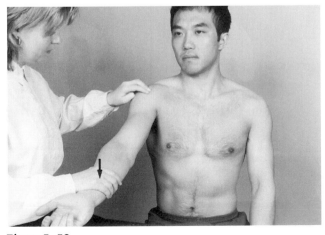

Figure 5–58
Speed's test (biceps or straight-arm test).

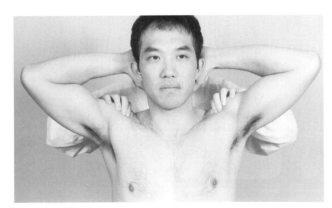

Figure 5–60
Ludington's test.

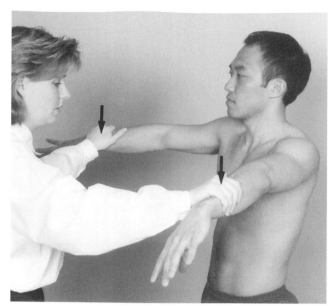

Figure 5–61
Supraspinatus test.

tendon in its resting position. The patient then alternately contracts and relaxes the biceps muscles. While the patient does the contractions and relaxations, the examiner palpates the biceps tendon, which will be felt on the uninvolved side but not on the affected side if the test result is positive. A positive result indicates rupture of the long head of biceps tendon.

Gilchrest's Sign.[50, 70] While standing, the patient lifts a 2- to 3-kg (5- to 7-lb) weight over the head. The arm is laterally rotated fully and lowered to the side in the coronal plane. A positive test is indicated by discomfort or pain in the bicipital groove. A positive test indicates bicipital tendinitis. In some cases, an audible snap or pain may be felt at between 100° and 90° abduction.

Lippman's Test.[71] The patient sits or stands while the examiner holds the arm flexed to 90° with one hand. With the other hand, the examiner palpates the biceps tendon 7 to 8 cm (2.5 to 3 inches) below the glenohumeral joint and moves the biceps tendon from side to side in the bicipital groove. A sharp pain is a positive test and indicates bicipital tendinitis.

Heuter's Sign.[70] Normally, if elbow flexion is resisted when the arm is pronated, some supination occurs as the biceps attempts to help the brachialis muscle flex the elbow. This supination movement is called Heuter's sign. If it is absent, the distal biceps tendon has been disrupted.

Supraspinatus ("Empty Can") Test.[72] The patient's shoulder is abducted to 90° with neutral (no) rotation, and resistance to abduction is provided by the examiner. The shoulder is then medially rotated and angled forward 30° (empty can position) so that the patient's thumbs point toward the floor (Fig. 5–61). Resistance to abduction is again given while the examiner looks for weakness or pain, reflecting a positive test result. A positive test result indicates a tear of the supraspinatus tendon or muscle, or neuropathy of the suprascapular nerve.

Drop-Arm (Codman's) Test. The examiner abducts the patient's shoulder to 90° and then asks the patient to slowly lower the arm to the side in the same arc of movement (Fig. 5–62). A positive test is indicated if the patient is unable to return the arm to the side slowly or has severe pain when attempting to do so. A positive result indicates a tear in the rotator cuff complex.[73]

Abrasion Sign.[11] The patient sits and abducts the arm to 90° with the elbow flexed to 90°. The patient then medially and laterally rotates the arm at the shoulder. Normally, there are no signs and symptoms. If crepitus occurs, it is a sign that the rotator cuff tendons are frayed and are abrading the acromion process and the coracoacromial ligament.

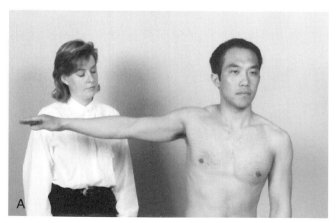
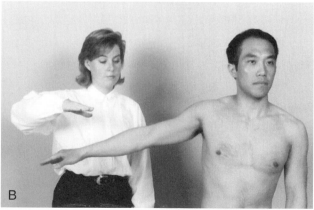

Figure 5–62
Drop-arm test. (A) The patient abducts the arm to 90°. (B) The patient tries to lower the arm slowly and is unable to do so; instead, the arm drops to his side. Examiner's hand illustrates the start position.

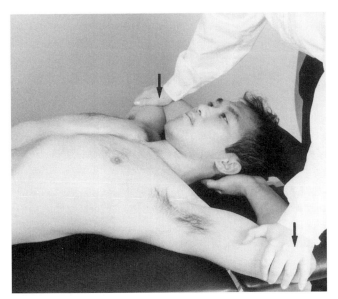

Figure 5–63
Pectoralis major flexibility test. Examiner is testing end feel.

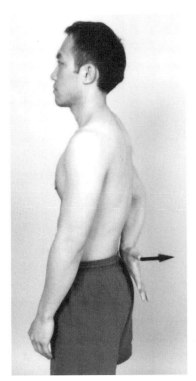

Figure 5–64
"Lift-off" sign.

Pectoralis Major Contracture Test. The patient lies supine and clasps the hands together behind the head. The arms are then lowered until the elbows touch the examining table (Fig. 5–63). A positive test occurs if the elbows do not reach the table and indicates a tight pectoralis major muscle.

Lift-off Sign.[74] The patient stands and places the dorsum of the hand on the back pocket (Fig. 5–64). The patient then lifts the hand away from the back. An inability to do so indicates a lesion of the subscapularis muscle. Abnormal motion in the scapula during the test may indicate scapular instability. The test may also be used to test the rhomboids. Medial border winging of the scapula during the test may indicate that the rhomboids are affected.

Tests for Impingement

Common Shoulder Impingement Tests

• Neer impingement test
• Hawkins-Kennedy impingement test

Neer Impingement Test.[75] The patient's arm is forcibly elevated through forward flexion by the examiner's causing a "jamming" of the greater tuberosity against the anteroinferior border of the acromion (Fig. 5–65). The patient's face shows pain, reflecting a positive test result (Fig. 5–66A). The test is indicative of an overuse injury to the supraspinatus muscle and sometimes to the biceps tendon.

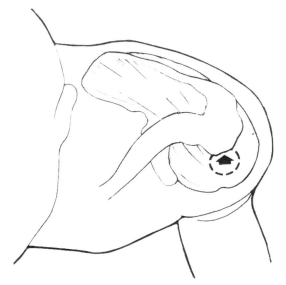

Figure 5–65
The functional arc of elevation of the proximal humerus is forward, as proposed by Neer. The greater tuberosity impinges against the anterior one third of the acromial surface. This critical area comprises the supraspinatus and bicipital tendons and the subacromial bursa. (From Hawkins, R.J., and J.S. Abrams: Impingement syndrome in the absence of rotator cuff tear [stage 1 and 2]. Orthop. Clin. North Am. 18:374, 1987.)

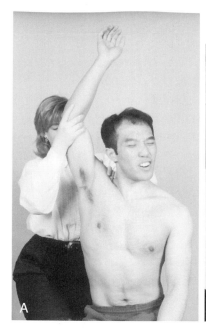
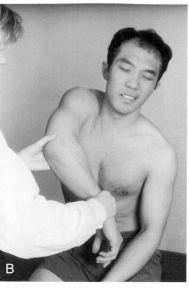

Figure 5–66

Impingement sign. (A) A positive Neer impingement sign is present if pain and its resulting facial expression are produced when the arm is forcibly flexed forward by the examiner, jamming the greater tuberosity against the anteroinferior surface of the acromion. (B) An alternative method (Hawkins-Kennedy impingement test) demonstrates the impingement sign by forcibly medially rotating the proximal humerus when the arm is forward flexed to 90°.

Hawkins-Kennedy Impingement Test.[76] The patient stands while the examiner forward flexes the arms to 90° and then forcibly medially rotates the shoulder (Fig. 5–66B). This movement pushes the supraspinatus tendon against the anterior surface of the coracoacromial ligament and coracoid process.[77] Pain indicates a positive test for supraspinatus tendinitis.

Impingement Test.[78] The patient is seated. The examiner takes the arm to 90° abduction and full lateral rotation. This is the same position as for the apprehension test. However, if there is no history of possible traumatic subluxation or dislocation, the movement also can cause anterior translation of the humerus, resulting in secondary impingement of the rotator cuff. Therefore, a positive test indicates a grade II or III shoulder lesion based on Jobe's classification.[40] A positive test depends on production of the patient's symptoms and anterior or posterior shoulder pain, or both.

Reverse Impingement Sign.[43] This test is used if the patient has a positive painful arc or pain on lateral rotation. The patient lies supine. The examiner pushes the head of the humerus inferiorly as the arm is abducted or laterally rotated. If the pain decreases or disappears, it is considered a positive test for mechanical impingement under the acromion (Fig. 5–67).

Tests for Neurological Function

> ### Neurological Function Tests
>
> - Upper limb tension tests

Upper Limb Tension (Brachial Plexus Tension) Test.[79] This test is the upper limb equivalent of the straight leg raising test of the lower limb. The patient is positioned to stress the neurological tissue entering the arm. The patient lies supine. The test may be performed by placing the joints of the upper limb in different positions to stress each of the neurological tissues differently (see Table 3–7 and Fig. 3–22). There are in effect four upper limb tension tests (ULTT 1–4).[80] Depending on the history, the examiner picks the ULTT that will stress the appropriate neurological tissue. Pain in the form of tin-

Figure 5–67

Reverse impingement sign.

gling or a stretch or ache in the cubital fossa indicates stretching of the dura mater in the cervical spine. The available range of passive movement at the elbow, when compared with the normal side, can give an indication of the restriction. Lateral or side flexion of the cervical spine to the opposite side can enhance the effect. If full ROM is not available in the shoulder, the test can still be performed by taking the shoulder to the point just short of pain in abduction and lateral rotation and performing the other maneuvers of the arm or by passively side flexing the cervical spine. It is important to understand that the upper limb tension tests put tension on the upper limb neurological tissues even in normal individuals. Therefore, reproduction of the patient's symptoms, rather than stretching, constitutes a positive sign.

Tinel's Sign (at the Shoulder). The area of the brachial plexus above the clavicle in the area of the scalene triangle is tapped. A positive sign is indicated by a tingling sensation in one or more of the nerve roots.

Tests for Thoracic Outlet Syndrome

Common Tests for Thoracic Outlet Syndrome

- Roos test
- Wright test
- Costoclavicular syndrome test

Thoracic outlet syndromes may combine neurological and vascular signs, or the signs and symptoms of neurological deficit, restriction of arterial flow, or restriction of venous flow may be seen individually. For this reason, a diagnosis of thoracic outlet syndrome is usually one of exclusion in which all other causes have been eliminated. In fact, neurogenic signs are rare in thoracic outlet syndrome, and there is poor correlation between the vascular signs of the condition and neurological involvement.

With thoracic outlet tests that involve taking the pulse, the examiner must find the pulse before positioning the patient's arm or cervical spine. Because the pulse may be diminished even in a "normal" individual, it is more important to look for the reproduction of symptoms than for diminution of the pulse.

Roos Test (EAST).[81] The patient stands and abducts the arms to 90°, laterally rotates the shoulder, and flexes the elbows to 90° so that the elbows are slightly behind the frontal plane. The patient then opens and closes the hands slowly for 3 minutes (Fig. 5–68). If the patient is unable to keep the arms in the starting position for 3 minutes or suffers ischemic pain, heaviness or profound weakness of the arm, or numbness and tingling of the hand during the 3 minutes, the test is considered positive for thoracic outlet syndrome on the affected

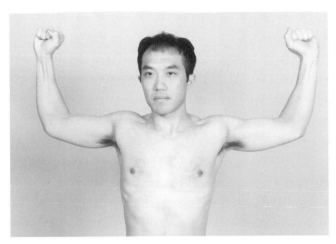

Figure 5–68
Roos test.

side. Minor fatigue and distress are considered negative tests. The test is sometimes called the positive abduction and external rotation (AER) position test, the "hands-up" test, or the **elevated arm stress test (EAST)**.[81-84]

Wright Test or Maneuver. Wright[85] advocated "hyperabducting" the arm so that the hand is brought over the head with the elbow and arm in the coronal plane. He advocated doing the test in the sitting and then the supine positions. Taking a breath or rotating or extending the head and neck may have an additional effect. The pulse is palpated for differences. This test is used to detect compression in the costoclavicular space.

Costoclavicular Syndrome (Military Brace) Test. The examiner palpates the radial pulse and then draws the patient's shoulder down and back (Fig. 5–69). A positive

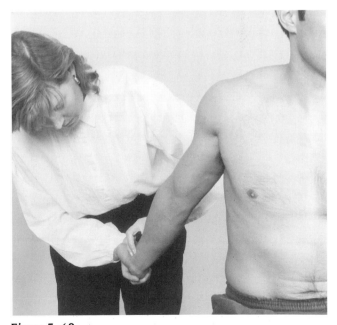

Figure 5–69
Costoclavicular syndrome test.

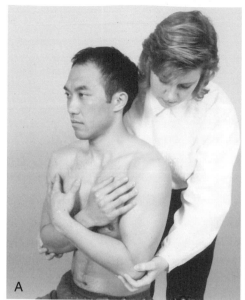
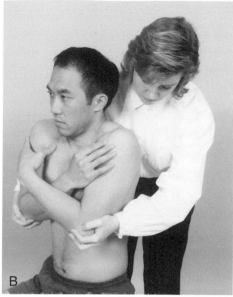

Figure 5–70
Shoulder girdle passive elevation.
(A) Start position. (B) Relief
position.

test is indicated by an absence of the pulse and implies possible thoracic outlet syndrome. This test is particularly effective in patients who complain of symptoms while wearing a backpack or heavy coat.

Provocative Elevation Test.[42] The patient elevates both arms above the horizontal and is asked to rapidly open and close the hands 15 times. If fatigue, cramping, or tingling occurs during the test, the test is positive for vascular insufficiency and thoracic outlet syndrome. This test is a modification of the Roos test.

Shoulder Girdle Passive Elevation.[43] This test is used on patients who already present with symptoms. The patient sits and the examiner grasps the patient's arms from behind and passively elevates the shoulder girdle up and forward into full elevation (a passive bilateral shoulder shrug), and the position is held for 30 or more seconds

(Fig. 5–70). Arterial relief is evidenced by stronger pulse, skin color change (more pink), and increased hand temperature. Venous relief is shown by decreased cyanosis and venous engorgement. Neurological signs go from numbness to pins and needles or tingling as well as some pain as the ischemia to the nerve is released. This is referred to as a **release phenomenon.**

Adson Maneuver.[86] This test is probably one of the most common methods of testing for thoracic outlet syndrome reported in the literature. The examiner locates the radial pulse. The patient's head is rotated to face the test shoulder (Fig. 5–71). The patient then extends the head while the examiner laterally rotates and extends the patient's shoulder. The patient is instructed to take a deep breath and hold it. A disappearance of the pulse indicates a positive test.

Allen Test.[87] The examiner flexes the patient's elbow to 90° while the shoulder is extended horizontally and rotated laterally (Fig. 5–72). The patient then rotates the

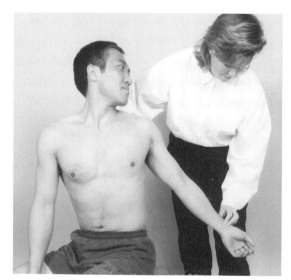

Figure 5–71
Adson maneuver.

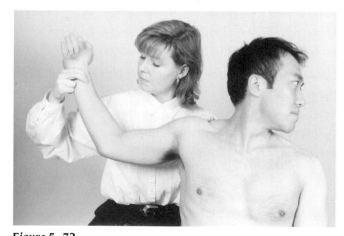

Figure 5–72
Allen maneuver.

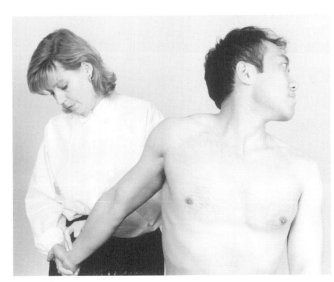

Figure 5–73
Halstead maneuver.

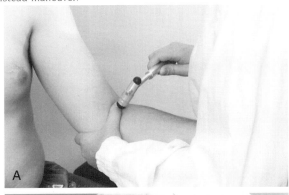

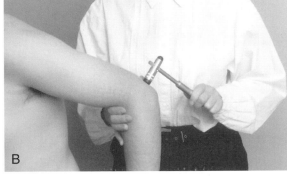

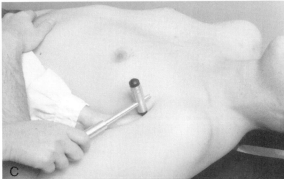

Figure 5–74
Positioning to test the reflexes around the shoulder. (A) Biceps.
(B) Triceps. (C) Pectoralis major.

head away from the test side. The examiner palpates the radial pulse, which becomes absent (disappears) when the head is rotated away from the test side. The pulse disappearance indicates a positive test result for thoracic outlet syndrome.

Halstead Maneuver. The examiner finds the radial pulse and applies a downward traction on the test extremity while the patient's neck is hyperextended and the head is rotated to the opposite side (Fig. 5–73). Absence or disappearance of a pulse indicates a positive test for thoracic outlet syndrome.

Reflexes and Cutaneous Distribution

The reflexes in the shoulder region that are often assessed include the pectoralis major, clavicular portion (C5–C6), sternocostal portion (C7–C8 and T1), the biceps (C5–C6), and the triceps (C7–C8) (Fig. 5–74).

The examiner must be aware of the dermatome patterns of the nerve roots (Fig. 5–75) as well as the cutaneous distribution of the peripheral nerves (Fig. 5–76). Dermatomes vary from person to person, so the diagrams are estimations only. A scanning test for altered sensa-

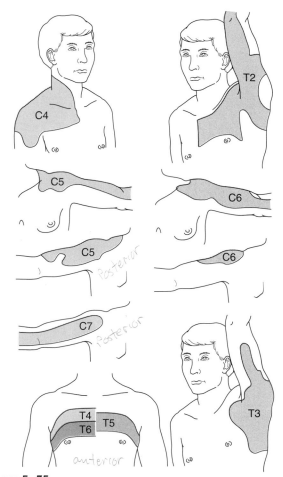

Figure 5–75
Dermatome pattern of the shoulder. Dermatomes on one side only are illustrated.

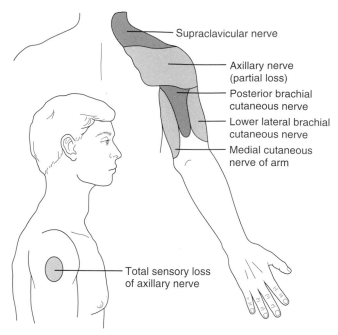

Figure 5–76
Cutaneous distribution of peripheral nerves around the shoulder.

tion is performed by running the relaxed hands and fingers over the neck, shoulders, and anterior and posterior chest area. Any difference in sensation between the two sides should be noted. These differences can be mapped more exactly using a pinwheel, a pin, a brush, and/or cotton batting. In this way, the examiner can use sensation to help differentiate between a peripheral nerve lesion and a nerve root lesion referred from the cervical spine.

True shoulder pain rarely extends below the elbow. Pain in the acromioclavicular or sternoclavicular joint tends to be localized to the affected joint and usually does not spread or radiate. Pain can be referred to the

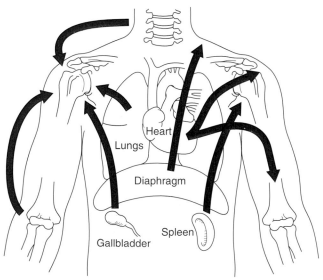

Figure 5–77
Structures referring pain to the shoulder.

Table 5–10
Shoulder Muscles and Referral of Pain

Muscle	Referral Pattern
Levator scapulae	Over muscle to posterior shoulder and along medial border of scapula
Latissimus dorsi	Inferior angle of scapula up to posterior and anterior shoulder into posterior arm; may refer to area above iliac crest
Rhomboids	Medial border of scapula
Supraspinatus	Over shoulder cap and above spine of scapula; sometimes down lateral aspect of arm to proximal forearm
Infraspinatus	Anterolateral shoulder and medial border of scapula; may refer down lateral aspect of arm
Teres minor	Near deltoid insertion, up to shoulder cap, and down lateral arm to elbow
Subscapularis	Posterior shoulder to scapula and down posteromedial and anteromedial aspects of arm to elbow
Teres major	Shoulder cap down lateral aspect of arm to elbow
Deltoid	Over muscle and posterior glenoid area of shoulder
Coracobrachialis	Anterior shoulder and down posterior arm

shoulder and surrounding tissues from many structures,[88] including the cervical spine, elbow, lungs, heart, diaphragm, gallbladder, and spleen (Fig. 5–77; Table 5–10).

Peripheral Nerve Injuries About the Shoulder

Axillary (Circumflex) Nerve (C5–C6). The axillary nerve is the most commonly injured nerve in the shoulder, and the most common cause of injury is anterior dislocation of the shoulder or fracture of the neck of the humerus.[89] The nerve injury may occur during the dislocation itself or during the reduction. Other traumatic events (e.g., fracture, bullet or stab wounds) or brachial plexus injuries, compression (e.g., crutches), or shoulder surgery also may affect the axillary nerve.

Motor loss (see Tables 5–2 and 5–5) includes an inability to abduct the arm (deltoid), although the patient may attempt to laterally rotate the arm and use the long head of biceps to abduct the arm (trick movement). There is some weakness of lateral rotation owing to the loss of teres minor. The patient may attempt to use scapular movement (i.e., trapezius or serratus anterior) to compensate for the muscle loss (trick movement). Atrophy of the deltoid leads to loss of the lateral roundness (flattening) of the shoulder. Sensory loss is over the deltoid, with the main loss being a small, 2- to 3-cm (1-inch) circular area at the deltoid insertion (see Fig. 5–4).

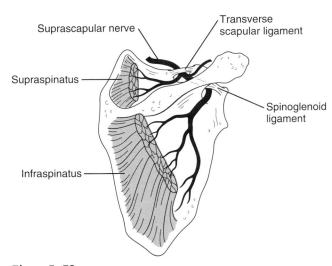

Figure 5–78
Suprascapular nerve.

Suprascapular Nerve (C5–C6). The suprascapular nerve may be injured by a fall on the posterior shoulder, stretching, repeated microtrauma, or fracture of the scapula. Commonly, the nerve is injured as it passes through the suprascapular notch under the transverse scapular (suprascapular) ligament or as it winds around the spine of the scapula[12] (Fig. 5–78). Often, it is hard to distinguish from rotator cuff syndrome, so the history and mechanism of injury become important for differential diagnosis. Most commonly, the condition is seen in people who work with their arms overhead or in activities involving cocking and following through (e.g., pitching).[90]

Signs and symptoms include persistent rear shoulder pain and paralysis of the supraspinatus (suprascapular notch) and infraspinatus (suprascapular notch and spine of scapula), leading to decreased strength of abduction (supraspinatus) and external rotation (infraspinatus) of the shoulder. Wasting may also be evident over the scapula.

Musculocutaneous Nerve (C5–C6). This nerve is not commonly injured, although it may be injured by trauma (e.g., humeral dislocation or fracture) or in conjunction with injury to the brachial plexus or adjacent axillary artery. Injury to this nerve (see Tables 5–2 and 5–5) results primarily in loss of elbow flexion (biceps and brachialis), shoulder forward flexion (biceps and coracobrachialis), and decreased supination strength (biceps). In addition, injury to its sensory branch, the antebrachial cutaneous nerve, leads to altered sensation in the anterolateral aspect of the forearm (see Fig. 5–5). This sensory branch is sometimes compressed as it passes under the distal biceps tendon, resulting in **musculocutaneous nerve tunnel syndrome**. The injury results in sensory loss in the forearm; it is usually the result of forced elbow hyperextension and/or repeated pronation (e.g., excessive screwdriving, backhand tennis strokes) and may be misdiagnosed as tennis elbow.

Long Thoracic Nerve (C5–C8). Injury to the long thoracic nerve, although not common, may occur from repetitive microtrauma with heavy effort above shoulder height, pressure on the nerve from backpacking, vigorous upper limb activities (e.g., shoveling, chopping), or wounds (see Tables 5–2 and 5–5). The result is paralysis of the serratus anterior, causing winging (medial border) of the scapula and pain and weakness on forward flexion of the extended arm.[12, 89] Abduction above 90° is difficult because of scapular winging. Stabilization of the scapula by the examiner enables the patient to further abduct the arm.

Spinal Accessory Nerve (C3–C4). The spinal accessory nerve is vulnerable to traumatic injury as it passes the posterior triangle of the neck; injury spares the sternocleidomastoid muscles but affects the trapezius muscle. A common example would be abnormal pressure from a poorly fitting backpack (see Tables 5–2 and 5–5). Shoulder drooping and scapular winging (medial superior portion), especially on resisted abduction, may be evident, along with "deepening" of the supraclavicular fossa as a result of trapezius atrophy.[12] The patient has difficulty abducting the arm above 90°.[89]

Joint Play Movements

Joint play movements[29, 91] are usually performed with the patient lying supine. The examiner compares the amount of available movement and end feel on the affected side with the movement on the unaffected side and notes whether the movements affect the patient's symptoms.

Joint Play Movements of the Shoulder Complex

- Backward glide of the humerus
- Forward glide of the humerus
- Lateral distraction of the humerus
- Caudal glide of the humerus (long arm traction)
- Backward glide of the humerus in abduction
- Lateral distraction of the humerus in abduction
- Anteroposterior and cephalocaudal movements of the clavicle at the acromioclavicular joint
- Anteroposterior and cephalocaudal movements of the clavicle at the sternoclavicular joint
- General movement of the scapula to determine mobility

To perform the backward joint play movement of the humerus, the examiner grasps the patient's upper limb, placing one hand over the anterior humeral head. The other hand is placed around the humerus above and near the elbow while the patient's hand is held against the examiner's thorax by the examiner's arm (Fig. 5–79A).

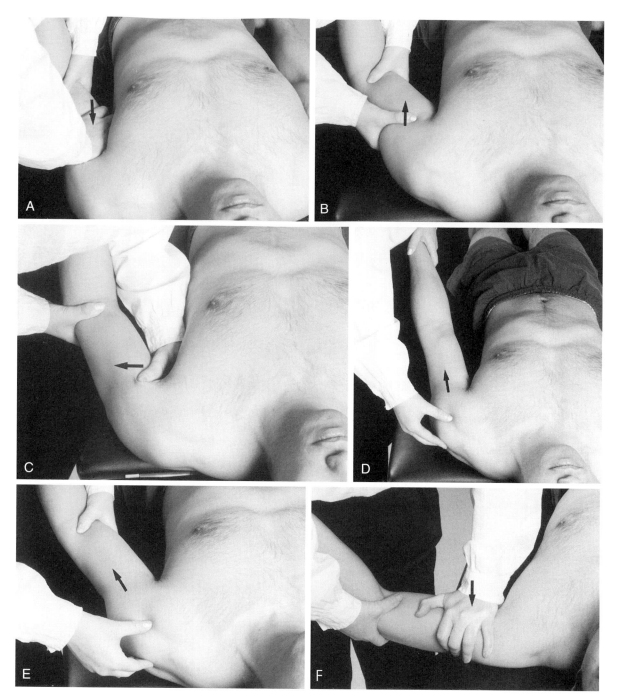

Figure 5–79

Joint play movements of the shoulder complex. (A) Backward glide of the humerus. (B) Forward glide
of the humerus. (C) Lateral distraction of the humerus. (D) Long arm traction applied below elbow.
(E) Long arm traction applied above elbow. (F) Backward glide of the humerus in abduction.

The examiner then applies a backward force, keeping the patient's arm parallel to the body so that no rotation or torsion occurs at the glenohumeral joint.

Forward joint play movement of the humerus is carried out in a similar fashion, with the examiner's hands placed as shown in Figure 5–79B. The examiner applies an anterior force (anterior drawer), keeping the patient's arm parallel to the body so that no rotation or torsion occurs at the glenohumeral joint.

To apply a lateral distraction joint play movement to the humerus, the examiner's hands are placed as shown in Figure 5–79C. A lateral distraction force is applied to the glenohumeral joint, with the patient's arm kept parallel to the body so that no rotation or torsion occurs at the glenohumeral joint.

Caudal glide (long arm traction) joint play movement is performed with the patient in the same supine position. The examiner grasps above the patient's wrist with one hand and palpates with the other hand, below the distal spine of the scapula posteriorly and below the distal clavicle anteriorly over the glenohumeral joint line (Fig. 5–79D). The examiner then applies a traction force to the shoulder while palpating to see whether the head of the humerus drops down (moves distally) in the glenoid cavity as it normally should. If the patient complains of pain in the elbow, the test may be done with the hands positioned as in Figure 5–79E.

The examiner then abducts the patient's arm to 90°, grasping above the patient's wrist with one hand while stabilizing the thorax with the other hand. The examiner applies a long arm traction force to determine joint play in this position.

With the patient's arm abducted to 90°, the examiner places one hand over the anterior humerus while stabilizing the patient's arm with the other hand and stabilizing the patient's hand against the thorax with the same arm. A backward force is then applied, keeping the patient's arm parallel to the body. This is a backward joint play movement of the humerus in abduction (Fig. 5–79F).

To assess the acromioclavicular and sternoclavicular joints (Figs. 5–79G and 5–79H, respectively), the examiner gently grasps the clavicle as close to the joint to be tested as possible and moves it in and out or up and down while palpating the joint with the other hand. A comparison of the amount of movement available is made between the two sides. Care should be taken not to "squeeze" the clavicle as it may cause pain.

For a determination of mobility of the scapula, the patient lies on one side to fixate the thorax with the arm relaxed and resting behind the back (hand by opposite back pocket). The uppermost scapula is tested in this position. The examiner faces the patient, placing the lower hand along the medial border of the patient's scapula. The hand of the examiner's other arm holds the upper (cranial) dorsal surface of the patient's scapula. To "relax" the scapula further, the examiner uses his or her body to push the patient's test shoulder posteriorly to obtain a better "hold" on the scapula. By holding the scapula in this way, the examiner is able to move it medially, laterally, caudally, cranially, and away from the thorax (Fig. 5–79I).

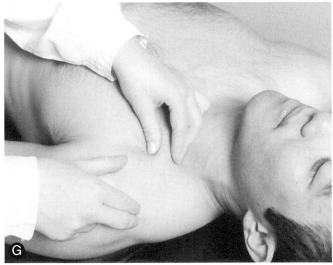

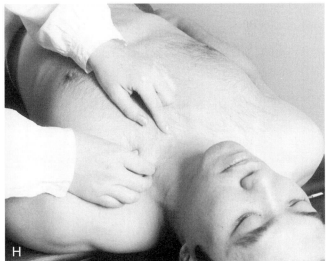

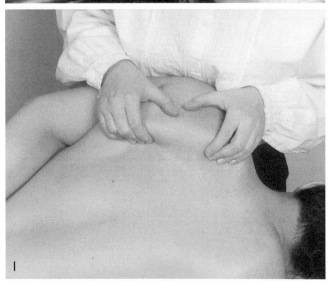

Figure 5–79 *Continued*
(G) Joint play of the acromioclavicular joint. (H) Joint play of the sternoclavicular joint. (I) General movement of the scapula to determine mobility.

Palpation

When palpating the shoulder complex, the examiner should note any muscle spasm, tenderness, abnormal "bumps," or other signs and symptoms that may indicate the source of pathology. The examiner should perform palpation in a systematic manner, beginning with the anterior structures and working around to the posterior structures. Findings on the injured side should be compared with those on the unaffected side. Any differences between the two sides should be noted, because they may give an indication of the cause of the patient's problems.

Anterior Structures

The anterior structures of the shoulder may be palpated with the patient in the supine lying or sitting position (Fig. 5–80A).

Clavicle. The clavicle should be palpated along its full length for tenderness or abnormal bumps, such as callus

formation after a fracture, and to ensure that it is in its resting position relative to the uninjured side. That is, it may be rotated anteriorly or posteriorly more than the unaffected side, or one end may be higher than that of the uninjured side, indicating a possible subluxation or dislocation at the sternoclavicular or acromioclavicular joint.

Sternoclavicular Joint. The sternoclavicular joint should be palpated for normal positioning in relation to the sternum and first rib. Palpation should also include the supporting ligaments and sternocleidomastoid muscle. Adjacent to the joint, the suprasternal notch may be palpated. From the notch, the examiner moves the fingers laterally and posteriorly to palpate the first rib. The examiner should apply slight caudal pressure to the first rib on both sides and note any difference. Spasm of the scalene muscles or pathology in the area may result in elevation of the first rib on the affected side.

Acromioclavicular Joint. Like the sternoclavicular joint, the acromioclavicular joint should be palpated for nor-

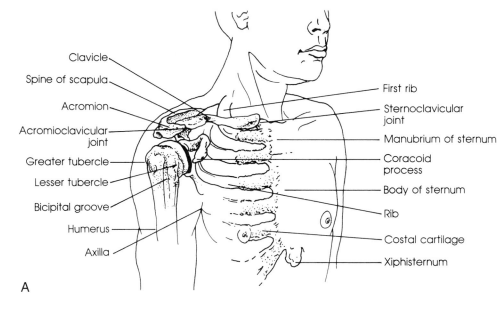

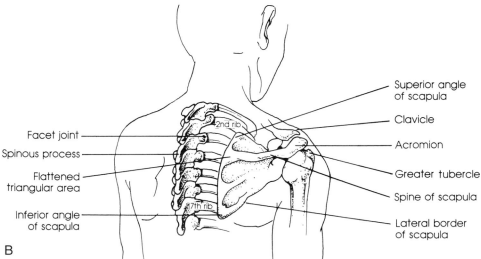

Figure 5–80

Landmarks of the shoulder region. (A) Anterior view. (B) Posterior view.

Figure 5–81
Palpation around the shoulder: greater tuberosity (A) and lesser tuberosity (B). The bicipital groove lies between these two landmarks.

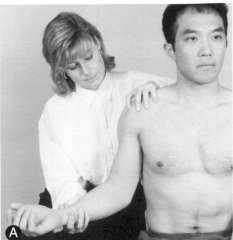
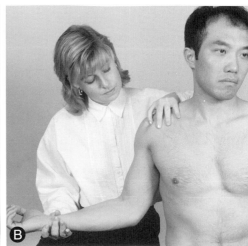

mal positioning and tenderness. Likewise, supporting ligaments (acromioclavicular and coracoclavicular) and the trapezius, subclavius, and deltoid (anterior, middle, and posterior fibers) muscles should be palpated for tenderness and spasm.

Coracoid Process. The coracoid process may be palpated approximately 2.5 cm (1 inch) below the junction of the lateral one third and medial two thirds of the clavicle. The short head of biceps and coracobrachialis muscles originate from, and the pectoralis minor inserts into, this process.

Sternum. In the midline of the chest, the examiner should palpate the three portions of the sternum (manubrium, body, and xiphoid process), noting any abnormality or tenderness.

Ribs and Costal Cartilage. Adjacent to the sternum, the examiner should palpate the sternocostal and costochondral articulations, noting any swelling, tenderness, or other abnormality. These "articulations" are sometimes sprained or subluxed, or a costochondritis (Tietze's syndrome) may be evident. The examiner should palpate the ribs as they extend around the chest wall, seeking any potential pathology.

Humerus and Rotator Cuff Muscles. Moving laterally from the chest and caudally from the acromion process, the examiner should palpate the humerus and its surrounding structures for potential pathology. The examiner first palpates the lateral tip of the acromion process and then moves inferiorly to the greater tuberosity of the humerus. The examiner should then laterally rotate the humerus. During palpation, the long head of the biceps in the bicipital groove will slip under the fingers, followed by the lesser tuberosity of the humerus (Fig. 5–81). As with all palpation, the testing should be done gently and carefully to prevent causing the patient undue pain. By rotating the humerus alternately laterally and medially, the smooth progression over the three structures is normally noted (**de Anquin test**), and the lesser tuberosity is felt at the level of the coracoid process. If the examiner then palpates along the lesser tuberosity and the lip of the bicipital groove, the fingers will rest on the tendon of subscapularis muscle. If the examiner places the thumb over the lesser tuberosity and "grips" the shoulder between the second, third, and fourth fingers as shown in Figure 5–1, the fingers will be over the insertion of the other three rotator cuff muscles—supraspinatus, infraspinatus, and teres minor. Moving laterally over the bicipital groove to its other lip, the examiner may palpate the insertion of the pectoralis major muscle. The patient is then asked to further medially rotate the humerus so that the forearm rests behind the back, and the examiner palpates 2 cm inferior to the anterior aspect of the acromion process for the supraspinatus tendon. Any tenderness of the tendon should be noted. The examiner then passively abducts the patient's shoulder to between 80° and 90° and palpates the notch formed by the acromion and spine of the scapula with the clavicle. In the notch, the examiner is palpating the musculotendinous junction of the supraspinatus muscle.

Axilla. With the shoulder slightly abducted (20 to 30°), the examiner palpates the structures of the axilla; latissimus dorsi muscle (posterior wall), pectoralis major muscle (anterior wall), serratus anterior muscle (medial wall), lymph nodes (palpable only if swollen), and brachial artery. The patient is then asked to lie prone "on the elbows" (sphinx position) with the shoulders slightly laterally rotated and the elbow slightly adducted in relation to the shoulder. The examiner then palpates just inferior to the most lateral aspect of the scapula for the insertion of the infraspinatus muscle. Just distal to this insertion, the examiner may be able to palpate the insertion of the teres minor.

Posterior Structures

To complete the palpation, the patient may be either sitting or lying prone with the upper limb by the trunk (see Fig. 5–80B).

Spine of Scapula. From the acromion process the examiner moves his or her hands along the spine of the scapula, noting any tenderness or abnormality.

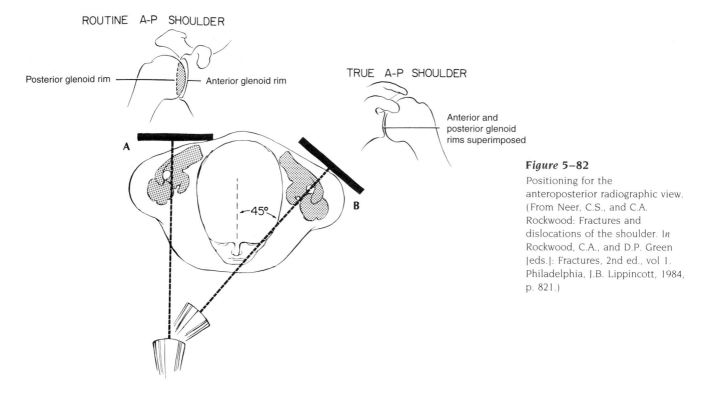

ROUTINE   A-P   SHOULDER

Posterior glenoid rim ——————— —— Anterior glenoid rim

A

—45°

TRUE   A-P   SHOULDER

Anterior and posterior glenoid rims superimposed

B

Figure 5–82
Positioning for the anteroposterior radiographic view. (From Neer, C.S., and C.A. Rockwood: Fractures and dislocations of the shoulder. In Rockwood, C.A., and D.P. Green (eds.): Fractures, 2nd ed., vol 1. Philadelphia, J.B. Lippincott, 1984, p. 821.)

Scapula. The examiner follows the spine of the scapula to the medial border of the scapula and then follows the outline of the scapula, which normally extends from the spinous process of T2 to the spinous process of T9, depending on the size of the scapula. The superior angle lies at the level of the T2 spinous process. The base or root of the spine of the scapula lies between T3 and T4, and the inferior angle lies between T7 and T9. The examiner then moves around the inferior angle of the scapula and along its lateral border. After the borders of the scapula have been palpated, the posterior surface (supraspinatus and infraspinatus muscles) may be palpated for tenderness, atrophy, or spasm.

Spinous Processes of Lower Cervical and Thoracic Spine. In the midline, the examiner may palpate the cervical and thoracic spinous processes for any abnormality or tenderness. This is followed by palpation of the trapezius muscle.

Triceps Tendon. Inferior to the posterior aspect of the acromion process, the examiner may palpate the tendon of the long head of triceps as it originates from the infraglenoid tubercle.

Diagnostic Imaging

Plain Film Radiography

Anteroposterior View. This may be a true anteriorposterior view or a tilt view (Fig. 5–82). With either view, a great deal of information can be obtained (Fig. 5–83).

Figure 5–83
Normal radiographic examination. (A) Lateral rotation. The greater tuberosity (GT) is seen in profile. The humeral head normally overlaps the glenoid on this view. The anterior (*black arrows*) and posterior (*arrowheads*) glenoid margins are well seen and do not overlap owing to the anterior tilt of the glenoid. The anatomic (*black A*) and surgical (S) necks of the humerus are indicated. White A = acromion process; CP = coracoid process. A vacuum phenomenon (*white arrow*) is present. (B) Medial rotation. The overlap of the greater tuberosity and the humeral head produces a rounded appearance of the proximal humerus. LT = lesser tuberosity. A small exostosis is noted projecting from the humeral metaphysis. (C) Posterior oblique. The glenohumeral cartilage space is seen in profile with no overlap of the humerus and glenoid. (D) Normal scapular Y view. This true lateral view of the scapula (anterior oblique of the shoulder) shows the humeral head centered over the glenoid (*arrows*). A = acromion; C = clavicle; CP = coracoid process. (E) Diagram of normal scapular Y view. (F) Axillary view. A = acromion; ANT = anterior; C = clavicle; CP = coracoid process. (G) Normal transthoracic view. The smooth arch formed by the inferior border of the scapula and the posterior aspect of the humerus is indicated (*arrowheads*). The coracoid process (CP) is faintly seen. The margins of the glenoid are indicated (*arrows*). This view is slightly oblique, allowing the glenoid to be seen more en face than usual. (From Weissman, B.N.W., and C.B. Sledge: Orthopedic Radiology. Philadelphia, W.B. Saunders Co., 1986, p. 219.)

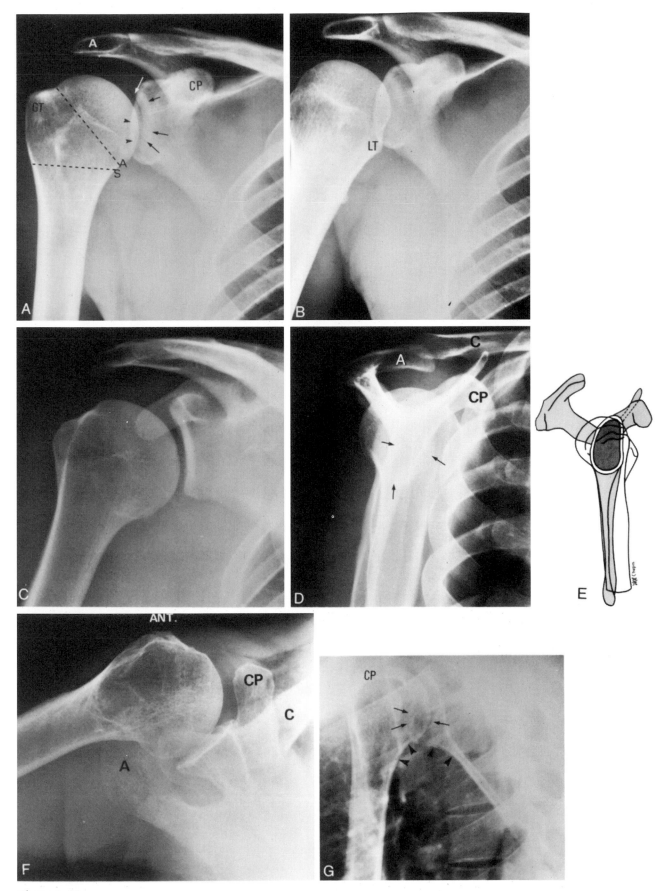

Figure 5–83

See legend on opposite page

Figure 5–84

"Empty glenoid" sign of posterior dislocation on anteroposterior radiograph. The head of the humerus fills the glenoid in the normal radiograph (*left*). With a posterior dislocation, the glenoid is "empty," especially in its anterior portion (*right*). (From Magee, D.J., and D.C. Reid: Shoulder injuries. In Zachazewski, J.E., D.J. Magee, and W.S. Quillen [eds.]: Athletic Injuries and Rehabilitation. Philadelphia, W.B. Saunders Co., 1996, p. 523.)

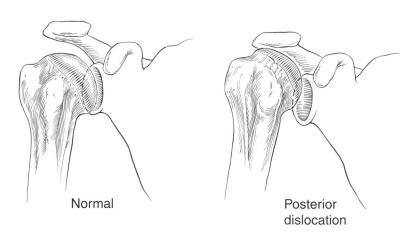

Normal

Posterior dislocation

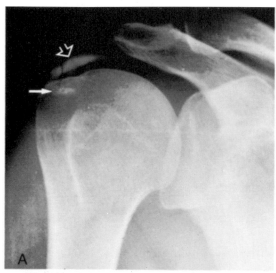

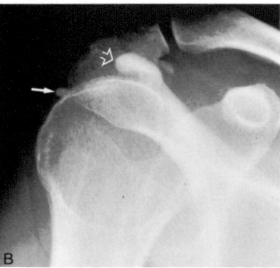

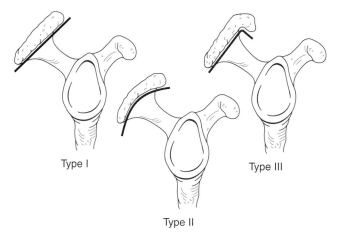

Type I

Type III

Type II

Figure 5–86

Acromion morphology.

Figure 5–85

Calcific tendinitis–supraspinatus and infraspinatus. (A) Lateral rotation view shows calcification projected over the base of the greater tuberosity (*white arrow*) and above the greater tuberosity (*open arrow*). (B) Medial rotation view projects the infraspinatus calcification (*white arrow*) in profile and documents its posterior location. The supraspinatus calcification (*open arrow*) is rotated medially and maintains its superior location. (From Weissman, B.N.W., and C.B. Sledge: Orthopedic Radiology. Philadelphia, W.B. Saunders Co., 1986, p. 227.)

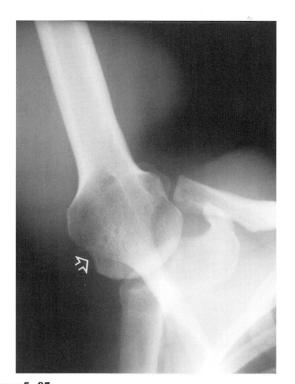

Figure 5–87

Hill-Sachs lesion (*arrow*).

1. The relation of the humerus to the glenoid cavity should be examined. Posterior dislocations may be recognized by the "empty glenoid" sign. Normally, the radiograph shows overlapping shadows of the humerus and glenoid. With a posterior dislocation, this shadow is reduced or absent (Fig. 5–84).[92]

2. The relation of the clavicle to the acromion process and the humerus to the glenoid should also be observed.

3. The examiner should determine whether the epiphyseal plate of the humeral head is present and, if so, whether it is normal.

4. The examiner should note whether there are any calcifications in any of the tendons (Fig. 5–85), especially those of the supraspinatus or infraspinatus muscles.

5. The examiner should note the configuration of the undersurface of the acromion (see Fig. 5–83D; Fig. 5–86)[93, 94] and the presence of any subacromial spurs. The possible configurations are type I (flat [17%]), type II (curved [43%]), and type III (hooked [39%]).

6. Medial rotation of the humerus with this view may show a defect on the lateral aspect of the humeral head from recurrent dislocations. This defect is called a Hill-Sachs lesion (Fig. 5–87).

7. The examiner should look at the acromiohumeral interval (the space between the acromion and the humerus) and see whether it is normal.[95] The normal interval is 7 to 14 mm (Fig. 5–88). If this distance decreases, it may be an indication of rotator cuff tears. Likewise, if

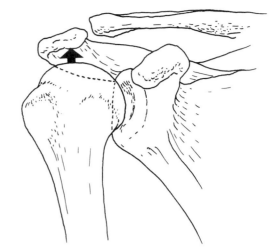

Figure 5–88
Acromiohumeral interval.

the arm is medially rotated and the view shows the coracohumeral distance of less than 11 mm, it is indicative of impingement and rotator cuff pathology.[96]

8. A stress anteroposterior radiograph may be used to "gap" the injured acromioclavicular joint to see whether there has been a third-degree sprain or to show an inferior laxity at the glenohumeral joint (Fig. 5–89). Equal weights of 9 kg (20 lbs) are tied to each hand of the patient to apply traction to the arms. If a third-degree acromioclavicular sprain has occurred, the coracoclavicular distance will increase step deformity.

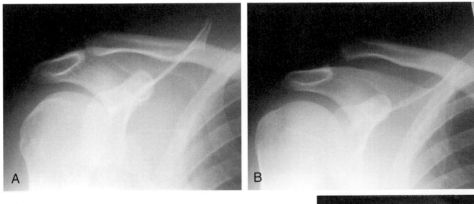

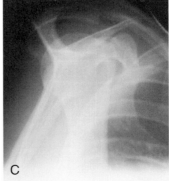

Figure 5–89
Stress radiograph for third-degree acromioclavicular sprain. (A) No stress. (B) Stress. Note the increase in the distance between the coracoid process and the clavicle. (C) Lateral view showing the complete separation.

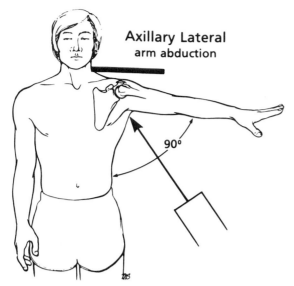

Figure 5–90
Axillary lateral view (From Rockwood, C.A., E.A. Szalay, R.J. Curtis, et al.: X-ray evaluation of shoulder problems. In Rockwood, C.A., and F.A. Matsen [eds.]: The Shoulder. Philadelphia, W.B. Saunders Co., 1990, p. 181.)

Axillary Lateral View. This view shows the relation of the humeral head to the glenoid. It is used to diagnose dislocations at the glenohumeral joint (Fig. 5–90) and to look for avulsion fractures of the glenoid or a Hill-Sachs lesion. It does, however, require the patient to be able to abduct the arm 70 to 90°. This view is the best for observation of the acromioclavicular joint. In addition, the examiner should note the relations of the glenoid cavity, humerus, scapula, and clavicle and any calcifications in the subscapularis, infraspinatus, or teres minor muscles.

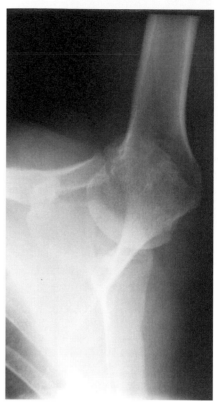

Figure 5–92
A Stryker notch view demonstrates a notch in the posterolateral aspect of the humeral head, representing a large Hill-Sachs lesion.

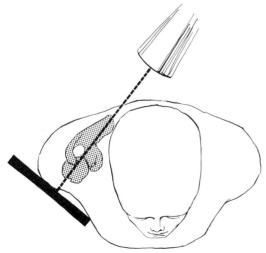

Figure 5–91
Positioning for transscapular (Y) lateral view. (From Rockwood, C.A., S.C. Thomas, and F.A. Matsen: Subluxations and dislocations about the glenohumeral joint. In Rockwood, C.A., D.P. Green, and R.W. Bucholz [eds.]: Fractures, 4th ed., vol. I. Philadelphia, Lippincott-Raven Publishers, 1996, p. 1225.)

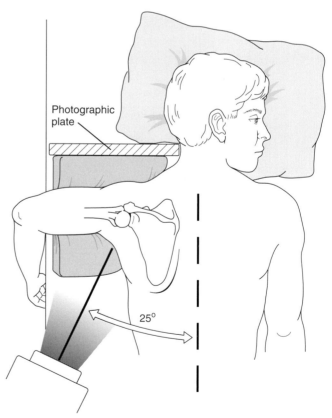

Figure 5–93
Positioning patient for West Point axillary view. The beam (bottom left) is also angled downward to form an angle of 25° from the horizontal plane.

Transscapular (**Y**) *Lateral View*. This view (Fig. 5–91) shows the position of the humerus relative to the glenoid and the acromion and coracoid processes. This view is the true lateral view of the scapula (see Fig. 5–83D and 5–83E).

Stryker Notch View. For this view, the patient lies supine with the arm forward flexed and the hand on top of the head. The radiograph centers on the coracoid process. This view is used to assess a Hill-Sachs lesion (Fig. 5–92) or a Bankart lesion.[97]

West Point View. The patient is positioned in prone (Fig. 5–93). This projection gives a good view of the glenoid to delineate glenoid fractures.[98]

Arch View. This lateral view is used to determine the width and height of the subacromial arch. It helps the examiner determine the type of acromial arch (Fig. 5–94).

Arthrography

An arthrogram of the shoulder is useful for delineating many of the soft tissues and recesses around the glenohumeral joint[99-101] (Figs. 5–95 and 5–96). For example, the glenohumeral joint can normally hold approximately

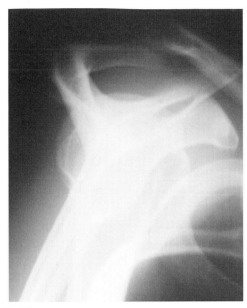

Figure 5–94

Arch view of acromioclavicular joint. Notice the separation of the clavicle and acromion. The view also shows the relation of the humerus to the glenoid (**Y** view).

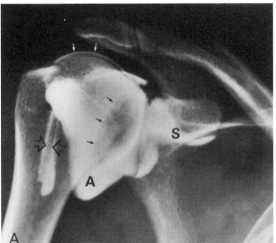
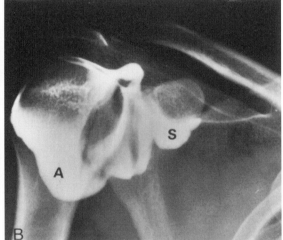
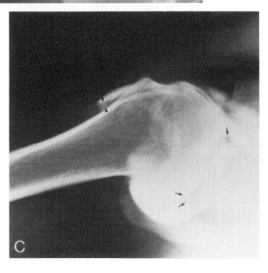

Figure 5–95

Normal single-contrast arthrogram. (A) Lateral rotation. (B) Medial rotation. A = axillary recess; S = subscapularis recess; *open arrows* = tendon of long head of biceps within biceps sheath. The humeral articular cartilage is coated with contrast medium (*white arrows*). There is no contrast agent in the subacromial-subdeltoid bursa. The defect created by the glenoid labrum (*black arrows*) is seen. Filling of the subscapularis recess is often poor on lateral rotation views because of bursal compression by the subscapularis muscle. In the axillary view (C), the anterior (*single arrow*), and posterior (*double arrows*) glenoid labral margins are seen. The biceps tendon (*arrowheads*) can be seen surrounded by contrast medium in the biceps tendon sheath. No contrast agent overlies the surgical neck of the humerus. (From Weissman, B.N.W., and C.B. Sledge: Orthopedic Radiology. Philadelphia, W.B. Saunders Co., 1986, p. 222.)

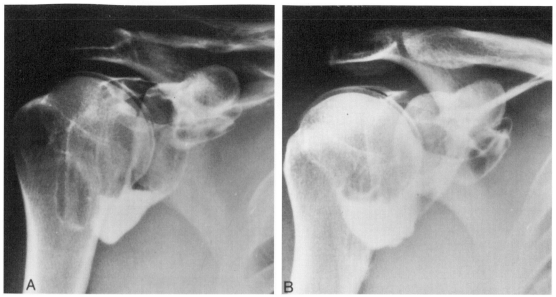

Figure 5–96

Normal double-contrast arthrogram. Upright views of the patient with a sandbag suspended from the wrist and the humerus in lateral rotation (A) and medial rotation (B) show the structures noted on single-contrast examination and allow better appreciation of the articular cartilages. (From Weissman, B.N.W., and C.B. Sledge: Orthopedic Radiology. Philadelphia, W.B. Saunders Co., 1986, p. 222.)

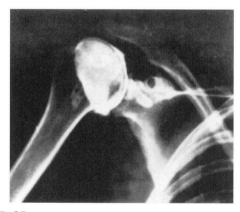

Figure 5–97

Typical arthrographic picture in adhesive capsulitis. Note the absence of a dependent axillary fold and poor filling of the biceps. (From Neviaser, J.S.: Arthrography of the shoulder joint: Study of the findings of adhesive capsulitis of the shoulder. J. Bone Joint Surg. Am. 44:1328, 1962.)

16 to 20 ml of solution. With adhesive capsulitis (idiopathic frozen shoulder), the amount the joint can hold may decrease to 5 to 10 ml. The arthrogram shows a decrease in the capacity of the joint and obliteration of the axillary fold. Also, there is an almost complete lack of filling of the subscapular bursa with adhesive capsulitis (Fig. 5–97). Tearing of any structures, such as the supraspinatus tendon and rotator cuff, may result in extravasation of the radiopaque dye.[102]

Computed Tomography

Computed tomography, especially when combined with radiopaque dye (**computed tomoarthrogram,** or CTA), is effective in diagnosing bone and soft-tissue anomalies and injuries around the shoulder, including tears of the labrum (Figs. 5–98, 5–99, and 5–100). This technique helps delineate capsular redundancy, glenoid rim abnormalities, and loose bodies.[103, 104]

Text continued on page 237

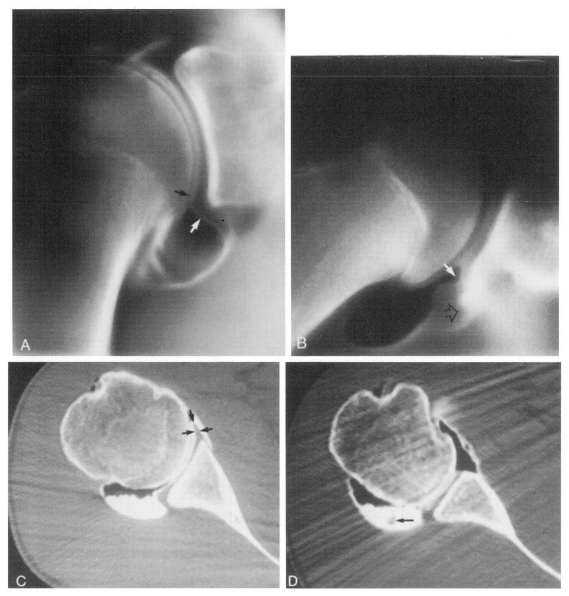

Figure 5-98

Tomogram and computed tomography scan of the glenoid labrum. (A) Normal glenoid labrum on posterior oblique double-contrast arthrotomography. Tomographic section through the anterior margin of the glenoid in the posterior oblique position shows smooth articular cartilage on the humeral head (*black arrow*) and glenoid and a smooth contour to the glenoid labrum (*white arrow*). (B) Abnormal glenoid labrum. Tomographic section shows a triangular defect in the labrum (*white arrow*). The bony margin of the glenoid is also irregular (*open arrow*). The patient had suffered a single anterior dislocation. (B, courtesy of Dr. Ethan Braunstein, Brigham and Women's Hospital, Boston, Massachusetts.) (C) Normal glenoid labrum on computed tomography after double-contrast arthrography. The sharply pointed anterior (*arrows*) and slightly rounder posterior margins of the labrum are well seen. (D) Computed tomoarthrogram shows absence of the anterior labrum and a loose body (*arrow*) posteriorly. (C and D, courtesy of Dr. Arthur Newberg, Boston, Massachusetts.) (From Weissman, B.N.W., and C.B. Sledge: Orthopedic Radiology. Philadelphia, W.B. Saunders Co., 1986, p. 257.)

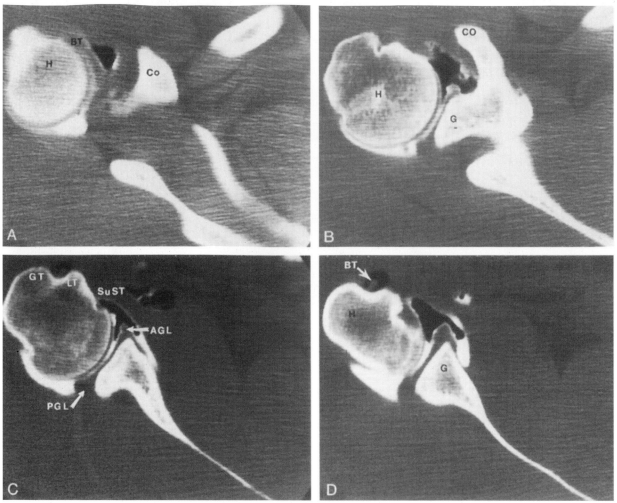

Figure 5-99

Normal shoulder, computed arthrotomography. Normal anatomy is demonstrated by computed arthrotomographic sections at the level of the bicipital tendon origin (A), the coracoid process (B), the subscapularis tendon (C), and the inferior joint level (D). Bt = bicipital tendon; H = humeral head; Co = coracoid process; G = glenoid process; GT = greater tuberosity; LT = lesser tuberosity; SuST = subscapularis tendon; AGL = anterior glenoid labrum; PGL = posterior glenoid labrum. (From De Lee, J.C., and D. Drez [eds.]: Orthopedic Sports Medicine: Principles and Practice. Philadelphia, W.B. Saunders Co., 1994, p. 721.)

Figure 5-100

Computed tomography scan of labral tear (*arrow*).

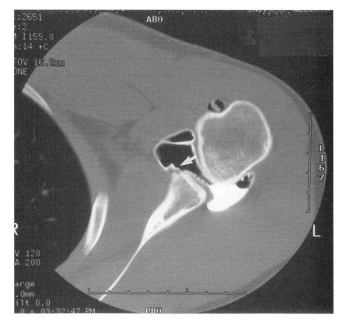

Magnetic Resonance Imaging

Magnetic resonance imaging (MRI) is proving to be useful in diagnosing soft-tissue injuries to the shoulder. It is possible to differentiate bursitis, tendinitis, and muscle strains, especially with injuries to the rotator cuff. It is also useful for differentially diagnosing causes of impingement syndrome. Labral tears and the state of bone marrow can also be diagnosed in the shoulder with the use of MRI (Figs. 5–101 through 5–104).

Angiography

In the case of thoracic outlet syndromes and other syndromes involving arterial impingement, angiograms are sometimes used to demonstrate blockage of the subclavian artery during certain moves (Fig. 5–105).

Text continued on page 240

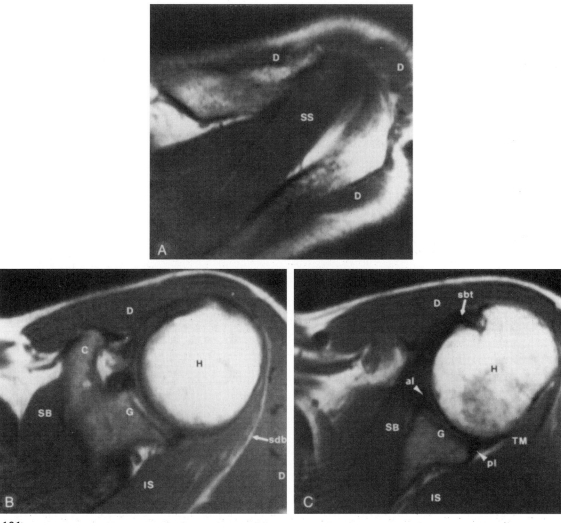

Figure 5–101
T1-weighted axial magnetic resonance images from cranial (A) to caudal (C). D = deltoid muscle; SS = supraspinatus muscle; C = coracoid; H = humerus; SB = subscapularis muscle; G = glenoid of scapula; sdb = subdeltoid-subacromial bursa; IS = infraspinatus muscle; sbt = subscapularis tendon; al = anterior labrum; TM = teres minor muscle; pl = posterior labrum. (From Meyer, S.J.F., and M.K. Dalinka: Magnetic resonance imaging of the shoulder. Orthop. Clin. North Am. 21:499, 1990.)

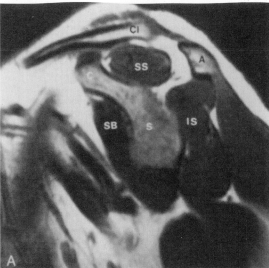

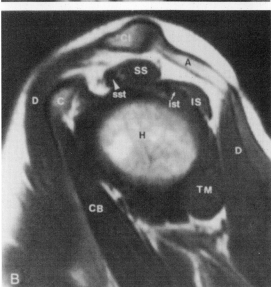

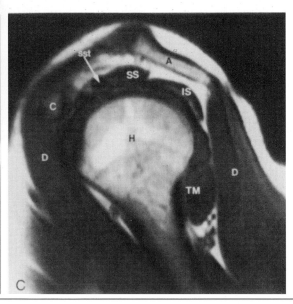

Figure 5–102

T1-weighted sagittal oblique magnetic resonance images from medial (A) to lateral (C). Cl = clavicle; C = coracoid; SS = supraspinatus muscle; A = acromion; SB = subscapularis muscle; s = scapula; IS = infraspinatus muscle; D = deltoid muscle; sst = supraspinatus tendon; ist = infraspinatus tendon; H = humerus; CB = coracobrachialis and biceps (short head) muscle; TM = teres minor muscle. (From Meyer, S.J.F., and M.K. Dalinka: Magnetic resonance imaging of the shoulder. Orthop. Clin. North Am. 21:501, 1990.)

Figure 5–103

Magnetic resonance imaging. (A) Midplane coronal oblique image (repetition time, 800 msec; echo time, 20 msec) of a normal shoulder, illustrating the intermediate signal intensity of the supraspinatus muscle (SSM) and the homogeneous signal void of the supraspinatus tendon (*black arrows*). The subacromial-subdeltoid peribursal fat plane, which has a high signal intensity, is also clearly defined (*open arrows*). (B) Anterior coronal oblique image (repetition time, 800 msec; echo time, 20 msec) showing tendinitis. Diffuse high signal intensity is seen in the distal portion of the supraspinatus tendon (*black arrow*). The tendon is neither thinned nor irregular. The peribursal fat plane is normal. A small acromial spur is present anteriorly (*open arrow*), and the capsule of the acromioclavicular joint is mildly hypertrophic (*white arrow*). (From Iannotti, J.P., M.B. Zlatkin, J.L. Esterhai, H.Y. Kressel, M.K. Dalinka, and K.P. Spindler: Magnetic resonance imaging of the shoulder. J. Bone Joint Surg. Am. 73:20, 1991.)

Figure 5–104

Midplane coronal oblique magnetic resonance images showing a small tear of the cuff. (A) On an image made with a short repetition time and echo time (800 and 20 msec), a small focus of discontinuity is seen in the supraspinatus tendon (*arrows*). The peribursal fat plane is lost. (B) On an image made with a long repetition time and echo time (2,500 and 70 msec), the intensity of the signal within the small region of discontinuity in the tendon is increased further (*black arrow*). High-signal-intensity fluid is seen in the subacromial-subdeltoid bursa (*white arrows*). (From Iannotti, J.P., M.B. Zlatkin, J.L. Esterhai, H.Y. Kresssel, M.K. Dalinka, and K.P. Spindler: Magnetic resonance imaging of the shoulder. J. Bone Joint Surg. Am. 73:20, 1991.)

Figure 5–105

Angiograms of the subclavian artery with the arm at rest (A) and abducted (B). Note complete obstruction of the subclavian artery (B). (From Brown, C.: Compressive, invasive referred pain to the shoulder. Clin. Orthop. 173:59, 1983.)

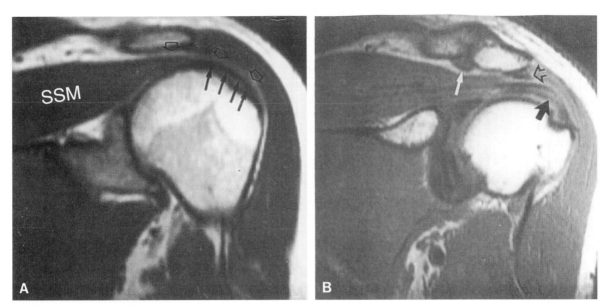

Figure 5–103
See legend on opposite page

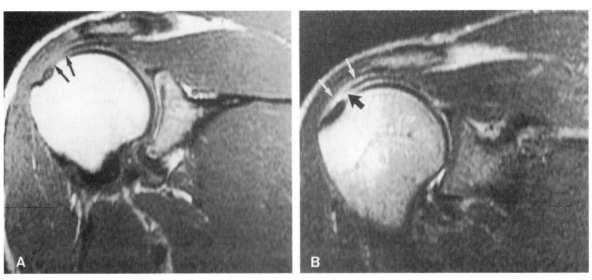

Figure 5–104
See legend on opposite page

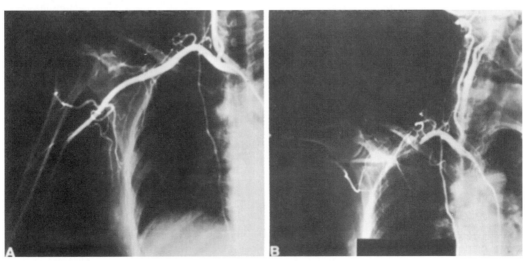

Figure 5–105
See legend on opposite page

Précis of the Shoulder Assessment*

History (sitting)
Observation (sitting or standing)
Examination
   Active movements (sitting or standing)
      Elevation through forward flexion of the arm
      Elevation through abduction of the arm
      Elevation through the plane of the scapula
         (scaption)
      Medial rotation of the arm
      Lateral rotation of the arm
      Adduction of the arm
      Horizontal adduction and abduction of the arm
      Circumduction of the arm
   Passive movements (sitting)
      Elevation through abduction of the arm
      Elevation through forward flexion of the arm
      Elevation through abduction at the glenohumeral
         joint only
      Lateral rotation of the arm
      Medial rotation of the arm
      Extension of the arm
      Adduction of the arm
      Horizontal adduction and abduction of the arm
   Special tests (sitting)
      Instability tests
         Load and shift test (anterior and posterior)
         Sulcus sign (multidirectional and inferior)
      Muscle/tendon pathology
         Speed's test (biceps)
         Yergason's test (biceps)
         Empty can test (supraspinatus)
         Lift-off sign (subscapularis)
      Impingement tests
         Neer test
         Hawkins-Kennedy test
      Thoracic outlet tests
         Roos test
         Wright test
         Costoclavicular syndrome test
   Reflexes and cutaneous distribution (sitting)
      Reflexes
      Sensory scan
      Peripheral nerves

      Axillary nerve
      Suprascapular nerve
      Musculocutaneous nerve
      Long thoracic nerve
      Spinal accessory nerve
   Palpation (sitting)
   Resisted isometric movements (supine lying)
      Forward flexion of the shoulder
      Extension of the shoulder
      Abduction of the shoulder
      Adduction of the shoulder
      Medial rotation of the shoulder
      Lateral rotation of the shoulder
      Flexion of the elbow
      Extension of the elbow
   Special tests (supine lying)
      Instability tests
         Crank (apprehension) and relocation tests
            (anterior)
         Norwood test (posterior)
         Push-pull test (posterior)
      Neurological tests
         Upper limb tension tests
   Joint play movements (supine lying)
      Backward glide of the humerus
      Forward glide of the humerus
      Lateral distraction of the humerus
      Long arm traction
      Backward glide of the humerus in abduction
      Anteroposterior and cephalocaudal movements of
         the clavicle at the acromioclavicular joint
      Anteroposterior and cephalocaudal movements of
         the clavicle at the sternoclavicular joint
      General movement of the scapula to determine
         mobility
   Diagnostic imaging

---

* The précis is shown in an order that limits the amount of movement that the patient has to do but ensures that all necessary structures are tested.

After any examination, the patient should be warned of the possibility of exacerbation of symptoms as a result of the assessment.

Case Studies

When doing these case studies, the examiner should list the appropriate questions to be asked and why they are being asked, what to look for and why, and what things should be tested and why. Depending on the answers of the patient (and the examiner should consider several different responses), several possible causes of the patient's problem may become evident (examples are given in parentheses). A differential diagnosis chart should be made up. The examiner can then decide how different diagnoses may affect the treatment plan. For example, a 23-year-old man comes to the clinic complaining of shoulder pain. He says that 2 days ago he was playing touch football. When his friend threw the ball, he reached for it, lost his balance, and fell on the tip of his shoulder but managed to hang onto the ball. How would you differentiate between acromioclavicular sprain and supraspinatus tendinitis? Table 5–11 demonstrates a differential diagnosis chart for the two conditions.

1. A 47-year-old man comes to you complaining of pain in the left shoulder. There is no history of overuse activity. The pain that occurs when he elevates his shoulder is referred to his neck and sometimes down the arm to his wrist. Describe your assessment plan for this patient (cervical spondylosis versus subacromial bursitis).

2. An 18-year-old woman recently had a Putti-Platt procedure for a recurring dislocation of the left shoulder. When you see her, her arm is still in a sling, but the surgeon wants you to begin treatment. Describe your assessment for this patient.

3. A 68-year-old woman comes to you complaining of pain and restricted ROM in the right shoulder. She tells you that 3 months ago she slipped on a rug on a tile floor and landed on her elbow. Both her elbow and shoulder hurt at

Table 5–11
Differential Diagnosis of Acromioclavicular Joint Sprain and Supraspinatus Tendinitis

	Acromioclavicular Joint Sprain	Supraspinatus Tendinitis
Observation	Step deformity (third-degree)	Normal
Active movement	Pain especially at extreme of motion (horizontal adduction and full elevation especially painful)	Pain on active movement, especially of abduction
Passive movement	Pain on horizontal adduction and elevation Muscle spasm end feel at end of ROM possible	No pain except if impingement occurs
Resisted isometric movement	May have some pain if test causes stress on joint (e.g., abduction)	Pain on abduction May have some pain on stabilizing for other movements
Functional tests	Pain on extremes of movement	Pain on any abduction movement
Special tests	Acromioclavicular shear test painful	Empty can test positive Impingement tests positive
Reflexes and cutaneous distribution	Negative	Negative
Joint play	Acromioclavicular joint play movements painful	Negative
Palpation	Acromioclavicular joint painful	Supraspinatus tendon and insertion tender or painful

ROM = range of motion.

that time. Describe your assessment plan for this patient (olecranon bursitis versus adhesive capsulitis).

4. A 5-year-old boy is brought to you by his parents. They state that he was running around the recreation room chasing a friend when he tripped over a stool and landed on his shoulder. He refuses to move his arm and is crying because the accident occurred only 2 hours ago. Describe your assessment plan for this patient (clavicular fracture versus humeral epiphyseal injury).

5. A 35-year-old female master swimmer comes to you complaining of shoulder pain. She states she has been swimming approximately 2,000 m per day in two training sessions; she recently increased her swimming from 1,500 m per day to get ready for a competition in 3 weeks. Describe your assessment plan for this patient (subacromial bursitis versus biceps tendinitis).

6. A 20-year-old male tennis player comes to you complaining that when he serves the ball, his arm "goes dead." He has had this problem for 3 weeks but never before. He has increased his training during the past month. Describe your assessment plan for this patient (thoracic outlet syndrome versus brachial plexus lesion).

7. A 15-year-old female competitive swimmer comes to you complaining of diffuse shoulder pain. She notices the problem most when she does the backstroke. She complains that her shoulder sometimes feels unstable when doing this stroke. Describe your assessment plan for this patient (anterior instability versus supraspinatus tendinitis).

8. A 48-year-old man comes to you complaining of neck and shoulder pain. He states that he has difficulty abducting his right arm. There is no history of trauma, but he remembers being in a car accident 10 years ago. Describe your assessment plan for this patient (cervical spondylosis versus adhesive capsulitis).

References

Cited References

1. Warner, J.J.: The gross anatomy of the joint surfaces, ligaments, labrum and capsule. In Matsen, F.A., F.H. Fu, and R.J. Hawkins (eds.): The Shoulder: A Balance of Mobility and Stability. Rosemont, Illinois, American Academy of Orthopedic Surgeons, 1993.
2. Hawkins, R.J., and G.W. Misamore: Overview of glenohumeral instability. In Hawkins, R.J., and G.W. Misamore (eds.): Shoulder Injuries in the Athlete. New York, Churchill Livingstone, 1996.
3. Kvitne, R.S., and F.W. Jobe: The diagnosis and treatment of anterior instability in the throwing athlete. Clin. Orthop. 291:107–123, 1993.
4. Cyriax, J.: Textbook of Orthopaedic Medicine, vol. 1: Diagnosis of Soft Tissue Lesions. London, Bailliere Tindall, 1982.
5. Nichols, H.M.: Anatomic structures of the thoracic outlet syndrome. Clin. Orthop. 51:17–25, 1967.
6. Riddell, D.H.: Thoracic outlet syndrome: Thoracic and vascular aspects. Clin. Orthop. 51:53–64, 1967.
7. Baker, C.L., and S.H. Liu: Neurovascular injuries to the shoulder. J. Orthop. Sports Phys. Ther. 18:360–364, 1993.
8. Priest, J.D., and D.A. Nagel: Tennis shoulder. Am. J. Sports Med. 4:28–42, 1976.
9. Hitchcock, H.H., and C.O. Bechtol: Painful shoulder: Observation on the role of the tendon of the long head of the biceps brachii in its causation. J. Bone Joint Surg. Am. 30:263–273, 1948.
10. Silliman, J.F., and M.T. Dean: Neurovascular injuries to the shoulder complex. J. Orthop. Sports Phys. Ther. 18:442–448, 1993.

11. Matsen, F.A., S.B. Lippitt, J.A. Sidles, and D.T. Harryman: Practical Evaluation and Management of the Shoulder. Philadelphia, W.B. Saunders Co., 1994.
12. Butters, K.P.: Nerve lesions of the shoulder. In De Lee, J.C., and D. Drez (eds.): Orthopedic Sports Medicine: Principles and Practice. Philadelphia, W.B. Saunders Co., 1994.
13. Bowen, M., and R. Warren: Ligamentous control of shoulder stability based on selective cutting and static translation. Clin. Sports Med. 10:757–782, 1991.
14. Makin, G.J., W.F. Brown, and G.C. Webers: C7 radiculopathy: Importance of scapular winging in clinical diagnosis. J. Neurol. Neurosurg. Psych. 49:640–644, 1986.
15. Saeed, M.A., P.F. Gatens, and S. Singh: Winging of the scapula. Am. Fam. Physician 24:139–143, 1981.
16. Fiddian, N.J., and R.J. King: The winged scapula. Clin. Orthop. 185:228–236, 1984.
17. Carson, W.C., W.W. Lovell, and T.E. Whitesides: Congenital elevation of the scapula. J. Bone Joint Surg. Am. 63:1199–1207, 1981.
18. Cavendish, M.E.: Congenital elevation of the scapula. J. Bone Joint Surg. Br. 54:395–408, 1972.
19. Perry, J.: Biomechanics of the shoulder. In Rowe, C.R. (ed.): The Shoulder. Edinburgh, Churchill Livingstone, 1988.
20. Kapandji, I.A.: The Physiology of Joints, vol. 1: Upper Limb. New York, Churchill Livingstone, 1970.
21. Boublik, M., and J.F. Silliman: History and physical examination. In Hawkins, R.J., and G.W. Misamore (eds.): Shoulder Injuries in the Athlete. New York, Churchill Livingstone, 1996.
22. Kessel, L., and M. Watson: The painful arc syndrome. J. Bone Joint Surg. Br. 59:166–172, 1977.
23. Reid, D.C.: The shoulder girdle: Its function as a unit in abduction. Physiotherapy 55:57–59, 1969.
24. Saha, S.K.: Mechanism of shoulder movements and a plea for the recognition of "zero position" of glenohumeral joint. Clin. Orthop. 173:3–10, 1983.
25. Davies, G.J., and S. Dickoff-Hoffman: Neuromuscular testing and rehabilitation of the shoulder complex. J. Orthop. Sports Phys. Ther. 18:449–458, 1993.
26. Poppen, N.K., and P.S. Walker: Normal and abnormal motion of the shoulder. J. Bone Joint Surg. Am. 58:195–201, 1976.
27. Kuhn, J.E., K.D. Plancher, and R.J. Hawkins: Scapular winging. J. Am. Acad. Orthop. Surg. 3:319–325, 1995.
28. Pagnani, M.J., B.J. Galinat, and R.F. Warren: Glenohumeral instability. In De Lee, J.C., and D. Drez (eds.): Orthopedic Sports Medicine: Principles and Practice. Philadelphia, W.B. Saunders Co., 1994.
29. Maitland, G.D.: Peripheral Manipulation. London, Butterworths, 1977.
30. Rowe, C.R.: Unusual shoulder conditions. In Rowe, C.R. (ed.): The Shoulder. Edinburgh, Churchill Livingstone, 1988.
31. MacConaill, M.A., and J.V. Basmajian: Muscles and Movements: A Basis for Human Kinesiology. Baltimore, Williams & Wilkins, 1969.
32. Corrigan, B., and G.D. Maitland: Practical Orthopedic Medicine. London, Butterworths, 1985.
33. Ellman, H., G. Hanker, and M. Bayer: Repair of the rotator cuff: End result study of factors influencing reconstruction. J. Bone Joint Surg. Am. 68:1136–1144, 1986.
34. Patte, D.: Directions for the use of the index of severity for painful and/or chronically disabled shoulder. Abstracts from First Open Congress, European Society of Surgery of the Shoulder and Elbow, Paris, France, 1987, pp. 36–41.
35. Rowe, C.R., D. Patel, and W.W. Southmayd: Bankart procedure: A long term end result study. J. Bone Joint Surg. Am. 60:1–6, 1978.
36. Macdonald, D.A.: The shoulder and elbow. In Pynsent, P.B., J.C. Fairbank, and A. Carr (eds.): Outcome Measures in Orthopedics, appendices 8-1 through 8-7. Oxford, Butterworth-Heinemann, 1993.
37. Constant, C.R., and A.H.G. Murley: A clinical method of functional assessment of the shoulder. Clin. Orthop. 214:160–164, 1987.
38. Lippitt, S.B., D.T. Harryman, and F.A. Matsen: A practical tool for evaluating function: The simple shoulder test. In Matsen, F.A., F.H. Fu, and R.J. Hawkins (eds.): The Shoulder: A Balance of Mobility and Stability. Rosemont, Illinois, American Academy of Orthopedic Surgeons, 1993.
39. Silliman, J.F., and R.J. Hawkins: Classification and physical diagnosis of instability of the shoulder. Clin. Orthop. 291:7–19, 1993.
40. Jobe, F.W., R.S. Kvitne, and C.E. Giangarra: Shoulder pain in the overhand or throwing athlete: The relationship of anterior instability and rotator cuff impingement. Orthop. Rev. 18:963–975, 1989.
41. Hawkins, R.J., and N.G. Mohtadi: Clinical evaluation of shoulder instability. Clin. J. Sports Med. 1:59–64, 1991.
42. Hawkins, R.J., and D.J. Bokor: Clinical evaluation of shoulder problems. In Rockwood, C.A., and F.A. Matsen (eds.): The Shoulder. Philadelphia, W.B. Saunders Co., 1990.
43. Kelley, M.J.: Evaluation of the shoulder. In Kelley, M.J., and W.A. Clark (eds.): Orthopedic Therapy of the Shoulder. Philadelphia, J.B. Lippincott Co., 1995.
44. Rockwood, C.A.: Subluxations and dislocations about the shoulder. In Rockwood, C.A., and D.P. Green (eds.): Fractures in Adults—I. Philadelphia, J.B. Lippincott Co., 1984.
45. Rowe, C.R.: Dislocations of the shoulder. In Rowe, C.R. (ed.): The Shoulder. Edinburgh, Churchill Livingstone, 1988.
46. Matsen, F.A., S.C. Thomas, and C.A. Rockwood: Glenohumeral instability. In Rockwood, C.A., and F.A. Matsen (eds.): The Shoulder. Philadelphia, W.B. Saunders Co., 1990.
47. Andrews, J.A., L.A. Timmerman, and K.E. Wilk: Baseball. In Pettrone, F.A. (ed.): Athletic Injuries of the Shoulder. New York, McGraw-Hill Inc., 1995.
48. Gerber, C., and R. Ganz: Clinical assessment of instability of the shoulder. J. Bone Joint Surg. Br. 66:551–556, 1984.
49. Protzman, R.R.: Anterior instability of the shoulder. J. Bone Joint Surg. Am. 62:909–918, 1980.
50. Davies, G.J., J.A. Gould, and R.L. Larson: Functional examination of the shoulder girdle. Phys. Sports Med. 9:82–104, 1981.
51. Leffert, R.D., and G. Gumley: The relationship between dead arm syndrome and thoracic outlet syndrome. Clin. Orthop. 223:20–31, 1987.
52. Evans, R.C.: Illustrated Essentials in Orthopedic Physical Assessment. St. Louis, Mosby–Year Book, 1994.
53. Pollack, R.G., and L.U. Bigliani: Recurrent posterior shoulder instability: Diagnosis and treatment. Clin. Orthop. 291:85–96, 1993.
54. Pagnani, M.J., and R.F. Warren: Multidirectional instability in the athlete. In Pettrone, F.A. (ed.): Athletic Injuries of the Shoulder. New York, McGraw-Hill Inc., 1995.
55. Norwood, L.A., and G.C. Terry: Shoulder posterior and subluxation. Am. J. Sports Med. 12:25–30, 1984.
56. Cofield, R.H., and J.F. Irving: Evaluation and classification of shoulder instability. Clin. Orthop. 223:32–43, 1987.
57. Helmig, P., J. Sojbjerg, P. Kjaersgaard-Andersen, S. Strange, and J. Ovesen: Distal humeral migration as a component of multidirectional shoulder instability. Clin. Orthop. 252:139–143, 1990.
58. Snyder, S.J., R.P. Karzel, W. Del Pizzo, R.D. Ferkel, and M.J. Friedman: SLAP lesions of the shoulder. Arthroscopy 6:274–279, 1990.
59. Andrews, J.R., and S. Gillogly: Physical examination of the shoulder in throwing athletes. In Zarins, B., J.R. Andrews, and W.G. Carson (eds.): Injuries to the Throwing Arm. Philadelphia, W.B. Saunders Co., 1985.
60. Walsh, D.A.: Shoulder evaluation of the throwing athlete. Sports Med. Update 4:24–27, 1989.
61. Kibler, W.B.: Clinical examination of the shoulder. In Pettrone, F.A. (ed.): Athletic Injuries of the Shoulder. New York, McGraw-Hill Inc., 1995.
62. Kibler, W.B.: Specificity and sensitivity of the anterior slide test in throwing athletes with superior glenoid labral tears. Arthroscopy 11:296–300, 1995.
63. Guidi, E.J., and J.D. Suckerman: Glenoid labral lesions. In Andrews, J.R., and K.E. Wilk (eds.): The Athlete's Shoulder. New York, Churchill Livingstone, 1994.

64. Kibler, W.B.: Role of the scapula in the overhead throwing motion. Contemp. Orthop. 22:525–533, 1991.

65. Petersen, S.A.: Arthritis and arthroplasty. In Hawkins, R.J., and G.W. Misamore (eds.): Shoulder Injuries in the Athlete. New York, Churchill Livingstone, 1996.

66. Ellman, H., E. Harris, and S.P. Kay: Early degenerative joint disease simulating impingement syndrome: arthroscopic findings. Arthroscopy 8:482–487, 1992.

67. Bell, R.H., and J.B. Noble: Biceps disorders. In Hawkins, R.J., and G.W. Misamore (eds.): Shoulder Injuries in the Athlete. New York, Churchill Livingstone, 1996.

68. Yergason, R.M.: Supination sign. J. Bone Joint Surg. 13:160, 1931.

69. Ludington, N.A.: Rupture of the long head of the biceps flexor cubiti muscle. Ann. Surg. 77:358–363, 1923.

70. Post, M.: Physical Examination of the Musculoskeletal System. Chicago, Year Book Medical Publishers Inc., 1987.

71. Lippman, R.K.: Frozen shoulder: Periarthritis, bicipital tendinitis. Arch. Surg. 7:283–296, 1943.

72. Jobe, F.W., and D.R. Moynes: Delineation of diagnostic criteria and a rehabilitation program for rotator cuff injuries. Am. J. Sports Med. 10:336–339, 1982.

73. Moseley, H.F.: Disorders of the shoulder. Clin. Symp. 12:1–30, 1960.

74. Gerber, C., and R.J. Krushell: Isolated ruptures of the tendon of the subscapularis muscle. J. Bone Joint Surg. Br. 73:389–394, 1991.

75. Neer, C.S., and R.P. Welsh: The shoulder in sports. Orthop. Clin. North Am. 8:583–591, 1977.

76. Hawkins, R.J., and J.C. Kennedy: Impingement syndrome in athletics. Am. J. Sports Med. 8:151–163, 1980.

77. Gerber, C., F. Terrier, and R. Ganz: The role of the coracoid process in the chronic impingement syndrome. J. Bone Joint Surg. Br. 67:703–708, 1985.

78. Miniaci, A., and P.A. Dowdy: Rotator cuff disorders. In Hawkins, R.J., and G.W. Misamore (eds.): Shoulder Injuries in the Athlete. New York, Churchill Livingstone, 1996.

79. Elvey, R.L.: The investigation of arm pain. In Grieve, G.P. (ed.): Modern Manual Therapy of the Vertebral Column. Edinburgh, Churchill Livingstone, 1986.

80. Butler, D.S.: Mobilisation of the Nervous System. Melbourne, Churchill Livingstone, 1991.

81. Roos, D.B.: Congenital anomalies associated with thoracic outlet syndrome. J. Surg. 132:771–778, 1976.

82. Liebenson, C.S.: Thoracic outlet syndrome: Diagnosis and conservative management. J. Manip. Physiol. Ther. 11:493–499, 1988.

83. Ribbe, E.B., S.H. Lindgren, and N.E. Norgren: Clinical diagnosis of thoracic outlet syndrome: Evaluation of patients with cervicobrachial symptoms. Manual Med. 2:82–85, 1986.

84. Sallstrom, J., and H. Schmidt: Cervicobrachial disorders in certain occupations, with special reference to compression in the thoracic outlet. Am. J. Ind. Med. 6:45–52, 1984.

85. Wright, I.S.: The neurovascular syndrome produced by hyperabduction of the arms. Am. Heart J. 29:1–19, 1945.

86. Adson, A.W., and J.R. Coffey: Cervical rib: A method of anterior approach for relief of symptoms by division of the scalenus anticus. Ann. Surg. 85:839–857, 1927.

87. Allen, E.V.: Thromboangiitis obliterans: Methods of diagnosis of chronic occlusive arterial lesions distal to the wrist with illustrative cases. Am. J. Med. Sci. 178:237–244, 1929.

88. Brown, C.: Compressive, invasive referred pain to the shoulder. Clin. Orthop. 173:55–62, 1983.

89. Kelly, J.J.: Neurologic problems in the athlete's shoulder. In Pettrone, F.A. (ed.): Athletic Injuries of the Shoulder. New York, McGraw-Hill Inc., 1995.

90. Pecina, M.M., J. Krmpotic-Nemanic, and A.D. Markiewitz: Tunnel Syndromes. Boca Raton, Florida, CRC Press, 1991.

91. Kaltenborn, E.M.: Mobilization of the Extremity Joints. Oslo, Olaf Norlis Bokhandle, 1980.

92. Magee, D.J., and D.C. Reid: Shoulder injuries. In Zachazewski, J.E., D.J. Magee, and W.S. Quillen (eds.): Athletic Injuries and Rehabilitation. Philadelphia, W.B. Saunders Co., 1996.

93. Epstein, R.E., M.E. Schweitzer, B.G. Frieman, J.M. Fenlin, and D.G. Mitchell: Hooked acromion: Prevalence on MR images of painful shoulders. Radiology 187:479–481, 1993.

94. Bigliani, L.U., J.B. Tucker, E.L. Flatow, L.J. Soslowsky, and V.C. Mow: The relationship of acromial architecture to rotator cuff disease. Clin. Sports Med. 10:823–838, 1991.

95. Weiner, D.S., and I. Macnab: Superior migration of the humeral head. J. Bone Joint Surg. Br. 52:524–527, 1970.

96. Bonutti, P.M., J.F. Norfray, R.J. Friedman, and B.M. Gomez: Kinematic MRI of the shoulder. J. Comput. Assist. Tomogr. 17:666–669, 1993.

97. Pavlov, H., R.F. Warren, C.B. Weiss, and D.M. Dines: The roentgenographic evaluation of anterior shoulder instability. Clin. Orthop. 194:153–158, 1985.

98. Engebretsen, L., and E.V. Craig: Radiologic features of shoulder instability. Clin. Orthop. 291:29–44, 1993.

99. Kernwein, G.A., B. Rosenberg, and W.R. Sneed: Arthrographic studies of the shoulder joint. J. Bone Joint Surg. Am. 39:1267–1279, 1957.

100. Neviaser, J.S.: Arthrography of the shoulder joint: Study of the findings of adhesive capsulitis of the shoulder. J. Bone Joint Surg. Am. 44:1321–1330, 1962.

101. Reeves, B.: Arthrography of the shoulder. J. Bone Joint Surg. Br. 48:424–435, 1966.

102. Nevasier, T.J., R.J. Nevasier, and J.S. Nevasier: Incomplete rotator cuff tears: A technique of diagnosis and treatment. Clin. Orthop. 306:12–16, 1994.

103. Collaghan, J.J., L.M. McNeish, J.P. Dehaven, C.G. Savory, and D.W. Polly: A prospective comparison study of double contrast computed tomography (CT) arthrography and arthroscopy of the shoulder. Am. J. Sports Med. 16:13–20, 1988.

104. Bernageau, J.: Roentgenographic assessment of the rotator cuff. Clin. Orthop. 254:87–91, 1990.

General References

Adams, J.C.: Outline of Orthopaedics. London, E & S Livingstone, 1968.

Albert, M.S., and M.J. Wooden: Isokinetic evaluation and treatment of the shoulder. In Physical Therapy of the Shoulder. Edinburgh, Churchill Livingstone, 1991.

American Orthopaedic Association: Manual of Orthopaedic Surgery. Chicago, 1972.

Anderson, J.E.: Grant's Atlas of Anatomy. Baltimore, Williams & Wilkins, 1983.

Arrigo, C.A., K.E. Wilk, and J.R. Andrews: Peak torque and maximum work repetition during isokinetic testing of the shoulder internal and external rotators. Isokin. Exerc. Sci. 4:171–175, 1994.

Bassett, L.W., R.H. Gold, and L.L. Seeger: MRI Atlas of the Musculoskeletal System. London, Martin Dunitz Ltd., 1989.

Bateman, J.E.: The Shoulder and Neck, 2nd ed. Philadelphia, W.B. Saunders Co., 1978.

Bateman, J.E.: Neurogenic painful conditions affecting the shoulder. Clin. Orthop. 173:44–54, 1983.

Beetham, W.P., H.F. Polley, C.H. Slocum, and W.F. Weaver: Physical Examination of the Joints. Philadelphia, W.B. Saunders Co., 1965.

Bennett, J.B., and T.L. Mehlhoff: Thoracic outlet syndrome. In De Lee, J.C., and D. Drez (eds.): Orthopedic Sports Medicine: Principles and Practice. Philadelphia, W.B. Saunders Co., 1994.

Bigg-Wither, G., and P. Kelly: Diagnostic imaging in musculoskeletal physiotherapy. In Refshauge, K., and E. Gass (eds.): Musculoskeletal Physiotherapy. Oxford, Butterworth-Heinemann, 1995.

Black, K.P., and J.A. Lombardo: Suprascapular nerve injuries with isolated paralysis of the infraspinatus. Am. J. Sports Med. 18:225–228, 1990.

Boissonnault, W.G., and S.C. Janos: Dysfunction, evaluation and treatment of the shoulder. In Donatelli, R.A., and M.J. Wooden (eds.): Orthopedic Physical Therapy. Edinburgh, Churchill Livingstone, 1989.

Booth, R.E., and J.P. Marvel: Differential diagnosis of shoulder pain. Orthop. Clin. North Am. 6:353–379, 1975.

Borsa, P.A., S.M. Lephart, M.S. Kocher, and S.P. Lephart: Functional assessment and rehabilitation of shoulder proprioception for glenohumeral instability. J. Sports Rehab. 3:84–104, 1994.

Boublik, M., and R.J. Hawkins: Clinical examination of the shoulder complex. J. Orthop. Sports Phys. Ther. 18:379–385, 1993.

Brown, L.P., S.L. Niehues, A. Harrah, P. Yavorsky, and H.P. Hirshman: Upper extremity range of motion and isokinetic strength of the internal and external shoulder rotators in major league baseball players. Am. J. Sports Med. 16:577–585, 1988.

Cailliet, R.: Shoulder Pain. Philadelphia, F.A. Davis Co., 1966.

Clarkson, H.M., and G.B. Gilewich: Musculoskeletal Assessment: Joint Range of Motion and Manual Muscle Strength. Philadelphia, Williams & Wilkins, 1989.

Cofield, R.H., J.P. Nessler, and R. Weinstabl: Diagnosis of shoulder instability by examination under anesthesia. Clin. Orthop. 291:45–53, 1993.

Collins, K., and K. Peterson: Case report: Diagnosing suprascapular neuropathy. Pinpointing a shoulder injury site. Phys. Sportsmed. 22:59–69, 1994.

Cone, R.O.: Imaging the glenohumeral joint. In De Lee, J.C., and D. Drez (eds.): Orthopedic Sports Medicine: Principles and Practice. Philadelphia, W.B. Saunders Co., 1994.

De Laat, E.A., C.P. Visser, L.N. Coene, P.V. Pahlplatz, and D.L. Tavy: Nerve lesions in primary shoulder dislocations and humeral neck fractures. J. Bone Joint Surg. Br. 76:381–383, 1994.

Dempster, W.T.: Mechanisms of shoulder movement. Arch. Phys. Med. Rehabil. 46:49–70, 1965.

Deutsch, A.L., D. Resnick, and J.H. Mink: Computed tomography of the glenohumeral and sternoclavicular joints. Orthop. Clin. North Am. 16:497–511, 1985.

Drez, D.: Suprascapular neuropathy in the differential diagnosis of rotator cuff injuries. Am. J. Sports Med. 4:43–45, 1976.

Drye, C., and J.E. Zachazewski: Peripheral nerve injuries. In Zachazewski, J.E., D.J. Magee, and W.S. Quillen (eds.): Athletic Injuries and Rehabilitation. Philadelphia, W.B. Saunders Co., 1996.

Duralde, X.A., and L.U. Bigliani: Neurologic disorders. In Hawkins, R.J., and G.W. Misamore (eds.): Shoulder Injuries in the Athlete. New York, Churchill Livingstone, 1996.

Fallcel, J.E., T.C. Murphy, and T.R. Malone: Shoulder injuries: Sports Injury Management. Baltimore, Williams & Wilkins, 1988.

Ferreti, A., G. Cerullo, and G. Russo: Suprascapular neuropathy in volleyball players. J. Bone Joint Surg. Am. 69:260–263, 1987.

Forrester, D.M., and J.C. Brown: The Radiology of Joint Disease. Philadelphia, W.B Saunders Co., 1987.

Foster, C.R.: Multidirectional instability of the shoulder in the athlete. Clin. Sports Med. 2:355–368, 1983.

Fowler, P.J.: Swimming. In Fu, F.H., and D.A. Stone (eds.): Sports Injuries: Mechanisms, Prevention, Treatment. Baltimore, Williams & Wilkins, 1994.

France, M.K.: Anatomy and biomechanics of the shoulder. In Donatelli, R.A. (ed.): Physical Therapy of the Shoulder. Edinburgh, Churchill Livingstone, 1991.

Francis. W.R.: Thoracic outlet syndrome. In Camins, M.B., and P.F. O'Leary (eds.): Disorders of the Cervical Spine. Baltimore, Williams & Wilkins, 1992.

Fritts, H.M., and C.R. Cooper: Magnetic resonance and shoulder imaging. In Hawkins, R.J., and G.W. Misamore (eds.): Shoulder Injuries in the Athlete. New York, Churchill Livingstone, 1996.

Garrick, J.G., and D.R. Webb: Sports Injuries: Diagnosis and Management. Philadelphia, W.B. Saunders Co., 1990.

Gartland, J.J.: Fundamentals of Orthopaedics. Philadelphia, W.B. Saunders Co., 1979.

Gerber, C.: Integrated scoring systems for the functional assessment of the shoulder. In Matsen, F.A., F.H. Fu, and R.J. Hawkins (eds.): The Shoulder: A Balance of Mobility and Stability. Rosemont, Illinois, American Academy of Orthopedic Surgeons, 1993.

Gilliman, J.F., and R.J. Hawkins: Clinical examination of the shoulder complex. In Andrews, J.R., and K.E. Wilk (eds.): The Athlete's Shoulder. New York, Churchill Livingstone, 1994.

Greenfield, B.H., R. Donatelli, M.J. Wooden, and J. Wilkes: Isokinetic evaluation of shoulder rotational strength between the plane of the scapula and the frontal plane. Am. J. Sports Med. 18:124–128, 1990.

Gregg, J.R., D. Labosky, M. Harty, et al.: Serratus anterior paralysis in the young athlete. J. Bone Joint Surg. Am. 61:825–832, 1997.

Halback, J.W., and R.T. Tank: The shoulder. In Gould, J.A. (ed.): Orthopedic and Sports Physical Therapy. St. Louis, C.V. Mosby Co., 1990.

Harryman, D.T., J.A. Sidles, J.M. Clark, K.J. McQuade, T.D. Gibb, and F.A. Matsen: Translation of the humeral head on the glenoid with passive glenohumeral motion. J. Bone Joint Surg. Am. 72:1334–1343, 1990.

Hawkins, R.J.: Musculoskeletal Examination. St. Louis, Mosby–Year Book Inc., 1995.

Hawkins, R.J., and J.S. Abrams: Impingement syndrome in the absence of rotator cuff tear (stage 1 and 2). Orthop. Clin. North Am. 18:373–382, 1987.

Hawkins, R.J., and P.E. Hobeika: Impingement syndrome in the athletic shoulder. Clin. Sports Med. 2:391–405, 1983.

Hershman, E.B., A.J. Wilbourn, and J.A. Bergfeld: Acute brachial neuropathy in athletes. Am. J. Sports Med. 17:655–659, 1989.

Hirayama, T., and Y. Takemitsa: Compression of the suprascapular nerve by a ganglion at the suprascapular notch. Clin. Orthop. 155:95–96, 1981.

Hollinshead, W.H., and D.B. Jenkins: Functional Anatomy of the Limb and Back. Philadelphia, W.B. Saunders Co., 1981.

Hoppenfeld, S.: Physical Examination of the Spine and Extremities. New York, Appleton-Century-Crofts, 1976.

Iannotti, J.P.: Lesions of the rotator cuff: pathology and pathogenesis. In Matsen, F.A., F.H. Fu, and R.J. Hawkins (eds.): The Shoulder: A Balance of Mobility and Stability. Rosemont, Illinois, American Academy of Orthopedic Surgeons, 1993.

Iannotti, J.P., M.B. Zlatkin, J.L. Esterhai, H.Y. Kressel, M.K. Dalinka, and K.P. Spindler: Magnetic resonance imaging of the shoulder. J. Bone Joint Surg. Am. 73:17–29, 1991.

Jobe, F.W., and J.P. Bradley: Rotator cuff injuries in basketball. Sports Med. 6:378–389, 1988.

Jobe, F.W., and C.M. Jobe: Painful athletic injuries of the shoulder. Clin. Orthop. 173:117–124, 1983.

Judge, R.D., G.D. Zuidema, and F.T. Fitzgerald: Clinical Diagnosis: A Physiological Approach. Boston, Little, Brown & Co., 1982.

Keskula, D.R., and D.H. Perrin: Effect of test protocol on torque production of the rotators of the shoulder. Isokin. Exerc. Sci. 4:176–181, 1994.

Leffert, R.D.: Clinical diagnoses, testing and electromyographic study in brachial plexus traction injuries. Clin. Orthop. 237:24–31, 1988.

Lippman, R.K.: Frozen shoulder; periarthritis; bicipital tenosynovitis. Arch. Surg. 47:283–296, 1943.

Maday, M.G., C.D. Harner, and J.J. Warner: Shoulder injuries. In Fu, F.H., and D.A. Stone (eds.): Sports Injuries: Mechanisms, Prevention, Treatment. Baltimore, Williams & Wilkins, 1994.

Maki, N.J.: Cineradiographic studies with shoulder instabilities. Am. J. Sports Med. 16:362–364, 1988.

Malerba, J.L., M.L. Adam, B.A. Harris, and D.E. Krebs: Reliability of dynamic and isometric testing of shoulder external and internal rotators. J. Orthop. Sports Phys. Ther. 18:543–552, 1993.

McIlveen, S.J., X.A. Duralde, D.F. D'Alessandro, and L.U. Bigliani: Isolated nerve injuries about the shoulder. Clin. Orthop. 306:54–63, 1994.

McMaster, W.C.: Painful shoulder in swimmers: A diagnostic challenge. Phys. Sportsmed. 14:108–122, 1986.

Meyer, S.J.F., and M.K. Dalinka: Magnetic resonance imaging of the shoulder. Orthop. Clin. North Am. 21:497–513, 1990.

Moran, C.A., and S.R. Saunders: Evaluation of the shoulder: A sequential approach. In Donatelli, R.A. (ed.): Physical Therapy of the Shoulder. Edinburgh, Churchill Livingstone, 1991.

Naffziger, H.C., and W.T. Grant: Neuritis of the brachial plexus mechanical in origin: The scalenus syndrome. Clin. Orthop. 51:7–15, 1967.

Neer, C.S.: Anterior acromioplasty for the chronic impingement syndrome in the shoulder. J. Bone Joint Surg. Am. 54:41–50, 1972.

Neer, C.S.: Impingement lesions. Clin. Orthop. 173:70–77, 1983.

Neer, C.S., and C.R. Foster: Inferior capsular shift for involuntary inferior and multidirectional instability of the shoulder. J. Bone Joint Surg. Am. 62:897–908, 1980.

Neiers, L., and T.W. Worrell: Assessment of scapular position. J. Sports Rehab. 2:20–25, 1993.

Neviaser, J.S.: Adhesive capsulitis and the stiff and painful shoulder. Orthop. Clin. North Am. 11:327–331, 1980.

Neviaser, R.J.: Anatomic considerations and examination of the shoulder. Orthop. Clin. North Am. 11:187–195, 1980.

Neviaser, R.J.: Lesions of the biceps and tendinitis of the shoulder. Orthop. Clin. North Am. 11:343–348, 1980.

Neviaser, R.J.: Painful conditions affecting the shoulder. Clin. Orthop. 173:63–69, 1983.

Neviaser, R.J.: Tears of the rotator cuff. Orthop. Clin. North Am. 11:295–306, 1980.

Norris, T.R.: History and physical examination of the shoulder. In Nicholas, J.A., and E.B. Hershman (eds.): The Upper Extremity in Sports Medicine. St. Louis, C.V. Mosby Co., 1990.

Norris, T.R., and A. Green: Imaging modalities in the evaluation of shoulder disorders. In Matsen, F.A., F.H. Fu, and R.J. Hawkins (eds.): The Shoulder: A Balance of Mobility and Stability. Rosemont, Illinois, American Academy of Orthopedic Surgeons, 1993.

O'Donoghue, D.H.: Treatment of Injuries to Athletes, 4th ed. Philadelphia, W.B. Saunders Co., 1984.

O'Driscoll, S.W.: Atraumatic instability: pathology and pathogenesis. In Matsen, F.A., F.H. Fu, and R.J. Hawkins (eds.): The Shoulder: A Balance of Mobility and Stability. Rosemont, Illinois, American Academy of Orthopedic Surgeons, 1993.

Overton, L.M.: The causes of pain in the upper extremities: A differential diagnosis study. Clin. Orthop. 51:27–44, 1967.

Palmer, M.L., and M. Epler: Clinical Assessment Procedures in Physical Therapy. Philadelphia, J.B. Lippincott Co., 1990.

Patla, C.E.: Upper extremity. In Payton, O.D., R.P.D. Fabio, S.V. Paris, et al. (eds.): Manual of Physical Therapy. Edinburgh, Churchill Livingstone, 1989.

Pellecchia, G.L., J. Paolino, and J. Connell: Intertester reliability of the Cyriax evaluation assessing patients with shoulder pain. J. Orthop. Sports Phys. Ther. 23:34–38, 1996.

Perry, J.: Anatomy and biomechanics of the shoulder in throwing, swimming, gymnastics, and tennis. Clin. Sports Med. 2:247–270, 1983.

Pink, M., J. Perry, A. Browne, M.L. Scovazzo, and J. Kerrigan: The normal shoulder during freestyle swimming: An electromyographic and cinemagraphic analysis of 12 muscles. Am. J. Sports Med. 19:569–576, 1991.

Pollack, R.G., and L.U. Bigliani: Glenohumeral instability: Evaluation and treatment. J. Am. Acad. Orthop. Surg. 1:24–32, 1993.

Post, M., and J. Mayer: Suprascapular nerve entrapment: Diagnosis and treatment. Clin. Orthop. 223:126–131, 1987.

Post, M., R. Silver, and M. Singh: Rotator cuff tear: Diagnosis and treatment. Clin. Orthop. 173:78–91, 1983.

Rathburn, J.B., and I. Macnab: The microvascular pattern of the rotator cuff. J. Bone Joint Surg. Br. 52:540–553, 1970.

Recht, M.P., and D. Resnick: Magnetic resonance imaging studies of the shoulder: Diagnosis of lesions of the rotator cuff. J. Bone Joint Surg. Am. 75:1244–1253, 1993.

Reid, D.C.: Focusing the diagnosis of shoulder pain. Pearls of practice. Phys. Sportsmed. 22:28–43, 1994.

Reid, D.C.: Sports Injury Assessment and Rehabilitation. New York, Churchill Livingstone, 1992.

Reid, D.C.: Functional Anatomy and Joint Mobilization. Edmonton, University of Alberta Press, 1970.

Ringel, S.P., M. Treihaft, M. Carry, R. Fisher, and P. Jacobs: Suprascapular neuropathy in pitchers. Am. J. Sports Med. 18:80–86, 1990.

Rockwood, C.A., E.A. Szalay, R.J. Curtis, D.C. Young, and S.P. Kay: X-ray evaluation of shoulder problems. In Rockwood, C.A., and F.A. Masten (eds.): The Shoulder. Philadelphia, W.B. Saunders Co., 1990.

Rowe, C.R.: Examination of the shoulder. In Rowe, C.R. (ed.): The Shoulder. Edinburgh, Churchill Livingstone, 1988.

Rowe, C.R.: Recurrent transient anterior subluxation of the shoulder: The "dead arm" syndrome. Clin. Orthop. 223:11–19, 1987.

St. John's Ambulance. First Aid. Ottawa, The Runge Press Ltd., 1963.

Sarrafian, S.K.: Gross and functional anatomy of the shoulder. Clin. Orthop. 173:11–19, 1983.

Schenkman, M., and V.R. de Cartaya: Kinesiology of the shoulder complex. J. Orthop. Sports Phys. Ther. 8:438–450, 1987.

Schob, C.J.: Suprascapular nerve entrapment. In Andrews, J.R., and K.E. Wilk (eds.): The Athlete's Shoulder. New York, Churchill Livingstone, 1994.

Schwartz, E., R.F. Warren, S.J. O'Brien, and J. Fronek: Posterior shoulder instability. Orthop. Clin. North Am. 18:409–419, 1987.

Schwartz, M.L.: Diagnostic imaging of the shoulder complex. In Andrews, J.R., and K.E. Wilk (eds.): The Athlete's Shoulder. New York, Churchill Livingstone, 1994.

Scovazzo, M.L., A. Browne, M. Pink, F.W. Jobe, and J. Kerrigan: The painful shoulder during freestyle swimming: An electromyographic cinematographic analysis of 12 muscles. Am. J. Sports Med. 19:577–582, 1991.

Seeger, L.L.: Magnetic resonance imaging of the shoulder. Clin. Orthop. 244:48–59, 1989.

Skurja, M., and J.H. Monlux: Case studies: The suprascapular nerve and shoulder dysfunction. J. Orthop. Sports Phys. Ther. 6:254–258, 1985.

Sobush, D.C., G.G. Simoneau, K.E. Dietz, J.A. Levene, R.E. Grossman, and W.B. Smith: The Lennie test for measuring scapular position in healthy young adult females: A reliability and validity study. J. Orthop. Sports Phys. Ther. 23:39–50, 1996.

Souza, T.A.: Sports Injuries of the Shoulder. New York, Churchill Livingstone, 1994.

Speer, K.P., and W.E. Garrett: Muscular control of motion and stability about the pectoral girdle. In Matsen, F.A., F.H. Fu, and R.J. Hawkins (eds.): The Shoulder: A Balance of Mobility and Stability. Rosemont, Illinois, American Academy of Orthopedic Surgeons, 1993.

Speer, K.P., B. Ghelman, and R.F. Warren: Computed tomography: Arthrography of the shoulder. In Andrews, J.R., and K.E. Wilk (eds.): The Athlete's Shoulder. New York, Churchill Livingstone, 1994.

Speer, K.P., J.A. Hannafin, D.W. Altchek, and R.F. Warren: An evaluation of the shoulder relocation test. Am. J. Sports Med. 22:177–183, 1994.

Starkey, C., and J. Ryan: Evaluation of Orthopedic and Athletic Injuries. Philadelphia, F.A. Davis, 1996.

Tank, R., and J. Halbach: Physical therapy evaluation of the shoulder complex in athletes. J. Orthop. Sports Phys. Ther. 3:108–120, 1982.

Tardiff, G.S.: Nerve injuries, testing and treatment tractics. Phys. Sportsmed. 23:61–72, 1995.

Tata, G.E., L. Ng, and J.F. Kramer: Shoulder antagonistic strength ratios during concentric and eccentric muscle actions in the scapular plane. J. Orthop. Sports Phys. Ther. 18:654–660, 1993.

Thompson, R.C., W. Schneider, and T. Kennedy: Entrapment neuropathy of the inferior branch of the suprascapular nerve by ganglion. Clin. Orthop. 166:185–187, 1982.

Tibone, J.E., and J.P. Bradley: Evaluation of treatment outcomes for the athlete's shoulder. *In* Matsen, F.A., F.H. Fu, and R.J. Hawkins (eds.): The Shoulder: A Balance of Mobility and Stability. Rosemont, Illinois, American Academy of Orthopedic Surgeons, 1993.

Travell, J.G., and D.G. Simons: Myofascial Pain and Dysfunction: The Trigger Point Manual. Baltimore, Williams & Wilkins, 1983.

Vastamaki, M., and H. Goransson: Suprascapular nerve entrapment. Clin. Orthop. 297:135–143, 1993.

Wadsworth, C.T.: Manual Examination and Treatment of the Spine and Extremities. Baltimore, Williams & Wilkins, 1988.

Warner, J.J., R.J. Krushell, A. Masquelet, and C. Gerber: Anatomy and relationships of the suprascapular nerve: Anatomical constraints to mobilization of the supraspinatus and infraspinatus muscles in the management of massive rotator cuff tears. J. Bone Joint Surg. Am. 74:36–45, 1992.

Wechsler, L.R., and N.A. Busis: Sports neurology. *In* Fu, F.H., and D.A. Stone (eds.): Sports Injuries: Mechanisms, Prevention, Treatment. Baltimore, Williams & Wilkins, 1994.

Weissman, B.N.W., and C.B. Sledge: Orthopedic Radiology. Philadelphia, W.B. Saunders Co., 1986.

White, S.M., and C.M. Witten: Long thoracic nerve palsy in a professional ballet dancer. Am. J. Sports Med. 21:626–628, 1993.

Wiles, P., and R. Sweetnam: Essentials or Orthopaedics. London, J.A. Churchill Ltd., 1965.

Williams, A., R. Evans, and P.D. Shirley: Imaging of Sports Injuries. London, Bailliere Tindall, 1989.

Williams, G.R., and J.P. Iannotti: Diagnostic tests and surgical techniques. *In* Kelley, M.J., and W.A. Clark (eds.): Orthopedic Therapy of the Shoulder. Philadelphia, J.B. Lippincott Co., 1995.

Wilson, R.W.: Entrapment neuropathy of the inferior suprascapular nerve in a weight lifter. J. Sports Rehab. 2:208–210, 1993.

Woo, S.L., P.J. McMahon, R.E. Debski, F.H. Fu, and G.L. Blomstrom: Factors limiting and defining shoulder motion: what keeps it from going farther? *In* Matsen, F.A., F.H. Fu, and R.J. Hawkins (eds.): The Shoulder: A Balance of Mobility and Stability. Rosemont, Illinois, American Academy of Orthopedic Surgeons, 1993.

Wood, V.E., and J. Brondi: Double crush nerve compression in thoracic outlet syndrome. J. Bone Joint Surg. Am. 72:85–87, 1990.

Wood, V.E., R. Twito, and J.M. Verska: Thoracic outlet syndrome. Orthop. Clin. North Am. 19:131–146, 1988.

Yocum, L.A.: Assessing the shoulder: History, physical examination, differential diagnosis, and special tests used. Clin. Sports Med. 2:281–289, 1983.

Yoon, T.N., M. Grabois, and M. Guillen: Suprascapular nerve injury following trauma to the shoulder. J. Trauma 21:652–655, 1981.

Zarins, B.: Anterior subluxation and dislocation of the shoulder. *In* AAOSS on Upper Extremity Injuries in Athletes. St. Louis, C.V. Mosby Co., 1986.

Zarins, B., M.S. McMahon, and C.R. Rowe: Diagnosis and treatment of traumatic anterior instability of the shoulder. Clin. Orthop. 291:75–84, 1993.

Zemek, M.J., and D.J. Magee: Comparison of glenohumeral joint laxity in elite and recreational swimmers. Clin. J. Sports Med. 6:40–47, 1996.

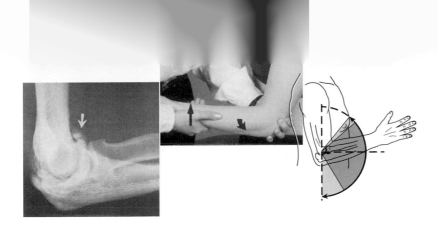

6

Elbow

The elbow's primary role in the upper limb complex is to help position the hand in the appropriate location to perform its function. Once the shoulder has positioned the hand in a gross fashion, the elbow allows for adjustments in height and length of the limb to position the hand correctly. In addition, the forearm rotates, in part at the elbow, to place the hand in the most effective position to perform its function.

Applied Anatomy

The elbow consists of a complex set of joints that require careful assessment for proper treatment. The treatment must be geared to the pathology of the condition, because the joint responds poorly to trauma, harsh treatment, or incorrect treatment.

Because they are closely related, the joints of the elbow complex make up a compound synovial joint, with injury to any one part affecting the other components as well. The elbow articulations are made up of the ulnohumeral joint and the radiohumeral joint. In addition, the complexity and intricate relation of the elbow articulations is further increased by the superior radioulnar joint, which has continuity with the elbow articulations. These three joints make up the **cubital articulations**. The capsule and joint cavity are continuous for all three joints. The combination of these joints allows two degrees of freedom at the elbow. The trochlear joint allows one degree of freedom (flexion-extension), and the radiohumeral and superior radioulnar joints allow the other degree of freedom (rotation).

The **ulnohumeral** or **trochlear joint** is found between the trochlea of the humerus and the trochlear notch of the ulna and is classified as a uniaxial hinge joint. The bones of this joint are shaped so that the axis of movement is not horizontal but instead passes downward and medially, going through an arc of movement. This position leads to the carrying angle at the elbow (Fig.

6–1). The resting position of this joint is with the elbow flexed to 70° and the forearm supinated 10°. The neutral position (0°) is midway between supination and pronation in the "thumb-up" position (Fig. 6–2). The capsular

Ulnohumeral (Trochlear) Joint

Resting position:	70° elbow flexion, 10° supination
Close packed position:	Extension with supination
Capsular pattern:	Flexion, extension

pattern is flexion more limited than extension, and the close packed position is extension with the forearm in supination. On full extension, the medial part of the olecranon process is not in contact with the trochlea; on full flexion, the lateral part of the olecranon process is not in contact with the trochlea. This change allows the side-to-side joint play movement necessary for supination and pronation. A small amount of rotation occurs at this joint. In early flexion, 5° of medial rotation occurs; in late flexion, 5° of lateral rotation occurs.

The **radiohumeral joint** is a uniaxial hinge joint between the capitulum of the humerus and the head of the radius. The resting position is with the elbow fully extended and the forearm fully supinated. The close packed position of the joint is with the elbow flexed to 90° and the forearm supinated 5°. As with the trochlear joint, the capsular pattern is flexion more limited than extension.

Radiohumeral Joint

Resting position:	Full extension and full supination
Close packed position:	Elbow flexed to 90°, forearm supinated to 5°
Capsular pattern:	Flexion, extension

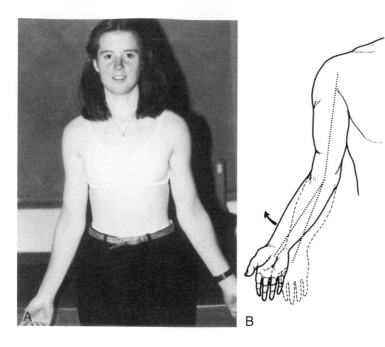

Figure 6–1
(A) Carrying angle of the elbow. (B) Excessive valgus carrying angle. (B, American Orthopaedic Association: Manual of Orthopaedic Surgery. Chicago, 1979, p. 146.)

The ulnohumeral and radiohumeral joints are supported medially by the **ulnar collateral ligament**, a fan-shaped structure, and laterally by the **radial collateral ligament**, a cordlike structure. The ulnar collateral ligament has two parts, which along with the flexor carpi ulnaris muscle form the **cubital tunnel** through which passes the ulnar nerve (Fig. 6–3). Any injury or blow to the area or injury that increases the carrying angle puts an abnormal stress on the nerve as it passes through the tunnel. This can lead to problems such as **tardy ulnar palsy**, the symptoms of which can occur many years after the original injury and may be caused by the "double crush" phenomena of a cubital tunnel problem combined with a cervical spine problem.

The **superior radioulnar joint** is a uniaxial pivot joint.

The head of the radius is held in proper relation to the ulna and humerus by the **annular ligament**, which makes up four fifths of the joint. The resting position of this joint is supination of 35° and elbow flexion of 70°. The close packed position is supination of 5°. The capsular pattern of this joint is equal limitation of supination and pronation.

Superior Radioulnar Joint

Resting position:	35° supination, 70° elbow flexion
Close packed position:	5° supination
Capsular pattern:	Equal limitation of supination and pronation

Figure 6–2
"Thumb-up" or neutral (zero) position between supination and pronation.

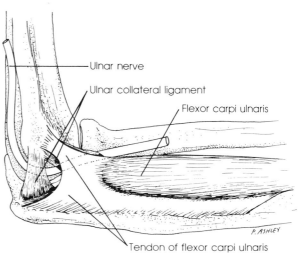

Figure 6–3
Cubital tunnel, through which passes the ulnar nerve.

The three elbow articulations are innervated by branches from the musculocutaneous, median, ulnar, and radial nerves.

The **middle radioulnar articulation** is not a true joint but is made up of the radius and ulna and the **interosseous membrane** between the two bones. The interosseous membrane is tense only midway between supination and pronation (neutral position). Although this "joint" is not part of the elbow joint complex, it is affected by injury to the elbow joints; conversely, injury to this area can affect the mechanics of the elbow articulations. The interosseous membrane prevents proximal displacement of the radius on the ulna. The displacement is most likely to occur with pushing movements. The **oblique cord** connects the radius and ulna, running from the lateral side of the **ulnar tuberosity** to the radius slightly below the **radial tuberosity**. Its fibers run at right angles to those of the interosseous membrane. The cord assists in preventing displacement of the radius on the ulna, especially during movements involving pulling.

Patient History

In addition to the questions listed under Patient History in Chapter 1, the examiner should obtain the following information from the patient:

1. How old is the patient? What is the patient's occupation? Tennis elbow (lateral epicondylitis) problems usually occur in persons 35 years of age or older and in those who use a great deal of wrist flexion and extension in their occupations. If the patient is a child who complains of pain in the elbow and lacks supination on examination, the examiner could suspect a dislocation of the head of the radius. This type of injury is often seen in young children. A parent may give the child a sharp "come-along" tug on the arm or the child may trip while the parent is holding the hand, leading to a dislocation of the head of the radius.

2. What was the mechanism of injury? Did the patient fall on the outstretched hand (FOOSH injury) or on the tip of the elbow? Were any repetitive activities involved? Does the patient's job involve any repetitive activities? Were there any unusual activities that the patient performed in the last week? Did the patient feel a "pop" when throwing or doing other activity? If the pop is followed by pain and swelling on the medial side of the elbow, it may be indicative of an ulnar collateral ligament sprain.[1] Such questions help determine the structure injured and the degree of injury.

3. How long has the patient had the problem? Does the condition come and go? What activities aggravate the problem? Such questions give an indication of the seriousness of the condition and how much it bothers the patient.

4. What are the details of the present pain and other symptoms? What are the sites and boundaries of the pain? Is the pain radiating, does it ache, and is it worse at night? Aching pain over the lateral epicondyle that radiates may be indicative of a "tennis elbow" problem. Depending on the age of the patient and past history, the examiner may want to consider referral of pain from the cervical spine or the possibility of a double crush neurological injury. Also, multiple joint diseases (e.g., rheumatoid arthritis, osteoarthritis) must be considered if the patient complains of pain in several joints.

5. Are there any activities that increase or decrease the pain? Does pulling (traction), twisting (torque), or pushing (compression) alter the pain? Such questions may give an indication of the tissues being stressed or the tissues injured.

6. Are there any positions that relieve the pain? Patients often protectively hold the elbow to the side (in the resting position) and hold the wrist for support, especially in acute conditions.

7. Is there any indication of deformity, bruising, wasting, or muscle spasm?

8. Are any movements impaired? Which movements does the patient feel are restricted? If flexion or extension is limited, two joints may be involved, the ulnohumeral and/or the radiohumeral. If supination or pronation is problematic, any one of five joints could be involved: the radiohumeral, superior radioulnar, middle radioulnar, inferior radioulnar, or ulnomeniscocarpal.

9. What is the patient unable to do functionally? Is the patient able to position the hand properly? Are abnormal movements of the upper limb complex necessary to position the hand? Questions such as these help the examiner determine how functionally limiting the condition is to the patient.

10. What is the patient's usual activity or pastime? Have any of these activities been altered or increased in the last month?

11. Does the patient complain of any abnormal nerve distribution pain? The examiner should note the presence and location of any tingling or numbness for reference when checking dermatomes and peripheral nerve distribution later in the examination.

12. Does the patient have any history of previous injury overuse or trauma? This question is especially important in regard to the elbow because the ulnar nerve may be affected by tardy ulnar palsy.

Observation

The patient must be suitably undressed so that both arms are exposed to allow comparison of the two sides. If the history has indicated an insidious onset of elbow problems, the examiner should take the time to observe full body posture, and especially the neck and shoulder area, for possible referral of symptoms.

The examiner first places the patient's arm in the anatomic position to determine whether there is a normal carrying angle[2] (see Fig. 6–1). It is the angle formed by the long axis of the humerus and the long axis of the ulna and is most evident when the elbow is straight and the forearm is fully supinated (Fig. 6–4). In the adult, this would be a slight valgus deviation between the humerus and the ulna when the forearm is supinated and the elbow is extended. In males, the normal carrying angle is 5 to 10°; in females, it is 10 to 15°. If the carrying angle is more than 15°, it is called **cubitus valgus**; if it is less than 5 to 10°, it is called **cubitus varus**. Because of the shape of the humeral condyles that articulate with the radius and ulna, the carrying angle changes linearly depending on the degree of extension or flexion. Cubitus valgus is greatest in extension. The angle decreases as the elbow flexes, reaching varus in full flexion.[3] If there has been a fracture or epiphyseal injury to the distal humerus and a cubitus varus results, a **gun stock deformity** may be seen in full extension (Fig. 6–5).

If swelling exists, all three joints of the elbow complex are affected because they have a common capsule. Joint swelling is often most evident in the triangular space between the radial head, tip of olecranon, and lateral epicondyle (Fig. 6–6). Swelling resulting from olecranon bursitis (student's elbow) is more discrete,

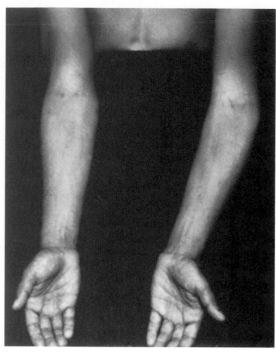

Figure 6–5

Cubitus varus with gun stock deformity on the left arm. (From Regan, W.D., and B.F. Morrey: The physical examination of the elbow. In Morrey, B.F. [ed.]: The Elbow and Its Disorders, 2nd ed. Philadelphia, W.B. Saunders Co., 1993, p. 74.)

being more sharply demarcated as a "goose egg" over the olecranon process (Fig. 6–7). With swelling, the joint would be held in its resting position, with the elbow held in approximately 70° of flexion, because it is in the resting position that the joint has maximum volume.

The examiner should look for normal bony and soft-tissue contours anteriorly and posteriorly. Often, athletes such as pitchers, other throwers, and rodeo riders have a much larger forearm on the dominant side.

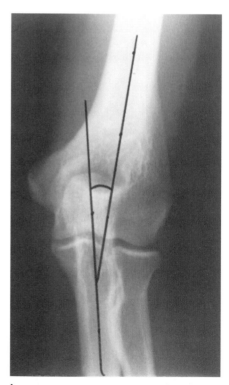

Figure 6–4

Carrying angle. The carrying angle may be determined by noting the angle of intersection between a line connecting midpoints in the distal humerus and a line connecting midpoints in the proximal ulna.

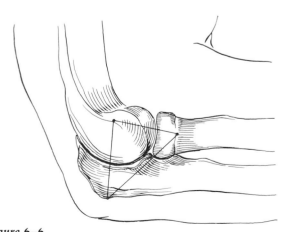

Figure 6–6

The triangular area in which intra-articular swelling is most evident in the elbow.

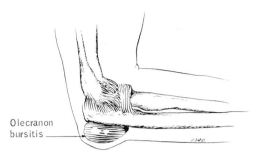

Figure 6–7
Olecranon bursitis. (From O'Donoghue, D.H.: Treatment of Injuries to Athletes, 4th ed. Philadelphia, W.B. Saunders Co., 1984, p. 243.)

The examiner should note whether the patient can assume the normal position of function of the elbow (Fig. 6–8). A normal functional position is 90° of flexion with the forearm midway between supination and pronation.[4] The forearm may also be considered to be in a functional position when slightly pronated, as in writing. From this position, forward flexion of the shoulder along with slightly more elbow flexion (up to 120°) enables the person to bring food to the mouth; supination of the forearm decreases the amount of shoulder flexion necessary to accomplish this. At 90° of elbow flexion, the olecranon process of the ulna and the medial and lateral epicondyles of the humerus normally form an isosceles triangle (Fig. 6–9). When the arm is fully extended, the three points normally form a straight line.[5] The isosceles triangle is sometimes called the **triangle sign**. If there is a fracture, dislocation, or degeneration leading to loss of bone and/or cartilage, the distance between the apex and the base decreases and the isosceles triangle no longer exists. The triangle can be measured on x-ray films.[3]

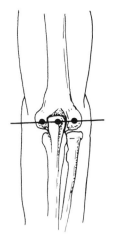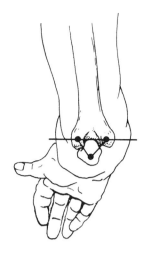

Figure 6–9
Relation of the medial and lateral epicondyles and the olecranon at the elbow in extension (*left*) and flexion (*right*).

Examination

If the history has indicated an insidious onset of elbow symptoms and if the patient has complained of weakness and pain, the examiner may consider performing an examination of the cervical spine, which includes the upper limb peripheral joint scanning examination and myotome testing. Because of the potential referral of symptoms from the cervical spine and the necessity of differentiating nerve root symptoms from peripheral nerve lesions, the consideration of including cervical assessment is essential.

Active Movements

The examination is performed with the patient in the sitting position. As always, active movements are done first, and it is important to remember that the most painful movements are done last.

Active elbow flexion is 140 to 150°. Movement is usually stopped by contact of the forearm with the muscles of the arm.

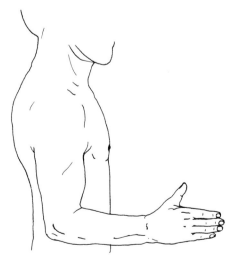

Figure 6–8
Position of function of the elbow—90° flexion, midway between supination and pronation.

Active Movements of the Elbow Complex

- Flexion of the elbow (140 to 150°)
- Extension of the elbow (0 to 10°)
- Supination of the forearm (90°)
- Pronation of the forearm (80 to 90°)
- Combined movements (if necessary)
- Repetitive movements (if necessary)
- Sustained positions (if necessary)

Active elbow extension is 0°, although up to a 10° hyperextension may be exhibited, especially in women. This hyperextension is considered normal if it is equal on both sides and there is no history of trauma. Normally, the movement is arrested by the locking of the olecranon process of the ulna into the olecranon fossa of the humerus. In some cases, under violent compressive loads (e.g., gymnastics, weight lifting), the olecranon process may act as a pivot, resulting in posterior dislocation of the elbow. This mechanism of injury is more likely to be seen in someone with hyperextended elbows. Loss of elbow extension is a sensitive indicator of intra-articular pathology. It is the first movement lost after injury to the elbow and the first regained with healing. However, terminal flexion loss is more disabling than the same degree of terminal extension loss because of the need of flexion for many activities of daily living. Loss of either motion affects the area of reach of the hand, which in turn affects function.

Active supination should be 90°, so that the palm faces up. The examiner should ensure that the shoulder is not adducted further in an attempt to give the appearance of increased supination or to compensate for a lack of sufficient supination[6] (Fig. 6–10).

For active pronation, the range of motion (ROM) is approximately the same (80 to 90°), so that the palm faces down. The examiner should be sure that the patient does not abduct the shoulder in an attempt to increase the amount of pronation or to compensate for a lack of

sufficient pronation.[6] However, for both supination and pronation, only about 75° of movement occurs in the forearm articulations. The remaining 15° is the result of wrist action.

If, in the history, the patient has complained that combined movements, repetitive movements, or sustained positions cause pain, these specific movements should also be included in the active movement assessment. If the patient has difficulty or cannot complete a movement, but it is pain free, the examiner must consider a severe injury to the contractile tissue (rupture) or a neurological injury, and further testing is necessary.

Passive Movements

If the ROM is full on active movements, overpressure may be gently applied to test the end feel in each direction. If the movement is not full, passive movements should be carried out to test the end feel.

> ### Passive Movements of the Elbow Complex and Normal End Feel
>
> - Elbow flexion (tissue approximation)
> - Elbow extension (bone-to-bone)
> - Forearm supination (tissue stretch)
> - Forearm pronation (tissue stretch)

It should be pointed out that although tissue approximation is the normal end feel of elbow flexion, in thin patients the end feel may be bone-to-bone as a result of the coronoid process' hitting in the coronoid fossa. Likewise, in thin individuals, pronation may be bone-to-bone.

In addition to the end feel tests during passive movements, the examiner should note whether a capsular pattern is present. The capsular pattern for the elbow complex as a whole is more limitation of flexion than extension.

Resisted Isometric Movements

For proper testing of the muscles of the elbow complex, the movement must be resisted and isometric. Muscle flexion power around the elbow is greatest in the range of 90 to 110° with the forearm supinated. At 45 and 135°, flexion power is only 75% of maximum.[4] Isometrically, it has been shown that men are two times stronger than women at the elbow; extension is 60% of flexion, and pronation is about 85% of supination.[7] To perform the resisted isometric tests, the patient is seated (Fig. 6–11). If the examiner finds that a particular movement or movements cause pain, Table 6–1 can be used to help differentiate the cause. It is also necessary to carry out wrist extension and flexion, because a large number of muscles act over the wrist as well as the elbow.

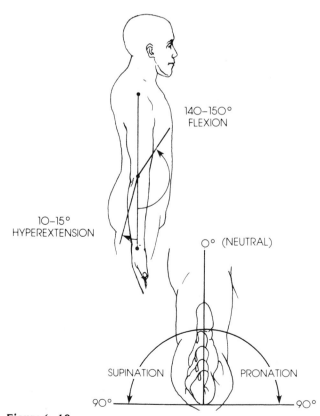

Figure 6–10
Range of motion at the elbow.

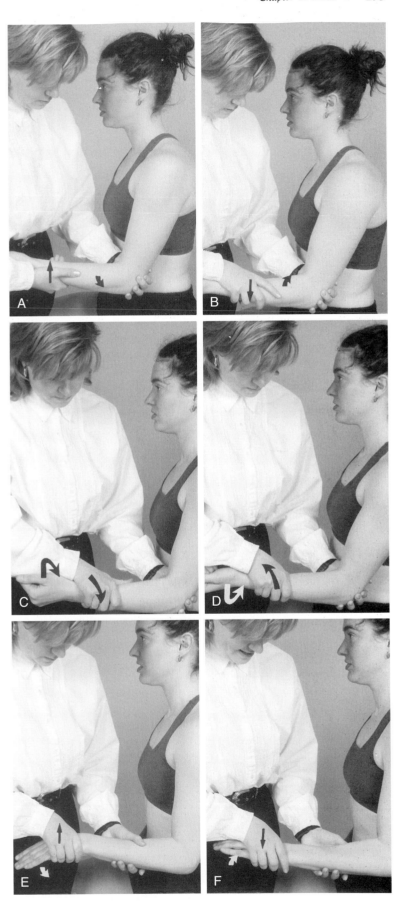

Figure 6–11
Positioning for resisted isometric movements. (A) Elbow
extension. (B) Elbow flexion. (C) Forearm pronation.
(D) Forearm supination. (E) Wrist flexion. (F) Wrist
extension.

Table 6–1
Muscles About the Elbow: Their Actions, Nerve Supply, and Nerve Root Derivation

Action	Muscles Acting	Nerve Supply	Nerve Root Derivation
Flexion of elbow	1. Brachialis	Musculocutaneous	C5–C6, (C7)
	2. Biceps brachii	Musculocutaneous	C5–C6
	3. Brachioradialis	Radial	C5–C6, (C7)
	4. Pronator teres	Median	C6–C7
	5. Flexor carpi ulnaris	Ulnar	C7–C8
Extension of elbow	1. Triceps	Radial	C6–C8
	2. Anconeus	Radial	C7–C8, (T1)
Supination of forearm	1. Supinator	Posterior interosseous (radial)	C5–C6
	2. Biceps brachii	Musculocutaneous	C5–C6
Pronation of forearm	1. Pronator quadratus	Anterior interosseous (median)	C8, T1
	2. Pronator teres	Median	C6–C7
	3. Flexor carpi radialis	Median	C6–C7
Flexion of wrist	1. Flexor carpi radialis	Median	C6–C7
	2. Flexor carpi ulnaris	Ulnar	C7–C8
Extension of wrist	1. Extensor carpi radialis longus	Radial	C6–C7
	2. Extensor carpi radialis brevis	Posterior interosseous (radial)	C7–C8
	3. Extensor carpi ulnaris	Posterior interosseous (radial)	C7–C8

Resisted Isometric
Movements of the Elbow Complex

- Elbow flexion
- Elbow extension
- Supination
- Pronation
- Wrist flexion
- Wrist extension

If, in the history, the patient has complained that combined movements under load, repetitive movements under load, or sustained positions under load cause pain, the examiner should carefully examine these resisted isometric movements and positions as well, but only after the basic movements have been tested isometrically. If the history has indicated that concentric, eccentric, or econcentric movements have caused symptoms, these movements should also be tested with load or no load, as required.

If the resisted isometric contraction is weak and pain free, the examiner must consider a major injury to the contractile tissue (third-degree strain) or neurological injury. If there is no history of trauma, the most likely cause is neurological, either a nerve root or peripheral nerve lesion. By selectively testing the muscles and sensory distribution (Table 6–2) and by having a knowledge of nerve compression sites (see section on reflexes and cutaneous distribution), the examiner should be able to determine the neurological tissue injured and where the injury has occurred.

Functional Assessment

When assessing the elbow, it is important to remember that the elbow is the middle portion of an integral upper limb kinetic chain. It allows the hand to be positioned

in space; it helps stabilize the upper extremity for power and detailed work activities; and it provides power to the arm for lifting activities.[8] Motion in the elbow allows the hand to be positioned so that daily functions can easily be performed. The full range of elbow movements is not necessary to perform these activities; most activities of daily living are performed at between 30° and 130° of flexion and between 50° of pronation and 50° of supination (Figs. 6–12 and 6–13). To reach the head,

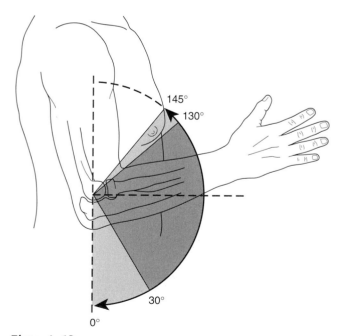

Figure 6–12

Normal range of elbow flexion is approximately 0 to 145°. However, the functional arc of motion is somewhat less, and most activities can be performed with flexion of 30 to 130°. (Redrawn from Regan, W.D., and B.F. Morrey: The physical examination of the elbow. In Morrey, B.F. [ed.]: The Elbow and Its Disorders, 2nd ed. Philadelphia, W.B. Saunders Co., 1993, p. 81.)

Table 6–2
Nerve Injuries About the Elbow

Nerve	Motor Loss	Sensory Loss	Functional Loss
Median nerve (C6–C8, T1)	Pronator teres Flexor carpi radialis Palmaris longus Flexor digitorum superficialis Flexor pollicis longus Lateral half of flexor digitorum profundus Pronator quadratus Thenar eminence Lateral two lumbricals	Palmar aspect of hand with thumb, index, middle, and lateral half of ring finger Dorsal aspect of distal third of index, middle, and lateral half of ring finger	Pronation weak or lost Weak wrist flexion and abduction Radial deviation at wrist lost Inability to oppose or flex thumb Weak thumb abduction Weak grip Weak or no pinch (ape hand deformity)
Anterior interosseous nerve (branch of median nerve)	Flexor pollicis longus Lateral half of flexor digitorum profundus Pronator quadratus Thenar eminence Lateral two lumbricals	None	Pronation weak especially at 90° elbow flexion Weak opposition and flexion of thumb Weak finger flexion Weak pinch (no tip-to-tip)
Ulnar nerve (C7–C8, T1)	Flexor carpi ulnaris Medial half of flexor digitorum profundus Palmaris brevis Hypothenar eminence Adductor pollicis Medial two lumbricals All interossei	Dorsal and palmar aspect of little and medial half of ring finger	Weak wrist flexion Loss of ulnar deviation at wrist Loss of distal flexion of little finger Loss of abduction and adduction of fingers Inability to extend second and third phalanges of little and ring fingers (benediction hand deformity) Loss of thumb adduction
Radial nerve (C5–C8, T1)	Anconeus Brachioradialis Extensor carpi radialis longus and brevis Extensor digitorum Extensor pollicis longus and brevis Abductor pollicis longus Extensor carpi ulnaris Extensor indices Extensor digiti minimi	Dorsum of hand (lateral two thirds) Dorsum and lateral aspect of thumb Proximal two thirds of dorsum of index, middle, and half of ring finger	Loss of supination Loss of wrist extension (wrist drop) Inability to grasp Inability to stabilize wrist Loss of finger extension Inability to abduct thumb
Posterior interosseous nerve (branch of ulnar nerve)	Extensor carpi radialis brevis Extensor digitorum Extensor pollicis longus and brevis Abductor pollicis longus Extensor carpi ulnaris Extensor indices Extensor digiti minimi	None	Weak wrist extension Weak finger extension Difficulty stabilizing wrist Difficulty with grasp Inability to abduct thumb

Figure 6–13

Pronation and supination motions average 75° and 85°, respectively. Most activities of daily living, however, can be accomplished with 50° of each motion. (Redrawn from Regan, W.D., and B.F. Morrey: The physical examination of the elbow. In Morrey, B.F. [ed.]: The Elbow and Its Disorders, 2nd ed. Philadelphia, W.B. Saunders Co., 1993, p. 81.)

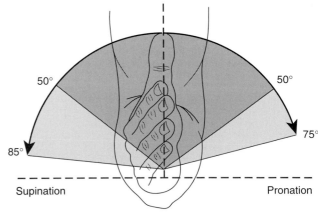

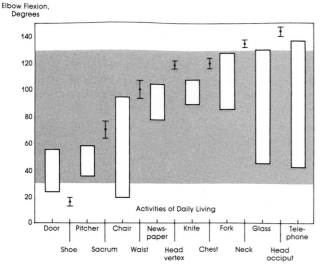

Figure 6–14

The arc and position of elbow flexion required to accomplish 15 daily activities. Most of these activities are accomplished within a flexion range of 30 to 130°. (Modified from Morrey, B.F., L.J. Askew, and E.Y. Chao: A biomechanical study of normal functional elbow motion. J. Bone Joint Surg. Am. 63:873, 1981.)

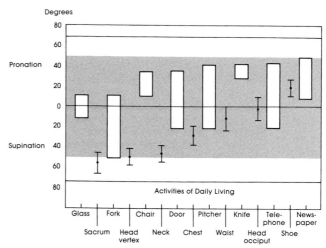

Figure 6–15

Fifteen activities of daily living accomplished with pronation and supination of up to 50° each. (Modified from Morrey, B.F., L.J. Askew, and E.Y. Chao: A biomechanical study of normal functional elbow motion. J. Bone Joint Surg. Am. 63:874, 1981.)

approximately 140° of flexion is needed. The activities of combing or washing the hair, reaching a back zipper, and walking with crutches require a greater ROM. Activities such as pouring fluid, drinking from a container, cutting with a knife, reading a newspaper, and using a screwdriver require an adequate range of supination and pronation. Figures 6–14 and 6–15 show the ROM or arc of movement necessary to do certain activities or the ROM needed to touch parts of the body. It must be

remembered that elbow injuries may preclude lifting objects as light as a cup of coffee, owing to lifting mechanics. Because of the length of the lever arm of the forearm when the elbow is at 90°, loads at the hand are magnified 10-fold at the elbow.[9] Figure 6–16 is a numerical scoring assessment form that can be used to assess the elbow and includes an important functional component. Table 6–3 demonstrates functional tests of strength for the elbow.

Table 6–3
Functional Testing of the Elbow

Starting Position	Action	Functional Test*
Sitting	Bring hand to mouth lifting weight (elbow flexion)	Lift 2.3–2.7 kg: Functional Lift 1.4–1.8 kg: Functionally fair Lift 0.5–0.9 kg: Functionally poor Lift 0 kg: Nonfunctional
Standing 90 cm from wall, leaning against wall	Push arms straight (elbow extension)	5–6 Repetitions: Functional 3–4 Repetitions: Functionally fair 1–2 Repetitions: Functionally poor 0 Repetitions: Nonfunctional
Standing, facing closed door	Open door starting with palm down (supination of arm)	5–6 Repetitions: Functional 3–4 Repetitions: Functionally fair 1–2 Repetitions: Functionally poor 0 Repetitions: Nonfunctional
Standing, facing closed door	Open door starting with palm up (pronation of arm)	5–6 Repetitions: Functional 3–4 Repetitions: Functionally fair 1–2 Repetitions: Functionally poor 0 Repetitions: Nonfunctional

* Younger patients should be able to lift more (2.7–4.5 kg) more often (6–10 repetitions). With age, weight and repetitions will decrease.

Data from Palmer, M.L., and M. Epler: Clinical Assessment Procedures in Physical Therapy. Philadelphia, J.B. Lippincott, 1990, pp. 109–111.

Elbow Evaluation

Name: _____   UH#: _____   Elbow: R/L

Procedure: _____   Date: _____   Dominant: R/L

Date of Exam (month/day/year)	/ /	/ /	/ /	/ /	/ /
Pain (maximum points) 5 = none (30); 4 = slight—with continuous activity, no medication (25); 3 = moderate—with occasional activity, some medication (15); 2 = moderately severe—much pain, frequent medication (10); 1 = severe—constant pain, markedly limited activity (5); 0 = complete disability (0)	____ ( )				
Motion degrees (37 points maximum) Extension Flexion Extension (8 pts max) Flexion (17 pts max) Pronation/Supination Pronation (pt) = 0.1 per degree—6 maximum Supination	Extension ____°( ) Flexion ____°( ) Pronation ____°( ) Supination ____°( )				
Strength (15 points maximum) 5 = normal; 4 = good; 3 = fair; 2 = poor; 1 = trace; 0 = paralysis; NA = not available					

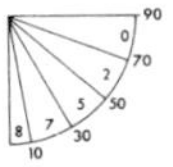

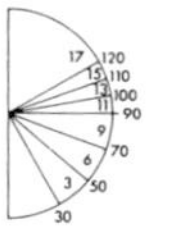

	Flex.	Ext.	Pro.	Sup.		
Normal	5	(5)	(4)	(3)	(3)	Extension ____( )
Good	4	(4)	(3)	(2)	(2)	Flexion ____( )
Fair	3	(3)	(2)	(1)	(1)	
Poor	2	(2)	(1)	(0)	(0)	Pronation ____( )
Trace	1	(1)	(0)	(0)	(0)	
None	0	(0)	(0)	(0)	(0)	Supination ____( )

Instability (6 points maximum)

	Ant./Post.	Med./Lat.		
None	3	3	Ant./Post.	_____
Mild <5 mm, <5°	2	2		
Moderate <10 mm, <10°	1	1	Med./Lat.	_____
Severe >10 mm, >10°	0	0		

Function (12 points maximum)

4 = normal (1); 3 = mild compromise (0.75); 2 = difficulty (0.5); 1 = with aid (0.25); 0 = unable (0); NA = not applicable

(Index—multiply × 0.25)

	/ /	/ /	/ /	/ /	/ /
1. Use back pocket	_____( )				
2. Rise from chair	_____( )				
3. Perineal care	_____( )				
4. Wash opposite axilla	_____( )				
5. Eat with utensil	_____( )				
6. Comb hair	_____( )				
7. Carry 10–15 pounds with arm at side	_____( )				
8. Dress	_____( )				
9. Pulling	_____( )				
10. Throwing	_____( )				
11. Do usual work Specify work:	_____( )				
12. Do usual sport Specify sport:	_____( )				
Patient Response 3 = much better; 2 = better; 1 = same; 0 = worse; NA = not available/not applicable	_____				
Completed By: Name of Examiner					
Index Key: 95–100 = excellent; 80–95 = good; 50–80 = fair; <50 = poor	( )	( )	( )	( )	( )

Figure 6–16

Clinically useful elbow evaluation sheet providing objective data retrieval and grading as well as information about function. The use of such a rating index in the clinical setting provides an objective means of comparing different treatment options. (From Morrey, B.F., K.N. An, and E.Y.S. Chao: Functional Evaluation of the Elbow. In Morrey, B.F. [ed.]: The Elbow and Its Disorders. Philadelphia, W.B. Saunders Co., 1985, pp. 88–89. Copyright Mayo Clinic Foundation, Rochester, Minnesota.)

Special Tests

Only those special tests that the examiner believes have relevance or will help to confirm the diagnosis should be performed. If the history has not indicated any trauma or repetitive movement that could be associated with problems, the examiner, depending on the age of the patient, may want to include some of the nerve root compression tests (see Chapter 3) to rule out the possibility of referred symptoms from the cervical spine or the possibility of a "double crush" injury.

Special Tests Commonly Performed on the Elbow

- Ligamentous instability test
- Lateral epicondylitis test (method 1 or 2)
- Elbow flexion test (ulnar nerve)
- Pinch grip test (median nerve and anterior interosseous nerve)

Ligamentous Test

Ligamentous Instability Test. The patient's arm is stabilized with one of the examiner's hands at the elbow and the other hand placed above the patient's wrist. With the patient's elbow slightly flexed (20 to 30°) and stabilized with the examiner's hand, an adduction or varus force is applied by the examiner to the distal forearm to test the lateral collateral ligament while the ligament is palpated (Fig. 6–17). Normally, the examiner feels the ligament tense when stress is applied. Regan and Morrey[9] advocate doing the varus stress test with the humerus in full medial rotation. The examiner applies the force several times with increasing pressure while noting any alteration in pain or ROM.

An abduction or valgus force at the distal forearm is then applied in a similar fashion to test the medial collateral ligament while the ligament is palpated. Regan and Morrey[9] advocate doing the valgus stress test with the humerus in full lateral rotation. The examiner should note any laxity, decreased mobility, or altered pain that may be present compared with the uninvolved elbow.

Tests for Epicondylitis

When testing for epicondylitis, whether medial or lateral, the examiner must keep in mind that there may be referral of pain from the cervical spine or peripheral nerve involvement. If the epicondylitis does not respond to treatment, the examiner would be wise to check for neurological pathology.

Lateral Epicondylitis (Tennis Elbow or Cozen's) Test (Method 1). The patient's elbow is stabilized by the examiner's thumb, which rests on the patient's lateral epicondyle (Fig. 6–18). The patient is then asked to make a fist, pronate the forearm, and radially deviate and extend the wrist while the examiner resists the motion. A positive sign is indicated by a sudden severe pain in the area of the lateral epicondyle of the humerus. The epicondyle may be palpated to indicate the origin of the pain.

Lateral Epicondylitis (Tennis Elbow or Mill's) Test (Method 2). While palpating the lateral epicondyle, the examiner pronates the patient's forearm, flexes the wrist fully, and extends the elbow (see Fig. 6–18). A positive test is indicated by pain over the lateral epicondyle of the humerus. The examiner may simultaneously palpate the epicondyle. This maneuver also puts stress on the radial nerve and, in the presence of compression of the radial nerve, causes symptoms very similar to those of tennis elbow.[10] Electrodiagnostic studies help differentiate the two conditions.

Lateral Epicondylitis (Tennis Elbow) Test (Method 3). The examiner resists extension of the third digit of the hand distal to the proximal interphalangeal joint, stressing the extensor digitorum muscle and tendon (see Fig. 6–18). A positive test is indicated by pain over the lateral epicondyle of the humerus.

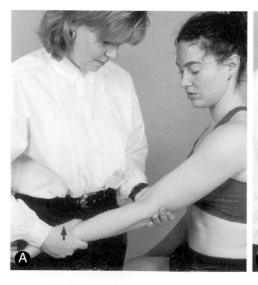
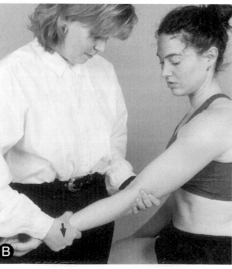

Figure 6–17
Testing the collateral ligaments of the elbow. (A) Lateral collateral ligament. (B) Medial collateral ligament.

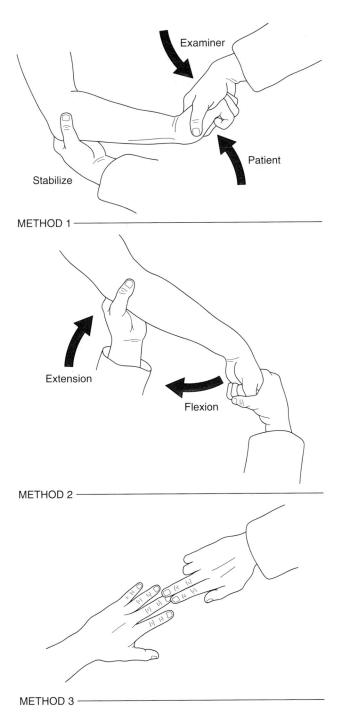

METHOD 1 ——————————

METHOD 2 ——————————

METHOD 3 ——————————

Figure 6–18
Tests for tennis elbow.

Medial Epicondylitis (Golfer's Elbow) Test. While the examiner palpates the patient's medial epicondyle, the patient's forearm is supinated and the elbow and wrist are extended by the examiner. A positive sign is indicated by pain over the medial epicondyle of the humerus.

Tests for Neurological Dysfunction

Tinel's Sign (at the Elbow). The area of the ulnar nerve in the groove (between the olecranon process and medial

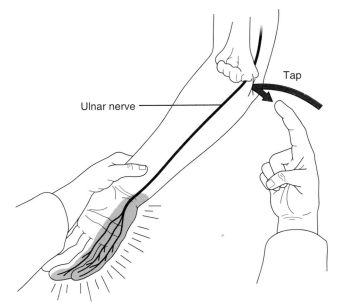

Figure 6–19
Tinel's sign at the elbow for the ulnar nerve.

epicondyle) is tapped. A positive sign is indicated by a tingling sensation in the ulnar distribution of the forearm and hand distal to the point of compression of the nerve (Fig. 6–19). The test indicates the point of regeneration of the sensory fibers of a nerve. The most distal point at which the abnormal sensation is felt represents the limit of nerve regeneration.

Wartenberg's Sign. The patient sits with his or her hands resting on the table. The examiner passively spreads the fingers apart and asks the patient to bring them together again. Inability to squeeze the little finger to the remainder of the hand indicates a positive test for ulnar neuropathy.[9]

Elbow Flexion Test. The patient is asked to fully flex the elbow with extension of the wrist and shoulder girdle abduction and depression[11, 12] and to hold this position for 3 to 5 minutes (Fig. 6–20). A positive test is indicated

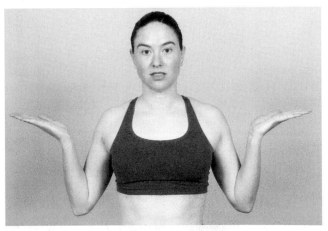

Figure 6–20
Elbow flexion test for ulnar nerve pathology.

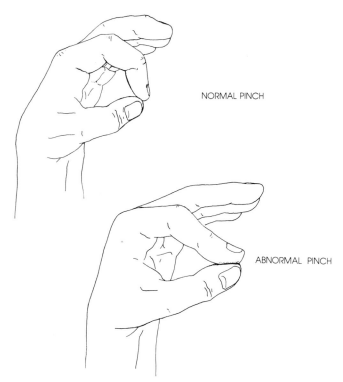

NORMAL PINCH

ABNORMAL PINCH

Figure 6–21
Normal pinch compared with the abnormal pinch seen in anterior interosseous nerve syndrome.

by tingling or paresthesia in the ulnar nerve distribution of the forearm and hand. The test helps to determine whether a cubital tunnel (ulnar nerve) syndrome is present.

Test for Pronator Teres Syndrome.[9] The patient sits with the elbow flexed to 90°. The examiner strongly resists pronation as the elbow is extended. A positive test is indicated by tingling or paresthesia in the median nerve distribution in the forearm and hand.

Pinch Grip Test. The patient is asked to pinch the tips of the index finger and thumb together. Normally, there should be a tip-to-tip pinch. If the patient is unable to pinch tip-to-tip and instead has an abnormal pulp-to-pulp pinch of the index finger and thumb, the test is indicative of a positive sign for pathology to the anterior interosseous nerve, a branch of the median nerve (Fig. 6–21). This finding may indicate an entrapment of the anterior interosseous nerve as it passes between the two heads of the pronator teres muscle.[13]

Reflexes and Cutaneous Distribution

The reflexes around the elbow that are often checked (Fig. 6–22) include the biceps (C5–C6), brachioradialis (C5–C6), and triceps (C7–C8). The examiner should also assess the dermatomes around the elbow and the cutaneous distribution of the various nerves, noting any difference (Figs. 6–23 and 6–24). When looking at the dermatomes, the examiner should realize there is a great deal of variability in the distribution patterns. Except for T2 dermatome, which ends at the elbow, all other dermatomes extend distally to the forearm, wrist, and hand; therefore, the elbow cannot be looked at in isolation when viewing dermatomes. Similarly, the peripheral nerves extend into the forearm, wrist, and hand, so testing for sensory loss must involve the whole upper limb, not just the elbow. Pain may be referred to the elbow and surrounding tissues from the neck (often mimicking tennis elbow), the shoulder, or the wrist (Fig. 6–25; Table 6–4).

In the extremities, the neurological tissues (nerve roots and peripheral nerves) play a significant role in function. Injury, pinching, or stress to these structures can have dire consequences functionally for the patient. The next section is a review of the peripheral nerves and how and where they may be traumatized about the elbow.

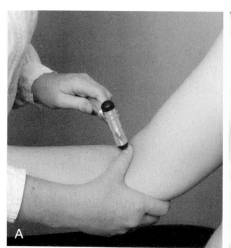
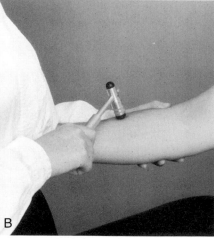
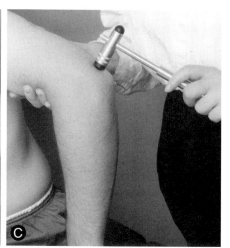

Figure 6–22
Reflexes around the elbow. (A) Biceps. (B) Brachioradialis. (C) Triceps.

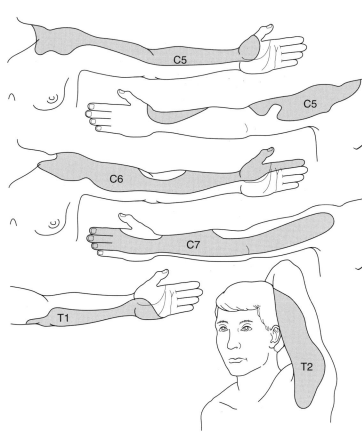

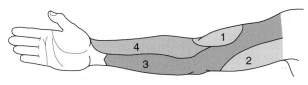

Anterior aspect

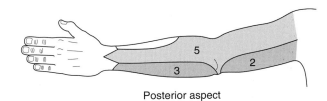

Posterior aspect

Figure 6–24
Sensory nerve distribution around the elbow. (1) Lower lateral cutaneous nerve of arm (radial). (2) Medial cutaneous nerve of arm. (3) Medial cutaneous nerve of forearm. (4) Lateral cutaneous nerve of forearm (musculocutaneous nerve). (5) Posterior cutaneous nerve of forearm (radial nerve).

Figure 6–23
Dermatomes around the elbow.

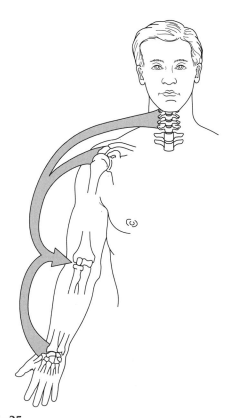

Figure 6–25
Pain referred to the elbow.

Table 6–4
Elbow Muscles and Referral of Pain

Muscles	Referral Pattern
Biceps	Upper shoulder (bicipital groove) to anterior elbow
Brachialis	Anterior arm, elbow to lateral thenar eminence
Triceps	Posterior shoulder, arm, elbow, and forearm to medial two fingers, medial epicondyle
Brachioradialis	Lateral epicondyle, lateral forearm to posterior web space between thumb and index finger
Anconeus	Lateral epicondyle area
Supinator	Lateral epicondyle and posterior web space between thumb and index finger
Pronator teres	Anterior forearm to wrist and part of anterior thumb
Extensor carpi ulnaris	Medial wrist
Extensor carpi radialis brevis	Posterior forearm to posterior wrist
Extensor carpi radialis longus	Lateral epicondyle to posterolateral wrist
Extensor indices	Posterior forearm to appropriate digit
Palmaris longus	Anterior forearm to palm
Flexor digitorum superficialis	Palm to appropriate digit
Flexor carpi ulnaris	Anteromedial wrist
Flexor carpi radialis	Anteromiddle wrist

Peripheral Nerve Injuries About the Elbow

Median Nerve (C6–C8, T1). In the elbow region, the median nerve proper can be injured by trauma (e.g., lacerations, fractures, dislocations), by systemic disease, and especially by compression and/or traction.[14, 15]

The median nerve may also be pinched or compressed above the elbow as it passes under the **ligament of Struthers,** an anomalous structure found in approximately 1% of the population[16] (Fig. 6–26). The ligament runs from an abnormal spur on the shaft of the humerus to the medial epicondyle of the humerus. Because the brachial artery sometimes accompanies the nerve through this tunnel, it may also be compressed, resulting in possible vascular as well as neurological symptoms. In this case, the neurological involvement would include weakness of the pronator teres muscle and of those muscles affected by the pronator syndrome (see later discussion). The condition may also be called the **humerus supracondylar process syndrome.**

Pressure in the ligament of Struthers area leads to motor loss (see Table 6–2) and sensory loss (see Fig. 7–55) of the median nerve. Initially, the patient complains of pain and paresthesia in the elbow and forearm; abnormality of motor function is secondary. With time, however, motor function is also affected, with wrist and finger flexion as well as thumb movements being most affected.

A second area of compression of the median nerve as it passes through the elbow occurs where it passes through the two heads of pronator teres (**pronator syndrome**). In this case, the pronator teres remains normal, but the other muscles supplied by the median nerve (see Table 6–2) are affected, as is its sensory distribution. Pronation is possible, but weakness is evident as pronation is loaded. If the elbow is flexed to 90° and pronation is tested, there will be noticeable weakness because, in this position, the action of pronator teres is minimized.

Butlers and Singer[17] report four possible ways of eliciting median nerve symptoms if the nerve is suffering from pathology: resisted pronation with elbow and wrist flexion for 30 to 60 seconds; resisted elbow flexion and supination; resisted long finger flexion at the proximal interphalangeal joint; and direct pressure over the proximal aspect of pronator teres during pronation. It is interesting to note that one of the tests is similar to Mill's test for lateral epicondylitis. The results should be compared with the good side, and production of the patient's symptoms is considered a positive test.

Anterior Interosseous Nerve. The anterior interosseous nerve, which is a branch of the median nerve, is sometimes pinched or entrapped as it passes between the two heads of the pronator teres muscle, leading to pain and functional impairment of flexor pollicis longus, the lateral half of the flexor digitorum profundus, and the pronator quadratus muscles. The condition is called an-

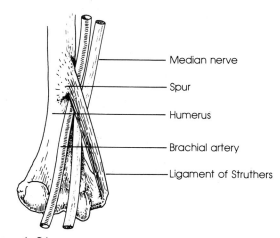

Figure 6–26
Compression of the median nerve by ligament of Struthers.

terior interosseous nerve syndrome or Kiloh-Nevin syndrome (Fig. 6–27)[18, 19] and is characterized by a pinch deformity (see Fig. 6–21). The deformity results from the paralysis of the flexors of the index finger and thumb. This leads to extension of the distal interphalangeal joint of the index finger and the interphalangeal joint of the thumb. The resulting pinch is pulp-to-pulp rather than tip-to-tip. It has been reported that the nerve may also be injured with a forearm fracture (Monteggia fracture).[20] With anterior interosseous syndrome, there is no sensory loss, because the anterior interosseous nerve is a motor

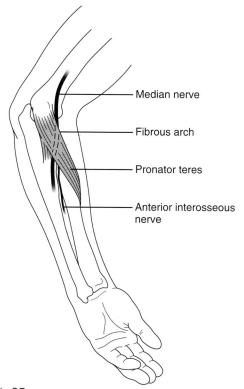

Figure 6–27
Anterior interosseous syndrome.

nerve; signs and symptoms of the condition are related to motor function.

Ulnar Nerve (C7–C8, T1). In the elbow region, the ulnar nerve is most likely to be injured, compressed, or stretched in the **cubital tunnel**[16, 21–24] (see Fig. 6–3). In fact, it is a common entrapment neuropathy, second only to carpal tunnel syndrome. The ulnar nerve may be injured or compressed as a result of swelling (e.g., trauma, pregnancy), osteophytes, arthritic diseases, trauma, or repeated microtrauma. This tunnel, which is relatively long, can cause compression of the nerve as the nerve passes through the tunnel or between the two heads of the flexor carpi ulnaris muscle. Compression is altered as the elbow moves from extension (decreased) to flexion (increased), causing traction on the nerve, and is further enhanced if a significant cubitus valgus is present.[25, 26] Symptoms therefore are more likely to occur when the elbow is flexed. It is usually in the cubital tunnel area that the ulnar nerve is affected, leading to tardy ulnar palsy.

Tardy ulnar palsy implies that the symptoms of nerve injury come on long after the patient has been injured; this delayed reaction seems to be unique to the ulnar nerve. Although most common in adults, it has been reported in children, and in children the delay has been up to 29 months.[27] In adults, the possibility of a double crush injury should always be considered.

Injury to the ulnar nerve in the cubital tunnel affects the flexor carpi ulnaris and the ulnar half of the flexor digitorum profundus in the forearm, the hypothenar eminence in the hand (flexor digiti minimi, abductor digiti minimi, opponens digiti minimi, and adductor pollicis), the interossei, and the third and fourth lumbricals (see Table 6–2). Although these muscles show weakness and atrophy over time, the earliest and most obvious symptoms are sensory, with pain and paresthesia in the medial elbow and forearm and paresthesia in the ulnar sensory distribution of the hand (see Fig. 7–55).

Radial Nerve (C5–C8, T1). The radial nerve may be injured near the elbow if there is a fracture of the shaft of the humerus. The nerve may be damaged as it winds around behind the humerus in the radial groove. Injury may occur at the time of the fracture, or the nerve may get "caught" in the callus of fracture healing. Because the radial nerve supplies all of the extensor muscles of the arm, only the triceps is spared with this type of injury, and even it may show some weakness.

The major branch of the radial nerve in the forearm is the **posterior interosseous nerve,** which is given off in front of the lateral epicondyle of the humerus.[16, 28] This branch may be compressed as it passes between the two heads of the supinator in the **arcade** or **canal of Frohse,** a fibrous arch in the supinator muscle occurring in 30% of the population (Fig. 6–28). Compression leads to functional involvement of the forearm extensor muscles (see Table 6–2) and functional wrist drop, so the patient has

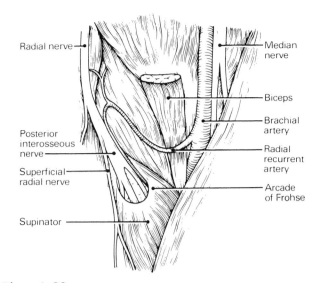

Figure 6–28

Canal or arcade of Frohse. (From Wadsworth, T.G.: The Elbow. New York, Churchill Livingstone, 1982, p. 264.)

difficulty or is unable to stabilize the wrist for proper hand function. Diagnosis of this condition is often delayed because there is no sensory deficit. This condition, called **radial tunnel syndrome,** may mimic tennis elbow.[10, 29–32] If the patient has a persistent form of tennis elbow, a possible nerve lesion or cervical problem should be considered.

A third area of pathology is compression of the superficial branch of the radial nerve as it passes under the tendon of the brachioradialis. This branch is sensory only, and the patient complains primarily of nocturnal pain along the dorsum of the wrist, thumb, and web space. The compression may be caused by trauma, a tight cast, or any swelling in the area. The condition is referred to as **cheiralgia paresthetica** or **Wartenberg's disease.**[24]

Joint Play Movements

When examining the joint play movements (Fig. 6–29), the examiner must compare the injured side with the normal side.

Joint Play Movements of the Elbow Complex

- Radial deviation of the ulna and radius on the humerus
- Ulnar deviation of the ulna and radius on the humerus
- Distraction of the olecranon from the humerus in 90° of flexion
- Anteroposterior glide of the radius on the humerus

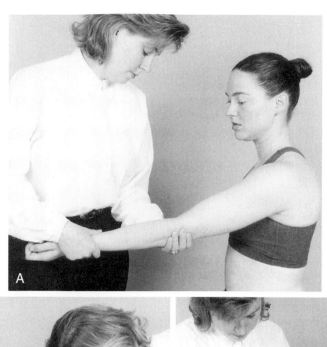

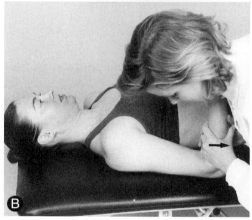

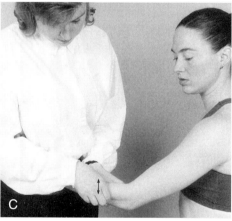

Figure 6–29
Joint play movements of the elbow complex. (A) Radial and ulnar deviation of the ulna on the humerus.
(B) Distraction of the olecranon process from the humerus. (C) Anteroposterior movement of the
radius.

Radial and ulnar deviations of the ulna and radius on the humerus are performed in a fashion similar to those in the collateral ligament tests. The examiner stabilizes the patient's elbow by holding the patient's humerus firmly and places the other hand above the patient's wrist, abducting and adducting the forearm (see Fig. 6–29A). The patient's elbow is almost straight (extended) during the movement, and the end feel should be bone-to-bone.

To distract the olecranon from the humerus, the examiner flexes the patient's elbow to 90°. Wrapping both hands around the patient's forearm close to the elbow, the examiner then applies a distractive force at the elbow, ensuring that no torque is applied (see Fig. 6–29B).

To test anteroposterior glide of the radius on the humerus, the examiner stabilizes the patient's forearm. The patient's arm is held between the examiner's body and arm. The examiner places the thumb of his or her hand over the anterior radial head while the index finger is over the posterior radial head. The examiner then pushes the radial head posteriorly with the thumb and anteriorly with the index finger (see Fig. 6–29C). This movement must be performed with care because it can be very painful as a result of pinching of the skin between the examiner's digits and the bone. In addition, pain may result from the force being applied even in the normal arm, so both sides must be compared.

Palpation

With the patient's arm relaxed, the examiner begins palpation on the anterior aspect of the elbow and moves to the medial aspect, the lateral aspect, and finally the posterior aspect (Fig. 6–30). The patient may sit or lie supine, whichever is more comfortable. The examiner is looking for any tenderness, abnormality, change in temperature or in texture of the tissues, or abnormal "bumps." As with all palpation, the injured side must be compared with the normal or uninjured side.

Anterior Aspect

Cubital Fossa. The fossa is bound by the pronator teres muscle medially, the brachioradialis muscle laterally, and an imaginary line joining the two epicondyles superiorly. Within the fossa, the biceps tendon and brachial artery may be palpated. After crossing the elbow joint, the **brachial artery** divides into two branches, the radial artery and the ulnar artery. The examiner must be aware of the brachial artery because it has the potential for being injured as a result of severe trauma (e.g., fracture, dislocation). Trauma to this area may lead to compartment syndromes such as **Volkmann's ischemic contracture**. The median and musculocutaneous nerves are also found in the fossa, but they are not palpable. Pressure on the median nerve may cause symptoms in its cutaneous distribution.

Coronoid Process and Head of Radius. Within the cubital fossa, if the examiner palpates carefully so as not to hurt the patient, the coronoid process of the ulna and the head of the radius may be palpated. Palpation of the radial head is facilitated by supination and pronation of the forearm. The examiner may palpate the head of the radius from the posterior aspect at the same time by placing the fingers over the head on the posterior aspect and the thumb over it on the anterior aspect. In addition to the muscles previously mentioned, the biceps and brachialis muscles may be palpated for potential abnormality.

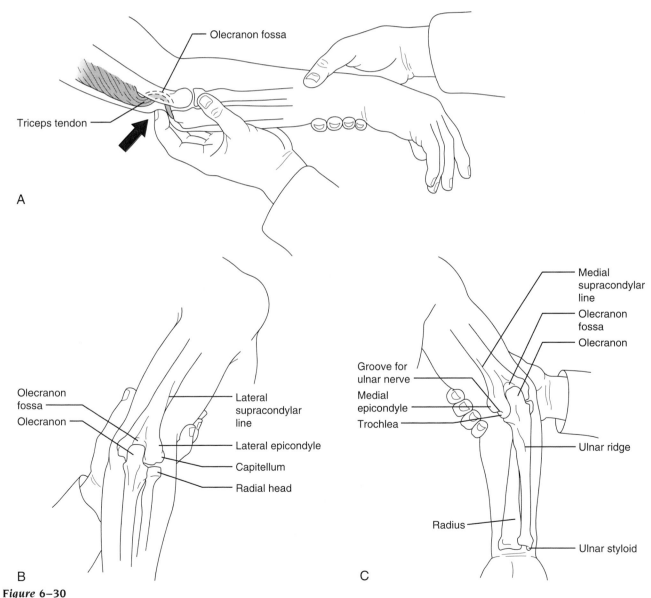

Figure 6–30
Palpation around the elbow. (A) Olecranon fossa. (B) Posterolateral aspect of the elbow. (C) Posteromedial aspect of the elbow.

Medial Aspect

Medial Epicondyle. Originating from the medial epicondyle are the **wrist flexor–forearm pronator** groups of muscles. Both the muscle bellies and their insertions into bone should be palpated. Tenderness over the epicondyle where the muscles insert is sometimes called golfer's elbow or tennis elbow of the medial epicondyle.

Medial (Ulnar) Collateral Ligament. This fan-shaped ligament may be palpated as it extends from the medial epicondyle to the medial margin of the coronoid process anteriorly and to the olecranon process posteriorly.

Ulnar Nerve. If the examiner moves posteriorly behind the medial epicondyle, the fingers will rest over the ulnar nerve in the cubital tunnel (proximal part). Usually, the nerve is not directly palpable, but pressure on the nerve often causes abnormal sensations in its cutaneous distribution. It is this nerve that is struck when someone hits his or her "funny bone."

Lateral Aspect

Lateral Epicondyle. The wrist extensor muscles originate from the lateral epicondyle, and their muscle bellies as well as their insertions into the epicondyle should be palpated. It is at this point of insertion of the common extensor tendon that lateral epicondylitis originates. When palpating, the examiner should remember that the extensor carpi radialis longus muscle inserts above the epicondyle along a short ridge extending from the epicondyle to the humeral shaft. The examiner palpates the brachioradialis and supinator muscles on the lateral aspect of the elbow at the same time.

Lateral (Radial) Collateral Ligament. This cordlike ligament may be palpated as it extends from the lateral epicondyle of the humerus to the annular ligament and lateral surface of the ulna.

Annular Ligament. Distal to the lateral epicondyle, the annular ligament and head of the radius may be palpated

if this has not previously been done. The palpation is facilitated by supination and pronation of the forearm.

Posterior Aspect

Palpation of posterior structures is shown in Figure 6–30.

Olecranon Process and Olecranon Bursa. The olecranon process is best palpated with the elbow flexed to 90°. If the examiner then grasps the skin overlying the process, the olecranon bursa can be palpated. The examiner should note any synovial thickening or the presence of any **rice bodies,** which are small seeds of fragmented fibrous tissue that can act as further irritants to the bursa should it be affected.

Triceps Muscle. The triceps muscle, which inserts into the olecranon process, should be palpated both at its insertion and along its length for any signs of abnormality.

Diagnostic Imaging

Plain Film Radiography

Anteroposterior View. The examiner should note the relation of the epicondyles, trochlea, capitulum, radial head, radial tuberosity, coronoid process, and olecranon process (Fig. 6–31). Any loose bodies, calcification, myositis ossificans, joint space narrowing, or osteophytes should be identified. If the patient is a young child, the epiphyseal plate should be checked to see if it is normal for each bone.

Lateral View. The examiner should note the relation of the epicondyles, trochlea, capitulum, radial head, radial tuberosity, coronoid process, and olecranon process. As with the anteroposterior view, any loose bodies, calcifications in or around the joint (Fig. 6–32), myositis ossificans, dislocations (Fig. 6–33), joint space narrowing, or osteophytes should be noted. The presence of the "fat pad" sign (Fig. 6–34) occurs with elbow joint effusion

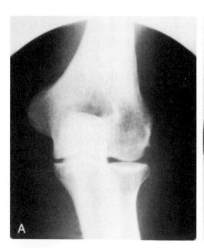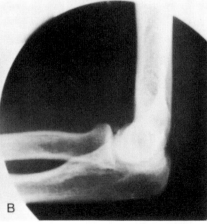

Figure 6–31

Posteroanterior (A) and lateral (B) radiographs of the elbow.

and may indicate, for example, a fracture, acute rheumatoid arthritis, infection, or osteoid osteoma.[33] Plain radiographs may also be used to visualize the cubital tunnel (Fig. 6–35) and to measure the carrying angle (see Fig. 6–4).

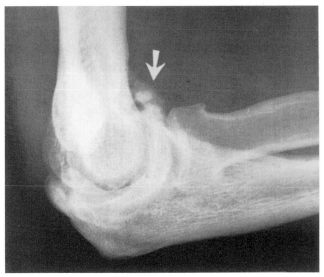

Figure 6–32
Excessive ossification (*arrow*) after dislocation of elbow treated by early active use. (From O'Donoghue, D.H.: Treatment of Injuries to Athletes, 4th ed. Philadelphia, W.B. Saunders Co., 1984, p. 232.)

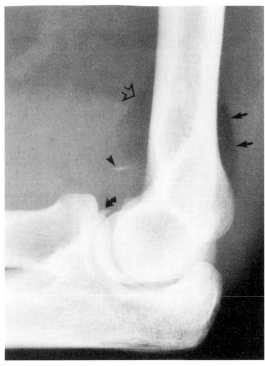

Figure 6–34
Coronoid process fracture with hemarthrosis. The posterior fat pad (*arrows*) is clearly seen on this lateral view with the arm flexed to 90°, indicating joint effusion. The anterior fat pad (*open arrow*) is clearly visible. There is a fracture of the coronoid process (*curved arrow*) and a loose body (*arrowhead*). (From Weissman, B.N.W., and C.B. Sledge: Orthopedic Radiology. Philadelphia, W.B. Saunders Co., 1986, p. 179.)

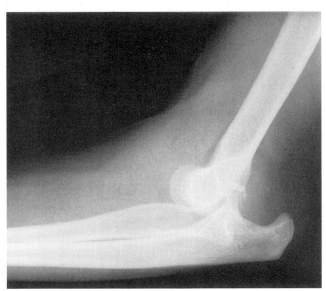

Figure 6–33
Lateral film of a dislocated elbow, showing the lower end of the humerus resting on the ulna in front of the coronoid. Note fragmentation of the coronoid. (From O'Donoghue, D.H.: Treatment of Injuries to Athletes, 4th ed. Philadelphia, W.B. Saunders Co., 1984, p. 227.)

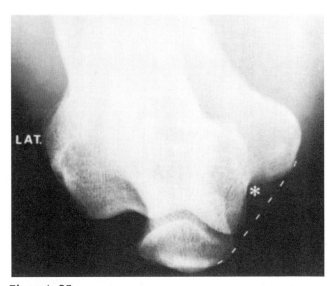

Figure 6–35
Cubital tunnel. The ulnar nerve (*asterisk*) lies in a tunnel bridged by the arcuate ligament (*dashed line*), which extends from the medial epicondyle to the olecranon process. LAT = lateral. (After Wadsworth, T.G.: The Elbow. Edinburgh, Churchill Livingstone, 1982.)

Axial View. This view is taken with the elbow flexed to 45°. It shows the olecranon process and epicondyles. It is useful for showing osteophytes and loose bodies.[13]

Arthrography

Figure 6–36 illustrates the views seen in normal elbow arthrograms.

Magnetic Resonance Imaging

Magnetic resonance imaging (MRI) is used to differentiate bone and soft tissues. Because of its high soft-tissue contrast, MRI, a noninvasive technique, is able to discriminate among bone marrow, cartilage, tendons, nerves, and vessels without the use of a contrast medium (Fig. 6–37).[34] The technique is used to demonstrate tendon ruptures, collateral ligament ruptures, cubital tunnel pathology, epicondylitis, and osteochrondritis dissecans.[35]

Xerography

Figure 6–38 illustrates the detailed borders of the various structures around the elbow.

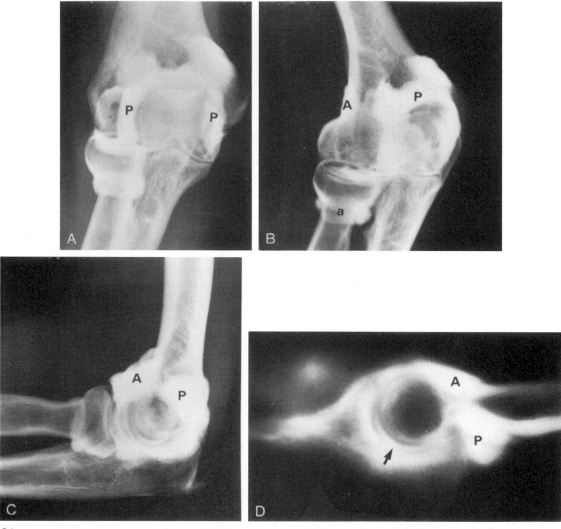

Figure 6–36

Normal elbow arthrogram. Anteroposterior (A), external oblique (B), and lateral (C) views in extension show the normal annular (a), anterior (A), and posterior (P) recesses. (D) Lateral tomogram with the arm extended. The area of the trochlea that is devoid of cartilage (*arrow*) is seen. (From Weissman, B.N.W., and C.B. Sledge: Orthopedic Radiology. Philadelphia, W.B. Saunders Co., 1986, p. 178.)

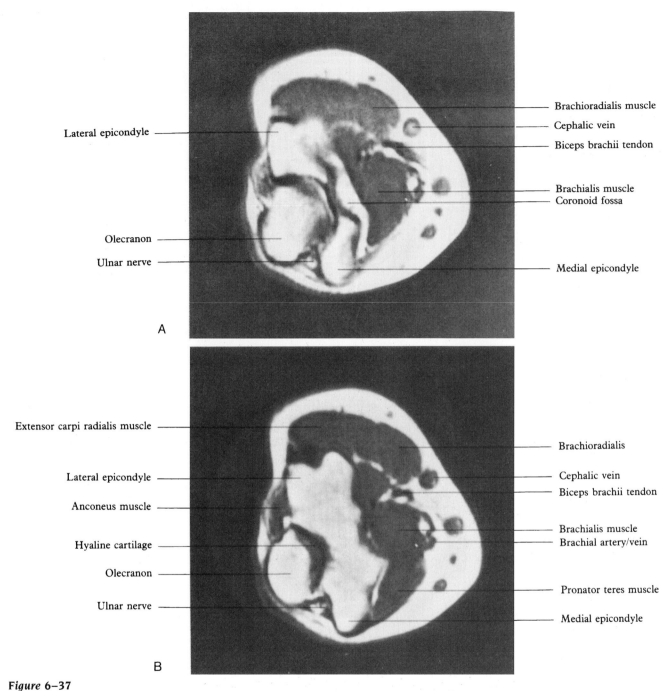

Lateral epicondyle

Olecranon

Ulnar nerve

Brachioradialis muscle

Cephalic vein

Biceps brachii tendon

Brachialis muscle
Coronoid fossa

Medial epicondyle

A

Extensor carpi radialis muscle

Lateral epicondyle

Anconeus muscle

Hyaline cartilage

Olecranon

Ulnar nerve

Brachioradialis

Cephalic vein
Biceps brachii tendon

Brachialis muscle
Brachial artery/vein

Pronator teres muscle

Medial epicondyle

B

Figure 6–37

(A *and* B) Normal MRI anatomy, axial view. Serial magnetic resonance (MR) images (SE 500/28) of the normal elbow joint from superior to inferior.

Illustration continued on following page

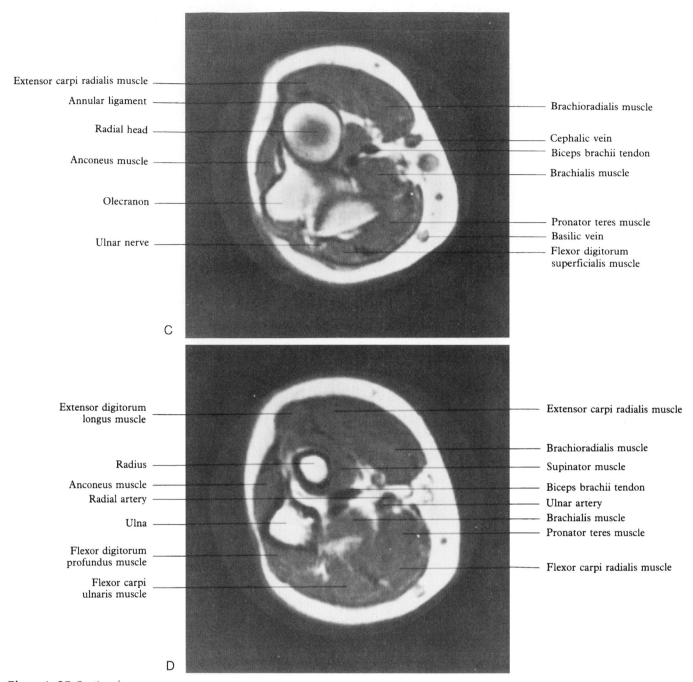

Extensor carpi radialis muscle

Annular ligament

Radial head

Anconeus muscle

Olecranon

Ulnar nerve

Brachioradialis muscle

Cephalic vein

Biceps brachii tendon

Brachialis muscle

Pronator teres muscle

Basilic vein

Flexor digitorum superficialis muscle

C

Extensor digitorum longus muscle

Radius

Anconeus muscle

Radial artery

Ulna

Flexor digitorum profundus muscle

Flexor carpi ulnaris muscle

Extensor carpi radialis muscle

Brachioradialis muscle

Supinator muscle

Biceps brachii tendon

Ulnar artery

Brachialis muscle

Pronator teres muscle

Flexor carpi radialis muscle

D

Figure 6–37 *Continued*
(C *and* D) Normal MRI anatomy, axial view. Serial magnetic resonance (MR) images (SE 500/28) of the normal elbow joint from superior to inferior.

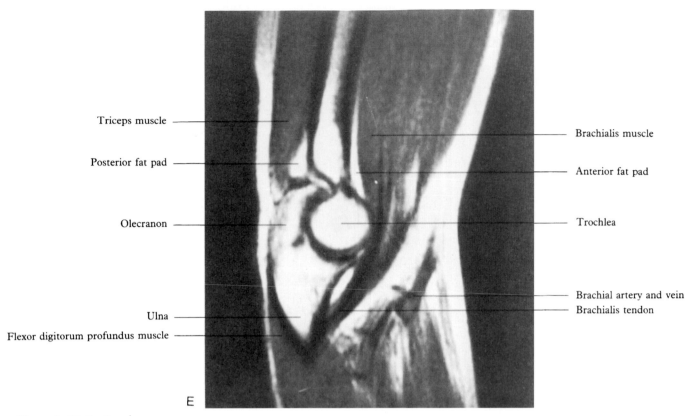

Triceps muscle —

Posterior fat pad —

Olecranon —

Ulna —

Flexor digitorum profundus muscle —

— Brachialis muscle

— Anterior fat pad

— Trochlea

— Brachial artery and vein
— Brachialis tendon

E

Figure 6–37 *Continued*
(E) Normal anatomy, sagittal view. Serial MR images (SE 500/28) of the normal elbow joint, from medial to lateral. (From Bassett, L.W., R.H. Gold, and L.L. Seeger: MRI Atlas of the Musculoskeletal System. London, Martin Dunitz Ltd., 1989, p. 133.)

Figure 6–38
Xerogram of the elbow demonstrating the fat pads and supinator fat stripe resulting from subtle radial head fracture. (From Berquist, T.H.: Diagnostic radiographic techniques of the elbow. *In* Morrey, B.F. [ed.]: The Elbow and Its Disorders. Philadelphia, W.B. Saunders Co., 1993, p. 106.)

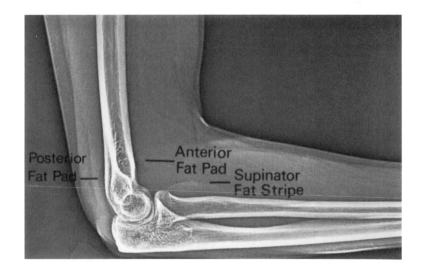

Posterior
Fat Pad —

Anterior
Fat Pad Supinator
Fat Stripe

Précis of the Elbow Assessment*

History
Observation
Examination
    Active movements
        Elbow flexion
        Elbow extension
        Supination
        Pronation
        Combined movements (if necessary)
        Repetitive movements (if necessary)
        Sustained positions (if necessary)
    Passive movements (as in active movements, if necessary)
    Resisted isometric movements
        Elbow flexion
        Elbow extension
        Supination
        Pronation
        Wrist flexion
        Wrist extension
    Special tests
    Reflexes and cutaneous distribution

Reflexes
Sensory scan
Peripheral nerves
    Median nerve and branches
    Ulnar nerve
    Radial nerve and branches
Joint play movements
    Radial deviation of ulna and radius on humerus
    Ulnar deviation of ulna and radius on humerus
    Distraction of olecranon process on humerus in 90°
        of flexion
    Anteroposterior glide of radius on humerus
Palpation
Diagnostic Imaging

---

* The entire assessment may be done with the patient in sitting position.

After any examination, the patient should be warned of the possibility of exacerbation of symptoms as a result of the assessment.

Case Studies

When doing these case studies, the examiner should list the appropriate questions to be asked and why they are being asked, what to look for and why, and what things should be tested and why. Depending on the answers of the patient (and the examiner should consider several different responses), several possible causes of the patient's problem may become evident (examples are given in parentheses). A differential diagnosis chart should be made up (see Table 6–5 as an example for question 1). The examiner can then decide how different diagnoses may affect the treatment plan.

1. A 24-year-old woman comes to you complaining of pain in her right elbow on the medial side. The pain sometimes extends into the forearm and is often accompanied by tingling into the little finger and half of the ring finger. The pain and paresthesia are particularly bothersome when she plays recreational volleyball, which she enjoys very much. Describe your assessment plan for this patient (ulnar neuritis versus medial epicondylitis).

Table 6–5
Differential Diagnosis of Ulnar Neuritis and Medial Epicondylitis

	Ulnar Neuritis	Medial Epicondylitis
History	May follow repetitive activity May follow bumped elbow May follow previously injured elbow Pain in forearm and into ulnar distribution of hand	Usually follows repetitive activity Pain in forearm, may radiate to wrist
Observation	Normal	Normal
Active movements	Weakness of ulnar deviation Weakness of little and ring finger flexion	Slight pain on wrist flexion
Passive movements	Normal, or pain may come on with elbow flexion and wrist flexion	Normal, but pain may occur with elbow extension and wrist extension
Resisted isometric movements	Weakness of ulnar deviation Weakness of little and ring finger flexion	Pain on wrist extension with elbow extension Pain on supination and wrist and finger flexion
Special tests	Tinel's sign positive Wartenberg's sign positive Elbow flexion test positive	Golfer's elbow test positive
Sensation	Paresthesia and pain in forearm, little finger, and half of ring finger	Pain in forearm, possibly to wrist

2. A 52-year-old man is referred to you with a history of right elbow pain. He complains of tenderness over the lateral epicondyle. He informs you that he has not been doing any repetitive forearm activity and does not play tennis. He has some restriction of neck movement. Describe your assessment plan for this patient (cervical spondylosis versus lateral epicondylitis).

3. A 26-year-old male football player is referred to you after surgery for a ruptured (third-degree strain) left biceps tendon at its insertion. His cast has been removed, and you have been asked to restore the patient to normal function. Describe your assessment plan for this patient.

4. A 4-year-old girl is brought to you by her parents. They state that about 2 hours previously they were out shopping and the mother was holding the little girl's arm. The little girl tripped, and the mother "yanked" her up as she fell. The little girl started to cry and would not move her elbow. Describe your assessment plan for this patient (radial head dislocation versus ligamentous sprain).

5. A 46-year-old man comes to you complaining of diffuse left elbow pain. When he carries a briefcase for three or four blocks, his elbow becomes stiff and sore. When he picks up things with his left hand, the pain increases dramatically. Describe your assessment plan for this patient (lateral epicondylitis versus osteoarthritis).

6. A 31-year-old man comes to you complaining of posterior elbow pain. He says he banged his elbow on the table 10 days ago, and he has had posterior swelling for 8 or 9 days. Describe your assessment plan for this patient (olecranon bursitis versus joint synovitis).

7. A 14-year-old female gymnast comes to you complaining of elbow pain. She explains she was doing a vault and bent her elbow backward when she heard a snap. The injury occurred 1 hour ago, and there is some swelling; she does not want to move the elbow. Describe your assessment plan for this patient (biceps tendon rupture versus epiphyseal fracture).

References

Cited References

1. Andrews, J.R., K.E. Wilk, Y.E. Satterwhite, and J.L. Tedder: Physical examination of the thrower's elbow. J. Orthop. Sports Phys. Ther. 17:296–304, 1993.
2. Beals, R.K.: The normal carrying angle of the elbow. Clin. Orthop. 1190:194–196, 1976.
3. Charton, A.: The Elbow: The Rheumatological Physical Examination. Orlando, Florida, Grune & Stratton, Inc., 1986.
4. Kapandji, A.I.: The Physiology of the Joints, vol. 1: Upper Limb. New York, Churchill Livingstone, 1970.
5. American Orthopaedic Association: Manual of Orthopaedic Surgery. Chicago, American Orthopaedic Association, 1972.
6. Tarr, R.R., A.I. Garfinkel, and A. Sarmiento: The effects of angular and rotational deformities of both bones of the forearm. J. Bone Joint Surg. Am. 66:65–70, 1984.
7. Askew, L.J., K.N. An, B.F. Morrey, and E.Y. Chao: Isometric elbow strength in normal individuals. Clin. Orthop. 222:261–266, 1987.
8. Morrey, B.F., K.N. An, and E.Y.S. Chao: Functional evaluation of the elbow. In Morrey, B.F. (ed.): The Elbow and Its Disorders. Philadelphia, W.B. Saunders Co., 1993.
9. Regan, W.D., and B.F. Morrey: The physical examination of the elbow. In Morrey, B.F. (ed.): The Elbow and Its Disorders. Philadelphia, W.B. Saunders Co., 1993.
10. Roles, N.C., and R.H. Maudsley: Radial tunnel syndrome. Resistant tennis elbow as a nerve entrapment. J. Bone Joint Surg. Br. 54:499–508, 1972.
11. Buehler, M.J., and D.T. Thayer: The elbow flexion test: A clinical test for the cubital tunnel syndrome. Clin. Orthop. 233:213–216, 1988.
12. Butler, D.S.: Mobilisation of the Nervous System. Melbourne, Churchill Livingstone, 1991.
13. Bigg-Wither, G., and P. Kelly: Diagnostic imaging in musculoskeletal physiotherapy. In Refshauge, K., and E. Gass (eds.): Musculoskeletal Physiotherapy: Clinical Science and Practice. Oxford, Butterworth-Heinemann, 1995.
14. Limb, D., S.L. Hodkinson, and R.F. Brown: Median nerve palsy after posterolateral elbow dislocation. J. Bone Joint Surg. Br. 76:987–988, 1994.
15. Conrad, R.W., and R.J. Spinner: Snapping brachialis tendon associated with median neuropathy. J. Bone Joint Surg. Am. 77:1891–1893, 1995.
16. Spinner, M., and P.S. Spencer: Nerve compression lesions of the upper extremity: A clinical and experimental review. Clin. Orthop. 104:46–67, 1974.
17. Butlers, K.P., and K.M. Singer: Nerve lesions of the arm and elbow. In De Lee, J.C., and D. Drez (eds.): Orthopedic Sports Medicine: Principles and Practice. Philadelphia, W.B. Saunders Co., 1994.
18. Rask, M.R.: Anterior interosseous nerve entrapment (Kiloh-Nevin Syndrome). Clin. Orthop. 142:176–181, 1979.
19. Wiens, E., and S.C.K. Lau: The anterior interosseous nerve syndrome. Can. J. Surg. 21:354–357, 1978.
20. Engher, W.D., and J.S. Keene: Anterior interosseous nerve palsy associated with a Monteggia fracture. Clin. Orthop. 174:133–137, 1983.
21. O'Driscoll, S.W., E. Horii, S.W. Carmichael, and B.F. Morrey: The cubital tunnel and ulnar neuropathy. J. Bone Joint Surg. Br. 73:613–617, 1991.
22. McPherson, S.A., and R.A. Meals: Cubital tunnel syndrome. Orthop. Clin. North Am. 23:111–123, 1992.
23. Wadsworth, T.G.: The external compression syndrome of the ulnar nerve at the cubital tunnel. Clin. Orthop. 124:189–204, 1977.
24. Pecina, M.M., J. Krmpotic-Nemanic, and A.D. Markiewitz: Tunnel Syndromes. Boca Raton, Florida, CRC Press, 1991.
25. Gelberman, R.H., R. Eaton, and J.R. Urbaniak: Peripheral nerve compression. J. Bone Joint Surg. Am. 75:1854–1878, 1993.
26. Apfelberg, D.B., and S.J. Larsen: Dynamic anatomy of the ulnar nerve by the deep flexor-pronator aponeurosis. Plast. Reconstr. Surg. 51:79–81, 1973.
27. Holmes, J.C., and J.E. Hall: Tardy ulnar nerve palsy in children. Clin. Orthop. 135:128–131, 1978.
28. Wadsworth, T.G.: The Elbow. New York, Churchill Livingstone, 1982.
29. Lutz, F.R.: Radial tunnel syndrome: An etiology of chronic lateral elbow pain. J. Orthop. Sports Phys. Ther. 14:14–17, 1991.
30. Ferlec, D.C., and B.F. Morrey: Evaluation of the painful elbow: The problem elbow. In Morrey, B.F. (ed.): The Elbow and Its Disorders. Philadelphia, W.B. Saunders Co., 1993.
31. Lister, G.D., R.B. Belsole, and H.E. Kleinert: The radial tunnel syndrome. J. Hand Surg. 4:52–59, 1979.
32. Van Rossum, J., O.J. Buruma, H.A. Kamphuisen, and G.J. Onvlee: Tennis elbow: A radial tunnel syndrome? J. Bone Joint Surg. Br. 60:197–198, 1978.
33. Quinton, D.N., D. Finlay, and R. Butterworth: The elbow fat pad sign: Brief report. J. Bone Joint Surg. Br. 69:844–845, 1987.
34. Herzog, R.J.: Efficacy of magnetic resonance imaging of the elbow. Med. Sci. Sports Exerc. 26:1193–1202, 1994.
35. Fritz, R.C., and G.A. Brody: MR imaging of the wrist and elbow. Clin. Sports Med. 14:315–352, 1995.

General References

Amir, D., U. Frankel, and H. Pogrund: Pulled elbow and hypermobility of joints. Clin. Orthop. 257:94–99, 1990.

An, K.N., and B.F. Morrey: Biomechanics of the elbow. In Morrey, B.F. (ed.): The Elbow and Its Disorders. Philadelphia, W.B. Saunders Co., 1993.

Anderson, T.E.: Anatomy and physical examination of the elbow. In Nicholas, J.A., and E.B. Hershman (eds.): The Upper Extremity in Sports Medicine. St. Louis, C.V. Mosby Co., 1990.

Andrews, J.R., and K. Meister: Overuse injuries of the athlete's elbow. In Griffin, L.Y. (ed.): Orthopedic Knowledge Update: Sports Medicine. Rosemont, Illinois, American Academy of Orthopaedic Surgeons, 1994.

Aeurbach, D.M., E.D. Collins, K.L. Kunkle, and E.H. Monsanto: The radial sensory nerve: An anatomic study. Clin. Orthop. 308:241–249, 1994.

Bassett, L.W., R.H. Gold, and L.L. Seeger: MRI Atlas of the Musculoskeletal System. London, Martin Dunitz Ltd., 1989.

Belhobek, G.H.: Roentgenographic evaluation of the elbow. In Nicholas, J.A., and E.B. Hershman (eds.): The Upper Extremity in Sports Medicine. St. Louis, C.V. Mosby Co., 1990.

Berquist, T.H.: Diagnostic radiographic techniques of the elbow. In Morrey, B.F. (ed.): The Elbow and Its Disorders. Philadelphia, W.B. Saunders Co., 1993.

Bledsoe, R.C., and J.L. Izenstark: Displacement of fat pads in disease and injury of the elbow. Radiology 73:717–724, 1959.

Booker, J.M., and G.A. Thibodeau: Athletic Injury Assessment. St. Louis, Times Mirror/Mosby, 1989.

Bowling, R.W., and P.A. Rockar: The elbow complex. In Gould, J.A. (ed.): Orthopedic and Sports Physical Therapy. St. Louis, C.V. Mosby Co., 1990.

Bunnell, D.H., D.A. Fisher, L.W. Bassett, R.H. Gold, and H. Ellman: Elbow joint: Normal anatomy on MR images. Radiology 165:527–531, 1987.

Cabrera, J.M., and F.C. McCue: Nonosseous athletic injuries of the elbow, forearm, and hand. Clin. Sports Med. 5:681–700, 1986.

Chusid, J.G., and J.J. McDonald: Correlative Neuroanatomy and Functional Neurology. Los Altos, California, Lange Medical Publications, 1961.

Clark, C.B.: Cubital tunnel syndrome. JAMA 241:801–802, 1979.

Clarkson, H.M., and G.B. Gilewich: Musculoskeletal Assessment: Joint Range of Motion and Manual Muscle Strength. Baltimore, Williams & Wilkins, 1989.

Conwell, H.E.: Injuries to the elbow. Clin. Symp. 22:35–54, 1970.

Cyriax, J.: Textbook of Orthopaedic Medicine, vol. 1: Diagnosis of Soft Tissue Lesions. London, Bailliere Tindall, 1982.

Del Pizzo, W., F.W. Jobe, and L. Norwood: Ulnar nerve entrapment in baseball players, Am. J. Sports Med. 5:182–185, 1977.

Dellon, A.L., and S.E. Mackinnon: Radial sensory nerve entrapment in the forearm. J. Hand Surg. 11:199–205, 1986.

Dilorenzo, C.E., J.C. Parker, and R.D. Chmelar: The importance of shoulder and cervical dysfunction in the etiology and treatment of athletic elbow injuries. J. Orthop. Sports Phys. Ther. 11:402–409, 1990.

Evans, R.C.: Illustrated Essentials in Orthopedic Physical Assessment. St. Louis, C.V. Mosby Co., 1994.

Forrester, D.M., and J.C. Brown: The Radiology of Joint Disease. Philadelphia, W.B. Saunders Co., 1987.

Garrick, J.G., and D.R. Webb: Sports Injuries: Diagnosis and Management. Philadelphia, W.B. Saunders Co., 1990.

Gunn, C.C., and W.E. Milbrandt: Tennis elbow and the cervical spine. Can. Med. Assoc. J. 114:803–809, 1976.

Hollinshead, W.H., and D.B. Jenkins: Functional Anatomy of the Limbs and Back. Philadelphia, W.B. Saunders Co., 1981.

Hoppenfeld, S.: Physical Examination of the Spine and Extremities. New York, Appleton-Century-Crofts, 1976.

Ishizuki, M.: Functional anatomy of the elbow joint and three-dimensional quantitative motion analysis of the elbow joint. J. Jpn. Orthop. Assoc. 53:989, 1979.

Jobe, F.W., G.S. Fanton, and N.S. Elaltrache: Ulnar nerve injury. In Morrey, B.F. (ed.): The Elbow and Its Disorders. Philadelphia, W.B. Saunders Co., 1993.

Johnson, R.K., M. Spinner, and M.M. Shrewsburg: Median nerve entrapment syndrome in the proximal forearm. J. Hand Surg. 4:48–51, 1979.

Judge, R.D., G.D. Zuidema, and F.T. Fitzgerald: Clinical Diagnosis: A Physiological Approach. Boston, Little, Brown & Co., 1982.

Kaltenborn, F.M.: Mobilization of the Extremity Joints. Oslo, Olaf Norlis Bokhandel, 1980.

Kiloh, L.G., and S. Nevin: Isolated neuritis of the anterior interosseous nerve. Br. Med. J. 1:850–851, 1952.

Leach, R.E., and J.K. Miller: Lateral and medial epicondylitis of the elbow. Clin. Sports Med. 6:259–272, 1987.

London, J.T.: Kinematics of the elbow. J. Bone Joint Surg. Am. 63:529–535, 1981.

Macdonald, D.A.: The shoulder and elbow. In Pynsent, P., J. Fairbank, and A. Carr (eds.): Outcome Measures in Orthopedics. Oxford, Butterworth-Heinemann Ltd., 1993.

Maitland, G.D.: The Peripheral Joints: Examination and Recording Guide. Adelaide, Australia, Virgo Press, 1973.

Morrey, B.F.: Loose bodies. In Morrey, B.F. (ed.): The Elbow and Its Disorders. Philadelphia, W.B. Saunders Co., 1993.

Morrey, B.F.: Physical examination of the elbow. In Post, M. (ed.): Physical Examination of the Musculoskeletal System. Chicago, Year Book Medical Publishers, 1987.

Moss, S.H., and H.E. Switzer: Radial tunnel syndrome: A spectrum of clinical presentations. J. Hand Surg. 8:414–420, 1983.

Newberg, A.H.: The radiographic examination of shoulder and elbow pain in the athlete. Clin. Sports Med. 6:785–809, 1987.

Nolan, R.: Cubital tunnel syndrome. Sports Med. Update 5:21–23, 1990.

O'Donoghue, D.H.: Treatment of Injuries to Athletes. Philadelphia, W.B. Saunders Co., 1976, 1984.

Omer, G.E.: Physical diagnosis of peripheral nerve injuries. Orthop. Clin. North Am. 12:207–228, 1981.

Palmer, M.L., and M. Epler: Clinical Assessment Procedures in Physical Therapy. Philadelphia, J.B. Lippincott Co., 1990.

Regan, W.D.: Lateral elbow pain in the athlete: A clinical review. Clin. J. Sports Med. 1:53–58, 1991.

Reid, D.C.: Sports Injury Assessment and Rehabilitation. New York, Churchill Livingstone, 1992.

Reid, D.C., and S. Kushner: The elbow region. In Donatelli, R., and M.J. Wooden (eds.): Orthopedic Physical Therapy. Edinburgh, Churchill Livingstone, 1989.

Roles, N.C., and R.H. Madusley: Radial tunnel syndrome: Resistant tennis elbow as a nerve entrapment. J. Bone Joint Surg. Br. 54:499–508, 1972.

Spinner, M., and R.L. Linscheld: Nerve entrapment syndromes. In Morrey, B.F. (ed.): The Elbow and Its Disorders. Philadelphia, W.B. Saunders Co., 1993.

Spinner, M.: The arcade of Frohse and its relationship to posterior interosseous nerve paralysis. J. Bone Joint Surg. Br. 50:809–812, 1968.

Sprofkin, B.E.: Cheiralgia paresthetica: Wartenberg's disease. Neurology 4:857–862, 1954.

Steinberg, B.D., and K.D. Plancher: Clinical anatomy of the wrist and elbow. Clin. Sports Med. 14:299–313, 1995.

Stroyan, M., and K.E. Wilk: The functional anatomy of the elbow complex. J. Orthop. Sports Phys. Ther. 17:279–288, 1993.

Terzis, J.K., and E.M. Noah: Anatomy and morphology of upper extremity nerves and frequent sites of compression. In Gordon, S.L., S.J. Blair, and L.J. Fine (eds.): Repetitive Motion Disorders of the Upper Extremity. Rosemont, Illinois, American Academy of Orthopaedic Surgeons, 1995.

Tomberlin, J.P., and H.D. Saunders: Evaluation, Treatment and Prevention of Musculoskeletal Disorders: The Extremities. Chaska, Minnesota, The Saunders Group, 1994.

Tullos, H.S., and W.J. Bryan: Examination of the throwing elbow. In Zarins, B., J.R. Andrews, and W.G. Carson (eds.): Injuries to the Throwing Arm. Philadelphia, W.B. Saunders Co., 1985.

Wadsworth, C.T.: Manual Examination and Treatment of the Spine and Extremities. Baltimore, Williams & Wilkins, 1988.

Weissman, B.N.W., and C.B. Sledge: Orthopedic Radiology. Philadelphia, W.B. Saunders Co., 1986.

Williams, P.L., and R. Warwick (eds.): Gray's Anatomy, 36th British ed. Edinburgh, Churchill Livingstone, 1980.

Yokum, L.A.: The diagnosis and nonoperative treatment of elbow problems in the athlete. Clin. Sports Med. 8:439–451, 1989.

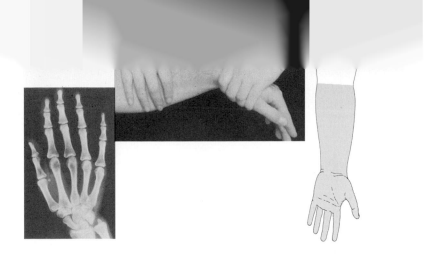

7

Forearm, Wrist, and Hand

The hand and wrist are the most active and intricate parts of the upper extremity. Because of this, they are vulnerable to injury and do not respond well to serious trauma. Their mobility is enhanced by a wide range of movement at the shoulder and complementary movement at the elbow. The 28 bones, numerous articulations, and 19 intrinsic and 20 extrinsic muscles of the wrist and hand provide a tremendous variability of movement. In addition to being an expressive organ of communication, the hand has a protective role and acts as both a motor and a sensory organ, providing information such as temperature, thickness, texture, depth, and shape as well as the motion of an object. It is this sensual acuity that enables the examiner to accurately examine and palpate during an assessment.

The assessment of the hand should be done with two objectives in mind. First, the injury or lesion should be assessed as accurately as possible to ensure proper treatment. Second, the examiner should evaluate the remaining function to determine whether the patient will have any incapacity in everyday life.

Although the joints of the forearm, wrist, and hand are discussed separately, it must be remembered that these joints act not in isolation but rather as functional groups. The position of one joint influences the position and action of the other joints. For example, if the wrist is flexed, the interphalangeal joints do not fully flex, primarily because of passive insufficiency of the finger extensors. Each articulation depends on balanced forces for proper positioning and control. If this balance or equilibrium is not present because of trauma, nerve injury, or other factors, the loss of counterbalancing forces results in deformities. In addition, the entire upper limb should be considered a kinetic chain so that the hand can be properly positioned. The actions of the shoulder, elbow, and wrist joints enable the hand to be placed on almost any area of the body.

Applied Anatomy

The **distal radioulnar joint** is a uniaxial pivot joint that has one degree of freedom. Although the radius moves over the ulna, the ulna does not remain stationary. It moves back and laterally during pronation and forward and medially during supination. The resting position of the joint is 10° of supination, and the close packed position is 5° of supination. The capsular pattern of the distal radioulnar joint is full range of motion (ROM) with pain at extreme of rotation.

Distal Radioulnar Joint	
Resting position:	10° of supination
Close packed position:	5° of supination
Capsular pattern:	Pain at extreme of rotation

The **radiocarpal (wrist) joint** is a biaxial ellipsoid joint. The radius articulates with the scaphoid and lunate. The distal radius is not straight but is angled toward the ulna (15 to 20°), and its posterior margin projects more distally to provide a "buttress effect."[1] The lunate and triquetrum also articulate with the triangular cartilaginous disc and not the ulna. The disc extends from the ulnar side of the distal radius and attaches to the ulna at the base of the ulnar styloid process. The disc adds stability to the wrist. It creates a close relation between the ulna and carpal bones and binds together the distal ends of the radius and ulna. With the disc in place, the radius bears 60% of the load and the ulna bears 40%. If the disc is removed, the radius transmits 95% of the axial load and the ulna transmits 5%.[2] Therefore, the cartilaginous disc acts as a cushion for the wrist joint and as a major stabilizer of the distal radioulnar joint.[1, 3] The disc can be damaged by forced extension and pronation. The distal end of the radius is concave and the proximal row of carpals is convex, but the curvatures are not equal. The joint has two degrees of freedom, and the resting position is neutral with slight ulnar deviation. The close packed position is extension, and the capsular pattern is equal limitation of flexion and extension.

Radiocarpal (Wrist) Joint

Resting position:	Neutral with slight ulnar deviation
Close packed position:	Extension
Capsular pattern:	Flexion and extension equally limited (works with midcarpal joint)

The **intercarpal joints** include the joints between the individual bones of the proximal row of carpal bones (scaphoid, lunate, and triquetrum) and the joints between the individual bones of the distal row of carpal bones (trapezium, trapezoid, capitate, and hamate). They are bound together by small intercarpal ligaments (dorsal, palmar, and interosseous), which allow only a slight amount of gliding movement between the bones. The close packed position is extension, and the resting position is neutral or slight flexion.

Intercarpal Joints

Resting position:	Neutral or slight flexion
Close packed position:	Extension
Capsular pattern:	None

---

tion is neutral or slight flexion. The **pisotriquetral joint** is considered separately because the pisiform sits on the triquetrum and does not take a direct part in the other intercarpal movements.

The **midcarpal joints** form a compound articulation between the proximal and distal rows of carpal bones, with the exception of the pisiform bone. On the medial side, the scaphoid, lunate, and triquetrum articulate with the capitate and hamate, forming a compound sellar (saddle-shaped) joint. On the lateral aspect, the scaphoid articulates with the trapezoid and trapezium, forming another compound sellar joint. As with the intercarpal joints, these articulations are bound together by dorsal and palmar ligaments; however, there are no interosseous ligaments between the proximal and distal rows of bones. Therefore, greater movement exists at the midcarpal joints than at the intercarpal joints. The close packed

position of these joints is extension with ulnar deviation, and the resting position is neutral or slight flexion with ulnar deviation.

Midcarpal Joints

Resting position:	Neutral or slight flexion with ulnar deviation
Close packed position:	Extension with ulnar deviation
Capsular pattern:	Equal limitation of flexion and extension (works with radiocarpal joints)

At the thumb, the **carpometacarpal joint** is a sellar joint that has three degrees of freedom, whereas the second to fifth carpometacarpal joints are plane joints.[4] The capsular pattern of the carpometacarpal joint of the thumb is abduction most limited, followed by extension. The resting position is midway between abduction and adduction and midway between flexion and extension. The close packed position of the carpometacarpal joint of the thumb is full opposition. For the second to fifth carpometacarpal joints, the capsular pattern of restriction is equal limitation in all directions. The bones of these joints are held together by dorsal and palmar ligaments. In addition, the thumb articulation has a strong lateral ligament extending from the lateral side of the trapezium to the radial side of the base of the first metacarpal, and the medial four articulations have an interosseous ligament similar to that found in the carpal articulation.

Carpometacarpal Joints

Resting position:	Thumb, midway between abduction and adduction, and midway between flexion and extension. Fingers, midway between flexion and extension
Close packed position:	Thumb, full opposition. Fingers, full flexion
Capsular pattern:	Thumb, abduction, then extension. Fingers, equal limitation in all directions

---

The carpometacarpal articulations of the fingers allow only gliding movement. The carpometacarpal articulation of the thumb is unique in that it allows flexion, extension, abduction, adduction, rotation, and circumduction. It is able to do this because the articulation is saddle shaped. Because of the many movements possible at this joint, the thumb is able to adopt any position relative to the palmar aspect of the hand.[4]

The plane **intermetacarpal joints** have only a small amount of gliding movement between them and do not include the thumb articulation. They are bound together by palmar, dorsal, and interosseous ligaments.

The **metacarpophalangeal joints** are condyloid joints. The second and third metacarpophalangeal joints tend to be immobile and are the primary stabilizing factor of the hand, whereas the fourth and fifth joints are more mobile. The collateral ligaments of these joints are tight on flexion and relaxed on extension. These articulations are also bound by palmar ligaments and deep transverse metacarpal ligaments. Each joint has two degrees of freedom. The first metacarpophalangeal joint has three degrees of freedom, thus facilitating the movement of the carpometacarpal joint of the thumb.[4] The close packed position of the first metacarpophalangeal joint is maximum opposition, and the close

packed position for the second through the fifth metacarpophalangeal joints is maximum flexion.[5] The resting position of the metacarpophalangeal joints is slight flexion, whereas the capsular pattern is more limitation of flexion than extension.

The **interphalangeal joints** are uniaxial hinge joints, each having one degree of freedom. The close packed position of the proximal interphalangeal joints and distal interphalangeal joints is full extension; the resting position is slight flexion. The capsular pattern of these joints

Interphalangeal Joints

Resting position:	Slight flexion
Close packed position:	Full extension
Capsular pattern:	Flexion, extension

is that flexion is more limited than extension. The bones of these joints are bound together by a fibrous capsule and by the palmar and collateral ligaments. During flexion, there is some rotation in these joints so that the pulp of the fingers face more fully the pulp of the thumb. If the metacarpophalangeal joints and the proximal interphalangeal joints of the fingers are flexed, they converge toward the scaphoid tubercle (Fig. 7–1). This is sometimes referred to as a **cascade sign**. If one or more fingers do not converge, it usually indicates trauma (e.g., fracture) to the digits that has altered their normal alignment.

Metacarpophalangeal Joints

Resting position:	Slight flexion
Close packed position:	Thumb, full opposition
	Fingers, full flexion
Capsular pattern:	Flexion, then extension

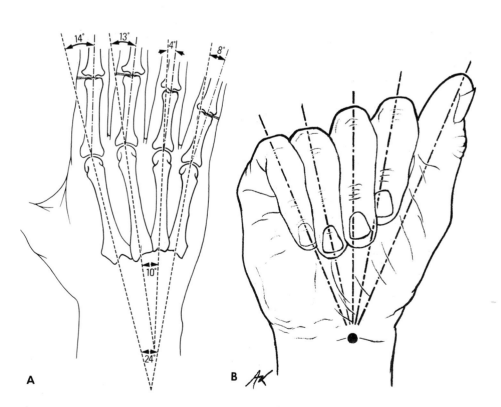

Figure 7–1
Alignment of the fingers. (A) Normal physiological alignment. (B) Oblique flexion of the last four digits. Only the index ray flexes toward the median axis. When the last four digits are flexed separately at the metacarpophalangeal and proximal interphalangeal joints, their axes converge toward the scaphoid tubercle. (From Tubiana, R.: The Hand. Philadelphia, W.B. Saunders Co., 1981, pp. 22, 197.)

A   B

Patient History

The assessment of the hand often takes longer than that of other joints of the body because of the importance of the hand to everyday function and because of the many structures and joints involved.

In addition to the questions listed under Patient History in Chapter 1, the examiner should obtain the following information from the patient:

1. What is the patient's age? Certain conditions are more likely to occur at different ages. For example, arthritic changes are most commonly seen in patients who are older than 40 years of age.

2. What is the patient's occupation? Certain occupations are more likely to affect the wrist and hand. For example, typists are more likely to suffer repetitive strain injuries, and mechanics are more likely to suffer traumatic injuries.

3. What was the mechanism of injury? For example, a fall on the outstretched hand (FOOSH) injury may lead to a lunate dislocation, or extension of the fingers may cause dislocation of the fingers. A rotational force applied to the wrist or near it may lead to a **Galleazzi fracture,** which is a fracture of the radius and dislocation of the distal end of the ulna.

4. What tasks is the patient able or unable to perform? For example, is there any problem with buttoning, dressing, tying shoelaces, or any other everyday activity? This type of question gives an indication of the patient's functional limitation.

5. When did the injury or onset occur, and how long has the patient been incapacitated? These questions are not necessarily the same; for instance, a burn may occur at a certain time, but incapacity may not occur until hypertrophic scarring appears. The wrist is commonly injured by weight bearing (e.g., gymnastics), by rotational stress combined with ulnar deviation (e.g., hitting a racquet), by twisting, and by impact loading (FOOSH injury).[6, 7]

6. Which hand is the patient's dominant hand? The dominant hand is more likely to be injured, and the functional loss, at least initially, is greater.

7. Has the patient ever injured the forearm, wrist, or hand before? Was it the same type of injury? Was the mechanism of injury the same? If so, how was it treated?

8. Which part of the forearm, wrist, or hand is injured? If the flexor tendons (which are round, have synovial sheaths, and have a longer excursion than the extensor tendons) are injured, they respond much more slowly to treatment than do extensor tendons (which are flat or ovoid). Within the hand, there is a surgical "no man's land" (Fig. 7–2), which is a region between the distal palmar crease and the midportion of the middle phalanx

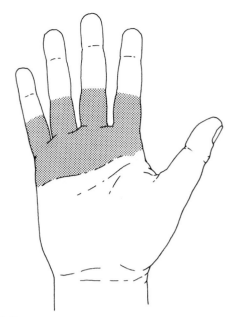

Figure 7–2
Surgical "no-man's land" (palmar view).

of the fingers. Damage to the flexor tendons in this area that requires surgical repair usually leads to the formation of adhesive bands that restrict gliding. In addition, the tendons may become ischemic, being replaced by scar tissue. Because of this, the prognosis after surgery in this area is poor.

Observation

While observing the patient and viewing the hands from both the anterior and posterior aspects, the examiner should note the patient's willingness and ability to use the hand. Normally, when the hand is in the resting position and the wrist is in the normal position, the fingers are progressively more flexed as one moves from the radial side of the hand to the ulnar side. Loss of this normal attitude may be caused by pathology affecting the hand, such as a lacerated tendon, or by a contracture such as **Dupuytren's contracture.**

The bone and soft-tissue contours of the forearm, wrist, and hand should be compared for both upper limbs, and any deviation should be noted. The cosmetic appearance of the hand is very important to some patients. The examiner should note the patient's reaction to the appearance of the hand and be prepared to provide a cosmetic evaluation. This evaluation should always be included with the more important functional assessment. The posture of the hand at rest often demonstrates common deformities. Are the normal skin creases present? Skin creases occur because of movement at the

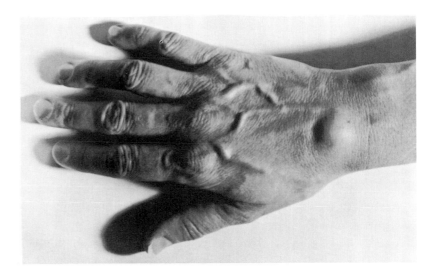

Figure 7–3

Ganglion or small cystic swelling on the dorsum of the right hand just distal to the wrist joint. (From Polley, H.F., and G.G. Hunder: Rheumatologic Interviewing and Physical Examination of the Joints. Philadelphia, W.B. Saunders Co., 1978, p. 96.)

various joints. The examiner should note any muscle wasting on the thenar eminence (median nerve), first dorsal interosseous muscle (C7 nerve root), or hypothenar eminence (ulnar nerve) that may be indicative of nerve or nerve root injury.

Any localized swellings (e.g., ganglion) that are seen on the dorsum of the hand should be recorded (Fig. 7–3). In the wrist and hand, effusion and synovial thickening are most evident on the dorsal and radial aspects. Swelling of the metacarpophalangeal and interphalangeal joints is most obvious on the dorsal aspect.

The dominant hand tends to be larger than the nondominant hand. If the patient has an area on the fingers that lacks sensation, this area will be avoided when the patient lifts or identifies objects, and the patient will instead use another finger with normal sensitivity. Therefore, the examiner should watch for abnormal or different patterns of movement, which may indicate adaptations or modifications necessitated by the presence of pathology.

Any vasomotor, sudomotor, pilomotor, and trophic changes should be recorded. These changes may be indicative of a peripheral nerve injury, peripheral vascular disease, diabetes mellitus, Raynaud's disease, or reflex neurovascular syndromes such as shoulder-hand syndrome or Sudeck's atrophy. The changes seen could include loss of hair on the hand, brittle fingernails, increase or decrease in sweating of the palm, shiny skin, radiographic evidence of osteoporosis, or any difference in temperature between the two limbs. Table 7–1 illustrates vasomotor, sudomotor, pilomotor, and trophic changes that occur in the hand when sympathetic nerve function has been affected.

The examiner should note any hypertrophy of the fingers. Hypertrophy of the bone may be seen in Paget's disease, neurofibromatosis, or arteriovenous fistula.

The presence of Heberden's or Bouchard's nodes (Fig. 7–4) should be recorded. Heberden's nodes appear on the dorsal surface of the distal interphalangeal joints and are associated with osteoarthritis. Bouchard's nodes

Table 7–1
Sympathetic Changes After Nerve Injury

Sympathetic Function	Feature	Early Changes	Late Changes
Vasomotor	Skin color	Rosy	Mottled or cyanotic
	Skin temperature	Warm	Cool
Sudomotor	Sweating	Dry skin	Dry or overly moist
Pilomotor	Gooseflesh response	Absent	Absent
Trophic	Skin texture	Soft, smooth	Smooth, nonelastic
	Soft-tissue atrophy	Slight	More pronounced, especially in finger pulps
	Nail changes	Blemishes	Curved in longitudinal and horizontal planes, "talonlike"
	Hair growth	May fall out or become longer and finer	May fall out or become longer and finer
	Rate of healing	Slowed	Slowed

From Hunter, J., L.H. Schneider, E.J. Mackin, and A.D. Callahan (eds.): Rehabilitation of the Hand: Surgery and Therapy. St. Louis, C.V. Mosby Co., 1990, p. 595.

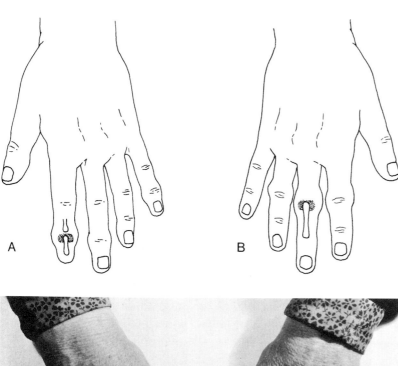

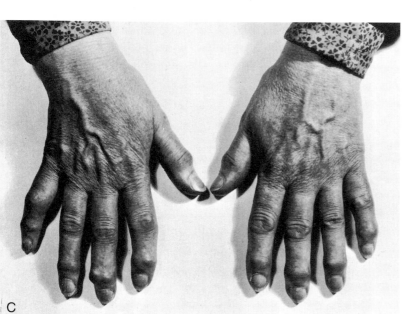

Figure 7–4

(A) Heberden's nodes. (B) Bouchard's nodes. (C) Degenerative joint disease (osteoarthritis) of both hands. Osteoarthritic enlargement of the distal interphalangeal joints (Heberden's nodes) and the proximal interphalangeal joints (Bouchard's nodes) is present. The metacarpophalangeal joints are not affected. (C, from Polley, H.F., and G.G. Hunder: Rheumatologic Interviewing and Physical Examination of the Joints. Philadelphia, W.B. Saunders Co., 1978, p. 120.)

are on the dorsal surface of the proximal interphalangeal joints. They are often associated with gastrectasis and rheumatoid arthritis.

Any ulcerations may indicate neurological or circulatory problems. Any alteration in the color of the limb with changes in position may indicate a circulatory problem.

The examiner should note any rotational or angulated deformities of the fingers, which may be indicative of previous fracture. The nail beds are normally parallel to one another. The fingers, when extended, are slightly rotated toward the thumb to aid pinch. Ulnar drift (Fig. 7–5) may be seen in rheumatoid arthritis owing to the shape of the metacarpophalangeal joints and the pull of the long tendons.

The presence of any wounds or scars should be noted, because they may indicate recent surgery or past trauma. If wounds are present, are they new or old? Are they healing properly? Is the scar red (new) or white (old)? Is the scar mobile or adherent? Is it normal, hypertrophic, or keloid? Palmar scars may interfere with finger extension. Web space scars may interfere with finger separation and metacarpophalangeal joint flexion.

The examiner should take time to observe the fingernails. "Spoon-shaped" nails (Fig. 7–6) are often the result of fungal infection, anemia, iron deficiency, long-term diabetes, local injury, developmental abnormality, chemical irritants, or psoriasis. They may also be a congenital or hereditary trait. "Clubbed" nails (Fig. 7–7) may result from hypertrophy of the underlying soft tissue or respiratory or cardiac problems such as chronic obstructive pulmonary disease, congenital heart defects, or cor pulmonale. Table 7–2 shows other pathological processes that may affect the fingernails.

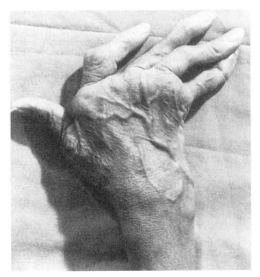

Figure 7–5

The most common deformities occurring in rheumatoid arthritis are ulnar drift and palmar subluxation at the metacarpophalangeal joints. Note swan-neck and boutonnière deformities present in digits. (From Swanson, A.B.: Pathomechanics of deformities in hand and wrist. *In* Hunter, J., L.H. Schneider, E.J. Mackin, and A.D. Callahan [eds.]: Rehabilitation of the Hand: Surgery and Therapy. St. Louis, C.V. Mosby Co., 1990, p. 895.)

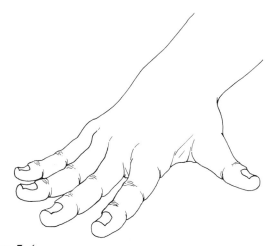

Figure 7–6

Spoon-shaped nails.

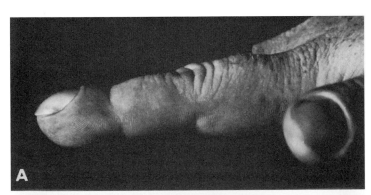

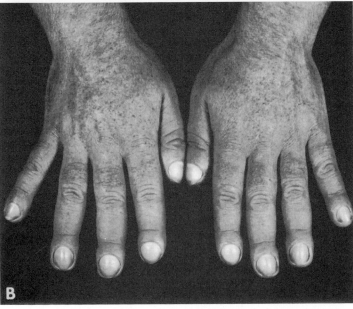

Figure 7–7

Clubbing of the distal interphalangeal joints and rounding of the nails in a patient with hypertrophic osteoarthropathy. (A) Close-up side view of index finger. (B) Dorsal aspect of both hands. (From Polley, H.F., and G.G. Hunder: Rheumatologic Interviewing and Physical Examination of the Joints. Philadelphia, W.B. Saunders Co., 1978, p. 122.)

Table 7–2
Glossary of Nail Pathology

Condition	Description	Occurrence
Beau's lines	Transverse lines or ridges marking repeated disturbances of nail growth	Systemic diseases, toxic or nutritional deficiency states of many types, trauma (from manicuring)
Defluvium unguium (onychomadesis)	Complete loss of nails	Certain systemic diseases such as scarlet fever, syphilis, leprosy, alopecia areata, and exfoliative dermatitis
Diffusion of lunula unguis	"Spreading" of lunula	Dystrophies of the extremities
Eggshell nails	Nail plate thin, semitransparent bluish-white, with a tendency to curve upward at the distal edge	Syphilis
Fragilitas unguium	Friable or brittle nails	Dietary deficiency, local trauma
Hapalonychia	Nails very soft, split easily	Following contact with strong alkalis; endocrine disturbances, malnutrition, syphilis, chronic arthritis
Hippocratic nails	"Watch-glass nails" associated with "drumstick fingers"	Chronic respiratory and circulatory diseases, especially pulmonary tuberculosis; hepatic cirrhosis
Koilonychia	"Spoon nails"; nails are concave on the outer surface	Dysendocrinisms (acromegaly), trauma, dermatoses, syphilis, nutritional deficiencies, hypothyroidism
Leukonychia	White spots or striations or rarely the whole nail may turn white (congenital type)	Local trauma, hepatic cirrhosis, nutritional deficiencies, and many systemic diseases
Mees' lines	Transverse white bands	Hodgkin's granuloma, arsenic and thallium toxicity, high fevers, local nutritional derangement
Moniliasis of nails	Infections (usually paronychial) caused by yeast forms (*Candida albicans*)	Occupational (common in food-handlers, dentists, dishwashers, and gardeners)
Onychatrophia	Atrophy or failure of development of nails	Trauma, infection, dysendocrinism, gonadal aplasia, and many systemic disorders
Onychauxis	Nail plate is greatly thickened	Mild persistent trauma, systemic diseases such as peripheral stasis, peripheral neuritis, syphilis, leprosy, hemiplegia, or at times may be congenital
Onychia	Inflammation of the nail matrix causing deformity of the nail plate	Trauma, infection, many systemic diseases
Onychodystrophy	Any deformity of the nail plate, nail bed, or nail matrix	Many diseases, trauma, or chemical agents (poisoning, allergy)
Onychogryposis	"Claw nails"—extreme degree of hypertrophy, sometimes with horny projections arising from the nail surface	May be congenital or related to many chronic systemic diseases (see onychauxis)
Onycholysis	Loosening of the nail plate beginning at the distal or free edge	Trauma, injury by chemical agents, many systemic diseases
Onychomadesis	Shedding of all the nails (defluvium unguium)	Dermatoses such as exfoliative dermatitis, alopecia areata, psoriasis, eczema, nail infection, severe systemic diseases, arsenic poisoning
Onychophagia	Nail biting	Neurosis
Onychorrhexis	Longitudinal ridging and splitting of the nails	Dermatoses, nail infections, many systemic diseases, senility, injury by chemical agents, hyperthyroidism
Onychoschizia	Lamination and scaling away of nails in thin layers	Dermatoses, syphilis, injury by chemical agents
Onychotillomania	Alteration of the nail structures caused by persistent neurotic picking of the nails	Neurosis
Pachyonychia	Extreme thickening of all the nails; the nails are more solid and more regular than in onychogryposis	Usually congenital and associated with hyperkeratosis of the palms and soles
Pterygium unguis	Thinning of the nail fold and spreading of the cuticle over the nail plate	Associated with vasospastic conditions such as Raynaud's phenomenon and occasionally with hypothyroidism

From Berry, T.J.: The Hand as a Mirror of Systemic Disease. Philadelphia, F.A. Davis Co., 1963.

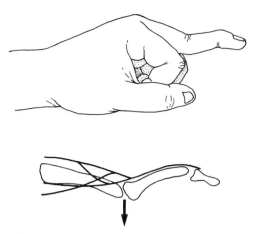

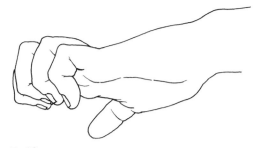

Figure 7–10
Claw fingers (intrinsic-minus hand). Fingers are hyperextended at the metacarpophalangeal joints and flexed at the interphalangeal joints.

Figure 7–8
Swan-neck deformity. Note the hyperextension at the proximal interphalangeal joint.

Common Hand and Finger Deformities

Swan-Neck Deformity. This deformity usually involves only the fingers. There is flexion of the metacarpophalangeal and distal interphalangeal joints. In addition, there is extension of the proximal interphalangeal joint. The condition is a result of contracture of the intrinsic muscles and is often seen in patients with rheumatoid arthritis or after trauma (Fig. 7–8).

Boutonnière Deformity. Extension of the metacarpophalangeal and distal interphalangeal joints and flexion of the proximal interphalangeal joint are seen with this deformity. The deformity is the result of a rupture of the central tendinous slip of the extensor hood and is most common after trauma or in rheumatoid arthritis (Fig. 7–9).

Ulnar Drift. This deformity, which is commonly seen in patients with rheumatoid arthritis but can occur with other conditions, results in ulnar deviation of the digits due to weakening of the capsuloligamentous structures of the metacarpophalangeal joints and the accompanying "bowstring" effect of the extensor communis tendons (see Fig. 7–5).

Extensor Plus Deformity. This deformity is caused by adhesions or shortening of the extensor communis tendon proximal to the metacarpophalangeal joint. It results in the inability to simultaneously flex the metacarpophalangeal and proximal interphalangeal joints, although they may be flexed individually.

Claw Fingers. This deformity results from the loss of intrinsic muscle action and the overaction of the extrinsic (long) extensor muscles on the proximal phalanx of the fingers. The metacarpophalangeal joints are hyperextended, and the proximal and distal interphalangeal joints are flexed (Fig. 7–10). If intrinsic function is lost, the hand is called an **intrinsic minus hand**. The normal cupping of the hand is lost, both the longitudinal and the transverse arches of the hand (Fig. 7–11) disappear, and there is intrinsic muscle wasting. The deformity is most often caused by a combined median and ulnar nerve palsy.

Trigger Finger. Also known as **digital tenovaginitis stenosans**, this deformity is the result of a thickening of the flexor tendon sheath, which causes sticking of the tendon when the patient attempts to flex the finger. A low-grade inflammation of the proximal fold of the flexor tendon leads to swelling and constriction (stenosis) in

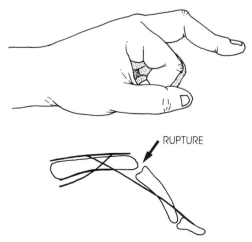

RUPTURE

Figure 7–9
Boutonnière deformity. Note the flexion deformity at the proximal interphalangeal joint.

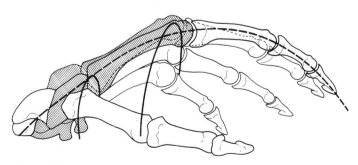

Figure 7–11
Longitudinal and transverse arches of the hand (lateral view). Shaded areas show the fixed or stable part of the hand. (From Tubiana, R.: The Hand. Philadelphia, W.B. Saunders Co., 1981, p. 25.)

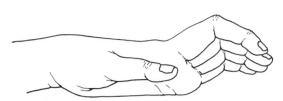

Figure 7–12
Ape hand deformity.

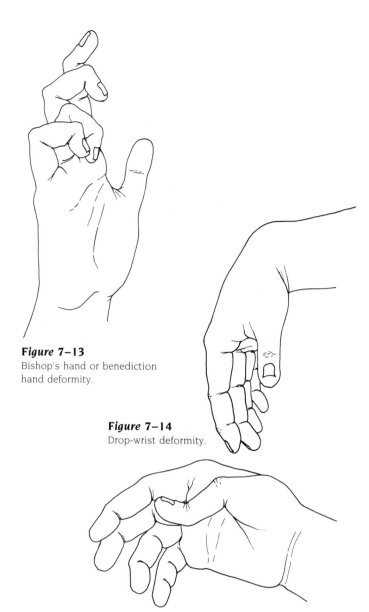

the digital flexor tendon. When the patient attempts to flex the finger, the tendon sticks, and the finger "lets go," often with a snap. As the condition worsens, eventually the finger will flex but not let go, and it will have to be passively extended. The condition is more likely to occur in middle-aged women, whereas "trigger thumb" is more common in young children. The condition usually occurs in the third or fourth finger. It is most often associated with rheumatoid arthritis and tends to be worse in the morning.

Ape Hand Deformity. Wasting of the thenar eminence of the hand occurs as a result of a median nerve palsy, and the thumb falls back in line with the fingers as a result of the pull of the extensor muscles. The patient is also unable to oppose or flex the thumb (Fig. 7–12).

Bishop's Hand or Benediction Hand Deformity. Wasting of the hypothenar muscles of the hand, the interossei muscles, and the two medial lumbrical muscles occurs because of ulnar nerve palsy (Fig. 7–13). Flexion of the fourth and fifth fingers is the most obvious resulting change.

Drop-Wrist Deformity. The extensor muscles of the wrist are paralyzed as a result of a radial nerve palsy, and the wrist and fingers cannot be extended (Fig. 7–14).

"Z" Deformity of the Thumb. The thumb is flexed at the metacarpophalangeal joint and hyperextended at the interphalangeal joint (Fig. 7–15). The deformity may be caused by heredity, or it may be associated with rheumatoid arthritis.

Figure 7–13
Bishop's hand or benediction hand deformity.

Figure 7–14
Drop-wrist deformity.

Figure 7–15
"Z" deformity of the thumb.

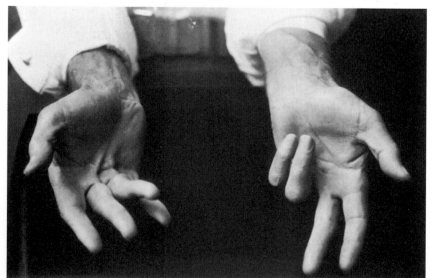

Figure 7–16
Dupuytren's contracture in both hands, showing flexion contractures of the fourth and fifth digits of the left hand and less severe contractures in the third, fourth, and fifth digits of the right hand. Note the puckering of palmar skin and the presence of bands extending from the concavity of the palm to the proximal interphalangeal joints of the third and fourth digits of the right hand. (From Polley, H.F., and G.G. Hunder: Rheumatologic Interviewing and Physical Examination of the Joints. Philadelphia, W.B. Saunders Co., 1978, p. 98.)

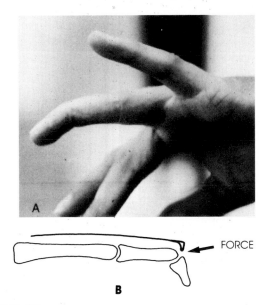

Figure 7–17
Mallet finger. (A) Patient actively attempting to extend finger.
(B) Mechanism of injury. Tendon is ruptured or avulsed from bone.

Dupuytren's Contracture. This condition is the result of contracture of the palmar fascia. There is a fixed flexion deformity of the metacarpophalangeal and proximal interphalangeal joints (Fig. 7–16). Dupuytren's contracture is usually seen in the ring or little finger, and the skin is often adherent to the fascia. It affects men more often than women and is usually seen in the 50- to 70-year-old age group.

Mallet Finger. A mallet finger deformity is the result of a rupture or avulsion of the extensor tendon where it inserts into the distal phalanx of the finger. The distal phalanx rests in a flexed position (Fig. 7–17).

Other Physical Findings

The hand is the terminal part of the upper limb. Many pathological conditions manifest themselves in this structure and may lead the examiner to suspect pathological conditions elsewhere in the body. It is important for the examiner to take the time to view the hands when assessing any joint, especially if an abnormal pattern is presented or the history gives an indication that more than one joint may be involved. For example, if a patient presents with insidious neck pain and also demonstrates nail changes that indicate psoriasis, the examiner should consider the possibility of psoriatic arthritis affecting the cervical spine. Some other conditions involving the hand include the following:

1. Generalized or continued body exposure to radiation produces brittle nails, longitudinal nail ridges, skin keratosis (thickening), and ulceration.

2. The Plummer-Vinson syndrome produces spoon-shaped nails (see Fig. 7–6). This condition is a dysphasia with atrophy in the mouth, pharynx, and upper esophagus.

3. Psoriasis may cause scaling, deformity, and fragmentation and detachment of the nails. Psoriasis may lead to psoriatic arthritis affecting spinal and peripheral joints.

4. Hyperthyroidism produces nail atrophy and ridging with warm, moist hands.

5. Vasospastic conditions produce a thin nail fold and pterygium (abnormal extension) of the cuticle.

6. Trauma to the nail bed, toxic radiation, acute illness, prolonged fever, avitaminosis, and chronic alcoholism produce transverse, or Beau's, lines in the nails (Fig. 7–18).

7. Many arterial diseases produce a lack of linear growth with thick, dark nails.

8. Lues (syphilis) produces a hypertrophic overgrowth of the nail plate. The nails break and crumple easily.

9. Chronic respiratory disorders produce clubbing of the nails (see Fig. 7–7).

10. Subacute bacterial endocarditis may produce Osler's nodes, which are small, tender nodes in the finger pads.

11. Congenital heart disease may produce cyanosis and nail clubbing.

12. Neurocirculatory aesthesia (loss of strength and energy) produces cold, damp hands.

13. Parkinson's disease produces a typical hand tremor known as "pill rolling hand" (Fig. 7–19).

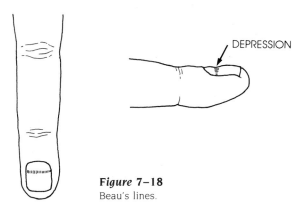

Figure 7–18
Beau's lines.

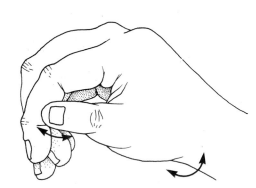

Figure 7–19
Pill rolling hand, seen in Parkinson's disease.

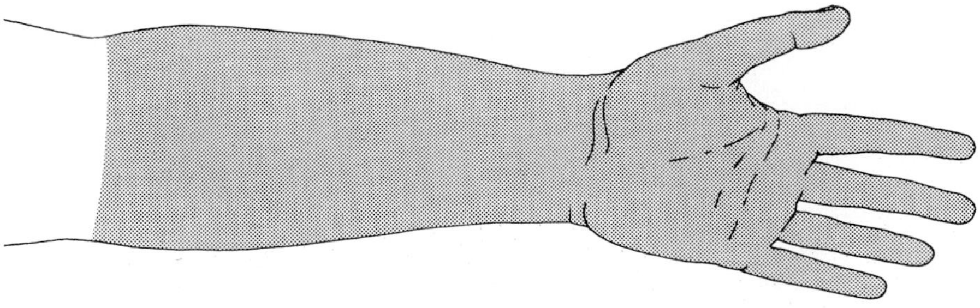

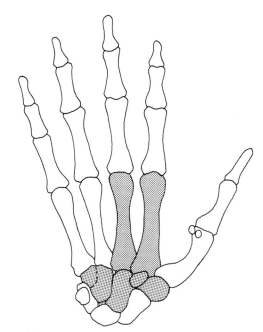

Figure 7–20
Opera glove anesthesia, showing area of abnormal sensation.

14. Causalgic states produce a painful, swollen, hot hand.

15. "Opera glove" anesthesia is seen in hysteria, leprosy, and diabetes. It is a condition in which there is numbness from the elbow to the fingers (Fig. 7–20).

16. Raynaud's disease produces a cold, mottled, painful hand. It is an idiopathic vascular disorder characterized by intermittent attacks of pallor and cyanosis of the extremities brought on by cold or emotion.

17. Rheumatoid arthritis produces a warm, wet hand as well as joint swelling, dislocations or subluxations, and ulnar deviation or drift of the wrist (see Fig. 7–5).

18. The deformed hand of Volkmann's ischemic contracture is one that is very typical for a compartment syndrome after a fracture or dislocation of the elbow (Fig. 7–21).

Table 7–3 gives further examples of physical findings of the hand.

Examination

The examination of the forearm, wrist, and hand may be very extensive, or it may be limited to one or two joints, depending on the area and degree of injury. Regardless, because of its functional importance, the examiner must take extra care when examining this area. Not only must clinical limitations be determined, but functional limita-tions brought on by trauma, nerve injuries, or other factors must be carefully considered to have an appropriate outcome functionally, cosmetically, and clinically.

Because there are so many joints, bones, muscles, and ligaments involved, the examiner must develop a working knowledge of all of these tissues and how they interact with one another. It is important for the examiner to remember that adduction of the hand (ulnar deviation) is greater than abduction (radial deviation) because of shortness of the ulnar styloid process. Supination of the forearm is stronger than pronation, whereas abduction has a greater ROM in supination than pronation. Adduction and abduction ROM is minimal when the wrist is fully extended or flexed. Both flexion and extension at the fingers are maximal when the wrist is in neutral (not abducted or adducted); flexion and extension of the wrist are minimal when the wrist is in pronation.

The wrist and hand have both a fixed and a mobile segment. The fixed segment consists of the distal row of carpal bones (trapezium, trapezoid, capitate, and hamate) and the second and third metacarpals. This is the stabilizing segment of the wrist and hand (Fig. 7–22),

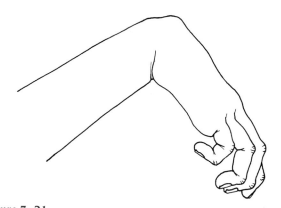

Figure 7–21
Deformity seen with Volkmann's ischemic contracture. Note clawed fingers.

Figure 7–22
Palmar view of hand, showing stable segment (stippled areas).

Table 7–3
Outline of Physical Findings of the Hand

I. Variations in size and shape of hand
  A. Large, blunt fingers (spade hand)
    1. Acromegaly
    2. Hurler's disease (gargoylism)
  B. Gross irregularity of shape and size
    1. Paget's disease of bone
    2. Maffucci's syndrome
    3. Neurofibromatosis
  C. Spider fingers, slender palm (arachnodactyly)
    1. Hypopituitarism
    2. Eunuchism
    3. Ehlers-Danlos syndrome, pseudoxanthoma
       elasticum
    4. Tuberculosis
    5. Asthenic habitus
    6. Osteogenesis imperfecta
  D. Sausage-shaped phalanges
    1. Rickets (beading of joints)
    2. Granulomatous dactylitis (tuberculosis, syphilis)
  E. Spindliform joints (fingers)
    1. Early rheumatoid arthritis
    2. Systemic lupus erythematosus
    3. Psoriasis
    4. Rubella
    5. Boeck's sarcoidosis
    6. Osteoarthritis
  F. Cone-shaped fingers
    1. Pituitary obesity
    2. Fröhlich's dystrophy
  G. Unilateral enlargement of hand
    1. Arteriovenous aneurysm
    2. Maffucci's syndrome
  H. Square, dry hands
    1. Cretinism
    2. Myxedema
  I. Single, widened, flattened distal phalanx
    1. Sarcoidosis
  J. Shortened fourth and fifth metacarpals
     (bradymetacarpalism)
    1. Pseudohypoparathyroidism
    2. Pseudopseudohypoparathyroidism
  K. Shortened, incurved fifth finger (symptom of Du
     Bois)
    1. Mongolism
    2. "Behavioral problem"
    3. Gargoylism (broad, short, thick-skinned hand)
  L. Malposition and abduction, fifth finger
    1. Turner's syndrome (gonadal dysgenesis, webbed
       neck, etc.)
  M. Syndactylism
    1. Congenital malformations of the heart, great
       vessels
    2. Multiple congenital deformities
    3. Laurence-Moon-Biedl syndrome
    4. In normal individuals as an inherited trait
  N. Clubbed fingers
    1. Subacute bacterial endocarditis
    2. Pulmonary causes
      a. Tuberculosis
      b. Pulmonary arteriovenous fistula
      c. Pulmonic abscess
      d. Pulmonic cysts
      e. Bullous emphysema

      f. Pulmonary hypertrophic osteoarthropathy
      g. Bronchogenic carcinoma
    3. Alveolocapillary block
      a. Interstitial pulmonary fibrosis
      b. Sarcoidosis
      c. Beryllium poisoning
      d. Sclerodermatous lung
      e. Asbestosis
      f. Miliary tuberculosis
      g. Alveolar cell carcinoma
    4. Cardiovascular causes
      a. Patent ductus arteriosus
      b. Tetralogy of Fallot
      c. Taussig-Bing complex
      d. Pulmonic stenosis
      e. Ventricular septal defect
    5. Diarrheal states
      a. Ulcerative colitis
      b. Tuberculous enteritis
      c. Sprue
      d. Amebic dysentery
      e. Bacillary dysentery
      f. Parasitic infestation (gastrointestinal tract)
    6. Hepatic cirrhosis
    7. Myxedema
    8. Polycythemia
    9. Chronic urinary tract infections (upper and lower)
      a. Chronic nephritis
    10. Hyperparathyroidism (telescopy of distal
        phalanx)
    11. Pachydermoperiostosis (syndrome of Touraine,
        Solente, and Golé)
  O. Joint disturbances
    1. Arthritides
      a. Osteoarthritis
      b. Rheumatoid arthritis
      c. Systemic lupus erythematosus
      d. Gout
      e. Psoriasis
      f. Sarcoidosis
      g. Endocrinopathy (acromegaly)
      h. Rheumatic fever
      i. Reiter's syndrome
      j. Dermatomyositis
    2. Anaphylactic reaction—serum sickness
    3. Scleroderma
II. Edema of the hand
  A. Cardiac disease (congestive heart failure)
  B. Hepatic disease
  C. Renal disease
    1. Nephritis
    2. Nephrosis
  D. Hemiplegic hand
  E. Syringomyelia
  F. Superior vena caval syndrome
    1. Superior thoracic outlet tumor
    2. Mediastinal tumor or inflammation
    3. Pulmonary apex tumor
    4. Aneurysm
  G. Generalized anasarca, hypoproteinemia
  H. Postoperative lymphedema (radical breast
     amputation)
  I. Ischemic paralysis (cold, blue, swollen, numb)

Table continued on following page

Table 7–3
Outline of Physical Findings of the Hand (Continued)

J. Lymphatic obstruction
  1. Lymphomatous masses in axilla
K. Axillary mass
  1. Metastatic tumor, abscess, leukemia, Hodgkin's disease
L. Aneurysm of ascending or transverse aorta, or of axillary artery
M. Pressure on innominate or subclavian vessels
N. Raynaud's disease
O. Myositis
P. Cervical rib
Q. Trichiniasis
R. Scalenus anticus syndrome
III. Neuromuscular effects
  A. Atrophy
    1. Painless
      a. Amyotrophic lateral sclerosis
      b. Charcot-Marie-Tooth peroneal atrophy
      c. Syringomyelia (loss of heat, cold, and pain sensation)
      d. Neural leprosy
    2. Painful
      a. Peripheral nerve disease
        1. Radial nerve (wrist drop)
          a. Lead poisoning, alcoholism, polyneuritis, trauma
          b. Diphtheria, polyarteritis, neurosyphilis, anterior poliomyelitis
        2. Ulnar nerve (benediction palsy)
          a. Polyneuritis, trauma
        3. Median nerve (claw hand)
          a. Carpal tunnel syndrome
            1. Rheumatoid arthritis
            2. Tenosynovitis at wrist
            3. Amyloidosis
            4. Gout
            5. Plasmacytoma
            6. Anaphylactic reaction
            7. Menopause syndrome
            8. Myxedema
  B. Extrinsic pressure on the nerve (cervical, axillary, supraclavicular, or brachial)
    1. Pancoast tumor (pulmonary apex)
    2. Aneurysms of subclavian arteries, axillary vessels, or thoracic aorta
    3. Costoclavicular syndrome
    4. Superior thoracic outlet syndrome
    5. Cervical rib
    6. Degenerative arthritis of cervical spine
    7. Herniation of cervical intervertebral disc
  C. Shoulder-hand syndrome
    1. Myocardial infarction
    2. Pancoast tumor
    3. Brain tumor
    4. Intrathoracic neoplasms
    5. Discogenetic disease

6. Cervical spondylosis
7. Febrile panniculitis
8. Senility
9. Vascular occlusion
10. Hemiplegia
11. Osteoarthritis
12. Herpes zoster
  D. Ischemic contractures (sensory loss in fingers)
    1. Tight plaster cast applications
  E. Polyarteritis nodosa
  F. Polyneuritis
    1. Carcinoma of lung
    2. Hodgkin's disease
    3. Pregnancy
    4. Gastric carcinoma
    5. Reticuloses
    6. Diabetes mellitus
    7. Chemical neuritis
      a. Antimony, benzene, bismuth, carbon tetrachloride, heavy metals, alcohol, arsenic, lead, gold, emetine
    8. Ischemic neuropathy
    9. Vitamin B deficiency
    10. Atheromata
    11. Arteriosclerosis
    12. Embolic
  G. Carpodigital (carpopedal spasm) tetany
    1. Hypoparathyroidism
    2. Hyperventilation
    3. Uremia
    4. Nephritis
    5. Nephrosis
    6. Rickets
    7. Sprue
    8. Malabsorption syndrome
    9. Pregnancy
    10. Lactation
    11. Osteomalacia
    12. Protracted vomiting
    13. Pyloric obstruction
    14. Alkali poisoning
    15. Chemical toxicity
      a. Morphine, lead, alcohol
  H. Tremor
    1. Parkinsonism
    2. Familial disorder
    3. Hypoglycemia
    4. Hyperthyroidism
    5. Wilson's disease (hepatolenticular degeneration)
    6. Anxiety
    7. Ataxia
    8. Athetosis
    9. Alcoholism, narcotic addiction
    10. Multiple sclerosis
    11. Chorea (Sydenham's, Huntington's)

Modified from Berry, T.J.: The Hand as a Mirror of Systemic Disease. Philadelphia, F.A. Davis Co., 1963.

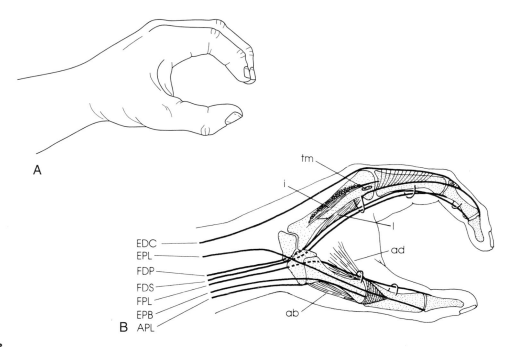

Figure 7–23
Position of function of the hand. (A) Normal view. (B) The hand is in the position of function. Notice in particular that a very small amount of motion in the thumb and fingers is useful motion in that it can be used in pinch and grasp. Notice the close relation of the tendons to bone. The flexor tendons are held close to bone by a pulley-like thickening of the flexor sheath as represented schematically. With the hand in this position, intrinsic and extrinsic musculature is in balance, and all muscles are acting within their physiological resting length. EDC = extensor digitorum communis; EPL = extensor pollicis longus; FDP = flexor digitorum profundus; FDS = flexor digitorum sublimis; FPL = flexor pollicis longus; EPB = extensor pollicis brevis; APL = abductor pollicis longus; I = interossei; tm = transverse metacarpal ligament; l = lumbrical; ad = adductor pollicis brevis; ab = abductor pollicis brevis. (B, from O'Donoghue, D.H.: Treatment of Injuries to Athletes. Philadelphia, W.B. Saunders Co., 1984, p. 287.)

and movement between these bones is less than that between the bones of the mobile segment. This arrangement allows stability without rigidity, enables the hand to move more discretely and with suppleness, and enhances the function of the thumb and fingers when they

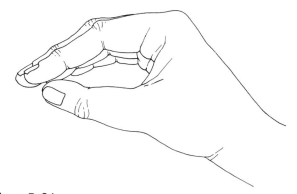

Figure 7–24
Position of immobilization.

are used for power and/or precision grip. The mobile segment is made up of the five phalanges and the first, fourth, and fifth metacarpal bones.

The **functional position** of the wrist is extension to between 20° and 35° with ulnar deviation of 10 to 15°.[5] This position, sometimes called the **position of rest**, minimizes the restraining action of the long extensor tendons and allows complete flexion of the fingers (Fig. 7–23). In this position, the pulps of the index finger and thumb come into contact to facilitate thumb-finger action. The position of **wrist immobilization** (Fig. 7–24) is further extension than is seen in the position of rest, with the metacarpophalangeal joints more flexed and the interphalangeal joints extended. In this way, when the joints are immobilized, the potential for contracture is kept to a minimum.

During extension at the wrist (Fig. 7–25), most of the movement occurs in the radiocarpal joint (approximately 50°) and less occurs in the midcarpal joint (approximately 35°). The motion of extension is accompanied by slight radial deviation and pronation of the forearm.

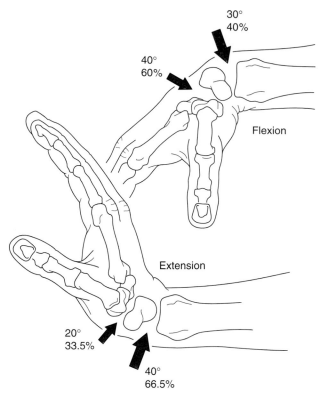

Figure 7–25
During flexion of the wrist, the motion is more midcarpal and less radiocarpal. During extension of the wrist, the motion is more radiocarpal and less midcarpal. (Adapted from Sarrafian, S.K., J.L. Melamed, and G.M. Goshgarian: Study of wrist motion in flexion and extension. Clin. Orthop. 126:156, 1977.)

During wrist flexion, most of the movement occurs in the midcarpal joint (approximately 50°) and less occurs in the radiocarpal joint (approximately 35°). This movement is accompanied by slight ulnar deviation and supination of the forearm. Radial deviation occurs primarily between the proximal and distal rows of carpal bones (0 to 20°), with the proximal row moving toward the ulna and the distal row moving radially. Ulnar deviation occurs primarily at the radiocarpal joint (0 to 37°).[5]

Active Movements

Active movements are sometimes referred to as physiological or anatomic movements. If there is pathology to only one area of the hand or wrist, only that area needs to be assessed, provided the examiner is satisfied that the pathology is not affecting or has not affected the function of the other areas of the forearm, wrist, and hand. For example, if the patient has suffered a FOOSH injury to the wrist, the examiner spends most of the examination looking at the wrist. However, because positioning of the wrist can affect the function of the rest of

the hand and forearm, the examiner must determine the functional effect of the injury to these other areas. Also, if the injury is chronic, adaptive changes may have occurred in adjacent joints.

Examination is accomplished with the patient in the sitting position. As always, the most painful movements are done last. When the examiner is determining the movements of the hand, the middle finger is considered to be midline (Fig. 7–26). Wrist flexion decreases as the fingers are flexed, and movements of flexion and extension are limited, usually by the antagonistic muscles and ligaments. The patient should actively perform the various movements. Initially, the active movements of the forearm, wrist, and hand may be performed in a "scanning" fashion by having the patient make a fist and then open the hand wide. As the patient does these two movements, the examiner notes any restrictions, deviations, or pain. Depending on the results, the examiner can then do a detailed examination of the affected joints. This detailed examination is initiated by selection of the appropriate active movements to be performed, keeping in mind the effect one joint can have on others.

Active Movements of the Forearm, Wrist, and Hand

- Pronation of the forearm (85 to 90°)
- Supination of the forearm (85 to 90°)
- Wrist abduction or radial deviation (15°)
- Wrist adduction or ulnar deviation (30 to 45°)
- Wrist flexion (80 to 90°)
- Wrist extension (70 to 90°)
- Finger flexion (MCP, 85 to 90°; PIP, 100 to 115°; DIP, 80 to 90°)
- Finger extension (MCP, 30 to 45°; PIP, 0°; DIP, 20°)
- Finger abduction (20 to 30°)
- Finger adduction (0°)
- Thumb flexion (CMC, 45 to 50°; MCP, 50 to 55°; IP, 85 to 90°)
- Thumb extension (MCP, 0°; IP, 0 to 5°)
- Thumb abduction (60 to 70°)
- Thumb adduction (30°)
- Opposition of little finger and thumb (tip-to-tip)
- Combined movements (if necessary)
- Repetitive movements (if necessary)
- Sustained positions (if necessary)

CMC = carpometacarpal; DIP = distal interphalangeal; IP = interphalangeal; MCP = metacarpophalangeal; PIP = proximal interphalangeal.

Active pronation and supination are approximately 85 to 90°, although there is variability between individu-

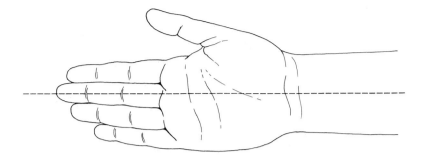

Figure 7–26
Axis or reference position of the hand.

als and it is more important to compare the movement with that of the normal side. Approximately 75° of supination or pronation occurs in the forearm articulations. The remaining 15° is the result of wrist action. The normal end feel of both movements is tissue stretch, although in thin patients the end feel of pronation may be bone-to-bone.

Radial and ulnar deviation of the wrist are 15° and 30 to 45°, respectively. The normal end feel of these movements is bone-to-bone. Wrist flexion is 80 to 90°; wrist extension is 70 to 90°. The end feel of each movement is tissue stretch.

Flexion of the fingers occurs at the metacarpophalangeal joints (85 to 90°), followed by the proximal interphalangeal joints (100 to 115°) and the distal interphalangeal joints (80 to 90°). This sequence enables the hand to grasp large and small objects. Extension occurs at the metacarpophalangeal joints (30 to 45°), the proximal interphalangeal joints (0°), and the distal interphalangeal joints (20°). Hyperextension at the proximal interphalangeal joints can lead to a swan-neck deformity. This hyperextension is usually prevented by the volar plates.[1] The end feel of finger flexion and extension is tissue stretch. Finger abduction occurs at the metacarpophalangeal joints (20 to 30°); the end feel is tissue stretch. Finger adduction (0°) occurs at the same joint.

The digits are medially deviated slightly in relation to the metacarpal bones (see Fig. 7–1). When the fingers are flexed, they should point toward the scaphoid tubercle. In addition, the metacarpals are at an angle to each other. These positions increase the dexterity of the hand and oblique flexion of the medial four digits but contribute to deformities (e.g., ulnar drift) in conditions such as rheumatoid arthritis.

Thumb flexion occurs at the carpometacarpal joint (45 to 50°), the metacarpophalangeal joint (50 to 55°), and the interphalangeal joint (80 to 90°). It is associated with medial rotation of the thumb as a result of the saddle shape of the carpometacarpal joint. Extension of the thumb occurs at the interphalangeal joint (0 to 5°); it is associated with lateral rotation. Flexion and extension take place in a plane parallel to the palm of the hand. Thumb abduction is 60 to 70°; thumb adduction is 30°. These movements occur in a

plane at right angles to the flexion-extension plane.[5] The thumb is controlled by three nerves, a situation that is unique among the digits. The radial nerve controls extension and opening of the hand as it does for the other digits. The ulnar nerve controls adduction, produces closure of pinch, and gives power to the grip; the median nerve controls flexion and opposition, producing precision with any grip.[1] The intrinsic muscles are stronger than the extrinsic muscles of the thumb; the opposite is true for the fingers.[1]

If the history has indicated that combined, repetitive, and/or sustained movements have resulted in symptoms, these movements should also be tested.

The examiner must be aware that active movements may be affected because of neurological as well as contractile tissue problems. For example, the median nerve is sometimes compressed as it passes through the carpal tunnel (Fig. 7–27), affecting its motor and sensory distribution in the hand and fingers. The condition is referred to as **carpal tunnel syndrome.**

If the patient does not have full active ROM and it is difficult to measure ROM because of swelling, pain, or contracture, the examiner can use a ruler or tape measure to record the distance from the fingertip to one of the palmar creases (Fig. 7–28).[8] This measurement provides baseline data for any effect of treatment. It is important to note on

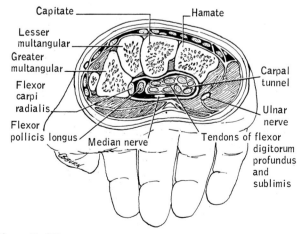

Figure 7–27
Cross section of the wrist showing the carpal tunnel. (From O'Donoghue, D.H.: Treatment of Injuries to Athletes. Philadelphia, W.B. Saunders Co., 1984, p. 285.)

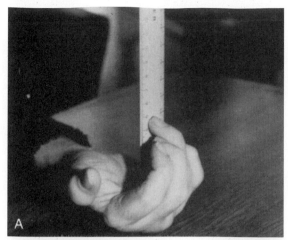

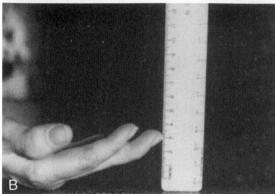

Figure 7–28
(A) Gross flexion is measured as the distance between fingertips and proximal palmar crease. (B) Gross extension is measured as the distance between fingertips and dorsal plane. (From Wadsworth, C.T.: Wrist and hand examination and interpretation. J. Orthop. Sports Phys. Ther. 5:115, 1983.)

the chart which crease was used in the measurement. The majority of functional activities of the hand require the fingers and thumb to open at least 5 cm (2 inches), and the fingers should be able to flex within 1 to 2 cm (0.4 to 0.8 inch) of the distal palmar crease.[9]

Passive Movements

If, when watching the patient perform the active movements, the examiner believes the ROM is full, overpressure can be gently applied to test the end feel of the joint in each direction. If the movement is not full, passive movements must be performed by the examiner to test the end feel. At the same time, the examiner must watch for the presence of a capsular pattern. The passive movements are the same as the active movements, and the examiner must remember to test each individual joint.

Passive Movements of the Forearm, Wrist, and Hand and Normal End Feel

---

- Pronation (tissue stretch)
- Supination (tissue stretch)
- Radial deviation (bone-to-bone)
- Ulnar deviation (bone-to-bone)
- Wrist flexion (tissue stretch)
- Wrist extension (tissue stretch)
- Finger flexion (tissue stretch)
- Finger extension (tissue stretch)
- Finger abduction (tissue stretch)
- Thumb flexion (tissue stretch)
- Thumb extension (tissue stretch)
- Thumb abduction (tissue stretch)
- Thumb adduction (tissue approximation)
- Opposition (tissue stretch)

The capsular pattern of the distal radioulnar joint is full ROM with pain at the extremes of supination and pronation. At the wrist, the capsular pattern is equal limitation of flexion and extension. At the metacarpophalangeal and interphalangeal joints, the capsular pattern is flexion more limited than extension. At the trapeziometacarpal joint of the thumb, the capsular pattern is abduction more limited than extension.

Resisted Isometric Movements

As with the active movements, the resisted isometric movements to the forearm, wrist, and hand are done with the patient in the sitting position. Not all resisted isometric movements need to be tested, but the examiner must keep in mind that the actions of the fingers and thumb and the wrist are controlled by extrinsic muscles (wrist, fingers, thumb) and intrinsic muscles (fingers,

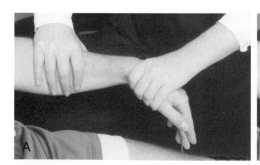

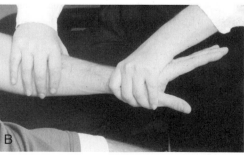

Figure 7–29
Resisted isometric movements of the wrist. (A) Flexion. (B) Extension.

Figure 7–30

Muscles and their actions at the wrist. (1) Flexor carpi ulnaris. (2) Flexor digitorum profundus. (3) Flexor digitorum superficialis. (4) Palmaris longus. (5) Flexor carpi radialis. (6) Abductor pollicis longus. (7) Extensor pollicis brevis. (8) Extensor carpi radialis longus. (9) Extensor carpi radialis brevis. (10) Extensor pollicis longus. (11) Extensor digitorum. (12) Extensor digiti minimi. (13) Extensor carpi ulnaris. (14) Flexor pollicis longus. (15) Extensor indices.

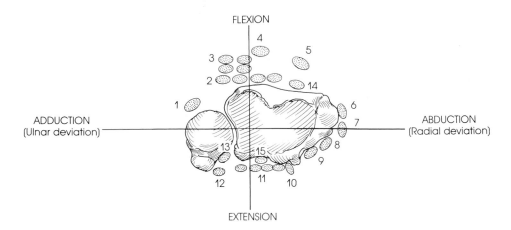

thumb), so injury affecting these structures requires testing of the appropriate muscles. The movements must be isometric and must be performed in the neutral position (Figs. 7–29 and 7–30). If the history has indicated that concentric, eccentric, or econcentric movements have caused symptoms, these different types of resisted movement should be tested, but only after the movements have been tested isometrically.

Resisted Isometric Movements of the Forearm, Wrist, and Hand

- Pronation of the forearm
- Supination of the forearm
- Wrist abduction (radial deviation)
- Wrist adduction (ulnar deviation)
- Wrist flexion
- Wrist extension
- Finger flexion
- Finger extension
- Finger abduction
- Finger adduction
- Thumb flexion
- Thumb extension
- Thumb abduction
- Thumb adduction
- Opposition of the little finger and thumb

Table 7–4 shows the muscles and their actions for differentiation during resisted isometric testing. If measured by test instruments, the strength ratio of wrist extensors to wrist flexors is approximately 50%, whereas the strength ratio of ulnar deviators to radial deviators is approximately 80%. The greatest torque is produced by the wrist flexors, followed by the radial deviators, ulnar deviators, and finally the wrist extensors.[10]

Functional Assessment (Grip)

Having completed the basic movement testing of active, passive, and resisted isometric movements, the examiner then assesses the patient's functional active movements. Functionally, the thumb is the most important digit. Because of its relation with the other digits, its mobility, and the force it can bring to bear, its loss can affect hand function greatly. The index finger is the second most important digit because of its musculature, its strength, and its interaction with the thumb. Its loss greatly affects lateral and pulp-to-pulp pinch and power grip. In flexion, the middle finger is strongest, and it is important for both precision and power grips. The ring finger has the least functional role in the hand. The little finger, because of its peripheral position, greatly enhances power grip, affects the capacity of the hand, and holds objects against the hypothenar eminence.[1] In terms of **functional impairment,** the loss of thumb function affects about 40 to 50% of hand function. The loss of index finger function accounts for about 20% of hand function; the middle finger, about 20%; the ring finger, about 10%; and the little finger, about 10%. Loss of the hand accounts for about 90% loss of upper limb function.[11]

Although the wrist, hand, and finger joints have the ability to move through a relatively large ROM, most functional daily tasks do not require full ROM. Brumfield and Champoux reported that the optimum functional ROM at the wrist was 10° flexion to 35° extension.[12] Normally, the wrist is held in slight extension (10 to 15°) and slight ulnar deviation and is stabilized in this position to provide maximum function for the fingers and thumb. Excessive radial deviation, like ulnar drift of the fingers, can affect grip strength adversely.[13] Functional flexion at the metacarpophalangeal and proximal interphalangeal joints is approximately 60°. Functional flexion at the distal interphalangeal joint is approximately 40°. For the thumb, functional flexion at the metacarpophalangeal

Table 7–4
Muscles of the Forearm, Wrist, and Hand: Their Actions, Nerve Supply, and Nerve Root Derivation

Action	Muscles Acting	Nerve Supply	Nerve Root Deviation
Supination of forearm	1. Supinator	Posterior interosseous (radial)	C5–C6
	2. Biceps brachii	Musculocutaneous	C5–C6
Pronation of forearm	1. Pronator quadratus	Anterior interosseous (median)	C8, T1
	2. Pronator teres	Median	C6–C7
	3. Flexor carpi radialis	Median	C6–C7
Extension of wrist	1. Extensor carpi radialis longus	Radial	C6–C7
	2. Extensor carpi radialis brevis	Posterior interosseous (radial)	C7–C8
	3. Extensor carpi ulnaris	Posterior interosseous (radial)	C7–C8
Flexion of wrist	1. Flexor carpi radialis	Median	C6–C7
	2. Flexor carpi ulnaris	Ulnar	C7–C8
Ulnar deviation of wrist	1. Flexor carpi ulnaris	Ulnar	C7–C8
	2. Extensor carpi ulnaris	Posterior interosseous (radial)	C7–C8
Radial deviation of wrist	1. Flexor carpi radialis	Median	C6–C7
	2. Extensor carpi radialis longus	Radial	C6–C7
	3. Abductor pollicis longus	Posterior interosseous (radial)	C7–C8
	4. Extensor pollicis brevis	Posterior interosseous (radial)	C7–C8
Extension of fingers	1. Extensor digitorum communis	Posterior interosseous (radial)	C7–C8
	2. Extensor indices (second finger)	Posterior interosseous (radial)	C7–C8
	3. Extensor digiti minimi (little finger)	Posterior interosseous (radial)	C7–C8
Flexion of fingers	1. Flexor digitorum profundus	Anterior interosseous (median)	C8, T1
		Anterior interosseous (median): lateral two digits	C8, T1
		Ulnar: medial two digits	C8, T1
	2. Flexor digitorum superficialis	Median	C7–C8, T1
	3. Lumbricals	First and second: median; third and fourth: ulnar (deep terminal branch)	C8, T1 / C8, T1
	4. Interossei	Ulnar (deep terminal branch)	C8, T1
	5. Flexor digiti minimi (little finger)	Ulnar (deep terminal branch)	C8, T1
Abduction of fingers (with fingers extended)	1. Dorsal interossei	Ulnar (deep terminal branch)	C8, T1
	2. Abductor digiti minimi (little finger)	Ulnar (deep terminal branch)	C8, T1
Adduction of fingers (with fingers extended)	1. Palmar interossei	Ulnar (deep terminal branch)	C8, T1
Extension of thumb	1. Extensor pollicis longus	Posterior interosseous (radial)	C7–C8
	2. Extensor pollicis brevis	Posterior interosseous (radial)	C7–C8
	3. Abductor pollicis longus	Posterior interosseous (radial)	C7–C8
Flexion of thumb	1. Flexor pollicis brevis	Superficial head: median (lateral terminal branch)	C8, T1
		Deep head: ulnar	C8, T1
	2. Flexor pollicis longus	Anterior interosseous (median)	C8, T1
	3. Opponens pollicis	Median (lateral terminal branch)	C8, T1
Abduction of thumb	1. Abductor pollicis longus	Posterior interosseous (radial)	C7–C8
	2. Abductor pollicis brevis	Median (lateral terminal branch)	C8, T1
Adduction of thumb	1. Adductor pollicis	Ulnar (deep terminal branch)	C8, T1
Opposition of thumb and little finger	1. Opponens pollicis	Median (lateral terminal branch)	C8, T1
	2. Flexor pollicis brevis	Superficial head: median (lateral terminal branch)	C8, T1
	3. Abductor pollicis brevis	Median (lateral terminal branch)	C8, T1
	4. Opponens digiti minimi	Ulnar (deep terminal branch)	C8, T1

and interphalangeal joints is approximately 20°.[9] Within these ROMs, the hand is able to perform most of its grip[5, 14] and other functional activities.

Stages of Grip

1. Opening of the hand, which requires the simultaneous action of the intrinsic muscles of the hand and the long extensor muscles
2. Closing of the fingers and thumb to grasp the object and adapt to the object's shape, which involves intrinsic and extrinsic flexor and opposition muscles
3. Exerted force, which varies depending on the weight, surface characteristics, fragility, and use of the object, again involving the extrinsic and intrinsic flexor and opposition muscles
4. Release, in which the hand opens to let go of the object, involving the same muscles as for opening of the hand

The thumb, although not always used in gripping, adds another important dimension when it is used. It gives stability and helps control the direction in which the object moves. Both of these factors are necessary for precision movements. The thumb also increases the power of a grip by acting as a buttress, resisting the pressure of an object held between it and the fingers.

The nerve distribution and the functions of the digits also present interesting patterns. Flexion and sensation of the ulnar digits are controlled by the ulnar nerve and are more related to power grip. Flexion and sensation of the radial digits are controlled by the median nerve and are more related to precision grip. The muscles of the thumb, often used in both types of grip, are supplied by both nerves. In all cases of gripping, opening of the hand or release of grip depends on the radial nerve.

Power Grip. A power grip requires firm control and gives greater flexor asymmetry to the hand (Fig. 7–31); it is a primary function of the ulnar side of the hand. The ulnar digits tend to work together to provide support and static control.[1, 5, 14, 15] This grip is used whenever strength or force is the primary consideration. With this

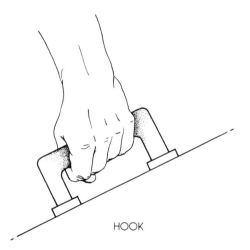

HOOK

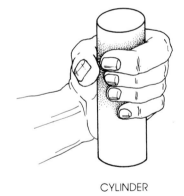

CYLINDER

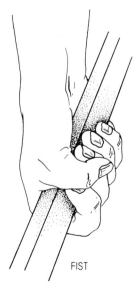

FIST

Figure 7–31

Types of power grips. (Based on concepts from Reid, D.C.: Functional Anatomy and Joint Mobilization. Edmonton, University of Alberta Press, 1970; and Tubiana, R.: The Hand. Philadelphia, W.B. Saunders Co., 1981.)

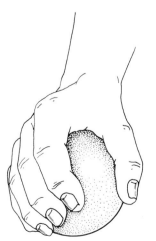

SPHERICAL

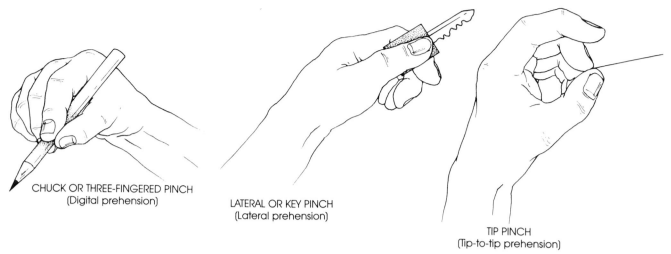

CHUCK OR THREE-FINGERED PINCH
(Digital prehension)

LATERAL OR KEY PINCH
(Lateral prehension)

TIP PINCH
(Tip-to-tip prehension)

Figure 7–32

Types of precision grips or pinches. (Based on concepts from Reid, D.C.: Functional Anatomy and Joint Mobilization. Edmonton, University of Alberta Press, 1970; and Tubiana, R.: The Hand. Philadelphia, W.B. Saunders Co., 1981.)

grip, the digits maintain the object against the palm; the thumb may or may not be involved, and the extrinsic (forearm) muscles are more important. The combined effect of joint position brings the hand into line with the forearm. For a power grip to be formed, the fingers are flexed and the wrist is in ulnar deviation and extended. Examples of power grips include the **hook grasp**, in which all or the second and third fingers are used as a hook controlled by the forearm flexors and extensors. The hook grasp may involve the interphalangeal joints only or the interphalangeal and metacarpophalangeal joints (the thumb is not involved). In the **cylinder grasp**, a type of **palmar prehension**, the thumb is used, and the entire hand wraps around an object. With the **fist grasp**, or **digital palmar prehension**, the hand moves around a narrow object. Another type of power grip is the **spherical grasp**, another type of palmar prehension, in which there is more opposition and the hand moves around the sphere.

Precision or Prehension Grip. The precision grip is an activity that is limited mainly to the metacarpophalangeal joints and involves primarily the radial side of the hand[5, 14, 15] (Fig. 7–32). This grip is used whenever accuracy and precision are required. The radial digits (index and long fingers) provide control by working in concert with the thumb to form a "dynamic tripod" for precision handling.[1] With precision grips, the thumb and fingers are used and the palm may or may not be involved; there is pulp-to-pulp contact between the thumb and fingers, and the thumb opposes the fingers. The intrinsic muscles are more important in precision than in power grips. The thumb is essential for precision grips because it provide stability and control of direction and can act as a buttress, providing power to the grip.[1] There are three types of **pinch grip**. The first is called a **three-point chuck, three-fingered,** or **digital prehension,** in

which palmar pinch, or subterminal opposition, is achieved. With this grip, there is pulp-to-pulp pinch, and opposition is necessary. An example is holding a pencil. This grip is sometimes called a **precision grip with power**. The second pinch grip is termed **lateral key, pulp-to-side pinch, lateral prehension,** or **subterminolateral opposition**. The thumb and lateral side of the index finger come into contact. No opposition is needed. An

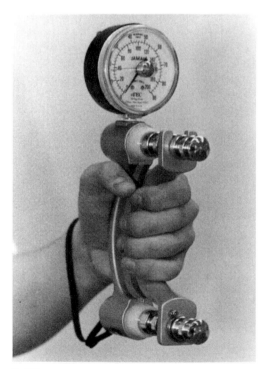

Figure 7–33

Jamar dynamometer. Arm should be held at the patient's side with elbow flexed at approximately 90° when grip is measured.

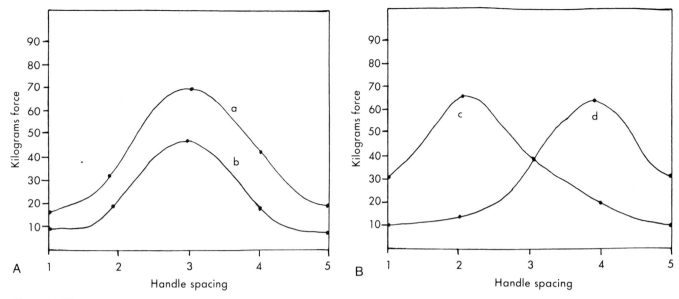

Figure 7–34

(A) The grip strengths of a patient's uninjured hand (a) and injured hand (b) are plotted. Despite the patient's decrease in grip strength because of injury, curve b maintains a bell-shaped pattern and parallels that of the normal hand. These curves are reproducible in repeated examinations, with minimal change in values. A great fluctuation in the size of the curve or absence of a bell-shaped pattern casts doubt on the patient's compliance with the examination and may indicate malingering. (B) If the patient has an exceptionally large hand, the curve shifts to the right (d); with a very small hand, the curve shifts to the left (c). In both cases, the bell-shaped pattern is maintained. (From Aulicino, P.L., and T.E. DuPuy: Clinical examination of the hand. In Hunter, J., L.H. Schneider, E.J. Mackin, and A.D. Callahan [eds.]: Rehabilitation of the Hand: Surgery and Therapy. St. Louis, C.V. Mosby Co., 1990, p. 45.)

example of this movement is holding keys or a card. The third pinch grip is called the **tip pinch, tip-to-tip prehension,** or **terminal opposition.** With this positioning, the tip of the thumb is brought into opposition with the tip of another finger. This pinch is used for activities requiring fine coordination rather than power.

Testing Grip Strength

When testing grip strength using the grip dynamometer, the examiner should use the five adjustable hand spacings in consecutive order with the patient grasping the dynamometer with maximum force (Fig. 7–33). Both hands are tested alternately, and each force is recorded.[16, 17] Care must be taken to ensure that the patient does not fatigue. The results normally form a bell curve (Fig. 7–34), with the greatest strength readings at the middle (second and third) spacings and the weakest at the beginning and at the end. There should be a 5 to 10% difference between the dominant and nondominant hands.[18] With injury, the bell curve should still be present, but the force exerted is less. If the patient does not exert maximum force for each test, the typical bell curve will not be produced, nor will the values obtained be consistent. Discrepancies of more than 20% in a test-retest situation indicate that the patient is not exerting maximal force.[17, 19] Usually, the mean value of three trials is recorded, and both hands are compared.[9] Table 7–5 gives normal values by age group and gender.

Table 7–5
Normal Values by Age Group (Years) and Gender for Combined Right and Left Hand Grip Strength (kg)

	Ages 15 to 19		Ages 20 to 29		Ages 30 to 39		Ages 40 to 49		Ages 50 to 59		Ages 60 to 69	
	Male	Female	Male	Female	Male	Female	Male	Female	Male	Female	Male	Female
Excellent	≥113	≥71	≥124	≥71	≥123	≥73	≥119	≥73	≥110	≥65	≥102	≥60
Above average	103–112	64–70	113–123	65–70	113–122	66–72	110–118	65–72	102–109	59–64	93–101	54–59
Average	95–102	59–63	106–112	61–64	105–112	61–65	102–109	59–64	96–101	55–58	86–92	51–53
Below average	84–94	54–58	97–105	55–60	97–104	56–60	94–101	55–58	87–95	51–54	79–85	48–50
Poor	≤83	≤53	≤96	≤54	≤96	≤55	≤93	≤54	≤86	≤50	≤78	≤47

Modified from Canadian Standardized Test of Fitness: Operations Manual. Ottawa, Fitness and Amateur Sport Canada, 1986, p. 36.

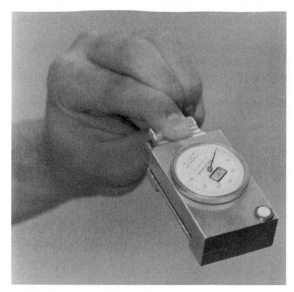

Figure 7–35
Commercial pinch meter to test pinch strength.

Testing Pinch Strength

The strength of the pinch may be tested with the use of a pinch meter (Fig. 7–35). Average values are given for pulp-to-pulp pinch of each finger with the thumb (Table 7–6), lateral prehension (Table 7–7), and pulp-to-pulp pinch (Table 7–8) for different occupational levels. Normally, the mean value of three trials is recorded, and both hands are compared.

Other Functional Testing Methods

In addition to testing grip and pinch strength, the examiner may want to perform a full functional assessment of the patient. Figures 7–36 and 7–37 give examples of functional assessment forms for the hand. These forms are not numerical scoring charts, but they do include some functional aspects. Levine and colleagues[20] have developed a severity questionnaire including a functional component to measure severity of symptoms and functional disability for a nerve, in this case the median nerve in the carpal tunnel (Fig. 7–38). Table 7–9 provides a functional testing method. These strength values would be considered normal for an average population. They would be considered low for an athletic population or for persons in occupations subjecting the forearm, wrist, and hand to high repetitive loads.

Functional coordinated movements may be tested by asking the patient to perform simple activities, such as fastening a button, tying a shoelace, or tracing a diagram. Different prehension patterns are used regularly during daily activities.[21]

Table 7–7
Average Strength of Lateral Prehension Pinch by Occupation (100 Subjects)

| | Lateral Prehension Pinch (kg) | | | |
| | Male Hand | | Female Hand | |
Occupation	Major	Minor	Major	Minor
Skilled	6.6	6.4	4.4	4.3
Sedentary	6.3	6.1	4.1	3.9
Manual	8.5	7.7	6.0	5.5
Average	7.5	7.1	4.9	4.7

From Hunter, J., L.H. Schneider, E.J. Mackin, and A.D. Callahan (eds.): Rehabilitation of the Hand: Surgery and Therapy. St. Louis, C.V. Mosby Co., 1990, p. 114.

Table 7–6
Average Strength of Chuck (Pulp-to-Pulp) Pinch With Separate Digits (100 Subjects)

| | Pulp-to-Pulp Pinch (kg) | | | |
| | Male Hand | | Female Hand | |
Digit	Major	Minor	Major	Minor
II	5.3	4.8	3.6	3.3
III	5.6	5.7	3.8	3.4
IV	3.8	3.6	2.5	2.4
V	2.3	2.2	1.7	1.6

From Hunter J., L.H. Schneider, E.J. Mackin, and A.D. Callahan (eds.): Rehabilitation of the Hand: Surgery and Therapy. St. Louis, C.V. Mosby Co., 1990, p. 115.

Table 7–8
Average Strength of Chuck (Pulp-to-Pulp) Pinch by Occupation (100 Subjects)

| | Pulp-to-Pulp Pinch (kg) | | | |
| | Male Hand | | Female Hand | |
Occupation	Major	Minor	Major	Minor
Skilled	7.3	7.2	5.4	4.6
Sedentary	8.4	7.3	4.2	4.0
Manual	8.5	7.6	6.1	5.6
Average	7.9	7.5	5.2	4.9

From Hunter, J., L.H. Schneider, E.J. Mackin, and A.D. Callahan (eds.): Rehabilitation of the Hand: Surgery and Therapy. St. Louis, C.V. Mosby Co., 1990, p. 114.

Rheumatoid Arthritis Evaluation Record
Preoperative Silastic Implants

Name _____ Sex: [ ] Male [ ] Female Date _____ Birth date _____

Address _____

Occupation _____ Dominant hand: [ ] R [ ] L Hospital _____ Examiner _____

Diagnosis: [ ] Juvenile rheumatoid [ ] Adult rheumatoid [ ] Erosive arthritis [ ] Osteoarthritis [ ] Psoriatic arthritis
[ ] Ankylosing spondylitis [ ] Sjögren's syndrome [ ] Systemic lupus erythematosus [ ] Trauma

Onset date: _____ Sedimentation rate: [ ] Wintrobe [ ] Westergren [ ] Rourke

Rheumatoid test [ ] (+) [ ] (−) Family Hx [ ] (+) [ ] (−)

Onset distribution: [ ] Peripheral [ ] Central [ ] Both: Remission [ ] Yes [ ] No: Anemia [ ] Yes [ ] No:

Check if the following has been completed: [ ] X-rays [ ] Photographs [ ] Movies [ ] Cineradiography

Range of motion (ROM): use neutral zero method of American Academy of Orthopedic Surgeons, 1965.
Codes 1–25 represent observed and measured abnormalities. Use as indicated in appropriate sections.
Severity indices mild, moderate, and severe are represented by a, b, and c and further categorize codes 1–25.
This evaluation record has been designed for computer analysis. Responses must be complete.

THUMB: Codes: 1, 2, 3, 9–14, 19, 22	Code R	Code L	Abd (degrees) Add (cm) Opp (cm)			
			Joints		ROM R	ROM L
			MC	Abd		
				Add		
				Opp		
			MP			
			IP			

FINGER: Codes: 3–15, 19, 22–25

Index			MP		
			PIP		
			DIP		
Flex DIP crease to palmar crease (cm)					
Middle			MP		
			PIP		
			DIP		
Flex DIP crease to palmar crease (cm)					
Ring			MP		
			PIP		
			DIP		
Flex DIP crease to palmar crease (cm)					
Little			MP		
			PIP		
			DIP		
Flex DIP crease to palmar crease (cm)					
WRIST: Codes: 3, 7–14, 19, 20, 22, 23			Flex		
			Ext		
			U. Dev		
			R. Dev		

Prehensile patterns: Check if able to perform

		R	L
GRASP: Cylinders	2.5 cm		
	5 cm		
	7.5 cm		
	10 cm		
Spheres	5 cm		
	7.5 cm		
	10 cm		
	12.5 cm		

STRENGTH: [ ] Lb [ ] Kg [ ] mm Hg

		R	L
Pulp pinch	Index		
	Middle		
	Ring		
	Little		
Lateral or key pinch			
Grip			

ADL: I: Independent A: Assisted U: Unable

Dress	I	A	U	Hygiene	I	A	U
Upper ext				Teeth			
Trunk				Hair			
Lower ext				Shave			
Bathe				Pick up coin			
Shower				Turn key			
Eat				Doorknob			
Toilet				Car door			
Telephone				Screw-top jar			
Typewrite				Aerosol can			
Write				Fasteners			

Ambulatory status:
[ ] Independent [ ] Wheelchair with partial walking
[ ] Assisted walk [ ] Bedfast

Code for clinical abnormality:
1—Swan-neck, thumb
2—Thumb boutonnière
3—Subluxation–dislocation
4—Swan-neck, finger
5—Boutonnière, finger
6—Intrinsic tightness
7—Ulnar drift
8—Radial drift
9—Ankylosis
10—Instability
11—Tendon rupture
12—Constrictive tenosynovitis
13—Synovial hypertrophy
14—Crepitation with motion
15—Extensor tendon subluxation
16—Varus angle

17—Valgus angle
18—Rotational deformity
19—Erosions
20—Joint narrowing
21—Subchondral sclerosis
22—Painful joint with motion
23—Nerve compression—M, U, R
24—Vasculitis
25—Nodules

Severity index:
a—Mild
b—Moderate
c—Severe

Sketch implant into appropriate site

Palm R   Palm L

Figure 7–36

Functional assessment form for the hand, designed for evaluation of rheumatoid and arthritic hands.
(Modified from Swanson, A.B.: Flexible Implant Resection Arthroplasty in the Hand and Extremities. St. Louis, C.V. Mosby Co., 1973.)

HAND EVALUATION RECORD

Name _____ Age _____ Date _____ Major hand _____
Occupation _____ X-rays _____ Photographs _____
History:

Shoulder:	L	R		Wrist:				Circ:		
For	____	____		DF	____	____		Biceps	____	____
Back	____	____		PF	____	____		Forearm	____	____
Abd	____	____		RD	____	____		Grip: L		
Add	____	____		UD	____	____		R	____	____
Rotation Int	____	____		Elbow: Ext	____	____		Forearm: Pro	____	____
Ext	____	____		Flex	____	____		Sup	____	____

		MP	IP			% Impairment
Thumb	Ext			Abd		
	Flex			Add		
	Ankylosis			Opp		

		MP	PIP	DIP	Flex pulp to midpalmar crease	
Index	Ext					
	Flex					
	Ankylosis					
Middle	Ext					
	Flex					
	Ankylosis					
Ring	Ext					
	Flex					
	Ankylosis					
Little	Ext					
	Flex					
	Ankylosis					

Chart:

1. Amputations
2. Scars
3. Skin—subcutaneous loss
4. Nail bed injury
5. Major nerve loss: R, M, U
6. Digital bundle loss
7. Neuroma
8. Pain and tenderness
9. Bone damage
10. Joint damage
11. Flexor tendon loss
12. Extensor tendon loss
13. Ligament injury
14. Sensibility—pickup
          two-point
          Ninhydrin
15. Prehension:
      Grasp—small
              large
      Pinch—pulp
              tip
              lateral
      Hook—distal
              proximal
      Scoop
16. Maximum improvement
17. Rehabilitation needed
18. Further treatment
19. Classification

NOTE: Degrees of motion recorded as left/right

Total % _____

Dorsum R hand
or
Palmar L hand

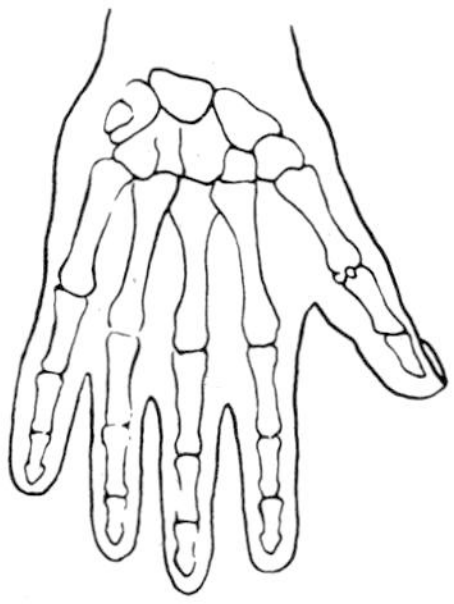

Dorsum L hand
or
Palmar R hand

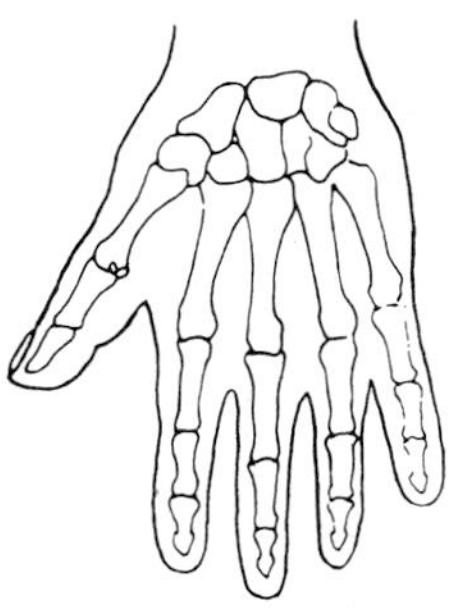

Figure 7–37

This form is designed for posttraumatic conditions and other disorders of the hand. (From Swanson, A.B.: Flexible Implant Resection Arthroplasty in the Hand and Extremities. St. Louis, C.V. Mosby Co., 1973.)

Table 7–9
Functional Testing of the Wrist and Hand

Starting Position	Action	Functional Test
1. Forearm supinated, resting on table	Wrist flexion	Lift 0 lb: Nonfunctional Lift 1 to 2 lb: Functionally poor Lift 3 to 4 lb: Functionally fair Lift 5+ lb: Functional
2. Forearm pronated, resting on table	Wrist extension lifting 1 to 2 lb	0 Repetitions: Nonfunctional 1 to 2 Repetitions: Functionally poor 3 to 4 Repetitions: Functionally fair 5+ Repetitions: Functional
3. Forearm between supination and pronation, resting on table	Radial deviation lifting 1 to 2 lb	0 Repetitions: Nonfunctional 1 to 2 Repetitions: Functionally poor 3 to 4 Repetitions: Functionally fair 5+ Repetitions: Functional
4. Forearm between supination and pronation, resting on table	Thumb flexion with resistance from rubber band* around thumb	0 Repetitions: Nonfunctional 1 to 2 Repetitions: Functionally poor 3 to 4 Repetitions: Functionally fair 5+ Repetitions: Functional
5. Forearm resting on table, rubber band around thumb and index finger	Thumb extension against resistance of rubber band*	0 Repetitions: Nonfunctional 1 to 2 Repetitions: Functionally poor 3 to 4 Repetitions: Functionally fair 5+ Repetitions: Functional
6. Forearm resting on table, rubber band around thumb and index finger	Thumb abduction against resistance of rubber band*	0 Repetitions: Nonfunctional 1 to 2 Repetitions: Functionally poor 3 to 4 Repetitions: Functionally fair 5+ Repetitions: Functional
7. Forearm resting on table	Thumb adduction, lateral pinch of piece of paper	Hold 0 sec: Nonfunctional Hold 1 to 2 sec: Functionally poor Hold 3 to 4 sec: Functionally fair Hold 5+ sec: Functional
8. Forearm resting on table	Thumb opposition, pulp-to-pulp pinch of piece of paper	Hold 0 sec: Nonfunctional Hold 1 to 2 sec: Functionally poor Hold 3 to 4 sec: Functionally fair Hold 5+ sec: Functional
9. Forearm resting on table	Finger flexion, patient grasps mug or glass using cylindrical grasp and lifts off table	0 Repetitions: Nonfunctional 1 to 2 Repetitions: Functionally poor 3 to 4 Repetitions: Functionally fair 5+ Repetitions: Functional
10. Forearm resting on table	Patient attempts to put on rubber glove keeping fingers straight	21+ sec: Nonfunctional 10 to 20 sec: Functionally poor 4 to 8 sec: Functionally poor 2 to 4 sec: Functional
11. Forearm resting on table	Patient attempts to pull fingers apart (finger abduction) against resistance of rubber band* and holds	Hold 0 sec: Nonfunctional Hold 1 to 2 sec: Functionally poor Hold 3 to 4 sec: Functionally fair Hold 5+ sec: Functional
12. Forearm resting on table	Patient holds piece of paper between fingers while examiner pulls on paper	Hold 0 sec: Nonfunctional Hold 1 to 2 sec: Functionally poor Hold 3 to 4 sec: Functionally fair Hold 5+ sec: Functional

* Rubber band should be at least 1 cm wide.

Data from Palmer, M.L., and M. Epler: Clinical Assessment Procedures in Physical Therapy. Philadelphia, J.B. Lippincott, 1990, pp. 140–144.

Carpal Tunnel (Median Nerve) Function Disability Form

Symptom Severity Scale

The following questions refer to your symptoms for a typical twenty-four-hour period during the past two weeks (circle one answer to each question)

How severe is the hand or wrist pain that you have at night? 1 I do not have hand or wrist pain at night 2 Mild pain 3 Moderate pain 4 Severe pain 5 Very severe pain	How long, on average, does an episode of pain last during the daytime? 1 I never get pain during the day 2 Less than 10 minutes 3 10 to 60 minutes 4 Greater than 60 minutes 5 The pain is constant throughout the day
How often did hand or wrist pain wake you up during a typical night in the past two weeks? 1 Never 2 Once 3 Two or three times 4 Four or five times 5 More than five times	Do you have numbness (loss of sensation) in your hand? 1 No 2 I have mild numbness 3 I have moderate numbness 4 I have severe numbness 5 I have very severe numbness
Do you typically have pain in your hand or wrist during the daytime? 1 I never have pain during the day 2 I have mild pain during the day 3 I have moderate pain during the day 4 I have severe pain during the day 5 I have very severe pain during the day	Do you have weakness in your hand or wrist? 1 No weakness 2 Mild weakness 3 Moderate weakness 4 Severe weakness 5 Very severe weakness
How often do you have hand or wrist pain during the daytime? 1 Never 2 Once or twice a day 3 Three to five times a day 4 More than five times a day 5 The pain is constant	Do you have tingling sensations in your hand? 1 No tingling 2 Mild tingling 3 Moderate tingling 4 Severe tingling 5 Very severe tingling

Figure 7–38

Carpal tunnel (median nerve) function disability form. (Modified from Levine, D.W., B.P. Simmons, M.J. Koris, et al.: A self-administered questionnaire for the assessment of severity of symptoms and functional status in carpal tunnel syndrome. J. Bone Joint Surg. Am. 75:1586–1587, 1993.)

Illustration continued on opposite page

Estimated Use of Grips for Activities of Daily Living[21]

Pulp-to-pulp pinch:	20%
Three lateral pinch:	20%
Five-finger pinch:	15%
Fist grip:	15%
Cylinder grip:	14%
Three-fingered (thumb, index finger, middle finger) pinch:	10%
Spherical grip:	4%
Hook grip:	2%

These tests may also be graded on a four-point scale.[21] This scale is particularly suitable if the patient has difficulty with one of the subtests, and the subtests can be scale-graded:

Unable to perform task:	0
Completes task partially:	1
Completes task but is slow and clumsy:	2
Performs task normally:	3

As part of the functional assessment, manual dexterity tests may be performed. Many standardized tests have been developed to assess manual dexterity and coordination. If comparison with other subjects is desired, the examiner must ensure that the patient is compared with a similar group of patients in terms of age, disability, and occupation. Each of these tests has its supporters and detractors. Some of the more common tests include the following.

Jebson-Taylor Hand Function Test. This easily administered test involves seven functional areas: (1) writing, (2) card turning, (3) picking up small objects, (4) simulated feeding, (5) stacking, (6) picking up large, light objects, and

---

Symptom Severity Scale *Continued*

How severe is numbness (loss of sensation) or tingling at night?	Do you have difficulty with the grasping and use of small objects such as keys or pens?
1 I have no numbness or tingling at night	1 No difficulty
2 Mild	2 Mild difficulty
3 Moderate	3 Moderate difficulty
4 Severe	4 Severe difficulty
5 Very severe	5 Very severe difficulty

How severe is numbness (loss of sensation) or tingling at night?
1 I have no numbness or tingling at night
2 Mild
3 Moderate
4 Severe
5 Very severe

How often did hand numbness or tingling wake you up during a typical night during the past two weeks?
1 Never
2 Once
3 Two or three times
4 Four or five times
5 More than five times

Do you have difficulty with the grasping and use of small objects such as keys or pens?
1 No difficulty
2 Mild difficulty
3 Moderate difficulty
4 Severe difficulty
5 Very severe difficulty

Functional Status Scale

Figure 7–38 Continued

On a typical day during the past two weeks have hand and wrist symptoms caused you to have any difficulty doing the activities listed below? Please circle one number that best describes your ability to do the activity.

Activity	No Difficulty	Mild Difficulty	Moderate Difficulty	Severe Difficulty	Cannot Do at All Due to Hand or Wrist Symptoms
Writing	1	2	3	4	5
Buttoning of clothes	1	2	3	4	5
Holding a book while reading	1	2	3	4	5
Gripping of a telephone handle	1	2	3	4	5
Opening of jars	1	2	3	4	5
Household chores	1	2	3	4	5
Carrying of grocery bags	1	2	3	4	5
Bathing and dressing	1	2	3	4	5

(7) picking up large, heavy objects. The subtests are timed for each limb. This test primarily measures gross coordination, assessing prehension and manipulative skills with functional tests. It does not test bilateral integration.[9, 22–24] Anyone wishing to do the test should consult the original article[25] for details of administration.

Minnesota Rate of Manipulation Test. This test involves five activities: (1) placing, (2) turning, (3) displacing, (4) one-hand turning and placing, and (5) two-hand turning and placing. The activities are timed for both limbs and compared with normal values. The test primarily measures gross coordination and dexterity.[9, 22, 23]

Purdue Pegboard Test. This test measures fine coordination with the use of small pins, washers, and collars. The assessment categories of the test are (1) right hand, (2) left hand, (3) both hands, (4) right, left, and both, and (5) assembly. The subtests are timed and compared with normal values based on gender and occupation.[9, 22, 23]

Crawford Small Parts Dexterity Test. This test measures fine coordination, including the use of tools such as tweezers and screwdrivers to assemble things, to adjust equipment, and to do engraving.[9, 22]

Simulated Activities of Daily Living Examination. This test consists of 19 subtests, including standing, walking, putting on a shirt, buttoning, zipping, putting on gloves, dialing a telephone, tying a bow, manipulating safety pins, manipulating coins, threading a needle, unwrapping a Band-Aid, squeezing toothpaste, and using a knife and fork. Each subtask is timed.[21]

Moberg's Pickup Test. An assortment of 9 or 10 objects (e.g., bolts, nuts, screws, buttons, coins, pens, paper clips, keys) is used. The patient is timed for the following tests:

1. Putting objects in a box with the affected hand
2. Putting objects in a box with the unaffected hand
3. Putting objects in a box with the affected hand with eyes closed

The examiner notes which digits are used for prehension. Digits with altered sensation are less likely to be used. The test is used for median or combined median and ulnar nerve lesions.[26]

Box and Block Test. This is a test for gross manual dexterity in which 150 blocks, each measuring 2.5 cm (1 inch) on a side, are used. The patient has 1 minute in which to individually transfer the blocks from one side of a divided box to the other. The number of blocks transferred is given as the score. Patients are given a 15-second practice trial before the test.[24]

Nine-Hole Peg Test. This test is used to assess finger dexterity. The patient places nine 3.2-cm (1.3-inch) pegs in a 12.7 by 12.7 cm (5 by 5 inch) board and then removes them. The score is the time taken to do this task. Each hand is tested separately.[24]

Special Tests

For the forearm, wrist, and hand, there are no special tests that are commonly done with each assessment. Depending on the history, observation, and examination to this point, certain special tests may be performed. The examiner picks the appropriate test or tests to help confirm the diagnosis. As with all special tests, however, the examiner must keep in mind that they are confirming tests. When they are positive, they are highly suggestive that the problem exists, but if they are negative, they do not rule out the problem. This is especially true for the tests of neurological dysfunction.

Tests for Ligament, Capsule, and Joint Instability

Ligamentous Instability Test for the Fingers. The examiner stabilizes the finger with one hand proximal to the joint to be tested. With the other hand, the examiner grasps the finger distal to the joint to be tested. The distal hand is then used to apply a varus or valgus stress to the joint (proximal or distal interphalangeal) to test the integrity of the collateral ligaments. The results are compared for laxity with those of the uninvolved hand, which is tested first.

Thumb Ulnar Collateral Ligament Laxity or Instability Test. The patient sits while the examiner stabilizes the patient's hand with one hand and takes the patient's thumb into extension with the other hand. While holding the thumb in extension, the examiner applies a valgus stress to the metacarpophalangeal joint of the thumb, stressing the ulnar collateral ligament. If the valgus movement is greater than 35°, it indicates a tear of the ulnar collateral and accessory collateral ligaments.[27] This is a test for gamekeeper's or skier's thumb (Fig. 7–39).

Test for Tight Retinacular Ligaments. This test tests the structures around the proximal interphalangeal joint. The proximal interphalangeal joint is held in a neutral position while the distal interphalangeal joint is flexed by the examiner (Fig. 7–40). If the distal interphalangeal joint does not flex, the retinacular (collateral) ligaments or capsule are tight. If the proximal interphalangeal joint is flexed and the distal interphalangeal joint flexes easily, the retinacular ligaments are tight and the capsule is normal. During the test, the patient remains passive and does no active movements.

Lunatotriquetral Ballottement (Reagan's) Test. The examiner grasps the triquetrum between the thumb and second finger of one hand and the lunate with the thumb and second finger of the other hand (Fig. 7–41). The examiner then moves the lunate up and down (anteriorly and posteriorly), noting any laxity, crepitus, or pain, which indicates a positive test for lunatotriquetral instability.[28, 29]

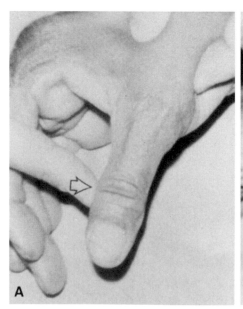
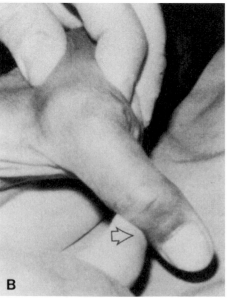

A   B

Figure 7–39

(A) and (B) Testing stability of the ulnar collateral ligament in the thumb of a normal individual. In extension, the thumb was stable, but in flexion, it appeared to be unstable. This was caused by the laxity of the dorsal capsule at the metacarpophalangeal joint. (From Nicholas, J.A., and E.B. Hershman (eds.): Upper Extremity in Sports Medicine. St. Louis, C.V. Mosby Co., 1989, p. 580.)

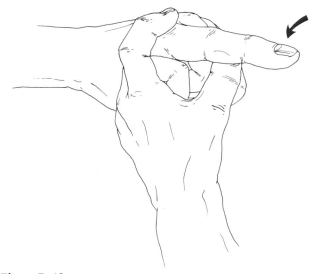

Figure 7–40
Test for retinacular ligaments.

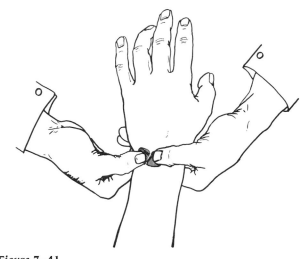

Figure 7–41
Lunatotriquetral ballottement test for lunatotriquetral interosseous membrane dissociations. (From Linschead, R.L., and J.H. Dobyns: Physical examination of the wrist. In Post, M. [ed.]: Physical Examination of the Musculoskeletal System. Chicago, Year Book Medical Pub., 1987, p. 87.)

Murphy's Sign. The patient is asked to make a fist. If the head of the third metacarpal is level with the second and fourth metacarpals, the sign is positive and indicative of a lunate dislocation.[30]

Watson (Scaphoid Shift) Test. The patient sits with the elbow resting on the lap and forearm pronated. With one hand, the examiner takes the patient's wrist into full ulnar deviation and slight extension. The examiner presses the thumb of the other hand against the distal pole of the scaphoid to prevent it from moving toward the palm. With the first hand, the examiner radially deviates and slightly flexes the patient's hand. If the scaphoid (and lunate) are unstable, the dorsal pole of the scaphoid subluxes over the dorsal rim of the radius and the patient complains of pain, indicating a positive test[7, 29, 31, 32] (Fig. 7–42).

Scaphoid Stress Test. The patient sits and the examiner holds the patient's wrist with one hand so that the thumb applies pressure over the distal pole of the scaphoid. The patient then attempts to radially deviate the wrist. Normally, the patient is unable to deviate the wrist. If

excessive laxity is present, the scaphoid is forced dorsally out of the scaphoid fossa of the radius with a resulting "clunk" and pain, indicating a positive test for scaphoid instability.[32, 33] This test is a modification of the Watson test, done actively by the patient.

"Piano Keys" Test. The patient sits with both arms in pronation. The examiner stabilizes the patient's arm with one hand so that the examiner's index finger can push down on the distal ulna. The examiner's other hand supports the patient's hand. The examiner pushes down on the distal ulna as one would push down on a piano key. The results are compared with the nonsymptomatic side. A positive test is indicated by a difference in mobility and the production of pain and/or tenderness. A positive test indicates instability of the distal radioulnar joint.[6]

Axial Load Test. The patient sits while the examiner stabilizes the patient's wrist with one hand. With the other hand, the examiner carefully grasps the patient's thumb and applies axial compression. Pain and/or crepi-

Figure 7–42
Watson (scaphoid shift) test. (A) Start position (ulnar deviation). (B) Radial deviation.

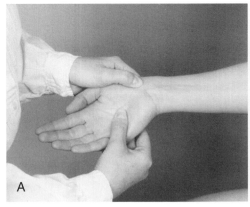
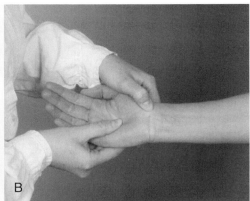

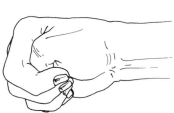
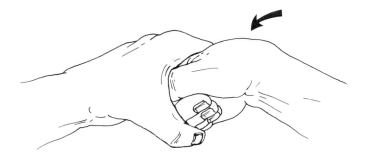

Figure 7–43
Finkelstein test.

tation indicates a positive test for a fracture of metacarpal or adjacent carpal bones or joint arthrosis. A similar test may be done for the fingers.

Pivot Shift Test of the Midcarpal Joint. The patient is seated with the elbow flexed to 90° and resting on a firm surface and the hand fully supinated. The examiner stabilizes the forearm with one hand and with the other hand takes the patient's hand into full radial deviation with the wrist in neutral. While the examiner maintains the patient's hand position, the patient's hand is taken into full ulnar deviation. A positive test results if the capitate "shifts" away from the lunate, indicating injury to the anterior capsule and interosseous ligaments.[1]

Grind Test. The examiner holds the patient's hand with one hand and grasps the patient's thumb below the metacarpophalangeal joint with the other hand. The examiner then applies axial compression and rotation to the metacarpophalangeal joint. If pain is elicited, the test is positive and indicative of degenerative joint disease in the metacarpophalangeal or metacarpotrapezial joint.[19]

Tests for Tendons and Muscles

Finkelstein Test. The Finkelstein test[34] is used to determine the presence of de Quervain's or Hoffmann's disease, a tenosynovitis in the thumb. The patient makes a fist with the thumb inside the fingers (Fig. 7–43). The examiner stabilizes the forearm and deviates the wrist toward the ulnar side. A positive test is indicated by pain over the abductor pollicis longus and extensor pollicis brevis tendons at the wrist and is indicative of a tenosynovitis in these two tendons. Because the test can cause some discomfort in normal individuals, the examiner should compare the pain caused on the affected side with that of the normal side and consider whether the patient's symptoms are reproduced.

Sweater Finger Sign. The patient is asked to make a fist. If the distal phalanx of one of the fingers does not flex, the sign is positive for a ruptured flexor digitorum profundus tendon (Fig. 7–44). It occurs most often to the ring finger.

Test for Extensor Hood Rupture.[35] The finger to be examined is flexed to 90° at the proximal interphalangeal joint over the edge of a table. The finger is held in position by the examiner. The patient is asked to carefully extend the proximal interphalangeal joint while the examiner palpates the middle phalanx. A positive test for a torn central extensor hood is the examiner's feeling little pressure from the middle phalanx while the distal interphalangeal joint is extending.

Boyes Test.[35, 36] This test also tests the central slip of the extensor hood. The examiner holds the finger to be examined in slight extension at the proximal interphalangeal joint. The patient is then asked to flex the distal interphalangeal joint. If the patient is unable or has difficulty flexing the distal interphalangeal joint, it is considered a positive test.

Bunnel-Littler (Finochietto-Bunnel) Test. This test tests the structures around the metacarpophalangeal joint. The metacarpophalangeal joint is held slightly extended while the examiner moves the proximal interphalangeal joint into flexion, if possible (Fig. 7–45).[37] If the test is positive, which is indicated by inability to flex the proxi-

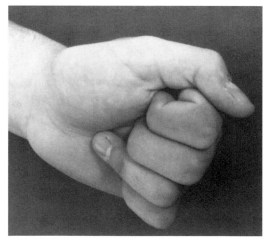

Figure 7–44
Sweater finger sign. Rupture of the flexor profundus tendon in the ring finger of a football player.

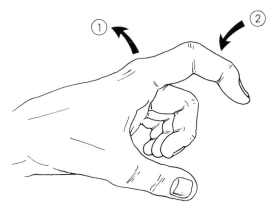

Figure 7–45
Positioning for the Bunnel-Littler test.

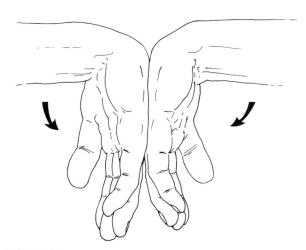

Figure 7–47
Phalen's test.

mal interphalangeal joint, there is a tight intrinsic muscle or contracture of the joint capsule. If the metacarpophalangeal joints are slightly flexed, the proximal interphalangeal joint flexes fully if the intrinsic muscles are tight, but it does not flex fully if the capsule is tight. The patient remains passive during the test. This test is also called the **intrinsic-plus test.**[1]

Linburg's Sign. The patient flexes the thumb maximally onto the hypothenar eminence and actively extends the index finger as far as possible. If limited index finger extension and pain are noted, the sign is positive for tendinitis at the interconnection between flexor pollicis longus and flexor indices (an anomalous tendon condition seen in 10 to 15% of hands).[28, 38]

Tests for Neurological Dysfunction

Tests for neurological dysfunction are highly suggestive of a particular nerve lesion if they are positive, but they do not rule out the problem if they are negative. In fact, they may be negative 50% of the time, or more, when the condition actually exists. Electrodiagnostic tests are more conclusive.

Tinel's Sign (at the Wrist).[34] The examiner taps over the carpal tunnel at the wrist (Fig. 7–46). A positive test causes tingling or paresthesia into the thumb, index

finger (forefinger), and middle and lateral half of the ring finger (median nerve distribution). Tinel's sign at the wrist is indicative of a carpal tunnel syndrome. The tingling or paresthesia must be felt distal to the point of pressure for a positive test. The test gives an indication of the rate of regeneration of sensory fibers of the median nerve. The most distal point at which the abnormal sensation is felt represents the limit of nerve regeneration.

Phalen's (Wrist Flexion) Test. The examiner flexes the patient's wrists maximally and holds this position for 1 minute by pushing the patient's wrists together (Fig. 7–47). A positive test is indicated by tingling in the thumb, index finger, and middle and lateral half of the ring finger and is indicative of carpal tunnel syndrome caused by pressure on the median nerve.[39]

Reverse Phalen's (Prayer) Test. The examiner extends the patient's wrist while asking the patient to grip the examiner's hand. The examiner then applies direct pressure over the carpal tunnel for 1 minute. A positive test produces the same symptoms as are seen in Phalen's test and is indicative of pathology of the median nerve.[28]

Carpal Compression Test.[40] The examiner holds the supinated wrist in both hands and applies direct, even pressure over the median nerve in the carpal tunnel for up

Figure 7–46
Tinel's sign at the wrist.

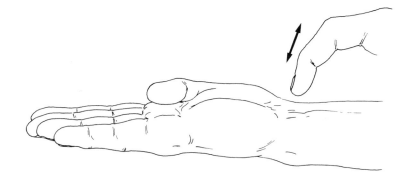

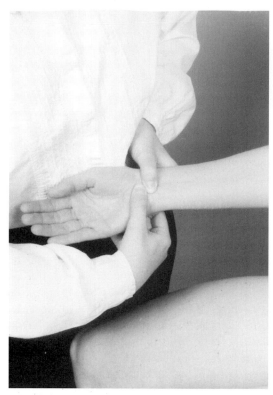

Figure 7–48
Carpal compression test.

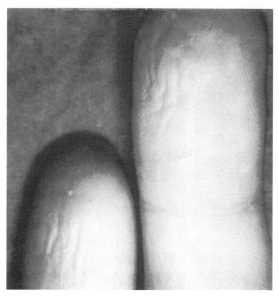

Figure 7–50
The wrinkle test may be reliable for digital nerve sympathetic function if the fingers (in this case, the radial digital nerve of the fourth and fifth digits) are completely denervated. (From Waylett-Rendall, J.: Sensibility evaluation and rehabilitation. Orthop. Clin. North Am. 19:48, 1988.)

to 30 seconds (Fig. 7–48). Production of the patient's symptoms is considered to be a positive test for carpal tunnel syndrome. This test is a modification of the reverse Phalen's test.

Froment's Sign. The patient attempts to grasp a piece of paper between the thumb and index finger (Fig. 7–49).[41] When the examiner attempts to pull away the paper, the terminal phalanx of the thumb flexes because of paralysis of the adductor pollicis muscle, indicating a positive test. If, at the same time, the metacarpophalangeal joint of the thumb hyperextends, the hyperexten-

sion is noted as a positive **Jeanne's sign.**[19] Both tests, if positive, are indicative of ulnar nerve paralysis.

Egawa's Sign. The patient flexes the middle digit and then alternately deviates the finger radially and ulnarly. If the patient is unable to do this, the interossei are affected. A positive sign is indicative of ulnar nerve palsy.

Wrinkle (Shrivel) Test. The patient's fingers are placed in warm water for approximately 5 to 20 minutes. The examiner then removes the patient's fingers from the water and observes whether the skin over the pulp is wrinkled (Fig. 7–50). Normal fingers show wrinkling, but denervated ones do not. The test is valid only within the first few months after injury.[42]

Ninhydrin Sweat Test. The patient's hand is cleaned thoroughly and wiped with alcohol. The patient then waits 5 to 30 minutes with the fingertips not in contact with any surface. This allows time for the sweating process to ensue. After the waiting period, the fingertips are pressed with moderate pressure against good-quality bond paper that has not been touched. The fingertips are held in place for 15 seconds and traced with a pencil. The paper is then sprayed with triketohydrindene (Ninhydrin) spray reagent and allowed to dry (24 hours). The sweat areas stain purple. If the change in color (from white to purple) does not occur, it is considered a positive test for a nerve lesion.[26, 43] The reagent must be fixed if a permanent record is required.

Weber's (Moberg's) Two-Point Discrimination Test. The examiner uses a paper clip, two-point discriminator, or

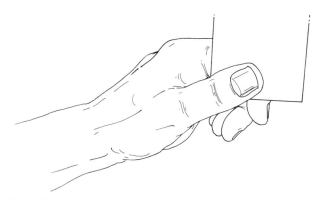

Figure 7–49
Froment's sign.

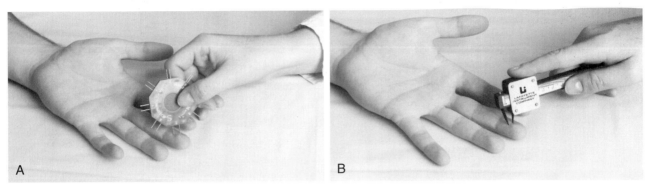

Figure 7–51
Devices used to test two-point discrimination. (A) The Disk-Criminator is a set of two plastic discs, each containing a series of metal rods at varying intervals from 1 to 25 mm apart. This device evaluates both moving and static two-point discrimination. (B) Two-point esthesiometer.

calipers (Fig. 7–51) to simultaneously apply pressure on two adjacent points in a longitudinal direction or perpendicular to the long axis of the finger; the examiner moves proximal to distal in an attempt to find the minimal distance at which the patient can distinguish between the two stimuli.[14] This distance is called the **threshold for discrimination**. Coverage values are shown in Figure 7–52). The patient must concentrate on feeling the points and must not be able to see the area being tested. Only the fingertips need to be tested. The patient's hand should be immobile on a hard surface. For accurate results, the examiner must ensure that the two points touch the skin simultaneously. There should be no blanching of the skin when the points are applied. The distance between the points is decreased or increased depending on the response of the patient. The starting distance between the points is one that the patient can easily distinguish (e.g., 15 mm). If the patient is hesitant to respond or becomes inaccurate, the patient is required to respond accurately on 7 or 8 of 10 trials before the distance is narrowed and the test repeated.[9, 26, 44, 45] Normal discrimination distance recognition is less than 6 mm, but this varies from person to person. This test is best for hand sensation involving static holding of an

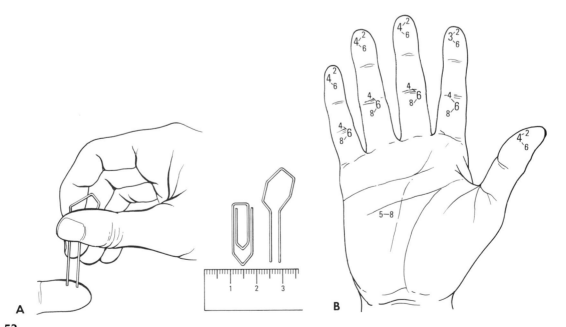

Figure 7–52
Two-point discrimination. (A) Technique of performing the two-point discrimination test of Weber (after Moberg). (B) Values of discrimination in the Weber test in millimeters in the different zones of the palm. The largest figure indicates the average values, the other two figures the minimum and maximum values (after Moberg). (From Tubiana, R.: The Hand. Philadelphia, W.B. Saunders Co., 1981, pp. 645–646.)

Table 7–10
Two-Point Discrimination Normal Values and
Discrimination Distances Required for Certain Tasks

Normal	Less than 6 mm
Fair	6 to 10 mm
Poor	11 to 15 mm
Protective	1 point perceived
Anesthetic	0 points perceived
Winding a watch	6 mm
Sewing	6 to 8 mm
Handling precision tools	12 mm
Gross tool handling	>15 mm

Adapted from Callahan, A.D.: Sensibility testing. In Hunter, J., L.H. Schneider, E.J. Mackin, and A.D. Callahan (eds.): Rehabilitation of the Hand: Surgery and Therapy. St. Louis, C.V. Mosby Co., 1990, p. 605.

object between the fingers and thumb and requiring pinch strength. Table 7–10 demonstrates some two-point discrimination normal values and distances required for certain tasks.

Dellon's Moving Two-Point Discrimination Test. This test is used to predict functional recovery; it measures the quickly adapting mechanoreceptor system.[14] The test is similar to Weber's two-point discrimination test except that the two points are moved during the test. This test is best for hand sensation related to activity and movement. The examiner moves two blunt points from proximal to distal along the long axis of the limb or digit, starting with a distance of 8 mm between the points. The distance between the points is increased or decreased, depending on the response of the patient, until the two points can no longer be distinguished. During the test, the patient's eyes are closed and the hand is cradled in

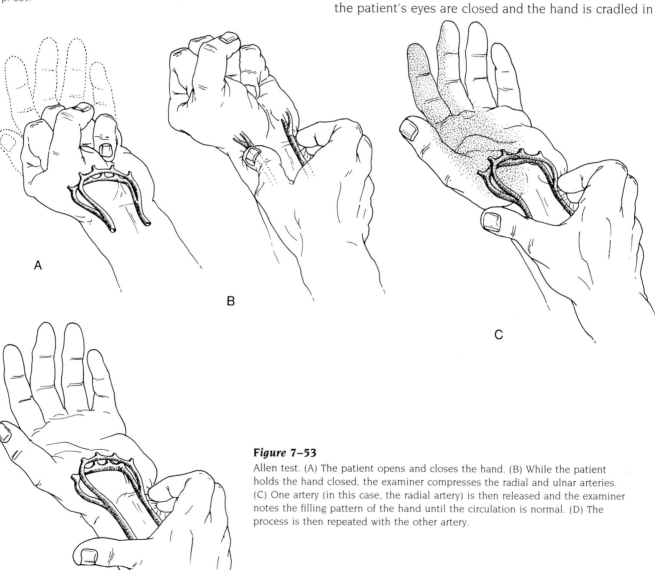

Figure 7–53
Allen test. (A) The patient opens and closes the hand. (B) While the patient holds the hand closed, the examiner compresses the radial and ulnar arteries. (C) One artery (in this case, the radial artery) is then released and the examiner notes the filling pattern of the hand until the circulation is normal. (D) The process is then repeated with the other artery.

the examiner's hand. The two smooth points, whether paper clip, two-point discriminator, or calipers, are gently placed longitudinally. There should be no blanching of the skin when the points are applied. The patient is asked whether one or two points are felt. If the patient is hesitant to respond or becomes inaccurate, the patient is required to respond accurately 7 or 8 of 10 times before the distance is narrowed and the test repeated.[9, 26, 44, 46]

Normal discrimination distance recognition is 2 to 5 mm.[45] The values obtained for this test are slightly lower than those obtained for Weber's static two-point discrimination test.[44] Although the entire hand may be tested, it is more common to test only the anterior digital pulp.

Tests for Circulation and Swelling

Allen Test. The patient is asked to open and close the hand several times as quickly as possible and then squeeze the hand tightly (Fig. 7–53).[39] The examiner's thumb and index finger are placed over the radial and ulnar arteries, compressing them. The patient then opens the hand while pressure is maintained over the arteries. One artery is tested by releasing the pressure over that artery to see if the hand flushes. The other artery is then tested in a similar fashion. Both hands should be tested for comparison. This test determines the patency of the radial and ulnar arteries and determines which artery provides the major blood supply to the hand.

Digit Blood Flow. To test distal blood flow, the examiner compresses the nail bed and notes the time taken for color to return to the nail. Normally, when the pressure is released, color should return to the nail bed within 3 seconds. If return takes longer, arterial insufficiency to the fingers should be suspected. Comparison with the normal side gives some indication of restricted flow.

Hand Volume Test. If the examiner is concerned about changes in hand size, a volumeter (Fig. 7–54) may be used. This device can be used to assess change in hand size resulting from localized swelling, generalized edema, or atrophy.[22] Comparisons with the normal limb give the examiner an idea of changes occurring in the affected hand. Care must be taken when doing this test to ensure accurate readings. There is often a 10-ml difference between right and left hands and between dominant and nondominant hands. If swelling is the problem, differences of 30 to 50 ml can be noted.[9, 47]

Measurement for Swelling. Swelling may also be measured with a tape measure, as long as the examiner is consistent with the measuring points. When assessing swelling, the examiner commonly measures around the proximal interphalangeal joints individually, around the metacarpophalangeal joints as a group, and around the palm and wrist. The values for both sides are compared.

Reflexes and Cutaneous Distribution

Although it is possible to obtain reflexes from the tendons crossing the wrist, this is not commonly done. In fact, no deep tendon reflexes are routinely tested in the forearm, wrist, and hand. The only reflex that may be tested in the hand is Hoffman's reflex, which is a pathological reflex. This reflex may be tested if an upper motor neuron lesion is suspected. To test the reflex, the examiner "flicks" the terminal phalanx of the index, middle, or ring finger. A positive test is indicated by reflex flexion of the distal phalanx of the thumb or a finger that was not "flicked."

The examiner must be aware of the sensory distribution of the ulnar, median, and radial nerves in the hand (Fig. 7–55) and must be prepared to compare peripheral

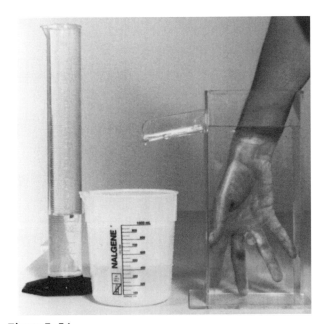

Figure 7–54
Volumeter used to measure hand volume.

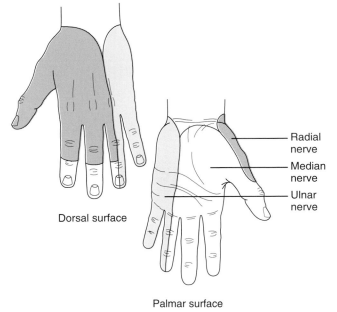

Radial nerve
Median nerve
Ulnar nerve

Dorsal surface

Palmar surface

Figure 7–55
Peripheral nerve distribution in the hand.

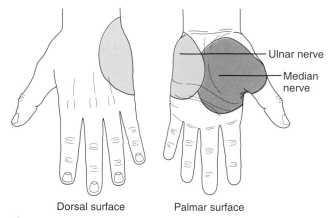

Dorsal surface   Palmar surface

Figure 7–56
Sensory distribution of branches of the ulnar and median nerves given off above the wrist.

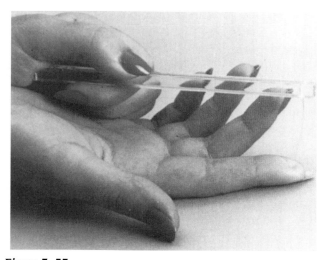

Figure 7–57
The Semmes-Weinstein monofilament is applied perpendicular to the skin for 1 to 1.5 seconds, held in place for 1 to 1.5 seconds, and lifted for 1 to 1.5 seconds. (From Waylett-Rendall, J.: Sensibility evaluation and rehabilitation. Orthop. Clin. North Am. 19:51, 1988.)

nerve sensory distribution with nerve root sensory (dermatome) distributions. As previously mentioned, there is variability in both distributions. It has been reported, however, that each peripheral nerve of the upper limb has a "constant" area in the hand that is always affected if the nerve is injured. For the radial nerve, it is on the dorsum of the thumb near the apex of the anatomical snuff box; for the median nerve, it is the tip of the index finger; and for the ulnar nerve, it is the tip of the little finger.[48]

The median nerve gives off a sensory branch above the wrist before it passes through the carpal tunnel. This sensory branch supplies the skin of the palm (Fig. 7–56). It is important to remember that carpal tunnel syndrome does not affect the median sensory distribution in the palm but results in altered sensation in the fingers.

Several sensation tests may be carried out in the hand. Table 7–11 illustrates the tests used and the sensa-

tion and nerve fibers tested. Pinprick is used to test for pain. Constant light touch, which is a component of fine discrimination, may be tested in the hand using a Semmes-Weinstein pressure esthesiometer (Von Frey test). This kit has 20 probes, each with different thicknesses of nylon monofilament (Fig. 7–57). The patient is blindfolded or otherwise unable to see the hand, and each filament is applied perpendicularly to the finger, with the smallest filament being used first. The filament is pushed against the finger until the filament bends. The next filament is then used, and so on until the patient feels one before or just as it bends.[9, 26] The test is repeated three times to ensure a positive result.[45] Normal values vary between 2.36 and 2.83 mg (Table 7–12). When doing the Semmes-Weinstein test, the hand

Table 7–11
Tests for Cutaneous Sensibility

Test	Sensation	Fiber/Receptor Type
Pin	Pain	Free nerve endings
Warm/cold	Temperature	Free nerve endings
Cotton wool	Moving touch	Quick adapting
Finger stroking	Moving touch	Quick adapting
Dellon's test	Moving touch	Quick adapting
Tuning fork	Vibration	Quick adapting
Von Frey	Constant touch	Slow adapting
Weber's test	Constant touch	Slow adapting
Pick-up test	Constant touch	Slow adapting
Precision sensory grip	Constant touch	Slow adapting
Gross grip	Constant touch	Slow adapting

Modified from Dellon, A.L.: The paper clip: Light hardware to evaluate sensibility in the hand. Contemp. Orthop. 1:40, 1979.

Table 7–12
Light Touch Testing Using Semmes-Weinstein Pressure Esthesiometer

Esthesiometer Probe No.	Calculated Pressure (g/mm²)	Interpretation
2.44–2.83	3.25–4.86	Normal light touch
3.22–4.56	11.1–47.3	Diminished light touch, point localization* intact
4.74–6.10	68.0–243.0	Minimal light touch, area localization† intact
6.10–6.65	243.0–439.0	Sensation but no localization sensibility

* Point localization: the dowel is in contact with the skin point stimulated.

† Area localization: the dowel is in contact with any point inside the zone of the area being tested (in the hand or foot).

From Omer, G.E.: Report of the Committee for Evaluation of the Clinical Result in Peripheral Nerve Injury. J. Hand Surg. Am. 8:755, 1983.

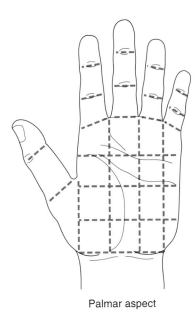

Palmar aspect

Figure 7–58
Grid pattern used for recording results of light touch sensation testing.

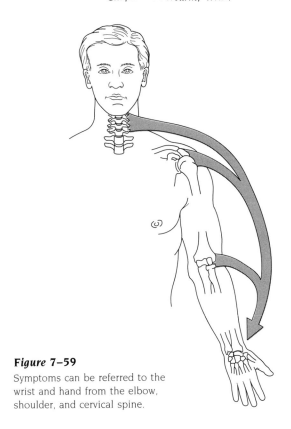

Figure 7–59
Symptoms can be referred to the wrist and hand from the elbow, shoulder, and cervical spine.

and fingers are commonly divided into a grid (Fig. 7–58), and only one point (usually in the center) is tested in each square. It is primarily the palmar aspect of the hand that is tested.

Stereognosis or tactile gnosis, which is the ability to identify common objects by touch, should also be tested. Objects are placed in the patient's hand while the patient is blindfolded or otherwise unable to see the object. The time taken to recognize the object is noted. Normal subjects can usually name the object within 3 seconds of contact.[44]

Vibratory sense is tested using a 256-cps (high-frequency) or 30-cps (low-frequency) tuning fork. The patient, who cannot see the test site, indicates when vibration is felt as the examiner touches the skin with the vibrating tuning fork and whether the vibration feels the same. The score is the number of correct responses divided by the total number of presentations.[49]

To test moving touch, the examiner's fingers stroke the patient's finger. The patient notes whether the stroking was felt and what it felt like.

It must be remembered that pain may be referred to the wrist and hand from the cervical or upper thoracic spine, shoulder, and elbow. Seldom is wrist or hand pain referred up the limb (Fig. 7–59). Table 7–13 shows the muscles acting on the forearm, wrist, and hand and their pain referral patterns when injured.

The examiner can attempt a differential diagnosis of paresthesia in the hand if altered sensation is present. A comparison with a normal dermatome chart should be made, and the examiner should remember that there is a fair amount of variability and overlap with derma-

Table 7–13
Forearm, Wrist, and Hand Muscles and Referral of Pain

Muscle	Referral Pattern
Brachioradialis	Lateral epicondyle, lateral forearm, and web space between thumb and index finger
Extensor carpi ulnaris	Medial side of dorsum of wrist
Extensor carpi radialis brevis	Middle of dorsum of wrist
Extensor carpi radialis longus	Lateral epicondyle, forearm, and lateral dorsum of hand
Extensor digitorum	Forearm, wrist to appropriate digit
Extensor indices	Dorsum of wrist to index finger
Palmaris longus	Anterior aspect of forearm to palm
Flexor carpi ulnaris	Anteromedial wrist into lateral palm
Flexor carpi radialis	Forearm to anterolateral wrist
Flexor digitorum superficialis	Palm into appropriate digit
Flexor pollicis longus	Thumb
Adductor pollicis	Anterolateral and posterolateral palm into thumb
Opponens pollicis	Anterolateral wrist into anterior thumb
Abductor digiti minimi	Dorsomedial surface of hand into little finger
Interossei	Into adjacent digit, and for first interossei, dorsum of hand

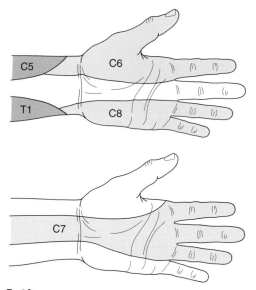

Figure 7–60

Dermatomes of the hand. Note overlap at dermatomes. Both views are palmar.

tomes (Fig. 7–60). In addition, there are areas of the hand where sensation is more important (Fig. 7–61). Abnormal sensation may mean the following:

1. Numbness in the thumb only may be caused by pressure on the digital nerve on the outer aspect of the thumb.

2. A "pins and needles" feeling in the thumb may be caused by a contusion of the thenar branch of the median nerve.

3. Paresthesia in the thumb and index finger may be caused by a C5 disc lesion or C6 nerve root palsy.

4. Paresthesia in the thumb, index finger, and middle finger may be caused by a C5 disc lesion, C6 nerve root palsy, or thoracic outlet syndrome.

5. Paresthesia of the thumb, index finger, middle finger, and half of the ring finger on the palmar aspect may be caused by an injury to the median nerve, possibly through the carpal tunnel; on the dorsal aspect, it could be caused by injury to the radial nerve.

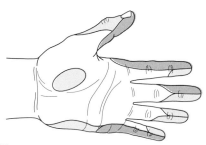

Figure 7–61

Importance of hand sensation. Darker areas indicate where sensation is most important; lighter areas, where sensation is a little less important; and white areas, where sensation is least important. (Redrawn from Tubiana, R.: The Hand. Philadelphia, W.B. Saunders Co., 1981, p. 74.)

6. Numbness of the thumb and middle finger may be caused by a tumor of the humerus.

7. Paresthesia on all five digits in one or both hands may be caused by a thoracic outlet syndrome. If it is in both hands, it may be caused by a central cervical disc protrusion. The level of protrusion would be indicated by the distribution of the paresthesia.

8. Paresthesia of the index and middle fingers may be caused by a trigger finger or "stick" palsy, if it is on the palmar aspect, or by a C6 disc lesion or C7 nerve root palsy. On the dorsal aspect of the hand, it may be caused by a carpal exostosis or subluxation. Stick palsy is the result of an inordinant amount of pressure from a cane or crutches on the ulnar nerve as it passes through the palm.

9. Paresthesia of the index, middle, and ring fingers may be caused by a C6 disc lesion, C7 nerve root injury, or carpal tunnel syndrome.

10. Paresthesia of all four fingers may be caused by a C6 disc lesion or injury to the C7 nerve root.

11. Paresthesia of the middle finger only may be caused by a C6 disc lesion or C7 nerve root lesion.

12. Paresthesia of the middle and ring fingers may be caused by a C6 disc lesion, C7 nerve root lesion, or stick palsy.

13. Paresthesia of the middle, ring, and little fingers may be caused by a C7 disc lesion or C8 nerve root palsy. The same would be true if there were paralysis of the ring and little fingers. This paresthesia may also be the result of a thoracic outlet syndrome.

14. Paresthesia on the ulnar side of the ring finger and the entire little finger may be caused by pressure of the ulnar nerve at the elbow or in the palm.

Peripheral Nerve Injuries of the Forearm, Wrist, and Hand

Carpal Tunnel Syndrome. The most common "tunnel" syndrome in the body is the carpal tunnel syndrome, in which the median nerve is compressed under the flexor retinaculum at the wrist (see Fig. 7–27). This compression may follow trauma (for example, a Colles fracture or lunate dislocation), flexor tendon tenosynovitis, a ganglion, arthritis (osteoarthritis or rheumatoid arthritis), or collagen disease. As many as 20% of pregnant women may experience median nerve symptoms, because compression of the nerve as a result of fluid retention causes swelling in the carpal tunnel. With carpal tunnel syndrome, the symptoms, which are primarily distal to the wrist, are usually worse at night and include burning, tingling, pins and needles, and numbness into the median nerve sensory distribution (Table 7–14). In severe cases, pain may be referred to the forearm. Symptoms are often aggravated by wrist movements, and long-standing cases show atrophy and weakness of the thenar muscles (flexor and abductor pollicis brevis, opponens pollicis)

Table 7–14
Nerve Injuries (Neuropathy) About the Wrist and Hand

Nerve	Motor Loss	Sensory Loss	Functional Loss
Median nerve (C6–C8, T1; carpal tunnel)	Flexor pollicis brevis Abductor pollicis brevis Opponens pollicis Lateral two lumbricals	Palmar and dorsal thumb, index, middle and lateral half of ring finger If lesion above carpal tunnel, palmar sensation also affected	Thumb opposition Thumb flexion Weak or no pinch Weak grip
Ulnar nerve (C7, C8, T1; pisohamate canal)	Flexor digiti minimi Abductor digiti minimi Opponens digiti minimi Adductor pollicis Interossei Medial two lumbricals Palmaris brevis	Little finger, half of ring finger Palm often not affected	Thumb adduction Inability to extend PIP and DIP joints of fourth and fifth fingers Finger abduction Finger adduction Flexion of little finger

DIP = distal interphalangeal; PIP = proximal interphalangeal.

and the lateral two lumbricals. The condition is most common in women between 40 and 60 years of age, and although it may occur bilaterally, it is seen most commonly in the dominant hand. It is also commonly seen in younger patients who use their wrists a great deal in repetitive manual labor or are exposed to vibration.[50] Because of the apparent connection between carpal tunnel syndrome and cervical lesions resulting in double crush syndromes, the examiner should take care to include cervical assessment if the history appears to warrant such inclusion.[51–53]

Guyon's (Pisohamate) Canal. The ulnar nerve is sometimes compressed as it passes through the pisohamate, or Guyon's canal (Fig. 7–62). The nerve may be com-

pressed from trauma (e.g., fractured hook of hamate), use of crutches, or chronic pressure, as in people who cycle long distances while leaning on the handlebars or who use pneumatic jackhammers. The ulnar nerve gives off two sensory branches above the wrist. These branches supply the palmar and dorsal aspects of the hand, as illustrated in Figure 7–56, and do not pass through Guyon's canal. Therefore, if the ulnar nerve is compressed in the canal, only the fingers show an altered sensation (see Table 7–14). Motor loss includes the muscles of the hypothenar eminence (flexor digiti minimi, abductor digiti minimi, opponens digiti minimi), adductor pollicis, the interossei, medial two lumbricals, and palmaris brevis.

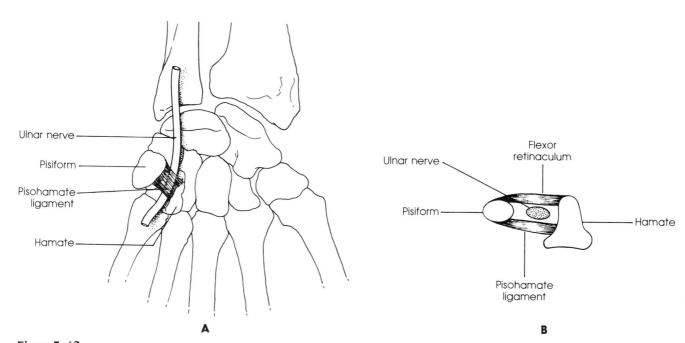

Figure 7–62
Guyon's canal. (A) Palmar view. (B) Section view showing position of nerve relative to pisohamate ligament and flexor retinaculum.

Joint Play Movements

When assessing joint play movements, the examiner should remember that if the patient complains of inability or pain on wrist flexion, the lesion is probably in the midcarpal joints. If the patient complains of inability or pain on wrist extension, the lesion is probably in the radiocarpal joints, because it is in these joints that most of the movement occurs during these actions. If the patient complains of pain or inability on supination and pronation, the lesion is probably in the ulnameniscocarpal joint or inferior radioulnar joint.

The amount of movement obtained by the joint play should be compared with that of the normal side and considered significant only if there is a difference between the two sides. Reproduction of the patient's symptoms would also give an indication of the joints at fault.

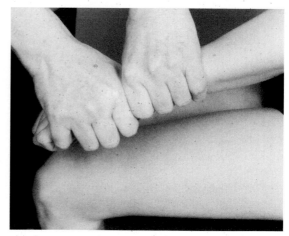

Figure 7–63
Position for testing joint play movements of the wrist.

Joint Play Movements of the Hand

Wrist	Intermetacarpal Joints	Fingers
• Long-axis extension (traction or distraction)	• Antero-posterior glide	• Long-axis extension (traction or distraction)
• Antero-posterior glide		• Antero-posterior glide
• Side glide		• Rotation
• Side tilt		• Side glide

Wrist

To perform **long-axis extension** at the wrist, the examiner stabilizes the radius and ulna with one hand (the patient's arm may be flexed to 90°, and stabilization may be applied at the elbow if there is no pathology at the elbow) and places the other hand just distal to the wrist. The examiner then applies a longitudinal traction movement with the distal hand.

Anteroposterior glide is applied at the wrist in two positions. The examiner first places the stabilizing hand around the distal end of the radius and ulna just proximal to the radiocarpal joint and then places the other hand around the proximal row of carpal bones. If the hands are positioned properly, they should touch each other (Fig. 7–63). The examiner applies an anteroposterior gliding movement of the proximal row of carpal bones on the radius and ulna. Then, the stabilizing hand is moved slightly distally (<1 cm) so that it is around the proximal row of carpal bones. The examiner places the

mobilizing hand around the distal row of carpal bones. An anteroposterior gliding movement is applied to the distal row of carpal bones on the proximal row. These movements are sometimes called the **anteroposterior drawer test** of the wrist.[1] If the examiner then moves the stabilizing hand slightly distally (<1 cm) again, the hand will be around the distal carpal bones. The mobilizing hand is then placed around the metacarpals, and an anteroposterior gliding movement is applied to the base of the metacarpals.

Side glide is performed in a similar fashion, except that a side-to-side movement is performed instead of an anteroposterior movement. To perform **side tilting** of the carpals on the radius and ulna, the examiner stabilizes the radius and ulna by placing the stabilizing hand around the distal radius and ulna just proximal to the radiocarpal joint and the mobilizing hand around the patient's hand and then radially and ulnarly deviating the hand on the radius and ulna.

The above joint play movements are general ones involving different "rows" of carpal bones. To check the joint play movements of the individual carpal bones, a technique such as **Kaltenborn's technique** should be used. Kaltenborn[54] suggested 10 tests to determine the mobility of each of the carpal bones. The movement of each of the bones is determined in a sequential manner, and both sides are tested for comparison. These tests are sometimes referred to as **ballottement tests** or **shear tests**.[1] The examiner may use Kaltenborn's order or any other order as long as each bone is tested individually. For example, some people start by testing the movement of the lunate relative to the radius, then move to the capitate (relative to the lunate), followed by scaphoid-radius, scaphoid-trapezoid/trapezium, triquetrum-radius, and triquetrum-hamate. Pisiform may be tested individually.

Kaltenborn's Carpal Mobilization

- Fixate the capitate and move the trapezoid
- Fixate the capitate and move the scaphoid
- Fixate the capitate and move the lunate
- Fixate the capitate and move the hamate
- Fixate the scaphoid and move the trapezoid and trapezium
- Fixate the radius and move the scaphoid
- Fixate the radius and move the lunate
- Fixate the ulna and move the triquetrum
- Fixate the triquetrum and move the hamate
- Fixate the triquetrum and move the pisiform

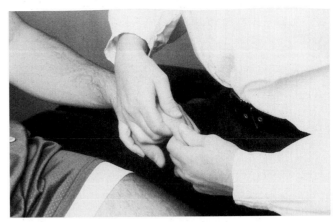

Figure 7–64
Position for testing joint play movements of the fingers.

Intermetacarpal Joints

To accomplish **anteroposterior glide** at the intermetacarpal joints, the examiner stabilizes one metacarpal bone and moves the adjacent metacarpal anteriorly and posteriorly in relation to the fixed bone. The process is repeated for each joint.

Fingers

The joint play movements for the fingers are the same for the metacarpophalangeal, proximal interphalangeal, and distal interphalangeal joints; the hand position of the examiner simply moves farther distally.

To perform **long-axis extension,** the examiner stabilizes the proximal segment or bone using one hand while placing the second hand around the distal segment or bone of the particular joint to be tested. With the mobilizing hand, the examiner applies a longitudinal traction to the joint.

Anteroposterior glide is accomplished by stabilizing the proximal bone with one hand. The mobilizing hand is placed around the distal segment of the joint, and the examiner applies an anterior and/or posterior movement to the distal segment, being sure to maintain the joint surfaces parallel to one another (Fig. 7–64). A minimal amount of traction may be applied to bring about slight separation of the joint surfaces.

Rotation of the joints of the fingers is accomplished by stabilizing the proximal segment with one hand. With the other hand, the examiner applies slight traction to the joint to distract the joint surfaces and then rotates the distal segment on the proximal segment.

To perform **side glide** joint play to the joints of the fingers, the proximal segment is stabilized with one hand, while the examiner applies slight traction to the joint with the mobilizing hand to distract the joint surfaces and then moves the distal segment sideways, keeping the joint surfaces parallel to one another.

Palpation

To palpate the forearm, wrist, and hand, the examiner starts proximally and works distally, first on the dorsal surface and then on the anterior surface (Fig. 7–65). The muscles of the forearm are palpated first for any signs of tenderness or pathology.

Dorsal Surface

On the dorsal aspect, the examiner begins on the thumb side of the hand and palpates the "snuff box," the carpal bones, and the metacarpal bones and phalanges.

Anatomic Snuff Box. The snuff box is located between the tendons of extensor pollicis longus and extensor pollicis brevis and can best be seen by having the patient actively extend the thumb. The scaphoid bone may be palpated inside the snuff box. Tenderness of the scaphoid bone is often treated as a fracture until proven otherwise because of the possibility of avascular necrosis of the bone. With the wrist in anatomic position, proximal palpation is used to find the radial styloid on the lateral aspect. Moving medially over the radius, the examiner comes to the radial (Lister's) tubercle. The extensor pol-

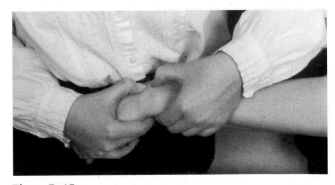

Figure 7–65
Palpation of the wrist using both hands.

licis longus tendon moves around the tubercle to enter the thumb, which gives it a different angle of pull from that of the extensor pollicis brevis. With the wrist in anatomic position, the ulnar styloid is palpated on the medial aspect. The radial styloid extends farther distally than the ulnar styloid. By palpating over the dorsum of the wrist, crossing the radius and ulna, the examiner should attempt to palpate the six extensor tendon tunnels (noting any crepitus or restriction to movement), moving lateral to medial (see Fig. 7–30):

> Tunnel 1: abductor pollicis longus and extensor pollicis brevis
> Tunnel 2: extensor carpi radialis longus and brevis
> Tunnel 3: extensor pollicis longus
> Tunnel 4: extensor digitorum and extensor indices
> Tunnel 5: extensor digiti minimi
> Tunnel 6: extensor carpi ulnaris

Carpal Bones. In the anatomic snuff box, the examiner can begin palpating the proximal row of carpal bones, starting with the scaphoid or lunate bone. When palpating the carpal bones, the examiner usually palpates them on the anterior and dorsal surfaces at the same time. The proximal row of carpal bones from lateral to medial (in the anatomic position) are the scaphoid, lunate, triquetrum (just below the ulnar styloid), and pisiform.

On the anterior aspect, the examiner should take care to ensure proper positioning of the lunate bone. If it dislocates or subluxes, it tends to move in an anterior direction into the carpal tunnel, which may lead to symptoms of carpal tunnel syndrome. The pisiform is often easier to palpate if the patient's wrist is flexed. The examiner may then palpate the pisiform where the flexor carpi ulnaris tendon inserts into it.

Returning to the anatomic snuff box and moving distally, the examiner palpates the trapezium bone. As this is done, the radial pulse is often palpated in the anatomic snuff box. The distal row of carpal bones from lateral to medial (in the anatomic position) are palpated individually: trapezium, trapezoid, capitate (distal to lunate and a slight indentation before the metacarpal), and hamate (distal to triquetrum; the hook of the hamate on the anterior surface is the easiest part to palpate).

Metacarpal Bones and Phalanges. The examiner returns to the trapezium bone and moves farther distally to palpate the first metacarpal joint and the first metacarpal bone. Moving medially, the examiner palpates each metacarpal bone on the anterior and dorsal surface in turn. A similar procedure is carried out for the metacarpophalangeal and interphalangeal joints and the phalanges. These structures are also palpated on their medial and lateral aspects for tenderness, swelling, altered temperature, or other signs of pathology (Fig. 7–66).

Anterior Surface

Pulses. Proximally, the radial and ulnar pulses are palpated first. The radial pulse on the anterolateral as-

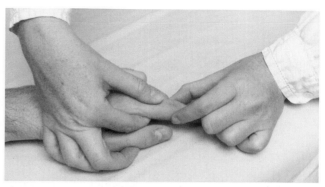

Figure 7–66
Palpation of the proximal interphalangeal joint of the left second finger.

pect of the wrist on top of the radius is easiest to palpate and is the one most frequently used when taking a pulse. It runs between the tendons of flexor carpi radialis and abductor pollicis longus. The ulnar pulse may be palpated lateral to the tendon of flexor carpi ulnaris. It is more difficult to palpate because it runs deeper and lies under the pisiform and the palmar fascia.

Tendons. Moving across the anterior aspect, the examiner may be able to palpate the long flexor tendons (see Fig. 7–30) in a lateral-to-medial direction: flexor carpi radialis, flexor pollicis longus, flexor digitorum superficialis, flexor digitorum profundus, palmaris longus, and flexor carpi ulnaris (inserts into pisiform). The palmaris longus (if present) lies over the tendons of the flexor digitorum superficialis, which lie over the tendons of the flexor digitorum profundus. The palmaris longus tendon may sometimes be used for tendon repairs or transfers.

Palmar Fascia and Intrinsic Muscles. The examiner should then move distally to palpate the palmar fascia and intrinsic muscles of the thenar and hypothenar eminences for indications of pathology.

Skin Flexion Creases. From an anatomic point of view, the examiner should note the various skin flexion creases of the wrist, hand, and fingers (Fig. 7–67). The flexion creases indicate lines of adherence between the skin and fascia with no intervening adipose tissue. The following creases should be noted:

1. The proximal skin crease of the wrist indicates the upper limit of the synovial sheaths of the flexor tendons.

2. The middle skin crease of the wrist indicates the wrist (radiocarpal) joint.

3. The distal skin crease of the wrist indicates the upper margin of the flexor retinaculum.

4. The radial longitudinal skin crease of the palm encircles the thenar eminence. (Palm readers refer to this line as the "life line.")

5. The proximal transverse line of the palm runs across the shafts of the metacarpal bones, indicating the

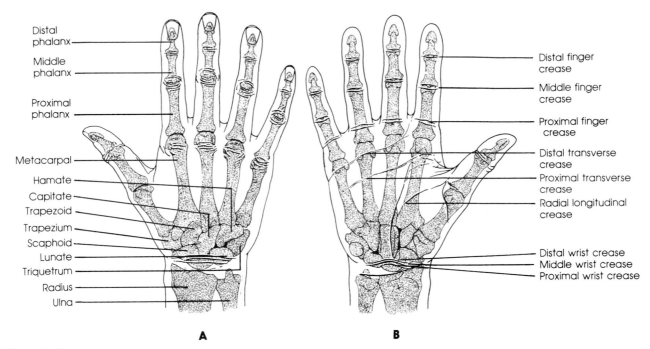

Distal phalanx
Middle phalanx
Proximal phalanx
Metacarpal
Hamate
Capitate
Trapezoid
Trapezium
Scaphoid
Lunate
Triquetrum
Radius
Ulna

Distal finger crease
Middle finger crease
Proximal finger crease
Distal transverse crease
Proximal transverse crease
Radial longitudinal crease
Distal wrist crease
Middle wrist crease
Proximal wrist crease

A　　　　**B**

Figure 7–67

Bony landmarks and skin creases of the hand and wrist. (A) Dorsal view. (B) Palmar view. (Adapted from Tubiana, R.: The Hand. Philadelphia, W.B. Saunders Co., 1981, p. 619.)

superficial palmar arterial arch. (Palm readers refer to this line as the "head line.")

6. The distal transverse line of the palm lies over the heads of the second to fourth metacarpals. (Palm readers refer to this line as the "love line.")

7. The proximal skin crease of the fingers is 2 cm (0.8 inch) distal to the metacarpophalangeal joints.

8. The middle skin crease of the fingers is made up of two lines and lies over the proximal interphalangeal joints.

9. The distal skin crease of the fingers lies over the distal interphalangeal joints.

10. On the flexor and extensor aspects, the skin creases over the proximal and distal interphalangeal joints lie proximal to the joint. On the extensor aspect, the metacarpophalangeal creases lie proximal to the joint; on the flexor aspect, they lie distal to the joint.

Arches. In addition, the examiner should ensure the viability of the arches of the hand (see Fig. 7–11). The **carpal transverse arch** is the result of the shape of the carpal bones, which in part forms the carpal tunnel. The flexor retinaculum forms the roof for the tunnel. The **metacarpal transverse arch** is formed by the metacarpal bones, and its shape can have great variability because of the mobility of these bones. This arch is most evident when the palm is cupped. The **longitudinal arch** is made of the carpal bones, metacarpal bones, and phalanges. The keystone of this arch is the metacarpophalangeal joints, which provide stability and support for the arch. Weakness or atrophy of the intrinsic muscles of the hand

leads to a loss of these arches. The deformity is most obvious with paralysis of the median and ulnar nerve, which results in an "ape hand" deformity.

Diagnostic Imaging

Plain Film Radiography

A routine wrist series of plane x-rays involves the following views; anteroposterior (AP), lateral, and scaphoid. Other possible views include the carpal tunnel view, clenched-fist (AP) view, and radial and ulnar deviation views. Motion views are sometimes taken, especially if instability is suspected.

Anteroposterior View. The examiner should note the shape and position of the bones (Fig. 7–68), watching for any evidence of fractures or displacement, decrease in the joint spaces, or change in bone density, which may be caused by avascular necrosis. The arcs of the wrist (Fig. 7–69) show the normal relation of the carpal bones in the AP view. If avascular necrosis is present, there is rarefaction and increased density of the bone and possibly sclerosis of the bone. Avascular necrosis is often seen in the scaphoid bone (Figs. 7–70 and 7–71A) after a fracture or in the lunate in Kienböck's disease (Fig. 7–71B).[24] In some cases, the triangular fibrocartilage or disc may be visualized (Fig. 7–72). The AP view may also be used to show dislocations of the lunate (Fig. 7–73A), the distal ulna (Fig. 7–73B), the lunatotriquetral relation (Fig. 7–73C), and ulnar variance (length of ulna in relation to radius).[55]

Text continued on page 322

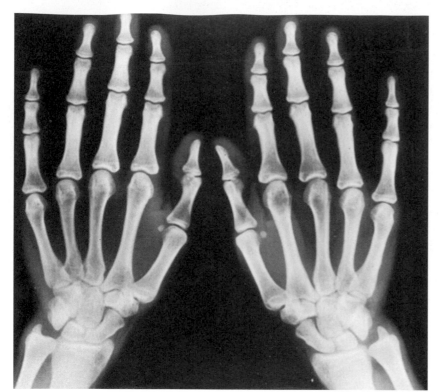

Figure 7–68

Radiograph showing the bones of both hands. The thumb metacarpal is the shortest, and the index metacarpal is by far the longest. The first and second phalanges of the middle and ring fingers are longer than those of the index finger. Note the interlocking design of the carpometacarpal articulations and the saddle shape in opposing planes of the articular surfaces of the trapezium and the base of the first metacarpal. (From Tubiana, R.: The Hand. Philadelphia, W.B. Saunders Co., 1981, p. 21.)

Figure 7–69

Wrist arcs. Three arcuate lines can normally be constructed along the carpal articular surfaces: (1) along the proximal margins of the scaphoid, lunate, and triquetrum; (2) along the distal aspects of these bones; and (3) along the proximal margins of the capitate and hamate. (From Weissman, B.N.W., and C.B. Sledge: Orthopedic Radiology. Philadelphia, W.B. Saunders Co., 1986, p. 117.)

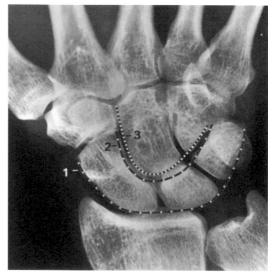

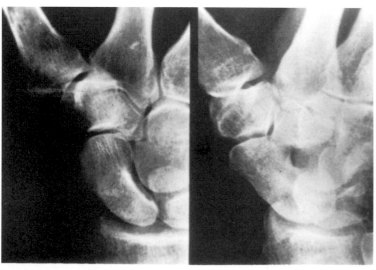

A   B

Figure 7–70

Radiographs of the normal scaphoid. (A) Posteroanterior view. (B) Lateral view. (From Tubiana, R.: The Hand. Philadelphia, W.B. Saunders Co., 1981, p. 659.)

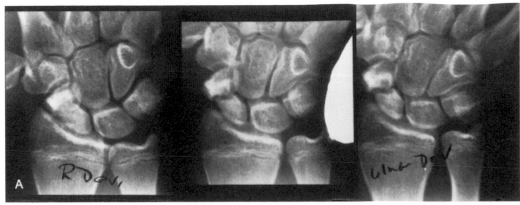

RADIAL
DEVIATION

NEUTRAL

ULNAR
DEVIATION

Figure 7–71

Avascular necrosis of the carpal bones. (A) Scaphoid fracture shown in three positions. (From Cooney, W.P., J.H. Dobyns, and R.L. Linscheid: Fractures of the scaphoid: A rational approach to management. Clin. Orthop. 149:92, 1980.) (B) Lunate fracture and sclerosis in Kienböck's disease. (From Beckenbaugh, R.D., T.C. Shives, J.H. Dobyns, and R.L. Linscheid: Kienböck's disease, the natural history of Kienböck's disease and consideration of lunate fractures. Clin. Orthop. 149:99, 1980.)

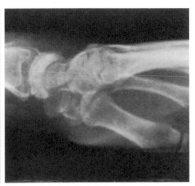

ANTEROPOSTERIOR
VIEW

LATERAL
VIEW

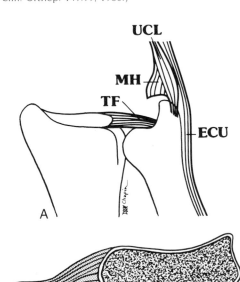

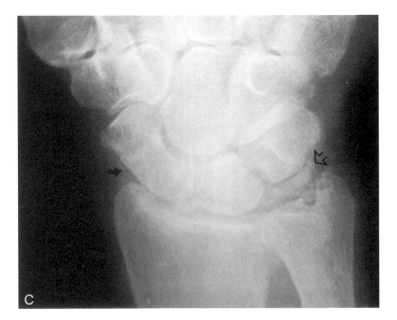

Figure 7–72

Triangular fibrocartilage complex. (A) This complex includes the triangular fibrocartilage (articular disc, TF), the meniscus homolog (MH), the ulnar collateral ligament (UCL), and the dorsal and volar radioulnar ligaments (not shown). The extensor carpi ulnaris tendon (ECU) is shown. (B) The triangular fibrocartilage (*dotted area*) attaches to the ulnar border of the radius and the distal ulna. The triangular shape is evident on this transverse section through the radius and ulnar styloid. The volar aspect of the wrist is at the top. (C) Chondrocalcinosis. There is heavy calcification of the articular cartilage (*curved arrow*) and the area of the triangular fibrocartilage complex (*open arrow*). (From Weissman, B.N.W., and C.B. Sledge: Orthopedic Radiology. Philadelphia, W.B. Saunders Co., 1986, p. 115.)

The AP view of the wrist and hand is also used to determine the skeletal age of a patient.[18] The left hand and wrist are used for study because they are thought to be less influenced by environmental factors. The method used in this technique is based on the fact that after an **ossification center** appears (Fig. 7–74), it changes its shape and size in a systematic manner as the ossification gradually spreads throughout the cartilaginous parts of the skeleton. The wrist and hand are studied because several bones are available for overall comparison, in-

cluding the carpal bones, the metacarpal growth plates (seen at distal end of bone), and the phalangeal growth plates (seen at proximal end of bone). The patient's hand is compared with standard plates[28] until one plate is found that best approximates that of the patient. There is one standard for males and another for females. In two thirds of the population, skeletal age is no more than 1 year above or below chronologic age. Acceleration or retardation of 3 years of more is considered abnormal. At birth, none of the carpal bones is visible (see Fig.

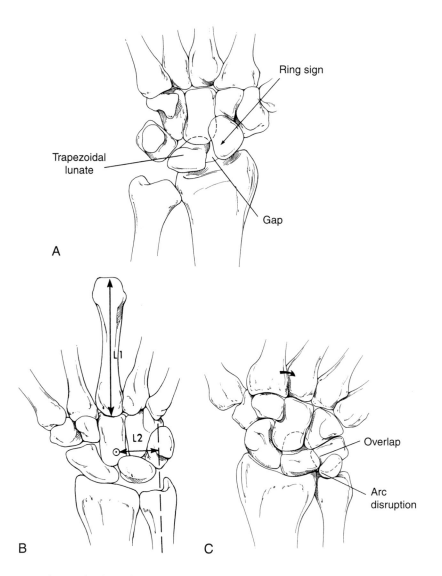

Figure 7–73

(A) Scapholunate dissociation. The scaphoid is palmar flexed, producing a cortical ring sign. A gap is present between the scaphoid and the lunate. The lunate appears trapezoidal. (B) Ulnar translocation can be identified radiographically from the ratio of the distance between the center of the capitate and a line along the longitudinal axis of the ulna (L2) divided by the length of the third metacarpal (L1). In normal wrists this ratio is 0.30 ± 0.03; it is decreased in wrists with ulnar translocation. (C) Lunatotriquetral instability. Shortened scaphoid and cortical ring sign are present without scapholunate widening. Lunate appears triangular. Lunatotriquetral widening is not present. (© 1993 American Academy of Orthopaedic Surgeons. Reprinted from the *Journal of the American Academy of Orthopaedic Surgeons: A Comprehensive Review*, Volume 1 (1), pp. 14–15 with permission.)

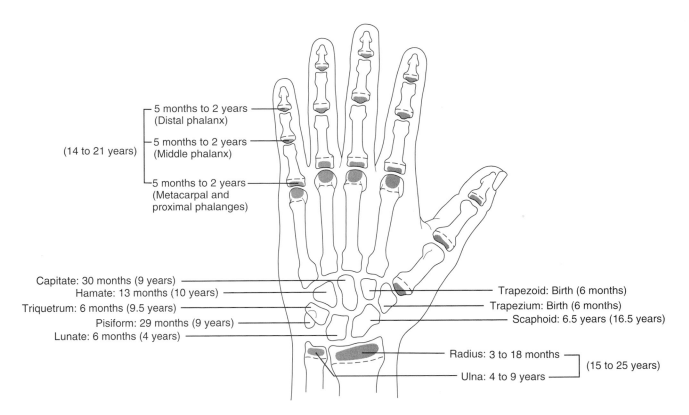

—5 months to 2 years—
(Distal phalanx)

—5 months to 2 years—
(Middle phalanx)

(14 to 21 years)

—5 months to 2 years—
(Metacarpal and
proximal phalanges)

Capitate: 30 months (9 years) ——————
Hamate: 13 months (10 years) ——————
Triquetrum: 6 months (9.5 years) ——————
Pisiform: 29 months (9 years) ——————
Lunate: 6 months (4 years) ——————

—————— Trapezoid: Birth (6 months)
—————— Trapezium: Birth (6 months)
—————— Scaphoid: 6.5 years (16.5 years)

—————— Radius: 3 to 18 months ——
                                                    (15 to 25 years)
—————— Ulna: 4 to 9 years ——

A

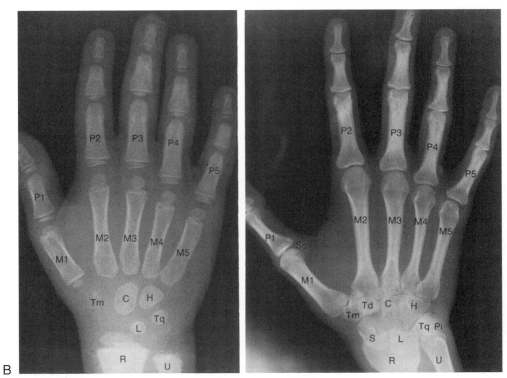

B

Figure 7–74

Ossification centers of the hand. (A) Dates of appearance of ossification centers are shown, with dates of fusion in parentheses. Note the different proximal and distal locations of growth plates. (Redrawn from Tubiana, R.: The Hand. Philadelphia: W.B. Saunders Co., 1981, p. 11.) (B) Radiographs of the hand and wrist of a 4- to 5-year-old boy or 3- to 4-year-old girl (*left*) and of an adult (*right*). C = capitate; H = hamate; L = lunate; M = metacarpal; P = phalanx; Pi = pisiform; R = radius; S = scaphoid; Td = trapezoid; Tm = trapezium; Tq = triquetrum; U = ulna. (B, from Liebgott, B.: The Anatomical Basis of Dentistry. St. Louis, C.V. Mosby Co., 1986.)

1–9). This method may be used up to age 20, when the bones of the hand and wrist have fused.

Lateral View. The examiner should note the shape and position of bones for any evidence of fracture and/or displacement (Fig. 7–75A). The lateral view is also useful in detecting swelling around the carpal bones and for measuring the relation of the scaphoid and lunate to the radius and metacarpals (Fig. 7–76).[55]

Scaphoid View. This view isolates the scaphoid to show a possible fracture (see Fig. 7–70).

Carpal Tunnel (Axial) View. This view is used to show the margins of the carpal tunnel and is useful for determining fractures of the hook of hamate and trapezium (Fig. 7–77).

Clenched-Fist (AP) View. This view is sometimes useful to show increased gapping between the carpal bones, indicating instability.[56]

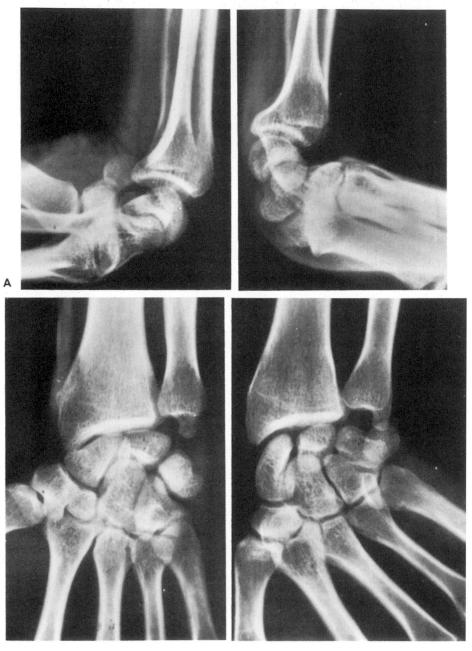

Figure 7–75

(A) Lateral radiographs showing wrist flexion (*left*) and extension (*right*). (B) Posteroanterior views of wrist in radial (*left*) and ulnar (*right*) deviation. Note the change in the form of the lunate, indicating a slipping toward the front in the radial slant and toward the rear in the ulnar slant. (From Tubiana, R.: The Hand. Philadelphia, W.B. Saunders Co., 1981, p. 655.)

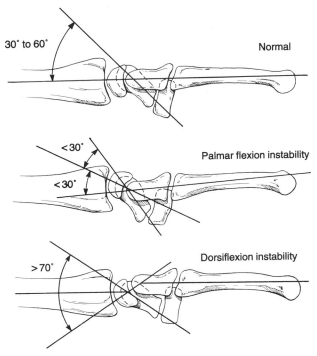

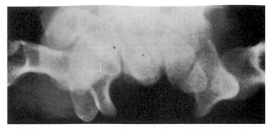

Figure 7–77

Carpal tunnel or axial radiographic view. (From Tubiana, R.: The Hand. Philadelphia, W.B. Saunders Co., 1981, p. 662.)

Figure 7–76

Scapholunate angle measurement in normal wrist and in carpal instability. (© 1993 American Academy of Orthopaedic Surgeons. Reprinted from the *Journal of the American Academy of Orthopaedic Surgeons: A Comprehensive Review*, Volume 1 (1), p. 14 with permission.)

Arthrography

If the history and clinical assessment suggest a ligament or fibrocartilage problem of the wrist, arthrography can help to confirm the diagnosis (Fig. 7–78). Arthrograms, especially of the wrist, can demonstrate compartment communication, tendon sheaths, synovial irregularity, loose bodies, and cartilage abnormalities.

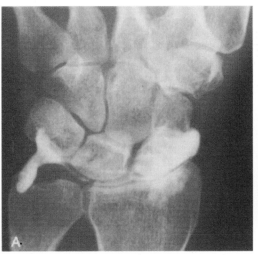

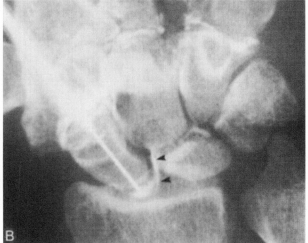

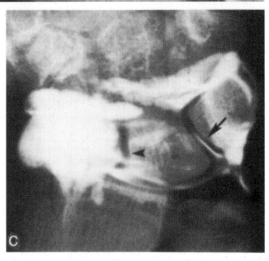

Figure 7–78

(A) Posteroanterior view of the wrist after a normal radiocarpal joint arthrogram. Contrast remains confined to the radiocarpal space. (B) After a radiocarpal joint space injection, contrast tracks (*arrowheads*) through a disrupted scapholunate ligament to fill the midcarpal and carpometacarpal joint spaces. (C) After a radiocarpal joint space arthrogram, the scapholunate ligament is intact because contrast has not yet filled the scapholunate space (*arrowhead*); however, contrast tracks through the lunatotriquetral joint space (*arrow*) as a result of lunatotriquetral ligament disruption. (From Lightman, D.M.: The Wrist and Its Disorders. Philadelphia, W.B. Saunders Co., 1988, p. 89.)

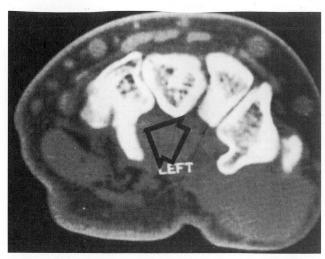

Figure 7–79
A fracture of the left hamate hook (*arrow*) as shown by a computed tomographic (CT) scan. In this instance, fracture was suspected on the carpal tunnel view but was not demonstrated as well as it was by CT scan. (From Zemel, N.P., and H.H. Stark: Fractures and dislocations of the carpal bones. Clin. Sports Med. 5:720, 1986.)

Computed Tomography

Computed tomography can be used to visualize bones and soft tissue; by making computer-assisted "slices," it allows tissues to be better visualized (Fig. 7–79).

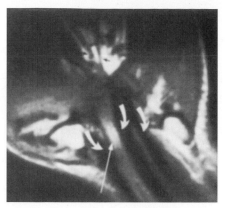

Figure 7–80
Magnetic resonance image (SETR = 1,500 msec; TE = 60 msec). Coronal section through palmar aspect of carpal tunnel clearly depicts median nerve (*long arrow*) coursing between the flexor tendons (*curved arrows*). Median nerve branches (*small arrows*) can also be delinated. (From Weiss, K.L., J. Beltran, and J.M. Lubbers: High-field MR surface-coil imaging of the hand and wrist: Pathologic correlations and clinical relevance. Radiology 160:150, 1986.)

Magnetic Resonance Imaging

Magnetic resonance imaging is a noninvasive technique that is useful for visualizing the soft tissues of the wrist and hand and provides the best means of delineating the soft tissues and bone. For example, it can show swelling of the median nerve in carpal tunnel syndrome, tears in the triangular fibrocartilage, and thickening of tendon sheaths (Fig. 7–80).

Précis of the Forearm, Wrist, and Hand Assessment*

History (sitting)
Observation (sitting)
Examination (sitting)
    Active movements
        Pronation of the forearm
        Supination of the forearm
        Wrist flexion
        Wrist extension
        Radial deviation of wrist
        Ulnar deviation of wrist
        Finger flexion (at MCP, PIP, and DIP joints)
        Flexion extension (at MCP, PIP, and DIP joints)
        Finger abduction
        Finger adduction
        Thumb flexion
        Thumb extension
        Thumb abduction
        Thumb adduction
        Opposition of the thumb and little finger
    Passive movements (as in active movements)
    Resisted isometric movements (as in active movements, in the
        neutral position)
    Functional testing
        Functional grip tests
        Pinch tests
        Coordination tests
    Special tests (sitting)

Reflexes and cutaneous distribution (sitting)
    Reflexes
    Sensory scan
    Nerve injuries
        Median nerve
        Ulnar nerve
        Radial nerve
Joint play movements (sitting)
    Long-axis extension at the wrist and fingers (MCP,
        PIP, and DIP joints)
    Anteroposterior glide at the wrist and fingers (MCP,
        PIP, and DIP joints)
    Side glide at the wrist and fingers (MCP, PIP, and
        DIP joints)
    Side tilt at the wrist
    Anteroposterior glide at the intermetacarpal joints
    Rotation at the MCP, PIP, and DIP joints
    Individual carpal bone mobility
Palpation (sitting)
Diagnostic imaging

---

* DIP = distal interphalangeal; MCP = metacarpophalangeal; PIP = proximal interphalangeal.

After any examination, the patient should be warned of the possibility of exacerbation of symptoms as a result of the assessment.

Case Studies

When doing these case studies, the examiner should list the appropriate questions to be asked and why they are being asked, what to look for and why, and what things should be tested and why. Depending on the answers of the patient (and the examiner should consider different responses), several possible causes of the patient's problem may become evident (examples are given in parentheses). A differential diagnosis chart should be made up. The examiner can then decide how different diagnoses may affect the treatment plan. For example, a 26-year-old man comes to you complaining of pain and clicking in his wrist. He is a carpenter, and it especially bothers him when he uses a screwdriver. See Table 7–15 for an example of a differential diagnosis chart for this patient.

1. A 31-year-old pregnant woman complains of pain in the right hand of 3 months' duration. The pain awakens her at night and is relieved only by vigorous rubbing of her hand and motion of the fingers and wrist. There is some tingling in the index and middle fingers. Describe your assessment for this patient (carpal tunnel syndrome versus lunate subluxation).

2. An 18-year-old man comes to you after suffering a right scaphoid fracture. He has been in a cast for 12 weeks, and clinical union has been achieved. Describe your assessment for this patient.

3. A 16-year-old girl comes to you complaining of thumb pain. She was skiing during the weekend and fell, landing on her ski pole. She hurt her thumb when she fell.

Describe your assessment for this patient (ulnar collateral ligament sprain versus Bennett's fracture).

4. A 48-year-old man comes to you complaining of a painful hand. He happened to hit it against a metal door jam as he was going outside. During the next few days, the hand became swollen and painful, and he has become very protective of it. Describe your assessment of this patient (Sudeck's atrophy versus hand aneurysm).

5. A 52-year-old woman who has rheumatoid arthritis comes to you because her hands hurt and she has difficulty doing things functionally. Describe your assessment of this patient.

6. A 14-year-old boy comes to you complaining of wrist pain with swelling on the dorsum of the hand. He says he tripped and fell on the outstretched hand. He states the wrist hurt, the pain decreased, and then the swelling came on over 2 or 3 days. Describe your assessment of this patient (scaphoid fracture versus ganglion).

7. A 28-year-old man was in an industrial accident and lacerated the flexor tendons in the palm of his hand. Describe your assessment of this patient.

8. A 37-year-old woman comes to you complaining of pain and grating on the radial side of the wrist. Describe your assessment of this patient (cartilaginous disc versus scaphoid fracture).

9. A 72-year-old woman comes to you with a left Colles fracture. Describe your assessment of this patient.

Table 7–15
Differential Diagnosis of Wrist Cartilaginous Disc and Degenerative Osteoarthritis

	Wrist Cartilaginous Disc	Degenerative Osteoarthritis
Mechanism of injury	Compression and pronation	Vibration, repetitive compression
Age affected	25 years and older	35 years and older
Active movement	Pain on compression and pronation Limited wrist extension more than flexion	Limited wrist flexion and extension
Passive movement	Pain on extension overpressure Pain on compression and pronation Tissue stretch end feel	Capsular pattern of wrist End feel is soft early, hard later
Resisted isometric movement	Pain on pronation	Possibly weak on wrist movements
Special tests	None	None
Reflexes and sensory distribution	Normal	Normal
Joint play	Pain on anteroposterior glide of radiocarpal joint	Pain on anteroposterior glide of radiocarpal and midcarpal joints
Palpation	Pain over lunate	Pain over affected carpal bones

References

Cited References

1. Tubiana, R., J.M. Thomiene, and E. Mackin: Examination of the Hand and Wrist. St. Louis, C.V. Mosby Co., 1996.
2. Palmer, A.D., and F.W. Werner: The triangular fibrocartilage complex of the wrist: Anatomy and function. J. Hand Surg. Am. 6:153–162, 1981.
3. Palmer, A.R., and F.W. Werner: Biomechanics of the distal radioulnar joint. Clin. Orthop. 187:26–35, 1984.
4. Sarrafian, S.K., J.L. Melamed, and G.M. Goshgarian: Study of wrist motion in flexion and extension. Clin. Orthop. 126:153–159, 1977.
5. Kapandji, I.A.: The Physiology of Joints, vol.1: Upper Limb. New York, Churchill Livingstone, 1970.
6. Rettig, A.C.: Wrist injuries: Avoid diagnostic pitfalls. Phys. Sportsmed. 22:33–39, 1994.
7. Burton, R.I., and R.G. Eaton: Common hand injuries in the athlete. Orthop. Clin. North Am. 4:309–338, 1975.

8. Wadsworth, C.T.: Wrist and hand examination and interpretation. J. Orthop. Sports Phys. Ther. 5:108–120, 1983.
9. Blair, S.J., E. McCormick, J. Bear-Lehman, E.E. Fess, and E. Rader: Evaluation of impairment of the upper extremity. Clin. Orthop. 221:42–58, 1987.
10. Vanswearingen, J.M.: Measuring wrist muscle strength. J. Orthop. Sports Phys. Ther. 4:217–228, 1983.
11. Hume, M.C., H. Gellman, H. McKellop, and R.H. Brumfield: Functional range of motion of the joints of the hand. J. Hand Surg. [Am.] 15:240–243, 1990.
12. Brumfield, R.H., and J.A. Champoux: A biomechanical study of normal functional wrist motion. Clin. Orthop. 187:23–25, 1984.
13. Lamereaux, L., and M.M. Hoffer: The effect of wrist deviation on grip and pinch strength. Clin. Orthop. 314:152–155, 1995.
14. Tubiana, R.: The Hand. Philadelphia, W.B. Saunders Co., 1981.
15. Reid, D.C.: Functional Anatomy and Joint Mobilization. Edmonton, University of Alberta Press, 1970.
16. Bechtal, C.D.: Grip test: The use of a dynamometer with adjustable handle spacing. J. Bone Joint Surg. Am. 36:820–832, 1954.
17. Mathiowetz, V., K. Weber, G. Volland, and N. Kashman: Reliability and validity of grip and pinch strength evaluations. J. Hand Surg. [Am.] 9:222–226, 1984.
18. Hansman, C.F., and M.M. Mresh: Appearance and fusion of ossification centers in the human skeleton. Am. J. Roentgenol. 88:476–482, 1962.
19. Aulicino, P.L., and T.E. DuPuy: Clinical examination of the hand. In Hunter, J., L.H. Schneider, E.J. Mackin, and A.D. Callahan (eds.): Rehabilitation of the Hand: Surgery and Therapy. St. Louis, C.V. Mosby Co., 1990.
20. Levine, D.W., B.P. Simmons, M.J. Koris, et al.: A self-administered questionnaire for the assessment of severity of symptoms and functional status in carpal tunnel syndrome. J. Bone Joint Surg. Am. 75:1585–1592, 1993.
21. McPhee, S.D.: Functional hand evaluations: A review. Am. J. Occup. Ther. 41:158–163, 1987.
22. Fess, E.E.: Documentation: Essential elements of an upper extremity assessment battery. In Hunter, J., L.H. Schneider, E.J. Mackin, and A.D. Callahan (eds.): Rehabilitation of the Hand: Surgery and Therapy. St. Louis, C.V. Mosby Co., 1990.
23. Baxter-Petralia, P.L., S.M. Blackmore, and P.M. McEntee: Physical capacity evaluation. In Hunter, J., L.H. Schneider, E.J. Mackin, and A.D. Callahan (eds.): Rehabilitation of the Hand: Surgery and Therapy. St. Louis, C.V. Mosby Co., 1990.
24. Beckenbaugh, R.D., T.C. Shives, J.H. Dobyns, and R.L. Linschied: Kienböck's disease: The natural history of Kienböck's disease and consideration of lunate fractures. Clin. Orthop. 149:98–106, 1980.
25. Jebson, R.H., N. Taylor, R.B. Trieschmann, M.J. Trotter, and L.A. Howard: An objective and standardized test of hand function. Arch. Phys. Med. Rehabil. 50:311–319, 1969.
26. Callahan, A.D.: Sensibility testing. In Hunter, J., L.H. Schneider, E.J. Mackin, and A.D. Callahan (eds.): Rehabilitation of the Hand: Surgery and Therapy. St. Louis, C.V. Mosby Co., 1990.
27. Heyman, P., R.H. Gelberman, K. Duncan, and J.A. Hipp: Injuries of the ulnar collateral ligament of the thumb metacarpophalangeal joint. Clin. Orthop. 292:165–171, 1993.
28. Post, M.: Physical Examination of the Musculoskeletal System. Chicago, Year Book Medical Pub., 1987.
29. Taliesnik, J.: Soft tissue injuries of the wrist. In Strickland, J.W., and A.C. Rettig (eds.): Hand Injuries in Athletes. Philadelphia, W.B. Saunders Co., 1992.
30. Booher, J.M., and G.A. Thibodeau: Athletic Injury Assessment. St. Louis, C.V. Mosby Co., 1989.
31. Taleisnik, J.: Carpal instability. J. Bone Joint Surg. Am. 70:1262–1268, 1988.
32. Watson, H.K., D. Ashmead, and M.V. Makhlouf: Examination of the scaphoid. J. Hand Surg. Am. 13:657–660, 1988.
33. Chidgey, L.K.: Chronic wrist pain. Orthop. Clin. North Am. 23:49–64, 1992.
34. Finkelstein, H.: Stenosing tendovaginitis at the radial styloid process. J. Bone Joint Surg. 12:509, 1930.
35. Elson, R.A.: Rupture of the central slip of the extensor hood of the finger: A test for early diagnosis. J. Bone Joint Surg. Br. 68:229–231, 1986.
36. Boyes, J.: Bunnell's Surgery of the Hand. Philadelphia, J.B. Lippincott Co., 1970.
37. Hoppenfeld, S.: Physical Examination of the Spine and Extremities. New York, Appleton-Century-Crofts, 1976.
38. Linburg, R.M., and B.E. Comstock: Anomalous tendon slips from the flexor pollicis longus to the flexor digitorum profundus. J. Hand Surg. Am. 4:79–83, 1979.
39. American Society for Surgery of the Hand: The Hand: Examination and Diagnosis. Aurora, Colorado, American Society for Surgery of the Hand, 1978.
40. Durkan, J.A.: A new diagnostic test for carpal tunnel syndrome. J. Bone Joint Surg. Am. 73:535–538, 1991.
41. Moldaver, J.: Tinel's sign: Its characteristics and significance. J. Bone Joint Surg. Am. 60:412–414, 1978.
42. O'Riain, S.: Shrivel test: A new and simple test of nerve function in the hand. Br. Med. J. 3:615–616, 1973.
43. Stromberg, W.B., R.M. McFarlane, J.L. Bell, S.L. Koch, and M.L. Mason: Injury of the median and ulnar nerves: 150 Cases with an evaluation of Moberg's ninhydrin test. J. Bone Joint Surg. Am. 43:717–730, 1961.
44. Jones, L.A.: The assessment of hand function: A critical review of techniques. J. Hand Surg. Am. 14:221–228, 1989.
45. Omer, G.E.: Report of the Committee for Evaluation of the Clinical Result in Peripheral Nerve Injury. J. Hand Surg. Am. 8:754–759, 1983.
46. Dellon, A.L., and C.H. Kallman: Evaluation of functional sensation in the hand. J. Hand Surg. Am. 8:865–870, 1983.
47. Bell-Krotoski, J.A., D.E. Breger, and R.B Beach: Application of biomechanics for evaluation of the hand. In Hunter, J., L.H. Schneider, E. J. Mackin, and A.D. Callahan (eds.): Rehabilitation of the Hand: Surgery and Therapy. St. Louis, C.V. Mosby Co., 1990.
48. Halpern, J.S.: Upper extremity peripheral nerve assessment. J. Emerg. Nurs. 15:261–265, 1989.
49. Trombly, C.A., and A.D. Scott: Evaluation of motor control. In Trombly, C.A. (ed.): Occupational Therapy for Physical Dysfunction. Baltimore, Williams & Wilkins, 1989.
50. Szabo, R.M., and M. Madison: Carpal tunnel syndrome. Orthop. Clin. North Am. 23:103–109, 1992.
51. Murray-Leslie, C.F., and V. Wright: Carpal tunnel syndrome, humeral epicondylitis and the cervical spine: A study of clinical and dimensional relations. Br. Med. J. 1:1439–1442, 1976.
52. Hurst, L.C., D. Weissberg, and R.E. Carroll: The relationship of the double crush to carpal tunnel syndrome. J. Hand Surg. [Br.] 10:202–204, 1985.
53. Massey, E.W., T.L. Riley, and A.B. Pleet: Co-existant carpal tunnel syndrome and cervical radiculopathy (double crush syndrome). South Med. J. 74:957–959, 1981.
54. Kaltenborn, F.M.: Mobilization of the Extremity Joints. Oslo, Olaf Norlis Bokhandel, 1980.
55. Bednar, J.M., and A.L. Osterman: Carpal instability: Evaluation and treatment. J. Am. Acad. Orthop. Surg. 1:10–17, 1993.
56. Weiss, A-P., and E. Akelman: Diagnostic imaging and arthroscopy for chronic wrist pain. Orthop. Clin. North Am. 26:759–767, 1995.

General References

American Orthopaedic Association: Manual of Orthopaedic Surgery. Chicago, 1972.
Aulicino, P.L.: Neurovascular injuries in the hands of athletes. Hand Clin. 6:455–466, 1990.
Backhouse, K.M.: Functional anatomy of the hand. Physiotherapy 4:114–117, 1968.
Balogun, J.A., S.A. Adenlola, and A.A. Akinloye: Grip strength normative data for the Harpenden dynamometer. J. Orthop. Sports Phys. Ther. 14:155–160, 1991.
Beach, R.B.: Measurement of extremity volume by water displacement. Phys. Ther. 57:286–287, 1977.
Beetham, W.P., H.F. Polley, C.H. Slocumb, and W.F. Weaver: Physical Examination of the Joints. Philadelphia, W.B. Saunders Co., 1965.

Bell-Krotoski, J., and E. Tomancik: The repeatability of testing with Semmes-Weinstein monofilaments. J. Hand Surg. [Am.] 12:155–161, 1987.

Bora, F.W., and A.L. Osterman: Compression neuropathy. Clin. Orthop. 163:20–37, 1982.

Boscheinen-Morrin, J., V. Davey, and W.B. Conolly: The Hand: Fundamentals of Therapy. Oxford, Butterworth-Heinemann Ltd., 1992.

Brand, P.W.: Clinical Mechanisms of the Hand. St. Louis, C.V. Mosby Co., 1985.

Brown, D.E., and D.M. Lightman: Physical examination of the wrist. In Lichtman, D. (ed.): The Wrist and Its Disorders. Philadelphia, W.B. Saunders Co., 1988.

Cailliet, R.: Hand Pain and Impairment. Philadelphia, F.A. Davis Co., 1971.

Canadian Standardized Test of Fitness: Operations Manual. Ottawa, Fitness and Amateur Sport Canada, 1986.

Clarkson, H.M., and G.B. Gilewich: Musculoskeletal Assessment: Joint Range of Motion and Manual Muscle Strength. Baltimore, Williams & Wilkins, 1989.

Clawson, D.K., W.A. Souter, C.J. Carthum, and M.L. Hymen: Functional assessment of the rheumatoid hand. Clin. Orthop. 77:203–210, 1971.

Coleman, H.M.: Injuries of the articular disc at the wrist. J. Bone Joint Surg. Br. 42:522–529, 1960.

Cooney, W.P., J.H. Dobyns, and R.L. Linschied: Fractures of the scaphoid: A rational approach to management. Clin. Orthop. 149:90–97, 1980.

Cooney, W.P., M.J. Lucca, E.Y.S. Chao, and R.L. Linscheid: Kinesiology of the thumb trapeziometacarpal joint. J. Bone Joint Surg. Am. 63:1371–1381, 1981.

Cyriax, J.: Textbook of Orthopaedic Medicine, vol. 1: Diagnosis of Soft Tissue Lesions. London, Bailliere Tindall, 1982.

Dellon, A.L.: Clinical use of vibratory stimuli to evaluate peripheral nerve injury and compression neuropathy. Plast. Reconstr. Surg. 65:466–475, 1980.

Dellon, A.L.: The paper clip: Light hardware to evaluate sensibility in the hand. Contemp. Orthop. 1:39–42, 1979.

Dellon, A.L.: The moving two point discrimination test: Clinical evaluation of the quickly adapting fiber/receptor system. J. Hand Surg. Am. 3:474–481, 1978.

Destouet, J.M., L.A. Gilula, and W.R. Reinus: Roentgenographic diagnosis of wrist pain and instability. In Lichtman, D. (ed.): The Wrist and Its Disorders. Philadelphia, W.B. Saunders Co., 1988.

Ellem, D.: Assessment of the wrist, hand and finger complex. J. Manip. Physiol. Ther. 3:9–14, 1995.

Ericson, W.B.: Computerized evaluation of the hand. Semin. Orthop. 7:58–67, 1992.

Evans, R.C.: Illustrated Essentials in Orthopedic Physical Assessment. St. Louis, C.V. Mosby Co., 1994.

Forrester, D.M., and J.C. Brown: The Radiology of Joint Disease. Philadelphia, W.B. Saunders Co., 1987.

Garrick, J.G., and D.R. Webb: Sports Injuries: Diagnosis and Treatment. Philadelphia, W.B. Saunders Co., 1990.

Gelberman, R.H., R. Eaton, and J.R. Urbaniak: Peripheral nerve compression. J. Bone Joint Surg. Am. 75:1854–1878, 1993.

Gelberman, R.H., R.M. Szabo, R.V. Williamson, and M.P. Dimick: Sensibility testing in peripheral nerve compression syndromes. J. Bone Joint Surg. Am. 65:632–637, 1983.

Gilula, L.A., J.M. Destouet, P.M. Wecks, L.V. Young, and R.C. Wray: Roentgenographic diagnosis of the painful wrist. Clin. Orthop. 187:52–64, 1984.

Gilula, L.A., and P.M. Weeks: Post-traumatic ligamentous instabilities of the wrist. Diagn. Radiol. 129:641, 1978.

Goodman, C.C., and T.E. Snyder: Differential Diagnosis in Physical Therapy. Philadelphia, W.B. Saunders Co., 1995.

Greulich, W.W., and S.U. Pyle: Radiographic Atlas of Skeletal Development of the Wrist and Hand. Stanford, California, Stanford University Press, 1959.

Hackel, M.E., G.A. Wolfe, S.M. Bang, and J.S. Canfield: Changes in hand function in the aging adult as determined by the Jebsen test of hand function. Phys. Ther. 72:373–377, 1992.

Henderson, W.R.: Clinical assessment of peripheral nerve injuries: Tinel's test. Lancet 2:801–805, 1948.

Hollinshead, W.H., and D.B. Jenkins: Functional Anatomy of the Limbs and Back. Philadelphia, W.B. Saunders Co., 1981.

Howard, F.M.: Controversies in the nerve entrapment syndrome in the forearm and wrist. Orthop. Clin. North Am. 17:375–381, 1986.

Jacobs, J.L.: Hand and wrist. In Richardson, J.K., and Z.A. Iglarsh (eds.): Clinical Orthopedic Physical Therapy. Philadelphia, W.B. Saunders Co., 1994.

Jacobs, P.: Atlas of Hand Radiographs. Baltimore, University Park Press, 1973.

Jacobsen, C., and L. Sperling: Classification of the hand grip: A preliminary study. J. Occup. Med. 18:395–398, 1976.

Johnson, R.P.: The acutely injured wrist and its residuals. Clin. Orthop. 149:33–44, 1980.

Judge, R.D., G.D. Zuidema, and F.T. Fitzgerald: Clincial Diagnosis: A Physiological Approach. Boston, Little, Brown & Co., 1982.

Kauer, J.M.G.: Functional anatomy of the wrist. Clin. Orthop. 149:9–20, 1980.

Kendall, E.P., and B.K. McCreary: Muscles: Testing and Function. Baltimore, Williams & Wilkins, 1983.

Koris, K., R.H. Gelberman, K. Duncan, M. Boublick, and B. Smith: Carpal tunnel syndrome: Evaluation of a quantitative provocational diagnostic test. Clin. Orthop. 251:157–161, 1990.

Kricum, M.E.: Wrist arthrography. Clin. Orthop. 187:65–71, 1984.

La Stayo, P.C., and D.L Wheeler: Reliability of passive wrist flexion and extension goniometric measurements: A multicentre study. Phys. Ther. 74:162–176, 1994.

Levin, S., G. Pearsall, and R.J. Ruderman: Von Frey's method of measuring pressure sensibility in the hand: An emergency analysis of the Weinstein-Semmes pressure aesthesiometer. J. Hand Surg. Am. 3:211–216, 1978.

Liebgott, B.: The Anatomical Basis of Dentistry. Philadelphia, W.B. Saunders Co., 1982.

Linn, M.R., F.A. Mann, and L.A. Gilula: Imaging the symptomatic wrist. Orthop. Clin. North Am. 21:515–543, 1990.

Long, C., P.W. Conrad, E.A. Hall, and S.L. Furler: Intrinsic-extrinsic muscle control of the hand in power grip and precision handling: An electromyographic study. J. Bone Joint Surg. Am. 52:853–867, 1970.

Macey, A., and C. Kelly: The hand. In Pynsent, P., J. Fairbank, and A. Carr (eds.): Outcome Measures in Orthopedics. Oxford, Butterworth-Heinemann Ltd., 1994.

Maitland, G.D.: The Peripheral Joints: Examination and Recording Guide. Adelaide, Australia, Virgo Press, 1973.

Mayer, V.: Evaluation and rehabilitation of athletic injuries of the hand and wrist: Hand and wrist injuries and treatment. Sports Injury Management 2:1–28, 1989.

Mayer, V., and J.H. Gieck: Rehabilitation of hand injuries in athletics. Clin. Sports Med. 5:783–794, 1986.

McCue, F.C., and J.F. Bruce: The wrist. In De Lee, J.C., and D. Drez (eds.): Orthopedic Sports Medicine: Principles and Practice. Philadelphia, W.B. Saunders Co., 1994.

McMurtry, R.Y.: The wrist. In Little, H. (ed.): The Rheumatological Physical Examination. Orlando, Florida, Grune & Stratton Inc., 1986.

McMurtry, R.Y., Y. Youm, A.E. Flatt, and T.E. Gillespie: Kinematics of the wrist, II: Clinical applications. J. Bone Joint Surg. Am. 60:955–961, 1978.

McRae, R.: Clinical Orthopaedic Examination. New York, Churchill Livingstone, 1976.

Mennell, J.M.: Joint Pain. Boston, Little, Brown & Co., 1964.

Mennell, J.M.: Manipulation of the joints of the wrist. Physiotherapy 57:246–254, 1971.

Middleton, W.D., J.B. Kneeland, G.M. Kellman, et al.: MRI imaging of the carpal tunnel: Normal anatomy and preliminary findings in the carpal tunnel syndrome. Am. J. Radiol. 148:307–316, 1987.

Mikic, Z.D.: Detailed anatomy of the articular disc of the distal radioulnar joint. Clin. Orthop. 245:123–132, 1989.

Mirabello, S.C., P.E. Loeb, and J.R. Andrews: The wrist: Field evaluation and treatment. Clin. Sports Med. 11:1–25, 1996.

Moberg, E.: Criticism and study of methods for examining sensibility in the hand. Neurology 12:8–19, 1962.

Mooney, J.F., D.B. Siegel, and L.A. Koman: Ligamentous injuries of the wrist in athletes. Clin. Sports Med. 11:129–139, 1992.

Moran, C.A., and A.D. Callahan: Sensibility measurement and management. In Moran, C. (ed.): Hand Rehabilitation. Clinics in Physical Therapy. Edinburgh, Churchill Livingstone, 1986.

Napier, J.R.: The prehensile movements of the human hand. J. Bone Joint Surg. Br. 38:902–913, 1956.

Newland, C.C.: Gamekeeper's thumb. Orthop. Clin. North Am. 23:41–48, 1992.

Nicholas, J.A., and E.B. Hershman (eds.): Upper Extremity in Sports Medicine. St. Louis, C.V. Mosby Co., 1989.

Nicholas, J.S.: The swollen hand. Physiotherapy 63:285–286, 1977.

Nuber, G.W., W.J. McCarthy, J.S. Yao, M.F. Schafer, and J.R. Suker: Arterial abnormalities of the hand in athletes. Am. J. Sports Med. 18:520–523, 1990.

O'Donoghue, D.H.: Treatment of Injuries to Athletes, 4th ed. Philadelphia, W.B. Saunders Co., 1984.

Omer, G.E.: Physical diagnosis of peripheral nerve injuries. Orthop. Clin. North Am. 12:207–228, 1981.

Omer, G.E.: Sensation and sensibility in the upper extremity. Clin. Orthop. 104:30–36, 1974.

Pagonis, J.F.: Imaging for the wrist and hand. Orthop. Phys. Ther. Clin. North Am. 4:95–121, 1995.

Palmer, A.K., and F.W. Werner: Biomechanics of the distal radioulnar joint. Clin. Orthop. 187:26–35, 1984.

Palmer, M.L., and M. Epler: Clinical Assessment Procedures in Physical Therapy. Philadelphia, J.B. Lippincott Co., 1990.

Philps, P.E., and E. Walker: Comparison of the finger wrinkling test results to established sensory tests in peripheral nerve injury. Am. J. Occup. Ther. 31:565–572, 1977.

Porter, R.W.: New test for finger-tip sensation. Br. Med. J. 2:927–928, 1966.

Reagan, D.S., R.L. Linscheid, J.H. Dobyns: Lunotriquetral sprains. J. Hand Surg. [Am.] 9:502–514, 1984.

Recht, M.P., D.L. Burk, and M.K. Dalinka: Radiology of wrist and hand injuries in athletes. Clin. Sports Med. 6:811–828, 1987.

Reid, D.C.: Sports Injury Assessment and Rehabilitation. New York, Churchill Livingstone, 1992.

Renfrew, S.: Fingertip sensation: A routine neurological test. Lancet 1:396–397, 1969.

Ruby, L.K.: Carpal instability. J. Bone Joint Surg. Am. 77:476–487, 1995.

Samman, P.D.: The Nails in Disease. London, Wm. Heinemann Medical Books Ltd., 1965.

Schuett, A.M., J. Gieck, and F.C. McCue: Evaluation and treatment of injuries to the thumb and fingers. Orthop. Phys. Ther. Clin. North Am. 3:367–383, 1994.

Schuind, F.G., R.L. Linscheid, K.N. An, and E.Y. Chio: A normal data base of posteroanterior roentgenographic measurements of the wrist. J. Bone Joint Surg. Am. 74:1418–1429, 1992.

Smith, H.B.: Smith hand function evaluation. Am. J. Occup. Ther. 27:244–251, 1973.

Smith, R.J.: Balance and kinetics of the fingers under normal and pathological conditions. Clin. Orthop. 104:92–111, 1974.

Sperling, L., and C. Jacobson-Sollerman: The grip pattern of the healthy hand during eating. Scand. J. Rehab. Med. 9:115–121, 1977.

Stanley, J.K., and I.A. Trail: Carpal instability. J. Bone Joint Surg. Br. 76:691–700, 1994.

Sunderland, S.: The nerve lesion in the carpal tunnel syndrome. J. Neurol. Neurosurg. Psych. 39:615–626, 1976.

Swanson, A.B., G. de Groof Swanson, and C. Goren-Hagert: Evaluation of impairment of hand function. In Hunter, J., L.H. Schneider, E.J. Mackin, and A.D. Callahan (eds.): Rehabilitation of the Hand: Surgery and Therapy. St. Louis, C.V. Mosby Co., 1990.

Swanson, A.B.: Pathomechanics of deformities in hand and wrist. In Hunter, J., L.H. Schneider, E.J. Mackin, and A.D. Callahan (eds.): Rehabilitation of the Hand: Surgery and Therapy. St. Louis, C.V. Mosby Co., 1990.

Szabo, R.M., and M. Madison: Carpal tunnel syndrome as a work-related disorder. In Gordon, S.L., S.J. Blair, and L.J. Fine: Repetitive Motion Disorders of the Upper Extremity. Rosemont, Illinois, American Academy of Orthopaedic Surgeons, 1995.

Szabo, R.M., and D.R. Steinberg: Nerve entrapment syndromes at the wrist. J. Am. Acad. Orthop. Surg. 2:115–123, 1994.

Tanzer, R.C.: The carpal tunnel syndrome. J. Bone Joint Surg. Am. 41:626–634, 1959.

Tardiff, G.S.: Nerve injuries: Testing and treatment tactics. Phys. Sportsmed. 23:61–72, 1995.

Terrono, A.L., P.G. Feldon, W. Hills, L.H. Millender, and E.A. Nalebuff: Evaluation and treatment of the rheumatoid wrist. J. Bone Joint Surg. Am. 77:1116–1128, 1995.

Thiru-Pathi, R.G., D.C. Ferlic, M.C. Clayton, and D.C. McClure: Arterial anatomy of the triangular fibrocartilage of the wrist and its surgical significance. J. Hand Surg. Am. 11:258–263, 1986.

Todd, T.W.: Atlas of Skeletal Maturation. St. Louis, C.V. Mosby Co., 1937.

Tucker, W.E.: Manipulative techniques employed in the treatment of injury and osteoarthritis of the fingers and hands. Physiotherapy 57:255–258, 1971.

Volz, R.G., M. Lieb, and J. Benjamin: Biomechanics of the wrist. Clin. Orthop. 149:112–117, 1980.

Wadsworth, C.T.: Elbow, forearm, wrist, and hand. In Myers, R.S. (ed.): Saunders Manual of Physical Therapy Practice. Philadelphia, W.B. Saunders Co., 1995.

Wadsworth, C.T.: The wrist and hand. In Gould, J.A. (eds.): Orthopedic and Sports Physical Therapy. St. Louis, C.V. Mosby Co., 1990.

Wadsworth, C.T.: Manual Examination and Treatment of the Spine and Extremities. Baltimore, Williams & Wilkins, 1988.

Wadsworth, C.T.: Wrist and hand examination and interpretation. J. Orthop. Sports Phys. Ther. 5:108–120, 1983.

Waylett-Rendall, J.: Sensibility evaluation and rehabilitation. Orthop. Clin. North Am. 19:43–56, 1988.

Weiss, K.L., J. Beltran, and L.M. Lubbers: High-field MR surface-coil imaging of the hand and wrist: Pathologic correlations and clinical relevance. Radiology 160:147–152, 1986.

Weissman, B.N.W., and C.B. Sledge: Orthopedic Radiology. Philadelphia, W.B. Saunders Co., 1986.

Williams, P., and R. Warwick: Gray's Anatomy, 36th British ed. Edinburgh, Churchill Livingstone, 1980.

Wynn Parry, C.B.: Rehabilitation of the Hand. London, Butterworths, 1981.

Youm, Y., R.Y. McMurtry, A.E. Flatt, and T.E. Gillespie: Kinematics of the wrist: I. An experimental study of radioulnar deviation and flexion-extension. J. Bone Joint Surg. Am. 60:423–431, 1978.

Zemel, N.P., and H.H. Stark: Fractures and dislocations of the carpal bones. Clin. Sports Med. 5:709–724, 1986.

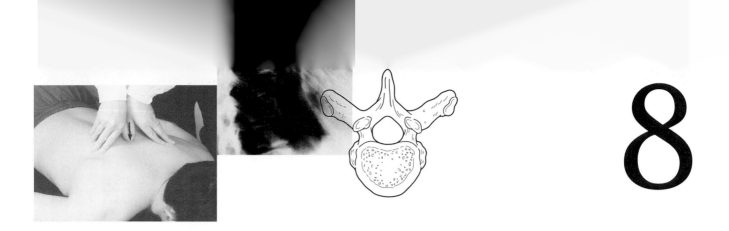

8

Thoracic (Dorsal) Spine

Assessment of the thoracic spine involves examination of the part of the spine that is most rigid because of the associated rib cage. The rib cage in turn provides protection for the heart and lungs. Normally, the thoracic spine, being one of the primary curves, exhibits a mild **kyphosis** (posterior curvature); the cervical and lumbar sections, being secondary curves, exhibit a mild **lordosis** (anterior curvature). When the examiner assesses the thoracic spine, it is essential that the cervical and/or lumbar spines be evaluated at the same time (Fig. 8–1).

Applied Anatomy

The **costovertebral joints** are synovial plane joints located between the ribs and the vertebral bodies (Fig. 8–2). There are 24 of these joints, and they are divided into two parts. Ribs 1, 10, 11, and 12 articulate with a single vertebra. The other articulations have no intra-articular ligament that divides the joint into two parts, so each of ribs 2 through 9 articulates with two adjacent vertebrae and the intervening intervertebral disc.

The **costotransverse joints** are synovial joints found between the ribs and the transverse processes of the vertebra of the same level for ribs 1 through 10 (see Fig. 8–2). Because ribs 11 and 12 do not articulate with the transverse processes, this joint does not exist for these two levels.

The **costochondral joints** lie between the ribs and

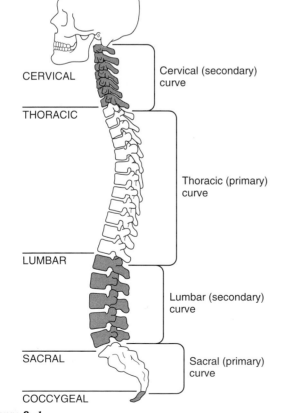

Figure 8–1
The articulated spine.

CERVICAL — Cervical (secondary) curve

THORACIC — Thoracic (primary) curve

LUMBAR — Lumbar (secondary) curve

SACRAL — Sacral (primary) curve

COCCYGEAL

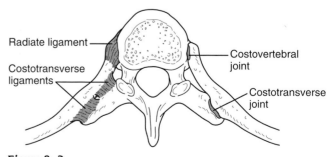

Radiate ligament

Costotransverse ligaments

Costovertebral joint

Costotransverse joint

Figure 8–2
Costovertebral and costotransverse joints, showing relation of ribs to thoracic vertebra.

331

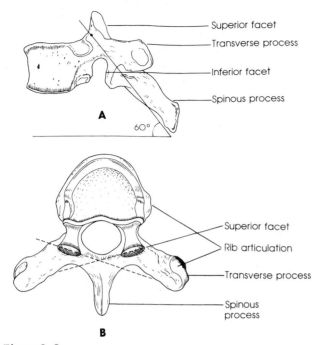

Figure 8-3

Thoracic vertebra. (A) Side view. (B) Superior view.

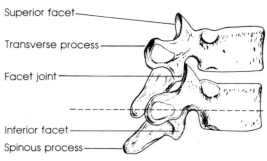

Figure 8-4

Spinous process of one thoracic vertebra at level of body of vertebra below (T7–T9).

the costal cartilage. The **sternocostal joints** are found between the costal cartilage and the sternum. Joints 2 through 6 are synovial, whereas the first costal cartilage is united with the sternum by a synchondrosis. Where a rib articulates with an adjacent rib or costal cartilage (ribs 5 through 9), a synovial interchondral joint exists.

The superior facet of the T1 vertebra is similar to a facet of the cervical spine. Because of this, T1 is classified as a **transitional vertebra.** The superior facet faces up and back; the inferior facet faces down and forward. The T2–T11 superior facets face up, back, and slightly laterally; the inferior facets face down, forward, and slightly medially (Fig. 8–3). This shape enables slight rotation in the thoracic spine. Thoracic vertebrae T11 and T12 are classified as transitional, and the facets of these vertebrae become positioned in a way similar to those of the lumbar facets. The superior facets of these two vertebrae face up, back, and more medially; the inferior facets face forward and slightly laterally. The close packed

Facet Joints of the Thoracic Spine

Resting position:	Midway between flexion and extension
Close packed position:	Extension
Capsular pattern:	Side flexion and rotation equally limited, then extension

position of the facet joints in the thoracic spine is extension.

Within the thoracic spine, there are 12 vertebrae, which diminish in size from T1 to T3 and then increase progressively in size to T12. These vertebrae are distinctive in having facets on the body and transverse processes for articulation with the ribs. The spinous processes of these vertebrae face obliquely downward (Fig. 8–4). T7 has the greatest spinous process angulation, whereas the upper three thoracic vertebrae have spinous processes that project directly posteriorly. In other words, the spinous process of these vertebrae are on the same plane as the transverse processes of the same vertebrae.

T4–T6 vertebrae have spinous processes that project downward slightly. In this case, the tips of the spinous processes are on a plane halfway between their own transverse processes and the transverse processes of the vertebrae below. For T7, T8, and T9 vertebrae, the spinous processes project downward, the tip of the spinous processes being on a plane of the transverse processes of the vertebrae below. For the T10 spinous process, the arrangement is similar to that of the T9 spinous process (i.e., the spinous process is level with the transverse process of the vertebra below). For T11, the arrangement is similar to that of T6 (i.e., the spinous process is halfway between the two transverse processes of the vertebra), and T12 is similar to T3 (i.e., the spinous process is level with the transverse process of the same vertebra). The location of the spinous processes becomes important if the examiner wishes to perform posteroanterior central vertebral pressures. For example, if the examiner pushes on the spinous process of T8, the body of T9 will also move. In fact, the vertebral body of T8 will probably arc, whereas T9 will move in an anterior direction. T7 is sometimes classified as a transitional vertebra because it is the point at which the lower limb axial rotation alternates with the upper limb axial rotation (Fig. 8–5).

The ribs, which help to stiffen the thoracic spine, articulate with the demifacets on vertebrae T2–T9. For

T1 and T10, there is a whole facet for ribs 1 and 10, respectively. The first rib articulates with T1 only, the second rib articulates with T1 and T2, the third rib articulates with T2 and T3, and so on. Ribs 1 through 7 articulate with the sternum directly and are classified as **true ribs**. Ribs 8 through 10 join directly with the costocartilage of the rib above and are classified as **false ribs**. Ribs 11 and 12 are classified as **floating ribs** because they do not attach to either the sternum or the costal cartilage at their distal ends. Ribs 11 and 12 articulate only with the bodies of the T11 and T12 vertebrae, not with the transverse processes of the vertebrae or with the costocartilage of the rib above. The ribs are held by ligaments to the body of the vertebra and to the transverse processes of the same vertebrae. Some of these ligaments also bind the rib to the vertebra above.

At the top of the rib cage, the ribs are relatively horizontal. As the rib cage descends, they run more and more obliquely downward. By the 12th rib, the ribs are more vertical than horizontal. With inspiration, the ribs are pulled up and forward; this increases the anteroposterior diameter of the ribs. The first six ribs increase the anteroposterior dimension of the chest, mainly by rotating around their long axes. Rotation downward of the rib neck is associated with depression, whereas rotation upward of the same portion is associated with elevation. These movements are known as a **pump handle action** and are accompanied by elevation of the manubrium sternum upward and forward (Fig. 8–6A).[1-3] Ribs 7 through 10 mainly increase in lateral, or transverse, dimension. To accomplish this, the ribs move upward, backward, and medially to increase the infrasternal angle or downward, forward, and laterally to decrease the angle. These movements are known as a **bucket handle action.** This action is also performed by ribs 2 through

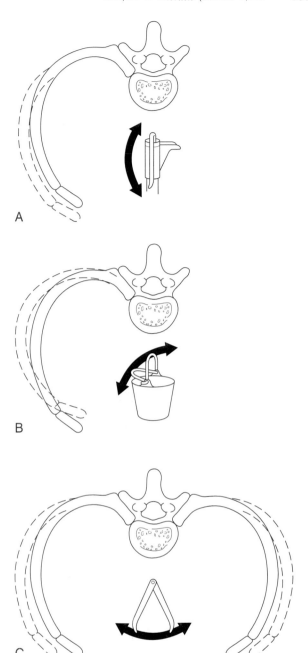

Figure 8–6
Actions of the ribs. (A) Pump handle action (T1–T6). (B) Bucket handle action (T7–T10). (C) Caliper action (T11–T12). (A and B, modified from Williams, P., and R. Warwick [eds.]: Gray's Anatomy, 37th British ed. Edinburgh, Churchill Livingstone, 1989, p. 498.)

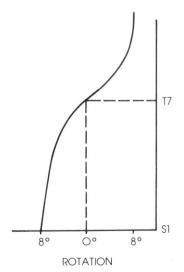

Figure 8–5
Axial rotation of the spine going from left to right on heel strike.

6 but to a much lesser degree (Fig. 8–6B). The lower ribs (ribs 8 through 12) move laterally, in what is known as a **caliper action,** to increase lateral diameter (Fig. 8–6C).[2]

The ribs are quite elastic in children, but they become increasingly brittle with age. In the anterior half of the chest, the ribs are subcutaneous; in the posterior half, they are covered by muscles.

Patient History

A thorough and complete history should include past and present problems. By listening carefully, the examiner is often able to identify the patient's problem and can then use the observation and examination to confirm or refute the impressions established from the history. All information concerning the present pain and its site, nature, and behavior is important. If any part of the history implicates the cervical or lumbar spine, the examiner must include these areas in the assessment as well.

In addition to the questions listed under Patient History in Chapter 1, the examiner should obtain the following information from the patient.

1. What are the patient's age and occupation? For example, conditions such as Scheuermann's disease occur in young people between 13 and 16 years of age. Idopathic scoliosis is most commonly seen in adolescent females.

2. What was the mechanism of injury? Most commonly, rib injuries are caused by trauma. Thoracic spine problems may result from disease processes (e.g., scoliosis) and may have an insidious onset. Pain from true thoracic trauma tends to be localized to the area of injury. Facet syndromes present as stiffness and local pain, which can be referred.[4, 5]

3. What are the details of the present pain and other symptoms? What are the sites and boundaries of the pain? Have the patient point to the location or locations. Is there any radiation of pain? The examiner should remember that many of the abdominal structures, such as the stomach, liver, and pancreas, may refer pain to the thoracic region. With thoracic disc lesions, because of the rigidity of the thoracic spine, active movements do not often show the characteristic pain pattern, and sensory and strength deficits are difficult if not impossible to detect.[6] Thoracic root involvement or spondylosis usually causes pain that follows the path of the ribs or a deep, "through-the-chest" pain.

4. Does the pain occur on inspiration, expiration, or both? Pain related to breathing may signal pulmonary problems or may be related to movement of the ribs. Pain referred around the chest wall tends to be costovertebral in origin. Does the patient have any difficulty in breathing? If a breathing problem exists, it may be caused by a structural deformity (e.g., scoliosis); thoracic trauma such as disc lesions, fractures, or contusions; or thoracic pathology such as pneumothorax, pleurisy, tumors, or pericarditis.

5. Is the pain deep, superficial, shooting, burning, or aching? Thoracic nerve root pain is often severe and is referred in a sloping band along an intercostal space. Pain between the scapulae may be the result of a cervical lesion. It has been reported that any symptoms above a line joining the inferior angles of the scapula should be considered of cervical origin until proven otherwise, especially if there is no history of trauma.[7]

6. Is the pain affected by coughing, sneezing, or straining? Dural pain is often accentuated by these maneuvers.

7. Which activities aggravate the problem? Active use of the arms sometimes irritates a thoracic lesion. Pulling and pushing activities can be especially bothersome to a patient with thoracic problems. Costal pain is often elicited by breathing and/or overhand arm motion.

8. Which activities ease the problem? For example, bracing the arms often makes breathing easier.

9. Is the condition improving, becoming worse, or staying the same?

10. Does any particular posture bother the patient?

11. Is there any paresthesia or other abnormal sensation that may indicate a disc lesion or radiculopathy?

12. Are the patient's symptoms referred to the legs, arms, or head and neck? If so, it is imperative that the examiner assess these areas as well. For example, shoulder movements may be restricted with thoracic spine problems.

13. Does the patient have any problems with digestion? Pain may be referred to the thoracic spine or ribs from pathological conditions within the thorax or abdomen. Visceral pain tends to be vague, dull, and indiscrete and may be accompanied by nausea and sweating. It tends to follow dermatome patterns in its referral. For example, cardiac pain is referred to the shoulder (C4) and posteriorly to T2. Stomach pain is referred to T6–T8 posteriorly. Ulcers may be referred to T4–T6 posteriorly.[4]

14. Is the skin in the thorax area normal? Conditions such as herpes zoster can cause unilateral, spontaneous pain. In the observation, the examiner should watch for erythema and grouped vesicles.[6]

Observation

The patient must be suitably undressed so that the body is exposed as much as possible. In the case of a female, the bra is often removed to provide a better view of the spine and rib cage. The patient is usually observed first standing and then sitting.

As with any observation, the examiner should note any alteration in the overall spinal posture (see Chapter 15) because it may lead to problems in the thoracic spine. It is important to observe the total body posture from the head to the toes and look for any deviation from normal (Fig. 8–7). Posteriorly, the spine of the scapula should be level with the T3 spinous process, whereas the inferior angle of the scapula is level with the T7–T9 spinous process, depending on the size of the scapula. The medial border of the scapula is parallel to the spine and approximately 5 cm lateral to the spinous processes.

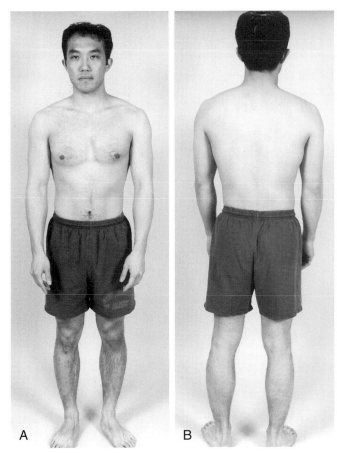

Figure 8–7
Normal posture. (A) Front view. (B) Posterior view.

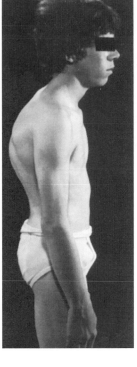

Figure 8–8
Congenital thoracic kyphosis. (From Bradford D.S., J.E. Lonstein, J.H. Moe, et al.: Moe's Textbook of Scoliosis and Other Spinal Deformities. Philadelphia, W.B. Saunders Co., 1987, p. 263.)

Kyphosis

Kyphosis is a condition that is most prevalent in the thoracic spine (Fig. 8–8). The examiner must ensure that a kyphosis is actually present, remembering that a slight kyphosis, or posterior curvature, is normal and is found in every individual. In addition, some people have "flat" scapulae, which give the appearance of an excessive kyphosis, as does winging of the scapulae. The examiner must ensure that it is actually the spine that has the excessive curvature. Types of kyphotic deformities are shown in Figure 8–9 and listed below[8]:

1. **Round back** is decreased pelvic inclination (20°) with a thoracolumbar or thoracic kyphosis (Fig. 8–10).

Figure 8–9
Kyphotic deformities.

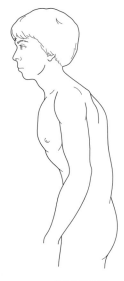

KYPHOSIS

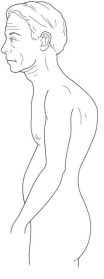

GIBBUS

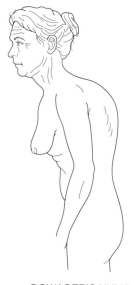

DOWAGER'S HUMP

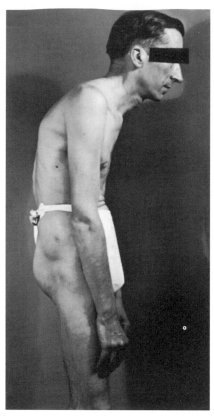

Figure 8–10
Lateral view of patient with ankylosing (rheumatoid) spondylitis showing forward protrusion of head, flattening of anterior chest wall, thoracic kyphosis, protrusion of abdomen, and flattening of lumbar lordosis. This patient also has slight flexion of the hips on the pelvis (From Polley, H.F., and G.G. Hunder: Rheumatologic Interviewing and Physical Examination of the Joints. Philadelphia, W.B. Saunders Co., 1978, p. 161.)

Most forms of kyphosis seen show a decreased pelvic inclination. To compensate and maintain the body's center of gravity, a structural kyphosis, usually caused by tight soft tissues from prolonged postural change or by a growth disturbance (e.g., Scheuermann's disease), results, causing a round back deformity.

2. **Hump back** is a localized, sharp, posterior angulation called **gibbus**. This kyphotic deformity is usually structural and often results from an anterior wedging of the body of one or two thoracic vertebrae. The wedging may be caused by a fracture, tumor, or bone disease. The pelvic inclination is usually normal (30°).

3. **Flat back** is decreased pelvic inclination (20°) with a mobile spine. This kyphotic deformity is similar to round back, except that the thoracic spine remains mobile and is able to compensate throughout its length for the altered center of gravity caused by the decreased pelvic inclination. Therefore, although a kyphosis is or should be present, it does not have the appearance of an excessive kyphotic curve.

4. **Dowager's hump** results from postmenopausal osteoporosis. Because of the osteoporosis, anterior wedge fractures occur to several vertebrae, usually in the upper to middle thoracic spine, causing a structural scoliosis that also contributes to a decrease in height.

Scoliosis

Scoliosis is a deformity in which there are one or more lateral curvatures of the lumbar or thoracic spine; it is this spinal deformity that was suffered by the "Hunchback of Notre Dame." (In the cervical spine, the condition is called **torticollis**.) The curvature may occur in the thoracic spine alone, in the thoracolumbar area, or in the lumbar spine alone (Fig. 8–11). Scoliosis may be nonstructural—in other words, relatively easily correctable once the cause is determined—or structural. Poor posture, hysteria, nerve root irritation, inflammation in the spine area, leg length discrepancy, or hip contracture can cause nonstructural scoliosis. Structural changes may be genetic, idiopathic, or caused by some congenital problem such as a wedge vertebra, hemivertebra, or failure of vertebral segmentation. In other words, there is a structural change in the bone, and normal flexibility of the spine is lost.[9]

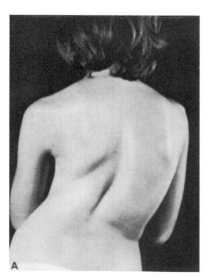
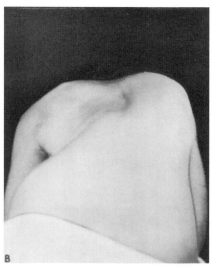

Figure 8–11
Idiopathic scoliosis. (A) Postural deformity caused by idiopathic thoracolumbar scoliosis. (B) Asymmetry of posterior thorax accentuated with patient flexed. Note "hump" on the right and "hollow" on the left. (From Gartland, J.J.: Fundamentals of Orthopedics. Philadelphia, W.B. Saunders Co., 1979, p. 341.)

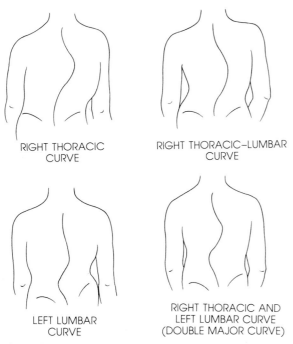

RIGHT THORACIC
CURVE

RIGHT THORACIC–LUMBAR
CURVE

LEFT LUMBAR
CURVE

RIGHT THORACIC AND
LEFT LUMBAR CURVE
(DOUBLE MAJOR CURVE)

Figure 8–12

Examples of scoliosis curve patterns.

A number of curve patterns may be present with scoliosis (Fig. 8–12).[9] The curve patterns are designated according to the level of the apex of the curve (Table 8–1). A right thoracic curve has a convexity toward the right, and the apex of the curve is in the thoracic spine. With a cervical scoliosis, or torticollis, the apex is between C1 and C6. For a cervicothoracic curve, the apex is at C7 or T1. For a thoracic curve, the apex is between T2 and T11. The thoracolumbar curve has its apex at T12 or L1. The lumbar curve has an apex between L2 and L4, and a lumbosacral scoliosis has an apex at L5 or S1. The involvement of the thoracic spine results in a very poor cosmetic appearance or defect as a result of deformation of the ribs along with the spine. The deformity can vary from a mild rib hump to a severe rotation of the vertebrae, causing a rib deformity called a **razorback spine**.

With a structural scoliosis, the vertebral bodies rotate to the convexity of the curve and become distorted.[10] If the thoracic spine is involved, this rotation causes the ribs on the convex side of the curve to push posteriorly, causing a rib "hump" and narrowing the thoracic cage on the convex side. As the vertebral body rotates to the convex side of the curve, the spinous process deviates

Table 8–1
Curve Patterns and Prognosis in Idiopathic Scoliosis

	Curve Pattern				
	Primary Lumbar	Thoracolumbar	Combined Thoracic and Lumbar	Primary Thoracic	Cervicothoracic
Incidence (%)	23.6	16	37	22.1	1.3
Average age curve noted (yr)	13.25	14	12.3	11.1	15
Average age curve stabilized (yr)	14.5	16	15.5	16.1	16
Extent of curve	T11–L3	T6 or T7–L1 or L1, L2	Thoracic, T6–T10 Lumbar, T11–L4	T6–T11	C7 or T1–T4 or T5
Apex of curve	L1 or L2	T11 or L2	Thoracic, T7 or T8 Lumbar, L2	T8 or T9 (rotation extreme, convexity usually to right)	T3
Average angular value at maturity (degrees)					
Standing	36.8	42.7	Thoracic, 51.9; lumbar, 41.4	81.4	34.6
Supine	29.1	35	Thoracic, 41.4; lumbar, 37.7	73.8	32.2
Prognosis	Most benign and least deforming of all idiopathic curves	Not severely deforming Intermediate between thoracic and lumbar curves	Good Body usually well aligned, curves even if severe tend to compensate each other High percentage of very severe scoliosis if onset before age of 10 yr	Worst Progresses more rapidly, becomes more severe, and produces greater clinical deformity than any other pattern Five years of active growth during which curve could increase	Deformity unsightly Poorly disguised because of high shoulder, elevated scapula, and deformed thoracic cage

Adapted from Ponseti, I.V., and B. Friedman: Prognosis in idiopathic scoliosis. J. Bone Joint Surg. Am. 32:382, 1950.

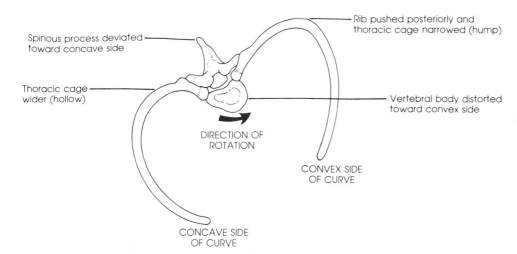

Figure 8–13

Pathological changes in the ribs and vertebra with idiopathic scoliosis in the thoracic spine.

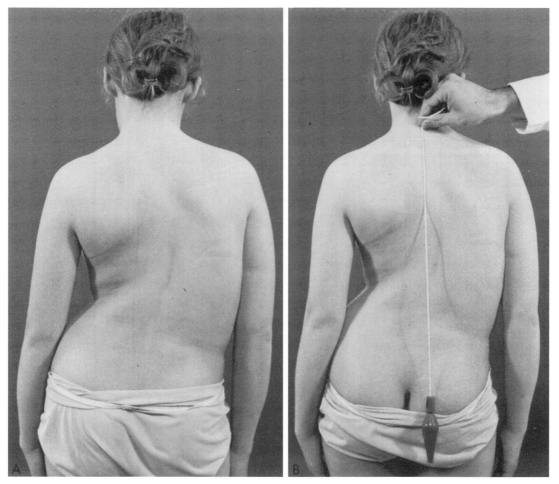

Figure 8–14

Right thoracic idiopathic scoliosis (posterior view). (A) The left shoulder is lower, and the right scapula is more prominent. Note the decreased distance between the right arm and the thorax, with the shift of the thorax to the right. The left iliac crest appears higher, but this results from the shift of the thorax, with fullness on the right and elimination of the waistline; the "high" hip is only apparent, not real. (B) Plumbline dropped from the prominent vertebra of C7 (vertebra prominens) measures the decompensation of the thorax over the pelvis. The distance from the vertical plumbline to the gluteal cleft is measured in centimeters and is recorded along with the direction of deviation. If there is a cervical or cervicothoracic curve, the plumb should fall from the occipital protuberance (inion). (From Moe, J.H., D.S. Bradford, R.B. Winter, and J.E. Lonstein: Scoliosis and Other Spinal Deformities. Philadelphia, W.B. Saunders Co., 1978, p. 14.)

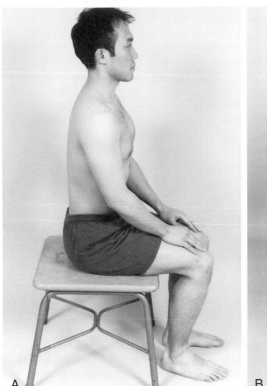
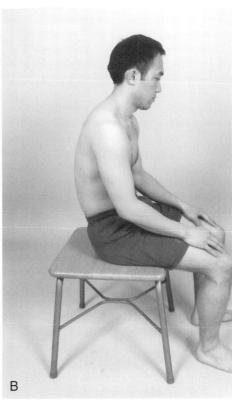

Figure 8–15

Sitting posture. (A) Normal position. (B) Sag sitting.

toward the concave side. The ribs on the concave side move anteriorly, causing a "hollow" and a widening of the thoracic cage on the concave side (Fig. 8–13). Lateral deviation may be more evident if the examiner uses a plumb bob (plumbline) from the C7 spinous process or external occipital protuberance (Fig. 8–14).

The examiner should note whether the ribs are symmetric and whether the rib contours are normal and equal on the two sides. In idiopathic scoliosis, the rib contours are not normal, and there is asymmetry of the ribs. Muscle spasm resulting from injury may also be evident. The bony and soft-tissue contours should be observed for equality on both sides or for any noticeable difference.

The examiner should note whether the patient sits up properly with the normal spinal curves present (Fig. 8–15A); whether the tip of the ear, tip of the acromion process, and high point of the iliac crest are in a straight line as they should be; and whether the patient sits in a slumped position (i.e., sag sitting, as in Fig. 8–15B).

The skin should be observed for any abnormality or scars (Fig. 8–16). If there are scars, are they a result of surgery or trauma? Are they new or old scars? If from surgery, what was the surgery for?

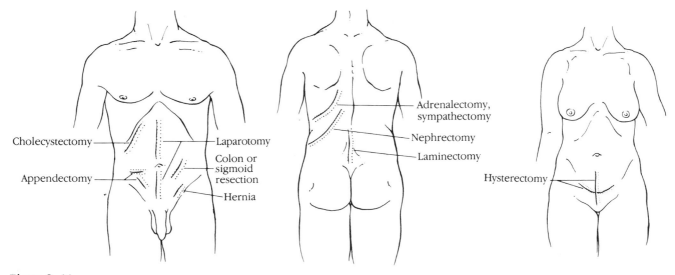

Figure 8–16

Common surgical scars of the abdomen and thorax. (From Judge, R.D., G.D. Zuidema, and F.T. Fitzgerald: Clinical Diagnosis: A Physiologic Approach. Boston, Little, Brown & Co., 1982, p. 295.)

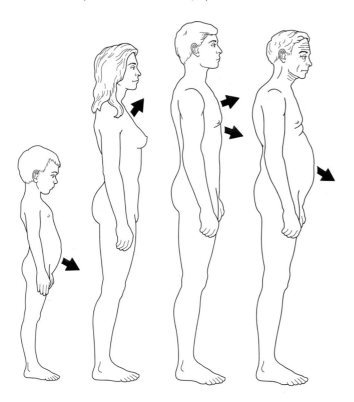

Figure 8–17

Normal breathing patterns for child, adult female, adult male, and elderly person.

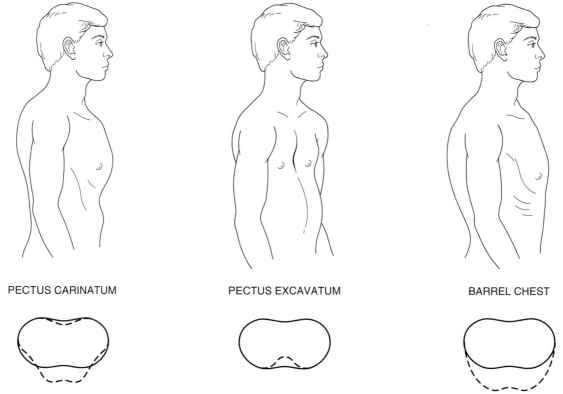

PECTUS CARINATUM   PECTUS EXCAVATUM   BARREL CHEST

Figure 8–18

Chest deformities. Lower vertical views show change in chest wall contours with deformity.

Breathing

As part of the observation, the examiner should note the patient's breathing pattern. Children tend to breathe abdominally, whereas women tend to do upper thoracic breathing. Men tend to be upper and lower thoracic breathers. In the aged, breathing tends to be in the lower thoracic and abdominal regions (Fig. 8–17). The examiner should note the quality of the respiratory movements as well as the rate, rhythm, and effort required to inhale and exhale. In addition, the presence of any coughing or noisy or abnormal breathing patterns should be noted. Because the chest wall movement that occurs during breathing displaces the pleural surfaces, thoracic muscles, nerve, and ribs, pain is accentuated by breathing and coughing if any one of these structures is injured.

Chest Deformities

In addition to rib movements during breathing, the examiner should note the presence of any chest deformities. The more common deformities are shown in Figure 8–18 and are listed below:

1. With a **pigeon chest** (pectus carinatum) deformity, the sternum projects forward and downward like the heel of a boot, increasing the anteroposterior dimension of the chest. This congenital deformity impairs the effectiveness of breathing by restricting ventilation volume.

2. The **funnel chest** (pectus excavatum) is a congenital deformity that results from the sternum's being pushed posteriorly by an overgrowth of the ribs.[11] The anteroposterior dimension of the chest is decreased, and the heart may be displaced. On inspiration, this deformity causes a depression of the sternum that affects respiration and may result in kyphosis.

3. With the **barrel chest** deformity, the sternum projects forward and upward so that the anteroposterior diameter is increased. It is seen in pathological conditions such as emphysema.

Examination

Although the assessment is primarily of the thorax and thoracic spine, if the history, observation, or examination indicates symptoms into or from the neck, upper limb, or lumbar spine and lower limb, these structures must be examined as well. Therefore, the examination of the thoracic spine may be an extensive one. Unless there is a history of specific trauma or injury to the thoracic spine, the examiner must be prepared to assess more than that area alone. If a problem is suspected above the thoracic spine, the scanning examination of the cervical spine and upper limb (as described in Chapter 3) should be performed. If a problem is suspected below the thoracic spine, the scanning examination of the lumbar spine and lower limb (as described in Chapter 9) should be done. Only examination of the thoracic spine is described here.

Active Movements

The active movements of the thoracic spine are usually done with the patient standing. It must be remembered that movement in the thoracic spine is limited by the rib cage and the long spinous processes of the thoracic spine. When assessing the thoracic spine, the examiner should be sure to note whether the movement occurs in the spine or in the hips. A patient can touch the toes with a completely rigid spine if there is sufficient range of motion (ROM) in the hip joints. Likewise, tight hamstrings may alter the results. The movements may be done with the patient sitting, in which case the effect of hip movement is eliminated or decreased. As with any examination, the most painful movements are done last.

The active movements to be carried out in the thoracic spine are shown in Figure 8–19.

Active Movements of the Thoracic Spine

- Forward flexion (20 to 45°)
- Extension (25 to 45°)
- Side flexion, left and right (20 to 40°)
- Rotation, left and right (35 to 50°)
- Costovertebral expansion (3 to 7.5 cm)
- Rib motion (pump handle, bucket handle, and caliper)
- Combined movements (if necessary)
- Repetitive movements (if necessary)
- Sustained postures (if necessary)

Forward Flexion

The normal ROM of forward flexion (forward bending) in the thoracic spine is 20 to 45° (Fig. 8–20). Because the ROM at each vertebra is difficult to measure, the examiner can use a tape measure to derive an indication of overall movement (Fig. 8–21). The examiner first measures the length of the spine from the C7 spinous process to the T12 spinous process with the patient in the normal standing posture. The patient is then asked to bend forward, and the spine is again measured. A 2.7-cm (1.1-inch) difference in tape measure length is considered normal.

If the examiner wishes, the spine may be measured from the C7 to S1 spinous process with the patient in the normal standing position. The patient is then asked

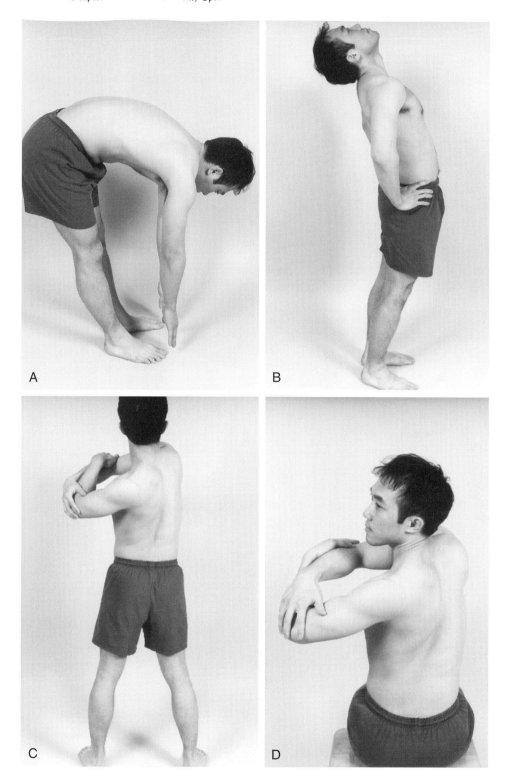

Figure 8–19
Active movement. (A) Forward
flexion. (B) Extension.
(C) Rotation (standing).
(D) Rotation (sitting).

to bend forward, and the spine is again measured. A 10-cm (4-inch) difference in tape measure length is considered normal. In this case, the examiner is measuring movement in the lumbar spine as well as in the thoracic spine; most movement, approximately 7.5 cm (3 inches), occurs between T12 and S1.

A third method of measuring spinal flexion is to ask the patient to bend forward and try to touch the toes while keeping the knees straight. The examiner then measures from the fingertips to the floor and records the distance. The examiner must keep in mind that with this method, in addition to the thoracic spine movement, the movement may also occur in the lumbar spine and hips; in fact, movement could occur totally in the hips.

Each of these methods is indirect. To measure the ROM at each vertebral segment, a series of radiographs

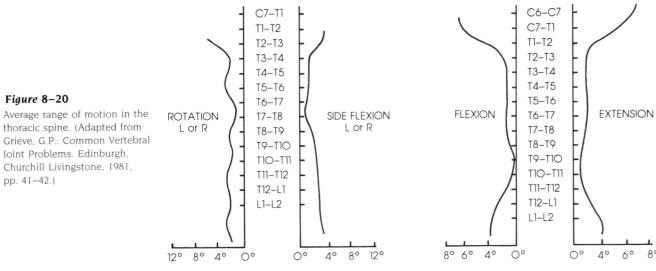

Figure 8–20

Average range of motion in the thoracic spine. (Adapted from Grieve, G.P.: Common Vertebral Joint Problems. Edinburgh, Churchill Livingstone, 1981, pp. 41–42.)

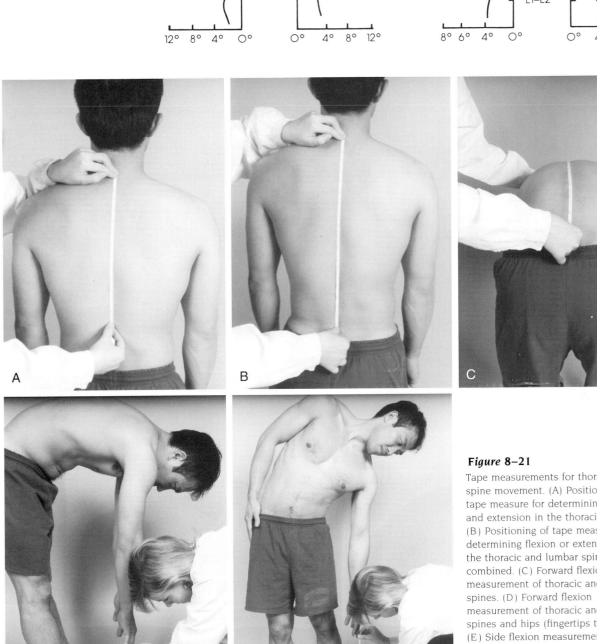

Figure 8–21

Tape measurements for thoracic spine movement. (A) Positioning of tape measure for determining flexion and extension in the thoracic spine. (B) Positioning of tape measure for determining flexion or extension in the thoracic and lumbar spines combined. (C) Forward flexion measurement of thoracic and lumbar spines. (D) Forward flexion measurement of thoracic and lumbar spines and hips (fingertips to floor). (E) Side flexion measurement (fingertips to floor).

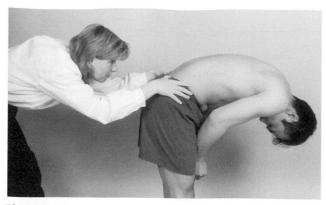

Figure 8-22

Examiner performing skyline view of spine for assessment of scoliosis.

would be necessary. The examiner can decide which method to use. It is of primary importance, however, to note on the patient's chart how the measuring was done and which reference points were used.

While the patient is flexed forward, the examiner can observe the spine from the "skyline" view (Fig. 8–22). With nonstructural scoliosis, the scoliotic curve disappears on forward flexion; with structural scoliosis, it remains. With the skyline view, the examiner is looking for a hump on one side (convex side of curve) and a hollow (concave side of curve) on the other. This "hump and hollow" sequence is caused by vertebral rotation in idiopathic scoliosis, which pushes the ribs and muscles out on one side and causes the paravertebral valley on the opposite side. The vertebral rotation is most evident in the flexed position.

When the patient flexes forward, the thoracic spine should curve forward in a smooth, even manner (Fig. 8–23). The examiner should look for any apparent tightness or sharp angulation such as a gibbus when the movement is performed. If the patient has an excessive kyphosis to begin with, very little forward flexion movement occurs in the thoracic spine. McKenzie advocates

doing flexion while sitting to decrease pelvic and hip movements. The patient puts the hands around the neck to apply overpressure at the end of flexion.[7]

Extension

Extension (backward bending) in the thoracic spine is normally 25 to 45°. Because this movement occurs over 12 vertebrae, the movement between the individual vertebrae is difficult to detect visually. As with flexion, the examiner can use a tape measure and obtain the distance between the same two points (the C7 and T12 spinous processes). Again a 2.5-cm (1-inch) difference in tape measure length between standing and extension is considered normal. McKenzie[7] advocates having the patient place the hands in the small of the back to add stability while performing the backward movement or to do extension while sitting or prone lying (sphinx position).

As the patient extends, the thoracic curve should curve backward or at least straighten in a smooth, even manner. The examiner should look for any apparent tightness or angulation when the movement is performed. If the patient shows excessive kyphosis (Fig. 8–24), the kyphotic curvature remains on extension, that is, the thoracic spine remains flexed, whether the movement is tested while the patient is standing or lying prone (see Fig. 8–24).

Side Flexion

Side (lateral) flexion is approximately 20 to 40° to the right and left in the thoracic spine. The patient is asked to run the hand down the side of the leg as far as possible without bending forward or backward. The examiner can then estimate the angle of side flexion or use a tape measure to determine the length from the fingertips to the floor and compare it with that of the other side (see Fig. 8–21E). Normally, the distances should be equal.

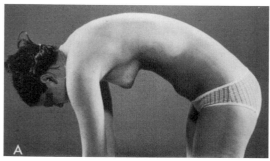 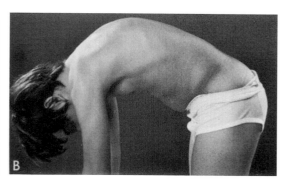

Figure 8-23

Side view in forward bending position for assessment of kyphosis. (A) Normal thoracic roundness is demonstrated with a gentle curve to the whole spine. (B) An area of increased bending is seen in the thoracic spine, indicating structural changes—Scheuermann's disease, in this example. (From Moe, J.H., D.S. Bradford, R.B. Winter, and J.E. Lonstein: Scoliosis and Other Spinal Deformities. Philadelphia, W.B. Saunders Co., 1978, p. 18.)

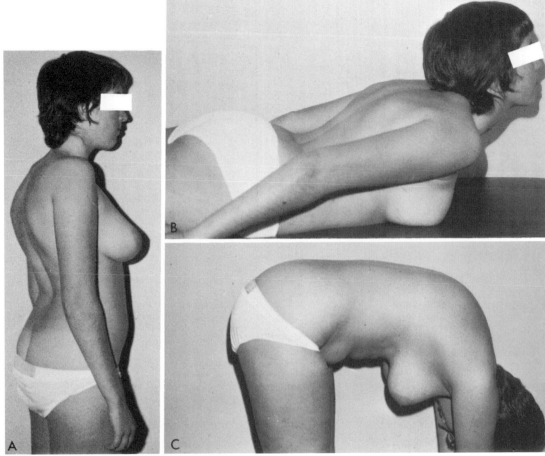

Figure 8–24

Kyphosis and lordosis. (A) On physical examination, definite increases in thoracic kyphosis and lumbar lordosis are visualized. (B) Thoracic kyphosis does not fully correct on thoracic extension. (C) Lumbar lordosis, on the other hand, usually corrects on forward bending; in this case, some lordosis remains. (From Moe, J.H., D.S. Bradford, R.B. Winter, and J.E. Lonstein: Scoliosis and Other Spinal Deformities. Philadelphia, W.B. Saunders Co., 1978, p. 339.)

In either case, the examiner must remember that movement in the lumbar spine as well as in the thoracic spine is being measured. As the patient bends sideways, the spine should curve sideways in a smooth, even, sequential manner. The examiner should look for any tightness or abnormal angulation, which may indicate hypomobility or hypermobility at a specific segment when the movement is performed. If on side flexion the ipsilateral paraspinal muscles tighten or their contracture is evident (**Forestier's bowstring sign**), ankylosing spondylitis should be considered.[12]

Rotation

Rotation in the thoracic spine is approximately 35 to 50°. The patient is asked to cross the arms in front or place the hands on opposite shoulders and then rotate to the right and left while the examiner looks at the amount of rotation, comparing both ways. Again, the examiner must remember that movement in the lumbar spine and hips as well as in the thoracic spine is occurring. To eliminate the hip movement, rotation may be done in sitting.

If the history indicated that repetitive motion, sustained postures, or combined movements caused aggravation of symptoms, then these movements should also be tested, but only after the original movements of flexion, extension, side flexion, and rotation have been completed.

Costovertebral Expansion

Costovertebral joint movement is usually determined by measuring chest expansion (Fig. 8–25). The examiner places the tape measure around the chest at the level of the fourth intercostal space. The patient is asked to exhale as much as possible, and the examiner takes a measurement. The patient is then asked to inhale as

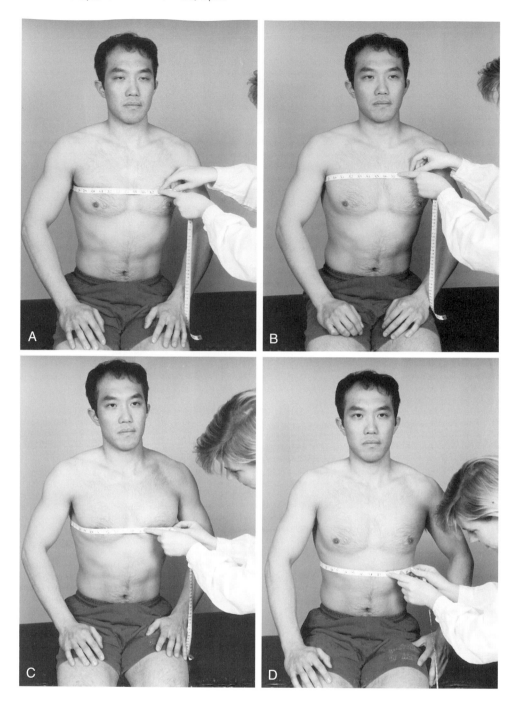

Figure 8–25
Measuring chest expansion.
(A) Fourth lateral intercostal
space. (B) Axilla. (C) Nipple line.
(D) Tenth rib.

much as possible and hold the breath while the second measurement is taken. The normal difference between inspiration and expiration is 3 to 7.5 cm (1 to 3 inches).

A second method of measuring chest expansion is to measure at three different levels. If this method is used, the examiner must take care to ensure that the levels of measurement are noted for consistency. The levels are (1) under the axillae for apical expansion, (2) at the nipple line or xiphisternal junction for midthoracic expansion, and (3) at the T10 rib level for lower thoracic expansion. As before, the measurements are taken at expiration and after inspiration.

After the measurement of chest expansion, it is worthwhile for the patient to take a deep breath and cough so that the examiner can determine whether this action causes or alters any pain. If it does, the examiner may suspect a respiratory-related problem.

Rib Motion

The patient is then asked to lie supine. The examiner's hands are placed in a relaxed fashion over the upper chest. In this position, the examiner is feeling anteroposterior movement of the ribs (Fig. 8–26). As the patient inhales and exhales, the examiner should compare to see whether the movement is equal on both sides. Any restriction or difference in motion should be noted. If a rib stops moving relative to the other ribs on inhalation, it is classified as a **depressed rib**. If a rib stops moving relative to the other ribs on exhalation, it is classified as an **elevated rib**. It must be remembered that restriction of one rib affects the adjacent ribs. If a depressed rib is implicated, it is usually the highest restricted rib that causes the greatest problem. If an elevated rib is present, it is usually the lowest restricted rib that causes the greatest problem.[3, 13] The examiner then moves his or her hands down the patient's chest, testing the movement in the middle and lower ribs in a similar fashion.

To test lateral movement of the ribs, the examiner's hands are placed around the sides of the rib cage approximately 45° to the vertical axis of the patient's body. The examiner begins at the level of the axilla and works down the lateral aspect of the ribs, feeling the movement of the ribs during inspiration and expiration and noting any restriction.

Passive Movements

Because passive movements in the thoracic spine are difficult to perform in a gross fashion, the movement between each pair of vertebrae may be assessed. With

> ### Passive Movements of the Thoracic Spine and Normal End Feel
>
> - Forward flexion (tissue stretch)
> - Extension (tissue stretch)
> - Side flexion, left and right (tissue stretch)
> - Rotation, left and right (tissue stretch)

the patient sitting, the examiner places one hand on the patient's forehead or on top of the head (Fig. 8–27). With the other hand, the examiner palpates over and between the spinous processes of the lower cervical and upper thoracic spines (C5–T3) and feels for movement between the spinous processes while flexing and extending the patient's head. Rotation and side flexion may be tested by rotating and side flexing the patient's head. To test the movement properly, the examiner places the middle finger over the spinous process of the vertebra being tested and the index and ring fingers on each side of it, between the spinous processes of the two adjacent vertebrae. The examiner should feel the movement occurring, assess its quality, and note whether the movement is hypomobile or hypermobile relative to the adjacent vertebrae. The hypomobility or hypermobility may be indicative of pathology.[13]

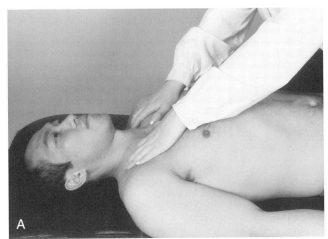
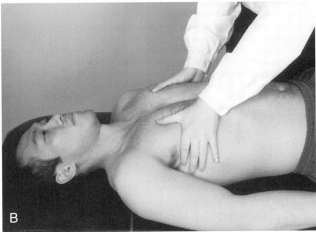
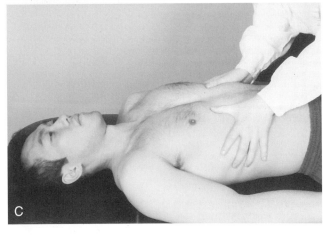

Figure 8–26
Feeling rib movement. (A) Upper ribs. (B) Middle ribs. (C) Lower ribs.

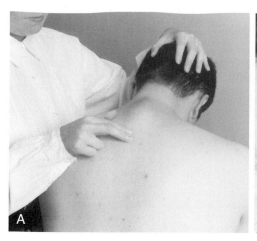
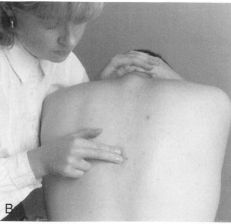

Figure 8–27
Passive movements of the thoracic spine. (A) Upper thoracic spine. (B) Middle and lower thoracic spine.

To test the movement of the vertebrae between T3 and T11, the patient sits with the fingers clasped behind the neck and the elbows together in front. The examiner places one hand and arm around the patient's elbows while palpating over and between the spinous processes, as previously described. The examiner then flexes and extends the spine by lifting and lowering the patient's elbows.

Side flexion and rotation of the trunk may be performed in a similar fashion to test these movements. The patient sits with the hands clasped behind the head. The examiner uses the thumb on one side of the spinous process and/or the index finger and/or the middle finger on the other side to palpate just lateral to the interspinous space. For side flexion, the examiner moves the patient into right side flexion and then left side flexion and by palpation compares the amount and quality of right and left movement including adjacent segments (Fig. 8–28A). For rotation, the examiner rotates the patient's shoulders to the right or left, comparing by palpa-tion the amount and quality of movement of each segment as well as that of adjacent segments (Fig. 8–28B).[13]

Resisted Isometric Movements

Resisted isometric movements are performed with the patient in the sitting position. The examiner places one leg behind the patient's buttocks and the upper limbs around the patient's chest and back (Fig. 8–29). The examiner then instructs the patient, "Don't let me move you," and isometrically tests the movements, noting any alteration in strength and occurrence of pain.

Resisted Isometric Movements of the Thoracic Spine

- Forward flexion
- Extension
- Side flexion, left and right
- Rotation, left and right

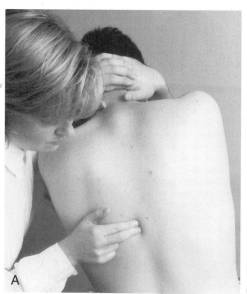
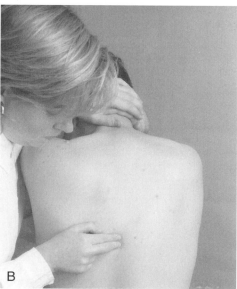

Figure 8–28
(A) Passive side flexion of the thoracic spine. (B) Passive rotation of the thoracic spine.

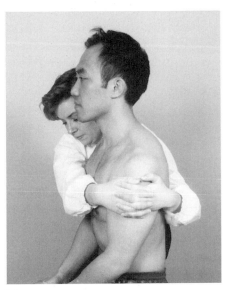

Figure 8–29
Positioning for resisted isometric movements.

The thoracic spine should be tested in a neutral position, and the most painful movements are done last. Table 8–2 lists the muscles of the thoracic spine, their actions, and their innervations. It must be remembered that the resisted isometric testing of the spine is in reality a very gross test, and subtle alterations in strength are almost impossible to detect. However, if the muscles being tested have been strained (1° or 2°), contraction produces pain. In some cases, the spine and thorax may have to be repositioned to isolate a particular muscle.

Functional Assessment

When doing specific activities, the thoracic spine primarily plays a stabilization role. Therefore, activities involving the cervical spine, lumbar spine, and shoulder may be impaired as a result of thoracic lesions. Functional activities involving these three areas should be reviewed or considered if functional impairment appears to be related to the thoracic spine. Activities such as lifting,

Table 8–2
Muscles of the Thorax and Abdomen: Their Actions and Nerve Root Derivation/Nerve Supply in the Thoracic Spine

Action	Muscles Active	Nerve Root Derivation
Flexion of thoracic spine	1. Rectus abdominis	T6–T12
	2. External abdominal oblique (both sides acting together)	T7–T12
	3. Internal abdominal oblique (both sides acting together)	T7–T12, L1
Extension of thoracic spine	1. Spinalis thoracis	T1–T12
	2. Iliocostalis thoracis (both sides acting together)	T1–T12
	3. Longissimus thoracis (both sides acting together)	T1–T12
	4. Semispinalis thoracis (both sides acting together)	T1–T12
	5. Multifidus (both sides acting together)	T1–T12
	6. Rotatores (both sides acting together)	T1–T12
	7. Interspinalis	T1–T12
Rotation and side flexion of thoracic spine	1. Iliocostalis thoracis (to same side)	T1–T12
	2. Longissimus thoracis (to same side)	T1–T12
	3. Intertransverse (to same side)	T1–T12
	4. Internal abdominal oblique (to same side)	T7–T12, L1
	5. Semispinalis thoracis (to opposite side)	T1–T12
	6. Multifidus (to opposite side)	T1–T12
	7. Rotatores (to opposite side)	T1–T12
	8. External abdominal oblique (to opposite side)	T7–T12
	9. Transverse abdominis (to opposite side)	T7–T12, L1
Elevation of ribs	1. Scalenus anterior (1st rib)	C4–C6
	2. Scalenus medius (1st rib)	C3–C8
	3. Scalenus posterior (2nd rib)	C6–C8
	4. Serratus posterior superior (2nd to 5th ribs)	2–5 intercostal
	5. Iliocostalis cervicis (1st to 6th rib)	C6–C8
	6. Levatores costarum (all ribs)	T1–T12
	7. Pectoralis major (if arm fixed)	Lateral pectoral (C6–C7) Medial pectoral (C7–C8, T1)
	8. Serratus anterior (lower ribs if scapula fixed)	Long thoracic (C5–C7)
	9. Pectoralis minor (2nd to 5th ribs if scapula fixed)	Lateral pectoral (C6–C7) Medial pectoral (C7–C8)
	10. Sternocleidomastoid (if head fixed)	Accessory C2–C3

Table continued on following page

Table 8–2
Muscles of the Thorax and Abdomen: Their Actions and Nerve Root Derivation/Nerve Supply in the Thoracic Spine *(Continued)*

Action	Muscles Active	Nerve Root Derivation
Depression of ribs	1. Serratus posterior inferior (lower 4 ribs)	T9–T12
	2. Iliocostalis lumborum (lower 6 ribs)	L1–L3
	3. Longissimus thoracis	T1–T12
	4. Rectus abdominis	T6–T12
	5. External abdominal oblique (lower 5 to 6 ribs)	T7–T12
	6. Internal abdominal oblique (lower 5 to 6 ribs)	T7–T12, L1
	7. Transverse abdominal (all acting to depress lower ribs)	T7–T12, L1
	8. Quadratus lumborum (12th rib)	T12, L1–L4
	9. Transversus thoracis	T1–T12
Approximation of ribs	1. Iliocostalis thoracis	T1–T12
	2. Intercostals (internal and external)	1–11 intercostal
	3. Diaphragm	Phrenic
Inspiration	1. External intercostals	1–11 intercostal
	2. Transverse thoracis (sternocostalis)	1–11 intercostal
	3. Diaphragm	Phrenic
	4. Sternocleidomastoid	Accessory C2–C3
	5. Scalenus anterior	C4–C6
	6. Scalenus medius	C3–C8
	7. Scalenus posterior	C6–C8
	8. Pectoralis major	Lateral pectoral (C5–C6) Medial pectoral (C7–C8, T1)
	9. Pectoralis minor	Lateral pectoral (C6–C7) Medial pectoral (C7–C8)
	10. Serratus anterior	Long thoracic (C5–C7)
	11. Latissimus dorsi	Thoracodorsal (C6–C8)
	12. Serratus posterior superior	2–5 intercostal
	13. Iliocostalis thoracis	T1–T12
Expiration	1. Internal intercostals	1–11 intercostal
	2. Rectus abdominis	T6–T12
	3. External abdominal oblique	T7–T12
	4. Internal abdominal oblique	T7–T12, L1
	5. Iliocostalis lumborum	L1–L3
	6. Longissimus	T1–L3
	7. Serratus posterior inferior	T9–T12
	8. Quadratus lumborum	T12, L1–L4

rotating the thorax, doing heavy work, any activity requiring stabilization of the thorax, or any activity increasing cardiopulmonary output are most likely to provoke thoracic symptoms.

Special Tests

If the examiner suspects a problem with movement of the spinal cord, any of the tests that stretch the cord may be performed. These include the straight leg raising test and the Kernig sign (see Chapter 9). Either neck

> **Special Tests Commonly Performed on the Thoracic Spine**
>
> • Slump test

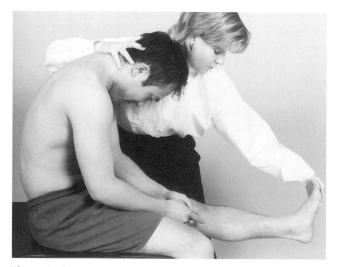

Figure 8–30
Slump test.

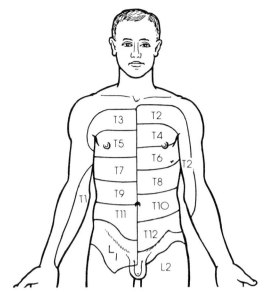

Figure 8–31

The cutaneous areas (dermatomes) supplied by the thoracic nerve roots. (After Foerster). By comparing both sides, the degree of overlapping and the area of exclusive supply of any individual nerve root may be estimated. (Adapted from Williams, P., and R. Warwick [eds.]: Gray's Anatomy, 37th British ed. Edinburgh, Churchill Livingstone, 1989, p. 1150.)

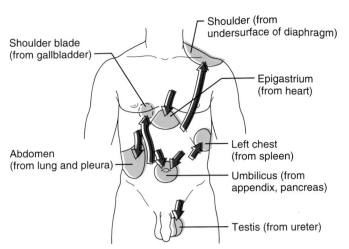

Figure 8–32

Referred pain in the thorax and chest. (Modified from Judge, R.D., G.D. Zuidema, and F.T. Fitzgerald: Clinical Diagnosis: A Physiologic Approach. Boston, Little, Brown & Co., 1982, p. 285.)

flexion from above or straight leg raising from below stretches the spinal cord within the thoracic spine. The following tests should be performed only if the examiner believes they are relevant.

Slump Test (Sitting Dural Stretch Test). The patient sits on the examining table and is asked to "slump" so that the spine flexes and the shoulders sag forward while the examiner holds the chin and head erect. The patient is asked if any symptoms are produced. If no symptoms are produced, the examiner flexes the patient's neck and holds the head down and shoulders slumped to see if symptoms are produced. If no symptoms are produced, the examiner passively extends one of the patient's knees to see if symptoms are produced. If no symptoms are produced, the examiner then passively dorsiflexes the foot of the same leg to see if symptoms are produced (Fig. 8–30). The process is repeated with the other leg. Symptoms of sciatic pain or reproduction of the patient's symptoms indicates a positive test, implicating impinge-

ment of the dura and spinal cord or nerve roots.[14] The pain is usually produced at the site of the lesion.

Passive Scapular Approximation. The patient lies prone while the examiner passively approximates the scapulae by lifting the shoulders up and back. Pain in the scapular area is indicative of a T1 or T2 nerve root problem on the side on which the pain is being experienced.[15]

First Thoracic Nerve Root Stretch. The patient abducts the arm to 90° and flexes the pronated forearm to 90°. No symptoms should appear in this position. The patient then fully flexes the elbow, putting the hand behind the neck. This action stretches the ulnar nerve and T1 nerve root. Pain into the scapular area or arm is indicative of a positive test for T1 nerve root.[15]

Reflexes and Cutaneous Distribution

Within the thoracic spine, there is a great deal of overlap of the dermatomes (Fig. 8–31). The dermatomes tend to follow the ribs, and the absence of only one dermatome may lead to no loss of sensation. Pain may be referred to the thoracic spine from various abdominal organs (Fig. 8–32; Table 8–3). Although there are no reflexes to test in conjunction with the thoracic spine, the examiner

Table 8–3
Differences in Pain Perception

Structure	Effective Stimulus*	Conscious Pain Perception
Skin	Discrete touch, prick, heat, cold	Precisely localized, superficial, burning, sharp
Chest wall (muscles, ribs, ligaments, parietal pleura)	Movement, deep pressure	Intermediate in localization and depth; aching, sharp, or dull
Thoracic viscera	Ischemia, distension, muscle spasm	Vague, diffuse, deep, aching, usually dull

* The effectiveness of all stimuli is heightened by the presence of inflammation.

From Levene, D.L.: Chest Pain: An Integrated Diagnostic Approach. Philadelphia, Lea & Febiger, 1977.

Table 8–4
Thoracic Muscles and Referral of Pain

Muscle	Referral Pattern
Levator scapulae	Neck shoulder angle to posterior shoulder and along medial edge of scapula
Latissimus dorsi	Inferior angle of scapula to posterior shoulder; iliac crest
Rhomboids	Medial border of scapula
Trapezius	Upper thoracic spine to medial border of scapula
Serratus anterior	Lateral chest wall to lower medial border of scapula
Serratus posterior	Medial border of arm to medial two fingers
Serratus superior	Scapular area to posterior and anterior arm down to little finger
Multifidi	Adjacent to spinal column
Iliocostalis	Spinal column to line along medial border of scapula

would be wise to test the lumbar reflexes—the patellar reflex (L3–L4), the medial hamstrings reflex (L5–S1), and the Achilles reflex (S1–S2)—because pathology in the thoracic spine can affect these reflexes.

Thoracic nerve root symptoms tend to follow the course of the ribs and may be referred as follows[16]:

T5:	Pain around nipple
T7–T8:	Pain in epigastric area
T10–T11:	Pain in umbilical area
T12:	Pain in the groin

Muscles of the thoracic spine may also refer pain into adjacent areas (Table 8–4).

Joint Play Movements

The joint play movements performed on the thoracic spine are specific ones that were developed by Maitland.[16] When testing joint play movements, the examiner should note any decreased ROM, muscle spasm, pain,

> **Joint Play Movements of the Thoracic Spine**
>
> - Posteroanterior central vertebral pressure
> - Posteroanterior unilateral vertebral pressure
> - Transverse vertebral pressure
> - Rib springing

or difference in end feel. The normal end feel is tissue stretch.

For the vertebral movements, the patient lies prone. The examiner palpates the thoracic spinous processes, starting at C6 and working down to L1 or L2. The occurrence of muscle spasm and/or pain on application of the vertebral pressure gives the examiner an indication of where the pathology may lie. The examiner must take care, however, because the pain and/or muscle spasm at one level may be the result of compensation for a lesion at another level. For example, if one level is hypomobile as a result of trauma, another level may become hypermobile to compensate for the decreased movement at the traumatized level. It is probable that both the hypomobile and the hypermobile segments will cause pain and/or muscle spasm. It is then important to determine which joint complex is hypomobile and which is hypermobile, because the treatment for each is different.

Posteroanterior Central Vertebral Pressure. The examiner's hands, fingers, and thumb are positioned as in Figure 8–33A. The examiner then applies pressure to the spinous process through the thumbs, pushing the vertebra forward. Care must be taken to apply pressure slowly and with careful control, so that the movement, which is minimal, can be felt. This springing test may be repeated several times to determine the quality of the movement. Each spinous process is done in turn, starting at C6 and working down to L1 or L2. When doing this test, the examiner must keep in mind that the thoracic spinous processes are not always at the level of the same vertebral body. For example, the spinous processes of T1, T2, T3, and T12 are at the same levels as the T1, T2, T3, and T12 vertebral bodies, but the spinous processes of T7, T8, T9, and T10 are at the same levels as the T8, T9, T10, and T11 vertebral bodies, respectively.

Posteroanterior Unilateral Vertebral Pressure. The examiner's fingers are moved laterally away from the tip of the spinous process so that the thumbs rest on the appropriate lamina or transverse process of the thoracic vertebra (Figs. 8–33B and 8–34). The same anterior springing pressure is applied as in the posteroanterior central vertebral pressure technique. Again, each vertebra is done in turn. The two sides should be examined and compared. It must be remembered that in the thoracic area, the spinous process is not necessarily at the same level as the transverse process on the same vertebra. For example, the T9 spinous process is at the level of the T10 transverse process. Therefore, it is necessary to move the fingers up and out from the tip of the T9 spinous process to the T9 transverse process, which is at the level of the T8 spinous process. This difference does not hold true for the entire thoracic spine. It is also important to realize that posteroanterior unilateral vertebral pressure applies a rotary force to the vertebra;

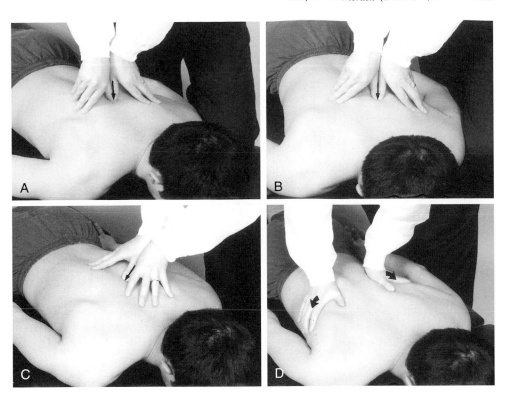

Figure 8–33
Hand, finger, and thumb positions for joint play movements. (A) Posteroanterior central vertebral pressure. (B) Posteroanterior unilateral vertebral pressure. (C) Transverse vertebral pressure. (D) Rib springing (prone).

it therefore places a greater stress at the costotransverse joints, because the ribs are also stressed where they attach to the vertebrae.

    Transverse Vertebral Pressure. The examiner's fingers are placed along the side of the spinous process, as shown in Figures 8–33C and 8–34. The examiner then applies a transverse springing pressure to the side of the spinous process, feeling for the quality of movement.

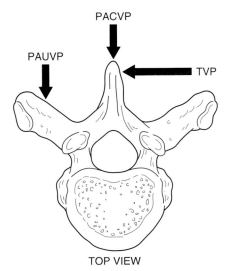

Figure 8–34
Direction of pressure during joint play movements. PACVP = posteroanterior central vertebral pressure; PAUVP = posteroanterior unilateral vertebral pressure; TVP = transverse vertebral pressure.

As before, each vertebra is assessed in turn, starting at C6 and working down to L1 or L2. Pressure should be applied to both sides of the spinous process to compare the movement.

    Rib Springing. The patient lies prone or on the side while the examiner's hands are placed around the posterolateral aspect of the rib cage (Fig. 8–33D). The examiner's hands are approximately 45° to the vertical axis of the patient's body. The examination begins at the top of the rib cage and extends inferiorly, springing the ribs by pushing in with the hands on each side in turn. The amount and quality of movement occurring on both sides should be noted. If one rib appears hypomobile or hypermobile in relation to the others being tested, it can be tested individually.

Palpation

As with any palpation technique, the examiner is looking for tenderness, muscle spasm, temperature alteration, swelling, or other signs that may indicate disease. Palpation should begin on the anterior chest wall, move around the lateral chest wall, and finish with the posterior structures (Fig. 8–35). Palpation is usually done with the patient sitting, although it may be done combining the supine and prone lying positions. At the same time, the thorax may be divided into sections (Fig. 8–36) to give some idea, in charting, where the pathology may lie.

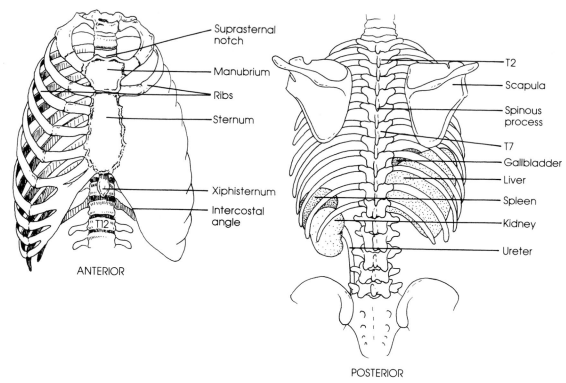

Figure 8–35
Landmarks of the thoracic spine.

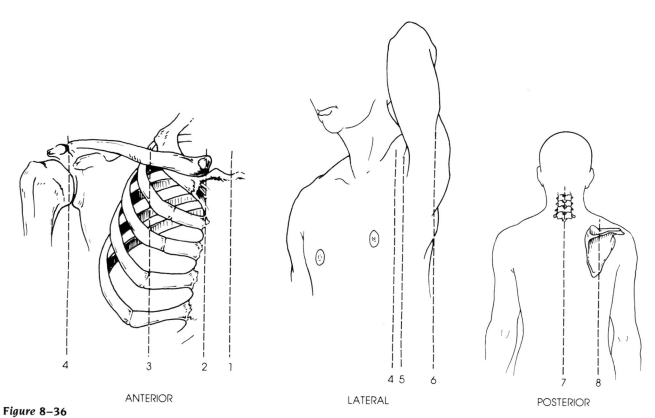

Figure 8–36
Lines of reference in the thoracic area: (1) midtarsal line; (2) parasternal line; (3) midclavicular line; (4) anterior axillary line; (5) midaxillary line; (6) posterior axillary line; (7) midspinal (vertebral) line; (8) midscapular line.

Anterior Aspect

Sternum. In the midline of the chest, the manubrium sternum, body of the sternum, and xiphoid process should be palpated for any abnormality or tenderness.

Ribs and Costal Cartilage. Adjacent to the sternum, the examiner should palpate the sternocostal and costochondral articulations, noting any swelling, tenderness, or abnormality. These "articulations" are sometimes sprained or subluxed, or a costochondritis (e.g., Tietze's syndrome) may be evident. The ribs should be palpated as they extend around the chest wall, with any potential pathology or crepitations (e.g., subcutaneous emphysema) noted.

Clavicle. The clavicle should be palpated along its length for abnormal bumps (e.g., fracture, callus) or tenderness.

Abdomen. The abdomen should be palpated for tenderness or other signs indicating pathology. The palpation is done in a systematic fashion, using the fingers of one hand to feel the tissues while the other hand is used to apply pressure. Palpation is carried out to a depth of 1 to 3 cm (0.5 to 1.5 inches) to reveal areas of tenderness and abnormal masses. Palpation is usually carried out using the quadrant or the nine-region system (Fig. 8–37).

Posterior Aspect

Scapula. The medial, lateral, and superior borders of the scapula should be palpated for any swelling or tenderness. The scapula normally extends from the spinous process of T2 to that of T7–T9. After the borders of the scapula have been palpated, the examiner palpates the posterior surface of the scapula. Structures palpated are the supraspinatus and infraspinatus muscles and the spine of the scapula.

Spinous Processes of the Thoracic Spine. In the midline, the examiner may posteriorly palpate the thoracic spinous processes for abnormality. The examiner then moves laterally approximately 2 to 3 cm (0.8 to 1.2 inches) to palpate the thoracic facet joints. Because of the overlying muscles, it is usually very difficult to palpate these joints, although the examiner may be able to palpate for muscle spasm and tenderness in the area. Muscle spasm may also be elicited if some internal structures are injured. For example, pathology affecting the following structures can cause muscle spasm in the surrounding area: gallbladder (spasm on the right side in the area of the eighth and ninth costal cartilages), spleen (spasm at the level of ribs 9 through 11 on the left side), and kidneys (spasm at the level of ribs 11 and 12 on both sides at the level of the L3 vertebra). Evidence of

RUQ
Liver
Gallbladder
Duodenum
Pancreas
(R) Kidney
Hepatic flexure

RLQ
Cecum
Appendix
(R) Ovary & tube

LUQ
Stomach
Spleen
(L) Kidney
Pancreas
Splenic flexure

LLQ
Sigmoid colon
(L) Ovary & tube

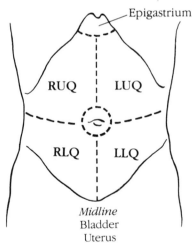

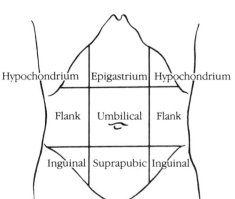

Figure 8–37
Superficial topography of the abdomen. (A) Four-quadrant system. RUQ = right upper quadrant; RLQ = right lower quadrant; LUQ = left upper quadrant; LLQ = left lower quadrant. (B) Nine-regions system. (From Judge, R.D., G.D. Zuidema, and F.T. Fitzgerald: Clinical Diagnosis: A Physiologic Approach. Boston, Little, Brown & Co., 1982, p. 284.)

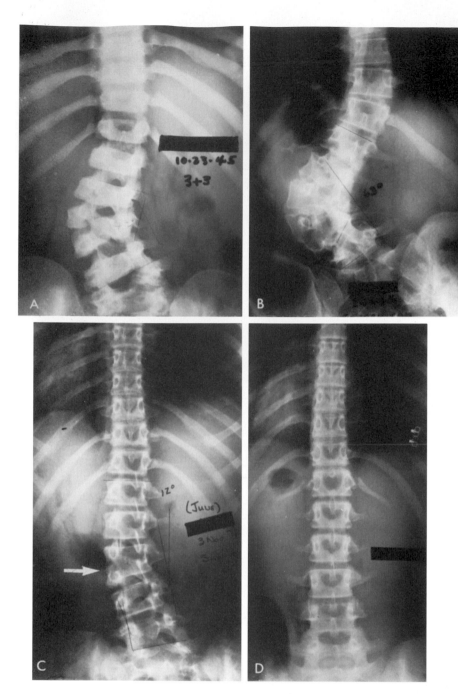

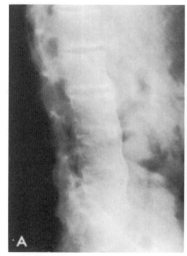
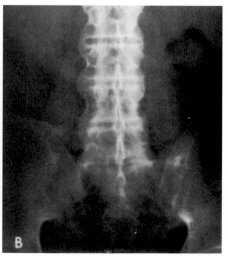

Figure 8–38

Structural scoliosis caused by congenital defect. (A) Left midlumbar and right lumbosacral hemivertebrae in a 3-year-old child (example of hemimetameric shift). (B) A first cousin also demonstrates a midlumbar hemivertebra as well as asymmetric development of the upper sacrum. (C) This girl has a semisegmented hemivertebra (*arrow*) in the midlumbar spine with a mild 12° curve. (D) Her identical twin sister showed no congenital anomalies of the spine. (From Moe, J.H., D.S. Bradford, R.B. Winter, and J.E. Lonstein: Scoliosis and Other Spinal Deformities. Philadelphia, W.B. Saunders Co., 1978, p. 134.)

Figure 8–39

Ankylosing spondylitis of spine. Note the bony encasement of vertebral bodies on the lateral view (A) and the bamboo effect on the anteroposterior view (B). (From Gartland, J.J.: Fundamentals of Orthopedics. Philadelphia, W.B. Saunders Co., 1979, p. 147.)

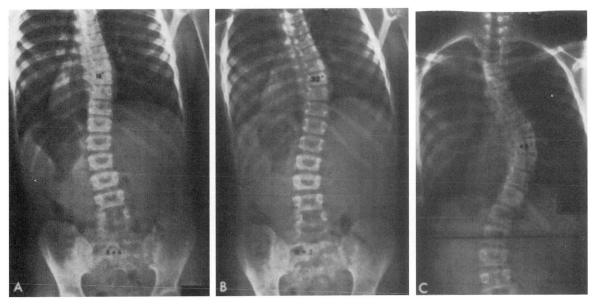

Figure 8–40
The natural history of idiopathic scoliosis. (A) Note the mild degree of vertebral rotation and curvature and the imbalance of the upper torso. (B) Note the rather dramatic increase in curvature and the increased rotation of the apical vertebrae 1 year later. (C) Further progression of the curvature has occurred, and the opportunity for brace treatment has been missed. (From Bunnel, W.P.: Treatment of idiopathic scoliosis. Orthop. Clin. North Am. 10:817, 1979.)

positive findings with no comparable history of musculo-skeletal origin could lead the examiner to believe the problem was not of a musculoskeletal origin.

Diagnostic Imaging

Plain Film Radiography

Anteroposterior View. With this view (Fig. 8–38), the examiner should note the following:

1. Any wedging of the vertebrae
2. Whether the disc spaces appear normal
3. Whether the ring epiphysis, if present, is normal
4. Whether there is a "bamboo" spine, indicative of ankylosing spondylitis (Fig. 8–39)
5. Any scoliosis (Fig. 8–40)
6. Malposition of heart and lungs
7. Normal symmetry of the ribs

Lateral View. The examiner should note the following:

1. A normal mild kyphosis
2. Any wedging of the vertebrae, which may be an indication of structural kyphosis resulting from conditions such as Scheuermann's disease or wedge fracture (Fig. 8–41)
3. Whether the disc spaces appear normal
4. Whether the ring epiphysis, if present, is normal
5. Whether there are any **Schmorl's nodules,** indicating herniation of the intervertebral disc into the vertebral body

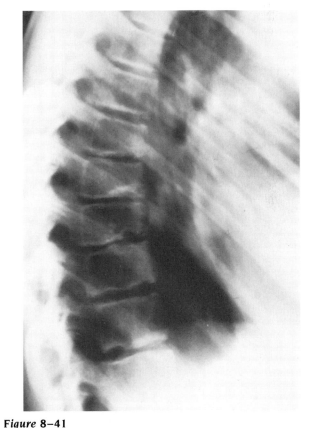

Figure 8–41
Classic radiographic appearance of the spine in a patient with Scheuermann's disease. Note the wedged vertebra, Schmorl's nodules, and marked irregularity of the vertebral end plates. (From Moe, J.H., D.S. Bradford, R.B. Winter, and J.E. Lonstein: Scoliosis and Other Spinal Deformities. Philadelphia, W.B. Saunders Co., 1978, p. 32.)

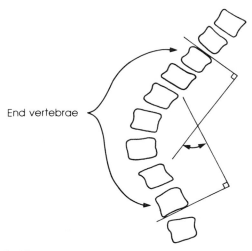

Figure 8–42
Cobb method of measuring scoliotic curve.

6. Angle of the ribs
7. Any osteophytes

Measurement of Spinal Curvature for Scoliosis. With the **Cobb method** (Fig. 8–42), an anteroposterior view is used.[9] A line is drawn parallel to the superior cortical plate of the proximal end vertebra and to the inferior cortical plate of the distal end vertebra. A perpendicular line is erected to each of these lines, and the angle of intersection of the perpendicular lines is the angle of spinal curvature resulting from scoliosis. Such techniques have led the Scoliosis Research Society to classify all forms of scoliosis according to the degree of curvature: group 1, 0 to 20°; group 2, 21 to 30°; group 3, 31 to 50°; group 4, 51 to 75°; group 5, 76 to 100°; group 6, 101 to 125°; and group 7, 126° or greater.[10] Other noninvasive methods of measuring the curve have been

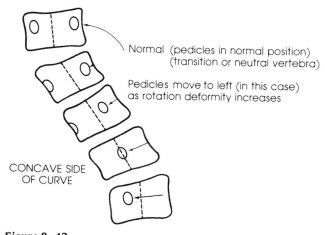

Figure 8–43
Rotation of vertebra in scoliosis. On radiography, the pedicles appear to be off center as the curve progresses.

advocated. However, the examiner should use the same method each time for consistency and reliability.[17, 18]

The rotation of the vertebrae may also be estimated from an anteroposterior view (Fig. 8–43). This estimation is best done by the **pedicle method,** in which the examiner determines the relation of the pedicles to the lateral margins of the vertebral bodies. The vertebra is in neutral position when the pedicles appear to be at equal distance from the lateral margin of the peripheral bodies on the film. If rotation is evident, the pedicles appear to move laterally toward the concavity of the curve.

Computed Tomography

Computed tomography is of primary use in evaluating the bony spine, the spinal contents, and the surrounding soft tissues in cross-sectional views.

Magnetic Resonance Imaging

Magnetic resonance imaging (MRI) is a noninvasive technique that is useful for delineating soft tissue, including herniated discs and intrinsic spinal cord lesions, as well as bony tissue (Fig. 8–44). However, MRI should be used only to confirm a clinical diagnosis, because conditions such as disc herniation have been demonstrated on MRI in the absence of clinical symptoms.[19]

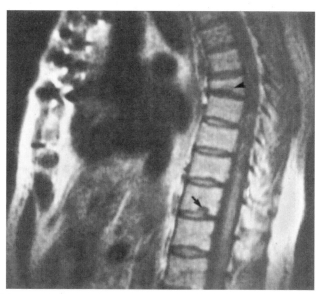

Figure 8–44
Osteoporotic compression fracture of thoracic spine. Midline sagittal T1-weighted magnetic resonance image (SE 500/30) shows compression fracture of upper thoracic vertebral body (*arrowhead*), indicated by anterior wedging. Marrow signal intensity is maintained (*arrowhead*). Schmorl's nodule is incidentally noted at a lower level (*arrow*). (From Bassett, L.W., R.H. Gold, and L.L. Seeger: MRI Atlas of the Musculoskeletal System. London, Martin Dunitz Ltd., 1989, p. 49.)

Précis of the Thoracic Spine Assessment*

History
Observation (standing)
Examination
    Active movements (standing or sitting)
        Forward flexion
        Extension
        Side flexion (left and right)
        Rotation (left and right)
        Combined movements (if necessary)
        Repetitive movements (if necessary)
        Sustained postures (if necessary)
    Passive movements (sitting)
        Forward flexion
        Extension
        Side flexion (left and right)
        Rotation (left and right)
    Resisted isometric movements (sitting)
        Forward flexion
        Extension
        Side flexion (left and right)
        Rotation (left and right)

Special tests (sitting)
Reflexes and cutaneous distribution (sitting)
    Reflex testing (?)
    Sensation scan
Special tests (prone lying)
Joint play movements (prone lying)
    Posteroanterior central vertebral pressure
    Posteroanterior unilateral vertebral pressure
    Transverse vertebral pressure
    Rib springing
Palpation (prone lying)
Palpation (supine lying)
Diagnostic imaging

---

* The précis is shown in an order that limits the amount of movement that the patient has to do but ensures that all necessary structures are tested.

After any assessment, the patient should be warned of the possibility of exacerbation of symptoms as a result of assessment.

Case Studies

When doing these case studies, the examiner should list the appropriate questions to be asked and why they are being asked, what to look for and why, and what things should be tested and why. Depending on the answers of the patient (and the examiner should consider different responses), several possible causes of the patient's problems may be evident (examples are given in parentheses). If so, a differential diagnosis chart (see Table 8–5 as an example) should be made up. The examiner can then decide how different diagnoses may affect the treatment plan.

1. A 33-year-old patient comes to you complaining of stiffness in the lower spine that is extending into the thoracic spine. Describe your assessment plan for this patient (ankylosing spondylitis versus thoracic spinal stenosis).

2. A 14-year-old boy presents complaining of a severe aching pain in the middorsal spine of several weeks' duration. He is neurologically normal. X-rays reveal a narrowing and anterior wedging at T5 with a Schmorl's nodule into T4. Describe your assessment plan for this patient (kyphosis versus Scheuermann's disease).

3. A 23-year-old woman has a structural scoliosis with a single C curve having its apex at T7. Describe your assessment plan before beginning treatment. How would you measure the curve and the amount of rotation?

Table 8–5
Differential Diagnosis of Ankylosing Spondylitis and Thoracic Spinal Stenosis

	Ankylosing Spondylitis	Thoracic Spinal Stenosis
History	Morning stiffness Male predominance Sharp pain → ache Bilateral sacroiliac pain may refer to posterior thigh	Intermittent aching pain Pain may refer to both legs with walking (neurogenic intermittant claudication)
Active movements	Restricted	May be normal
Passive movements	Restricted	May be normal
Resisted isometric movements	Normal	Normal
Special tests	None	Bicycle test of van Gelderen may be positive Stoop test may be positive
Reflexes	Normal	May be affected in long-standing cases
Sensory deficit	None	Usually temporary
Diagnostic imaging	Plain films are diagnostic	Computed tomography scans are diagnostic

4. A 38-year-old woman comes to your clinic complaining of chest pain with tenderness at the costochondral junction of two ribs on the left side. Describe your assessment plan for this patient (Tietze's syndrome versus rib hypomobility).

5. A 26-year-old male ice hockey player comes to you complaining of back pain that is referred around the chest. He explains that he was "boarded" (hit between another player and the boards). He did not notice the pain and stiffness until the next day. He has had the problem for 2 weeks. Describe your assessment plan for this patient (rib hypomobility versus ligament sprain).

6. A 21-year-old female synchronized swimmer comes to you complaining of pain in her side. She says she was kicked when she helped boost another athlete out of the water 5 days ago. Describe your assessment plan for this patient (rib fracture versus rib hypomobility).

References

Cited References

1. Williams, P., and R. Warwick (eds.): Gray's Anatomy, 36th British ed. Edinburgh, Churchill Livingstone, 1980.
2. MacConaill, M.A., and J.V. Basmajian: Muscles and Movements: A Basis for Human Kinesiology. Baltimore, Williams & Wilkins, 1969.
3. Mitchell, F.L., P.S. Moran, and N.A. Pruzzo: An Evaluation and Treatment Manual of Osteopathic Muscle Energy Procedures. Valley Park, Missouri, Mitchell, Moran & Pruzzo, Assoc., 1979.
4. Henderson, J.M.: Ruling out danger: Differential diagnosis of thoracic spine. Phys. Sportsmed. 20:124–132, 1992.
5. Dreyfuss, P., C. Tibiletti, and S.J. Dreyer: Thoracic zygapophyseal joint pain patterns: A study in normal volunteers. Spine 19:807–811, 1994.
6. Ombregt, L., P. Bisschop, H.J. ter Veer, and T. Van de Velde: A System of Orthopedic Medicine. London, W.B. Saunders Co., 1995.
7. McKenzie, R.A.: The Cervical and Thoracic Spine: Mechanical Diagnosis and Therapy. Waikanae, New Zealand, Spinal Publications Ltd., 1981.
8. Wiles, P., and R. Sweetnam: Essentials of Orthopaedics. London, J.A. Churchill, 1965.
9. Keim, H.A.: Scoliosis. Clin. Symposia 25:1–25, 1973.
10. Keim, H.A.: The Adolescent Spine. New York, Springer-Verlag, 1982.
11. Sutherland, I.D.: Funnel chest. J. Bone Joint Surg. Br. 40:244–251, 1958.
12. Evans, R.C.: Illustrated Essentials in Orthopedic Physical Assessment. St. Louis, C.V. Mosby Co., 1994.
13. Stoddard, A.: Manual of Osteopathic Technique. London, Hutchinson Medical Publications, 1959.
14. Maitland, G.D.: The slump test: Examination and treatment. Aust. J. Physiother. 31:215–219, 1985.
15. Cyriax, J.: Textbook of Orthopaedic Medicine, vol. 1: Diagnosis of Soft Tissue Lesions. London, Bailliere Tindall, 1982.
16. Maitland, G.D.: Vertebral Manipulation. London, Butterworths, 1973.
17. Pearsall, D.J., J.G. Reid, and D.M. Hedden: Comparison of three noninvasive methods for measuring scoliosis. Phys. Ther. 72:648–657, 1992.
18. Pun, W.K., K.D. Luk, W. Lee, and J.C. Leong: A simple method to estimate the rib hump in scoliosis. Spine 12:342–345, 1987.
19. Wood, K.B., T.A. Garvey, C. Gundry, and K.B. Heithoff: Magnetic resonance imaging of the thoracic spine. J. Bone Joint Surg. Am. 77:1631–1638, 1995.

General References

Adams, J.C.: Outline of Orthopaedics. London, E & S Livingstone, 1968.
American Orthopaedic Association: Manual of Orthopaedic Surgery. Chicago, 1972.
Bassett, L.W., R.H. Gold, and L.L. Seeger: MRI Atlas of the Musculoskeletal System. London, Martin Dunitz Ltd., 1989.
Beetham, W.P., H.F. Polley, C.H. Stocumb, and W.F. Weaver: Physical Examination of the Joints. Philadelphia, W.B. Saunders Co., 1965.
Blair, J.M.: Examination of the thoracic spine. In Grieve, G.P. (ed.): Modern Manual Therapy of the Vertebral Column. Edinburgh, Churchill Livingstone, 1986.
Bourdillon, J.R.: Spinal Manipulation, 4th ed. New York, Appleton-Century-Crofts, 1987.
Bowling, R.W., and P. Rockar: Thoracic spine. In Richardson, J.K., and Z.A. Iglarsh: Clinical Orthopedic Physical Therapy. Philadelphia, W.B. Saunders Co., 1994.
Bradford, D.S.: Juvenile kyphosis. Clin. Orthop. 128:45–55, 1977.
Bradford, D.S., J.E. Lonstein, J.H. Moe, J.W. Ogilvie, and R.B. Winter: Moe's Textbook of Scoliosis and Other Spinal Deformities. Philadelphia, W.B. Saunders Co., 1987.
Brashear, H.R., and R.B. Raney: Shand's Handbook of Orthopaedic Surgery. St. Louis, C.V. Mosby Co., 1978.
Bunnel, W.P.: Treatment of idopathic scoliosis. Orthop. Clin. North Am. 10:813–827, 1979.
Burwell, R.G., N.J. James, F. Johnson, J.K. Webb, and Y.G. Wilson: Standardized trunk asymmetry scores: A study of back contour in healthy school children. J. Bone Joint Surg. Br. 65:452–463, 1983.
Cacayorin, E.D., L. Hochhauser, and G.R. Petro: Lumbar and thoracic spine pain in the athlete: Radiographic evaluation. Clin. Sports Med. 6:767–783, 1987.
Cailliet, R.: Scoliosis: Diagnosis and Management. Philadelphia, F.A. Davis Co., 1975.
Drummond, D.S., E. Rogala, and J. Gurr: Spinal deformity: Natural history and the role of school screening. Orthop. Clin. North Am. 10:751–759, 1979.
Duval-Beaupre, G.: Rib hump and supine angle as prognostic factors for mild scoliosis. Spine 17:103–107, 1992.
Edgelow, P.E., A.C. Lescak, and M. Jewell: Trunk. In Myers, R.S. (ed.): Saunders Manual of Physical Therapy Practice. Philadelphia, W.B. Saunders Co., 1995.
Gartland, J.J.: Fundamentals of Orthopaedics. London, E & S Livingstone, 1968.
Goldstein, L.A., and T.R. Waugh: Classification and terminology of scoliosis. Clin. Orthop. 93:10–22, 1973.
Goodman, C.C., and T.E. Snyder: Differential Diagnosis in Physical Therapy. Philadelphia, W.B. Saunders Co., 1995.
Gould, J.A.: The spine. In Gould, J.A. (ed.): Orthopedic and Sports Physical Therapy. St. Louis, C.V. Mosby Co., 1990.
Gregersen, G.G., and D.B. Lucas: An in vivo study of the axial rotation of the human thoracolumbar spine. J. Bone Joint Surg. Am. 49:247–262, 1967.
Grieve, G.P.: Common Vertebral Joint Problems. Edinburgh, Churchill Livingstone, 1981.
Grieve, G.P.: Mobilisation of the Spine. Edinburgh, Churchill Livingstone, 1979.
Grieve, G.P.: Thoracic musculoskeletal problems. In Boyling, J.D., and N. Palastanga (eds.): Grieve's Modern Manual Therapy of the Vertebral Column. Edinburgh, Churchill Livingstone, 1994.

Hollingshead, W.H., and D.R. Jenkins: Functional Anatomy of the Limbs and Back. Philadelphia, W.B. Saunders Co., 1981.

Hoppenfeld, S.: Physical Examination of the Spine and Extremities. New York, Appleton-Century-Crofts, 1976.

Houpt, J.B.: The shoulder girdle. In Little, H. (ed.): The Rheumatological Physical Examination. Orlando, Florida, Grune & Stratton, 1986.

Howley, P.: The thoracic and abdominal region. In Zulauga, M., C. Briggs, J. Carlisle, et al. (eds.): Sports Physiotherapy: Applied Science and Practice. Melbourne, Churchill Livingstone, 1995.

James, J.J.P.: The etiology of scoliosis. J. Bone Joint Surg. Br. 52:410–419, 1970.

Judge, R.D., G.D. Zuidema, and F.T. Fitzgerald: Clinical Diagnosis: A Physiologic Approach. Boston, Little, Brown & Co., 1982.

Kapandji, I.A.: The Physiology of the Joints, vol. 3: The Trunk and Vertebral Column. New York, Churchill Livingstone, 1974.

Levene, D.L.: Chest Pain: An Integrated Diagnostic Approach. Philadelphia, Lea & Febiger, 1977.

Liebgott, B.: The Anatomical Basis of Dentistry. Philadelphia, W.B. Saunders Co., 1982.

Loder, R.T., A. Urquhart, H. Steen, et al.: Variability in Cobb angle measurements in children with congenital scoliosis. J. Bone Joint Surg. Br. 77:768–773, 1995.

Love, R.M., and R.R. Brodeur: Inter- and intra-examiner reliability of motion palpation for the thoracolumbar spine. J. Manip. Physiol. Ther. 10:1–4, 1987.

Maigne, R.: Orthopaedic Medicine: A New Approach to Vertebral Manipulation. Springfield, Illinois, Charles C. Thomas, 1972.

Maigne, R.: Diagnosis and Treatment of Pain of Vertebral Origin: A Manual Medicine Approach. Baltimore, Williams & Wilkins Co., 1996.

Margarey, M.E.: Examination of the cervical and thoracic spine. In Grant, R. (ed.): Physical Therapy of the Cervical and Thoracic Spine, Clinics in Physical Therapy. Edinburgh, Churchill Livingstone, 1988.

Moll, J.H., and V. Wright: Measurement of spinal movement. In Jayson, M. (ed.): Lumbar Spine and Back Pain. New York, Grune & Stratton, Inc., 1976.

Moll, J.M.H., and V. Wright: An objective clinical study of chest expansion. Ann. Rheum. Dis. 31:1, 1972.

Nash, C.L., and J.H. Moe: A study of vertebral rotation. J. Bone Joint Surg. Am. 51:223–229, 1969.

O'Donoghue, D.H.: Treatment of Injuries to Athletes, 4th ed. Philadelphia, W.B. Saunders Co., 1984.

Papaioannu, T., L. Stokes, and J. Kenwright: Scoliosis associated with limb length inequality. J. Bone Joint Surg. Am. 64:59–62, 1982.

Raine, S., and L.T. Twomey: Validation of a non-invasive method of measuring the surface curvature of the erect spine. J. Man. Manip. Ther. 2:11–21, 1994.

Rothman, R.H., and F.A. Simeone: The Spine. Philadelphia, W.B. Saunders Co., 1982.

Simmons, E.H.: Kyphotic deformity of the spine in ankylosing spondylitis. Clin. Orthop. 128:65–77, 1977.

Sturrock, R.D., J.A. Wojtulewski, and F.D. Hart: Spondylometry in a normal population and in ankylosing spondylitis. Rheumatol. Rehabil. 12:135–142, 1973.

Travell, J.G., and D.G. Simons: Myofascial Pain and Dysfunction: The Trigger Point Manual. Baltimore, Williams & Wilkins Co., 1983.

Tsou, P.M.: Embryology of congenital kyphosis. Clin. Orthop. 128:18–25, 1977.

Tsou, P.M., A. Yau, and A.R. Hodgson: Embryogenesis and prenatal development of congenital vertebral anomalies and their classification. Clin. Orthop. 152:211–231, 1980.

Watkins, R.G.: Thoracic pain syndromes. In Watkins, R.C. (ed.): The Spine in Sports. St. Louis, C.V. Mosby Co., 1996.

White, A.A.: Kinematics of the normal spine as related to scoliosis. J. Biomech. 4:405–411, 1971.

Whiteside, T.E.: Traumatic kyphosis of the thoracolumbar spine. Clin. Orthop. 128:78–92, 1977.

Wyke, B.: Morphological and functional features of the innervation of the costovertebral joints. Folia Morphol. (Warsz) 23:296, 1975.

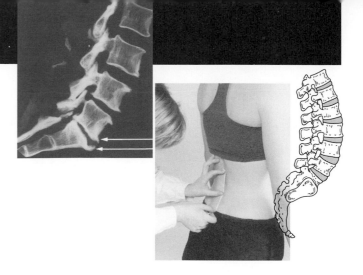

9

Lumbar Spine

Back pain is one of the great human afflictions. Almost anyone born today in Europe or North America has a great chance of suffering a disabling back injury regardless of occupation. The lumbar spine furnishes support for the upper body and transmits the weight of the upper body to the pelvis and lower limbs. Because of the strategic location of the lumbar spine, this structure should be included in any examination of the spine as a whole (i.e., posture) or in any examination of the hip and/or sacroiliac joints. Unless there is a definite history of trauma, it is often very difficult to determine whether an injury originates in the lumbar spine, sacroiliac joints, or hip joints; therefore, all three should be examined in a sequential fashion.

Applied Anatomy

There are 10 (five pairs) of facet joints in the lumbar spine (Fig. 9–1). These diarthrodial joints consist of superior and inferior facets and a capsule. The facets are located on the vertebral arches. Injury, degeneration, or trauma may lead to **spondylosis** (degeneration of the intervertebral disc), **spondylolysis** (a defect in the pars

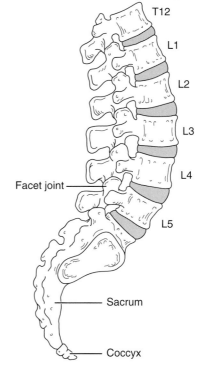

Figure 9–1
Lateral view of the lumbar spine.

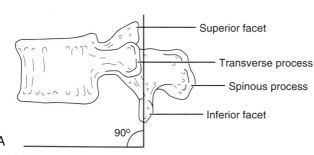

Figure 9–2
Lumbar vertebra. (A) Side view. (B) Superior view.

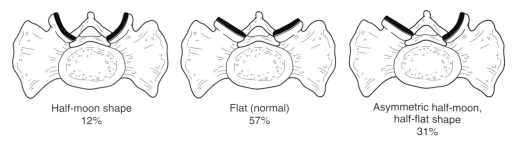

Half-moon shape
12%

Flat (normal)
57%

Asymmetric half-moon,
half-flat shape
31%

Figure 9–3
Facet anomalies (tropisms) at L5–S1.

interarticularis or the arch), or **spondylolisthesis** (a forward displacement of one vertebra over another). The superior facets, or articular processes, face medially and backward and in general are concave; the inferior facets face laterally and forward and are convex (Fig. 9–2). There are, however, abnormalities, or **tropisms,** that can occur in the shape of the facets, especially at the L5–S1 level (Fig. 9–3).[1]

These posterior, apophyseal, or facet joints direct the movement that occurs in the lumbar spine. Because of the shape of the facets, rotation in the lumbar spine is minimal and is accomplished only by a shearing force. Side flexion, extension, and flexion can occur in the lumbar spine, but the direction of movement is controlled by the facet joints. The close packed position of the facet joints in the lumbar spine is extension. Normally, the facet joints are not weight bearing; with increased extension, however, they begin to have a weight-bearing function. The resting position is midway between flexion and extension. The capsular pattern is side flexion and rotation equally limited, followed by extension. However, if only one facet joint in the lumbar spine has a capsular restriction, the amount of observable restriction is minimal. The first sacral segment is usually included in discussions of the lumbar spine, and it is at this joint that the fixed segment of the sacrum joins with the mobile segments of the lumbar spine. In some cases, the S1 segment may be mobile. This occurrence is called **lumbarization** of S1, and it results in a sixth "lumbar" vertebra. At other times, the fifth lumbar segment may be fused to the sacrum and ilium, resulting in a **sacralization** of that vertebra. Sacralization results in four mobile lumbar vertebrae.

The intervertebral discs make up approximately 20 to 25% of the total length of the vertebral column. The function of the intervertebral disc is to act as a shock absorber distributing and absorbing some of the load applied to the spine, to hold the vertebrae together and allow movement between the bones, to separate the vertebra as part of a functional segmental unit acting in concert with the facet joints (Fig. 9–4), and, by separating the vertebrae, to allow the free passage of the nerve roots out from the spinal cord through the intervertebral foramina. With age, the percentage of spinal length attributable to the discs decreases as a result of disc degeneration and loss of hydrophilic action in the disc.

The **annulus fibrosus,** the outer laminated portion of the disc, consists of three zones: (1) an outer zone made up of fibrocartilage (classified as **Sharpey's fibers**) that attaches to the outer or peripheral aspect of the vertebral body and contains increasing numbers of carti-

	Lumbar Spine	
Resting position:	Midway between flexion and extension	
Close packed position:	Extension	
Capsular pattern:	Side flexion and rotation equally limited, extension	

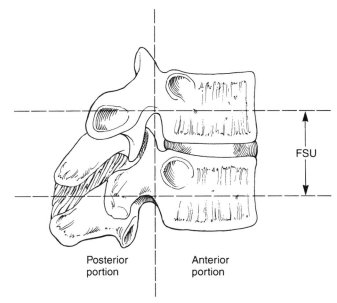

FSU

Posterior portion

Anterior portion

Figure 9–4
Functional segmental unit (three-joint complex) in the thoracic spine. Such a complex may also be seen in the cervical and lumbar spines. (From Dyrek, D.A., L.J. Micheli, and D.J. Magee: Injuries to the Thoracolumbar Spine and Pelvis. In Zachazewski, J.E., D.J. Magee, and W.S. Quillen [eds.]: Athletic Injuries and Rehabilitation. Philadelphia, W.B. Saunders Co., 1996, p. 468.)

lage cells in the fibrous strands with increasing depth; (2) an intermediate zone made up of another layer of fibrocartilage; and (3) an inner zone primarily made up of fibrocartilage and containing the largest number of cartilage cells.[2] The annulus fibrosus contains 20 concentric, collarlike rings of collagenous fibers that criss-cross each other to increase their strength and accommodate torsion movements.[3]

The **nucleus pulposus** is well developed in both the cervical and the lumbar spines. At birth, it is made up of a hydrophilic mucoid tissue, which is gradually replaced by fibrocartilage. With increasing age, the nucleus pulposus increasingly resembles the annulus fibrosus. The water-binding capacity of the disc decreases with age, and degenerative changes (spondylosis) begin to occur after the second decade of life. Initially, the disc contains approximately 85 to 90% water, but the amount decreases to 65% with age.[4] In addition, the disc contains a high proportion of mucopolysaccharides, which cause the disc to act as an incompressible fluid. However, these mucopolysaccharides decrease with age and are replaced with collagen. The nucleus pulposus lies slightly posterior to the center of rotation of the disc in the lumbar spine.

The shape of the disc corresponds to that of the body to which it is attached. The disc adheres to the vertebral body by means of the cartilaginous end plate. The end plates consist of thin layers of cartilage covering the inferior and superior surfaces of the vertebral body. The cartilaginous end plates are approximately 1 mm thick and allow fluid to move between the disc and the vertebral body. The discs are primarily avascular, with only the periphery receiving a blood supply. The remainder of the disc receives nutrition by diffusion, primarily through the cartilaginous end plate. Until the age of 8 years, the intervertebral discs have some vascularity; however, this vascularity decreases with age.

Usually, the intervertebral disc has no nerve supply, although the peripheral posterior aspect of the annulus fibrosus may be innervated by a few nerve fibers from the sinuvertebral nerve.[5, 6] The lateral aspects of the disc are innervated peripherally by the branches of the anterior rami and gray rami communicantes. The pain-sensitive structures around the intervertebral disc are the anterior longitudinal ligament, posterior longitudinal ligament, vertebral body, nerve root, and cartilage of the facet joint.

With the movement of fluid vertically through the cartilaginous end plate, the pressure on the disc is decreased as the patient assumes the natural lordotic posture in the lumbar spine. Direct vertical pressure on the disc can cause the disc to push fluid into the vertebral body. If the pressure is great enough, defects may occur in the cartilaginous end plate, resulting in **Schmorl's nodules,** which are herniations of the nucleus pulposus into the vertebral body. Normally, an adult is 1 to 2 cm (0.4 to 0.8 inch) taller in the morning than in the evening. This change results from fluid movement in and out of the disc during the day through the cartilaginous end plate. This fluid shift acts as a safety valve to protect the disc.

If there is an injury to the disc, four problems can result. There may be a **protrusion** of the disc, in which the disc bulges posteriorly without rupture of the annulus fibrosus. In the case of a disc **prolapse,** only the outermost fibers of the annulus fibrosus contain the nucleus. With a disc **extrusion,** the annulus fibrosus is perforated, and discal material (part of the nucleus pulposus) moves into the epidural space. The fourth problem is a **sequestrated** disc, or a formation of discal fragments from the annulus fibrosus and nucleus pulposus outside the disc proper (Fig. 9–5).[7]

Within the lumbar spine, different postures can increase the pressure on the intervertebral disc (Fig. 9–6). This information is based on the work of Nachemson and coworkers,[8, 9] who performed studies of intradiscal pressure changes in the L3 disc with changes in posture. The pressure in the standing position is classified as the

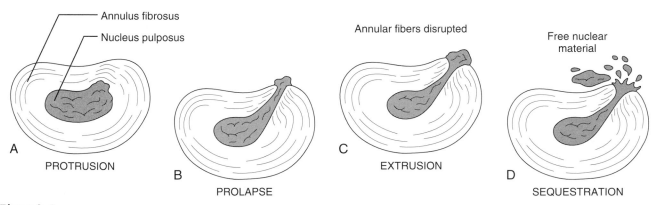

Figure 9–5
Types of disc herniations.

A   PROTRUSION

B   PROLAPSE

C   EXTRUSION

D   SEQUESTRATION

Annulus fibrosus
Nucleus pulposus

Annular fibers disrupted

Free nuclear material

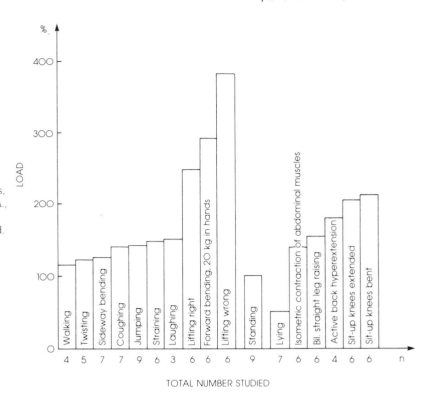

Figure 9-6

Mean change in load on L3 disc with various activities, compared with upright standing. (From Nachemson, A., and C. Elfstrom: Intravital dynamic pressure measurements in lumbar discs. Scand. J. Rehabil. Med. [Suppl. 1]:31, 1970.)

norm, and the values given are increases or decreases above or below this norm that occur with the change in posture.

Activity and Percentage Increase in Disc Pressure at L3

Coughing or straining:	5 to 35%
Laughing:	40 to 50%
Walking:	15%
Side bending:	25%
Small jumps:	40%
Bending forward:	150%
Rotation:	20%
Lifting a 20-kg weight with the back straight and knees bent:	73%
Lifting a 20-kg weight with the back bent and knees straight:	169%

In the lumbar spine, the nerve roots exit through relatively large intervertebral foramina, and each one is named for the vertebra above it. For example, the L4 nerve root exits between the L4 and L5 vertebrae. Because of this arrangement and the course of the nerve root, the L4 disc (between L4 and L5) only rarely compresses the L4 nerve root; it is more likely to compress the L5 nerve root (Fig. 9-7).

In general, the L5-S1 segment is the most common

site of problems in the vertebral column because this level bears more weight than any other vertebral level. The center of gravity passes directly through this vertebra, which is of benefit because it may decrease the shearing stresses to this segment. There is a transition

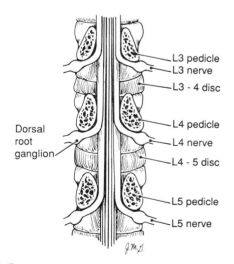

Figure 9-7

A coronal schematic view of the exiting lumbar spinal nerve roots. Note that the exiting root takes the name of the vertebral body under which it travels into the neural foramen. Because of the way the nerve roots exit, L4-L5 disc pathology usually affects the L5 root rather than the L4 root. (From Borenstein, D.G., S.W. Wiesel, and S.D. Boden: Low Back Pain: Medical Diagnosis and Comprehensive Management. Philadelphia, W.B. Saunders Co., 1995, p. 5.)

from the mobile segment, L5, to the stable or fixed segment of the sacrum, which can increase the stress on this area. Because the angle between L5 and S1 is greater than those between the other vertebrae, this joint has a greater chance of having stress applied to it. Another factor that increases the amount of stress on this area is the relatively greater amount of movement that occurs at this level compared with other levels of the lumbar spine.

Patient History

In addition to the questions listed under Patient History in Chapter 1, the examiner should obtain the following information from the patient:

1. What is the patient's age? Different conditions affect patients at different ages. For example, disc prob-

Table 9–1
Some Implications of Painful Reactions

Activity	Reaction of Pain	Possible Structural and Pathological Implications
Lying sleeping	↓	Decreased compressive forces—low intradiscal pressures Absence of forces produced by muscle activity
	↑	Change of position—noxious mechanical stress Decreased mechanoreceptor input Motor segment "relaxed" into a position compromising affected structure Poor external support (bed) Nonmusculoskeletal cause
First rising (stiffness)	↑	Nocturnal imbibition of fluid, disc volume greatest Mechanical inflammatory component Prolonged stiffness, active inflammatory disease (e.g., ankylosing spondylitis)
Sitting	↑	Compressive forces High intradiscal pressure
With extension	↓	Intradiscal pressure reduced Decreased paraspinal muscle activity
	↑	Greater compromise of structures of lateral and central canals Compressive forces on lower apophyseal joints
With flexion	↓	Little compressive load on lower apophyseal joints Greater volume lateral and central canals Reduced disc bulge posteriorly
	↑	Very high intradiscal pressures Increased compressive loads upper and mid apophyseal joints
Prolonged sitting	↑	Gradual creep of tissues
Sitting to standing	↑	Creep, time for reversal, difficulty in straightening up Extension of spine, increase disc bulge posteriorly

Walking	↑	Shock loads greater than body weight
		Compressive loads (vertical creep)
		Leg pain
		   Neurological claudication
		   Vascular claudication

Driving	↑	Sitting: compressive forces Vibration: vibro creep repetitive loading, decreased hysteresis loading, decreased hysteresis Increased dural tension sitting with legs extended Short hamstrings: pull lumbar spine into greater flexion
Coughing, sneezing, straining	↑	Increased pressure subarachnoid space (increased blood flow, Batson's plexus, compromises space in lateral and central canal) Increased intradiscal pressure Mechanical "jarring" of sudden uncontrolled movement

From Jull, G.A.: Examination of the lumbar spine. In Grieve, G.P. (ed.): Modern Manual Therapy of the Vertebral Column. Edinburgh, Churchill Livingstone, 1986, p. 553.

lems usually occur between the ages of 15 and 40 years, and ankylosing spondylitis is evident between 18 and 45 years. Osteoarthritis and spondylosis are more evident in people older than 45 years of age, and malignancy of the spine is most common in people older than 50 years of age.

2. What is the patient's occupation? Back pain tends to be more prevalent in people with strenuous occupations. For example, truck drivers and warehouse workers have a very high incidence of back injury.

3. What is the patient's sex? Lower back pain has a higher incidence in women. Female patients should be asked about any changes that occur with menstruation, such as altered pain patterns, irregular menses, and swelling of the abdomen or breasts. Knowledge of the date of the most recent pelvic examination is also useful. Ankylosing spondylitis is more common in men.

4. What was the mechanism of injury? Lifting commonly causes low back pain (Tables 9–1 and 9–2). This is not surprising when one considers the forces exerted on the lumbar spine and disc. For example, a 77-kg (170-lb) man lifting a 91-kg (200-lb) weight approximately 36 cm (14 inches) from the intervertebral disc exerts a force of 940 kg (2,072 lb) on that disc. The force exerted on the disc can be calculated as roughly 10 times the weight being lifted. Pressure on the intervertebral discs varies depending on the position of the spine. Nachemson and colleagues[8, 9] showed that pressure on the disc can be decreased by increasing the supported inclination of the back rest (e.g., an angle of 130° decreases the pressure on the disc by 50%). Using the arms for support can also decrease the pressure on the disc. When one is standing, the disc pressure is approximately 35% of the pressure that occurs in the relaxed sitting position. The examiner should also keep in mind that stress on the lower back tends to be 15 to 20% higher in men than in women because men are taller and their weight is distributed higher in the body.

5. Where are the sites and boundaries of pain? Have the patient point to the location or locations. Note whether the patient indicates a specific joint or whether the pain is more general. The more specific the pain, the easier it is to localize the area of pathology.

6. Is there any radiation of pain? If so, it is helpful for the examiner to remember and correlate this information with dermatome findings when evaluating sensation.

7. Is the pain deep? Superficial? Shooting? Burning? Aching? Questions related to the depth and type of pain often help to locate the structure injured and the source of pain.

8. Is the pain improving? Worsening? Staying the same? These questions give an indication of whether the condition is acute or chronic.

9. Is there any increase in pain with coughing? Sneezing? Deep breathing? Laughing? All of these actions increase the **intrathecal pressure** (the pressure inside the covering of the spinal cord).

10. Are there any postures or actions that specifically increase or decrease the pain or cause difficulty?[10, 11] For example, if sitting increases the pain and other symptoms, the examiner may suspect that sustained flexion is causing mechanical deformation of the spine. If standing increases the pain and other symptoms, the examiner may suspect that extension, especially relaxed standing, is the cause. If walking increases the pain and other symptoms, extension is probably causing the mechanical deformation, because walking accentuates extension. If lying (especially prone lying) increases the pain and other symptoms, extension may be the cause. Persistent pain or progressive increase in pain while the patient is in the supine position may lead the examiner to suspect neurogenic or space-occupying lesions, such as an infection or tumor. It must be remembered that pain may radiate to the lumbar spine from pathological conditions in other areas as well as from direct mechanical problems. For example, tumors of the pancreas refer pain to the low back. Stiffness and/or pain after rest may be indicative of ankylosing spondylitis or Scheuermann's disease. Pain from mechanical breakdown tends to increase with activity and decrease with rest. Discogenic pain increases if the patient maintains a single posture (especially flexion) for a long period. Pain arising from the spine almost always is influenced by posture and movement.

Table 9–2
Some Mechanisms of Musculoskeletal Pain

Behavior of Pain	Possible Mechanisms
Constant ache	Inflammatory process, venous hypertension
Pain on movement	Noxious mechanical stimulus (stretch, pressure, crush)
Pain accumulates with activity	Repeated mechanical stress Inflammatory process Degenerative disc—hysteresis decreased, less protection from repetitive loading
Pain increases with sustained postures	Fatigue of supporting muscles Gradual creep of tissues may stress affected part of motor unit
Latent nerve root pain	Movement has produced an acute and temporary neurapraxia

From Jull, G.A.: Examination of the lumbar spine, In Grieve, G.P. (ed.): Modern Manual Therapy of the Vertebral Column. Edinburgh, Churchill-Livingstone, 1986, p. 553.

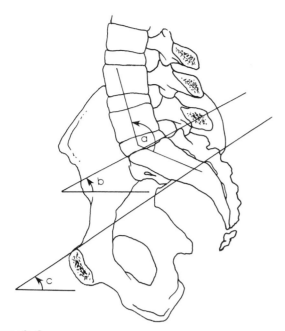

Figure 9–8

Normal angles of the spine and sacrum. a = Lumbosacral angle (140°); b = sacral angle (30°); c = pelvic angle (30°).

The normal lumbosacral angle in the standing position is 140°, the normal sacral angle is 30° (Fig. 9–8), and the normal pelvic angle is 30°. The pelvis is the key to proper back posture. For the pelvis to "sit" properly on the femora, the abdominal, hip flexor, hip extensor, and back extensor muscles must be strong, supple, and balanced (Fig. 9–9). Any deviation in the normal alignment should be noted and recorded. What types of shoes does the patient wear? Heel heights can modify the pelvic angle and lumbar curve, altering the stress on the spine.[12]

11. Is the pain worse in the morning or evening? Does the pain get better or worse as the day progresses? For example, osteoarthritis of the facet joints leads to morning stiffness, which in turn is relieved by activity.

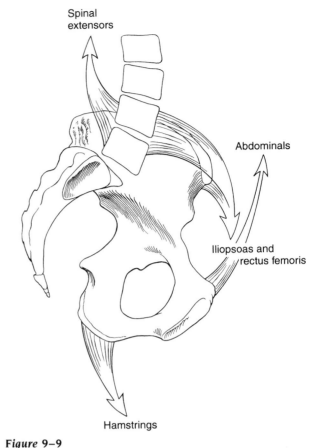

Figure 9–9

Muscles "balancing" the pelvis. (From Dyrek, D.A., L.J. Micheli, and D.J. Magee: Injuries to the Thoracolumbar Spine and Pelvis. In Zachazewski, J.E., D.J. Magee, and W.S. Quillen [eds.]: Athletic Injuries and Rehabilitation. Philadelphia, W.B. Saunders Co., 1996, p. 470.)

12. Which movements hurt? Which movements are stiff? Table 9–3 demonstrates some of the causes of mechanical low back pain and their symptoms. The ex-

Table 9–3
Differential Diagnosis of Mechanical Low Back Pain

	Muscle Strain	Herniated Nucleus Pulposus	Osteoarthritis	Spinal Stenosis	Spondylolisthesis	Scoliosis
Age (yr)	20–40	30–50	>50	>60	20	30
Pain pattern						
Location	Back (unilateral)	Back, leg (unilateral)	Back (unilateral)	Leg (bilateral)	Back	Back
Onset	Acute	Acute (prior episodes)	Insidious	Insidious	Insidious	Insidious
Standing	↑	↓	↑	↑	↑	↑
Sitting	↓	↑	↓	↓	↓	↓
Bending	↑	↑	↓	↓	↑	↑
Straight leg raise	−	+	−	+ (stress)	−	−
Plain x-ray	−	−	+	+	+	+

From Borenstein, D.G., S.W. Wiesel, and S.D. Boden: Low Back Pain: Medical Diagnosis and Comprehensive Management. Philadelphia, W.B. Saunders Co., 1995, p. 189.

aminer must help the patient differentiate between true pain and discomfort that is caused by stretching. **Postural**, or **static, muscles** (e.g., iliopsoas) tend to respond to pathology with tightness in the form of spasm or adaptive shortening; **dynamic**, or **phasic, muscles** (e.g., abdominals) tend to respond with atrophy. Does the patient describe a painful arc of movement on forward or side flexion? If so, it may indicate a disc protrusion with a nerve root riding over the bulge.[11] Patients with lumbar instability or lumbar muscle spasm have trouble moving to the seated position, whereas patients with discogenic pain usually have increased pain in flexion (e.g., sitting).

13. Is paresthesia (a "pins and needles" feeling) or anesthesia present? A sensation or a lack of sensation may be experienced if there is pressure on a nerve root. Paresthesia occurs if pressure is relieved from a nerve trunk; while the pressure is on the nerve trunk, a numb sensation is felt. Does the patient experience any paresthesia or tingling and numbness in the extremities, perineal (saddle) area, or pelvic area? Abnormal sensations in the perineal area often have associated micturition (urination) problems. These symptoms may indicate a myelopathy and are considered by many to be an emergency surgical situation because of potential long-term bowel and bladder problems if the pressure on the spinal cord is not relieved as soon as possible. The examiner

must remember that the adult spinal cord ends at the bottom of the L1 vertebra and becomes the cauda equina within the spinal column. The nerve roots extend in such a way that it is rare for the disc to pinch on the nerve root of the same level. For example, the L5 nerve root is more likely to be compressed by the L4 intervertebral disc than by the L5 intervertebral disc (Fig. 9–10). Seldom is the nerve root compressed by the disc at the same level, except when the protrusion is more lateral.

14. What is the patient's usual activity or pastime? Before the injury, did the patient modify or perform any unusual repetitive or high-stress activity? Such questions help the examiner determine whether the cause of injury was macrotrauma, microtrauma, or a combination of both.

15. Which activities aggravate the pain? Is there anything in the patient's lifestyle that increases the pain? Many common positions assumed by patients are similar to those in some of the provocative special tests. For example, getting into and sitting in a car is similar to the slump test and straight leg raise test. Long sitting in bed is a form of straight leg raise. Reaching up into a cupboard can be similar to an upper limb tension test.

16. Which activities ease the pain? If there are positions that relieve the pain, the examiner should use an understanding of anatomy to determine which tissues

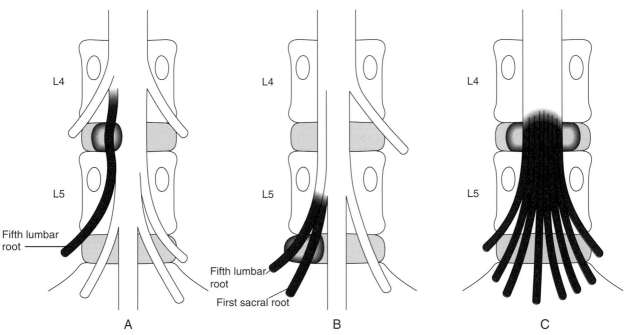

Figure 9–10

Possible effects of disc herniation. (A) Herniation of the disc between L4 and L5 compresses the fifth lumbar root. (B) Large herniation of the L5–S1 disc compromises not only the nerve root crossing it (first sacral nerve root) but also the nerve root emerging through the same foramen (fifth lumbar nerve root). (C) Massive central sequestration of the disc at the L4–L5 level involves all of the nerve roots in the cauda equina and may result in bowel and bladder paralysis. (Redrawn from MacNab, I.: Backache. Baltimore, Williams & Wilkins, 1977, pp. 96–97.)

would have stress taken off them in the pain-relieving postures, and these postures may later be used as resting postures during the treatment.

17. What is the patient's sleeping position? Is there any problem sleeping? What type of mattress is used (hard, soft)? The best sleeping position is in side lying with the legs bent in a semifetal position. If the patient lies prone, the lumbar spine often falls into extension increasing the stress on the posterior elements of the vertebrae. In supine lying, the spine tends to flatten out, decreasing the stress on the posterior elements.

18. Does the patient have any difficulty with micturition? If so, the examiner should proceed with caution, because the condition may involve more than the lumbar spine (e.g., a myelopathy, cauda equina syndrome, tabes dorsalis, tumor, multiple sclerosis). Conversely, these symptoms may result from a disc protrusion or spinal stenosis with minimal or no back pain or sciatica. A disc derangement can cause total urinary retention; chronic, longstanding partial retention; vesicular irritability; or the loss of desire or awareness of the necessity to void.

19. Is the patient receiving any medication? For example, long-term use of steroid therapy can lead to osteoporosis. Also, if the patient has taken medication just before the assessment, the examiner may not get a true reading of the pain.

Observation

The patient must be suitably undressed. Males must wear only shorts, and females must wear only a bra and shorts. When doing the observation, the examiner should note the willingness of the patient to move and the pattern of movement. The patient should be observed for the following traits, first in standing and then sitting position.

Body Type

There are three general body types (see Fig. 15–19): **ectomorphic**—thin body build, characterized by relative prominence of structures developed from the embryonic ectoderm; **mesomorphic**—muscular or sturdy body build, characterized by relative prominence of structures developed from the embryonic mesoderm; and **endomorphic**—heavy (fat) body build, characterized by relative prominence of structures developed from the embryonic endoderm.

Gait

Does the gait appear to be normal when the patient walks into the area, or is it altered in some way? If it is

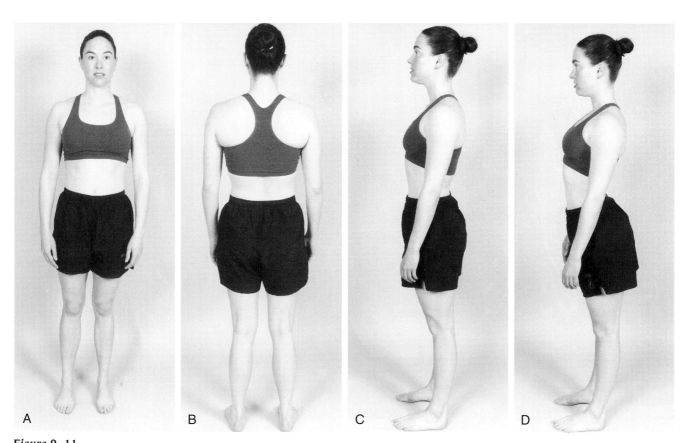

A   B   C   D

Figure 9–11
Views of the patient in the standing position. (A) Anterior view. (B) Posterior view. (C) Lateral view. (D) Lateral view with excessive lordosis.

altered, the examiner must take time to find out whether the problem is in the limb or whether the gait is altered to relieve symptoms elsewhere.

Attitude

Is the patient tense? Bored? Lethargic? What is the appearance of the patient? Healthy looking? Emaciated? Overweight?

Total Spinal Posture

The patient should be examined in the habitual relaxed posture (see Chapter 15) that is usually adopted. With acute back pain, the patient presents with some degree of antalgic (painful) posturing. Usually, a loss of lumbar lordosis and a lateral shift or scoliosis is present. This posturing is involuntary and cannot be reduced because of the muscle spasm.[13, 14]

The patient should be observed anteriorly, laterally, and posteriorly (Fig. 9–11). Anteriorly, the head should be straight on the shoulders, and the nose should be in line with the manubrium sternum and xiphisternum or umbilicus. The shoulders and clavicle should be level and equal, although the dominant side may be slightly lower. The waist angles should be equal. The arbitrary "high" points on both iliac crests should be the same height. If they are not, the possibility of unequal leg length should be considered. The difference in height would indicate a functional limb length discrepancy. This discrepancy could be caused by altered bone length, altered mechanics (e.g., pronated foot on one side), or joint dysfunction (Table 9–4). The anterior superior iliac spines (ASISs) should be level on each side. The patellae should point straight ahead. The lower limbs should be straight and not in genu varum or genu valgum. The heads of the fibulae should be level. The medial malleoli should be level, as should be the lateral malleoli. The medial longitudinal arches of the feet should be evident, and the feet should angle out equally. The arms should be an equal distance from the trunk and equally medially or laterally rotated. Any protrusion or depression of the sternum, ribs, or costocartilage, as well as any bowing of

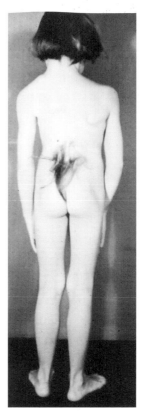

Figure 9–12
Congenital scoliosis and a diastematomyelia in a 9-year-old girl. This type of hairy patch strongly indicates a congenital maldevelopment of the neural axis. (From Rothman, R.H., and F.A. Simeone: The Spine. Philadelphia, W.B. Saunders Co., 1982, p. 371.)

bones, should be noted. The bony or soft-tissue contours should be equal on both sides.

From the side, the examiner should look at the head to ensure that the ear lobe is in line with the tip of the shoulder (acromion process) and the arbitrary high point of the iliac crest. Each segment of the spine should have a normal curve. Are any of the curves exaggerated or decreased? Is lordosis present? Kyphosis? Do the shoulders droop forward? Normally, the ASISs are lower than the posterior superior iliac spines (PSISs). Are the knees straight, flexed, or in recurvatum (hyperextended)?

From behind, the examiner should note the level of the shoulders, spines and inferior angles of the scapula, and any deformities (e.g., a Sprengel's deformity). Any lateral spinal curve (scoliosis) should be noted (Fig. 9–12). The waist angles should be equal from the posterior aspect, as they were from the anterior aspect. The PSISs should be level. The examiner should note whether the PSISs are higher or lower than the ASISs. The gluteal folds and knee joints should be level. The Achilles tendons and heels should appear to be straight. The examiner should note whether there is any protrusion of the ribs or bowing of bones. Does the pelvic angle appear to

Table 9–4
Functional Limb Length Difference

Joint	Functional Lengthening	Functional Shortening
Foot	Supination	Pronation
Knee	Extension	Flexion
Hip	Lowering Extension Lateral rotation	Lifting Flexion Medial rotation
Sacroiliac	Anterior rotation	Posterior rotation

From Wallace, L.A.: Lower quarter pain: Mechanical evaluation and treatment. In Grieve, G.P. (ed.): Modern Manual Therapy of the Vertebral Column. Edinburgh, Churchill Livingstone, 1986, p. 467.

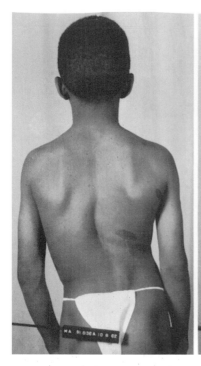
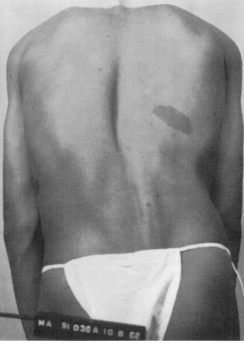

Figure 9–13
Neurofibromatosis with scoliosis. Note the café au lait spots on the right side of the trunk. (From Tachdjian, M.O.: Pediatric Orthopedics. Philadelphia, W.B. Saunders Co., 1990, p. 1290.)

be normal? Any deviation in the normal spinal postural alignment should be noted and recorded. The various possible sources of pathology related to posture are discussed in Chapter 15.

Markings

A "faun's beard" (tuft of hair) may indicate a spina bifida occulta or diastematomyelia (see Fig. 9–12).[15] Café au lait spots may indicate neurofibromatosis or collagen disease (Fig. 9–13). Unusual skin markings or the presence of skin lesions in the midline may lead the examiner to consider the possibility of underlying neural and mesodermal anomalies.

Step Deformity

A step deformity in the lumbar spine may indicate a spondylolisthesis.

Examination

The examiner must remember that when assessing the lumbar spine, referral of symptoms or the presence of neurological symptoms often makes it necessary to "clear" the lower limb. Many of the symptoms that occur in the lower limb may originate in the lumbar spine. Unless there is a history of definitive trauma to a peripheral joint, a screening examination must accompany assessment of that joint to rule out problems within the

lumbar spine referring symptoms to that joint. It is often helpful at this stage to ask the patient to demonstrate the movements that produce or have produced the pain. If the patient is asked to do this, time must be allowed for symptoms to disappear before the remainder of the examination is carried out.

Active Movements

Active movements are performed with the patient standing (Fig. 9–14). The examiner is looking for differences in range of motion (ROM) and the patient's willingness to do the movement. The ROM taking place during the active movement is normally the summation of the movements of the entire lumbar spine, not just movement at one level. The most painful movements are done last.

While the patient is doing the active movements, the examiner looks for limitation of movement and its possible causes, such as pain, spasm, stiffness, or blocking. As the patient reaches the full range of active movement, passive overpressure may be applied, but only if the active movements appear to be full and pain free. The overpressure must be applied with extreme care, because the upper body weight is already being applied to the lumbar joints by virtue of their position and gravity. If the patient reports that a sustained position increases the symptoms, then the examiner should consider having the patient maintain the position (e.g., flexion) at the end of the ROM for 10 to 20 seconds to see whether symptoms increase. Likewise, if repetitive motion or combined movements have been reported

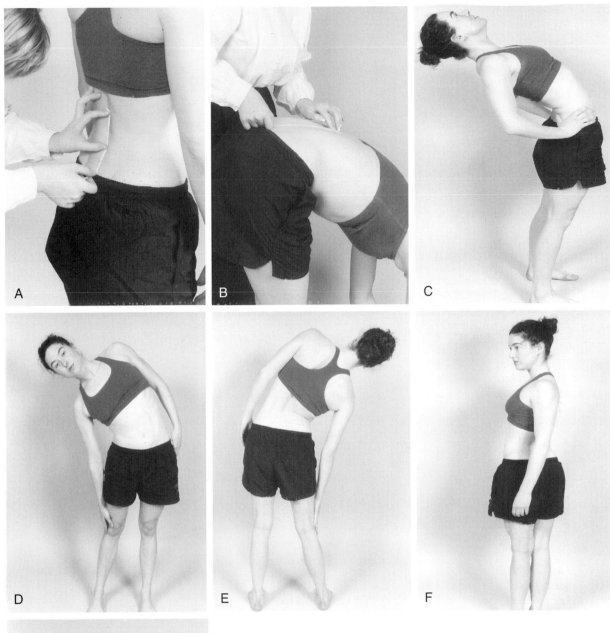

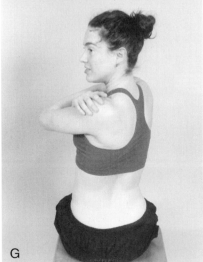

Figure 9–14

Active movements of the lumbar spine. (A and B) Measuring forward flexion using tape measure. (C) Extension. (D) Side flexion (anterior view). (E) Side flexion (posterior view). (F) Rotation (standing). (G) Rotation (sitting).

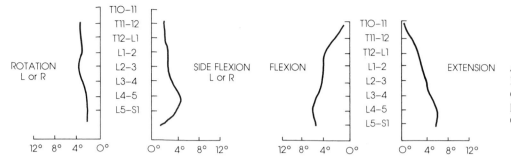

jure 9–15

Average range of motion in the lumbar spine. (Adapted from Grieve, G.P.: Common Vertebral Joint Problems. Edinburgh, Churchill Livingstone, 1981.)

in the history as causing symptoms, these movements should be performed as well, but only after the patient has completed the basic movements.

Active Movements of the Lumbar Spine

- Forward flexion (40 to 60°)
- Extension (20 to 35°)
- Side (lateral) flexion, left and right (15 to 20°)
- Rotation, left and right (3 to 18°)
- Sustained postures (if necessary)
- Repetitive motion (if necessary)
- Combined movements (if necessary)

The greatest motion in the lumbar spine occurs between the L4 and L5 vertebrae and between L5 and S1. There is considerable individual variability in the ROM of the lumbar spine (Fig. 9–15).[16–20] In reality, little obvious movement occurs in the lumbar spine because of the shape of the facet joints, tightness of the ligaments, presence of the intervertebral discs, and size of the vertebral bodies.

For flexion (forward bending), the maximum ROM is 40 to 60°. The examiner must ensure that the movement is occurring in the lumbar spine and not in the hips or thoracic spine. It must be remembered that a patient can touch his or her toes even if no movement occurs in the spine. On forward flexion, the lumbar spine should move from its normal lordotic curvature to at least a straight or slightly flexed curve (Fig. 9–16). If it does not do this, there is probably some hypomobility in the lumbar spine. If the patient bends one or both knees on forward flexion, the examiner should watch for nerve root symptoms or tight hamstrings, especially if spinal flexion is decreased when the knees are straight. When returning to the upright posture from forward flexion, the patient with no back pain first rotates the hips and pelvis to about 45° of flexion; during the last 45° of extension, the low back resumes its lordosis. In patients with back pain, almost all movement occurs in the hips, accompanied by knee flexion, and sometimes with hand support working up the thighs. As with the thoracic spine, the examiner may use a tape measure to

determine the increase in spacing of the spinous processes on forward flexion. Normally, the measurement should increase 7 to 8 cm (2.8 to 3.1 inches) if it is taken between the T12 spinous process and S1 (see Fig. 9–14A and B). The examiner should note how far forward the patient is able to bend (i.e., to midthigh, knees, midtibia, or floor) and compare this finding with the results of straight leg raising tests. Straight leg raising, especially if bilateral, is essentially the same movement done passively, except that it is a movement occurring from below upward instead of from above downward.

Maigne[13] describes an active movement flexion maneuver to help confirm lumbar movement and control. In this "**happy round maneuver**," the patient bends forward and places the hands on a bed or on the back of a chair. The patient then attempts to arch or hunch the back. Most patients with lumbar pathology are unable to sustain the hunched position.

Extension (backward bending) is normally limited to 20 to 35° in the lumbar spine. While performing the movement, the patient is asked to place the hands in the small of the back to help stabilize the back. Bourdillon and Day[21] advocate doing this movement in the prone lying position to hyperextend the spine. They called the resulting position the **sphinx position**. The patient hyperextends the spine by resting on the elbows with the hands holding the chin (Fig. 9–17) and allows the ab-

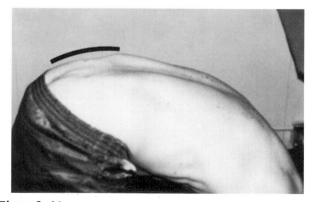

Figure 9–16

On forward flexion, the lumbar curve should normally flatten or go into slight flexion, as shown.

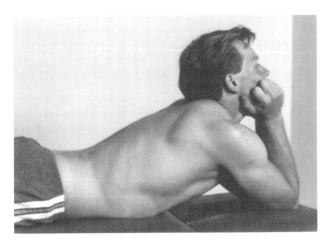

Figure 9–17
The sphinx position.

dominal wall to relax. The position is held for 10 to 20 seconds.

Side (lateral) flexion is approximately 15 to 20° in the lumbar spine. The patient is asked to run the hand down the side of the leg and not to bend forward or backward while performing the movement. The examiner can then "eyeball" the movement and compare it with that of the other side. The distance from the fingertips to the floor on both sides may also be measured, noting any difference. As the patient side flexes, the examiner should watch the lumbar curve. Normally, the lumbar curve forms a smooth curve on side flexion, and there should be no obvious sharp angulation at only one level. If angulation does occur, it may indicate hypomobility below the level or hypermobility above the level in the lumbar spine (Fig. 9–18).

Rotation in the lumbar spine is normally 3 to 18° to the left or right, and it is accomplished by a shearing movement of the lumbar vertebrae on each other. Although the patient is usually in the standing position, rotation may be performed while sitting to eliminate pelvic and hip movement. If the patient stands, the examiner must take care to watch for this accessory movement and try to eliminate it by stabilizing the pelvis.

If a movement such as side flexion toward the painful side increases the symptoms, the lesion is intra-articular, because the muscles and ligaments on that side are relaxed. If a disc protrusion is present and lateral to the nerve root, side flexion to the painful side increases the pain and radicular symptoms on that side. If a movement such as side flexion away from the painful side alters the symptoms, the lesion may be articular or muscular in origin, or it may be a disc protrusion medial to the nerve root (Fig. 9–19).

McKenzie[10] advocates repeating the active movements, especially flexion and extension, 10 times to see whether the movement increases or decreases the symptoms. He also advocates a side gliding movement in

which the head and feet remain in position and the patient shifts the pelvis to the left and to the right.

If the examiner finds that side flexion and rotation have been equally limited, and extension has been limited to a lesser extent, a capsular pattern may be suspected. A capsular pattern in one lumbar segment, however, may be difficult to detect.

Because back injuries rarely occur during a "pure" movement such as flexion, extension, side flexion, or rotation, it has been advocated that combined movements of the spine should be included in the examination.[22, 23] The examiner may want to test the following more habitual combined movements: lateral flexion in flexion; lateral flexion in extension; flexion and rotation; and extension and rotation. These combined movements (Fig. 9–20) may cause signs and symptoms different from those produced by pure movements and are definitely indicated if the patient has shown that a combined movement is what causes the symptoms. For example, if the patient is suffering from a facet syndrome, combined extension and rotation is the movement most likely to exacerbate symptoms.[24] Other symptoms that would indicate facet involvement include absence of radicular signs or neurological deficit, hip and buttock pain, and sometimes leg pain above the knee, no paresthesia, and low back stiffness.[25, 26]

While the patient is standing, a **"quick test"** may be performed (Fig. 9–21). The patient squats as far as possible, bounces two or three times, and returns to the

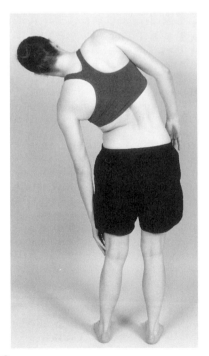

Figure 9–18
Lateral (side) flexion. Note that lower lumbar spine stays straight and upper lumbar and lower thoracic spine side flexes. This finding would indicate hypomobility in the lower lumbar spine.

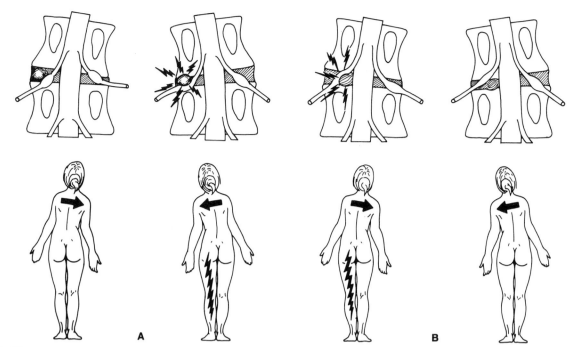

Figure 9–19

Patients with herniated disc problems may sometimes list to one side. This is a voluntary or involuntary mechanism to alleviate nerve root irritation. The list in some patients is toward the side of the sciatica; in others, it is toward the opposite side. A reasonable hypothesis suggests that when the herniation is lateral to the nerve root (A), the list is to the side opposite the sciatica because a list to the same side would elicit pain. Conversely, when the herniation is medial to the nerve root (B), the list is toward the side of the sciatica because tilting away would irritate the root and cause pain. (From White, A.A., and M.M. Panjabi: Clinical Biomechanics of the Spine, 2nd ed. Philadelphia, J.B. Lippincott, 1990, p. 415.)

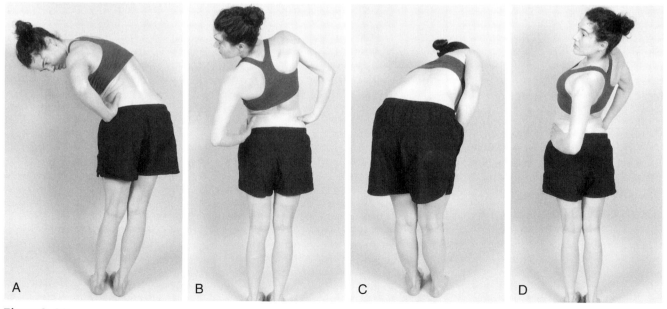

Figure 9–20

Combined active movements. (A) Lateral flexion in flexion. (B) Lateral flexion in extension. (C) Rotation and flexion. (D) Rotation and extension.

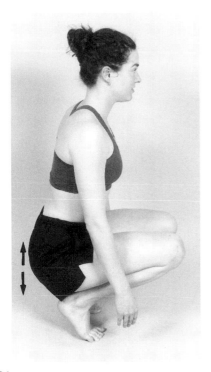

Figure 9–21
Quick test.

standing position. This action quickly tests the ankles, knees, and hips as well as the sacrum for any pathological condition. If the patient can fully squat and bounce without any signs and symptoms, these joints are probably free of pathology related to the complaint. However, this test should be used only with caution and should not be done with patients suspected of having arthritis in the lower limb joints, pregnant patients, or older patients who exhibit weakness and hypomobility. If this test is negative, there is no need to test the peripheral joints (peripheral joint scan) with the patient in the lying position.

The patient is then asked to balance on one leg and to go up and down on the toes four or five times. While the patient does this, the examiner should watch for **Trendelenburg's sign** (Fig. 9–22). A positive sign may be caused by a weak gluteus medius muscle or a coxa vara. If the patient is unable to complete the movement by going up and down on the toes, the examiner may suspect an **S1 nerve root** lesion. Both legs are tested.

McKenzie advocates doing flexion movements with the patient in the supine lying position as well.[10] In the standing position, flexion takes place from above downward, so pain at the end of the ROM indicates that

Figure 9–22
Trendelenburg and S1 nerve root test. (A) Anterior view, negative test. (B) Side view, negative test. (C) Posterior view, positive test for a weak left gluteus medius.

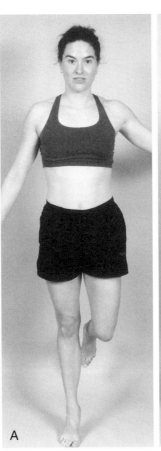

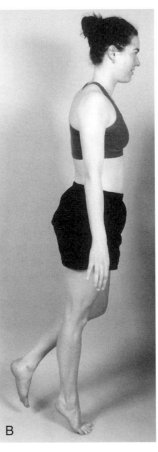

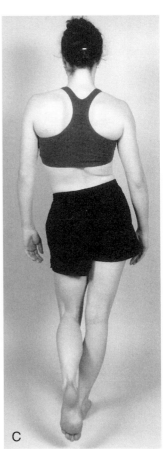

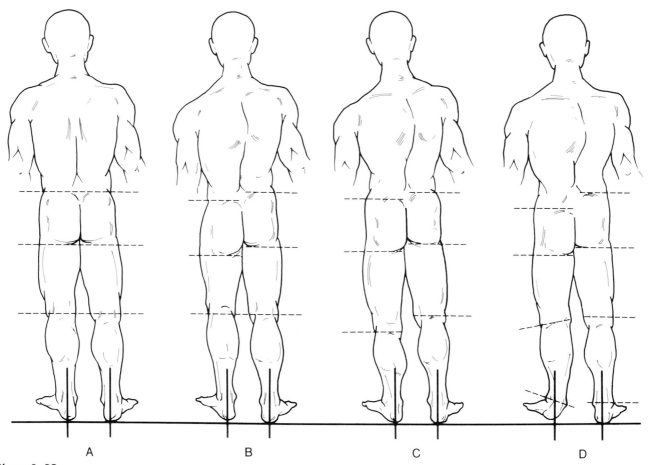

Figure 9–23
Effect of different leg lengths and posture. Note presence of scoliosis on the side with the "short" limb.
(A) Normal. (B) Short left femur. (C) Short left tibia. (D) Pronation of left foot.

L5–S1 is affected. When the patient is in the supine lying position, with the knees being lifted to the chest, flexion takes place from below upward so that pain at the beginning of movement indicates that L5–S1 is affected. It must also be remembered that greater stretch is placed on L5–S1 when the patient is in the lying position.

During the observation stage of the assessment, the examiner will have noted any changes in functional limb length (see Table 9–4). Wallace[27] developed a method for measuring **functional leg length**. The patient is first assessed in a relaxed stance. In this position, the examiner palpates the ASISs and the PSISs, noting any asymmetry. The examiner then places the patient in a symmetric stance, ensuring that the subtalar joint is in the neutral position (see Chapter 13), the toes are straight ahead, and the knees are extended. The ASISs and PSISs are again assessed for asymmetry. If differences are still noted, the examiner should check for structural leg length differences (see Chapters 10 and 11), sacroiliac joint dysfunction, and weak gluteus medius and quadratus lumborum (Fig. 9–23). The pelvis may also be leveled with the use of calibrated blocks or cards so that the functional length difference can be recorded.

Passive Movements

In the lumbar spine, passive movements are very difficult to perform because of the weight of the body. If active movements are full and pain free, overpressure can be attempted with care. However, it is safer to check the end feel of the individual vertebrae in the lumbar spine during the assessment of joint play movements. The end feel is the same, but the examiner has better control of the patient and is less likely to overstress the joints.

> ### Passive Movements of the Lumbar Spine and Normal End Feel
>
> • Flexion (tissue stretch)
> • Extension (tissue stretch)
> • Side flexion (tissue stretch)
> • Rotation (tissue stretch)

Resisted Isometric Movements

The patient is seated. The contraction must be resisted and isometric so that no movement occurs (Fig. 9–24).

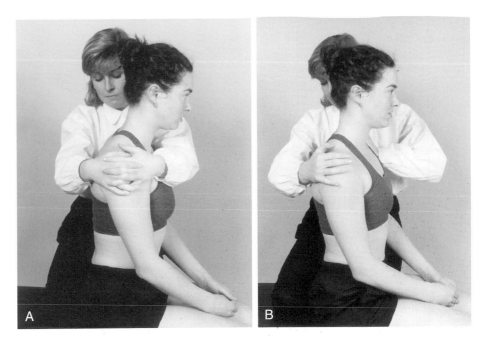

Figure 9–24
Positioning for resisted isometric movements of the lumbar spine. (A) Flexion, extension, and side flexion. (B) Rotation to right.

Resisted Isometric Movements of the Lumbar Spine

- Forward flexion
- Extension
- Side flexion (left and right)
- Rotation (left and right)

Because of the strength of the trunk muscles, the examiner should say, "Don't let me move you," so that minimal movement occurs. The examiner tests flexion, extension, side flexion, and rotation. Figure 9–25 shows the axes of movement of the lumbar spine. The lumbar spine should be in a neutral position, and the painful movements should be done last. The examiner should keep in mind that strong abdominal muscles help to reduce the load on the lumbar spine by approximately 30%, and

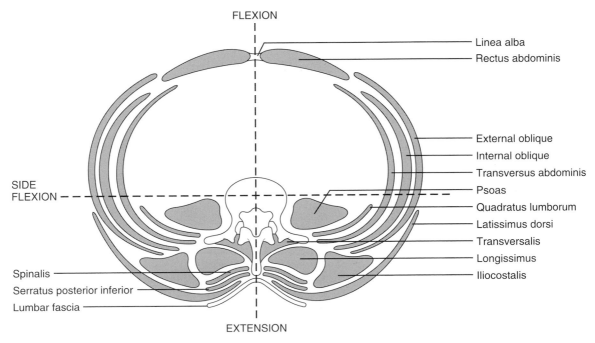

Figure 9–25
Diagram of relations of the lumbar spine showing movement.

Table 9–5
Muscles of the Lumbar Spine:
Their Actions and Nerve Root Derivation

Action	Muscles Acting	Nerve Root Derivation
Forward flexion	1. Psoas major	L1–L3
	2. Rectus abdominis	T6–T12
	3. External abdominal oblique	T7–T12
	4. Internal abdominal oblique	T7–T12, L1
	5. Transversus abdominis	T7–T12, L1
Extension	1. Latissimus dorsi	Thoracodorsal (C6–C8)
	2. Erector spinae	L1–L3
	3. Transversospinalis	L1–L5
	4. Interspinales	L1–L5
	5. Quadratus lumborum	T12, L1–L4
Side flexion	1. Latissimus dorsi	Thoracodorsal (C6–C8)
	2. Erector spinae	L1–L3
	3. Transversalis	L1–L5
	4. Intertransversarii	L1–L5
	5. Quadratus lumborum	T12, L1–L4
	6. Psoas major	L1–L3
	7. External abdominal oblique	T7–T12
Rotation*	—	—

* Very little rotation occurs in the lumbar spine because of the shape of the facet joints. Any rotation would be a result of shearing movement. If shear does occur, the transversalis muscles would be responsible for the movement.

on the thoracic spine by approximately 50%, as a result of the increased intrathoracic and intra-abdominal pressures caused by the contraction of these muscles. Table 9–5 lists the muscles acting on the lumbar vertebrae.

If tested isokinetically, the extensors are stronger than the flexors. Men produce a force equal to approximately 65% of body weight in flexion, whereas women produce approximately 65 to 70% of their body weight in flexion. In extension, men produce approximately 90 to 95% of their body weight, and women 80 to 95%, depending on the speed tested. In rotation, men produce approximately 55 to 65% of their body weight, whereas women produce approximately 40 to 55%, depending on the speed tested.[28]

Peripheral Joint Scanning Examination

After the resisted isometric movements of the lumbar spine have been completed, if the examiner did not use the "quick test" to test the peripheral joints or is unsure of the findings, the peripheral joints should be quickly

scanned to rule out obvious pathology in the extremities. Any deviation from normal could lead the examiner to do a detailed examination of that joint. The following joints are scanned.[29]

Lower Limb Scanning Examination

- Sacroiliac joints
- Hip joints
- Knee joints
- Ankle joints
- Foot joints

Sacroiliac Joints. With the patient standing, the examiner palpates the PSIS on one side with one thumb and one of the sacral spines with the other thumb. The patient then fully flexes the hip on that side, and the examiner notes whether the PSIS drops as it normally should or whether it elevates, indicating fixation of the sacroiliac joint on that side (Fig. 9–26). The examiner then compares the other side. The examiner next places one thumb on one of the patient's ischial tuberosities and one thumb on the sacral apex. The patient is then asked to flex the hip on that side again. If the movement is normal, the thumb on the ischial tuberosity moves laterally. If the sacroiliac joint on that side is fixed, the thumb moves up. The other side is then tested for comparison.

Hip Joints. These joints are actively moved through flexion, extension, abduction, adduction, and medial and lateral rotation in as full a ROM as possible. Any pattern of restriction or pain should be noted. As the patient flexes the hip, the examiner may palpate the ilium, sacrum, and lumbar spine to determine when movement begins at the sacroiliac joint on that side and at the lumbar spine. The two sides should be compared.

Knee Joints. The patient actively moves the knee joints through as full a range of flexion and extension as possible. Any restriction of movement or abnormal signs and symptoms should be noted.

Foot and Ankle Joints. Plantar flexion, dorsiflexion, supination, and pronation of the foot and ankle as well as flexion and extension of the toes are actively performed through a full ROM. Again, any alteration in signs and symptoms should be noted.

Myotomes

Having completed the scanning examination of the peripheral joints, the examiner next tests the patient's muscle power and possible neurological weakness (Table 9–6).[29] With the patient lying supine, the myotomes are assessed individually (Fig. 9–27). When testing myotomes (Table 9–7), the examiner should place the test

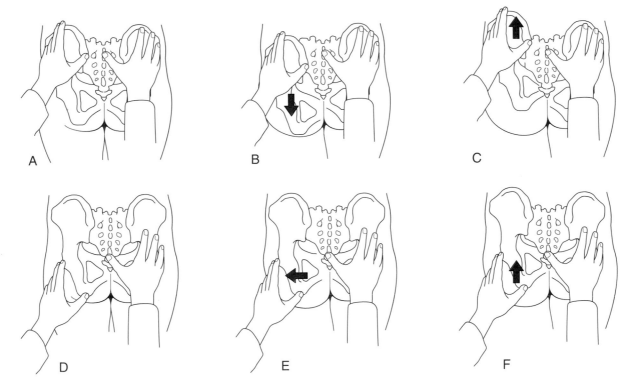

Figure 9–26

Tests to demonstrate left sacroiliac fixation. (A) Examiner places the left thumb on the posterior superior iliac spine and the right thumb over one of the sacral spinous processes. (B) With normal movement, the examiner's left thumb moves downward as the patient raises the left leg with full hip flexion. (C) If the joint is fixed, the examiner's left thumb moves upward as the patient raises the left leg. (D) The examiner places the left thumb over the ischial tuberosity and the right thumb over the apex of the sacrum. (E) With normal movement, the examiner's left thumb moves laterally as the patient raises the left leg with full hip flexion. (F) If the joint is fixed, the examiner's left thumb moves slightly upward as the patient raises the left leg. (Modified from Kirkaldy-Willis, W.H.: Managing Low Back Pain. New York, Churchill Livingstone, 1983, p. 94.)

joint or joints in a neutral or resting position and then apply a resisted isometric pressure. The contraction should be held for **at least 5 seconds** to show any weakness. If feasible, the examiner should test the two sides simultaneously to provide a comparison. The simultaneous bilateral comparison is not possible for movements involving the hip and knee joints, so both sides must be done individually. The examiner should not apply pressure over the joints, because this action may mask symptoms.

Myotomes of the Lumbar and Sacral Spines

- L2: Hip flexion
- L3: Knee extension
- L4: Ankle dorsiflexion
- L5: Great toe extension
- S1: Ankle plantar flexion, ankle eversion, hip extension
- S2: Knee flexion

It should be remembered that the examiner has previously tested the S1 myotome with the patient standing and has tested for a positive Trendelenburg's sign; these movements are repeated here only if the examiner is unsure of the result and wants to test again. The ankle movements should be tested with the knee flexed approximately 30°, especially if the patient complains of sciatic pain, because full dorsiflexion is considered a provocative maneuver for stretching of neurological tissue. Likewise, the extended knee increases the stretch on the sciatic nerve and may result in false signs, such as weakness that results from pain rather than from pressure on the nerve root.

If the patient is in extreme pain, all tests with the patient in the supine position should be completed before the patient is tested in prone. This reduces the amount of movement the patient must do, decreasing the patient's discomfort. Ideally, all tests in the standing position should be performed first, followed by tests in the sitting, supine, side lying, and prone positions. This procedure is shown in the précis at the end of the chapter.

Table 9–6
Lumbar Root Syndromes

Root	Dermatome	Muscle Weakness	Reflexes/Special Tests Affected	Paresthesias
L1	Back, over trochanter, groin	None	None	Groin, after holding posture, which causes pain
L2	Back, front of thigh to knee	Psoas, hip adductors	None	Occasionally front of thigh
L3	Back, upper buttock, front of thigh and knee, medial lower leg	Psoas, quadriceps—thigh wasting	Knee jerk sluggish, PKB positive, pain on full SLR	Inner knee, anterior lower leg
L4	Inner buttock, outer thigh, inside of leg, dorsum of foot, big toe	Tibialis anterior, extensor hallucis	SLR limited, neck-flexion pain, weak knee jerk; side flexion limited	Medial aspect of calf and ankle
L5	Buttock, back and side of thigh, lateral aspect of leg, dorsum of foot, inner half of sole and first, second, and third toes	Extensor hallucis, peroneals, gluteus medius, ankle dorsiflexors, hamstrings—calf wasting	SLR limited to one side, neck-flexion pain, ankle jerk decreased, crossed-leg raising—pain	Lateral aspect of leg, medial three toes
S1	Buttock, back of thigh, and lower leg	Calf and hamstrings, wasting of gluteals, peroneals, plantar flexors	SLR limited	Lateral two toes, lateral foot, lateral leg to knee, plantar aspect of foot
S2	Same as S1	Same as S1 except peroneals	Same as S1	Lateral leg, knee, heel
S3	Groin, inner thigh to knee	None	None	None
S4	Perineum, genitals, lower sacrum	Bladder, rectum	None	Saddle area, genitals, anus, impotence

Manipulation and traction are contraindicated if S4 or massive posterior displacement causes bilateral sciatica and S3 pain.

PKB = prone knee bendings; SLR = straight leg raising.

Table 9–7
Myotomes of the Lower Limb

Nerve Root	Test Action	Muscles
L1–L2	Hip flexion	Psoas, iliacus, sartorius, gracilis, pectineus, adductor longus, adductor brevis
L3	Knee extension	Quadriceps, adductor longus, magnus, and brevis
L4	Ankle dorsiflexion	Tibialis anterior, quadriceps, tensor fasciae latae, adductor magnus, obturator externus, tibialis posterior
L5	Toe extension	Extensor hallucis longus, extensor digitorum longus, gluteus medius and minimus, obturator internus, semimembranosus, semitendinosus, peroneus tertius, popliteus
S1	Ankle plantar flexion Ankle eversion Hip extension Knee flexion	Gastrocnemius, soleus, gluteus maximus, obturator internus, piriformis, biceps femoris, semitendinosus, popliteus, peroneus longus and brevis, extensor digitorum brevis
S2	Knee flexion	Biceps femoris, piriformis, soleus, gastrocnemius, flexor digitorum longus, flexor hallucis longus, intrinsic foot muscles
S3		Intrinsic foot muscles (except abductor hallucis), flexor hallucis brevis, flexor digitorum brevis, extensor digitorum brevis

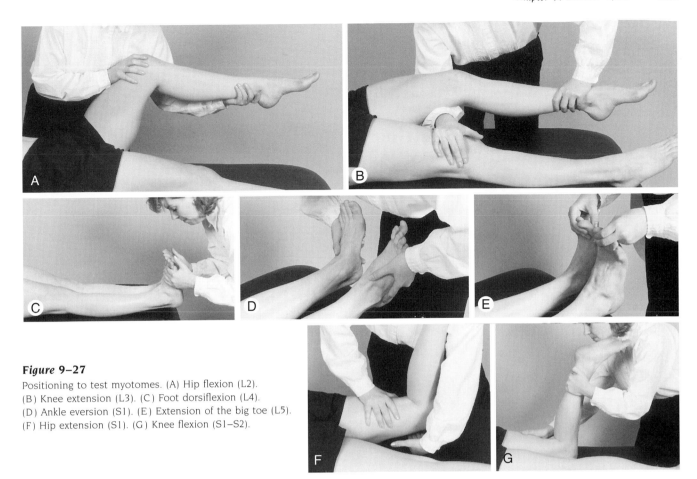

Figure 9–27

Positioning to test myotomes. (A) Hip flexion (L2).
(B) Knee extension (L3). (C) Foot dorsiflexion (L4).
(D) Ankle eversion (S1). (E) Extension of the big toe (L5).
(F) Hip extension (S1). (G) Knee flexion (S1–S2).

Hip flexion (L2 myotome) is tested by flexing the patient's hip to 30 to 40°. The examiner then applies a resisted force into extension proximal to the knee while ensuring that the heel of the patient's foot is not resting on the examining table (see Fig. 9–27A). The other side is then tested for comparison. To prevent excessive stress on the lumbar spine, the examiner must ensure that the patient does not increase the lumbar lordosis while doing the test and that only one leg at a time is tested.

To test knee extension or the L3 myotome, the examiner flexes the patient's knee to 25 to 35° and then applies a resisted flexion force at the midshaft of the tibia (see Fig. 9–27B). The other side is tested for comparison.

Ankle dorsiflexion (L4 myotome) is tested by asking the patient to place the feet at 90° relative to the leg. The examiner applies a resisted force to the dorsum of each foot and compares the two sides (see Fig. 9–27C). Ankle plantar flexion (S1 myotome) is compared in a similar fashion, but the resistance is applied to the sole of the foot. Because of the strength of the plantar flexor muscles, it is better to test this myotome with the patient standing. The patient slowly moves up and down on the toes of each foot in turn, and the examiner compares the differences as previously described. Ankle eversion (S1 myotome) is tested with the patient in the supine lying position, and the examiner applies a force to move the foot into inversion (see Fig. 9–27D).

Toe extension (L5 myotome) is tested with the patient holding both big toes in a neutral position. The examiner applies resistance to the nails of both toes and compares the two sides (see Fig. 9–27E). It is imperative that the resistance be isometric, so the amount of force in this case is less than that applied during knee extension, for example.

Hip extension (S1 myotome) is tested with the patient lying prone. This test needs to be done only if the patient is unable to do plantar flexion testing in standing or ankle eversion. The knee is flexed to 90°. The examiner then lifts the patient's thigh slightly off the examining table while stabilizing the leg. A downward force is applied to the patient's posterior thigh with one hand while the other hand ensures that the patient's thigh is not resting on the table (see Fig. 9–27F).

Knee flexion (S1–S2 myotomes) is tested in the same position with the knee flexed to 90°. An extension isometric force is applied just above the ankle (see Fig. 9–27G). Although it is possible to test both knee flexors at the same time, it is not advisable to do this because the stress on the lumbar spine may be too great.

Functional Assessment

Injury to the lumbar spine can greatly affect the patient's ability to function. Activities such as standing, walking, bending, lifting, traveling, socializing, dressing, and sexual intercourse can be affected. Numerical scoring tables may be used to determine the degree of pain caused by lumbar spine pathology or disability. Care must be taken when selecting one of these scales to ensure that it measures the disability from the patient's perspective.[30, 31] Examples are the Oswestry Disability Index (Fig. 9–28) and the Hendler 10-Minute Screening Test for Chronic Back Pain Patients (Fig. 9–29).[31–33] It has been reported that the Hendler test helps to differentiate or-

---

Oswestry Disability Index

Section 1 - Pain intensity
☐ I have no pain at the moment.
☐ The pain is very mild at the moment.
☐ The pain is moderate at the moment.
☐ The pain is fairly severe at the moment.
☐ The pain is very severe at the moment.
☐ The pain is the worst imaginable at the moment.

Section 2 - Personal care (washing, dressing, etc.)
☐ I can look after myself normally without causing extra pain.
☐ I can look after myself normally but it is very painful.
☐ It is painful to look after myself and I am slow and careful.
☐ I need some help but manage most of my personal care.
☐ I need help every day in most aspects of self care.
☐ I do not get dressed, wash with difficulty and stay in bed.

Section 3 - Lifting
☐ I can lift heavy weights without extra pain.
☐ I can lift heavy weights but it gives extra pain.
☐ Pain prevents me from lifting heavy weights off the floor but I can manage if they are conveniently positioned, e.g. on a table.
☐ Pain prevents me from lifting heavy weights but I can manage light to medium weights if they are conveniently positioned.
☐ I can lift only very light weights.
☐ I cannot lift or carry anything at all.

Section 4 - Walking
☐ Pain does not prevent me walking any distance.
☐ Pain prevents me walking more than 1 mile.
☐ Pain prevents me walking more than 1/4 of a mile.
☐ Pain prevents me walking more than 100 yards.
☐ I can only walk using a stick or crutches.
☐ I am in bed most of the time and have to crawl to the toilet.

Section 5 - Sitting
☐ I can sit in any chair as long as I like.
☐ I can sit in my favorite chair as long as I like.
☐ Pain prevents me from sitting for more than 1 hour.
☐ Pain prevents me from sitting for more than 1/2 an hour.
☐ Pain prevents me from sitting for more than 10 minutes.
☐ Pain prevents me from sitting at all.

Section 6 - Standing
☐ I can stand as long as I want without extra pain.
☐ I can stand as long as I want but it gives me extra pain.

☐ Pain prevents me from standing for more than 1 hour.
☐ Pain prevents me from standing for more than 1/2 an hour.
☐ Pain prevents me from standing for more than 10 minutes.
☐ Pain prevents me from standing at all.

Section 7 - Sleeping
☐ My sleep is never disturbed by pain.
☐ My sleep is occasionally disturbed by pain.
☐ Because of pain I have less than 6 hours sleep.
☐ Because of pain I have less than 4 hours sleep.
☐ Because of pain I have less than 2 hours sleep.
☐ Pain prevents me from sleeping at all.

Section 8 - Sex life (if applicable)
☐ My sex life is normal and causes no extra pain.
☐ My sex life is normal but causes some extra pain.
☐ My sex life is nearly normal but is very painful.
☐ My sex life is severely restricted by pain.
☐ My sex life is nearly absent because of pain.
☐ Pain prevents any sex life at all.

Section 9 - Social life
☐ My social life is normal and causes me no extra pain.
☐ My social life is normal but increases the degree of pain.
☐ Pain has no significant effect on my social life apart from limiting my more energetic interests, e.g., sport.
☐ Pain has restricted my social life and I do not go out as often.
☐ Pain has restricted social life to my home.
☐ I have no social life because of pain.

Section 10 - Traveling
☐ I can travel anywhere without pain.
☐ I can travel anywhere but it gives extra pain.
☐ Pain is bad but I manage journeys of over two hours.
☐ Pain restricts me to journeys of less than one hour.
☐ Pain restricts me to short necessary journeys under 30 minutes.
☐ Pain prevents me from traveling except to receive treatment.

Section 11 - Previous treatment
Over the past three months have you received treatment, tablets or medicines of any kind for your back or leg pain? Please tick the appropriate box.
☐ No
☐ Yes (if yes, please state the type of treatment you have received)

Figure 9–28
Oswestry Disability Index. (Redrawn from Fairbank, J.C., J. Couper, J.B. Davies, and J.P. O'Brien. The Oswestry low back pain disability questionnaire. Physiotherapy 66:271–273, 1980.)

Hendler 10-Minute Screening Test for Chronic Back Pain Patients

Instructions: Each question is asked by an examiner, and the patient is given points according to the response that he makes. The number of points to be awarded for the various responses is shown in the column at the right. At the end of the test, the examiner calculates the total number of points. The results are interpreted as explained in the Key.

Points

I How did the pain that you now experience occur?
(a) Sudden onset with accident or definable event — 0
(b) Slow, progressive onset without acute exacerbation — 1
(c) Slow, progressive onset with acute exacerbation without accident or event — 2
(d) Sudden onset without an accident or definable event — 3

II Where do you experience the pain?
(a) One site, specific, well-defined, consistent with anatomical distribution — 0
(b) More than one site, each well-defined and consistent with anatomical distribution — 1
(c) One site, inconsistent with anatomical considerations, or not well-defined — 2
(d) Vague description, more than one site, of which one is inconsistent with anatomical considerations, or not well-defined or anatomically explainable — 3

III Do you ever have trouble falling asleep at night, or are you ever awakened from sleep?

If the answer is "no," score 3 points and go to question IV. If the answer is "yes," proceed:

What keeps you from falling asleep, or what awakens you from sleep?

IIIA (a) Trouble falling asleep every night due to pain — 0
(b) Trouble falling asleep due to pain more than three times a week — 1
(c) Trouble falling asleep due to pain less than three times a week — 2
(d) No trouble falling asleep due to pain — 3
(e) Trouble falling asleep which is not related to pain — 4

IIIB (a) Awakened by pain every night — 0
(b) Awakened from sleep by pain more than three times a week — 1
(c) Not awakened from sleep by pain more than twice a week — 2
(d) Not awakened from sleep by pain — 3
(e) Restless sleep, or early morning awakening with or without being able to return to sleep, both unrelated to pain — 4

IV Does weather have any effect on your pain?
(a) The pain is always worse in both cold and damp weather. — 0
(b) The pain is always worse with damp weather or with cold weather. — 1
(c) The pain is occasionally worse with cold or damp weather. — 2
(d) The weather has no effect on the pain. — 3

V How would you describe the type of pain that you have?
(a) Burning; or sharp, shooting pain; or pins and needles; or coldness; or numbness — 0

Points

(b) Dull, aching pain, with occasional sharp, shooting pains not helped by heat; or, the patient is experiencing hyperesthesia — 1
(c) Spasm-type pain, tension-type pain, or numbness over the area, relieved by massage or heat — 2
(d) Nagging or bothersome pain — 3
(e) Excruciating, overwhelming, or unbearable pain, relieved by massage or heat — 4

VI How frequently do you have your pain?
(a) The pain is constant. — 0
(b) The pain is nearly constant, occurring 50–80% of the time. — 1
(c) The pain is intermittent, occurring 25–50% of the time. — 2
(d) The pain is only occasionally present, occurring less than 25% of the time. — 3

VII Does movement or position have any effect on the pain?
(a) The pain is unrelieved by position change or rest, and there have been previous operations for the pain. — 0
(b) The pain is worsened by use, standing, or walking; and is relieved by lying down or resting the part. — 1
(c) Position change and use have variable effects on the pain. — 2
(d) The pain is not altered by use or position change, and there have been no previous operations for the pain. — 3

VIII What medications have you used in the past month?
(a) No medications at all — 0
(b) Use of non-narcotic pain relievers; non-benzodiazepine tranquilizers; or use of antidepressants — 1
(c) Less than three-times-a-week use of a narcotic, hypnotic, or benzodiazepine — 2
(d) Greater than four-times-a-week use of a narcotic, hypnotic, or benzodiazepine — 3

IX What hobbies do you have, and can you still participate in them?
(a) Unable to participate in any hobbies that were formerly enjoyed — 0
(b) Reduced number of hobbies or activities relating to a hobby — 1
(c) Still able to participate in hobbies but with some discomfort — 2
(d) Participate in hobbies as before — 3

X How frequently did you have sex and orgasms before the pain, and how frequently do you have sex and orgasms now?
(a^1) Sexual contact, prior to pain, three to four times a week, with no difficulty with orgasm; now sexual contact is 50% or less than previously, and coitus is interrupted by pain — 0

Figure 9–29

Hendler 10-Minute Screening Test for Chronic Back Pain Patients. (Redrawn from Hendler N., M. Vierstein, P. Gucer, and D. Long: A preoperative screening test for chronic back pain patients. Psychosomatics 20:806–808, 1979. Copyright © Nelson Hendler, M.D., 1979.)

Points

(a²) (For people over 45) Sexual contact twice a week, with a 50% reduction in frequency since the pain 0

(a³) (For people over 60) Sexual contact once a week, with a 50% reduction in frequency of coitus since the onset of pain 0

(b) Pre-pain adjustment as defined above (a¹–a³), with no difficulty with orgasm; now loss of interest in sex and/or difficulty with orgasm or erection 1

(c) No change in sexual activity now as opposed to before the onset of pain 2

(d) Unable to have sexual contact since the onset of pain, and difficulty with orgasm or erection prior to the pain 3

(e) No sexual contact prior to the pain, or absence of orgasm prior to the pain 4

XI Are you still working or doing your household chores?

(a) Works every day at the same pre-pain job or same level of household duties 0

(b) Works every day but the job is not the same as pre-pain job, with reduced responsibility or physical activity 1

(c) Works sporadically or does a reduced amount of household chores 2

(d) Not at work, or all household chores are now performed by others 3

XII What is your income now compared with before your injury or the onset of pain, and what are your sources of income?

(a) Any one of the following answers scores 0
1. Experiencing financial difficulty with family income 50% or less than previously
2. Was retired and is still retired
3. Patient is still working and is not having financial difficulties

(b) Experiencing financial difficulty with family income only 50–75% of the pre-pain income 1

(c) Patient unable to work, and receives some compensation so that the family income is at least 75% of the pre-pain income 2

(d) Patient unable to work and receives no compensation, but the spouse works and

Points

family income is still 75% of the pre-pain income 3

(e) Patient doesn't work, yet the income from disability or other compensation sources is 80% or more of gross pay before the pain; the spouse does not work 4

XIII Are you suing anyone, or is anyone suing you, or do you have an attorney helping you with compensation or disability payments?

(a) No suit pending, and does not have an attorney 0

(b) Litigation is pending, but is not related to the pain 1

(c) The patient is being sued as the result of an accident 2

(d) Litigation is pending or workmen's compensation case with a lawyer involved 3

XIV If you had three wishes for anything in the world, what would you wish for?

(a) "Get rid of the pain" is the only wish. 0

(b) "Get rid of the pain" is one of the three wishes. 1

(c) Doesn't mention getting rid of the pain, but has specific wishes usually of a personal nature such as for more money, a better relationship with spouse or children, etc. 2

(d) Does not mention pain, but offers general, nonpersonal wishes such as for world peace 3

XV Have you ever been depressed or thought of suicide?

(a) Admits to depression; or has a history of depression secondary to pain and associated with crying spells and thoughts of suicide 0

(b) Admits to depression, guilt, and anger secondary to the pain 1

(c) Prior history of depression before the pain or a financial or personal loss prior to the pain; now admits to some depression 2

(d) Denies depression, crying spells, or "feeling blue" 3

(e) History of a suicide attempt prior to the onset of pain 4

POINT TOTAL

Key to Hendler Screening Test for Chronic Back Pain

A score of 18 pts or less suggests that the patient is an objective pain patient and is reporting a normal response to chronic pain. One may proceed surgically if indicated, and usually finds the patient quite willing to participate in all modalities of therapy, including exercise and psychotherapy. Occasionally, a person with conversion reaction or posttraumatic neurosis will score less than 18 points; this is because subjective distress is being experienced on an unconscious level. Persons scoring 14 points or less can be considered objective pain patients with more certainty than those at the upper range (14–18) of this group.

A score of 15–20 points suggests that the patient has features of an objective pain patient as well as of an exaggerating pain patient. This implies that a person with a poor premorbid adjustment has an organic lesion that has produced the normal response to pain; however, because of the person's poor pre-pain adjustment, the chronic pain produces a more extreme response than would otherwise occur.

A score of 19–31 points suggests that the patient is an exaggerating pain patient. Surgical or other interventions may be carried out with caution. This type of patient usually has a premorbid (pre-pain) personality that may increase his likelihood of using or benefiting from the complaint of chronic pain. The patient may show improvement after treatment in a chronic pain treatment center, where the main emphasis is placed on an attitude change toward the chronic pain.

A score of 32 points or more suggests that a psychiatric consultation is needed. These patients freely admit to a great many pre-pain problems, and show considerable difficulty in coping with the chronic pain they now experience. Surgical or other interventions should not be carried out without prior approval of a psychiatric consultant. Severe depression, suicide, and psychosis are potential problems in this group of affective pain patients.

Test copyright 1979 by Nelson Hendler, M.D., M.S.

Figure 9–29 Continued

ganic from functional low back pain.[34] The Oswestry Disability Index is a good functional scale because it deals with activities of daily living and therefore is based on the patient's response and concerns. The disability index is calculated by dividing the total score (each section is worth from 1 to 6 points) by the number of sections answered and multiplying by 100. Other numerical back pain scales include the Dallas Pain Questionnaire,[35] the Million Index,[36] the Japanese Orthopedic Association Scale,[37] and the Iowa Low Back Rating Scale.[38] Thomas[31] provides a good review of these and other scales. Lehman and colleagues[38] developed a rating scale for lumbar dysfunction (Fig. 9–30) that includes assessment criteria, physician criteria, and, equally important, patient criteria for determining the degree of dysfunction. These criteria can be evaluated during the normal assessment for the patient.

Waddell[39] developed a series of tests to differentiate between organic and nonorganic back pain. Each test counts +1 if positive or 0 if negative:

1. Superficial skin tenderness to light pinch over wide area of lumbar spine
2. Deep tenderness over wide area, often extending to thoracic spine, sacrum, and/or pelvis
3. Low back pain on axial loading of spine in standing
4. Straight leg raising test positive when specifically tested, but not when patient is seated with knee extended to test Babinski reflex
5. Abnormal neurological (motor and/or sensory) patterns
6. Overreaction.

Positive findings of +3 or more should be investigated for nonorganic cause; these patients may also have social and psychological components to their complaint.

Special Tests

When the examiner performs special tests in the lumbar assessment, the straight leg raising test, the prone knee bending test, and the slump test should always be done. The other tests need be done only if the examiner believes they are relevant or to confirm a diagnosis.

Tests for Neurological Dysfunction (Neurodynamic Tests)

Neurodynamic Tests Commonly Performed on the Lumbar Spine

- Slump test
- Straight leg raising test
- Prone knee bending test

FUNCTIONAL RATING SCALE FOR THE LUMBAR SPINE

A. Physical criteria ____
B. Patient's perception ____
C. Physician's perception ____
   TOTAL ____

A. PHYSICAL CRITERIA (Max: 30)
  1. Range of motion—Total flexion and extension in degrees ____
    Points (1 point for every 10 degrees— 15 points maximum) ____
  2. Trunk strength—Total flexion and extension in kilograms ____
    Points (1 point for every 8 kg, male patients—15 points maximum)
    Points (1 point for every 4 kg, female patients—15 points maximum)

B. PATIENT'S PERCEPTION (Max: 40)
  1. Average pain (visual-analog scale) (15) ____
  2. How disabled:
    No disability, able to work full-time (10) ____
    Able to work full-time but at a lower level (8)
    Able to work part-time but at usual level (6)
    Able to work only part-time and at lower level (4)
    Not able to work at all (0)
  3. Activities you can perform—1 point for each **Yes** answer ____

C. PHYSICIAN'S PERCEPTION (Max: 30)
  1. How much pain would you expect for this patient at this time? (visual-analog scale) ____
  2. At the present time, what is the degree of impairment? ____
    None (10)
    Mild but should not affect most activities (8)
    Moderate, cannot perform some strenuous activities (6)
    Only light activities, cannot perform any strenuous activities (2)
    Severely limited, cannot perform most light activities or some activities of daily living (0)
  3. Current drugs and daily doses (quantity): ____
    Analgesics (occasional) use = less than 5 times per week)
    Major narcotic, regular use (0)
    Major narcotic, occasional use (2)
    Minor narcotic, regular use (4)
    Minor narcotic, occasional use (6)
    Nonnarcotic, regular use (8)
    Nonnarcotic, occasional use (10)

TOTAL ____

Figure 9–30
Functional rating scale for the lumbar spine. (Modified from Lehmann, T.R., R.A. Brand, and T.W. German: A low back rating scale. Spine 8:309, 1983.)

Neurodynamic tests are performed to test the mechanical movement of the neurological tissues and to test their sensitivity to mechanical stress or compression.[40, 41] Most of the special tests for neurological involvement are progressive or sequential tests. The patient is positioned and one maneuver is tried; if no symptoms result, a second provocative, enhancing, or sensitizing maneuver is carried out, and so on, while the examiner watches for reproduction of the patient's symptoms. The order in which these maneuvers are done also makes a difference. For example, with straight leg raising, the results are different if the hip is flexed with the knee extended than if the hip is flexed with the knee first flexed and then extended after the hip is in position.

Because of **tension points,** the neurological tissues move in different directions (Fig. 9–31) depending on where the stress is applied,[41, 42] and the direction of movement varies depending on where movement is initiated. For example, when doing the straight leg raising test, movement is toward the hip; with dorsiflexion as a sensitizing maneuver, the neurological tissue moves toward the ankle. If knee extension is performed in the slump test, the neurological tissue moves toward the knee.[40] This movement in different directions or in convergence toward the joint being moved can lead to production of different symptoms depending on where and in what direction the movement occurs. The neurological tissue may move in one direction for one part of the test and in another direction for the next part of the test. Pathology may restrict this normal movement. Tension points are areas where there is minimal movement of the neuro-

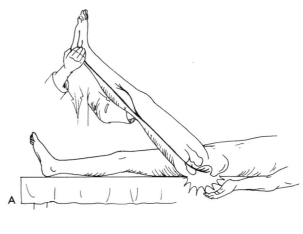

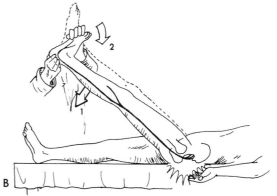

Figure 9–32
Straight leg raising. (A) Radicular symptoms are precipitated on the same side with straight leg raising. (B) The leg is lowered slowly until pain is relieved. The foot is then dorsiflexed, causing a return of symptoms; this indicates a positive test. (From Reilly, B.M.: Practical Strategies in Outpatient Medicine. Philadelphia, W.B. Saunders Co., 1991, p. 912.)

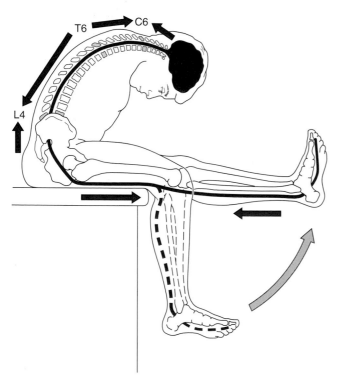

Figure 9–31
Postulated neurobiomechanics that occur with movement. The approximate points C6, T6, L4, and knee are where the neural tissue does not move in relation to the movements of the spinal canal. It is important to understand, however, that movement of neurological tissue is toward the joint where movement was initiated. (Adapted from Butler, D.S.: Mobilisation of the Nervous System. Melbourne, Churchill Livingstone, 1991, pp. 41–42.)

logical tissue. According to Butler,[41] these areas are C6, the elbow, the shoulder, T6, L4, and the knee. It is important to realize, however, that the amount of tension placed on these points depends on the position of the extremity.

For a neurodynamic test to be positive, it must reproduce the patient's symptoms. Because these tests are provocative tests designed to put stress on the neurological tissue, they often cause discomfort and/or pain, which may be bilateral. However, if the patient's symptoms are not reproduced, the test is considered negative. As a second check for a positive test, the symptoms which have been produced may be increased or decreased by adding or taking away the sensitizing parts of the test.[43]

Straight Leg Raising Test. Also known as Lasègue's test (Fig. 9–32), the straight leg raising test is done by the examiner with the patient completely relaxed.[44–51] It is a passive test, and each leg is tested individually. With the patient in the supine position, the hip medially rotated and adducted, and the knee extended, the examiner flexes the hip until the patient complains of pain or tightness in the back or back of the leg.[41] The examiner

Table 9–8
Straight Leg Raising (SLR) Test and Its Modifications

	SLR (Basic)	SLR2	SLR3	SLR4	Cross (Well Leg) SLR5
Hip	Flexion and adduction	Flexion	Flexion	Flexion and medial rotation	Flexion
Knee	Extension	Extension	Extension	Extension	Extension
Ankle	Dorsiflexion	Dorsiflexion	Dorsiflexion	Plantar flexion	Dorsiflexion
Foot	—	Eversion	Inversion	Inversion	—
Toes	—	Extension			
Nerve bias	Sciatic nerve and tibial nerve	Tibial nerve	Sural nerve	Common peroneal nerve	Nerve root (disc prolapse)

Data from Butler, D.A.: Mobilisation of the Nervous System. Melbourne, Churchill Livingstone, 1991.

then slowly and carefully drops the leg back slightly until the patient feels no pain or tightness. The patient is then asked to flex the neck so the chin is on the chest, or the examiner may dorsiflex the patient's foot, or both actions may be done simultaneously. Most commonly, foot dorsiflexion is done first. Both of these maneuvers are con-

sidered to be provocative or sensitizing tests for neurological tissue. Table 9–8 and Figure 9–33 show modifications of the straight leg raising test that can be used to stress different peripheral nerves to a greater degree; these are referred to as straight leg raising tests with a particular nerve bias.

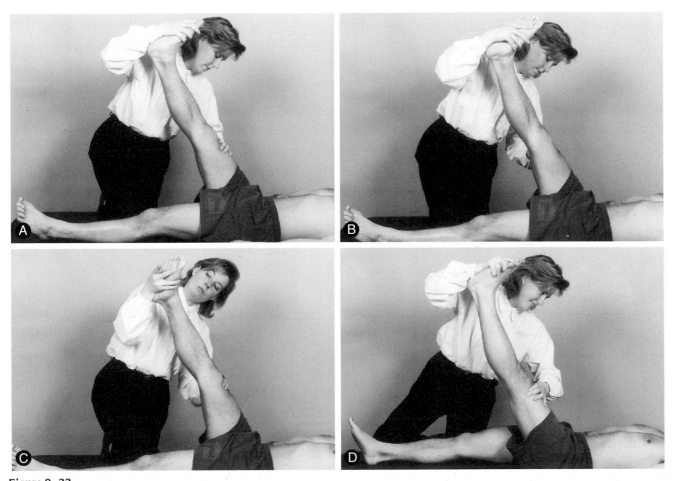

Figure 9–33
Modifications to straight leg raising (SLR) to stress specific nerve. (A) Basic SLR and SLR2 (sciatic and tibial nerves). (B) SLR3 (sural nerve). (C) SLR4 (common peroneal nerve). (D) SLR5 (intervertebral disc and nerve root). See Table 9–8 for movements at each joint.

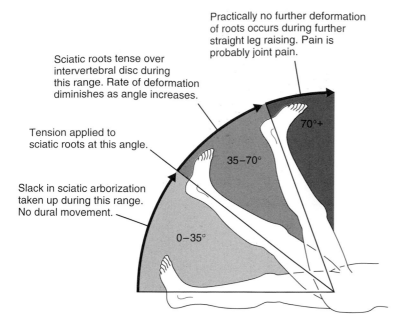

Sciatic roots tense over intervertebral disc during this range. Rate of deformation diminishes as angle increases.

Practically no further deformation of roots occurs during further straight leg raising. Pain is probably joint pain.

Tension applied to sciatic roots at this angle.

Slack in sciatic arborization taken up during this range. No dural movement.

70°+

35–70°

0–35°

Figure 9–34

Dynamics of single straight leg raising test in most people. (Modified from Fahrni, W.S.: Observations on straight leg raising with special reference to nerve root adhesions. Can. J. Surg. 9:44, 1966.)

The neck flexion movement has also been called **Hyndman's sign, Brudzinski's sign, Lidner's sign,** and the **Soto-Hall test.** If the examiner desires, neck flexion may be done by itself as a passive movement (passive neck flexion). Tension in the cervicothoracic junction is normal and should not be considered a production of symptoms. If lumbar, leg, or arm symptoms are produced, the neurological tissue is involved. The ankle dorsiflexion movement has also been called the **Bragard's test.** Pain that increases with neck flexion, ankle dorsiflexion, or both indicates stretching of the dura mater of the spinal cord or a lesion within the spinal cord (e.g., disc herniation, tumor, meningitis). Pain that does not increase with neck flexion may indicate a lesion in the hamstring area (tight hamstrings) or in the lumbosacral or sacroiliac joints. **Sicard's test** involves straight leg raising and then extension of the big toe instead of foot dorsiflexion. **Turyn's test** involves only extension of the big toe.[52]

With unilateral straight leg raising, the nerve roots, primarily the L5, S1, and S2 nerve roots (sciatic nerve), are normally completely stretched at 70°, having an excursion of approximately 2 to 6 mm (0.8 to 2.4 inches).[49] Pain after 70° is probably joint pain from the lumbar area (e.g., facet joints) or sacroiliac joints (Fig. 9–34). However, if the examiner suspects hamstring tightness, the hamstrings must also be cleared (see Chapter 11). The examiner should compare the two legs for any differences. It is important to realize that the ROM for straight leg raising and the stress placed on the neurological tissue vary greatly from person to person. For example, patients who are very hypermobile (e.g., gymnasts, syn-

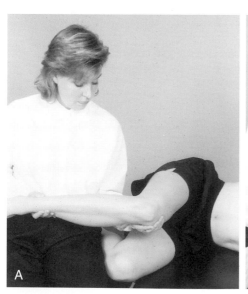

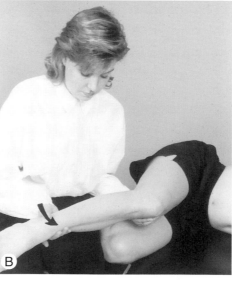

Figure 9–35

Modified straight leg raising for patients who cannot lie supine. (A) Starting position with knee flexed to 90°. (B) Knee is extended as far as possible.

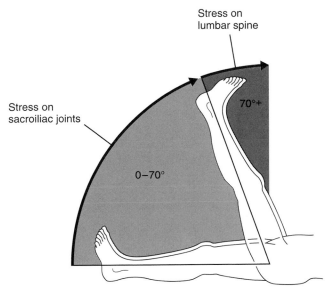

Figure 9–36
Dynamics of the bilateral straight leg raise.

chronized swimmers) may not show a positive straight leg raising test until 110 to 120° of hip flexion, even in the presence of nerve root pathology. It is more important to compare left and right sides for symptoms before deciding whether a lesion is caused by stretching of the neurological tissue or arises from the joints or other soft tissues.

During the unilateral straight leg raising test, tension develops in a sequential manner. It first develops in the greater sciatic foramen, then over the ala of the sacrum, next in the area where the nerve crosses over the pedicle, and finally in the intervertebral foramen. The test causes traction on the sciatic nerve, lumbosacral nerve roots, and dura mater. Adhesions within these areas may result from herniation of the intervertebral disc or extradural or meningeal irritation. Pain comes from the dura mater, nerve root, adventitial sheath of the epidural veins, or synovial facet joints. The test is positive if pain extends from the back down into the leg in the sciatic nerve distribution.

A central protrusion of an intervertebral disc leads to pain primarily in the back with the possibility of bowel and bladder symptoms; a protrusion in the intermediate area causes pain in the posterior aspect of the lower limb and low back; and a lateral protrusion causes pain primarily in the posterior leg.

For patients who have difficulty lying supine, a **modified straight leg raising test** has been suggested.[53] The patient is in side lying with the test leg uppermost and the hip and knee at 90°. The lumbosacral spine is in neutral but may be positioned in slight flexion or extension if this is more comfortable for the patient. The examiner then passively extends the patient's knee (Fig. 9–35), noting pain, resistance, and reproduction of the patient's symptoms for a positive test. The knee position (amount of flexion remaining) on the affected side is compared with that on the good side.

The examiner should then test both legs simultaneously (**bilateral straight leg raising,** Fig. 9–36). This test must be done with care, because the examiner is lifting the weight of both lower limbs and thereby placing a large stress on his or her lumbar spine. With the patient relaxed in the supine position and knees extended, the examiner lifts both of the legs by flexing the patient's hips until the patient complains of pain or tightness. If the test causes pain before 70° of hip flexion, the lesion is probably in the sacroiliac joints; if the test causes pain after 70°, the lesion is probably in the lumbar spine.

With the unilateral straight leg raising test, 80 to 90° of hip flexion is normal. If one leg is lifted and the patient complains of pain on the opposite side, it is an indication of a space-occupying lesion (e.g., a herniated disc). This finding of pain when the examiner is testing the opposite (good) leg may be called the **well leg raising test of Fajersztajn** (Fig. 9–37), a **prostrate leg raising test,** a **sciatic phenomenon, Lhermitt's test,** or the **crossover sign.**[49, 54, 55] It is usually indicative of a rather large intervertebral disc protrusion, usually medial to the nerve root (see Fig. 9–37).[49] The test causes stretching of the ipsilateral as well as the contralateral nerve root, pulling laterally on the dural sac. If the examiner finds this test

Figure 9–37
Well leg raising test of Fajersztajn. (A) Movement of nerve roots occurs when the leg on the opposite side is raised. (B) Position of disc and nerve root before opposite leg is lifted. (C) When the leg is raised on the unaffected side, the roots on the opposite side slide slightly downward and toward the midline. In the presence of a disc lesion, this movement increases the root tension resulting in radicular signs in the affected leg, which remains on the table. (Modified from DePalma, A.F., and R.H. Rothman: The Intervertebral Disc. Philadelphia, W.B. Saunders Co., 1970.)

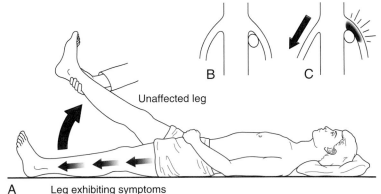

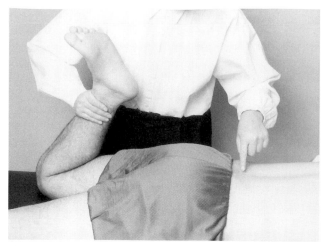

Figure 9–38
Prone knee bending test. Examiner is pointing to where pain may be expected in the lumbar spine with a positive test.

positive, careful questioning about bowel and bladder symptoms is in order. Most, but not all, patients with a central protrusion are candidates for surgery, especially if there are bowel and bladder symptoms.

Prone Knee Bending (Nachlas) Test. The patient lies prone while the examiner passively flexes the knee as far as possible so that the patient's heel rests against the buttock.[56, 57] At the same time, the examiner should ensure that the patient's hip is not rotated. If the examiner is unable to flex the patient's knee past 90° because of a pathological condition in the hip, the test may be

performed by passive extension of the hip while the knee is flexed as much as possible. Unilateral pain in the lumbar area, buttock, and/or posterior thigh may indicate an L2 or L3 nerve root lesion (Fig. 9–38).

This test also stretches the femoral nerve. Pain in the anterior thigh indicates tight quadriceps muscles or stretching of the femoral nerve. A careful history helps

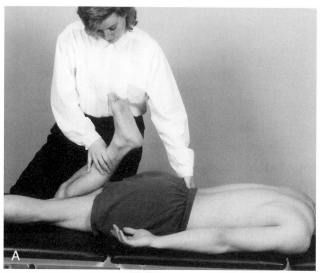

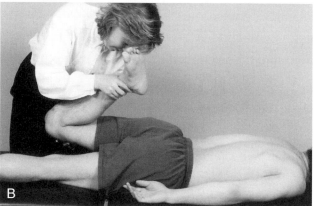

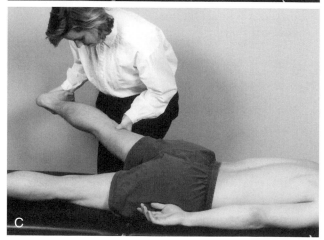

Figure 9–39
Modifications to the prone knee bending (PKB) test to stress specific nerve. (A) PKB1 (femoral nerve, L2–L4 nerve root). (B) PKB2 (lateral femoral cutaneous nerve). (C) Prone knee extension, or PKE (saphenous nerve). See Table 9–9 for movements at each joint.

Table 9–9
Prone Knee Bending (PKB) Test and Its Modifications

	Basic Prone Knee Bending (PKB1)	Prone Knee Bending (PKB2)	Prone Knee Extension (PKE)
Cervical spine	Rotation to test side	Rotation to test side	—
Thoracic and lumbar spine	Neutral	Neutral	Neutral
Hip	Neutral	Extension, adduction	Extension, abduction, lateral rotation
Knee	Flexion	Flexion	Extended
Ankle	—	—	Dorsiflexion
Foot	—	—	Eversion
Toes	—	—	—
Nerve bias	Femoral nerve, L2–L4 nerve root	Lateral femoral cutaneous nerve	Saphenous nerve

Data from Butler, D.A.: Mobilisation of the Nervous System. Melbourne, Churchill Livingstone, 1991.

delineate the problem. If the rectus femoris is tight, the examiner should remember that taking the heel to the buttock may cause anterior torsion to the ilium, which could lead to sacroiliac or lumbar pain. The flexed knee position should be maintained for 45 to 60 seconds. Butler[41] has suggested a modification of the prone knee bending test to stress individual peripheral nerves (Table 9–9 and Fig. 9–39).

Slump Test. The slump test has become the most common neurological test for the lower limb. The patient is seated on the edge of the examining table with the legs supported, the hips in neutral position (i.e., no rotation, abduction, or adduction), and the hands behind the back (Fig. 9–40). The examination is performed in sequential steps. First, the patient is asked to "slump" the back into thoracic and lumbar flexion. The examiner

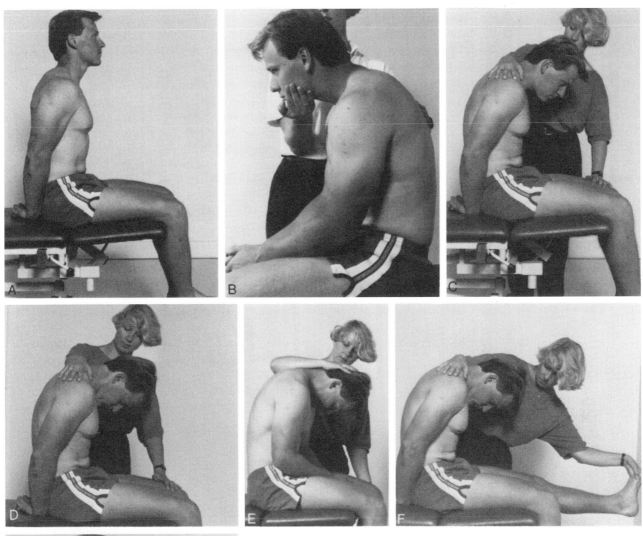

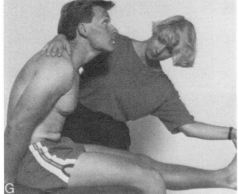

Figure 9–40
Sequence of subject postures in the slump test. (A) Patient sits erect. (B) Patient slumps lumbar and thoracic spine while examiner holds head in neutral.
(C) Examiner pushes down on shoulders while patient holds head in neutral.
(D) Patient flexes head. (E) Examiner carefully applies overpressure to cervical spine. (F) Examiner extends patient's knee and dorsiflexes foot. (G) Patient extends head. If symptoms are reproduced at any stage, further sequential movements are not attempted.

maintains the patient's chin in the neutral position to prevent neck and head flexion. The examiner then uses one arm to apply overpressure across the shoulders to maintain flexion of the thoracic and lumbar spines. While this position is held, the patient is asked to actively flex the cervical spine and head as far as possible (i.e., chin to chest). The examiner then applies overpressure to maintain flexion of all three parts of the spine (cervical, thoracic, and lumbar) using the hand of the same arm to maintain overpressure in the cervical spine. With the other hand, the examiner then holds the patient's foot in maximum dorsiflexion. While the examiner holds these positions, the patient is asked to actively straighten the knee as much as possible. The test is repeated with the other leg and then with both legs at the same time. If the patient is unable to fully extend the knee because of pain, the examiner releases the overpressure to the cervical spine and the patient actively extends the neck. If the knee extends further, the symptoms decrease with neck extension, or the positioning of the patient increases the patient's symptoms, then the test is considered positive for increased tension in the neuromeningeal tract.[58-60] Some clinicians modify the test to make the knee extension of the test passive. Once the patient is positioned with the three parts of the spine in flexion, the examiner first passively extends the knee. If symptoms do not result, then the examiner passively dorsiflexes the foot. A positive test would indicate the same lesion.

Butler[41] advocates doing bilateral knee extension in the slump position. Any asymmetry in the amount of knee extension is noted. Also, the effect of releasing neck flexion on the patient's symptoms should be noted.

In hypermobile patients, more hip flexion and hip adduction and medial rotation may be required to elicit a positive response.[41]

It is important to understand that if symptoms are produced in any phase of the sequence, the provocative maneuvers are stopped to prevent undue discomfort to the patient.

Butler[41] has suggested modifications to the slump test to stress individual nerves (Table 9–10 and Fig. 9–41).

When doing the slump test, it is important to look for reproduction of the patient's symptoms and to realize that the test does place stress on certain tissues, so some discomfort or pain is not necessarily symptomatic for the problem. For example, nonpathological responses include pain or discomfort in the area of T8–T9 (in 50% of normal patients), pain or discomfort behind the extended knee and hamstrings, symmetric restriction of knee extension, symmetric restriction of ankle dorsiflexion, and symmetric increased range of knee extension and ankle dorsiflexion on release of neck flexion.[41]

Brudzinski-Kernig Test. The patient is supine with the hands cupped behind the head (Fig. 9–42).[61-64] The patient is instructed to flex the head onto the chest. The patient raises the extended leg actively by flexing the hip until pain is felt. The patient then flexes the knee, and if the pain disappears, it is considered a positive test. The mechanics of the Brudzinski-Kernig test are similar to those of the straight leg raising test except that the movements are done actively by the patient. Pain is a positive sign and may indicate meningeal irritation, nerve root involvement, or dural irritation. The neck flexion aspect of the test was originally described by Brudzinski, and the hip flexion component was described by Kernig. The two parts of the test may be done individually, in which case they are described as the test of the original author.

Naffziger's Test. The patient lies supine while the examiner gently compresses the jugular veins (which lie

Table 9–10
Slump Test and Its Modifications

	Slump Test (ST1)	Slump Test (ST2)	Side Lying Slump Test (ST3)	Long Sitting Slump Test (ST4)
Cervical spine	Flexion	Flexion	Flexion	Flexion, rotation
Thoracic and lumbar spine	Flexion (slump)	Flexion (slump)	Flexion (slump)	Flexion (slump)
Hip	Flexion (90°+)	Flexion (90°+), abduction	Flexion (20°)	Flexion (90°+)
Knee	Extension	Extension	Flexion	Extension
Ankle	Dorsiflexion	Dorsiflexion	Plantar flexion	Dorsiflexion
Foot	—	—	—	—
Toes	—	—	—	—
Nerve bias	Spinal cord, cervical and lumbar nerve roots, sciatic nerve	Obturator nerve	Femoral nerve	Spinal cord, cervical and lumbar nerve roots, sciatic nerve

Data from Butler, D.A.: Mobilisation of the Nervous System. Melbourne, Churchill Livingstone, 1991.

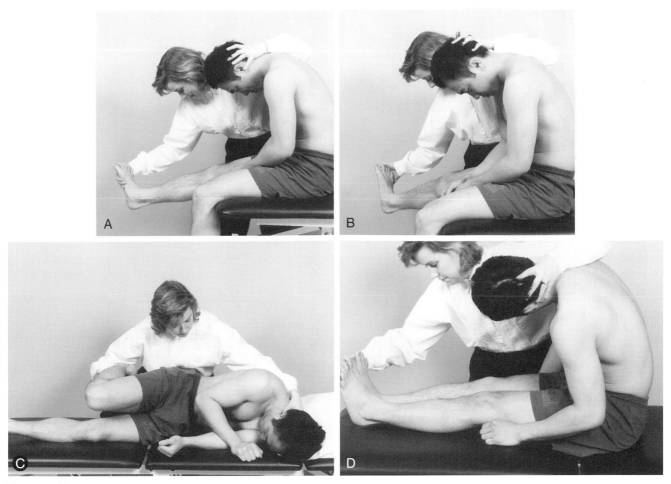

Figure 9–41
Modifications of the slump test (ST) to stress specific nerve. (A) Basic ST1 test (spinal cord, nerve roots). (B) ST2 (obturator nerve). (C) ST3 (femoral nerve). (D) ST4 (spinal cord, nerve roots). See Table 9–10 for movements at each joint.

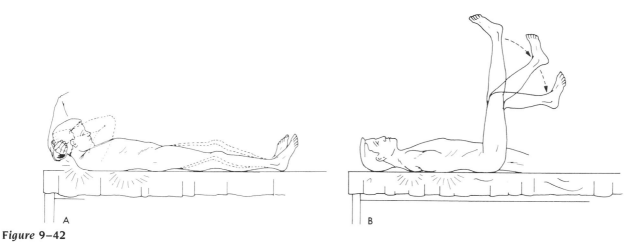

Figure 9–42
Brudzinski-Kernig test. (A) In Brudzinki's portion of the test, the patient lies supine, and the head is elevated from the table. The patient complains of neck and low back discomfort and attempts to relieve the meningeal irritation by involuntary flexion of the knees and hips. (B) In the Kernig portion of the test, the patient lies supine with the hip and knee flexed. Complaints of pain in the lower back, neck, and/or head on knee extension are suggestive of meningeal irritation. Knee flexion relieves pain. (Modified from Reilly, B.M.: Practical Strategies in Outpatient Medicine. Philadelphia, W.B. Saunders Co., 1991, p. 95.)

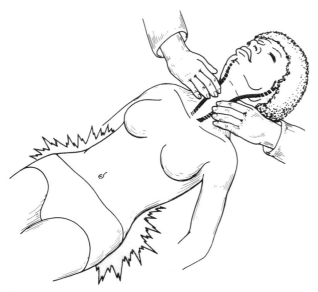

Figure 9–43
Naffziger's test. This test may be done while the patient is standing or lying down. The test is based on the hypothesis that bilateral jugular compression increases cerebral spinal fluid pressure. The pressure increase in the subarachnoid space in the root canal may cause back or leg pain by irritating a local mechanical or inflammatory condition. (From White, A.A., and M.M. Panjabi: Clinical Biomechanics of the Spine, 2nd ed. Philadelphia, J.B. Lippincott, 1990, p. 416.)

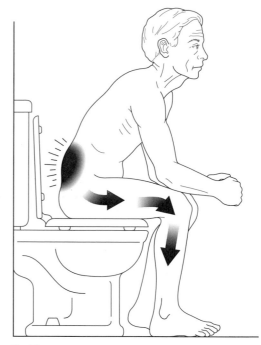

Figure 9–44
The Valsalva maneuver. Increased intrathecal pressure leads to symptoms in the sciatic nerve distribution in a positive test.

beside the carotid artery) for approximately 10 seconds (Fig. 9–43). The patient's face flushes, and then the patient is then asked to cough. If coughing causes pain in the low back, the spinal theca is being compressed, leading to an increase in intrathecal pressure. The theca is the covering (pia mater, arachnoid mater, and dura mater) around the spinal cord.

Valsalva Maneuver. The seated patient is asked to take a breath, hold it, and then bear down as if evacuating the bowels (Fig. 9–44). If pain increases, it is an indication of increased intrathecal pressure. The symptoms may be accentuated by having the patient first flex the hip to a position just short of that causing pain.[49]

Femoral Nerve Traction Test. The patient lies on the unaffected side with the unaffected limb flexed slightly at the hip and knee (Fig. 9–45).[65] The patient's back should be straight, not hyperextended. The patient's

head should be slightly flexed. The examiner grasps the patient's affected or painful limb and extends the knee while gently extending the hip approximately 15°. The patient's knee is then flexed on the affected side; this movement further stretches the femoral nerve. Pain radiates down the anterior thigh if the test is positive.

This is also a traction test for the nerve roots at the midlumbar area (L2–L4). As with the straight leg raising test, there may also be a contralateral positive test. Pain in the groin and hip that radiates along the anterior medial thigh indicates an L3 nerve root problem; pain extending to the midtibia indicates an L4 nerve root problem.

This test is similar to Ober's test for a tight iliotibial band, so the examiner must be able to differentiate between the two conditions. If the iliotibial band is tight, the test leg does not adduct but remains elevated away from the table as the tight tendon riding over the greater trochanter keeps the leg abducted. Femoral nerve injury

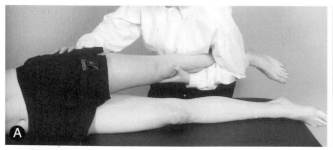
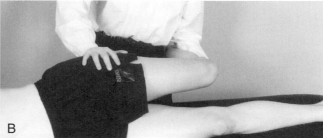

Figure 9–45
Femoral nerve traction test. (A) Hip and knee are extended. (B) Then knee is flexed.

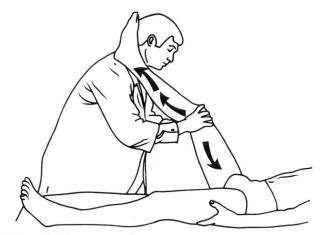

Figure 9–46
Bowstring sign. (From MacNab, I.: Backache. Baltimore, Williams & Wilkins, 1977, p. 175.)

presents with a different history, and the referred pain (anteriorly) tends to be stronger.

"Bowstring" Test (Cram Test or Popliteal Pressure Sign). The examiner carries out a straight leg raising test, and pain results (Fig. 9–46).[7, 66] While maintaining the thigh in the same position, the examiner flexes the knee slightly (20°), reducing the symptoms. Thumb or finger pressure is then applied to the popliteal area to reestablish the painful radicular symptoms. The test is an indication for tension or pressure on the sciatic nerve and is a modification of the straight leg raising test.

The test may also be done in the sitting position with the examiner passively extending the knee to produce pain. The examiner then slightly flexes the knee so that the pain and symptoms disappear. The examiner holds this slightly flexed position by clasping the patient's leg between the examiner's knees. The examiner then presses the fingers of both hands into the popliteal space. Pain resulting from these maneuvers indicates a positive test and pressure or tension on the sciatic nerve. In this case, the test is called the **sciatic tension test** or Deyerle's sign.[14, 63, 67]

Sitting Root Test. This test is a modification of the slump test. The patient sits with a flexed neck. The knee is actively extended while the hip remains flexed at 90°. Increased pain indicates tension on the sciatic nerve. This test is sometimes used to catch the patient unaware. In this case, the examiner passively extends the knee while pretending to examine the foot. Patients with true sciatic pain arch backward and complain of pain into the buttock, posterior thigh, and calf when the leg is straightened, indicating a positive test.[68] The **Bechterewis test**[54] follows a similar pattern. The patient is asked to extend one knee at a time. If no symptoms result, the patient is asked to extend both legs simultaneously. A positive response is indicated by symptoms in the back or leg.[69]

Flip Sign. While the patient is sitting, the examiner extends the patient's knee and looks for symptoms. The patient is then placed supine, and a unilateral straight leg raising test is performed. For the sign to be positive, both tests must cause pain in the sciatic nerve distribution. If only one test is positive, the examiner should suspect problems in the lower lumbar spine. This is a combination of the classic Lasègue test and the sitting root test.

Knee Flexion Test.[70] The patient who has complained of sciatica is in a standing position. The patient is asked to bend forward to touch the toes. If the patient bends the knee on the affected side while forward flexing the spine, the test is positive for sciatic spinal nerve root compression. Likewise, if the patient is not allowed to bend the knee, spinal flexion is decreased.

Babinski Test. The examiner runs a pointed object along the plantar aspect of the patient's foot.[71] A positive Babinski test or reflex suggests an upper motor neuron lesion and is demonstrated by extension of the big toe and abduction (splaying) of the other toes. In an infant up to a few weeks old, a positive test is normal. The test is often performed to determine the pathological reflex.

Oppenheim Test. The examiner runs a fingernail along the crest of the patient's tibia.[71] A negative Oppenheim test is indicated by no reaction or no pain. A positive test is indicated by a positive Babinski sign (positive pathological reflex) and suggests an upper motor neuron lesion.

Gluteal Skyline Test. The patient is relaxed in a prone position with the head straight and arms by the sides.[72] The examiner stands at the patient's feet and observes the buttocks from the level of the buttocks. The affected gluteus maximus muscle appears flat as a result of atrophy. The patient is asked to contract the gluteal muscles. The affected side may show less contraction, or it may be atonic and remain flat. If this occurs, the test is positive and may indicate damage to the inferior gluteal nerve or pressure on the L5, S1, and/or S2 nerve roots.

Tests for Joint Dysfunction

Schober Test. The Schober test may be used to measure the amount of flexion occurring in the lumbar spine. A point is marked midway between the two PSISs ("dimples of the pelvis"), which is the level of S2; then, points 5 cm (2 inches) below and 10 cm (4 inches) above that level are marked. The distance between the three points is measured, the patient is asked to flex forward, and the distance is remeasured. The difference between the two measurements is an indication of the amount of flexion occurring in the lumbar spine. Little[73] reported a modification of the Schober test to measure extension as well. After completion of the flexion movement, the patient extends the spine, and the distance between the marks is noted. Little also advocated using four marking points (one below the "dimples" and three above), with 10 cm (4 inches) between them.

Yeoman's Test. The patient lies prone while the examiner stabilizes the pelvis and extends each of the patient's hips in turn with the knees extended. The examiner then extends each of the patient's legs in turn with the knee flexed. In both cases, the patient remains passive. A positive test is indicated by pain in the lumbar spine during both parts of the test.

Milgram's Test. The patient lies supine and simultaneously actively lifts both legs off the examining table 5 to 10 cm (2 to 4 inches), holding this position for 30 seconds. The test is positive if the limbs or affected limb cannot be held for 30 seconds or if symptoms are reproduced in the affected limb.[54, 69] This test should always be performed with caution because of the high stress load placed on the lumbar spine.

McKenzie's Side Glide Test. The patient stands with the examiner standing to one side. The examiner grasps the patient's pelvis with both hands and places a shoulder against the patient's lower thorax. Using the shoulder as a "block," the examiner pulls the pelvis toward the examiner's body (Fig. 9–47). The position is held for 10 to 15 seconds, and then the test is repeated on the opposite side.[10, 69] If the patient has an evident scoliosis, the side to which the scoliosis curves should be tested first. A positive test is indicated by increased symptoms on the affected side. It also indicates whether the symptoms are actually causing the scoliosis.

One-Leg Standing (Stork Standing) Lumbar Extension Test. The patient stands on one leg and extends the

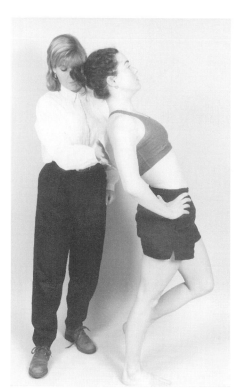

Figure 9–48
One-leg standing lumbar extension test.

spine while balancing on the leg (Fig. 9–48). The test is repeated with the patient standing on the opposite leg. A positive test is indicated by pain in the back and is associated with a pars interarticularis stress fracture (spondylolisthesis). If the stress fracture is unilateral, standing on the ipsilateral leg causes more pain.[74–76] If rotation is combined with extension and pain results, it is an indication of possible facet joint pathology on the side to which rotation occurs.

Pheasant Test. The patient lies prone. With one hand, the examiner gently applies pressure to the posterior aspect of the lumbar spine. With the other hand, the

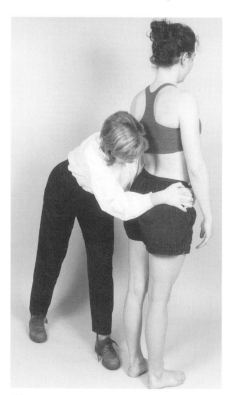

Figure 9–47
McKenzie's side glide test.

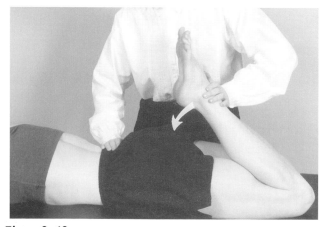

Figure 9–49
Pheasant test.

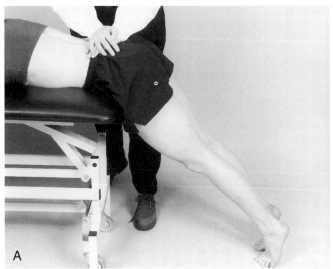
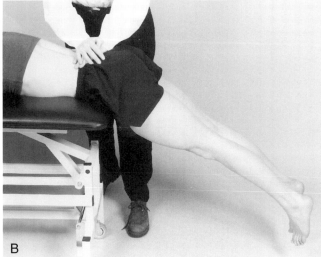

Figure 9–50
Segmental instability test. (A) Toes on floor. (B) Feet lifted off floor.

examiner passively flexes the patient's knees until the heels touch the buttocks (Fig. 9–49). If pain is produced in the leg by this hyperextension of the spine, the test is considered positive and indicates an unstable spinal segment.[77]

Segmental Instability Test. The patient lies prone with the body on the examining table and the legs over the edge resting on the floor (Fig. 9–50). The examiner applies pressure to the posterior aspect of the lumbar spine while the patient rests in this position. The patient then lifts the legs off the floor, and the examiner again applies posterior compression to the lumbar spine. If pain is elicited in the resting position only, the test is positive, because the muscle action masks the instability.[78]

Treadmill Test for Instability.[79] The patient is asked to walk on a treadmill beginning at 0.6 mph and gradually accelerating to 1.8 mph for up to 10 minutes or until symptoms are produced (low back pain, pain into lower extremities, intermittent claudication). The treadmill surface is horizontal to the floor. Production of symptoms is considered a positive test.

Quadrant Test. The patient stands with the examiner standing behind. The patient extends the spine while the examiner controls the movement by holding the patient's shoulders. The examiner may use his or her shoulders to hold the occiput and take the weight of the head. Overpressure is applied in extension while the patient side flexes and rotates to the side of pain. The movement is continued until the limit of range is reached or until symptoms are produced (Fig. 9–51). The position causes maximum narrowing of the intervertebral foramen and stress on the facet joint to the side which rotation occurs. The test is positive if symptoms are produced.[80] Cipriano[52] describes a similar test as **Kemp's test.**

Tests for Muscle Dysfunction

Beevor's Sign. The patient lies supine. The patient flexes the head against resistance, coughs, or attempts to sit up with the hands resting behind the head.[54, 81] The sign is positive if the umbilicus does not remain in a straight line when the abdominals contract, indicating pathology in the abdominal muscles (i.e., paralysis).

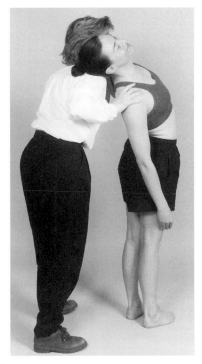

Figure 9–51
Quadrant test for the lumbar spine.

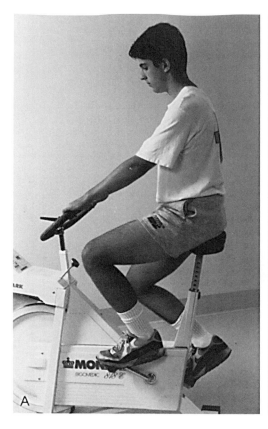
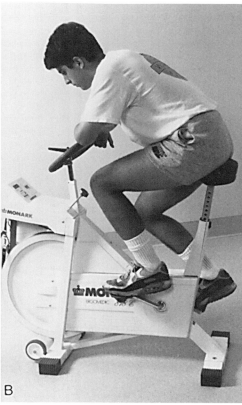

Figure 9–52
Bicycle test of van Gelderen. (A) Sitting erect. (B) Sitting flexed.

Tests for Intermittent Claudication

Stoop Test. The stoop test is done to assess neurogenic intermittent claudication to determine whether a relation exists among neurogenic symptoms, posture, and walking.[82] When the patient with neurogenic intermittent claudication walks briskly, pain ensues in the buttock and lower limb within a distance of 50 m (165 feet). To relieve the pain, the patient flexes forward. These symptoms may also be relieved when the patient is sitting and forward flexing. If flexion does not relieve the symptoms, the test is negative. Extension may also be used to bring the symptoms back.

Bicycle Test of van Gelderen.[83] The patient is seated on an exercise bicycle and is asked to pedal against resistance. The patient starts pedaling while leaning backward to accentuate the lumbar lordosis (Fig. 9–52). If pain into the buttock and posterior thigh occurs, followed by tingling in the affected lower extremity, the first part of the test is positive. The patient is then asked to lean forward while continuing to pedal. If the pain subsides over a short period of time, the second part of the test is positive; if the patient sits upright again, the pain returns. The test is used to determine whether the patient has neurogenic intermittent claudication.

Tests for Malingering

Hoover Test. The patient lies supine. The examiner places one hand under each calcaneus while the patient's

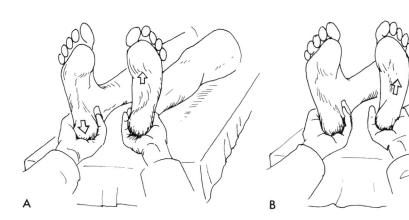

Figure 9–53
The Hoover test. (A) Normally, attempts to elevate one leg are accompanied by downward pressure by the opposite leg. (B) When the "weak" leg attempts to elevate but the opposite (asymptomatic) leg does not "help," at least some of the weakness is probably feigned. (From Reilly, B.M.: Practical Strategies in Outpatient Medicine. Philadelphia, W.B. Saunders Co., 1991, p. 946.)

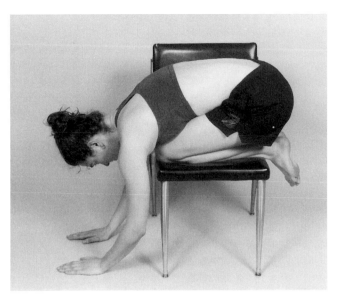

Figure 9–54
Burns test.

legs remain relaxed on the examining table (Fig. 9–53).[84–86] The patient is then asked to lift one leg off the table, keeping the knees straight, as for active straight leg raising. If the patient does not lift the leg or the examiner does not feel pressure under the opposite heel, the patient is probably not really trying or may be a malingerer. If the lifted limb is weaker, however, pressure under the normal heel increases, because of the increased effort to lift the weak leg. The two sides are compared for differences.

Burns Test. The patient is asked to kneel on a chair and then bend forward to touch the floor with the fingers (Fig. 9–54). The test is positive for malingering if the patient is unable to perform the test or the patient overbalances.[69]

Other Tests

Sign of the Buttock. The patient lies supine,[39] and the examiner performs a passive unilateral straight leg raising test. If there is unilateral restriction, the examiner then flexes the knee to see whether hip flexion increases. If the problem is in the lumbar spine or hamstrings, hip flexion increases. This finding indicates a negative sign of the buttock test. If hip flexion does not increase when the knee is flexed, it is a positive sign of the buttock test and indicates pathology in the buttock, such as a bursitis, tumor, or abscess. The patient should also exhibit a noncapsular pattern of the hip.

Reflexes and Cutaneous Distribution

After the special tests, the reflexes should be checked for differences between the two sides (Fig. 9–55).

Reflexes of the Lumbar Spine

- Patellar (L3–L4)
- Medial hamstring (L5–S1)
- Lateral hamstring (S1–S2)
- Posterior tibial (L4–L5)
- Achilles (S1–S2)

The deep tendon reflexes are tested with a reflex hammer, with the patient's muscles and tendons relaxed. The patellar reflex may be performed with the patient sitting or lying, and the hammer strikes the tendon directly. To test the patellar reflex, the knee should be flexed to 30° (supine lying) or 90° (sitting). The Achilles reflex may be tested in prone, sitting, or kneeling position. To test the Achilles reflex, the ankle should be at 90° or slightly dorsiflexed. It is important to ensure that

Figure 9–55
Reflexes of the lower limb.
(A) Patellar (L3) in sitting position. (B) Patellar (L3) in lying position.
Illustration continued on following page

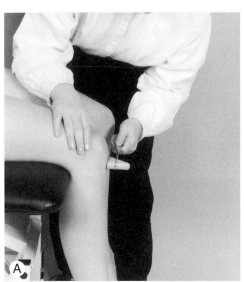

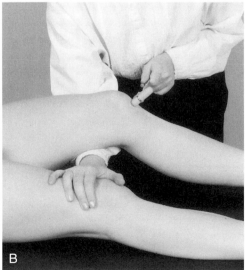

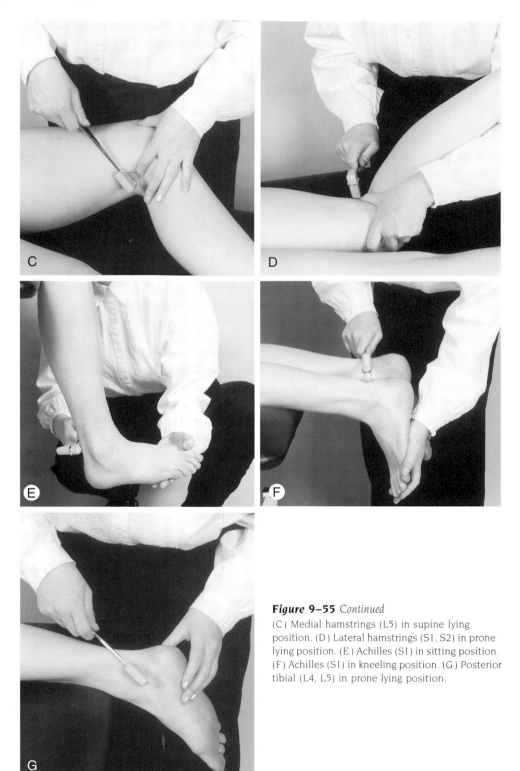

Figure 9–55 *Continued*
(C) Medial hamstrings (L5) in supine lying position. (D) Lateral hamstrings (S1, S2) in prone lying position. (E) Achilles (S1) in sitting position. (F) Achilles (S1) in kneeling position. (G) Posterior tibial (L4, L5) in prone lying position.

the patient's dorsiflexors are relaxed before doing the test; otherwise, the test will not work. This is done by passively dorsiflexing the foot and feeling for the "springing back" of the foot into plantar flexion. If this does not occur, the dorsiflexors are not relaxed. To test the hamstring reflex (semitendinosus and biceps femoris), the examiner places the thumb over the tendon and taps the thumbnail to elicit the reflex. Again, the knee should be slightly flexed with the hamstrings relaxed to perform the test.

It is also important to check the dermatome patterns of the nerve roots as well as the peripheral sensory distribution of the peripheral nerves (Table 9–11 and Fig. 9–56). It should be remembered that dermatomes vary

Table 9–11
Peripheral Nerve Lesions

Nerve (Root Derivation)	Sensory Supply	Sensory Loss	Motor Loss	Reflex Change	Lesion
Lateral cutaneous nerve of thigh (L2–L3)	Lateral thigh	Lateral thigh; often intermittent	None	None	Lateral inguinal entrapment
Posterior cutaneous nerve of thigh (S1–S2)	Posterior thigh	Posterior thigh	None	None	Local (buttock) trauma Pelvic mass Hip fracture
			(N.B. Sciatic nerve often involved, too)		
Saphenous branch of femoral nerve (L2–L4)	Anteromedial knee and medial leg	Medial leg	None	None	Local trauma Entrapment above medial epicondyle
			(N.B. Positive Tinel sign 5 to 10 cm above medial femoral epicondyle of knee)		
Obturator nerve (L2–L4)	Medial thigh	Often none ± medial thigh	Thigh adduction	None	Pelvic mass
Femoral nerve (L2–L4)	Anteromedial thigh and leg	Anteromedial thigh and leg	Knee extension ± hip flexion	Diminished knee jerk	Retroperitoneal or pelvic mass Femoral artery aneurysm (or puncture) Diabetic mononeuritis
Sciatic nerve (L4–L5, S1)	Anterior and posterior leg Sole and dorsum of foot	Entire foot	Foot dorsiflexion Foot inversion ± plantar flexion ± knee flexion	Diminished ankle jerk	Pelvic mass Hip fracture Piriformis entrapment Misplaced buttock injection
Common peroneal nerve (division of sciatic nerve)	Anterior leg, dorsum of foot	None or dorsal foot	Foot dorsiflexion, inversion, and eversion	None	Entrapment pressure at neck of fibula Rarely, diabetes, vasculitis, leprosy
			(N.B. Positive Tinel sign at lateral fibular neck)		

From Reilly, B.M.: Practical Strategies in Outpatient Medicine. Philadelphia, W.B. Saunders Co., 1991, p. 928.

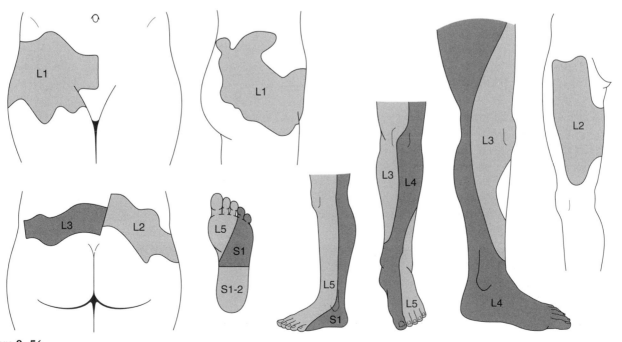

Figure 9–56
Lumbar dermatomes.

from person to person, and the accompanying representations are estimations only. The examiner tests for sensation by running relaxed hands over the back, abdomen, and lower limbs (front, sides, and back), being sure to cover all aspects of the leg and foot. If any difference between the sides is noted during this "sensation scan," the examiner may then use a pinwheel, pin, cotton ball, and/or brush to map out the exact area of sensory difference and determine the peripheral nerve or nerve root affected.

Pain may be referred from the lumbar spine to the sacroiliac joint and down the leg as far as the foot. Seldom is pain referred up the spine (Fig. 9–57). Pain may be referred to the lumbar spine from the abdominal organs, the lower thoracic spine, and the sacroiliac joints. Muscles may also refer pain to the lumbar area (Table 9–12).[87]

The examiner must remember that neurogenic intermittent claudication may cause the reflexes to be absent

Table 9–12
Lumbar Muscles and Referral of Pain

Muscle	Referral Pattern
Iliocostalis lumborum	Below T12 ribs lateral to spine down to buttock
Longissimus	Beside spine down to gluteal fold
Multifidus	Lateral to spine, sacrum to gluteal cleft, posterior leg, and lower abdomen
Abdominals	Below xiphisternum and along anterior rib cage down along inguinal ligament to genitals
Serratus posterior inferior	Lateral to spine in T9–T12 posterior rib area

Data from Travell, J.G., and D.G. Simons: Myofascial Pain and Dysfunction: The Trigger Point Manual. Baltimore, Williams & Wilkins, 1983.

soon after exercise (Table 9–13).[88, 89] If neurogenic intermittent claudication is suspected, it is necessary to test the reflexes immediately, because reflexes may return within 1 to 3 minutes after stopping the activity.

Another reflex that may be tested is the **superficial cremasteric reflex,** which occurs in males only (Fig. 9–58). The patient lies supine while the examiner strokes the inner side of the upper thigh with a pointed object. The test is negative if the scrotal sac on the tested side pulls up. Absence or reduction of the reflex bilaterally suggests an upper motor neuron lesion. A unilateral absence suggests a lower motor neuron lesion between L1 and L2. Absences have increased significance if they are associated with increased deep tendon reflexes.[90]

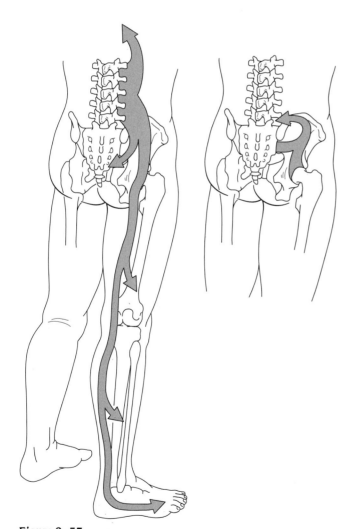

Figure 9–57
Referral of pain from and to the lumbar spine.

Table 9–13
Differential Diagnosis of Intermittent Claudication

	Vascular	Neurogenic
Pain	Related to exercise; occurs at various sites simultaneously	Related to exercise; sensations spread from area to area
Pulse	Absent after exercise	Present after exercise
Protein content of cerebrospinal fluid	Normal	Raised
Sensory change	Variable	Follows more specific dermatomes
Reflexes	Normal	Decreased but returns quickly

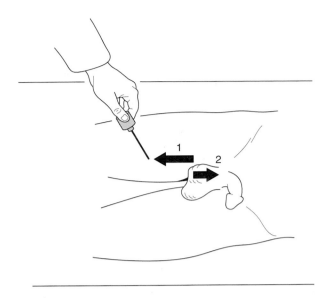

Figure 9–58
Cremasteric reflex. 1. The examiner runs a sharp object along the inner thigh. 2. A negative reflex is indicated by the scrotum's rising on that side.

Two other superficial reflexes are the **superficial abdominal reflex** (Fig. 9–59) and the **superficial anal reflex**. To test the superficial abdominal reflex, the examiner uses a pointed object to stroke each quadrant of the abdomen of the supine patient in a triangular fashion around the umbilicus. Absence of the reflex (reflex movement of the skin) indicates an upper motor neuron lesion; unilateral absence indicates a lower motor neuron

lesion from T7 to L2, depending on where the absence is noted, as a result of the segmental innervation. The examiner tests the superficial anal reflex by touching the perianal skin. A normal result is shown by contraction of the anal sphincter muscles (S2–S4).

Finally, the examiner should perform one or more of the pathological reflex tests (see Table 1–23) used to determine upper motor lesions or pyramidal tract disease, such as the Babinski or Oppenheim tests, which were described previously. The presence of these reflexes indicates the possible presence of disease, whereas their absence reflects the normal situation.

Peripheral Nerve Injuries of the Lumbar Spine

Lumbosacral Tunnel Syndrome. This syndrome involves compression of the L5 nerve root as it passes under the iliolumbar ligament in the iliolumbar canal (Fig. 9–60). The usual cause of compression is trauma (inflammation), osteophytes, or a tumor. Symptoms are primarily sensory (L5 dermatome) and pain. There is minimal or no effect on the L5 myotome.[91]

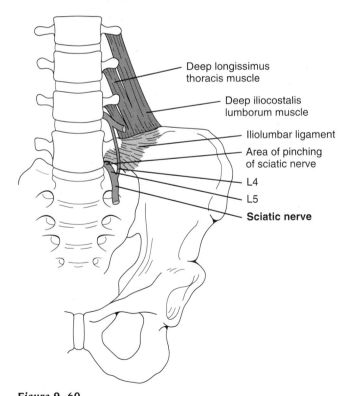

Deep longissimus thoracis muscle

Deep iliocostalis lumborum muscle

Iliolumbar ligament

Area of pinching of sciatic nerve

L4

L5

Sciatic nerve

Figure 9–60
Lumbosacral tunnel syndrome. This syndrome involves compression of the L5 nerve root as it passes under the iliolumbar ligament in the iliolumbar canal.

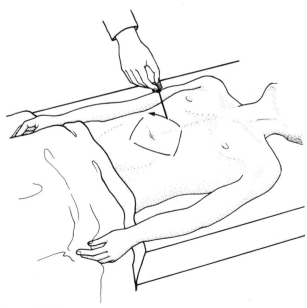

Figure 9–59
Superficial abdominal reflex.

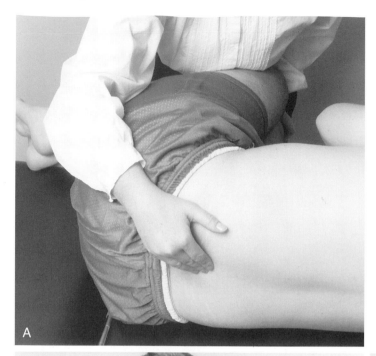

Figure 9–61
Joint play movements of the lumbar spine. (A) Flexion.
(B) Extension. (C) Side flexion. (D) Posteroanterior central
vertebral pressure. (E) Posteroanterior unilateral vertebral
pressure. (F) Transverse vertebral pressure.

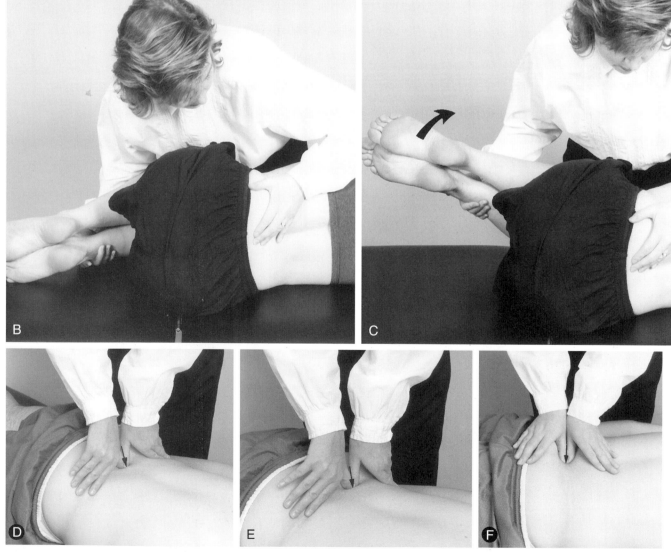

Joint Play Movements

The joint play movements have special importance in the lumbar spine because they are used to determine the end feel of joint movement as well as the presence of joint play. They are often used to replace passive movements in the lumbar spine, which are difficult to perform because of the need to move the heavy trunk and/or lower limbs. As the joint play movements are performed, any decreased ROM, pain, or difference in end feel should be noted.

Joint Play Movements of the Lumbar Spine

- Flexion
- Extension
- Side flexion
- Posteroanterior central vertebral pressure
- Posteroanterior unilateral vertebral pressure
- Transverse vertebral pressure

Flexion, Extension, and Side Flexion. Flexion is accomplished with the patient in the side lying position. The examiner flexes both of the patient's hips toward the chest with the knees bent (Fig. 9–61A). While palpating between the spinous processes of the lumbar vertebrae with one hand (one finger on the spinous process, one finger above, and one finger below the process), the examiner passively flexes and releases the patient's hips; the examiner's body weight is used to cause the movement. The examiner should feel the spinous processes "gap" or move apart on flexion. If this gapping does not occur between two spinous processes, or if it is excessive in relation to the other gapping movements, the segment is hypomobile or hypermobile, respectively.

Extension (Fig. 9–61B) and side flexion (Fig. 9–61C) are tested in a similar fashion, except that the movement is passive extension or passive side flexion rather than passive flexion. Side flexion is most easily accomplished by grasping the patient's uppermost leg and rotating the leg upward, which causes side flexion in the lumbar spine. Hip pathology must be ruled out before this is performed.

Central, Unilateral, and Transverse Vertebral Pressure. To perform the last three joint play movements, the patient lies prone.[92] The lumbar spinous processes are palpated beginning at L5 and working up to L1.

The examiner positions the hands, fingers, and thumbs as shown in Figure 9–61D to perform **posteroanterior central vertebral pressure**. Pressure is applied through the thumbs, with the vertebrae being pushed anteriorly (see Fig. 8–33). The examiner must take care to apply the pressure slowly and carefully so

that the feel of the movement can be recognized. In reality, the movement is minimal. This "springing test" may be repeated several times to determine the quality of the movement.

To perform **posteroanterior unilateral vertebral pressure**, the examiner moves the fingers laterally away from the tip of the spinous process so that the thumbs rest on the lamina or on the transverse process of the lumbar vertebra (Fig. 9–61E). The same anterior springing pressure is applied as in the central pressure technique. The two sides should be evaluated and compared.

To perform **transverse vertebral pressure**, the examiner's fingers are placed along the side of the spinous process of the lumbar spine (Fig. 9–61F). The examiner then applies a transverse springing pressure to the side of the spinous process, feeling for the quality of movement. Pressure should be applied to both sides of the spinous process to compare the quality of movement.

Palpation

If the examiner, having completed the examination of the lumbar spine, decides that the problem is in another joint, palpation should not be done until that joint is completely examined. However, when palpating the lumbar spine, any tenderness, altered temperature, muscle spasm, or other signs and symptoms that may indicate the source of pathology should be noted. If the problem is suspected to be in the lumbar spine area, palpation should be carried out in a systematic fashion, starting on the anterior aspect and working around to the posterior aspect.

Anterior Aspect

With the patient lying supine, the following structures are palpated anteriorly (Fig. 9–62).

Umbilicus. The umbilicus lies at the level of the L3–L4 disc space and is the point of intersection of the abdominal quadrants. It is also the point at which the aorta divides into the common iliac arteries. With some patients, the examiner may be able to palpate the anterior aspects of the L4, L5, and S1 vertebrae along with the discs and anterior longitudinal ligament. The abdomen may also be carefully palpated for symptoms (e.g., pain, muscle spasm) arising from internal organs. For example, the appendix is palpated in the right lower quadrant and the liver in the right upper quadrant; the kidneys are located in the left and right upper quadrants, and the spleen is found in the left upper quadrant.

Inguinal Area. The inguinal area is located between the ASIS and the symphysis pubis. The examiner should carefully palpate for symptoms of a hernia, abscess, infection (lymph nodes), or other pathological conditions in the area.

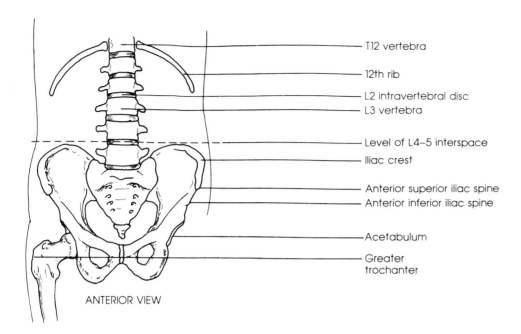

T12 vertebra

12th rib

L2 intravertebral disc

L3 vertebra

Level of L4–5 interspace

Iliac crest

Anterior superior iliac spine

Anterior inferior iliac spine

Acetabulum

Greater trochanter

ANTERIOR VIEW

Figure 9–62
Bony landmarks of the lumbar spine (anterior view).

Iliac Crest. The examiner palpates the iliac crest from the ASIS, moving posteriorly and looking for any symptoms (e.g., hip pointer or apophysitis).

Symphysis Pubis. The symphysis pubis is palpated by the examiner using both thumbs. Standing at the patient's side, the examiner pushes both thumbs down onto the symphysis pubis so that the thumbs rest on the superior aspect of the pubic bones (see Fig. 10–4). In this way, one can ensure that the two pubic bones are level at any joint. The symphysis pubis may also be palpated for any tenderness (e.g., osteitis pubis).

Posterior Aspect

The patient is then asked to lie prone, and the following structures are palpated posteriorly (Fig. 9–63).

Spinous Processes of the Lumbar Spine. The examiner palpates a point in the midline which is on a line joining the high point of the two iliac crests. This point is the L4–L5 interspace. After moving down to the first hard mass, the fingers will be resting on the spinous process of L5. Moving toward the head, the interspaces and spinous processes of the remaining lumbar vertebrae can be pal-

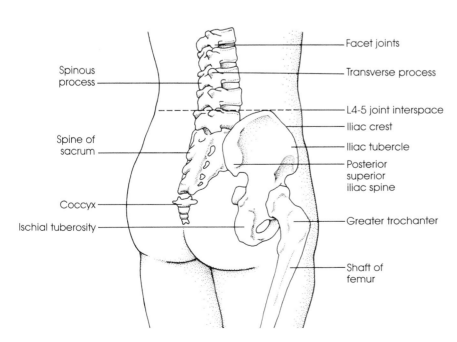

Spinous process

Spine of sacrum

Coccyx

Ischial tuberosity

Facet joints

Transverse process

L4-5 joint interspace

Iliac crest

Iliac tubercle

Posterior superior iliac spine

Greater trochanter

Shaft of femur

Figure 9–63
Bony landmarks of the lumbar spine (posterior view).

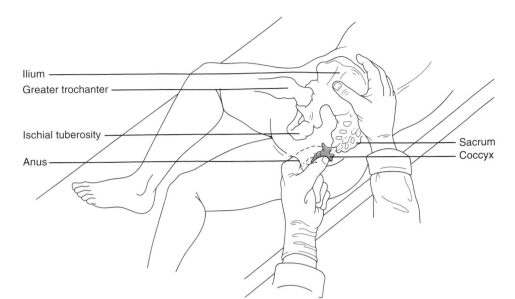

Ilium

Greater trochanter

Ischial tuberosity

Anus

Sacrum
Coccyx

Figure 9–64
Palpation of the coccyx.

pated. In addition to looking for tenderness, muscle spasm, and other signs of pathology, the examiner should watch for signs of a spondylolisthesis, which is most likely to occur at L4–L5 or L5–S1. A visible or palpable dip from one spinous process to another may be evident, depending on the type of spondylolisthesis present. Absence of a spinous process may be seen in a spina bifida. If the examiner moves laterally 2 to 3 cm (0.8 to 1.2 inches) from the spinous processes, the fingers will be resting over the lumbar facet joints. These joints should also be palpated for signs of pathology. Because of the depth of these joints, the examiner may have difficulty palpating them. However, pathology in this area results in spasm of the overlying paraspinal muscles, which can be palpated.

Sacrum, Sacral Hiatus, and Coccyx. If the examiner returns to the spinous process of L5 and moves caudally, the fingers will be resting on the sacrum. Like the lumbar spine, the sacrum has spinous processes, but they are much harder to distinguish because there are no interposing soft-tissue spaces between them. The S2 spinous process is at the level of a line joining the two PSISs ("posterior dimples"). Moving distally, the examiner's fingers may palpate the sacral hiatus, which is the caudal portion of the sacral canal. It has an inverted **U** shape and lies approximately 5 cm (2 inches) above the tip of the coccyx. The two bony prominences on each side of the hiatus are called the **sacral cornua** (see Fig. 10–38). As the examiner's fingers move farther distally, they eventually rest on the posterior aspect of the coccyx. Proper palpation of the coccyx requires a rectal examination using a surgical rubber glove (Fig. 9–64). The index finger is lubricated and inserted into the anus while the patient's sphincter muscles are relaxed. The finger is inserted as far as possible and then rotated so that the

pulpy surface rests against the anterior surface of the coccyx. The examiner then places the thumb of the same hand against the posterior aspect of the sacrum. In this way, the coccyx can be moved back and forth. Any major tenderness (e.g., coccyodynia) should be noted.

Iliac Crest, Ischial Tuberosity, and Sciatic Nerve. Beginning at the PSISs, the examiner moves along the iliac crest, palpating for signs of pathology. Then, moving slightly distally, the examiner palpates the gluteal muscles for spasm, tenderness, or the presence of abnormal nodules. Just under the gluteal folds, the examiner should palpate the ischial tuberosities on both sides for any abnormality. As the examiner moves laterally, the greater trochanter of the femur is palpated. It is often easier to palpate if the hip is flexed to 90°. Midway between the ischial tuberosity and the greater trochanter, the examiner may be able to palpate the path of the sciatic nerve. The nerve itself is not usually palpable. Deep to the gluteal muscles, the piriformis muscle should also be palpated for potential pathology. This muscle is in a line dividing the PSIS of the pelvis and greater trochanter of the femur from the ASIS and ischial tuberosity of the pelvis.

Diagnostic Imaging [93–101]

Plain Film Radiography

It is imperative when viewing plain films to correlate clinical findings with x-ray findings, because many anomalies, congenital abnormalities, and aging changes may be present that are not related to the patient's problems. Normally, anteroposterior and lateral views are taken. In some cases, two lateral views may be taken, one that shows the whole lumbar spine, and one that focuses on the lower two segments. Oblique views are taken if spondylolysis or spondylolisthesis is suspected.[31]

Anteroposterior View. With this view (Fig. 9–65), the examiner should note the following:

1. Shape of the vertebrae.
2. Any wedging of the vertebrae, possibly resulting from fracture (Fig. 9–66).
3. Disc spaces. Do they appear normal, or are there height decreases, as are seen in spondylosis?
4. Any vertebral deformity, such as a hemivertebra or other anomalies (Figs. 9–67 through 9–70).

5. The presence of a bamboo spine, as seen in ankylosing spondylitis.
6. Any evidence of lumbarization of S1, making S1–S2 the first mobile segment rather than L5–S1. Lumbarization is seen in 2 to 8% of the population (Fig. 9–71).
7. Any evidence of sacralization of L5, making the L4–L5 level the first mobile segment rather than L5–S1. This anomaly is seen in 3 to 6% of the population (Fig. 9–72).
8. Any evidence of spina bifida occulta, seen in 6 to 10% of the population (see Fig. 9–69).

Text continued on page 415

Figure 9–65

Anteroposterior radiograph of the lumbar spine. (A) Film tracing.

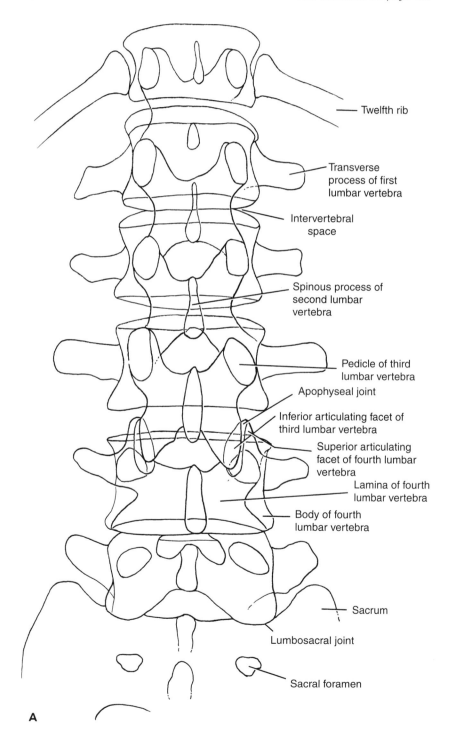

Twelfth rib

Transverse process of first lumbar vertebra

Intervertebral space

Spinous process of second lumbar vertebra

Pedicle of third lumbar vertebra

Apophyseal joint

Inferior articulating facet of third lumbar vertebra

Superior articulating facet of fourth lumbar vertebra

Lamina of fourth lumbar vertebra

Body of fourth lumbar vertebra

Sacrum

Lumbosacral joint

Sacral foramen

A

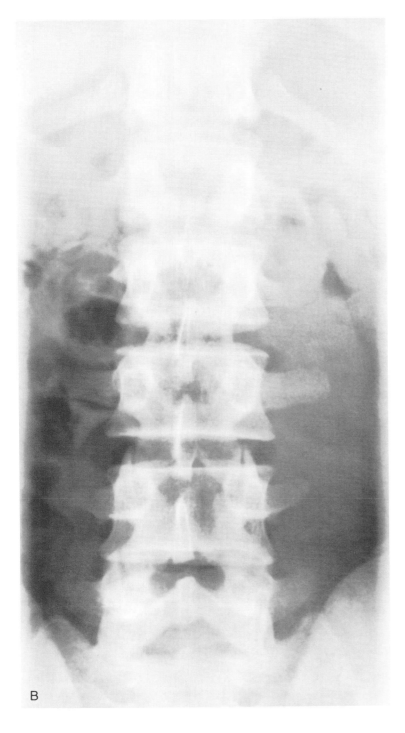

B

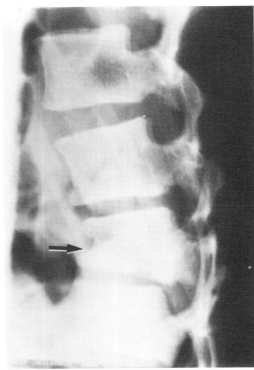

Figure 9–65 *Continued*
(B) Radiograph. (From Finneson, B.E.: Low Back Pain. Philadelphia, J.B. Lippincott, 1973, pp. 52–53.)

Figure 9–66
Wedging (*arrow*) of a vertebral body. Some wedging may also be seen in the vertebra above.

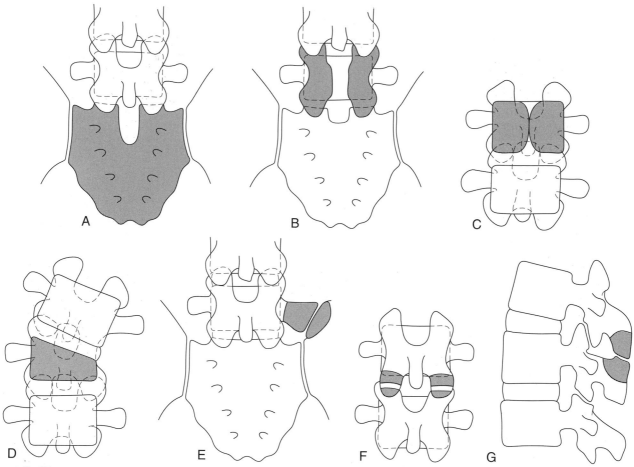

Figure 9–67

Diagrammatic representation of the x-ray appearance of common anatomic anomalies in the lumbosacral spine. (A) Spina bifida occulta, S1. (B) Spina bifida, L5. (C) Anterior spina bifida ("butterfly vertebra"). (D) Hemivertebra. (E) Iliotransverse joint (transitional segments). (F) Ossicles of Oppenheimer. These are free ossicles seen at the tip of the inferior articular facets and are usually found at the level of L3. (G) "Kissing" spinous processes. (Redrawn from MacNab, I.: Backache. Baltimore, Williams & Wilkins, 1977, pp. 14–15.)

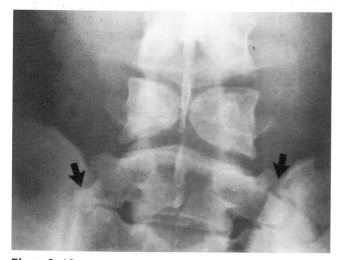

Figure 9–68

Butterfly vertebra. Also note transitional segments (*large arrows*). (Modified from Jaeger, S.A.: Atlas of Radiographic Positioning; Normal Anatomy and Developmental Variants. Norwalk, Appleton & Lange, 1988, p. 333.)

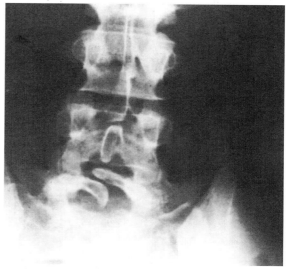

Figure 9–69

Spina bifida occulta. (From Jaeger, S.A.: Atlas of Radiographic Positioning: Normal Anatomy and Developmental Variants. Norwalk, Appleton & Lange, 1988, p. 317.)

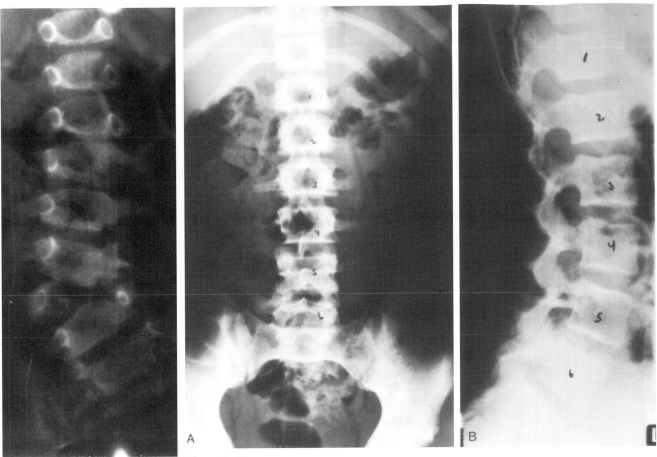

Figure 9–70
Hemivertebra shown on an anteroposterior radiograph.

Figure 9–71
Lumbarization of the S1 vertebra seen on anteroposterior (A) and lateral (B) radiographs.

Figure 9–72
Unilateral sacralization of the fifth lumbar vertebra. (A) Note the massive formation of sacral ala on the left side with a relatively normal transverse process on the right (anteroposterior view). (B) Lateral view showing the very narrow disc space and the massive arches. (From O'Donoghue, D.H.: Treatment of Injuries to Athletes, 4th ed. Philadelphia, W.B. Saunders Co., 1984, p. 403.)

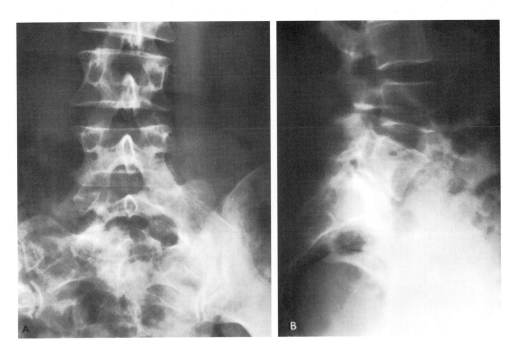

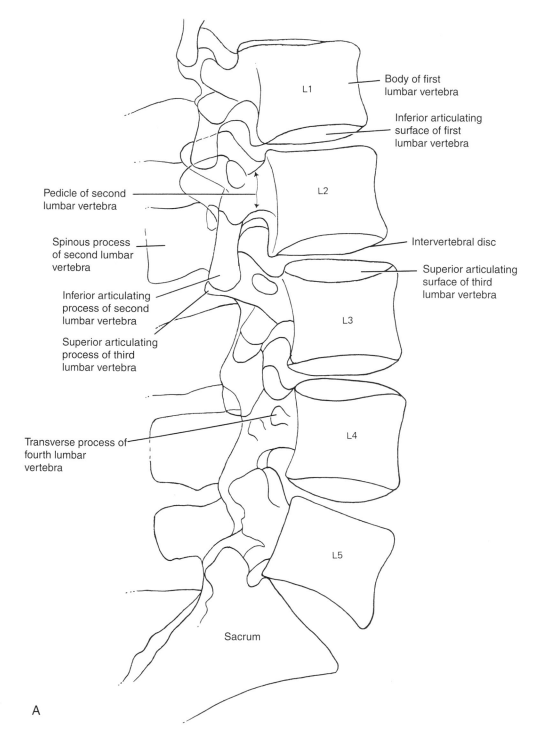

Body of first
lumbar vertebra

Inferior articulating
surface of first
lumbar vertebra

Pedicle of second
lumbar vertebra

Intervertebral disc

Spinous process
of second lumbar
vertebra

Superior articulating
surface of third
lumbar vertebra

Inferior articulating
process of second
lumbar vertebra

Superior articulating
process of third
lumbar vertebra

Transverse process of
fourth lumbar
vertebra

Sacrum

L1

L2

L3

L4

L5

Figure 9–73

Lateral radiograph of the lumbar
spine. (A) Film tracing.

A

Lateral View. With this view (Fig. 9–73), the examiner should note the following:

1. Any evidence of spondylosis or spondylolisthesis, which is seen in 2 to 4% of the population (Fig. 9–74). The degree of slipping can be graded as shown in Figure 9–75.
2. A normal lordosis. Do the intervertebral foramina appear normal?
3. Any wedging of the vertebrae.

4. Normal disc spacing.
5. Alignment of the vertebrae should be noted. Disruption of the curve may indicate spinal instability.
6. Any osteophyte formation or traction spurs (Fig. 9–76).[100] Traction spurs indicate an unstable lumbar intervertebral segment. A traction spur occurs approximately 1 mm from the disc border; an osteophyte occurs at the disc border with the vertebral body.

Text continued on page 420

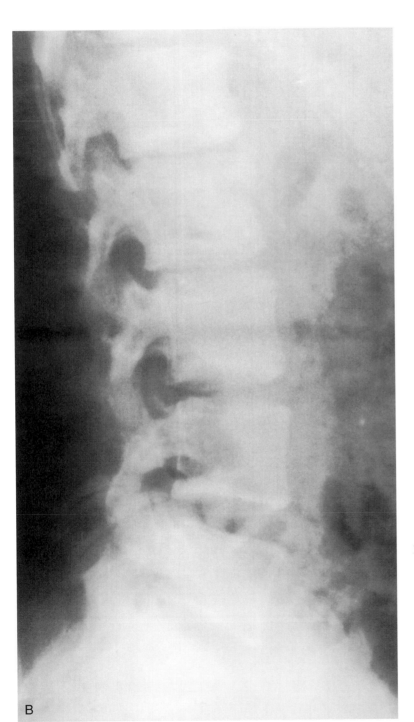

B

Figure 9–73 *Continued*
(B) Radiograph. (From Finneson, B.E.: Low Back Pain. Philadelphia, J.B. Lippincott, 1973, pp. 54–55.)

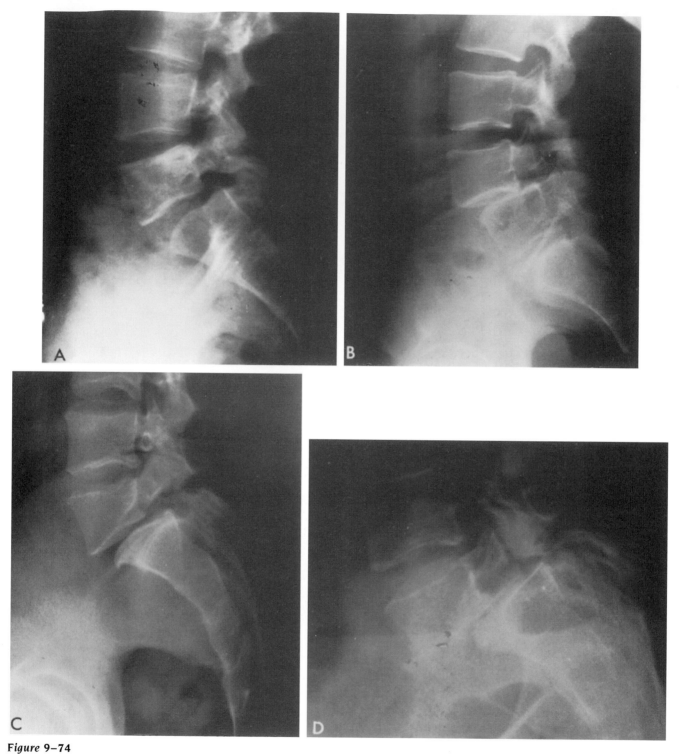

Figure 9–74

Spondylolisthesis. (A) Grade 1: arch defect in L5 with mild forward displacement of L5 on S1; backache but no gross disability. (B) Grade 2: there is more forward slipping between L4 and L5 with collapse of the intervertebral disc; definite symptomatic back with restriction of motion, muscle spasm, and curtailment of activities. (C) Grade 3: more extensive slipping combined with a wide separation at the arch defect and degenerative changes of the disc; grossly symptomatic. (D) Grade 4: vertebrae slipped forward more than halfway; severe disability. (From O'Donoghue, D.H.: Treatment of Injuries to Athletes, 4th ed. Philadelphia, W.B. Saunders Co., 1984, p. 402.)

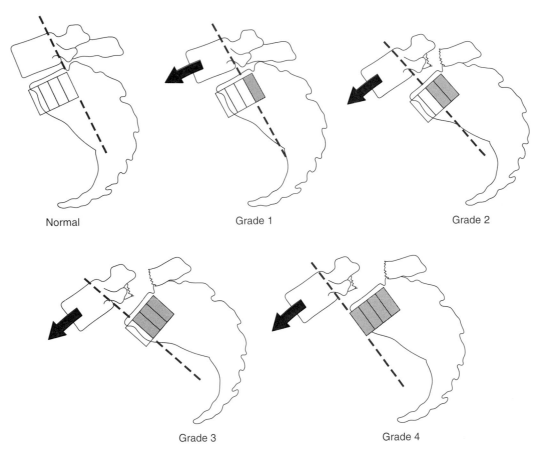

Figure 9–75
Meyerding grading system for slipping in spondylolisthesis.

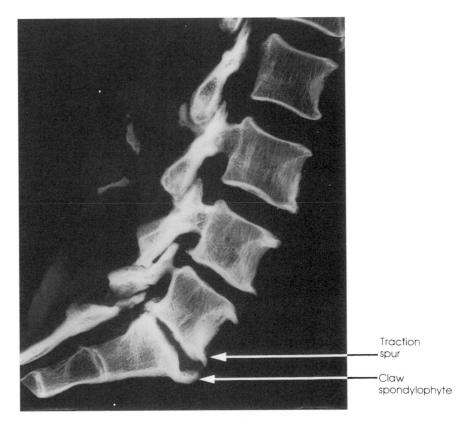

Figure 9–76
Lateral radiograph of a thin-slice pathological section of lumbar spine. Note traction spur and claw spondylophyte. (From Rothman, R.H., and F.A. Simeone: The Spine. Philadelphia, W.B. Saunders Co., 1982, p. 512.)

Traction spur

Claw spondylophyte

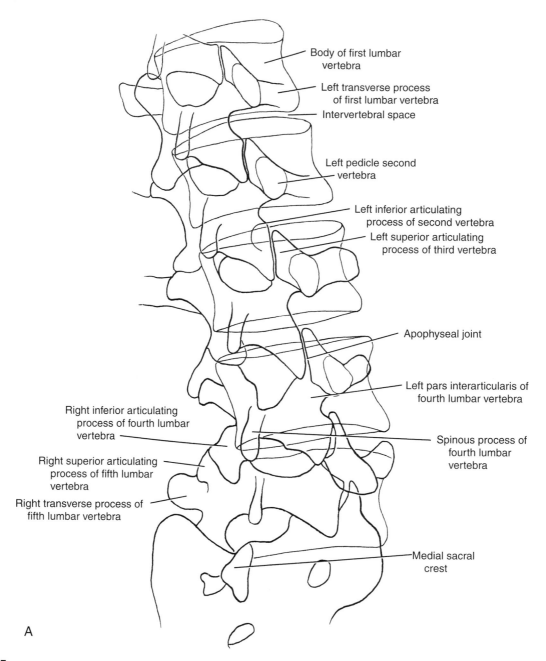

Body of first lumbar
vertebra

Left transverse process
of first lumbar vertebra

Intervertebral space

Left pedicle second
vertebra

Left inferior articulating
process of second vertebra

Left superior articulating
process of third vertebra

Apophyseal joint

Left pars interarticularis of
fourth lumbar vertebra

Right inferior articulating
process of fourth lumbar
vertebra

Spinous process of
fourth lumbar
vertebra

Right superior articulating
process of fifth lumbar
vertebra

Right transverse process of
fifth lumbar vertebra

Medial sacral
crest

A

Figure 9–77
Left posterior oblique radiograph of the lumbar spine. (A) Film tracing.

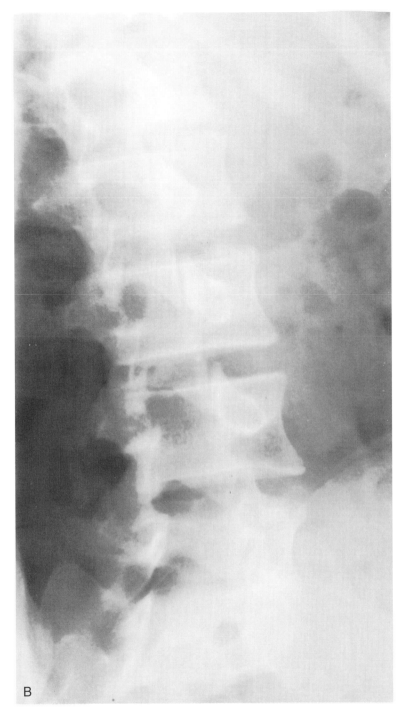

Figure 9-77 *Continued*
(B) Radiograph. (From Finneson, B.E.: Low Back Pain. Philadelphia, J.B. Lippincott, 1973, pp. 56-57.)

Oblique View. With the oblique view (Fig. 9–77), the examiner should look for any evidence of spondylolisthesis (sometimes referred to as a "Scottie dog decapitated") or spondylolysis (sometimes referred to as a "Scottie dog with a collar"; Fig. 9–78).

Motion Views. In some cases, motion views may be used to demonstrate abnormal spinal motion or structural abnormalities. These are usually lateral views showing flexion and extension to demonstrate instability or spondylolisthesis (Fig. 9–79), but they may also include anteroposterior views with side bending.[43, 102, 103]

Myelography

A myelogram can confirm the presence of a protruding intervertebral disc, osteophytes, a tumor, or spinal ste-

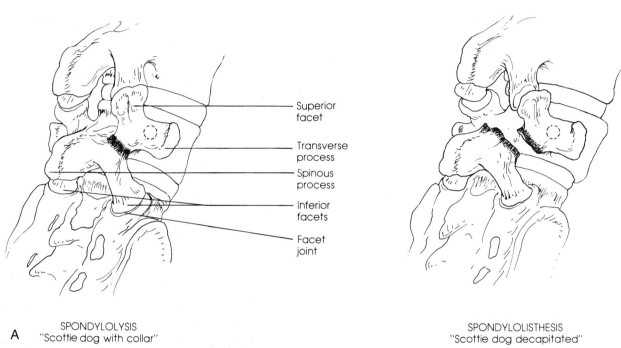

A   SPONDYLOLYSIS
"Scottie dog with collar"

SPONDYLOLISTHESIS
"Scottie dog decapitated"

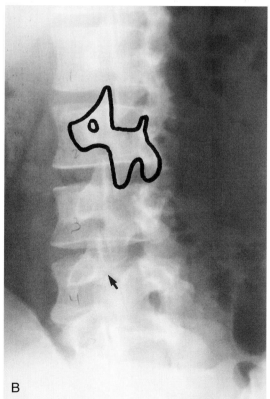

B

Figure 9–78

(A) Diagrammatic representation (posterior oblique view) of spondylolysis and spondylolisthesis. (B) Posterior oblique film showing "Scottie dog" at L2. L4 shows Scottie dog with a "collar" (*arrow*), indicating spondylolysis.

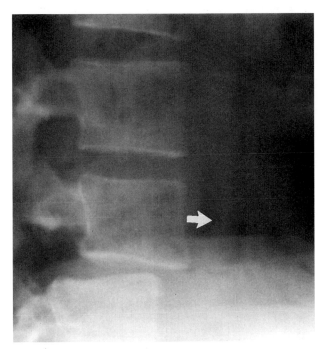

Figure 9–79

Lumbar spine in flexion. Note forward slipping of one vertebra on the one below (*arrow*).

nosis (Figs. 9–80 through 9–82). The examiner must be careful of the side effects of myelograms, which include headache, stiffness, low back pain, cramps, and paresthesia in the lower limbs. Although side effects do occur, no permanent injuries have been noted.

Radionuclide Imaging (Bone Scans)

Bone scans are useful for detecting active bone disease processes and areas of high bone turnover. In children, the epiphyseal and metaphyseal areas of the long bones show increased uptake. In adults, only the metaphyseal area is so affected. Traumatic bone injuries, tumors, metabolic abnormalities (e.g., Paget's disease), infection, and arthritis may be detected on bone scan.[31]

Computed Tomography

A computed tomography (CT) scan may be used to delineate a fracture or to show the presence of spinal stenosis caused by protrusion or a tumor (Figs. 9–83 through 9–85). As with plain x-rays, results must be correlated with clinical findings, because the anatomic changes seen are often unassociated with the patient's symp-

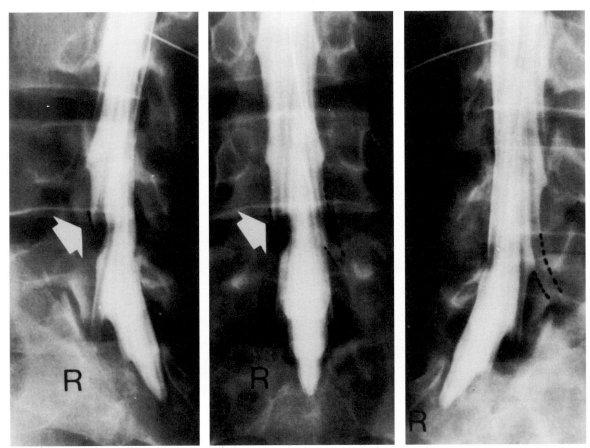

Figure 9–80

Metrizamide myelograms illustrating a herniated disc at L4–L5 on the right. Note lack of filling of the nerve root sleeve and indentation (*arrow*) of the dural sac. (From Rothman, R.H., and F.A. Simeone: The Spine. Philadelphia, W.B. Saunders Co., 1982, p. 550.)

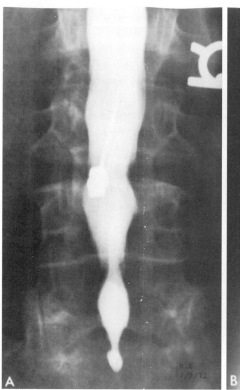
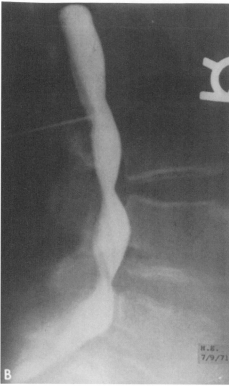

Figure 9–81

Oil myelograms showing the characteristic appearance of chronic disc degeneration and spinal stenosis with diffuse posterior bulging of the annulus and osteophyte formation. (A) There is symmetric wasting of the dye column in the anteroposterior view. Note the hourglass configuration. (B) Indentation of the dye column of the annulus anteriorly and the buckled ligamentum flavum and facet joints posteriorly (lateral view). (From Rothman, R.H., and F.A. Simeone: The Spine. Philadelphia, W.B. Saunders Co., 1982, p. 553.)

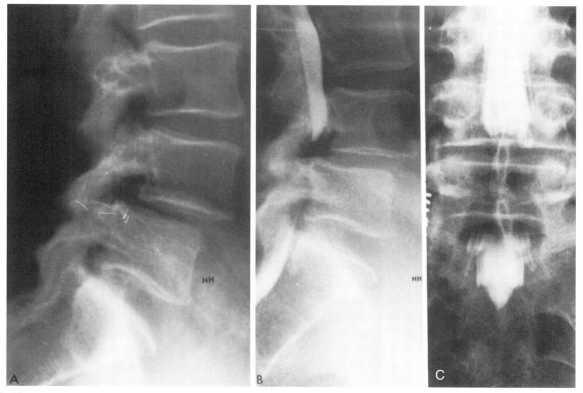

Figure 9–82

Metrizamide myelograms showing stenotic block at the L4–L5 level as a result of degenerative spondylolisthesis and spinal stenosis at the L4–L5 level. (A) Note the 4-mm anterior migration of L4 on L5 caused by the degenerative spondylolisthesis. (B) and (C) The extensive block on the myelogram is caused by spinal stenosis. (From Rothman, R.H., and F.A. Simeone: The Spine. Philadelphia, W.B. Saunders Co., 1982, p. 553.)

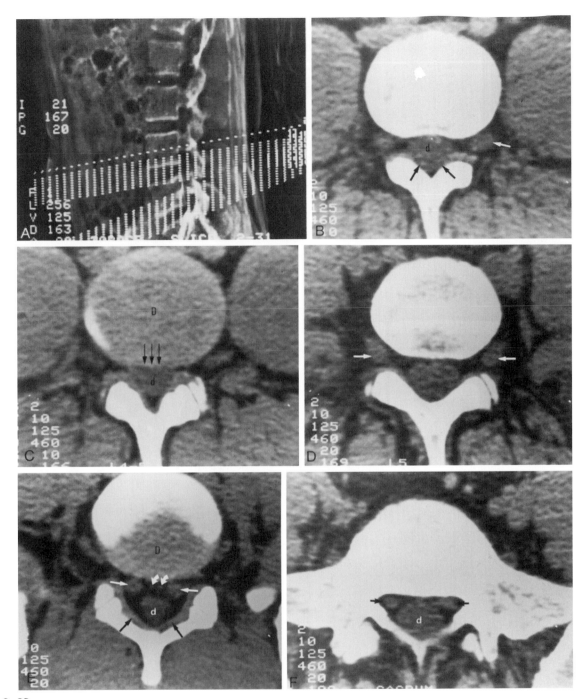

Figure 9–83

Normal disc anatomy on computed tomography (CT). (A) Scout view. The chosen sections (*dashed lines*) can be planned and angled along the planes of the discs. (B) CT scan through the L4 vertebral body shows the neural foramina and the L4 nerve root ganglia (white arrow indicates left ganglion). The dural sac (d) and ligamenta flava (*black arrows*) are shown. (C) CT scan through the L4–L5 disc (labeled D) shows very little fat between the posterior margin of the disc (*arrows*) and the dural sac (d). The nerve roots are not clearly seen. (D) CT scan through the L5 vertebral body and foramina shows the L5 nerve root ganglia (*arrows*). (E) CT scan through the L5–S1 disc space (labeled D) shows the L5 nerve roots (*straight white arrows*), the dural sac (d), and the ligamenta flava (*black arrows*). Small epidural veins are noted (*curved arrows*). (F) At the S1 level, the S1 nerve roots (*arrows*) and dural sac (d) are clearly visualized. (From Weissman, B.N.W., and C.B. Sledge: Orthopedic Radiology. Philadelphia, W.B. Saunders Co., 1986, p. 306.)

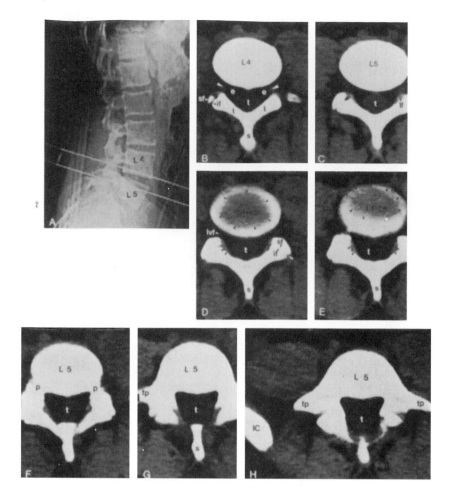

Figure 9–84

Soft-tissue detail of the L4–L5 intervertebral disc space on computed tomography (CT). (A) Lateral digital scout view obtained through the lumbosacral spine. The upper and lower scan limits through the L4–L5 region are designated with an electronic cursor. Scan collimation is 5 mm thick; incrementation is 3 mm (2-mm overlap). (B) Axial CT section of L4. The L4 root ganglia and spinal nerves are seen within the intervertebral foramina (*white arrowheads*) surrounded by abundant epidural fat (e). The thecal sac (t) is bounded anterolaterally by fat in the lateral recess. The posterior arch of L4 consists of inferior facets (if), laminae (l), and spinous process (s). The superior facet of L5 (sf) is just visible. (C) The next lower axial section demonstrates the L4–L5 facet articulations. The ligamentum flavum (lf) is contiguous with the facet joint capsule. Again, the thecal sac (t) is readily apparent; it is slightly higher in density than the adjacent epidural fat. Note that without subarachnoid contrast media, the intrathecal contents cannot be discerned. (D) Axial CT section of the L4–L5 disc space. The disc (*multiple black arrowheads*) is a region of central hypodensity surrounded by the cortical margin of L4. The posterior arch of L4 projects below the disc level. The intervertebral foramina (ivf) have begun to close. The cartilaginous articular surfaces (*white arrowhead*) between superior (sf) and inferior (if) facets are poorly demonstrated with these window settings. The ligamentum flavum (*double black arrowheads*) is noted medial to the facet joints. t = thecal sac; s = spinous process. (E) The next inferior CT section demonstrates the disc (*multiple arrowheads*) positioned somewhat more anteriorly, marginated posteriorly at this level by the posterosuperior cortical rim of the L5 body. The ligamentum flavum (*double arrowheads*) normally maintains a flat medial surface adjacent to the thecal sac (t). The posterior arch of L4 and its spinous process (s) are still in view. (F) Axial CT section through the L5 body at the level of the pedicles (p). The canal now completely encloses the thecal sac (t). (G) Immediately below, only the spinous process (s) of the posterior arch of L4 is visible. The transverse process (tp) of L5 is noted. t = thecal sac. (H) At the level of the iliac crest (IC), the posterior arch of L5 (*small arrowheads*) has just begun to form. The transverse processes (tp) are quite large at this level. t = thecal sac. (From LeMasters, D.L., and R.L. Dowart: High-resolution, cross-sectional computed tomography of the normal spine. Orthop. Clin. North Am. 16:359, 1985.)

toms. It is a technique that provides an axial projection of the spine, showing the anatomy of not only the spine but also the paravertebral muscles, vascular structures, and organs of the body cavity. In doing so, it shows more precisely the relation among the intervertebral discs, spinal canal, facet joints, and intervertebral foramina. It may be used to evaluate spinal stenosis, the shape of the spinal canal, epidural scarring (after surgery), facet joint arthritis, tumors, and trauma.[31] It may be used in conjunction with a water-soluble contrast medium (computer-assisted myelography) to further delineate the structures.

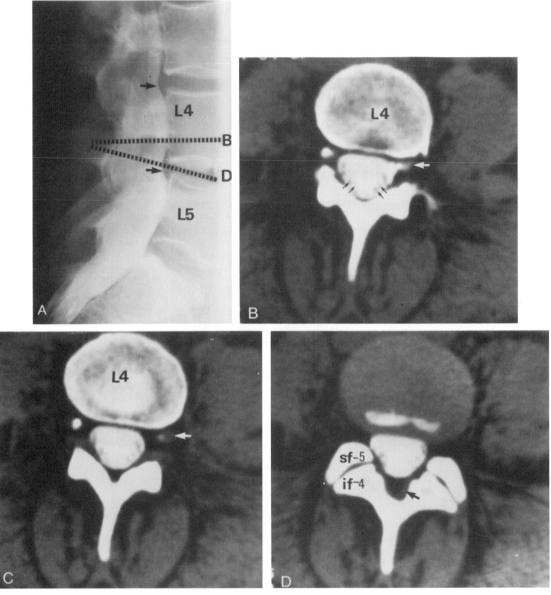

Figure 9–85

Computed tomography (CT) anatomy of L4 nerve roots. (A) Lateral view during metrizamide myelography showing indentations on the anterior aspect of the contrast column (*arrows*) at L3–L4 and L4–L5 resulting from bulging intervertebral discs. The levels for subsequent CT sections B and D are marked. (B) CT section through the L4 vertebra and L4–L5 foramina 1 hour after a metrizamide myelogram. Contrast agent fills the left axillary pouch (*white arrow*) and the right nerve root sleeve. Small arrows indicate the filling defects produced by the remaining nerve roots. (C) CT section slightly more distal than B shows the L4 nerve root ganglia (left ganglion is indicated by arrow). (D) Section through the L4–L5 disc and the posterior inferior body of L4 shows an abnormally bulging disc without compression of the subarachnoid space. The ligamentum flavum on the left (*arrow*), the superior facet of L5 (sf-5), and the inferior facet of L4 (if-4) are indicated. (From Weissman, B.N.W., and C.B. Sledge: Orthopedic Radiology. Philadelphia, W.B. Saunders Co., 1986, p. 284.)

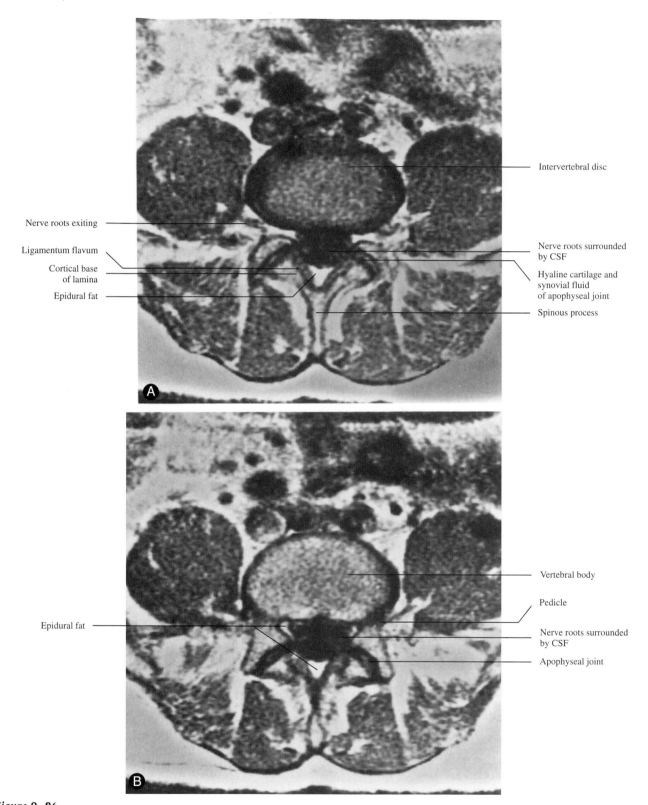

Intervertebral disc

Nerve roots exiting

Ligamentum flavum

Cortical base
of lamina

Epidural fat

Nerve roots surrounded
by CSF

Hyaline cartilage and
synovial fluid
of apophyseal joint

Spinous process

Epidural fat

Vertebral body

Pedicle

Nerve roots surrounded
by CSF

Apophyseal joint

Figure 9–86
Magnetic resonance imaging of normal lumbar spine. (A) Level of neural canal. (B) Level of pedicle.
CSF = cerebrospinal fluid. (From Bassett, L.W., R.H. Gold, and L.L. Seeger: MRI Atlas of the
Musculoskeletal System. London, Martin Dunitz, 1989, p. 40.)

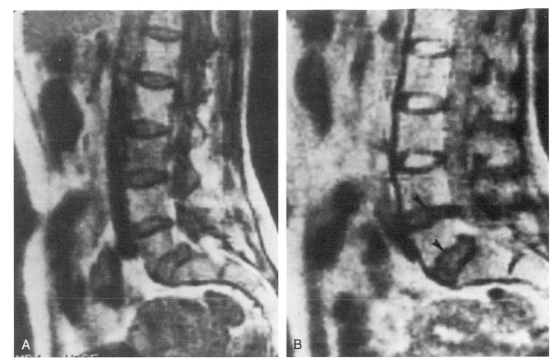

Figure 9–87

Disc degeneration viewed by magnetic resonance imaging. (A) T1-weighted image. There is little difference in intensity between the intervertebral discs. A grade 1 spondylolisthesis is present at L5–S1. (B) T2-weighted image. The L4–L5 and L5–S1 discs (*arrowheads*) are darker than the other, normal discs. A degenerating disc dehydrates, which shortens the T2 and consequently decreases the signal intensity on a T2-weighted image. (From Gillespy, T., H.K. Genant, and N.I. Chafetz: Magnetic Resonance Imaging Atlas of the Lumbar Spine. In Jayson, M. [ed.]: The Lumbar Spine and Back Pain. Edinburgh, Churchill Livingstone, 1987, p. 292.)

Magnetic Resonance Imaging

Magnetic resonance imaging (MRI) is a noninvasive technique that can be used in several planes (transaxial, coronal, or sagittal) to delineate bony and soft tissues. This technique is commonly used to diagnose tumors, to view the spinal cord within the spinal canal, and to assess for syringomyelia, cord infarction, or traumatic injury.[31] The delineation of soft tissues is much greater with MRI than with CT. For example, with MRI, the nucleus pulposus and the annulus fibrosis are easier to differentiate because of their different water contents,

making it the preferred imaging modality for disc disease (Figs. 9–86 and 9–87). As with other diagnostic imaging techniques, clinical findings must support what is seen before the structural abnormalities can be considered the source of the problem.

Discography

For discography, radiopaque dye is injected into the nucleus pulposus. It is not a commonly used technique but may be used to see whether injection of dye reproduces the patient's symptoms, making it diagnostic.

Précis of the Lumbar Spine Assessment*

History (*sitting*)
Observation (*standing*)
Examination
    Active movements (*standing*)
        Forward flexion
        Extension
        Side flexion (left and right)
        Rotation (left and right)
        Quick test
        Trendelenburg's test and S1 nerve root test

Passive movements (*only with care and caution*)
Peripheral joint scan (*standing*)
    Sacroiliac joints
Resisted isometric movements (*sitting*)
    Forward flexion
    Extension
    Side flexion (left and right)
    Rotation (left and right)

Peripheral joint scan (supine lying)
    Hip joints (flexion, abduction, adduction, and medial and lateral rotation)
    Knee joints (flexion and extension)
    Ankle joints (dorsiflexion and plantar flexion)
    Foot joints (supination, pronation)
    Toe joints (flexion, extension)
Myotomes (supine lying)
    Hip flexion (L2)
    Knee extension (L3)
    Ankle dorsiflexion (L4)
    Toe extension (L5)
    Ankle eversion and/or plantar flexion (S1)
Special tests (supine lying)
Reflexes and cutaneous distribution (anterior and side aspects)
Palpation (supine lying)
Joint play movements
    Flexion (side lying)
    Posteroanterior central vertebral pressure (prone lying)

Posteroanterior unilateral vertebral pressure (prone lying)
Transverse vertebral pressure (prone lying)
Peripheral joint scan (prone lying)
    Hip joints (extension, medial and lateral rotation)
Myotomes (prone lying)
    Hip extension (S1)
    Knee flexion (S1–S2)
Special tests (prone lying)
Reflexes and cutaneous distribution (prone lying) (posterior aspect)
Palpation (prone lying)
Diagnostic imaging

---

* The précis is shown in an order that limits the amount of moving the patient must do but ensures that all necessary structures are tested.

After any examination, the patient should be warned of the possibility of exacerbation of symptoms as a result of the assessment.

Case Studies

When doing these case studies, the examiner should list the appropriate questions to be asked and why they are being asked, what to look for and why, and what things should be tested and why. Depending on the answers of the patient (and the examiner should consider different responses), several possible causes of the patient's problem may become evident (examples given in parentheses). A differential diagnosis chart should be made up. The examiner can then decide how different diagnoses may affect the treatment plan. For example, an 18-year-old female synchronized swimmer was "boosting" another swimmer out of the water and felt a sharp pain in her back. She found that she could no longer swim because of the pain. She demonstrated paresthesia on the dorsum of the foot and lateral aspect of the leg. Describe your assessment plan for this patient (acute disc herniation versus lumbar strain) (Table 9–14).

1. A 23-year-old man comes to you complaining of a low backache. He works as a dishwasher, and although the pain has been present for 5 months, he has not missed any work. The pain gets worse as the day progresses and is

Table 9–14
Differential Diagnosis of Lumbar Strain and Posterolateral Lumbar Disc Herniation at L5–S1

	Lumbar Strain	Lumbar Disc (L5–S1)
History	Mechanism of injury: flexion, side flexion and/or rotation under load or without control	Quick movement into flexion, rotation, side flexion, or extension (may or may not be under load)
Pain	In lumbar spine, may be referred into buttocks May increase with extension (muscle contraction) or flexion (stretch)	In lumbar spine with referral into posterior leg to foot (radicular pain) Increases with extension
Observation	Scoliosis may be present Muscle spasm	Scoliosis may be present Muscle guarding
Active movement	Pain especially on stretch (flexion, side flexion, and rotation) Pain on unguarded movement Limited range of motion	Pain especially on extension and flexion Side flexion and rotation may be affected Limited range of motion
Resisted isometric movement	Pain on muscle contraction (often minimal pain) Myotomes normal	Minimal pain unless large protrusion L5–S1 myotomes may be affected
Special tests	Neurological tests negative	SLR and slump test often positive
Sensation	Normal	L5–S1 dermatomes may be affected
Reflexes	Normal	L5–S1 reflexes may be affected
Joint play	Muscle guarding	Muscle guarding

SLR = straight leg raising.

relieved by rest. X-rays reveal some sclerosis in the area of the sacroiliac joints. Describe your assessment plan for this patient (ankylosing spondylitis versus lumbar sprain).

2. A 36-year-old woman comes to you complaining of a chronic backache of 6 months' duration. The pain has been gradually increasing in severity and is worse at rest and in the morning on arising from bed. When present, the pain is centered in her low back and radiates into her buttocks and posterior left thigh. Describe your assessment plan for this patient (lumbar stenosis versus lumbar disc lesion).

3. A 13-year-old female gymnast comes to you complaining of low back pain. The pain increases when she extends the spine. Like most gymnasts, she is hypermobile in most of her joints. Describe your assessment plan for this patient (spondylolisthesis versus lumbar sprain).

4. A 56-year-old male steel worker comes to you complaining of low back pain that was brought on when he slipped on ice and twisted his trunk while trying to avoid falling. The injury occurred 2 days ago, and he has right-sided sciatica. X-rays show some lipping at L4–L5 and L5–S1 with slight narrowing of the L5 disc. He has difficulty bending forward. Describe your assessment plan for this patient (lumbar spondylosis versus acute lumbar disc herniation).

5. A 28-year-old man had a laminectomy for a herniated L5 disc 2 days ago. He is still an inpatient. Describe your assessment plan for this patient.

6. A 32-year-old man comes to you complaining of back pain and stiffness, especially with activity. He has a desk job and has no history of unusual activity. Describe your assessment plan for this patient (chronic lumbar sprain versus lumbar spina bifida occulta).

7. A 39-year-old male electrician comes to you complaining of back pain after a motor vehicle accident in which he was hit from behind while stopped for a red light. The accident occurred 3 days ago. Describe your assessment program for this patient (lumbar sprain versus lumbar stenosis).

8. A 26-year-old woman comes to you complaining of low back pain. She appears to have a functional leg length difference. Describe your assessment plan for this patient (lumbar sprain versus congenital anomaly).

References

Cited References

1. Taylor, J.R., and L.T. Twomey: Structure and function of lumbar zygapophyseal (facet) joints. In Boyling, J.D., and N. Palastanga (eds.): Grieve's Modern Manual Therapy: The Vertebral Column, 2nd ed. Edinburgh, Churchill Livingstone, 1994.
2. Kramer, J.: Intervertebral Disk Disease: Causes, Diagnosis, Treatment and Prophylaxis. Chicago, Year Book Medical Publishers, 1981.
3. Farfan, H.F.: Mechanical Disorders of the Low Back. Philadelphia, Lea & Febiger, 1973.
4. Coventry, M.B., R.K. Ghormley, and J.W. Kernohan: The intervertebral disc: Its microscopic anatomy and pathology. Part I: Anatomy, development and physiology; Part II: Changes in the intervertebral disc concomitant with age; Part III: Pathological changes in the intervertebral disc. J. Bone Joint Surg. 27:105 (Part I), 233 (Part II), 460 (Part III), 1945.
5. Bogduk, N.: The innervation of the lumbar spine. Spine 8:286–293, 1983.
6. Edgar, M.A., and J.A. Ghadially: Innervation of the lumbar spine. Clin. Orthop. 115:35–41, 1976.
7. Macnab, I.: Backache. Baltimore, Williams & Wilkins, 1977.
8. Nachemson, A., and J.M. Morris: In vivo measurements of intradiscal pressure. J. Bone Joint Surg. Am. 46:1077–1092, 1964.
9. Nachemson, A., and C. Elfstrom: Intravital dynamic pressure measurements in lumbar discs. Scand. J. Rehabil. Med. (Suppl. 1):5–40, 1970.
10. McKenzie, R.A.: The Lumbar Spine: Mechanical Diagnosis and Therapy. Waikanae, New Zealand, Spinal Publications Ltd., 1981.
11. Stoddard, A.: Manual of Osteopathic Practice. New York, Harper & Row, 1970.
12. Bendix, T., S.S. Sorenson, and K. Klausen: Lumbar curve, trunk muscles, and line of gravity with different heel heights. Spine 9:223–227, 1984.
13. Maigne, R.: Diagnosis and Treatment of Pain of Vertebral Origin. Baltimore, Williams & Wilkins, 1996.
14. Evans, R.C.: Illustrated Essentials in Orthopedic Physical Assessment. St. Louis, C.V. Mosby Co., 1994.
15. Matson, D.D., R.P. Woods, J.B. Campbell, and F.D. Ingraham: Diastematomyelia (congenital clefts of the spinal cord). Pediatrics 6:98–112, 1950.
16. Allbrook, D.: Movements of the lumbar spinal column. J. Bone Joint Surg. Br. 39:339–345, 1957.
17. Moll, J.M.H., and V. Wright: Normal range of spinal mobility: An objective clinical study. Ann. Rheum. Dis. 30:381–386, 1971.
18. Moll, J., and V. Wright: Measurement of spinal movement. In Jayson, M. (ed.): The Lumbar Spine and Back Pain. New York, Grune & Stratton, Inc., 1976.
19. Pennal, G.F., G.S. Conn, G. McDonald, et al.: Motion studies of the lumbar spine. J. Bone Joint Surg. Br. 54:442–452, 1972.
20. Tanz, S.S.: Motion of the lumbar spine: A roentgenologic study. Am. J. Roentgenol. 69:399–412, 1953.
21. Bourdillon, J.F., and E.A. Day: Spinal Manipulation. London, Wm. Heinemann Medical Books, 1987.
22. Edwards, B.C.: Clinical assessment: The use of combined movements in assessment and treatment. In Twomey, L.T., and J.R. Taylor (eds.): Physical Therapy of the Low Back: Clinics in Physical Therapy. Edinburgh, Churchill Livingstone, 1987.
23. Brown, L.: An introduction to the treatment and examination of the spine by combined movements. Physiotherapy 74:347–353, 1988.
24. Watkins, R.G.: Lumbar spine injuries. In Watkins, R.G. (ed.): The Spine in Sports. St. Louis, C.V. Mosby Co., 1996.
25. Hourigan, C.L., and J.M. Bassett: Facet syndrome: Clinical signs, symptoms, diagnosis, and treatment. J. Manip. Physiol. Ther. 12:293–297, 1989.
26. Lippitt, A.B.: The facet joint and its role in spine pain management with facet joint injections. Spine 9:746–750, 1984.
27. Wallace, L.A.: Limb length difference and back pain. In Grieve, G.P. (ed.): Modern Manual Therapy of the Vertebral Column. Edinburgh, Churchill Livingstone, 1986.
28. Smith, S.S., T.G. Mayer, R.J. Gatchel, and T.J. Becker: Quantification of lumbar function: Isometric and multispeed isokinetic trunk strength measures in sagittal and axial planes in normal subjects. Spine 10:757–764, 1985.
29. Cyriax, J.: Textbook for Orthopaedic Medicine, Vol. I: Diagnosis of Soft Tissue Lesions. London, Balliere Tindall, 1975.
30. Mayer, T.G.: Assessment of lumbar function. Clin. Orthop. 221:99–109, 1987.
31. Thomas, A.M.: The spine. In Pynsent, P., J. Fairbank, and A. Carr (eds.): Outcome Measures in Orthopedics. Oxford, Butterworth Heinemann, 1994.
32. Borenstein, D.G., S.W. Wiesel, and S.D. Boden: Low Back Pain: Medical Diagnosis and Comprehensive Management. Philadelphia, W.B. Saunders Co., 1995.

33. Fairbank, J.C., J. Couper, J.B. Davies, and J.P. O'Brien: The Oswestry low back pain disability questionnaire. Physiotherapy 66:217–273, 1980.

34. Hendler, N., A. Mollett, S. Talo, and S. Levin: A comparison between the Minnesota Multiphasic Personality Inventory and the Mensana Clinic Back Pain Test for validating the complaint of chronic back pain. J. Occup. Med. 30:98–102, 1988.

35. Lawlis, G.F., R. Cuencas, D. Selby, and C.E. McCoy: The development of the Dallas Pain Questionnaire. Spine 14:511–516, 1989.

36. Million, R., W. Hall, K. Haavick-Nilsen, R.D. Baker, and M.I. Jayson: Assessment of the progress of the back pain patient. Spine 7:204–212, 1982.

37. Japanese Orthopedic Association: Assessment of treatment of low back pain. J. Jap. Orthop. Assoc. 60:909–911, 1986.

38. Lehmann, T.R., R.A. Brand, and T.W. German: A low back rating scale. Spine 8:308–315, 1983.

39. Waddell, G., J. McCulloch, and E. Kummel: Nonorganic physical signs in low back pain. Spine 5:117–125, 1980.

40. Shacklock, M.: Neurodynamics. Physiotherapy 81:9–16, 1995.

41. Butler, D.A.: Mobilisation of the Nervous System. Melbourne, Churchill Livingstone, 1991.

42. Slater, H., D.S. Butler, and M.D. Shacklock: The dynamic central nervous system: examination and assessment using tension tests. In Boyling, J.D., and N. Palastanga (eds.): Grieve's Modern Manual Therapy: The Vertebral Column, 2nd ed. Edinburgh, Churchill Livingstone, 1994.

43. Butler, D., and L. Gifford: The concept of adverse mechanical tension in the nervous system. Physiotherapy 75:622–636, 1989.

44. Breig, A., and J.D.G. Troup: Biomechanical considerations in straight-leg-raising test: Cadaveric and clinical studies of the effects of medical hip rotation. Spine 4:242–250, 1979.

45. Charnley, J.: Orthopedic signs in the diagnosis of disc protrusion with special reference to the straight-leg-raising test. Lancet 1:186–192, 1951.

46. Edgar, M.A., and W.M. Park: Induced pain patterns on passive straight-leg-raising in lower lumbar disc protrusion. J. Bone Joint Surg. Br. 56:658–667, 1974.

47. Fahrni, W.H.: Observations on straight-leg-raising with special reference to nerve root adhesions. Can. J. Surg. 9:44–48, 1966.

48. Goddard, B.S., and J.D. Reid: Movements induced by straight-leg-raising in the lumbosacral roots, nerves, and plexus and in the intrapelvic section of the sciatic nerve. J. Neurol. Neurosurg. Psychiatry 28:12–18, 1965.

49. Scham, S.M., and T.K.F. Taylor: Tension signs in lumbar disc prolapse. Clin. Orthop. 75:195–204, 1971.

50. Urban, L.M.: The straight-leg-raising test: A review. J. Orthop. Sports Phys. Ther. 2:117–133, 1981.

51. Wilkins, R.H., and I.A. Brody: Lasègue's sign. Arch. Neurol. 21:219–220, 1969.

52. Cipriano, J.J.: Photographic Manual of Regional Orthopedic Tests. Baltimore, Williams & Wilkins, 1985.

53. Hall, T., M. Hepburn, and R.L. Elvey: The effect of lumbosacral posture on a modification of the straight leg raise test. Physiotherapy 79:566–570, 1993.

54. Hudgins, W.R.: The crossed-straight-leg raising test. N. Engl. J. Med. 297:1127, 1977.

55. Woodhall, R., and G.J. Hayes: The well-leg-raising test of Fajersztajn in the diagnosis of ruptured lumbar intervertebral disc. J. Bone Joint Surg. Am. 32:786–792, 1950.

56. Herron, L.D., and H.C. Pheasant: Prone knee-flexion provocative testing for lumbar disc protrusion. Spine 5:65–67, 1980.

57. Postacchini, F., G. Cinotti, and S. Gumina: The knee flexion test: A new test for lumbosacral root tension. J. Bone Joint Surg. Br. 75:834–835, 1993.

58. Maitland, G.D.: The slump test: Examination and treatment. Aust. J. Physiother. 31:215–219, 1985.

59. Philip, K., P. Lew, and T.A. Matyas: The inter-therapist reliability of the slump test. Aust. J. Physiother. 35:89–94, 1989.

60. Maitland, G.D.: Negative disc exploration: Positive canal signs. Aust. J. Physiother. 25:129–134, 1979.

61. Wartenberg, R.: The signs of Brudzinski and of Kernig. J. Pediatr. 37:679–684, 1950.

62. Brody, I.A., and R.H. Williams: The signs of Kernig and Brudzinski. Arch. Neurol. 21:215, 1969.

63. Brudzinski, J.: A new sign of the lower extremities in meningitis of children (neck sign). Arch. Neurol. 21:217, 1969.

64. Kernig, W.: Concerning a little noted sign of meningitis. Arch. Neurol. 21:216, 1969.

65. Dyck, P.: The femoral nerve traction test with lumbar disc protrusion. Surg. Neurol. 6:163–166, 1976.

66. Cram, R.H.: A sign of sciatic nerve root pressure. J. Bone Joint Surg. Br. 35:192–195, 1953.

67. Deyerle, W.M., and V.R. May: Sciatic tension test. South. Med. J. 49:999–1005, 1956.

68. Spengler, D.M.: Low Back Pain: Assessment and Management. Orlando, Florida, Grune & Stratton, 1982.

69. Palmer, M.L., and M. Epler: Clinical Assessment Procedures in Physical Therapy. Philadelphia, J.B. Lippincott, 1990.

70. Rask, M.: Knee flexion test and sciatica. Clin. Orthop. 134:221, 1978.

71. Dommisse, G.F., and L. Grobler: Arteries and veins of the lumbar nerve roots and cauda equina. Clin. Orthop. 115:22–29, 1976.

72. Katznelson, A., J. Nerubay, and A. Level: Gluteal skyline (G.S.L.): A search for an objective sign in the diagnosis of disc lesions of the lower lumbar spine. Spine 7:74–75, 1982.

73. Little, H.: The Neck and Back: The Rheumatological Physical Examination. Orlando, Florida, Grune & Stratton, 1986.

74. Garrick, J.G., and D.R. Webb: Sports Injuries: Diagnosis and Management. Philadelphia, W.B. Saunders Co., 1990.

75. Jackson, D.W., and J.V. Ciullo: Injuries of the spine in the skeletally immature athlete. In Nicholas, J.A., and E.B. Hershmann (eds.): The Lower Extremity and Spine in Sports Medicine, vol. 2. St. Louis, C.V. Mosby Co., 1986.

76. Jackson, D.W., L.L. Wiltse, R.D. Dingeman, and M. Hayes: Stress reactions involving the pars interarticularis in young athletes. Am. J. Sports Med. 9:304–312, 1981.

77. Kirkaldy-Willis, W.H.: Managing Low Back Pain. Edinburgh, Churchill Livingstone, 1983.

78. Wadsworth, C.T., R.F. DeFabio, and D. Johnson: The spine. In Manual Examination and Treatment of the Spine and Extremities. Baltimore, Williams & Wilkins, 1988.

79. Tokuhashi, Y., H. Matsuzaki, and S. Sano: Evaluation of clinical lumbar instability using the treadmill. Spine 18:2321–2324, 1993.

80. Corrigan, B., and G.D. Maitland: Practical Orthopedic Medicine. London, Butterworths, 1985.

81. Post, M.: Physical Examination of the Musculoskeletal System. Chicago, Year Book Medical Publishers, 1987.

82. Dyck, P.: The stoop-test in lumbar entrapment radiculopathy. Spine 4:89–92, 1979.

83. Dyck, P., and J.B. Doyle: "Bicycle test" of van Gelderen in diagnosis of intermittent cauda equina compression syndrome. J. Neurosurg. 46:667–670, 1977.

84. Archibald, K.C., and F. Wiechec: A reappraisal of Hoover's test. Arch. Phys. Med. Rehabil. 51:234–238, 1970.

85. Arieff, A.J., E.I. Tigay, J.F. Kurtz, and W.A. Larmon: The Hoover sign: An objective sign of pain and/or weakness in the back or lower extremities. Arch. Neurol. 5:673–678, 1961.

86. Hoover, C.F.: A new sign for the detection of malingering and functional paresis of the lower extremities. JAMA 51:746–747, 1908.

87. Travell, J.G., and D.G. Simons: Myofascial Pain and Dysfunction: The Trigger Point Manual. Baltimore, Williams & Wilkins, 1983.

88. Dyck, P., H.C. Pheasant, J.B. Doyle, and J.J. Reider: Intermittent cauda equina compression syndrome. Spine 2:75–81, 1977.

89. Joffe, R., A. Appleby, and V. Arjona: Intermittent ischemia of the cauda equina due to stenosis of the lumbar canal. J. Neurol. Neurosurg. Psychiatry 29:315–318, 1966.

90. Hoppenfeld, S.: Physical Examination of the Spine and Extremities. New York, Appleton-Century-Crofts, 1976.

91. Pecina, M.M., J. Krmpotic-Nemanic, and A.D. Markiewitz: Tunnel Syndromes. Boca Raton, Florida, CRC Press, 1991.

92. Maitland, G.D.: Examination of the lumbar spine. Aust. J. Physiother. 17:5–11, 1971.

93. Fullenlove, T.M., and A.J. Williams: Comparative roentgen findings in symptomatic and asymptomatic backs. Radiology 68:572–574, 1957.

94. Gillespie, H.W.: The significance of congenital lumbosacral abnormalities. Br. J. Radiol. 22:270–275, 1949.

95. Magora, A., and A. Schwartz: Relation between the low back pain syndrome and x-ray findings. Scand. J. Rehabil. Med. 10:135–145, 1978.

96. Southworth, J.D., and S.R. Bersack: Anomalies of the lumbosacral vertebrae in five hundred and fifty individuals without symptoms referable to the low back. Am. J. Roentgenol. 64:624–634, 1950.

97. Tulsi, R.S.: Sacral arch defect and low backache. Australas. Radiol. 18:43–50, 1974.

98. Willis, T.A.: An analysis of vertebral anomalies. Am. J. Surg. 6:163–168, 1929.

99. Willis, T.A.: Lumbosacral anomalies. J. Bone Joint Surg. Am. 41:935–938, 1959.

100. Macnab, I.: The traction spur: An indicator of segmental instability. J. Bone Joint Surg. Am. 53:663–670, 1971.

101. Friberg, O.: Functional radiography of the lumbar spine. Ann. Med. 21:341–346, 1989.

102. Bigg-Wither, G., and P. Kelly: Diagnostic imaging in musculoskeletal physiotherapy. In Refshauge, K., and E. Gass: Musculoskeletal Physiotherapy: Clinical Science and Practice. Oxford, Butterworth Heinemann, 1995.

103. Wood, K.B., C.A. Popp, E.E. Transfeldt, and A.E. Geissele: Radiographic evaluation of instability in spondylolisthesis. Spine 19:1697–1703, 1994.

General References

Adams, M.A., and W.C. Hutton: The mechanical function of the lumbar apophyseal joints. Spine 8:327–330, 1983.

Anderson, B.J., G.R. Ortengren, A.L. Nachemson, et al.: The sitting posture: An electromyographic and discometric study. Orthop. Clin. North Am. 6:105–120, 1975.

Barasch, E., and R. DeMaro: Typical MRI findings in sports medicine evaluation for degenerative disc disease. J. Orthop. Sports Phys. Ther. 10:290–296, 1989.

Bassett, L.W., R.H. Gold, and L.L. Seeger: MRI Atlas of the Musculoskeletal System. London, Martin Dunitz Ltd., 1989.

Boden, S.D.: The use of radiographic imaging studies in the evaluation of patients who have degenerative disorders of the lumbar spine. J. Bone Joint Surg. Am. 78:114–124, 1996.

Brown, L.: Treatment and examination of the spine by combined movements. Physiotherapy 76:66–74, 1990.

Brown, M.D.: Diagnosis of pain syndromes of the spine. Orthop. Clin. North Am. 6:233–248, 1975.

Cacayorin, E.D., L. Hockhauser, and G.R. Petro: Lumbar and thoracic spine pain in the athlete: Radiographic evaluation. Clin. Sports Med. 6:767–783, 1987.

Cameron, D.M., R.W. Bohannon, and S.V. Owen: Influence of hip position on measurements of the straight leg raise test. J. Orthop. Sports Phys. Ther. 19:168–172, 1994.

Carmichael, S.W., and S.L. Buckart: Clinical anatomy of the lumbosacral complex. Phys. Ther. 59:966–968, 1979.

Cavanaugh, J.M.: Neural mechanisms of lumbar pain. Spine 20:1804–1809, 1995.

Chadwick, P.R.: Examination, assessment and treatment of the lumbar spine. Physiotherapy 70:2–7, 1984.

Crock, H.V.: Normal and pathological anatomy of the lumbar spinal nerve root canals. J. Bone Joint Surg. Br. 63:487–490, 1981.

Crock, H.V., and H. Yoshizawa: The blood supply of the lumbar vertebral column. Clin. Orthop. 115:6–21, 1976.

Crouch, J.E.: Functional Human Anatomy. Philadelphia, Lea & Febiger, 1972.

Crow, N.E.: The "normal" lumbosacral spine. Radiology 72:97, 1959.

Cyriax, J.: Examination of the spinal column. Physiotherapy 56:2–6, 1970.

Davies, E.M.: Backache and its treatment by active exercise. Physiotherapy 49:81–84, 1963.

Davis, P.R.: The mechanics and movements of the back in working situations. Physiotherapy 53:44–47, 1967.

Deyo, R.A.: Measuring the functional status of patients with low back pain. Arch. Phys. Med. Rehabil. 69:1044–1053, 1988.

Deyo, R.A.: Comparative validity of the sickness impact profile and shorter scales for functional assessment in low back pain. Spine 11:951–954, 1986.

Deyo, R.A., G. Andersson, C. Bombardier, et al.: Outcome measures for studying patients with low back pain. Spine 19:2032S–2036S, 1994.

Deyo, R.A., J. Haselkorn, R. Hoffman, and D.L. Kent: Designing studies of diagnostic tests for low back pain or radiculopathy. Spine 19:2057S–2065S, 1994.

Dixon, A. St.: Diagnosis of low back pain: Sorting the complainers. In Jayson, M. (ed.): The Lumbar Spine and Back Pain. New York, Grune & Stratton, Inc., 1976.

Dohrmann, G.J., and W.J. Norwack: The upgoing great toe: Optimal method of elicitation. Lancet 799:339–341, 1973.

Dommisse, G.F., and L. Grobler: Arteries and veins of the nerve roots and cauda equina. Clin. Orthop. 115:22–29, 1976.

Doug, G., and R.W. Porter: Walking and cycling tests in neurogenic and intermittent claudications. Spine 14:965–969, 1989.

Edgelow, P.I.: Physical examination of the lumbosacral complex. Phys. Ther. 59:974–977, 1979.

Evans, J.H., and A. Kagan: The development of a functional rating scale to measure the treatment outcome of chronic spinal patients. Spine 11:277–281, 1986.

Evanski, P.M., D. Carver, A. Nehemkis, and T.R. Waugh: The Burns test in low back pain: Correlation with the hysterical personality. Clin. Orthop. 140:42–44, 1979.

Fairbank, J.C.T., H. Hall, P.F. van Akkerveeken, B.L. Rydevik, D.L. Spencer, and S. Haldemann: Diagnoses and neuromechanisms: History taking and physical examination. In Weinstein, J.N., and S.W. Wiesel (eds.): The Lumbar Spine. Philadelphia, W.B. Saunders Co., 1990.

Finneson, B.E.: Low Back Pain, 2nd ed. Philadelphia, J.B. Lippincott Co., 1981.

Fisk, J.W.: The straight leg raising test: its relevance to possible disc pathology. N. Z. Med. J. 81:557–560, 1975.

Floman, Y., S.W. Wiesel, and R.H. Rothman: Cauda equina syndrome presenting as a herniated lumbar disc. Clin. Orthop. 147:234–237, 1980.

Forrester, D.M., and J.C. Brown: The Radiology of Joint Disease. Philadelphia, W.B. Saunders Co., 1987.

Forst, J.J.: Contribution to the clinical study of sciatica. Arch. Neurol. 21:220–221, 1969.

Friberg, O.: Clinical symptoms and biomechanics of lumbar spine and hip joint in leg length inequality. Spine 8:643–651, 1983.

Frymoyer, J.W., R.M. Nelson, E. Spangford, and G. Waddell: Clinical tests applicable to the study of chronic low back disability. Spine 16:681–682, 1991.

Garfin, S.R., B. Rydevik, B. Lind, and J. Massie: Spinal nerve root compression. Spine 20:1810–1820, 1995.

Gartland, J.J.: Fundamentals of Orthopedics. Philadelphia, W.B. Saunders Co., 1979.

Gill, K., M.H. Krag, G.B. Johnson, L.D. Haugh, and M.H. Pope: Repeatability of four clinical methods for assessment of lumbar spinal motion. Spine 13:50–53, 1988.

Golub, B.S., and B. Silverman: Transforaminal ligaments of the lumbar spine. J. Bone Joint Surg. Am. 51:947–956, 1969.

Gould, J.A.: The Spine: Orthopedic and Sports Physical Therapy. St. Louis, C.V. Mosby Co., 1990.

Grieve, G.P.: Common Vertebral Joint Problems. Edinburgh, Churchill Livingstone, 1981.

Grieve, G.P.: Mobilisation of the Spine. Edinburgh, Churchill Livingstone, 1979.

Gutrecht, J.A., P.A. Espinosa, and P.J. Dyck: Early descriptions of common neurologic signs. Mayo Clin. Proc. 43:807–814, 1968.

Hall, G.W.: Neurologic signs and their discoveries. JAMA 95:703–707, 1930.

Helfet, A.J., and D.M. Lee: Disorders of the Lumbar Spine. Philadelphia, J.B. Lippincott Co., 1978.

Hirsch, C., R.O. Ingelmark, and M. Miller: The anatomical bases for low back pain. Acta. Orthop. Scand. 33:1–17, 1963.

Hollinshead, W.H., and D.B. Jenkins: Functional Anatomy of the Limbs and Back. Philadelphia, W.B. Saunders Co., 1981.

Jackson, H.C., R.K. Winkelmann, and W.H. Bickel: Nerve endings in the human lumbar spinal column and related structures. J. Bone Joint Surg. Am. 48:1272–1281, 1966.

Jaeger, S.A.: Atlas of Radiographic Positioning: Normal Anatomy and Development Variants. Norwalk, Connecticut, Appleton & Lange, 1988.

Jayson, M.: The Lumbar Spine and Back Pain. New York, Grune & Stratton, 1987.

Jensen, G.M.: Biomechanics of the lumbar intervertebral disk: A review. Phys. Ther. 60:765–773, 1980.

Jonck, L.M.: The mechanical disturbances resulting from lumbar disc space narrowing. J. Bone Joint Surg. Br. 43:362–375, 1961.

Jull, G.A.: Examination of the lumbar spine. In Grieve, G.P. (ed.): Modern Manual Therapy of the Vertebral Column. Edinburgh, Churchill Livingstone, 1986.

Kapandji, L.A.: The Physiology of Joints, vol. 3: The Trunk and Vertebral Column. New York, Churchill Livingstone, 1974.

Keim, H.A.: Low back pain. Clin. Symp. 26:2–32, 1974.

Keim, H.A.: The Adolescent Spine. New York, Springer-Verlag, 1982.

Kingston, R.S.: Radiology of the spine. In Watkins, R.G. (ed.): The Spine in Sports. St. Louis, C.V. Mosby Co., 1996.

Kirkaldy-Willis, W.H.: Diagnosis and treatment of lumbar spinal stenosis. American Academy of Orthopaedic Surgeons Symposium on the Lumbar Spine. St. Louis, C.V. Mosby Co., 1976.

Kirkaldy-Willis, W.H.: Managing Low Back Pain. New York, Churchill Livingstone, 1983.

Kirkaldy-Willis, W.H.: The relationship of structural pathology to the nerve root. Spine 9:49–52, 1984.

Koreska, J., D. Robertson, R.H. Mills, D.A. Gibson, and A.M. Albisser: Biomechanics of the lumbar spine and its clinical significance. Orthop. Clin. North Am. 8:121–133, 1977.

Kosteljanetz, M., F. Bang, and S. Schmidt-Olsen: The clinical significance of straight leg raising (Lasègue's sign) in the diagnosis of prolapsed lumbar disc. Spine 13:393–395, 1988.

Lamb, D.W.: The neurology of spinal pain. Phys. Ther. 59:971–973, 1979.

Lucas, D.B.: Mechanics of the spine. Hospital for Joint Diseases (New York Bulletin) 31:115–131, 1970.

Maher, C., and R. Adams: Reliability of pain and stiffness assessments in clinical manual lumbar spine examination. Phys. Ther. 74:801–811, 1994.

Maigne, R.: Orthopaedic Medicine: A New Approach to Vertebral Manipulation. Springfield, Illinois, Charles C. Thomas, 1972.

Maitland, G.D.: The Maitland concept: Assessment, examination, and treatment by passive movement. In Twomey, L.T., and J.R. Taylor (eds.): Physical Therapy of the Low Back. Edinburgh, Churchill Livingstone, 1987.

Mayer, T., R. Gatchel, J. Keeley, H. Mayer, and D. Richling: A male incumbent worker industrial database: Lumbar/cervical functional testing. Spine 19:765–770, 1994.

McCall, I.W.: Radiologic assessment of back pain. Semin. Orthop. 1:71–85, 1986.

McLean, I.P.: Tests for lumbar root tension. J. Bone Joint Surg. Br. 76:678, 1994.

McRae, R.: Clinical Orthopaedic Examination. New York, Churchill Livingstone, 1976.

Mierau, D., J.D. Cassidy, and K. Yong-Hing: Low back pain and straight leg raising in children and adolescents. Spine 14:526–528, 1989.

Mitchell, F.L., P.S. Moran, and N. A. Pruzzo: An Evaluation and Treatment Manual of Osteopathic Muscle Energy Procedures. Valley Park, Missouri, Mitchell, Moran & Pruzzo, 1979.

Mooney, V., and G.B. Andersson: Trunk strength testing in patient evaluation and treatment. Spine 19:2483–2485, 1994.

Morris, J.M.: Biomechanics of the spine. Arch. Surg. 107:418–423, 1973.

Murphy, R.W.: Nerve roots and spinal nerves in degenerative disc disease. Clin. Orthop. 129:46–60, 1977.

Nachemson, A.: Towards a better understanding of low back pain: A review of the mechanics of the lumbar disc. Rheumatol. Rehabil. 14:129–143, 1975.

O'Donoghue, D.H.: Treatment of Injuries to Athletes, 4th ed. Philadelphia, W.B. Saunders Co., 1984.

Ombregt, L., B. Bisschop, H.J. ter Veer, and T. Van de Velde: A System of Orthopedic Medicine. London, W.B. Saunders Co., 1995.

Paris, S.V.: Anatomy as related to function and pain. Orthop. Clin. North Am. 14:475–489, 1983.

Porter, R.W., and I.F. Trailescu: Diurnal changes in straight leg raising. Spine 15:103–106, 1990.

Porterfield, J.A., and C. DeRosa: Mechanical Low Back Pain: Perspectives in Functional Anatomy. Philadelphia, W.B. Saunders Co., 1991.

Quick Reference Guide for Physicians: Acute Low Back Problems in Adults. Assessment and Treatment. Rockville, Maryland, U.S. Department of Health and Human Services, 1994.

Ramsey, R.H.: The anatomy of the ligamentum flava. Clin. Orthop. 44:129–140, 1966.

Rauschnig, W., K.B. Heithoff, D.W. Stoller, et al.: Radiology. In Weinstein, J.N., and S.W. Weisel (eds.): The Lumbar Spine. Philadelphia, W.B. Saunders Co., 1990.

Reilly, B.M.: Practical Strategies in Outpatient Medicine. Philadelphia, W.B. Saunders Co., 1984.

Richardson, J.K., and Z.A. Iglarsh: Clinical Orthopedic Physical Therapy. Philadelphia, W.B. Saunders Co., 1994.

Rose, K., and P. Balasubramaniam: Nerve root canals in the lumbar spine. Spine 9:16–18, 1984.

Rothman, R.H., and F.A. Simeone: The Spine. Philadelphia, W.B. Saunders Co., 1982.

Rydevik, B., M.D. Brown, and G. Lundberg: Pathoanatomy and pathophysiology of nerve root compression. Spine 9:7–15, 1984.

Saal, J.S.: The role of inflammation in lumbar pain. Spine 20:1821–1827, 1995.

Saunders, H.D., and R. Saunders: Evaluation, Treatment and Prevention of Musculoskeletal Disorders. Chaska, Minnesota, Saunders Group, 1993.

Seimen, L.P.: Low Back Pain: Clinical Diagnosis and Management. Norwalk, Connecticut, Appleton-Century-Crofts, 1983.

Selby, D.K.: When to operate and what to operate on. Orthop. Clin. North Am. 14:577–588, 1983.

Shacklock, M.O., D.S. Butler, and H. Slater: The dynamic central nervous system: Structure and clinical neurobiomechanics. In Boyling, J.D., and N. Palastanga (eds.): Grieve's Modern Manual Therapy. Edinburgh, Churchill Livingstone, 1994.

Shiqing, X., Z. Quanzhi, and F. Dehao: Significance of the straight leg raise test in the diagnosis and clinical evaluation of lower lumbar intervertebral disc protrusion. J. Bone Joint Surg. Am. 69:517–522, 1987.

Simmons, E.D., R.D. Guyer, A. Graham-Smith, and R. Herzog: Radiographic assessments for patients with low back pain. Spine 20:1839–1841, 1995.

Smith, S.A., J.B. Massie, R. Chesnut, and S.R. Garfin: Straight leg raising: Anatomical effects on the spinal nerve root with and without fusion. Spine 18:992–999, 1993.

Snook, S.H.: Low back pain in industry. American Academy of Orthopaedic Surgeons Symposium on Idiopathic Low Back Pain. St. Louis, C.V. Mosby Co., 1982, pp. 23–38.

Supik, L.F., and M.J. Broom: Sciatic tension signs and lumbar disc herniation. Spine 19:1066–1069, 1994.

Tachdjian, M.O.: Pediatric Orthopedics. Philadelphia, W.B. Saunders Co., 1972.

Thelander, U., M. Fagerlund, S. Friberg, and S. Larsson: Straight leg raising test versus radiologic size, shape, and position of lumbar disc hernias. Spine 17:395–399, 1992.

Van Wijmen, P.M.: The use of repeated movements in the McKenzie method of spinal examination. In Boyling, J.D., and N. Palastanga (eds.): Grieve's Modern Manual Therapy: The Vertebral Column, 2nd ed. Edinburgh, Churchill Livingstone, 1994.

Vanharanta, H., B.L. Sachs, M. Spivey, et al.: A comparison of CT/discography, pain response and radiographic disc height. Spine 13:321–324, 1988.

Waddell, G.: Clinical assessment of lumbar impairment. Clin. Orthop. 221:110–120, 1987.

Waddell, G., and C.J. Main: Assessment of severity in low back disorders. Spine 9:204–208, 1984.

Watkins, R.G.: History, physical examination, and diagnostic tests for back and lower extremity problems. In Watkins, R.G. (ed.): The Spine in Sports. St. Louis, C.V. Mosby Co., 1996.

Weise, M.D., S.R. Garfin, R.H. Gelberman, M.M. Katz, and R.P. Thorne: Lower extremity sensibility testing in patients with herniated lumbar intervertebral discs. J. Bone Joint Surg. Am. 67:1219–1224, 1985.

Weissman, B.N.W., and C.B. Sledge: Orthopedic Radiology. Philadelphia, W.B. Saunders Co., 1986.

White, A.A., and M.M. Panjabi: Clinical Biomechanics of the Spine. Philadelphia, J.B. Lippincott Co., 1978.

Wiesel, S.W., P. Bernini, and R.H. Rothman: The Aging Lumbar Spine. Philadelphia, W.B. Saunders Co., 1982.

Williams, P.L., and Warwick, R. (eds.): Gray's Anatomy, 36th British ed. Edinburgh, Churchill Livingstone, 1980.

Yong-Hing, K., and W.H. Kirkaldy-Willis: The pathophysiology of degenerative disease of the lumbar spine. Orthop. Clin. North Am. 14:491–504, 1983.

10

Pelvis

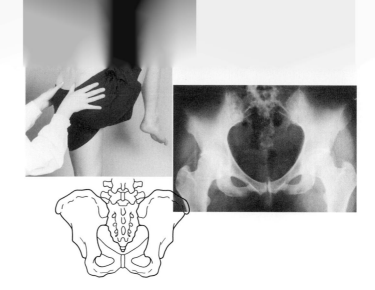

The sacroiliac joints form the "key" of the arch between the two pelvic bones; with the symphysis pubis, they help to transfer the weight from the spine to the lower limbs and provide elasticity to the pelvic ring. This triad of joints also acts as a buffer to decrease the force of jars and bumps to the spine and upper body caused by contact of the lower limbs with the ground. Because of this shock-absorbing function, the structure of the sacroiliac and symphysis pubis joints is different from that of most joints that are assessed. Assessment of the sacroiliac joints and symphysis pubis should be included in the examination of the lumbar spine and/or hips if there is no direct trauma to either one of these joints. Normally, a comprehensive examination of the sacroiliac joints is not made until examination of the lumbar spine and/or hip has been completed. If both of these joints are examined and the problem still appears to be present and remains undiagnosed, an examination of the pelvis should be initiated.

Applied Anatomy

The **sacroiliac joints** are part synovial joint and part syndesmosis. A syndesmosis is a type of fibrous joint in which the intervening fibrous connective tissue forms an interosseous membrane or ligament. The synovial portion of the joint is **C**-shaped, with the convex iliac surface of the **C** facing anteriorly and inferiorly. Kapandji[1] states that the greater or the more acute the angle of the **C**, the more stable the joint and the less the likelihood of a lesion to the joint. The sacral surface is slightly concave.

The size, shape, and roughness of the articular surfaces vary greatly among individuals. In the child, these surfaces are smooth. In the adult, they become irregular depressions and elevations that fit into one another; by so doing, they restrict movement at the joint and add strength to the joint for transferring weight from the lower limb to the spine. The articular surface of the ilium is covered with fibrocartilage; the articular surface of the sacrum is covered with hyaline cartilage that is three times thicker than that of the ilium. In older persons, parts of the joint surfaces may be obliterated by adhesions.

Sacroiliac Joint

Resting position:	Neutral
Capsular pattern:	Pain when joints are stressed

Although the sacroiliac joints are relatively mobile in young people, they become progressively stiffer with age. In some cases, ankylosis results. It must be remembered that the movements occurring in the sacroiliac and symphysis pubis joints are slight compared with the movements occurring in the spinal joints.

The **symphysis pubis** is a cartilaginous joint. There is a disc of fibrocartilage between the two joint surfaces called the **interpubic disc**.

The sacroiliac joints and symphysis pubis have no muscles that control their movements directly. However, they are influenced by the action of the muscles moving the lumbar spine and hip, because many of these muscles attach to the sacrum and pelvis.

The **sacrococcygeal joint** is usually a fused line (symphysis) united by a fibrocartilaginous disc. It is found between the apex of the sacrum and the base of the coccyx. Occasionally, the joint is freely movable and synovial. With advanced age, the joint may fuse and be obliterated.

Patient History

In addition to the questions listed under Patient History in Chapter 1, the examiner should obtain the following information from the patient:

1. Was there any known mechanism of injury? For example, the sacroiliac joints are commonly injured by a sudden jar caused by inadvertently stepping off a curb, an overzealous kick (either missing the object or hitting the ground), a fall on the seat of the pants, or a lift and twist maneuver.[2] Has the patient experienced any recent falls, twists, or strains? These movements increase the chance of sacroiliac joint sprains.

2. Where is the pain, and does it radiate? With a lesion of the sacroiliac joint, deep, dull, undefined pain tends to be unilateral and can be referred to the posterior thigh, iliac fossa, and buttock on the affected side.

3. When does the pain occur? Pain that is caused by sacroiliac joint problems is usually felt when turning in bed, getting out of a bed, or stepping up with the affected leg. Often, the pain is constant and unrelated to position. Symphysis pubis pain tends to be localized and increases with any movement involving the adductor or rectus abdominus muscles.

4. What is the patient's habitual working stance? Is a great deal of sitting or twisting involved? The examiner should look for postures that potentially increase the stress on the sacroiliac joints (e.g., standing, especially on one leg).

5. What is the patient's usual activity or pastime? Again, would any of these activities stress the sacroiliac joints?

6. Is there any particular position or activity that aggravates the condition? Climbing or descending stairs, walking, and standing from a sitting position all stress the sacroiliac joint.

7. What is the patient's age? Ankylosing spondylitis is found primarily in men between the ages of 15 and 35 years. Hypomobility is likely to be seen in men between 40 and 50 and in women after 50 years of age.[3]

8. Does the patient have or feel any weakness in the lower limbs? Neurological deficit in the limbs can be present if the sacroiliac joint is affected.

9. Has there been a recent pregnancy? Sprain of the sacroiliac ligaments can be the result of increased laxity of the ligaments caused by hormonal changes. It may take 3 to 4 months or longer for the ligaments to return to their normal state after a pregnancy.

10. Does the patient have a past history of rheumatoid arthritis, Reiter's disease, or ankylosing spondylitis? Each of these conditions can involve the sacroiliac joints.

Observation

The patient must be suitably undressed. For the sacroiliac joints to be observed properly, the patient is often required to be nude from the midchest to the toes. If he or she wishes to wear shorts, they must be rolled down as far as possible so that the sacroiliac joints are visible. The patient stands and is viewed from the front, side, and back. The examiner should note the following:

1. Whether the posture (see Chapter 15) and gait (see Chapter 14) are normal. If **contranutation**[4] (Fig. 10–1) occurs at the sacroiliac joint, indicating an anterior

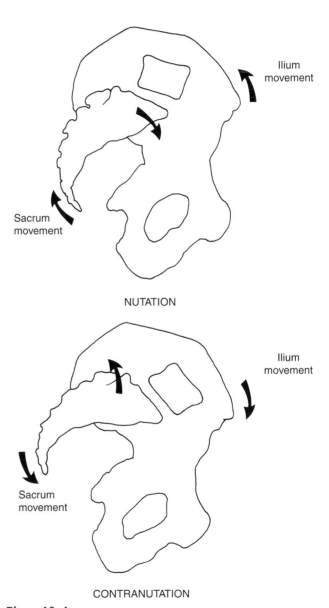

NUTATION

CONTRANUTATION

Figure 10–1
Movements of nutation and contranutation occurring at the sacroiliac joint.

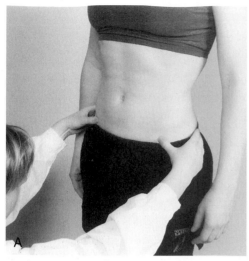
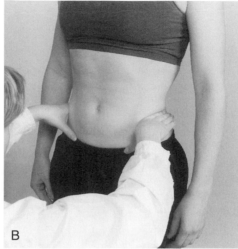

Figure 10–2
Anterior observational view.
(A) Level of anterior superior iliac spines. (B) Level of iliac crests.

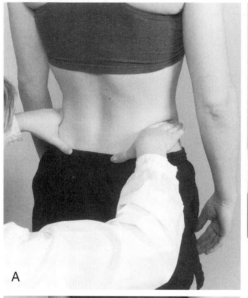
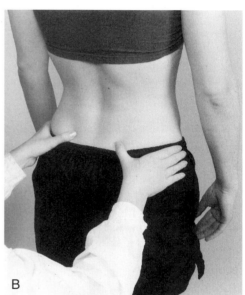

Figure 10–3
Posterior observational view.
(A) Level of iliac crests. (B) Level of posterior superior iliac spines.
(C) Level of ischial tuberosities.
(D) Level of gluteal folds.

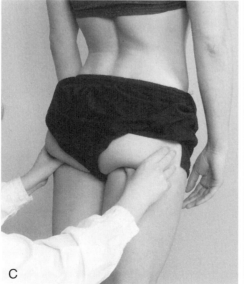
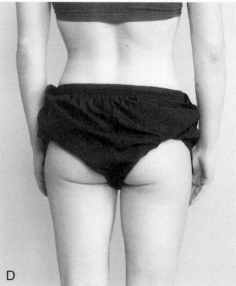

torsion of the joint or posterior rotation of the sacrum on the ilium on one side, the lower limb on that side will probably be medially rotated. Contranutation occurs when the anterior superior iliac spine (ASIS) is lower and the posterior superior iliac spine (PSIS) is higher on one side.[4] The iliac bones move apart, and the ischeal tuberosities approximate.[3] Contranutation is limited by the posterior sacroiliac ligaments. **Nutation**[4] is the backward rotation of the ilium on the sacrum (see Fig. 10–1). If nutation occurs on only one side, the ASIS is higher and the PSIS is lower on that side.[4] The iliac innominate bones move together, and the ischeal tuberosities move apart.[3] The result is an apparent or functional short leg on the same side.[5] Nutation is limited by the anterior sacroiliac ligaments, the sacrospinous ligament, and the sacrotuberous ligament. Nutation occurs when a person assumes a "pelvic tilt" position. Contranutation occurs when a person assumes a "lordotic" or "anterior pelvic tilt" position.

Gait is often affected if the pathology involves the pelvis. If the sacroiliac joints are not free to move, the stride length is decreased and a vertical limp may be present.[2] A painful sacroiliac joint may also cause reflex inhibition of the gluteus medius, leading to a Trendelenburg's gait or lurch.

2. Whether the ASISs are level when viewed anteriorly (Fig. 10–2). On the affected side, the ASIS tends to be higher and slightly forward. The examiner must remember this difference, if present, when the patient is viewed from behind (Fig. 10–3). If the ASIS and PSIS on one side are higher than the ASIS and PSIS on the other side, this indicates an **upslip** of the ilium on the sacrum on the high side, a short leg, or muscle spasm caused by lumbar pathology (e.g., disc lesion).[6, 7] If the ASIS is higher on one side and the PSIS is lower at the same time, it indicates an anterior **torsion** of the sacrum on that side.[6] This torsion may result in a spinal scoliosis or an altered functional leg length, or both. The sacrum is lower on the side of the pelvis that has rotated backward. The most common rotation of the innominate bones is left posterior rotation. The posterior rotational dysfunctions are usually the result of falling on an ischeal tuberosity, lifting when forward flexed with the knees straight, repeated standing on one leg, vertical thrusting onto an extended leg, or sustaining hyperflexion and abduction of hips. Anterior rotational dysfunction is seen most frequently in posterior horizontal thrust of the femur (dashboard injury), golf or baseball swing, or any forced anterior diagonal pattern.[7]

3. Whether both pubic bones are level at the symphysis pubis. The examiner tests for level equality by placing one finger or thumb on the superior aspect of each pubic bone and comparing the heights (Fig. 10–4). If the ASIS on one side is higher, the pubic bone on that side is suspected to be higher, and this can be confirmed by this procedure, indicating a backward torsion problem

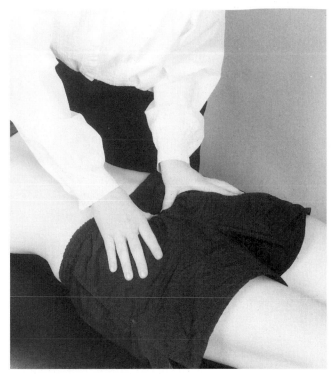

Figure 10–4
Determining level of pubic bones.

of the ilium on that side. This procedure is usually done with the patient lying supine.

4. Whether the patient stands with equal weight on both feet, favors one leg, or has a lateral pelvic tilt. This finding may indicate pathology in the sacroiliac joints, the leg, or the spine, or a short leg.

5. Whether the ASISs are equidistant from the center line of the body.

6. What type of pelvis the patient has. Gynecoid and android types are the most common (as described in Fig. 10–5 and Table 10–1).

7. Whether the sacrovertebral or lumbosacral angle is normal (140°).

8. Whether the pelvic angle or inclination is normal (30°).

9. Whether the sacral angle is normal (30°) (Fig. 10–6).

10. Whether the iliac crests are level. Altered leg length may alter their height.

11. Whether the PSISs are level.

12. Whether the buttock contours or gluteal folds are normal. The painful side is often flatter if there is loss of tone in the gluteus maximus muscle.

13. Whether there is any unilateral or bilateral spasm of the erector spinae muscles.

14. Whether the ischial tuberosities are level. If one tuberosity is higher, it may indicate an upslip of the ilium on the sacrum on that side.[6]

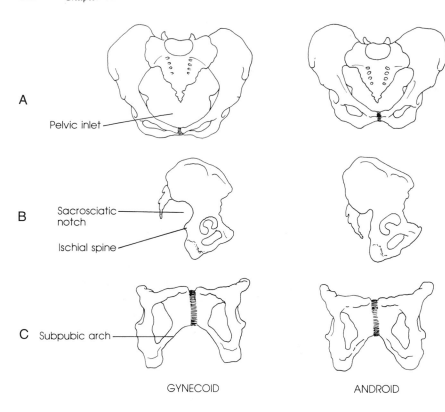

A — Pelvic inlet

B — Sacrosciatic notch — Ischial spine

C — Subpubic arch

GYNECOID   ANDROID

Figure 10–5
Gynecoid (predominantly female) and android (primarily male) pelvises. (A) Anterior view. (B) Lateral view. (C) Anterior view of the pubis and ischium.

15. Whether there is excessive lumbar lordosis. Forward or backward sacral torsion may increase or decrease the lordosis.

16. Whether the PSISs are equidistant from the center line of the body.

17. Whether the sacral sulci are equal. If one is deeper, it may indicate a sacral torsion.

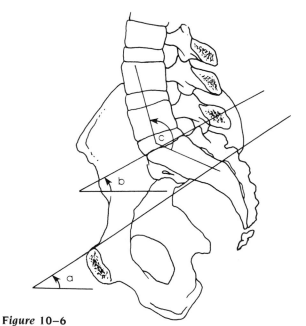

Figure 10–6
Normal angles of the pelvic joints. a, Pelvic angle (30°). b, Sacral angle (30°). c, Lumbosacral angle (140°).

Table 10–1
A Comparison of the Two Most Common Types of Pelvises

Feature	Gynecoid	Android
Inlet	Round	Triangular
Sacrosciatic notch	Average size	Narrow
Sacrum	Average	Forward
Subpubic arch	Inclination well curved	Inclination straight

18. Whether the feet face forward to the same degree. Often, the affected limb is medially rotated. With spasm of the piriformis muscle, the limb is laterally rotated on the affected side.

Examination

Before assessing the pelvic joints, the examiner should first assess the lumbar spine and hip, unless the history definitely indicates that one of the pelvic joints is at fault. The lumbar spine and hip can, and frequently do, refer pain to the sacroiliac joint area. Because the sacroiliac joints are in part a syndesmosis, movements at these joints are minimal compared with those of the other peripheral joints. It should also be remembered that any condition that alters the position of the sacrum relative to the ilium causes a corresponding change in the position of the symphysis pubis.

Active Movements

Unlike other peripheral joints, the sacroiliac joints do not have muscles that directly control their movement. However, because contraction of the muscles of the other joints may stress these joints or the symphysis pubis, the examiner must be careful during the active or resisted isometric movements of other joints and be sure to ask the patient about the exact location of the pain on each movement. For example, resisted abduction of the hip can cause pain in the sacroiliac joint on the same side if the joint is injured, because the gluteus medius muscle pulls the ilium away from the sacrum when it contracts strongly. In addition, side flexion to the same side increases the shearing stress to the sacroiliac joint on that side. The examiner is attempting to reproduce the patient's symptoms rather than just looking for pain.

The sacroiliac joints move in a "nodding" fashion of anteroposterior rotation. The sacrum moves forward on the ilia when the patient changes from a standing to a lying position. On forward flexion, the L5 vertebra moves on the sacrum, then the sacrum moves forward on the innominate bones (**kinetic forward flexion test**). The opposite occurs for movements in the opposite direction. Normally, the PSISs approximate when the patient stands and separate when the patient lies prone. When he or she stands on one leg, the pubic bone on the supported side moves forward in relation to the pubic bone on the opposite side as a result of rotation at the sacroiliac joint.

During the active movements of the pelvic joints, the examiner looks for unequal movement, loss of or increase in movement (hypomobility or hypermobility), tissue contracture, tenderness, or inflammation.

Active Movements That Stress the Sacroiliac Joints

- Forward flexion of the spine (40 to 60°)
- Extension of the spine (20 to 35°)
- Rotation of the spine, left and right (3 to 18°)
- Side flexion of the spine, left and right (15 to 20°)
- Flexion of the hip (100 to 120°)
- Abduction of the hip (30 to 50°)
- Adduction of the hip (30°)
- Extension of the hip (0 to 15°)
- Medial rotation of the hip (30 to 40°)
- Lateral rotation of the hip (40 to 60°)

The movements of the spine put a stress on the sacroiliac joints as well as on the lumbar and lumbosacral joints. Forward flexion movement while standing tests the movement of the ilia on the sacrum. During forward flexion, the innominate bones rotate anteriorly, so the two PSISs should move upward equally in relation to the sacrum and should move toward each other or approximate. During extension, the opposite movements occur.[2, 8] Side flexion normally produces a torsion movement between the ilia and the sacrum. If this torsion movement does not occur (e.g., in hypomobility), the patient finds that more effort is required to side flex and it is harder to maintain balance.[2]

The hip movements performed are also affected by sacroiliac lesions. As the patient flexes each hip maximally, the examiner should observe the range of motion present, the pain produced, and the movement of the PSISs. The examiner first notes whether the PSISs are level before the patient flexes the hip. Normally, flexion of the hip with the knee flexed to 90° or more causes the sacroiliac joint on that side to drop or move caudally in relation to the other sacroiliac joint. If this drop does not occur, it may indicate hypomobility on the flexed side. The examiner can observe this movement by placing one thumb over the PSIS and the other thumb over the spinous process of S2 (Fig. 10–7A). In the patient with a normal sacroiliac joint, the thumb on the PSIS drops (Fig. 10–7B). If it is hypomobile, the thumb moves up on hip flexion. The two sides are compared.

The examiner then leaves the one thumb over the sacral spinous process and moves the other thumb over the ischial tuberosity (Fig. 10–7C). The patient is again asked to flex the hip as far as possible. Normally, the thumb over the ischial tuberosity moves laterally (Fig. 10–7D). With a fixed or hypomobile joint, the thumb moves superiorly or toward the head. Again, the two sides are compared.

Passive Movements

The passive movements of the pelvic joints involve stressing of the ligaments and the joints themselves. They are not true passive movements, like those done at other joints, but are in reality stress tests. Because of their anatomic makeup, the pelvic joints do not move to the same degree or in the same fashion as other joints of the body. When testing passive movement, the examiner is looking for the **reproduction of the patient's symptoms,** not just pain or discomfort.[9, 10]

Common Stress Tests (Passive Movements) of the Sacroiliac Joints

- Ipsilateral prone kinetic test
- Passive extension and medial rotation of ilium on sacrum
- Passive flexion and lateral rotation of ilium on sacrum
- Gapping test
- Approximation test
- Knee-to-shoulder test

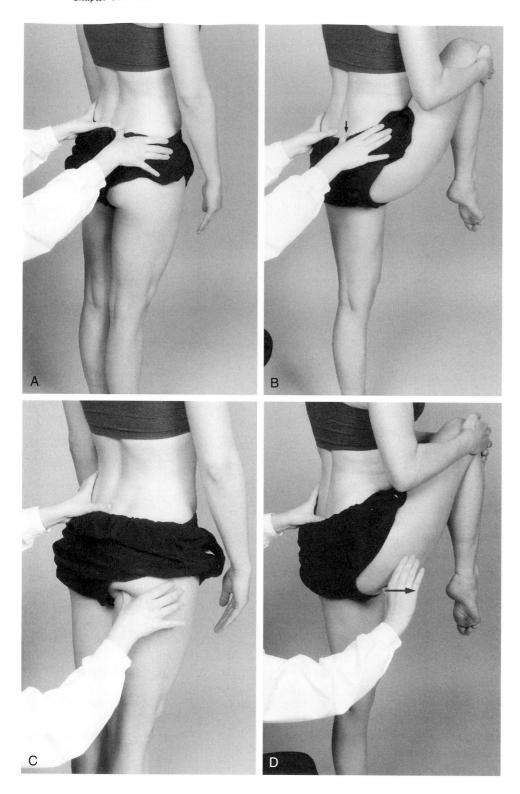

Figure 10–7
Active movements demonstrating how to show hypomobility of the sacroiliac joints. (A) Starting position for sacral spine and posterior superior iliac spine. (B) Hip flexion; the ilium drops as it normally should (*arrow*). (C) Starting position for sacral spine and ischial tuberosity. (D) Hip flexion. Ischial tuberosity moves laterally (*arrow*), as expected.

Ipsilateral Prone Kinetic Test.[2, 8] This test is designed to assess the ability of the ilium to flex and to rotate laterally or posteriorly. The patient lies prone while the examiner places one thumb on the PSIS and the other thumb parallel to it on the sacrum. The patient is then asked to actively extend the leg on the same side (Fig. 10–8).

Normally, the PSIS should move superiorly and laterally. If it does not, it indicates hypomobility with a posterior rotated ilium, or **outflare**.

Passive Extension and Medial Rotation of Ilium on Sacrum.[2, 8] The patient is in side lying position on the nontest side. The examiner places one hand over the

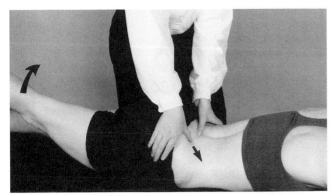

Figure 10–8
Ipsilateral prone kinetic test. On extension, the posterior superior iliac spine and sacral crest move superiorly and laterally.

ASIS area of the anterior ilium. The other hand is placed over the PSIS in such a way that the fingers of the hand palpate the posterior ilium and sacrum. The examiner then pulls the ilium forward with the hand over the ASIS and pushes the posterior ilium forward with the other hand while feeling the relative movement of the ilium on the sacrum (Fig. 10–9). The unaffected side is then tested for comparison. If the affected side moves less, it indicates hypomobility and a posterior rotated ilium, or **outflare.**

Passive Flexion and Lateral Rotation of Ilium on Sacrum. The patient is positioned as for the previous test. In this case, the examiner pushes the anterior ilium backward with the anterior hand, and the posterior hand and arm pull the ilium posteriorly while palpating the relative movement (Fig. 10–10). The unaffected side is then tested for comparison. If the affected side moves less,

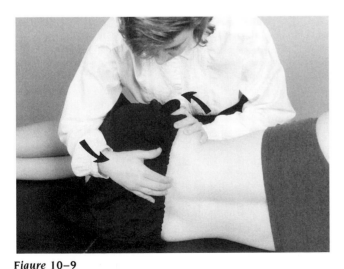

Figure 10–9
Passive extension and medial rotation of the ilium on the sacrum. The innominate bone is held in extension and medial rotation. The examiner palpates the sacrum and ilium with the fingers while rotating the ilium forward. With hypomobility, the relative movement is less than on the unaffected side, indicating an outflare.

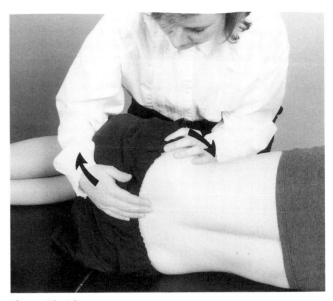

Figure 10–10
Passive flexion and lateral rotation of the ilium on the sacrum. The innominate bone is held in flexion and lateral rotation. The examiner palpates the sacrum and ilium with the left fingers while rotating the ilium backward. With hypomobility, the relative movement is less than on the unaffected side, indicating an inflare.

it is a sign of hypomobility and an anterior rotated ilium, or **inflare.**

If both this test and the previous one are positive, it means an upslip has occurred to the ilium relative to the sacrum.

Passive Lateral Rotation of the Hip. The patient lies supine. The examiner flexes the hip and knee to 90° and then laterally rotates the hip. This movement, provided the hip is normal, stresses the sacroiliac joint on the test side.[3]

Gapping (Transverse Anterior Stress) Test.[8] The patient lies supine while the examiner applies crossed-arm pressure to the ASIS (Fig. 10–11A). The examiner pushes down and out with the arms. The test is positive only if unilateral gluteal or posterior leg pain is produced, indicating a sprain of the anterior sacroiliac ligaments. Care must be taken when performing this test. The examiner's hands pushing against the ASIS can elicit pain because the soft tissue is being compressed between the examiner's hands and the patient's pelvis.

Prone Gapping (Hibb's) Test. The posterior sacroiliac ligaments may be stressed with the patient in the prone position (Fig. 10–11B). To perform the test, the patient's hips must have full range of motion and be pathology free. The patient lies prone, and the examiner stabilizes the pelvis with his or her chest. The patient's knee is flexed to 90° or greater, and the hip is medially rotated as far as possible. While pushing the hip into the very end of medial rotation, the examiner palpates the sacroiliac joint on the same side. The test is repeated on the other side, with the examiner comparing the degree of opening and the quality of the movement at each sacroil-

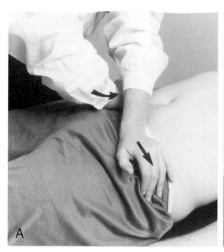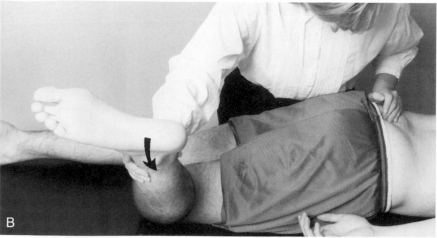

Figure 10–11
Gapping test. (A) Done in supine. (B) Done in prone.

iac joint as well as stressing the posterior sacroiliac ligaments.

Approximation (Transverse Posterior Stress) Test.[8] The patient is in the side lying position and the examiner's hands are placed over the upper part of the iliac crest, pressing toward the floor (Fig. 10–12). The movement causes forward pressure on the sacrum. An increased feeling of pressure in the sacroiliac joints indicates a possible sacroiliac lesion or a sprain of the posterior sacroiliac ligaments, or both.

"Squish" Test. With the patient in the supine position, the examiner places both hands on the patient's ASISs

and iliac crests and pushes down and in at a 45° angle (Fig. 10–13). This movement tests the posterior sacroiliac ligaments. A positive test is indicated by pain.

Sacroiliac Rocking (Knee-to-Shoulder) Test. This test is also called the **sacrotuberous ligament stress test.** The patient is in a supine position (Fig. 10–14). The examiner flexes the patient's knee and hip fully and then adducts the hip; both the hip and knee must demonstrate no pathology and have full range of motion. The sacroiliac joint is "rocked" by flexion and adduction of the patient's hip. To do the test properly, the knee is moved toward the patient's opposite shoulder. Some authors[8, 11] be-

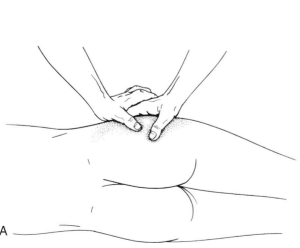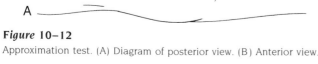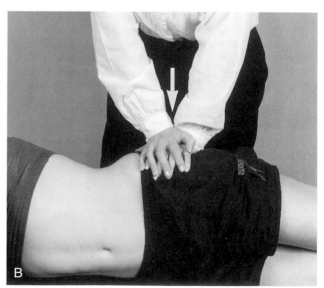

Figure 10–12
Approximation test. (A) Diagram of posterior view. (B) Anterior view.

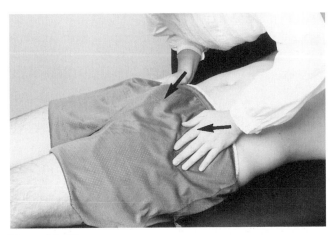

Figure 10–13
"Squish" test.

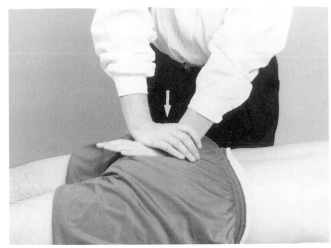

Figure 10–15
Sacral apex pressure test. Patient is lying prone.

lieve that the hip should be medially rotated as it is flexed and adducted to increase the stress on the sacroiliac joint. Simultaneously, the sacrotuberous ligament may be palpated for tenderness. Pain in the sacroiliac joints indicates a positive test. Care must be taken, because the test places a great deal of stress on the hip and sacroiliac joints. If a longitudinal force is applied through the hip in a slow, steady manner (for 15 to 20 seconds) in an oblique and lateral direction, further stress is applied to the sacrotuberous ligament.[8] While performing the test, the examiner may palpate the sacroiliac joint on the test side to feel for the slight amount of movement that normally is present.

Sacral Apex Pressure (Prone Springing) Test. The patient lies in a prone position on a firm surface while the examiner places the base of his or her hand at the apex of the

patient's sacrum (Fig. 10–15). Pressure is then applied to the apex of the sacrum, causing a shear of the sacrum on the ilium. The test may indicate a sacroiliac joint problem if pain is produced over the joint. The test causes a rotational shift of the sacroiliac joints.

Torsion Stress Test.[8] The patient lies prone. The examiner palpates the spinous process of L5, with one thumb holding it stable. The examiner's other hand is placed around the anterior ilium on the opposite side and lifts the contralateral ilium up (Fig. 10–16). This rotational movement stresses the lumbosacral junction, the iliolumbar ligament, the anterior sacroiliac ligament, and the sacroiliac joint.

Femoral Shear Test. The patient lies in the supine position. The examiner slightly flexes, abducts, and laterally rotates the patient's thigh at approximately 45° from the midline. The examiner then applies a graded force through the long axis of the femur, which causes an

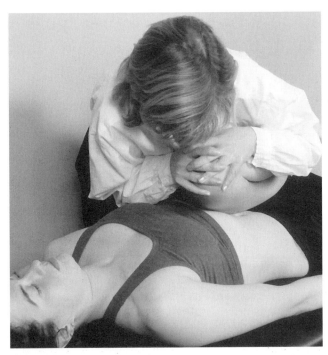

Figure 10–14
Sacroiliac rocking (knee-to-shoulder) test.

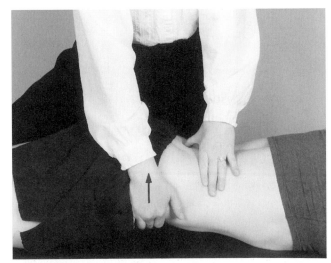

Figure 10–16
Torsion stress test. Patient is lying prone.

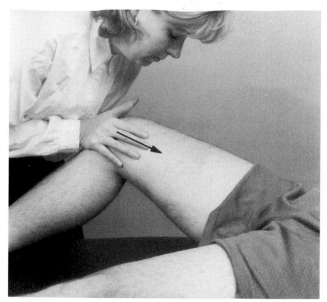

Figure 10–17
Femoral shear test.

anterior-to-posterior shear stress to the sacroiliac joint on the same side (Fig. 10–17).[11]

Superoinferior Symphysis Pubic Stress Test.[2, 8] The patient lies supine. The examiner places the heel of one hand over the superior pubic ramus of one pubic bone and the heel of the other hand over the inferior pubic ramus of the other pubic bone. The examiner then squeezes the hands together, applying a shearing force to the symphysis pubis (Fig. 10–18). Production of pain in the symphysis pubis is considered a positive test.

Resisted Isometric Movements

As previously stated, there are no specific muscles acting directly on the sacroiliac joints and symphysis pubis. However, contraction of adjacent muscles can stress

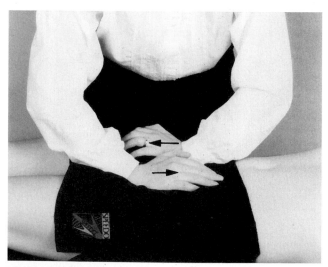

Figure 10–18
Superoinferior symphysis pubis stress test. Patient is lying supine.

these joints. The examiner performs these movements with the patient supine and attempts to reproduce the patient's symptoms.

> *Resisted Isometric Movements Stressing the Sacroiliac Joints*
>
> - Forward flexion of spine (the abdominals stress the symphysis pubis)
> - Flexion of hip (the iliacus stresses the sacroiliac joint)
> - Abduction of hip (the gluteus medius stresses the sacroiliac joint)
> - Adduction of the hip (the adductors stress the symphysis pubis)
> - Extension of hip (the gluteus maximus stresses the sacroiliac joints)

Functional Assessment

Functional assessment of the pelvic joints by themselves is very difficult because these joints do not work in isolation. Functionally, they should be considered part of the lumbar spine or part of the hip joint, depending on the area that the presenting pathology most affects.

Special Tests

The examiner should use only those special tests that are considered necessary to confirm the diagnosis. When doing these tests, especially the stress tests, the examiner is attempting to reproduce the patient's symptoms.

> *Special Tests Commonly Performed on the Pelvis*
>
> - Straight leg raising test
> - Sign of the buttock
> - Leg length tests
> - Trendelenburg's test
> - Flamingo test

Tests for Neurological Involvement

Straight Leg Raising (Lasègue's) Test. Although the Lasègue sign is primarily considered a test of the neurological tissue around the lumbar spine, this test also places a stress on the sacroiliac joints. With the patient in the supine position (Fig. 10–19), the examiner passively flexes the patient's hip with the knee extended. Pain occurring after 70° is usually indicative of joint pain. However, in hypermobile persons, joint pain is often not experienced until after 120° of hip flexion. Therefore, it is more important to watch for the production of the

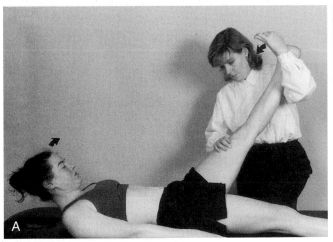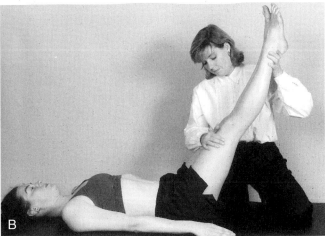

Figure 10–19
Straight leg raising test. (A) Unilateral (head may be flexed, ankle may be dorsiflexed, or both).
(B) Bilateral.

patient's symptoms than for the actual range of motion. In addition, the range of motion obtained should be compared with the unaffected side. If the examiner then does a passive bilateral straight leg raising test in a similar fashion, pain occurring before 70° is usually indicative of sacroiliac joint problems. A more detailed description of the straight leg raising test is given in Chapter 9.

Prone Knee Bending (Nachlas) Test. Normally, this is used to test for a tight rectus femoris, an upper lumbar joint lesion, an upper spine nerve root lesion, or a hypomobile sacroiliac joint. The patient lies prone, and the examiner flexes the knee so that the heel is brought to

the buttocks. If pain is felt in the front of the thigh before full range is reached, the problem is in the rectus femoris muscle. If the pain is in the lumbar spine, the problem is in the lumbar spine, usually the L3 nerve root, especially if these are radicular symptoms. If the problem is a hypomobile sacroiliac joint, the ipsilateral pelvic rim rotates forward, usually before the knee reaches 90° flexion.[11, 12]

Tests for Sacroiliac Joint Involvement

Piedallu's Sign. The patient is asked to sit on a hard, flat surface (Fig. 10–20). This position keeps the muscles

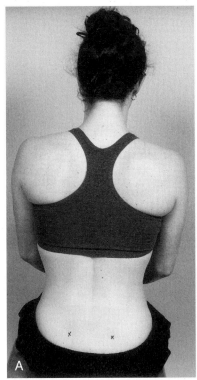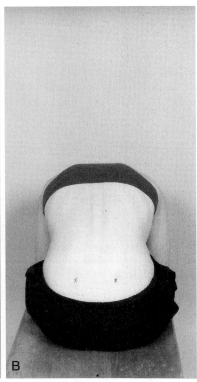

Figure 10–20
Piedallu's sign (A) Starting position. (B) Test position.

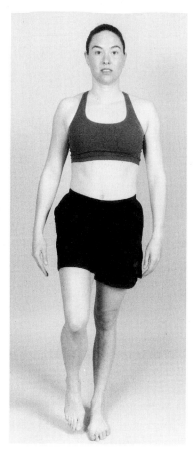

Figure 10–21
Flamingo test.

(e.g., hamstrings) from affecting the pelvic flexion symmetry and increases the stability of the ilia. In effect, it is a test of the sacrum on the ilia. The examiner palpates the PSISs and compares their heights. If one PSIS, usually the painful one, is lower than the other, the patient is asked to forward flex while remaining seated. If the lower PSIS becomes the higher one on forward flexion, the test is positive; it is that side that is affected. Because the affected joint does not move properly and is hypomobile, it goes from a low to a high position. This indicates an abnormality in the torsion movement at the sacroiliac joint.

Flamingo Test or Maneuver. The patient is asked to stand on one leg (Fig. 10–21). When the patient is standing on one leg, the weight of the trunk causes the sacrum to shift forward and distally (caudally) with forward rotation. The ilium moves in the opposite direction. On the non–weight-bearing side, the opposite occurs, but the stress is greatest on the stance side.[3] Pain in the symphysis pubis or sacroiliac joint indicates a positive test for lesions in whichever structure is painful. The stress may be increased by having the patient hop on one leg. This position is also used to take a stress x-ray of the symphysis pubis.

Gaenslen's Test. The patient lies on the side with the upper leg (test leg) hyperextended at the hip (Fig. 10–22A). The patient holds the lower leg flexed against the chest. The examiner stabilizes the pelvis while extending the hip of the uppermost leg. Pain indicates a positive test. The pain may be caused by an ipsilateral sacroiliac joint lesion, hip pathology, or an L4 nerve root lesion.

Gaenslen's test is sometimes done with the patient supine (Fig. 10–22B), but this position may limit the amount of hyperextension available. The patient is positioned so that the test hip extends beyond the edge of the table. The patient draws both legs up onto the chest and then slowly lowers the test leg into extension. The other leg is tested in a similar fashion for comparison. Pain in the sacroiliac joints is indicative of a positive test.

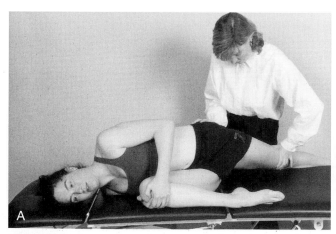
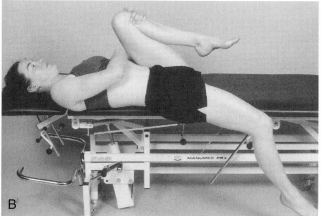

Figure 10–22
Gaenslen's test. (A) With patient in side lying position, examiner extends test leg. (B) With patient supine, test leg is extended over edge of table.

Mazion's Pelvic Maneuver.[13] The patient stands in a straddle position with the limb on the unaffected side forward so that the feet are 0.5 to 1 m (2 to 3 feet) apart. The patient bends forward, trying to touch the floor, until the heel of the back leg lifts off the floor. If pain is produced in the lower trunk on the affected side, it is considered a positive test for unilateral forward displacement of the ilium relative to the sacrum.

Laguere's Sign. The patient lies supine (Fig. 10–23). To test the right sacroiliac joint, the examiner flexes, abducts, and laterally rotates the patient's right hip, applying an overpressure at the end of the range of motion. The examiner must stabilize the pelvis on the opposite side by holding the opposite ASIS down. Pain in the right sacroiliac joint constitutes a positive test. The other side is tested for comparison. This test should be performed with caution for patients with hip pathology, because hip pain may ensue.

Gillet's (Sacral Fixation) Test.[7] While the patient stands, the examiner palpates the PSISs. The patient is then asked to stand on one leg while pulling the opposite knee up toward the chest. The test is repeated with the other leg. If the sacroiliac joint on the side on which the knee is flexed moves minimally or up, the joint is hypomobile, or "blocked," indicating a positive test. On the normal side, the test PSIS moves down or inferiorly

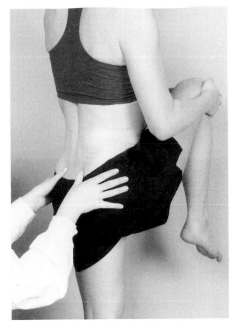

Figure 10–24
Gillet's (sacral fixation) test.

(Fig. 10–24). This test is similar to the test performed during hip flexion in active movement; the only difference is the points of palpation during the movement.

Supine-to-Sit (Long Sitting) Test. The patient lies supine with the legs straight. The examiner ensures that the medial malleoli are level. The patient is asked to sit up, and the examiner observes whether one leg moves up (proximally) farther than the other leg (Figs. 10–25 and 10–26). If one leg moves up farther than the other, there is a functional leg length difference resulting from a pelvic dysfunction caused by pelvic torsion or rotation.[11, 14, 15]

Goldthwait's Test. The patient lies supine. The examiner places one hand under the lumbar spine so that each finger is in an interspinous space (i.e., L5–S1, L4–L5, L3–L4, and L2–L3 interspaces). The examiner uses the other hand to perform straight leg raising. If pain is elicited before movement occurs at the interspaces, the problem is in the sacroiliac joint. Pain during interspace movement indicates a lumbar spine dysfunction. As with the straight leg raising test, pain may be referred along the course of the sciatic nerve if there is neurological (e.g., nerve root) involvement.[12]

Yeoman's Test. The patient lies prone. The examiner flexes the patient's knee to 90° and extends the hip (Fig. 10–27). Pain localized to the sacroiliac joint indicates pathology in the anterior sacroiliac ligaments. Lumbar pain indicates lumbar involvement.[12] Anterior thigh paresthesia may indicate a femoral nerve stretch.

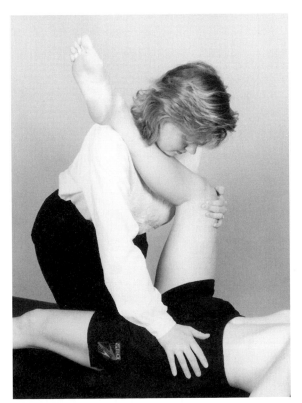

Figure 10–23
Laguere's sign.

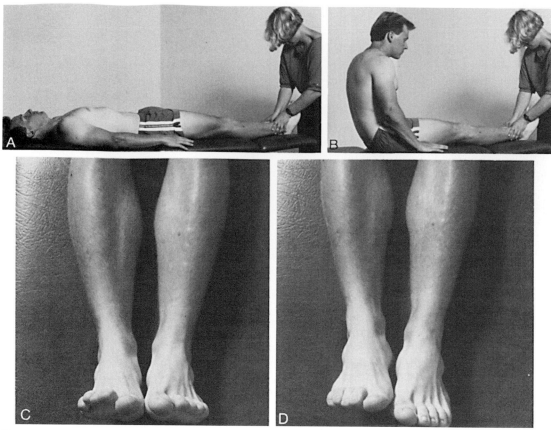

Figure 10–25

Supine-to-sit test for functional leg length discrepancy. (A) Initial position. (B) Final position.
(C) Symmetric leg lengths. (D) Asymmetric leg lengths.

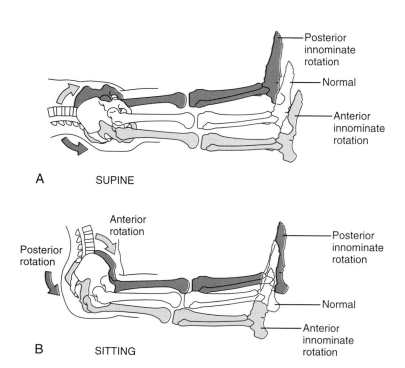

Figure 10–26

Supine-to-sit test. Leg length reversal; supine (A) versus sitting (B). If the lower limb on the affected side appears longer when a patient lies supine but shorter when sitting, the test is positive, implicating anterior innominate rotation of the affected side. (Redrawn from Wadsworth, C.T. [ed.]: Manual Examination and Treatment of the Spine and Extremities. Baltimore: Williams & Wilkins, 1988, p. 82.)

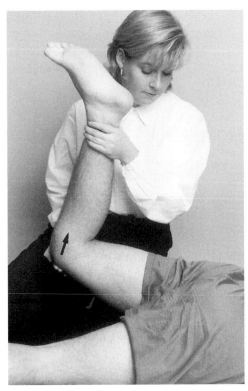

Figure 10–27
Yeoman's test.

Tests for Limb Length

Leg Length Test. The leg length test, described in detail in Chapter 11, should always be performed if the examiner suspects a sacroiliac joint lesion. Nutation (backward rotation) of the ilium on the sacrum results in a decrease in leg length, as does contranutation (anterior rotation) on the opposite side. If the iliac bone on one side is lower, the leg on that side is usually longer. True leg length is measured by placing the patient in a supine position with the ASISs level and the patient's lower limbs perpendicular to the line joining the ASISs (Fig. 10–28). Using a flexible tape measure, the examiner obtains the distance from the ASIS to the medial or lateral malleolus on the same side. The measurement is repeated on the other side, and the results are compared. A difference of 1 to 1.3 cm (0.5 to 1 inch) is considered normal. It should be remembered, however, that leg length differences within this range may also be pathological.

Functional Limb Length Test.[16] The patient stands relaxed while the examiner palpates the ASISs and the PSISs, noting any asymmetry. The patient is then placed in the correct stance (subtalar joints neutral, knees fully extended, and toes facing straight ahead), and the ASISs and PSISs are palpated, with the examiner noting whether the asymmetry has been corrected. If the asymmetry has been corrected by correct positioning of the

limb, the leg is structurally normal (i.e., the bones have proper length) but abnormal joint mechanics (functional deficit) are producing a functional leg length difference. Therefore, if the asymmetry is corrected by proper positioning, the test is positive for a functional leg length difference.

Other Tests

Sign of the Buttock Test. With the patient supine, the examiner performs a passive unilateral straight leg raising test as done previously (Fig. 10–29). If restriction or pain is found on one side, the examiner flexes the patient's knee while holding the patient's thigh in the same position. Once the knee is flexed, the examiner tries to flex the hip further. If the problem is in the lumbar spine or hamstrings, hip flexion increases. This finding indicates a negative sign of the buttock test. If hip flexion does not increase when the knee is flexed, it is a positive sign of the buttock test and indicates pathology in the buttock, such as a bursitis, tumor, or abscess. The patient with this pathology would also exhibit a noncapsular pattern of the hip.

Trendelenburg's Test or Sign. The patient is asked to stand or balance first on one leg and then on the other leg (Fig. 10–30). While the patient is balancing on one leg, the examiner watches the movement of the pelvis. If the pelvis on the side of the nonstance leg rises, the test is considered negative, because the gluteus medius muscle on the opposite (stance) side lifts it up as it normally does in one-legged stance. If the pelvis on the side of the nonstance leg falls, the test is considered positive and is an indication of weakness or instability of the hip abductor muscles, primarily the gluteus medius on the stance side. Therefore, although the examiner is watching what happens on the nonstance side, it is the stance side that is being tested.

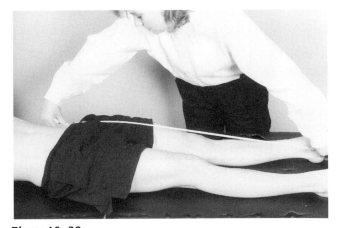

Figure 10–28
Measuring leg length (anterior superior iliac spine to medial malleolus).

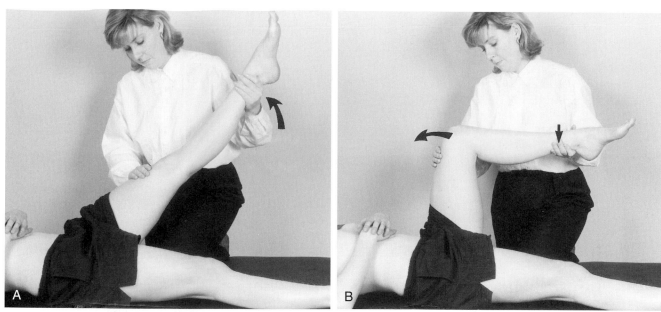

Figure 10–29

Sign of the buttock test. (A) Hip is flexed with knee straight until resistance or pain is felt. (B) Then knee is flexed to see whether further hip flexion can be achieved. If further hip flexion can be achieved, the test is negative.

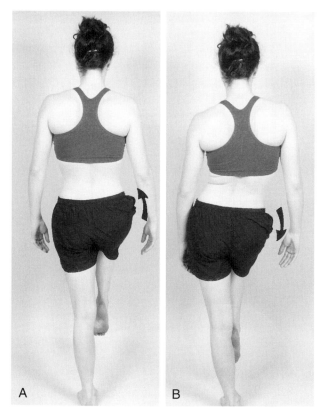

Figure 10–30

Trendelenburg's sign. (A) Negative test. (B) Positive test.

Reflexes and Cutaneous Distribution

There are no reflexes to test for the pelvic joints. However, the examiner must be aware of the dermatomes from the sacral nerve roots (Fig. 10–31). Pain may be

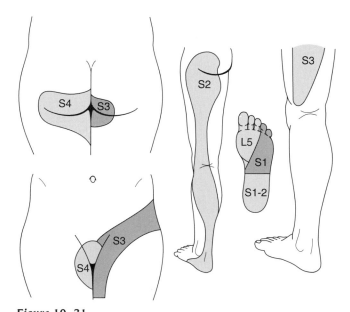

Figure 10–31

Posterior sacral dermatomes. Representation in the lower left is an anterior view.

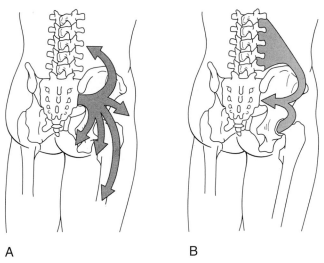

A   **B**

Figure 10–32
Referred pain from sacroiliac joint (A) and to sacroiliac joint (B).

referred to the sacroiliac joints from the lumbar spine and the hip (Fig. 10–32). In addition, the sacroiliac joint may refer pain to these same structures or along the courses of the superior gluteal and obturator nerves. The muscles of the spine may also refer pain to the sacral area (Table 10–2).

Peripheral Nerve Injuries About the Pelvis

Meralgia Paresthetica.[17] This condition is the result of pressure or entrapment of the lateral femoral cutaneous nerve near the ASIS as the nerve passes under the inguinal ligament. It may result from trauma such as that caused by a seat belt in a car accident, during delivery (in stirrups), by tight clothing, or as a complication of surgery (e.g., hernia). This nerve is sensory only, so the patient experiences sensory alteration and/or burning pain on the lateral aspect of the thigh (Fig. 10–33).

Ilioinguinal Nerve.[18] This nerve, which lies within the transverse abdominus muscle, may be compressed by spasm of the muscle (Fig. 10–34). The nerve is sensory only, and the sensory alteration and/or pain occur in the superior aspect of the anterior thigh (in the L1 dermatome area) as well as in the scrotum or labia.

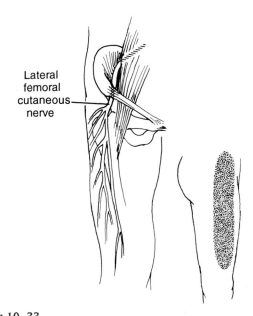

Figure 10–33
Meralgia paresthetica. The lateral femoral cutaneous nerve supplies the skin of the lateral thigh. An area from the inguinal ligament to the knee may be affected. (From Borenstein, D.G., S.W. Wiesel, and S.D. Boden: Low Back Pain: Medical Diagnosis and Comprehensive Management. Philadelphia, W.B. Saunders Co., 1995, p. 506.)

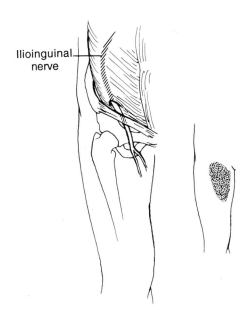

Figure 10–34
Ilioinguinal syndrome. The ilioinguinal nerve lies within the transversus abdominis and emerges below the inguinal ligament. An area of skin on the medial thigh near the genitalia is affected. (From Borenstein, D.G., S.W. Wiesel, and S.D. Boden: Low Back Pain: Medical Diagnosis and Comprehensive Management. Philadelphia, W.B. Saunders Co., 1995, p. 506.)

Table 10–2
Muscles and Referral of Pain to Pelvic Area

Muscle	Referral Pattern
Longissimus thoracis	From lower thoracic spine to posterior iliac crest and gluteal area
Iliocostalis lumborum	From area lateral to lumbar spine to sacral and gluteal area
Multifidi	Sacral area

Joint Play Movements

The joint play movements (Fig. 10–35) are minimal for the sacroiliac joints and are similar to the passive movements in that they are stress tests.

Joint Play Movements of the Sacroiliac Joints

- Cephalad movement of the sacrum with caudal movement of the ilium (left and right)
- Cephalad movement of the ilium with caudal movement of the sacrum (left and right)
- Anterior movement of the sacrum on the ilium

To test each of these movements, the patient is in the prone position. For the first joint play movement, the examiner places the heel of one hand over the iliac crest and the heel of the other hand over the apex of the sacrum. The ilium is pushed down or caudally with one hand while the sacrum is pushed up or cephalad with the other hand. The test is repeated for the other ilium (see Fig. 10–35A). The examiner should feel only minimal movement, and there should be no pain if the joint is normal. In an affected sacroiliac joint, there is usually pain over the joint and little or no movement. This positioning tests for cephalad movement of the sacrum and caudal movement of the ilium.

To test caudal movement of the sacrum and cephalad movement of the ilium, the examiner places the heel of one hand over the base of the sacrum and the heel of the other hand over the ischial tuberosity (see Fig. 10–35B). The examiner then pushes the pelvis cephalad and the sacrum caudally. The test is repeated with the other half of the pelvis being moved. The movement and amount of pain are compared.

The anterior movement of the sacrum on the ilium is tested with the patient lying prone (see Fig. 10–35C). The examiner places the heel of one hand over the sacrum and places the other hand under the iliac crest in the area of the ASIS on one side. The hand is then pushed down on the sacrum while the other hand lifts up. The process is repeated on the other side, and the results are compared. Similarly, with the patient supine, a wedge may be used against the sacrum with the patient's body weight acting to push the sacrum forward.

Palpation

Because many structures are included in the assessment of the pelvic joints, palpation of this area may be extensive, beginning on the anterior aspect and concluding posteriorly. While palpating, the examiner should note any tenderness, muscle spasm, or other signs that may indicate the source of pathology.

Anterior Aspect

The following structures should be carefully and thoroughly palpated (Fig. 10–36).

Iliac Crest and Anterior Superior Iliac Spine. The palpating fingers are placed on the iliac crests on both sides and gently moved anteriorly until each ASIS is reached. The inguinal ligament attaches to the ASIS and runs downward and medially to the symphysis pubis.

McBurney's Point and Baer's Point. The examiner may then draw an imaginary line from the right ASIS to the umbilicus. **McBurney's point** lies along this line approximately one third of the distance from the ASIS and is especially tender in the presence of acute appendicitis. **Baer's point** is located in the right iliac fossa anterior to the right sacroiliac joint and slightly medial to McBurney's point. It is tender in the presence of infection or when there are sprains of the right sacroiliac ligament

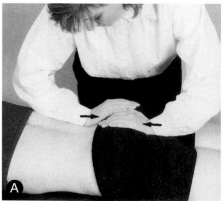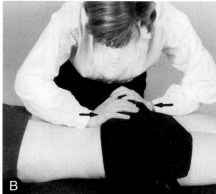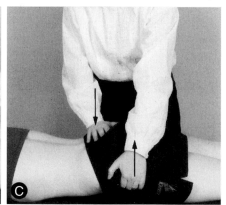

Figure 10–35

Joint play movements of the sacroiliac joints (A) Cephalad movement of sacrum with caudal movement of ilium. (B) Cephalad movement of ilium with caudal movement of sacrum. (C) Anterior movement of sacrum on ilium (left side demonstrated).

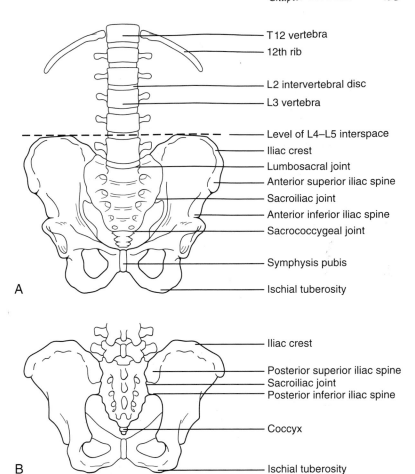

Figure 10-36
Landmarks of the sacroiliac joints and symphysis pubis. (A) Anterior view. (B) Posterior view.

and indicates spasm and tenderness of the iliacus muscle.

Lymph Nodes, Symphysis Pubis (Pubic Tubercles), Greater Trochanter of the Femur, Trochanteric Bursa, Femoral Triangle, and Surrounding Musculature. The examiner returns to the ASIS and gently palpates the length of the inguinal ligament, feeling for any tenderness or swelling of the lymph nodes or possible inguinal hernia. At the distal end of the inguinal ligament, the examiner comes to the pubic tubercles and symphysis pubis, which should be palpated for tenderness or signs of pathology.

The examiner then places the thumbs over the pubic tubercles and moves the fingers laterally until the bony greater trochanter of the femur is felt. The trochanters are usually level. The trochanteric bursa lies over the greater trochanter and is palpable only if it is swollen.

Returning to the ASIS, the examiner can move on to palpate the **femoral triangle,** which has as its boundaries the inguinal ligament superiorly, the adductor longus muscle medially, and the sartorius muscle laterally. It is in the superior aspect of the triangle that the examiner palpates for swollen lymph nodes. The **femoral pulse** can be palpated deeper in the triangle. Although almost impossible to palpate, the femoral nerve lies lateral to the artery, whereas the femoral vein lies medial to it.

The psoas bursa may also be palpated within the femoral triangle, but only if it is swollen. Before moving on to the posterior structures, the examiner should determine whether the adjacent musculature—the abductor, flexor, and adductor muscles—shows any indication of pathology (e.g., muscle spasm, pain).

Posterior Aspect

To complete the posterior palpation, the patient lies in the prone position, and the following structures are palpated.

Iliac Crest and Posterior Superior Iliac Spine. Again, the examiner places the fingers on the iliac crest and moves posteriorly until they rest on the PSIS, which is at the level of the S2 spinous process. On many patients, dimples indicate the position of the PSIS.

Ischial Tuberosity. If the examiner then moves distally from the PSIS and down to the level of the gluteal folds, the ischial tuberosities may be palpated. It is important that they be palpated, because the hamstring muscles attach here, and the bony prominences are what one "sits on."

Sacral Sulcus and Sacroiliac Joints. Returning to the PSIS as a starting point, the examiner should palpate slightly

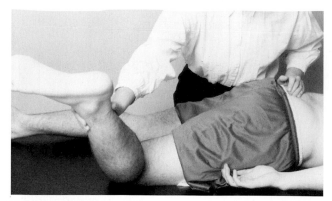

Figure 10–37
Palpation of the right sacroiliac joint.

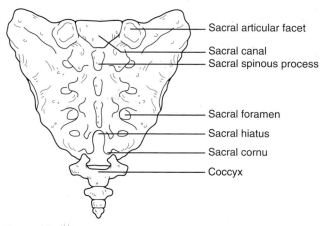

Figure 10–38
Posterior view of the sacrum and coccyx.

below it on the sacrum adjacent to the ilium. (This area is sometimes referred to as the **sacral sulcus**.) The depth on the right side should be compared with that on the left side. If one side is deeper than the other, sacral torsion or rotation on the ilium around the horizontal plane may be indicated.

If the examiner then moves slightly medially and distal to the PSIS, the fingers will rest adjacent to the sacroiliac joints. To palpate these joints, the patient's knee is flexed to 90° or greater and the hip is passively medially rotated while the examiner palpates the sacroiliac joint on the same side (Fig. 10–37). This procedure is identical to the prone gapping test previously described under Passive Movements. The procedure is repeated on the other side, and the two results are compared.

Sacrum, Lumbosacral Joint, Coccyx, Sacral Hiatus, Sacral Cornua, and Sacrotuberous and Sacrospinous Ligaments. The examiner again returns to the PSIS and moves to the midline of the sacrum, where the S2 spinous process can be palpated.

Moving superiorly over two spinous processes, the fingers now rest on the spinous process of L5. As a check, the examiner may look to see if the fingers rest just below a horizontal line drawn from the high point of the iliac crests. This horizontal line normally passes through the interspace between L4 and L5. Having found the L5 spinous process, the examiner then palpates between the spinous processes of L5 and S1, feeling for signs of pathology at the lumbosacral joint. Moving laterally approximately 2 to 3 cm (0.8 to 1.2 inches), the fingers lie over the lumbosacral facet joints, which are not palpable. However, the overlying structures may be palpated for tenderness or spasm, which may indicate pathology of these joints or related structures. In a similar fashion, the spinous processes and facet joints of the other lumbar spines and intervening structures can be palpated.

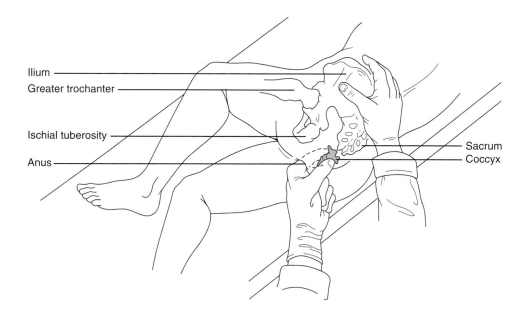

Figure 10–39
Palpation of the coccyx.

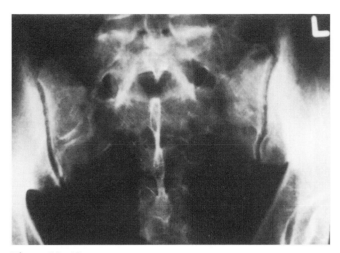

Figure 10–40
Anteroposterior radiograph of the sacroiliac joint.

then palpates the anterior surface of the coccyx while the thumb of the same hand palpates its posterior aspect. While holding the coccyx between the finger and thumb, the examiner is able to move it back and forth, rocking it at the sacrococcygeal joint. Normally, this action should not cause pain.

The examiner then returns to the PSIS. Moving straight down or distally from the PSIS, the fingers follow the path of the **sacrotuberous ligament,** which should be palpated for tenderness. Slightly more than halfway between the PSIS and ischial tuberosity and slightly medially, the fingers pass over the **sacrospinous ligament,** which is deep to the sacrotuberous ligament. Tenderness in this area may indicate pathology of this ligament.

Diagnostic Imaging

Plain Film Radiography

On plain film radiography, anteroposterior view (Figs. 10–40 and 10–41), the examiner should look for or note the following:

The examiner then returns to the S2 spinous process or tubercle. Carefully palpating farther distally, just before the coccyx, the examiner may be able to palpate the sacral hiatus lying in the midline. If the fingers are moved slightly laterally, the sacral cornua, which constitute the distal aspect of the sacrum, may be palpated (Fig. 10–38).

To palpate the coccyx properly, the examiner performs a rectal examination (Fig. 10–39). A rubber glove is put on, and the index finger is lubricated. The index finger is then carefully pushed into the rectum as the patient relaxes the sphincter muscles. The index finger

1. Ankylosis of sacroiliac joints (e.g., ankylosing spondylitis; Fig. 10–42).
2. Displacement of one sacroiliac joint and/or the symphysis pubis (Fig. 10–43).
3. Demineralization, sclerosis, or periosteal reaction of one or both pubic bones at the symphysis pubis (e.g., osteitis pubis; Fig. 10–44).
4. Any fracture.
5. Relation of the sacrum to the ilium.

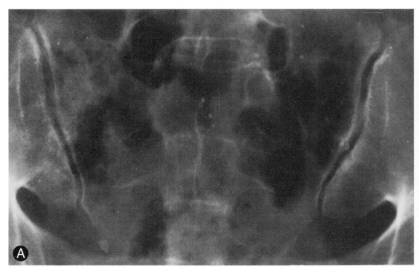

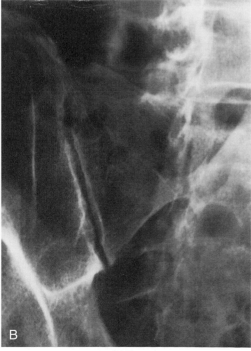

Figure 10–41
Normal sacroiliac joints. Angled (A) and oblique (B) anteroposterior views show normally maintained cortices and cartilage spaces. (From Weissman, B.N.W., and C.B. Sledge: Orthopedic Radiology. Philadelphia, W.B. Saunders Co., 1986, p. 347.)

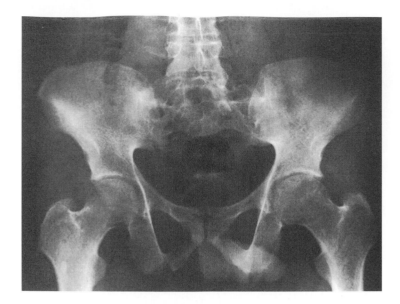

Figure 10–42
Fusion of sacroiliac joint spaces in the late stage of sacroiliitis of ankylosing spondylitis (anteroposterior view). The sclerosis has resorbed, and there is slight narrowing of the left hip joint. (From Rothman, R.H., and F.A. Simeone: The Spine. Philadelphia, W.B. Saunders Co., 1982, p. 921.)

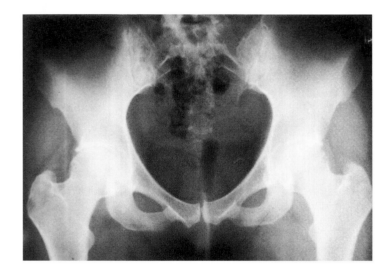

Figure 10–43
Anteroposterior radiograph of the pelvis. Note higher left pubic bone.

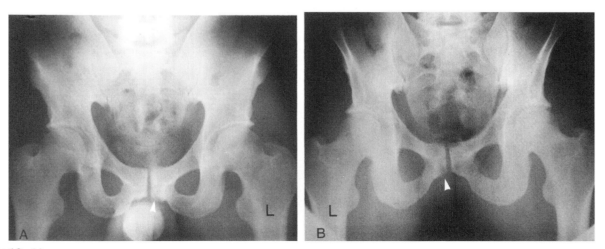

Figure 10–44
Osteitis pubis. (A) Anteroposterior view of pelvis showing well-concealed bony lesion at inferior corner of left pubis at the symphysis (*arrowhead*). (B) Posterior view of same pelvis; bony fragment is well delineated in this view. (From Wiley, J.J.: Traumatic osteitis pubis: The gracilis syndrome. Am. J. Sports Med. 11:361, 1983.)

Précis of the Pelvis Assessment*

History (sitting)
Observation (standing)
Examination
    Active moments (standing)
        Flexion of the spine
        Extension of the spine
        Rotation of the spine (left and right)
        Side flexion of the spine (left and right)
        Flexion of the hip
        Abduction of the hip
        Adduction of the hip
        Extension of the hip
        Medial rotation of the hip
        Lateral rotation of the hip
    Special tests (standing)
    Special tests (sitting)
    Passive movements (supine)
        Gapping test
        Rocking (knee-to-shoulder) test
        Sacral apex pressure test
    Resisted isometric movements (supine)**
        Forward flexion of the spine
        Flexion of the hip
        Abduction of the hip
        Adduction of the hip
        Extension of the hip
    Special tests (supine)
    Passive movements (side lying)
        Approximation test
        Passive extension and medial rotation of ilium on
            sacrum

        Passive flexion and lateral rotation of ilium on
            sacrum
    Reflexes and cutaneous distribution (supine, then prone)
    Passive movements (prone)
        Ipsilateral prone kinetic test
        Sacral apex pressure test
    Special tests (prone)
    Joint play movements (prone)
        Cephalad movement of the sacrum with caudal
            movement of the ilium
        Cephalad movement of the ilium with caudal
            movement of the sacrum
    Palpation (prone, then supine)
    Diagnostic imaging

---

* The précis is shown in an order that will limit the amount of moving or changing position that the patient has to do but ensure that all necessary structures are tested.
** If not done in standing.

As previously stated, assessment of the sacroiliac joints and symphysis pubis is done only after an assessment of the lumbar spine and hips, unless there has been specific trauma to the sacroiliac joints or symphysis pubis. Completion of the examination of the sacroiliac joints and symphysis pubis therefore may involve only passive movements, special tests, joint play movements, and palpation, because the other tests would have been completed when assessing the other joints.

After any examination, the patient should be warned of the possibility of exacerbation of symptoms as a result of the assessment.

Case Studies

When doing these case studies, the examiner should list the appropriate questions to be aked and why they are being asked, what to look for and why, and what things should be tested and why. Depending on the answers of the patient (and the examiner should consider different responses), several possible causes of the patient's problem may become evident (examples are given in parentheses). A differential diagnosis chart (Table 10–3) should be made up. The examiner can then decide how different diagnoses may affect the treatment plan.

Table 10–3
Differential Diagnosis Between Ankylosing Spondylitis and Sacroiliac Arthritis

	Ankylosing Spondylitis	**Sacroiliac Arthritis**
History	Bilateral sacroiliac pain that may refer to posterior thigh Morning stiffness Male predominance	Bilateral sacroiliac pain referring to gluteal area (S1–S2 dermatomes) Morning stiffness (prolonged) Coughing painful
Observation	Stiff, controlled movement of pelvis	Controlled movement of pelvis
Active movement	Decreased	Side flexion and extension full Slight limitation of flexion
Passive movement	Decreased	Normal
Resisted isometric movement	Pain and weakness, especially if sacroiliac joints are stressed	Pain, especially if sacroiliac joints are stressed
Special tests	Sacral stress tests probably positive	Sacral stress tests probably positive
Sensation and reflexes	Normal	Normal
Palpation	Tender over sacroiliac joints	Tender over sacroiliac joints
Diagnostic imaging	X-rays diagnostic	X-rays diagnostic
Lab tests	Erythrocyte sedimentation rate increased HLA-B27 human leukocyte antigen present in 80%	Normal

1. A 26-year-old male soccer player presents complaining of lower abdominal pain that is referred into the right groin. Sit-ups are painful, and he experiences pain when he kicks the ball. Describe your assessment plan for this patient (abdominal strain versus osteitis pubis).

2. A 35-year-old man presents complaining of "back pain." He complains that his back is stiff and sore when he gets up in the morning and that the stiffness remains for most of the day. Sclerosis of the sacroiliac is evident on x-ray. Describe your assessment plan for this patient (ankylosing spondylitis versus osteoarthritis of the sacroiliac joints).

3. An 18-year-old female figure skater presents complaining of back pain that increases when she is skating; the pain is prominent on one leg. The ASIS and PSIS are higher on the right side. Describe your assessment plan for this patient (sacroiliac dysfunction versus short leg syndrome).

References

Cited References

1. Kapandji, L.A.: The Physiology of the Joints, vol. 3: The Trunk and Vertebral Column. New York, Churchill Livingstone, 1974.
2. Lee, D.G.: Clinical manifestations of pelvic girdle dysfunction. In Boyling, J.D., and N. Palastanga (eds.): Grieve's Modern Manual Therapy: The Vertebral Column, 2nd ed. Edinburgh, Churchill Livingstone, 1994.
3. Ombregt, L., B. Bisschop, H.J. ter Veer, and T. Van de Velde: A System of Orthopedic Medicine. London, W.B. Saunders Co., 1995.
4. Maigne, R.: Orthopaedic Medicine: A New Approach to Vertebral Manipulation. Springfield, Illinois, Charles C Thomas, 1972.
5. Maigne, R.: Diagnosis and Treatment of Pain of Vertebral Origin. Baltimore, Williams & Wilkins, 1996.
6. Mitchell, F.L., P.S. Moran, and N.A. Pruzzo: An Evaluation and Treatment Manual of Osteopathic Muscle Energy Procedures. Valley Park, Missouri, Mitchell, Moran & Pruzzo, 1979.
7. Woerman, A.L.: Evaluation and treatment of dysfunction in the lumbar-pelvic-hip complex. In Donatelli, R., and M.J. Wooden (eds.): Orthopedic Physical Therapy. Edinburgh, Churchill Livingstone, 1989.
8. Lee, D.: The Pelvic Girdle. Edinburgh, Churchill Livingstone, 1989.
9. Dreyfus, P., S. Dreyer, J. Griffin, J. Hoffman, and N. Walsh: Positive sacroiliac screening tests in asymptomatic adults. Spine 19:1138–1143, 1994.
10. Laslett, M., and M. Williams: The reliability of selected pain provocation tests for sacroiliac joint pathology. Spine 19:1243–1249, 1994.
11. Porterfield, J.A., and C. DeRosa: Mechanical Low Back Pain: Perspectives in Functional Anatomy. Philadelphia, W.B. Saunders Co., 1991.
12. Cipriano, J.J.: Photographic Manual of Regional Orthopedic Tests. Baltimore, Williams & Wilkins, 1985.
13. Evans, R.C.: Illustrated Essentials in Orthopedic Physical Assessment. St. Louis, C.V. Mosby Co., 1994.
14. Palmer, M.C., and M. Epler: Clinical Assessment Procedures in Physical Therapy. Philadelphia, J.B. Lippincott, 1990.
15. Bemis, T., and M. Daniel: Validation of the long sitting test on subjects with iliosacral dysfunction. J. Orthop. Sports Phys. Ther. 8:336–345, 1987.
16. Wallace, L.A.: Limb length difference and back pain. In Grieve, G.P. (ed.): Modern Manual Therapy of the Vertebral Column. Edinburgh, Churchill Livingstone, 1986.
17. Pecina, M.M., J. Krmpotic-Nemanic, and A.D. Markiewitz: Tunnel Syndromes. Boca Raton, Florida, CRC Press, 1991.
18. Borenstein, D.G., S.W. Wiesel, and S.D. Boden: Low Back Pain: Medical Diagnosis and Comprehensive Management. Philadelphia, W.B. Saunders Co., 1995.

General References

Alderink, G.J.: The sacroiliac joint: Review of anatomy, mechanics, and function. J. Orthop. Sports Phys. Ther. 13:71–84, 1991.
Bourdillon, J.F.: Spinal Manipulation, 3rd ed. New York, Appleton-Century-Crofts, 1982.
Bowen, V., and J.D. Cassidy: Macroscopic and microscopic anatomy of the sacroiliac joint from embryonic life until the eighth decade. Spine 6:620–628, 1981.
Brooke, R.: The sacro-iliac joint. J. Anat. 58:299–305, 1924.
Carmichael, J.P.: Inter- and intra-examination reliability of palpation for sacroiliac joint dysfunction. J. Manip. Physiol. Ther. 10:164–171, 1987.
Cassidy, J.D.: The pathoanatomy and clinical significance of the sacroiliac joints, J. Manip. Physiol. Ther. 15:41–42, 1992.
Cohen, A.S., J.M. McNeill, E. Calkins, et al.: The "normal" sacroiliac joint: Analysis of 88 sacroiliac roentgenograms. Am. J. Roentgenol. 100:559–563, 1967.
Cyriax, J.: Textbook of Orthopaedic Medicine, vol. 1: Diagnosis of Soft Tissue Lesions. London, Bailliere Tindall, 1975.
DeRosa, C., and J.A. Porterfield: Lumbar spine and pelvis. In Richardson, J.K., and Z.A. Iglarsh (eds.): Clinical Orthopedic Physical Therapy. Philadelphia, W.B. Saunders Co., 1994.
Dietrichs, E.: Anatomy of the pelvic joints: A review. Scand. J. Rheumatol. Suppl. 88:4–6, 1991.
Dykstra, P.F.: Radiology of the normal SI joint. J. Man. Manip. Ther. 1:87–94, 1993.
Dyrek, D.A., L.J. Micheli, and D.J. Magee: Injuries to the thoracolumbar spine and pelvis. In Zachazewski, J.E., D.J. Magee, and W.S. Quillen (eds.): Athletic Injuries and Rehabilitation. Philadelphia, W.B. Saunders Co., 1996.
Fickel, T.E.: "Snapping hip" and sacroiliac sprain: Example of a cause-effect relationship. J. Manip. Physiol. Ther. 12:390–392, 1989.
Finneson, B.E.: Low Back Pain. Philadelphia, J.B. Lippincott Co., 1981.
Forrester, D.M., and J.C. Brown: The Radiology of Joint Disease. Philadelphia, W.B. Saunders Co., 1987.
Frigerio, N.A., R.R. Stowe, and J.W. Howe: Movement of the sacroiliac joint. Clin. Orthop. 100:370–377, 1974.
Gajdosik, R.L., C.R. Alberta, and J.J. Mitman: Influence of hamstring length on the standing position and flexion range of motion of the pelvic angle, lumbar angle, and thoracic angle. J. Orthop. Sports Phys. Ther. 20:213–219, 1994.
Gamble, J.G., S.C. Simmons, and M. Freedman: The symphysis pubis: Anatomic and pathologic considerations. Clin. Orthop. 203:261–272, 1986.
Gilliam, J., D. Brunt, M. MacMillan, R.E. Kinard, and W.J. Montgomery: Relationship of the pelvic angle to the sacral angle: Measurement of clinical reliability and validity. J. Orthop. Sports Phys. Ther. 20:193–199, 1994.
Gitelman, R.: A chiropractic approach to biomechanical disorders of the lumbar spine and pelvis. In Haldeman, S. (ed.): Modern Developments in the Principles and Practice of Chiropractic. New York, Appleton-Century-Crofts, 1980.
Gray, H.: Sacro-iliac joint pain: The finer anatomy. New International Clinics 2:54–64, 1938.

Grieve, G.P.: Mobilisation of the Spine. Edinburgh, Churchill Livingstone, 1979.

Grieve, G.P.: The sacro-iliac joint. Physiotherapy 62:384–400, 1976.

Grieve, G.P.: Common Vertebral Joint Problems. Edinburgh, Churchill Livingstone, 1981.

Gross, M.L., S. Nasser, and G.A. Finerman: Hip and pelvis. In DeLee, J.C., and D. Drez (eds.): Orthopedic Sports Medicine. Philadelphia, W.B. Saunders Co., 1994.

Hanson, P.G., M. Angevine, and J.H. Juhl: Osteitis pubis in sports activities. Phys. Sportsmed. 6:111–114, 1978.

Hollinshead, W.H., and D.R. Jenkins: Functional Anatomy of the Limbs and the Trunk and Vertebral Column. New York, Churchill Livingstone, 1981.

Kirkaldy-Willis, W.H.: Managing Low Back Pain. New York, Churchill Livingstone, 1983.

Klinefelter, F.W.: Osteitis pubis. Am. J. Roentgenol. 63:368–371, 1950.

Lee, D.G.: Kinematics of the pelvic joints. In Boyling, J.D., and N Palastanga (eds.): Grieve's Modern Manual Therapy: The Vertebral Column, 2nd ed. Edinburgh, Churchill Livingstone, 1994.

Macnab, I.: Backache. Baltimore, Williams & Wilkins, 1977.

McGillivray, D.: The pelvic girdle. In Little, H. (ed.): Rheumatological Physical Examination. Orlando, Grune & Stratton, 1986.

McRae, R.: Clinical Orthopedic Examination. New York, Churchill Livingstone, 1976.

Nicholas, J.A.: Football injuries. In Nicholas, J.A., and E.B. Hershsmann (eds.): The Lower Extremity and Spine in Sports Medicine, vol. 2. St. Louis, C.V. Mosby Co., 1986.

Oldreive, W.L.: A critical review of the literature on tests of the sacroiliac joint. J. Man. Manip. Ther. 3:157–161, 1995.

Osterbauer, P.J., K.F. De Boer, A. Widmaier, E. Petermann, and A.W. Fuhr: Treatment and biomechanical assessment of patients with chronic sacroiliac joint syndrome. J. Manip. Physiol. Ther. 15:82–90, 1993.

Pitkin, H.C., and H.C. Pheasant: Sacrathrogenetic telalgia: A study of referred pain. J. Bone Joint Surg. 18:111–133, 1936.

Porterfield, J.A., and C. DeRosa: The sacroiliac joint. In Gould, J.A. (ed.): Orthopedic and Sports Physical Therapy. St. Louis, C.V. Mosby Co., 1990.

Post, M.: Examination of the thoracic and lumbar spine. In Post, M. (ed.): Physical Examination of the Musculoskeletal System. Chicago, Year Book Medical Publishers, 1987.

Reilly, B.M.: Practical Strategies in Outpatient Medicine. Philadelphia, W.B. Saunders Co., 1984.

Rothman, R.H., and F.A. Simeone: The Spine. Philadelphia, W.B. Saunders Co., 1982.

Rudge, S.R., A.J. Swannell, D.H. Rose, and J.H. Todd: The clinical assessment of sacro-iliac joint involvement in ankylosing spondylitis. Rheumatol. Rehabil. 21:15–20, 1982.

Schwarzer, A.C., C.N. Aprill, and N. Bogduk: The sacroiliac joint in chronic low back pain. Spine 20:31–37, 1995.

Stoddard, A.: Manual of Osteopathic Practice. New York, Harper & Row, 1970.

Stoddard, A.: Manual of Osteopathic Technique. Atlantic Highlands, New Jersey, Humanities Press, 1969.

Toomey, M.: The pelvis, hip, and thigh. In Zuluaga, M., C. Briggs, J. Carlisle, et al. (eds.): Sports Physiotherapy: Applied Science and Practice. Melbourne, Churchill Livingstone, 1995.

Travell, J.G., and D.G. Simons: Myofascial Pain and Dysfunction: The Trigger Point Manual. Baltimore, Williams & Wilkins, 1983.

Wadsworth, C.T., R.P. DeFabio, and D. Johnson: The spine. In Wadsworth, C.T. (ed.): Manual Examination and Treatment of the Spine and Extremities. Baltimore, Williams & Wilkins, 1988.

Walker, J.M.: The sacroiliac joint: A critical review. Phys. Ther. 72:903–916, 1992.

Weissman, B.N.W., and C.B. Sledge: Orthopedic Radiology. Philadelphia, W.B. Saunders Co., 1986.

Wells, P.E.: The examination of the pelvic joints. In Grieve, G.P. (eds.): Modern Manual Therapy of the Vertebral Column. Edinburgh, Churchill Livingstone, 1986.

Wiley, J.J.: Traumatic osteitis pubis: The gracilis syndrome. Am. J. Sports Med. 11:360–363, 1983.

Williams, P.L., and R. Warwick (eds.): Gray's Anatomy, 36th British ed. Edinburgh, Churchill Livingstone, 1980.

Willis, T.A.: Lumbosacral anomalies. J. Bone Joint Surg. Am. 41:935–938, 1959.

Woerman, A.L.: Evaluation and treatment of pelvic girdle dysfunction. In Saunders, H.D., and R.S. Saunders (eds.): Evaluation, Treatment, and Prevention of Musculoskeletal Disorders, Chaska, Minnesota, Saunders Group, 1995.

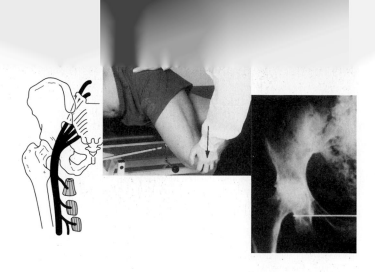

11

Hip

The hip joint is one of the largest and most stable joints in the body. If it is injured or exhibits pathology, the lesion is usually immediately perceptible during walking. Because pain from the hip can be referred to the sacroiliac joint or the lumbar spine, it is imperative, unless there is evidence of direct trauma to the hip, that these joints be examined along with the hip.

Applied Anatomy

The hip joint is a multiaxial ball-and-socket joint that has maximum stability because of the deep insertion of the head of the femur into the acetabulum. It has a strong capsule and very strong muscles that control its actions. The acetabulum is formed by fusion of the ilium, ischium, and pubis and is deepened by a labrum. The acetabulum opens outward, forward, and downward. It is half of a sphere, and the femoral head is two thirds of a sphere. The hip, already a stable joint because of its bony configuration, is supported by three strong liga-

ments: the iliofemoral, the ischiofemoral, and the pubofemoral ligaments (Fig. 11–1). The iliofemoral ligament (**Y** ligament of Bigelow) is considered to be the strongest ligament in the body. It is positioned to prevent excessive extension and plays a significant role in maintaining upright posture at the hip. The ischiofemoral ligament, the weakest of the three, winds tightly on extension, helping to stabilize the hip in extension. The pubofemoral ligament prevents excessive abduction of the femur and limits extension. All three ligaments also limit medial rotation of the femur.

Hip Joint	
Resting position:	30° flexion, 30° abduction, slight lateral rotation
Close packed position:	Extension, medial rotation, and abduction
Capsular pattern:	Flexion, abduction, medial rotation (order may vary)

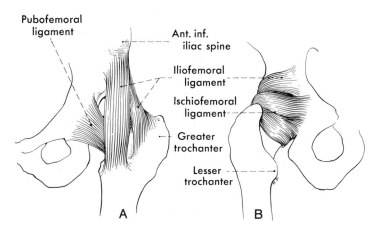

Pubofemoral ligament

Ant. inf. iliac spine

Iliofemoral ligament

Ischiofemoral ligament

Greater trochanter

Lesser trochanter

A   B

Figure 11–1
Ligaments of the hip. (A) Anterior view. (B) Posterior view. (From Jenkins, D.B.: Hollinshead's Functional Anatomy of the Limbs and Back, 6th ed. Philadelphia, W.B. Saunders Co., 1991, p. 230.)

Under low loads, the joint surfaces are incongruous; under heavy loads, they become congruous, providing maximum surface contact. The maximum contact brings the load per unit area down to a tolerable level.

Forces on the Hip

Standing:	0.3 times the body weight
Standing on one limb:	2.4 to 2.6 times the body weight
Walking:	1.3 to 5.8 times the body weight
Walking up stairs:	3 times the body weight
Running:	4.5+ times the body weight

Patient History

In addition to the questions listed under Patient History in Chapter 1, the examiner should obtain the following information from the patient.

1. What is the age of the patient? Different conditions occur in different age groups, and range of motion decreases with age. For example, congenital hip dysplasia is seen in infancy, primarily in girls; Legg-Calvé-Perthes disease is more common in boys 3 to 12 years old; and elderly women are more prone to osteoporotic femoral neck fractures.

2. If trauma was involved, what was the mechanism of injury? Did the patient land on the outside of the hip (e.g., trochanteric bursitis) or land on or hit the knee, jarring the hip (e.g., subluxation, acetabular labral tear)? Was the patient involved in repetitive loading activity (e.g., femoral stress fracture)? A careful determination of the mechanism of injury often leads to a diagnosis of the problem.

3. What are the details of the present pain and other symptoms? Hip pain is felt mainly in the groin and along the front or medial side of the thigh. In this position, the pain may simulate L4 nerve root pain; therefore, the back should also be examined for problems. Hip pain may also be referred to the knee or back and may increase on walking. **Snapping** in and around the hip (coxa saltans) can result from many causes. First, it may be caused by slipping of the iliopsoas tendon over the osseous ridge of the lesser trochanter or anterior acetabulum, or the iliofemoral ligament may be riding over the femoral head.[1,2] Some call this **internal snapping**. It often occurs at approximately 45° of flexion when the hip is moving from flexion to extension. The snap, which may be accompanied by pain or a jerk, is palpated anteriorly.[3] Second, the snapping may be caused by a tight iliotibial band or gluteus maximus tendon riding over the greater tuberosity of the femur.[1,2] This is sometimes called **external snapping**. This snapping or popping occurs during hip flexion and extension, especially if the hip is held in medial rotation, and may be made worse if the trochanteric bursa is inflamed.[3] The third cause of a snapping hip is acetabular labral tears or loose bodies.[2] This is sometimes referred to as **intra-articular snapping**. In this case, the patient complains of a sharp pain into the groin and anterior thigh, especially on pivoting movements. Passively, clicking may be felt and heard when the extended hip is adducted and laterally rotated.[2,3] Each of these conditions may be referred to as **snapping hip syndrome**.

4. Is the condition improving? Worsening? Staying the same? Such a question gives the examiner some idea of the present state of the joint and pathology.

5. Does any type of activity ease the pain or make it worse? For example, trochanteric bursitis often results from abnormal running mechanics with the feet crossing midline (increased adduction), wide pelvis and genu valgum, or running on tracks with no banking.[3]

6. Are there any movements that the patient feels are weak or abnormal? For example, in **piriformis syndrome**, the sciatic nerve may be compressed, the piriformis muscle is tender, and hip abduction and lateral rotation are weak.

7. What is the patient's usual activity or pastime? By listening to the patient, the examiner should be able to tell whether repetitive or sustained positions have contributed to the problem. Also, the examiner can develop some idea of the functional impairment felt by the patient.

Observation

As the patient comes into the assessment area, the gait should be observed. If the hip is affected, the weight is lowered carefully on the affected side and the knee bends slightly to absorb the shock. The length of the step on the affected side is shorter so that weight can be taken off the leg quickly. If the hip is stiff, the entire trunk and affected leg swing forward together. It is also important to watch for "balance" of the pelvis on the hip. If there is an imbalance of the flexors or extensors in the sagittal plane, the forward-backward motion of the trunk is altered to help maintain balance. For example, a bilateral hip flexion contracture causes the lumbar spine to extend to a greater degree (increased lordosis) as a compensating mechanism. Weak extensors cause the patient to move the trunk backward to maintain balance and avoid falling as a result of the unopposed action of the flexors. If the lateral rotators are significantly stronger than the medial rotators, as is normally the case, excessive toe-out can result. In addition, the patellae may have a "frog eyes" appearance (turn-out). Contracture of either of the rotators may lead to a pivoting at the hip during gait.[4] The different types of gait are discussed in greater detail in Chapter 14.

If the patient uses a cane, it should be held in the hand opposite the affected side to negate some of the force of gravity on the affected hip. The use of a cane can decrease the load on the hip as much as 40%.[5]

The patient should be standing and suitably undressed for the examiner to do a proper observation. The following aspects are noted from the front, side, and behind.

1. Posture. The examiner should watch for pelvic obliquity caused by, for example, unequal leg length, muscle contractures, or scoliosis (see Chapter 15 for more details). It must be remembered that injury to iliopsoas may also affect the spine. Therefore, when asking patients to do movements involving these muscles, the examiner must watch the effect on the spine and spinal movement (see Thomas test). Tightness of the iliopsoas can cause deviation of the spine to the same side.[6]

2. Whether the patient can or will stand on both legs. Two bathroom scales may be used to check symmetry of weight bearing.

3. Balance. It is important to check the patient's proprioceptive control in the joints being assessed. This control may be evaluated by asking the patient to balance first on one leg (the good one) and then the other leg— first with the eyes open, and then with the eyes closed. Differences should be noted through comparison. Loss of proprioceptive control is especially obvious when the patient's eyes are closed. The use of the **stork standing test**[4] (Fig. 11–2) has also been advocated for testing proprioception. With both methods, the examiner should watch for a positive Trendelenburg's sign, which would negate the proprioceptive tests.

4. Whether the limb positions are equal and symmetric. The position of the limb may indicate the type of injury. With traumatic posterior hip dislocation, the limb is shortened, adducted, and medially rotated, and the greater trochanter is prominent. With an anterior hip dislocation, the limb is abducted and laterally rotated and may appear cyanotic or swollen owing to pressure in the femoral triangle. With intertrochanteric fractures, the limb is shortened and laterally rotated.

5. Any obvious shortening of a leg. Shortening of the leg may be demonstrated by a spinal scoliosis if the shortening is present in only one lower limb. Shortening may be structural or functional. If the hips are unstable (e.g., bilateral unreduced congenital dislocation of the hip), an increased lumbar lordosis may be evident because the head of the femur usually rests above and

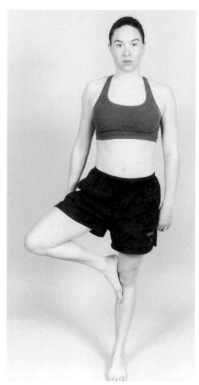

Figure 11–2
Stork standing test.

behind the acetabulum, causing the patient to have an increased lordosis to maintain the center of gravity.

6. Color and texture of the skin.

7. Any scars or sinuses.

8. The patient's willingness to move. If the hip is painful, the patient has an antalgic gait (see Chapter 14) and does not want to move the hip. If the hip is unstable, the patient has more difficulty controlling its movement.

Anterior View

The examiner should note any abnormality of the bony and soft-tissue contours. With many patients, differences in these contours are difficult to detect because of muscle bulk and other soft-tissue deposition around the hips. The examiner must therefore look closely. The same is true for swelling. Swelling in the hip joint itself is virtually impossible to detect by observation, and swelling resulting from a psoas or trochanteric bursitis can easily be missed if the examiner is not carefully observant.

Lateral View

While the patient is viewed from the side, the contour of the buttock should be observed for any abnormality (gluteus maximus atrophy or atonia). In addition, a hip flexion deformity is best observed from this position.

The examiner should take the time to compare the two sides and note any subtle differences.

Posterior View

The position of the hip and the effect, if any, of this position on the spine should be noted. For example, a hip flexion contracture may lead to an increased lumbar lordosis. Any differences in bony and soft-tissue contours should again be noted.

Examination

When doing an examination of the hip, the examiner must keep in mind that pain may be referred to the hip from the sacroiliac joints or the lumbar spine, and vice versa. Therefore, the examination may be an extensive one. If there is any doubt as to the location of the lesion, an assessment of the lumbar spine and sacroiliac joints should be performed. It is only through a careful examination of the three areas that the examiner can discern the location of the lesion.

As with any examination, the examiner should compare one side of the body with the other, noting any differences. This comparison is necessary because of the individual differences among normal people.

Active Movements

The active movements (Fig. 11–3) are done in such a way that the most painful ones are done last. To keep movement of the patient to a minimum, some movements are tested with the patient in the supine position, and others are tested using the prone position. For ease of description, the movements are described together. The examiner should follow the order as stated in the précis at the end of the chapter when examining the patient. If the history has indicated that repetitive move-

---

Active Movements of the Hip

- Flexion (110 to 120°)
- Extension (10 to 15°)
- Abduction (30 to 50°)
- Adduction (30°)
- Lateral rotation (40 to 60°)
- Medial rotation (30 to 40°)
- Sustained postures (if necessary)
- Repetitive movements (if necessary)
- Combined movements (if necessary)

---

ments, sustained postures, or combined movements have caused symptoms, the examiner should ensure that these movements are tested as well. For example, sustained extension of the hip may provoke gluteal pain in the presence of claudication in the common or internal iliac artery.[7]

Flexion of the hip normally ranges from 110 to 120° with the knee flexed. The patient's knee is flexed during the test to prevent limitation of movement caused by hamstring tightness.

Extension of the hip normally ranges from 0 to 15°. The patient is in the prone position, and the examiner must ensure that only hip movement is occurring. Patients often have a tendency to extend the lumbar spine, giving the appearance of increased hip extension. This lumbar extension should not be allowed to occur.

Hip abduction normally ranges from 30 to 50° and is tested with the patient in the supine position. Before asking the patient to do the abduction or adduction movement, the examiner should ensure that the patient's pelvis is "balanced," with the anterior superior iliac spines (ASISs) level and the legs perpendicular to a line joining the two ASISs. The patient is then asked to abduct one leg at a time. Abduction is stopped when the pelvis begins to move. Pelvic motion is detected by palpation of the ASIS and by telling the patient to stop the movement as soon as the ASIS on either side starts to move. When the patient abducts the leg, the opposite ASIS moves first; with an **adduction contracture**, this occurs earlier in the range of movement.

Hip adduction is normally 30° and is measured from the same starting position as abduction. The patient is asked to adduct one leg over the other leg while the examiner ensures that the pelvis does not move. An alternative method is for the patient to flex the opposite hip and hold the limb in flexion with the arms; the patient then adducts the test leg under the other leg. This method is useful only for thin patients. When the patient adducts the leg, the ASIS on the same side moves first. This movement occurs earlier in the range of motion if there is an **abduction contracture**. Adduction may also be measured by asking the patient to abduct one leg and leave it abducted; the other leg is then tested for the amount of adduction present. The advantage of this method is that the test leg does not have to be flexed to clear the other leg before doing the adduction movement.

Rotation movements may be performed with the patient supine or prone. Medial rotation normally ranges from 30 to 40°, and lateral rotation from 40 to 60°. In the supine position, the patient simply rotates the straight leg on a balanced pelvis. Turning the foot or leg outward tests lateral rotation; turning the foot or leg inward tests medial rotation. In another supine test (see

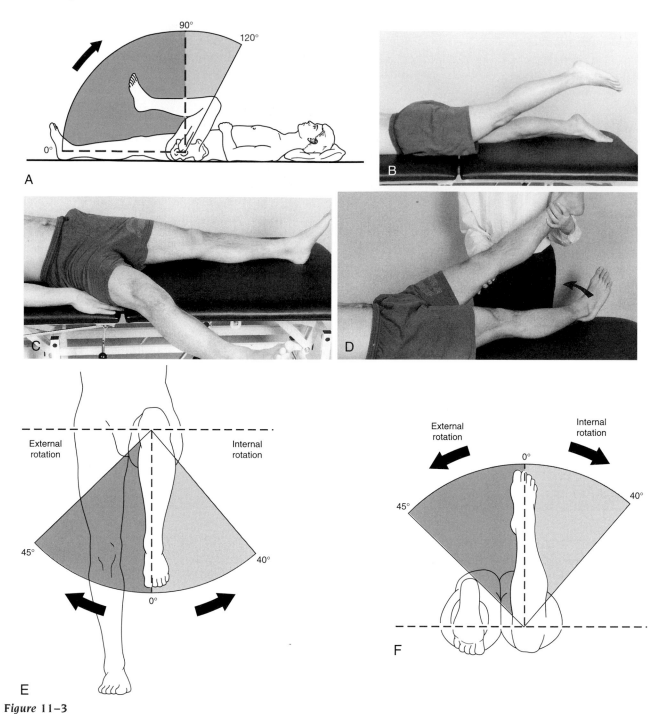

Figure 11–3

Active movements of the hip. (A) Flexion. (B) Extension. (C) Abduction. (D) Adduction. (E) Rotation in the supine position. (F) Rotation in the prone position. (A, E, and F redrawn from Beetham, W.P., H.F. Polley, C.H. Slocumb, and W.F. Weaver: Physical Examination of the Joints. Philadelphia, W.B. Saunders Co., 1965, pp. 134, 137, and 138, respectively.)

Fig. 11–3E), the patient is asked to flex both the hip and knee to 90°. When using this method, it must be recognized that having the patient rotate the leg outward tests medial rotation, whereas having the patient rotate the leg inward tests lateral rotation. With the patient prone, the pelvis is balanced by aligning the legs at right angles to a line joining the posterior superior iliac spines (PSISs). The patient then flexes the knee to 90°. Again, medial rotation is being tested when the leg is rotated outward, and lateral rotation is being tested when the leg is rotated inward (see Fig. 11–3F). Usually, one of these last two methods is used to measure hip rotation, because it is easier to measure the angle when performing the test.

Passive Movements

If the range of movement was not full and the examiner was unable to test end feel during the active movements, passive movements should be performed to determine the end feel and passive range of motion. The passive movements are the same as the active movements. All the movements except extension can be tested with the patient in the supine lying position.

The capsular pattern of the hip is flexion, abduction, and medial rotation. These movements are always the ones most limited in a capsular pattern, although the order of restriction may vary. For example, medial rotation may be most limited, followed by flexion and abduction. The hip joint is the only joint to exhibit this altered pattern of the same movements.

Passive Movements of the Hip and Normal End Feel

- Flexion (tissue approximation or tissue stretch)
- Extension (tissue stretch)
- Abduction (tissue stretch)
- Adduction (tissue approximation or tissue stretch)
- Medial rotation (tissue stretch)
- Lateral rotation (tissue stretch)

Intra-abdominal inflammation in the lower pelvis, as in the case of an abscess, may cause pain on passive medial and lateral rotation of the hip when the patient is supine with the hip and knee at 90°.

The pelvis should not move during hip movements. Groin discomfort and a limited range of motion on me-

dial rotation are good indications of hip problems. Passive hip flexion, adduction, and medial rotation, if painful, may indicate acetabular rim problems or labral tears, especially if clicking and pain into the groin is elicited.[8]

Resisted Isometric Movements

The resisted isometric movements are performed with the patient in the supine position (Fig. 11–4). Because the hip muscles are very strong, the examiner should position the patient's hip properly and say to the patient, "Don't let me move your hip," to ensure that the movement is isometric. By carefully noting which movements cause pain or show weakness when the tests are done isometrically, the examiner should be able to determine which muscle, if any, is at fault (Table 11–1). For example, the gluteus maximus is the only muscle that is involved in all of the following movements: extension, adduction, and lateral rotation. Therefore, if pain resulted from only these three movements, the examiner would suspect the gluteus maximus muscle. As with active movements, the most painful movements are performed last.

Resisted Isometric Movements of the Hip

- Flexion of the hip
- Extension of the hip
- Abduction of the hip
- Adduction of the hip
- Medial rotation of the hip
- Lateral rotation of the hip
- Flexion of the knee
- Extension of the knee

Resisted isometric flexion and extension of the knee must be performed, because there are two joint muscles (hamstrings and rectus femoris) that act over the knee as well as the hip. If the history has indicated that concentric, eccentric, or econcentric movement causes symptoms, these movements should also be tested, but only after the isometric tests have been completed. The examiner must be aware that intra-abdominal inflammation in the area of the psoas muscle may cause pain on resisted hip flexion. Intra-abdominal inflammation may also result in a rigid abdominal wall. It has been reported that hip flexors and hip extensors are almost equal in strength[9] and that the adductors are 2.5 times as strong as the abductors.[10] These ratios may vary depending on the speed tested.

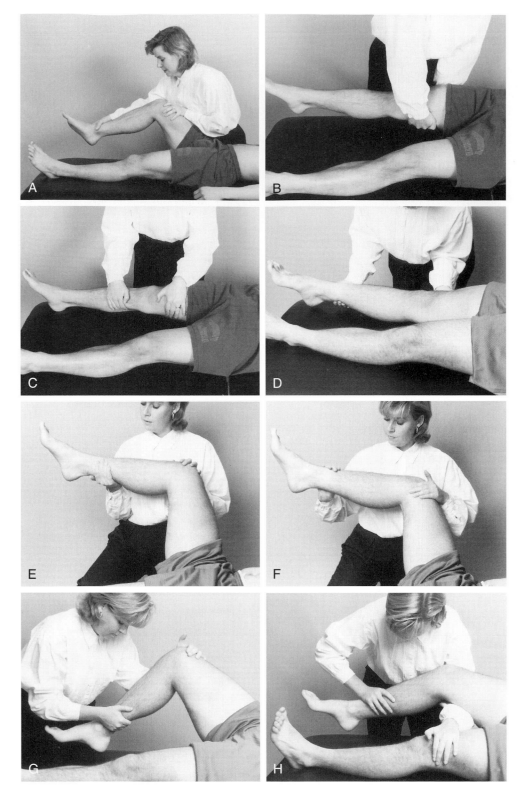

Figure 11–4
Resisted isometric movements around the hip. (A) Flexion. (B) Extension. (C) Adduction.
(D) Abduction. (E) Medial rotation. (F) Lateral rotation. (G) Knee flexion. (H) Knee extension.

Table 11-1
Muscles of the Hip: Their Actions, Innervation, and Nerve Root Deviation

Action	Muscle Acting	Innervation	Nerve Root Deviation
Flexion of hip	1. Psoas	L1–L3	L1–L3
	2. Iliacus	Femoral	L2–L3
	3. Rectus femoris	Femoral	L2–L4
	4. Sartorius	Femoral	L2–L3
	5. Pectineus	Femoral	L2–L3
	6. Adductor longus	Obturator	L2–L4
	7. Adductor brevis	Obturator	L2–L3, L5
	8. Gracilis	Obturator	L2–L3
Extension of hip	1. Biceps femoris	Sciatic	L5, S1–S2
	2. Semimembranosus	Sciatic	L5, S1–S2
	3. Semitendinosus	Sciatic	L5, S1–S2
	4. Gluteus maximus	Inferior gluteal	L5, S1–S2
	5. Gluteus medius (posterior part)	Superior gluteal	L5, S1
	6. Adductor magnus (ischiocondylar part)	Sciatic	L2–L4
Abduction of hip	1. Tensor fasciae latae	Superior gluteal	L4–L5
	2. Gluteus minimus	Superior gluteal	L5, S1
	3. Gluteus medius	Superior gluteal	L5, S1
	4. Gluteus maximus	Inferior gluteal	L5, S1–S2
	5. Sartorius	Femoral	L2–L3
Adduction of hip	1. Adductor longus	Obturator	L2–L4
	2. Adductor brevis	Obturator	L2–L4
	3. Adductor magnus (ischiofemoral part)	Obturator	L2–L4
	4. Gracilis	Obturator	L2–L3
	5. Pectineus	Femoral	L2–L3
Medial rotation of hip IR	1. Adductor longus	Obturator	L2–L4
	2. Adductor brevis	Obturator	L2–L4
	3. Adductor magnus	Obturator and sciatic	L2–L4
	4. Gluteus medius (anterior part)	Superior gluteal	L5, S1
	5. Gluteus minimus (anterior part)	Superior gluteal	L5, S1
	6. Tensor fasciae latae	Superior gluteal	L4–L5
	7. Pectineus	Femoral	L2–L3
	8. Gracilis	Obturator	L2–L3
Lateral rotation of hip ER	1. Gluteus maximus	Inferior gluteal	L5, S1–S2
	2. Obturator internus	N. to obturator internus	L5, S1
	3. Obturator externus	Obturator	L3–L4
	4. Quadratus femoris	N. to quadratus femoris	L5, S1
	5. Piriformis	L5, S1–S2	L5, S1–S2
	6. Gemellus superior	N. to obturator internus	L5, S1
	7. Gemellus inferior	N. to quadratus femoris	L5, S1
	8. Sartorius	Femoral	L2–L3
	9. Gluteus medius (posterior part)	Superior gluteal	L5, S1

Functional Assessment

Hip motion is necessary for more activities than just ambulation. In fact, more hip range of motion is required for daily living activities than is required for gait; activities such as shoe tying, sitting, getting up from a chair, and picking things up from the floor all require a greater range of motion. Table 11–2 illustrates the ranges of motion necessary for various activities. Ideally, the patient should have functional ranges of 120° of flexion, 20° of abduction, and 20° of lateral rotation.

There are several numerical rating scales with which to rate hip function. These rating methods are based primarily on pain, mobility, and gait. Tables 11–3 through 11–5 and Figures 11–5 and 11–6 illustrate three different rating scales. D'Aubigné and Postel[11] (Tables 11–3

Text continued on page 471

Table 11–2
Range of Motion Necessary at the Hip for Selected Activities

Activity	Average Range of Motion Necessary
Shoe tying	120° of flexion
Sitting (average seat height)	112° of flexion
Stooping	125° of flexion
Squatting	115° of flexion/20° of abduction/20° of medial rotation
Ascending stairs (average stair height)	67° of flexion
Descending stairs (average stair height)	36° of flexion
Putting foot on opposite thigh	120° of flexion/20° of abduction/20° of lateral rotation
Putting on trousers	90° of flexion

Table 11–3
Method of Grading Functional Value of Hip*

Grade	Pain	Mobility	Ability to Walk
0	Pain is intense and permanent	Ankylosis with bad position of the hip	None
1	Pain is severe, even at night	No movement; pain or slight deformity	Only with crutches
2	Pain is severe when walking; prevents any activity	Flexion less than 40°	Only with canes
3	Pain is tolerable with limited activity	Flexion between 40° and 60°	With one cane, for less than 1 hour; very difficult without a cane
4	Pain is mild when walking; it disappears with rest	Flexion between 60° and 80°; patient can reach own foot	A long time with a cane; a short time without cane and with limp
5	Pain is mild and inconstant; normal activity	Flexion between 80° and 90°; abduction at least 15°	Without cane but with slight limp
6	No pain	Flexion more than 90°; abduction to 30°	Normal

* Values used in conjunction with Table 11–4.

From D'Aubigné, R.M., and M. Postel: Functional results of hip arthroplasty with acrylic prosthesis. J. Bone Joint Surg. Am. 36:459, 1954.

Table 11–4
D'Aubigné and Postel Scale for Functional Grading of the Hip

Pain (P)	Ability to Walk (W)	Mobility Normal or Nearly Normal	Grade
		Very Good	P + W = 11 or 12
6	6	Walk without cane, with no pain and no limp	
6	5	Walk without cane, with no pain but slight limp	
5	6	Walk without cane, with no limp but slight pain when starting	
		Good	P + W = 10
5	5	Walk without cane, with slight pain and slight limp	
4	6	Walk without cane, with pain but no limp	
6	4*	Walk without cane, without pain; a cane used to go outdoors	
		Medium	P + W = 9
5	4	Slight pain; a cane is used outdoors	
4	5	Pain after walking some minutes; no cane is used, but there is a slight limp	
6	3†	No pain; a cane is used all the time	
		Fair	P + W = 8
5	3	Slight pain; a cane is used all the time	
4	4	Pain after walking; a cane is used outdoors	
≤3	≤3	*Poor*	P + W = 7 or less

* If the mobility is reduced to 4, the result is classified one grade lower.

† If the mobility is reduced to 3 or less, the result is classified two grades lower.

Adapted from D'Aubigné, R.M., and M. Postel: Functional results of hip arthroplasty with acrylic prosthesis. J. Bone Joint Surg. Am. 36:460, 1954.

Table 11–5

Method of Evaluating Improvement Brought About by Operation in Problems of the Hip (Relative Result)

	Preoperative Grading	Postoperative Grading	Difference	Improvement
Pain	3	5	$2 \times 2 = 4$	
Mobility	2	5	$3 = 3$	$= 9$
Ability to walk	3	4	$1 \times 2 = 2$	

Very great improvement = 12 or more, great improvement = 7 to 11, fair improvement = 3 to 7, failure = less than 3.

From D'Aubigné, R.M., and M. Postel: Functional results of hip arthroplasty with acrylic prosthesis. J. Bone Joint Surg. Am. 36:461, 1954.

Harris Hip Function Scale

(Circle one in each group)

Pain (44 points maximum)

None/ignores	44
Slight, occasional, no compromise in activity	40
Mild, no effect on ordinary activity, pain after unusual activity, uses aspirin	30
Moderate, tolerable, makes concessions, occasional codeine	20
Marked, serious limitations	10
Totally disabled	0

Function (47 points maximum)

Gait (walking maximum distance) (33 points maximum)

1. Limp:
   - None — 11
   - Slight — 8
   - Moderate — 5
   - Unable to walk — 0
2. Support:
   - None — 11
   - Cane, long walks — 7
   - Cane, full time — 5
   - Crutch — 4
   - Two canes — 2
   - Two crutches — 0
   - Unable to walk — 0
3. Distance walked:
   - Unlimited — 11
   - Six blocks — 8
   - Two to three blocks — 5
   - Indoors only — 2
   - Bed and chair — 0

Functional Activities (14 points maximum)

1. Stairs:
   - Normally — 4
   - Normally with banister — 2
   - Any method — 1
   - Not able — 0
2. Socks and tie shoes:
   - With ease — 4
   - With difficulty — 2
   - Unable — 0
3. Sitting:
   - Any chair, 1 hour — 5
   - High chair, ½ hour — 3
   - Unable to sit ½ hour any chair — 0
4. Enter public transport
   - Able to use public transportation — 1
   - Not able to use public transportation — 0

Absence of Deformity (requires all four) (4 points maximum)

1. Fixed adduction <10° — 4
2. Fixed internal rotation in extension <10° — 0
3. Leg length discrepancy less than 1¼"
4. Pelvic flexion contracture <30°

Range of Motion (5 points maximum)

Instructions

Record 10° of fixed adduction as "—10° abduction, adduction to 10°"

Similarly, 10° of fixed external rotation as "—10° internal rotation, external rotation to 10°"

Similarly, 10° of fixed external rotation with 10° further external rotation as "—10° internal rotation, external rotation to 20°"

Permanent flexion
(1) _____ °

	Range	Index Factor	Index Value*
A. Flexion to	_____ °		
(0–45°)		1.0	
(45–90°)		0.6	
(90–120°)		0.3	
(120–140°)	_____ °	0.0	
B. Abduction to			
(0–15°)		0.8	
(15–30°)		0.3	
(30–60°)		0.0	
C. Adduction to			
(0–15°)	_____ °	0.2	
(15–60°)		0.0	
D. External rotation in extension to	_____ °		
(0–30°)		0.4	
(30–60°)		0.0	
E. Internal rotation in extension to	_____ °		
(0–60°)		0.0	

*Index Value = Range × Index Factor

Total index value (A + B + C + D + E) _____

Total range of motion points
(multiply total index value × 0.05) _____

Pain points:	_____
Function points:	_____
Absence of Deformity points:	_____
Range of Motion points:	_____
Total points (100 points maximum)	_____

Comments:

Figure 11–5

Harris hip function scale. (Modified from Harris, W.H.: Traumatic arthritis of the hip after dislocation and acetabular fractures: Treatment by mold arthroplasty. An end result study using a new method of result evaluation. J. Bone Joint Surg. Am. 51:737–755, 1969.)

Iowa Functional Hip Evaluation

Chart 1	Chart 2

Chart 1

Date _____

Name _____   Age _____

100-Point Scale for Hip Evaluation

Total points _____

Function (35 points)
Does most of housework or job that
  requires moving about 5
Dresses unaided (includes tying shoes and
  putting on socks) 5
Walks enough to be independent 5
Sits with difficulty at table or toilet 4
Picks up objects from floor by squatting 3
Bathes without help 3
Negotiates stairs foot over foot......................... 3
Carries objects comparable to suitcase................... 2
Gets into car or public conveyance unaided and rides
  comfortably 2
Drives a car 1

                     _____

Freedom From Pain (35 points) (circle 1 only)
No pain. 35
Pain only with fatigue 30
Pain only with weight-bearing.......................... 20
Pain at rest but not with weight-bearing................. 15
Pain sitting or in bed 10
Continuous pain. 0

                     _____

Gait (10 points) (circle 1 only)
No limp; no support 10
No limp using cane.................................... 8
Abductor limp 8
Short leg limp. 8
Needs two canes 6
Needs two crutches.................................... 4
Cannot walk 0

                     ____

Absence of Deformity (10 points)
No fixed flexion over 30° 3
No fixed adduction over 10°............................ 3
No fixed rotation over 10° 2
Not over 1″ shortening (ASIS-MM)* 2

                     ____

Range of Motion (10 points)
Flexion-extension (normal 140°) .... ____°
Abduction-adduction (normal 80°) .... ____°
External-internal rotation (normal 80°) .... ____°
       Total degrees. .... ____°
       Points (1 point/30°) .... ____°

                     ____

Muscle Strength (no points)
Straight leg raising:
  Less than gravity _____Gravity _____
  Gravity + resistance _____
Abduction:
  Less than gravity _____Gravity _____
  Gravity + resistance _____
Extension:
  Less than gravity _____Gravity _____
  Gravity + resistance _____
        TOTAL (100 points maximum) _____

Chart 2

Name _____ Diagnosis _____
Age _____ Sex _____ Date of operation _____
Date of follow-up _____
Previous surgery: Date _____ Type _____
Subsequent surgery: Date _____ Type _____

Pain   40%
  None. 40
  Pain with fatigue 35
  Pain with weight-bearing:
    Mild. 30
    Moderate 20
    Severe. 10
  Persistence with non–weight-bearing. ...... 10 (less than above)
  Continuous pain. 0

Ability to Function   30%
  Work and household duties:
    Full day, usual occupation 10
    Modified work or duties 6
    Severe restriction of work or duties 2

  Walking tolerances:
    Long distances 10
    Short distances. 6
    Two blocks or less. 1

  Self-reliance:
    Dresses self unaided 3
    Help with shoes and socks 2
    Sit at table and toilet 3

  Stairs:
    Normal 2
    One at a time 1
    Gets into car or public conveyance without
      difficulty. 2

Gait   15%
  No limp, no support 15
  No limp, with cane 12
  Limp, mild, without cane 12
  Limp, mild, with cane 9
  Limp, moderate, without cane or crutch 9
  Limp, moderate, with cane or crutch 6
  Limp, severe, without cane or crutch. 3
  Limp, severe, with cane or crutch. 2
  Two canes or crutches 1

Anatomic Assessment   15%
A. Motion:
  Flexion—up to 80° in range 0–100° × 0.1 ... 8
  Abduction—up to 20° in range 0–30° × 0.1 .. 2
B. Shortening:
  None—½″. 3
  ½″–1″. 2
  1″–2″. 1
C. Trendelenburg—absent 2

                     100%

Figure 11–6

Iowa functional hip evaluation form. ASIS–MM = anterior superior iliac spine to medial malleolus.
(Modified from Larson, C.B.: Rating scale for hip disabilities. Clin. Orthop. 31:86, 1963.)

through 11–5) developed one of the first hip rating scales based on pain, mobility, and ability to walk.[12] The Harris hip function scale[13] (see Fig. 11–5) is useful for rating hips before and after surgery. This scale is most often used because it emphasizes pain and function. The Iowa scale (see Fig. 11–6) provides a single rating value. The Mayo hip score[14] for hip arthroplasty makes use of greater patient (functional) input and radiographic input (to predict long-term results). This score correlates well with the Harris scale.[12, 14] Johanson and colleagues[15] developed a numerical scale that is related to what patients are able to do functionally after total hip replacement. Its value comes from its focus on the outcome from the patient's perspective (Fig. 11–7). As Burton and coworkers[16] pointed out, the notion of expectations is more important than the notion of success. Table 11–6 gives a functional strength and endurance testing scheme for the hip.

If the patient is able to perform normal active movements with little difficulty, the examiner may use a series of functional tests to determine whether increased inten-

---

Functional Tests of the Hip

- Squatting
- Going up and down stairs one at a time
- Crossing the legs so that the ankle of one foot rests on the knee of the opposite leg
- Going up and down stairs two or more at a time
- Running straight ahead
- Running and decelerating
- Running and twisting
- One-legged hop (time, distance, crossover)
- Jumping

---

sity of activity produces pain or other symptoms. These tests must be geared to the individual patient. Older persons should not be expected to perform the last six activities unless they have been doing these movements or similar ones in the recent past.

Table 11–6
Functional Testing of the Hip

Starting Position	Action	Functional Test
Standing	Lift foot onto 20-cm step and return (hip flexion-extension)	5 to 6 Repetitions: Functional 3 to 4 Repetitions: Functionally fair 1 to 2 Repetitions: Functionally poor 0 Repetitions: Nonfunctional
Standing	Sit in chair and return to standing (hip extension-flexion)	5 to 6 Repetitions: Functional 3 to 4 Repetitions: Functionally fair 1 to 2 Repetitions: Functionally poor 0 Repetitions: Nonfunctional
Standing	Lift leg to balance on one leg keeping pelvis straight (hip abduction)	Hold 1 to 1.5 minutes: Functional Hold 30 to 59 seconds: Functionally fair Hold 1 to 29 seconds: Functionally poor Cannot hold: Nonfunctional
Standing	Walk sideways 6 m (hip adduction/abduction)	6 to 8 m one way: Functional 3 to 6 m one way: Functionally fair 1 to 3 m one way: Functionally poor 0 m: Nonfunctional
Standing	Test leg off floor (patient may hold onto something for balance) medially rotate non–weight-bearing hip	10 to 12 Repetitions: Functional 5 to 9 Repetitions: Functionally fair 1 to 4 Repetitions: Functionally poor 0 Repetitions: Nonfunctional
Standing	Test leg off floor (patient may hold onto something for balance) laterally rotate non–weight-bearing hip	10 to 12 Repetitions: Functional 5 to 9 Repetitions: Functionally fair 1 to 4 Repetitions: Functionally poor 0 Repetitions: Nonfunctional

Data from Palmer, M.L., and M. Epler: Clinical Assessment Procedures in Physical Therapy. Philadelphia, J.B. Lippincott, 1990, pp. 251–254.

A SELF-ADMINISTERED HIP-RATING QUESTIONNAIRE

Which hip is affected by arthritis? (circle one)

Left   Right   Both

Please answer the following questions about the hip(s) you have just indicated.

1. Considering all of the ways that your hip arthritis affects you, mark (X) on the scale for how well you are doing.

0	25	50	75	100
very well	well	fair	poor	very poor

Circle one response for each question (The score here is determined by subtraction of the number marked from 100, with the number being interpolated, if necessary, if the mark is between printed numbers. The result is divided by 4, and the answer then rounded off to the nearest integer. The maximum is 25 points.)

2. During the past month, how would you describe the usual arthritis pain in your hip? (maximum, 10 points)
   a. Very severe (2 points)
   b. Severe (4 points)
   c. Moderate (6 points)
   d. Mild (8 points)
   e. None (10 points)

3. During the past month, how often have you had to take medication for your arthritis? (maximum, 5 points)
   a. Always (1 point)
   b. Very often (2 points)
   c. Fairly often (3 points)
   d. Sometimes (4 points)
   e. Never (5 points)

4. During the past month, how often have you had severe arthritis pain in your hip? (maximum, 5 points)
   a. Every day (1 point)
   b. Several days per week (2 points)
   c. One day per week (3 points)
   d. One day per month (4 points)
   e. Never (5 points)

5. How often have you had hip arthritis pain at rest, either sitting or lying down? (maximum, 5 points)
   a. Every day (1 point)
   b. Several days per week (2 points)
   c. One day per week (3 points)
   d. One day per month (4 points)
   e. Never (5 points)

6. How far can you walk without resting because of your hip arthritis pain? (maximum, 15 points)
   a. Unable to walk (3 points)
   b. Less than one city block (6 points)
   c. 1 to <10 city blocks (9 points)
   d. 10 to 20 city blocks (12 points)
   e. Unlimited (15 points)

7. How much assistance do you need for walking? (maximum, 10 points)
   a. Unable to walk (1 point)
   b. Walk only with someone's help (2 points)
   c. Two crutches or walker every day (3 points)
   d. Two crutches or walker several days per week (4 points)
   e. Two crutches or walker once per week or less (5 points)
   f. Cane or one crutch every day (6 points)
   g. Cane or one crutch several days per week (7 points)
   h. Cane or one crutch once per week (8 points)
   i. Cane or one crutch once per month (9 points)
   j. No assistance (10 points)

8. How much difficulty do you have going up or down one flight of stairs because of your hip arthritis? (maximum, 5 points)
   a. Unable (1 point)
   b. Require someone's assistance (2 points)
   c. Require crutch or cane (3 points)
   d. Require banister (4 points)
   e. No difficulty (5 points)

9. How much difficulty do you have putting on your shoes and socks because of your hip arthritis? (maximum, 5 points)
   a. Unable (1 point)
   b. Require someone's assistance (2 points)
   c. Require long shoehorn and reacher (3 points)
   d. Some difficulty, but no devices required (4 points)
   e. No difficulty (5 points)

10. Are you able to use public transportation? (maximum, 3 points)
    a. No, because of my hip arthritis (1 point)
    b. No, for some other reason (2 points)
    c. Yes (3 points)

11. When you bathe—either a sponge bath or in a tub or shower—how much help do you need? (maximum, 3 points)
    a. No help at all (3 points)
    b. Help with bathing one part of my body, like back or leg (2 points)
    c. Help with bathing more than one part of my body (1 point)

12. If you had the necessary transportation, under what circumstances could you go shopping for groceries or clothes? (maximum, 3 points)
    a. Without help (taking care of all shopping needs myself) (3 points)
    b. With some help (need someone to go with me to help on all shopping trips) (2 points)
    c. Completely unable to do any shopping (1 point)

13. If you had household tools and appliances (vacuum, mops, and so on) could you do your own housework? (maximum, 3 points)
    a. Without help (can clean floors, windows, refrigerator, and so on) (3 points)
    b. With some help (can do light housework, but need help with some heavy work) (2 points)
    c. Completely unable to do any housework (1 point)

14. How well are you able to move around? (maximum, 3 points)
    a. Able to get in and out of bed or chair without the help of another person (3 points)
    b. Need the help of another person to get in and out of bed or chair (2 points)
    c. Not able to get out of bed (1 point)

This is the end of the Hip-Rating Questionnaire. Thank you for your cooperation

Figure 11–7

A self-administered hip-rating questionnaire. The maximum score is 100 points and the minimum is 16 points. The point values of the answers are not shown in the questionnaire that is administered to patients. (From Johanson, N.A., M.E. Charlson, T.P. Szatrowski, and C.S. Ranawat: A self-administered hip-rating questionnaire for the assessment of outcome after total hip replacement. J. Bone Joint Surg. Am. 74:589, 1992.)

Special Tests

Only those tests that the examiner believes are necessary should be performed when assessing the hip. Most tests are done primarily to confirm a diagnosis or to determine pathology. As with all special tests, if the test is positive, it is highly suggestive that the problem exists, but if it is negative, it does not necessarily rule out the problem. Therefore, special tests should not be taken in isolation but should be used to support the history, observation, and clinical examination.

Special Tests Commonly Performed on the Hip

- Patrick (Faber) test
- Trendelenburg's sign
- Leg length tests
- Thomas test
- Rectus femoris test
- Ober's test
- Hamstring contracture test
- Sign of the buttock (straight leg raising)

Tests for Hip Pathology

Patrick's Test (Faber or Figure-Four Test). The patient lies supine, and the examiner places the patient's test leg so that the foot of the test leg is on top of the knee of the opposite leg (Fig. 11–8). The examiner then slowly lowers the test leg in abduction toward the examining table. A negative test is indicated by the test leg's falling to the table or at least being parallel with the opposite leg. A positive test is indicated by the test leg's remaining above the opposite straight leg. If positive, the test indicates that the hip joint may be affected, there may be iliopsoas spasm, or the sacroiliac joint may be affected. **Faber** (which stands for **f**lexion, **ab**duction, and **e**xternal **r**otation) is the position of the hip when the patient begins the test. The test is also sometimes referred to as Jansen's test.[17]

Trendelenburg's Sign. This test assesses the stability of the hip and the ability of the hip abductors to stabilize the pelvis on the femur. The patient is asked to stand on one lower limb. Normally, the pelvis on the opposite side should rise; this finding indicates a negative test (Fig. 11–9). If the pelvis on the opposite side drops when the patient stands on the affected leg, a positive test is indicated. The test should always be performed on the normal side first so that the patient understands what to do. If the pelvis drops on the opposite side, it indicates a weak gluteus medius or an unstable hip on the affected side (e.g., as a result of hip dislocation).

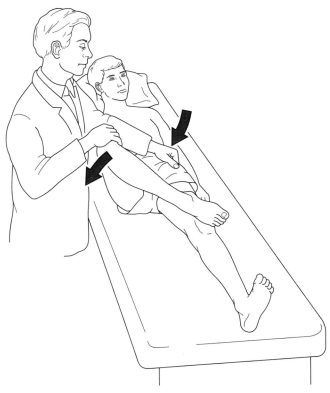

Figure 11–8
Patrick's test (Faber or figure-4 test) for the detection of limitation of motion in the hip. (Redrawn from Beetham, W.P., H.F. Polley, C.H. Slocumb, and W.F. Weaver: Physical Examination of the Joints. Philadelphia: W.B. Saunders Co., 1965, p. 139.)

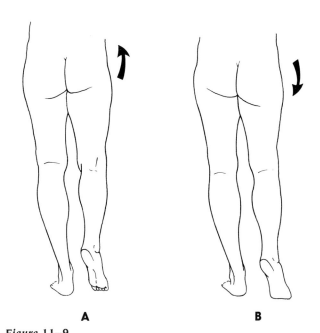

A   **B**

Figure 11–9
Trendelenburg's sign. (A) Negative test. (B) Positive test.

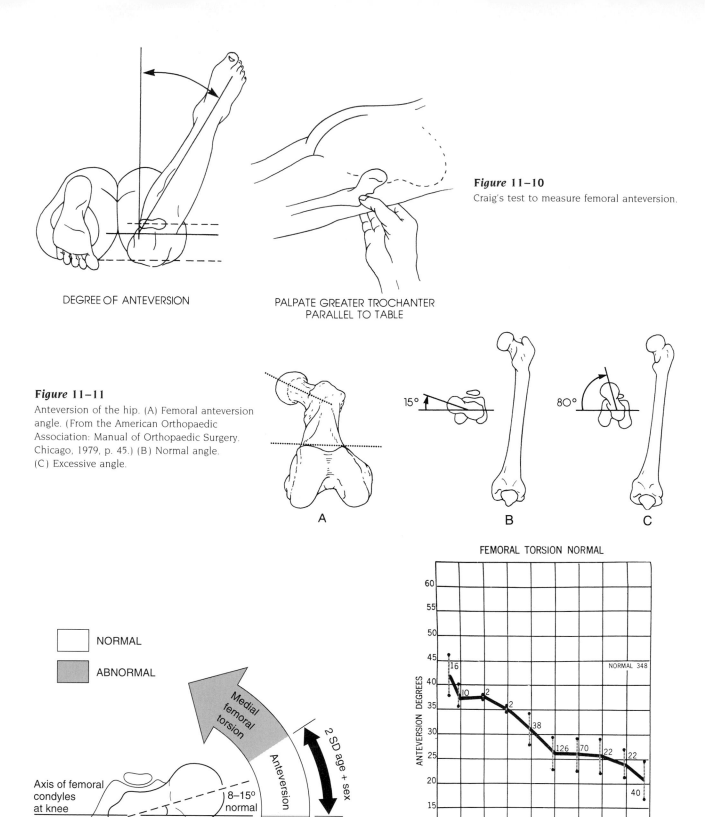

Figure 11–10

Craig's test to measure femoral anteversion.

DEGREE OF ANTEVERSION

PALPATE GREATER TROCHANTER
PARALLEL TO TABLE

Figure 11–11

Anteversion of the hip. (A) Femoral anteversion angle. (From the American Orthopaedic Association: Manual of Orthopaedic Surgery. Chicago, 1979, p. 45.) (B) Normal angle. (C) Excessive angle.

A   B   C

FEMORAL TORSION NORMAL

NORMAL

ABNORMAL

Medial femoral torsion

Anteversion

2 SD age + sex

Lateral femoral torsion

Axis of femoral condyles at knee

8–15° normal

Axis of femoral head

Retroversion

Figure 11–12

Axial view of right femur showing approximately normal angle of anteversion and torsional deformity beyond. (Redrawn from Staheli, L.T.: Medial femoral torsion. Orthop. Clin. North Am. 11:40, 1980.)

NORMAL 348

Figure 11–13

The degree of normal femoral torsion in relation to age. Solid lines represent the mean, vertical lines the standard deviation. (From Crane, L.: Femoral torsion and its relation to toeing-in and toeing-out. J. Bone Joint Surg. Am. 41:423, 1959.)

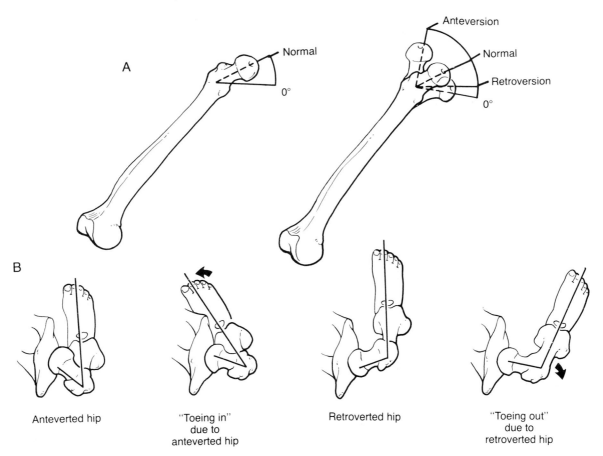

Figure 11–14
Torsion angles of the hip. (A) Positions of femoral neck. (B) Different foot positions with anteversion and retroversion at the hip (coronal views). (Redrawn from Echternach, J. [ed.]: Physical Therapy of the Hip. New York, Churchill Livingstone, 1990, p. 25.)

Craig's Test. Craig's test measures femoral **anteversion** or forward torsion of the femoral neck (Fig. 11–10). Anteversion of the hip is measured by the angle made by the femoral neck with the femoral condyles (Fig. 11–11). It is the degree of forward projection of the femoral neck from the coronal plane of the shaft (Fig. 11–12), and it decreases with age. At birth, the mean angle is approximately 30°; in the adult, the mean angle is 8 to 15° (Fig. 11–13). Increased anteversion leads to squinting patellae and toeing-in (Fig. 11–14). Excessive anteversion is twice as common in girls as in boys. A common clinical finding of excessive anteversion is excessive medial hip rotation (more than 60°) and decreased lateral rotation. In **retroversion,** the plane of the femoral neck rotates backward in relation to the coronal condylar plane (see Fig. 11–14).[18–21]

For Craig's test, the patient lies prone with the knee flexed to 90°. The examiner palpates the posterior aspect of the greater trochanter of the femur. The hip is then passively rotated medially and laterally until the greater trochanter is parallel with the examining table or reaches its most lateral position. The degree of anteversion can then be estimated, based on the angle of the lower leg with the vertical. The test is also called the **Ryder** method for measuring anteversion or retroversion.

Torque Test. The patient lies supine close to the edge of the examining table with the femur of the test leg extended over the edge of the table (Fig. 11–15). The test leg is extended until the pelvis begins to move. The examiner uses one hand to medially rotate the femur to the end of range and the other hand to apply a slow posterolateral pressure along the line of the neck of femur for 20 seconds to stress the capsular ligaments and test the stability of the hip joint.[22]

Stinchfield Test.[23] The patient lies supine and flexes the hip with the knee straight to 30° of hip flexion against

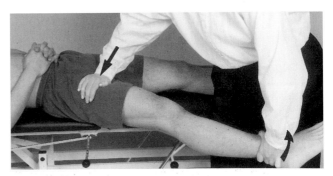

Figure 11–15
Torque test.

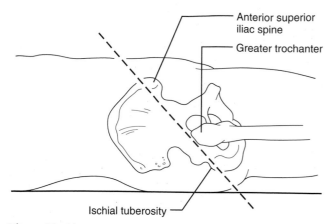

Figure 11–16
Nelaton's line.

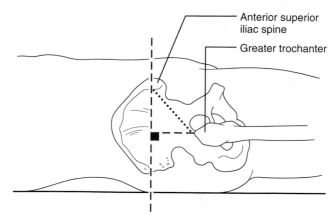

Figure 11–17
Bryant's triangle.

resistance. Hip or groin pain is a positive test for hip pathology. Posterior hip pain or back pain indicates lumbar or sacroiliac pathology. This test stresses the hip, sacroiliac joint, and lumbar spine.

Nelaton's Line. Nelaton's line is an imaginary line drawn from the ischial tuberosity of the pelvis to the ASIS of the pelvis on the same side (Fig. 11–16).[18] If the greater trochanter of the femur is palpated well above the line, it is an indication of a dislocated hip or coxa vara. The two sides should be compared.

Bryant's Triangle. With the patient lying supine, the examiner drops an imaginary perpendicular line from the ASIS of the pelvis to the examining table.[20] A second imaginary line is projected up from the tip of the greater trochanter of the femur to meet the first line at a right

angle (Fig. 11–17). This line is measured, and the two sides are compared. Differences may indicate conditions such as coxa vara or congenital dislocation of the hip. This measurement can be done with radiographs, in which case the lines may be drawn on the radiograph.

Rotational Deformities. Rotational deformities can occur anywhere between the hip and the foot (Table 11–7). Many of these deformities are hereditary. The patient lies supine with the lower limbs straight while the examiner looks at the patellae.[19] If the patellae face in (squinting patellae), it is a possible indication of medial rotation of the femur or the tibia. If the patellae face up, out, and away from each other ("frog eyes" or "grasshopper eyes"), it is a possible indication of lateral rotation of the femur or the tibia. If the tibia is affected, the feet

Table 11–7
Hip Malalignment

Malalignment	Related Posture	Possible Compensating Postures
Excessive anteversion	Toeing-in Subtalar pronation Lateral patellar subluxation Medial tibial torsion Medial femoral torsion	Lateral tibial torsion Lateral rotation at knee Lateral rotation of tibia, femur, and/or pelvis Lumbar rotation on same side
Excessive retroversion	Toeing-out Subtalar supination Lateral tibial torsion Lateral femoral torsion	Medial rotation at knee Medial rotation of tibia, femur, and/or pelvis Lumbar rotation on opposite side
Coxa vara	Pronated subtalar joint Medial rotation of leg Short ipsilateral leg Anterior pelvic rotation	Ipsilateral subtalar supination Contralateral subtalar pronation Ipsilateral plantar flexion Contralateral genu recurvatum Contralateral hip and/or knee flexion Ipsilateral posterior pelvic rotation and ipsilateral lumbar rotation
Coxa valga	Supinated subtalar joint Lateral rotation of leg Long ipsilateral leg Posterior pelvic tilt	Ipsilateral subtalar pronation Contralateral subtalar supination Contralateral plantar flexion Ipsilateral genu recurvatum Ipsilateral hip and/or knee flexion Ipsilateral anterior pelvic rotation and contralateral lumbar rotation

Adapted from Reigger-Krugh, C., and J.J. Keysor: Skeletal malalignments of the lower quarter: Correlated and compensatory motions and postures. J. Orthop. Sports Phys. Ther. 23:166–167, 1996.

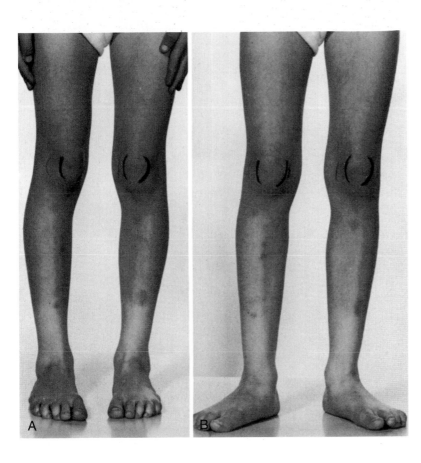

Figure 11–18

Clinical appearance of excessive femoral torsion in a girl. (A) With the knees in full extension and the feet aligned (pointing straight forward), the legs appear bowed and the patellae face inward (squinting patella). (B) On lateral rotation of the hips so that the patellae are facing to the front, the feet and legs point outward and the bowleg appearance is corrected. (From Tachdjian, M.O.: Pediatric Orthopedics. Philadelphia, W.B. Saunders Co., 1990, p. 2802.)

face in ("pigeon toes") for medial rotation and face out more than 10° for excessive lateral rotation of the tibia (Fig. 11–18). Normally, the feet angle out 5 to 10° (**Fick angle**) for better balance.

Pediatric Tests for Hip Pathology

Orthopedic tests are commonly performed in newborns to detect problems, especially congenital dislocation of the hip, which may be amenable to conservative treatment if caught early.[24]

Ortolani's Sign. Ortolani's test can determine whether an infant has a congenital dislocation of the hip (Fig. 11–19A and B).[19] With the infant supine, the examiner flexes the hips and grasps the legs so that the examiner's thumbs are against the insides of the knees and thighs and the fingers are placed along the outsides of the thighs to the buttocks. With gentle traction, the thighs are abducted, and pressure is applied against the greater trochanters of the femora. Resistance to abduction and lateral rotation begins to be felt at approximately 30 to 40°. The examiner may feel a click, clunk, or jerk, which indicates a positive test and that the hip has reduced; in addition, increased abduction of the hip is obtained. The femoral head has slipped over the acetabular ridge into the acetabulum, and normal abduction of 70 to 90° can be obtained.

This test is valid only for the first few weeks after birth and only for dislocated and lax hips, not for disloca-

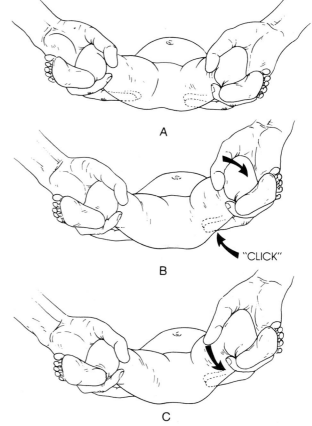

Figure 11–19

Ortolani's sign and Barlow's test. (A) In the newborn, the two hips can be equally flexed, abducted, and laterally rotated without producing a "click." (B) Ortolani's sign or first part of Barlow's test. (C) Second part of Barlow's test.

tions that are difficult to reduce. The examiner should take care to feel the quality of the click. Soft clicks may occur without dislocation and are thought to be caused by the iliofemoral ligament's clicking over the anterior surface of the head of the femur as it is laterally rotated. Soft clicking usually occurs without the prior resistance that is seen with dislocations. By repeated rotation of the hip, the exact location of the click can be palpated. However, Ortolani's test should not be repeated too often because it could lead to damage of the articular cartilage of the femoral head. As with all clinical tests, if the test is positive, it is highly suggestive that the problem (i.e., congenital dislocation of the hip) exists, but if it is negative, it does not necessarily rule out the problem.

Barlow's Test. Barlow's test is a modification of Ortolani's test[19] (see Fig. 11–19). The infant lies supine with the legs facing the examiner. The hips are flexed to 90°, and the knees are fully flexed. Each hip is evaluated individually while the examiner's other hand steadies the opposite femur and the pelvis. The examiner's middle finger of each hand is placed over the greater trochanter, and the thumb is placed adjacent to the inner side of the knee and thigh opposite the lesser trochanter. The hip is taken into abduction while the examiner's middle finger applies forward pressure behind the greater trochanter. If the femoral head slips forward into the acetabulum with a click, clunk, or jerk, the test is positive, indicating that the hip was dislocated. This part of the test is identical to Ortolani's test. The examiner then uses the thumb to apply pressure backward and outward on the inner thigh. If the femoral head slips out over the posterior lip of the acetabulum and then reduces again when pressure is removed, the hip is classified as unstable. The hip is not dislocated but is dislocatable. The procedure is repeated for the other hip.

This test may be used for infants up to 6 months of age. It should not be repeated too often because it may result in a dislocated hip as well as articular damage to the head of the femur.[25]

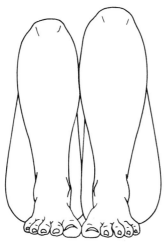

Figure 11–20
Galeazzi sign (Allis test).

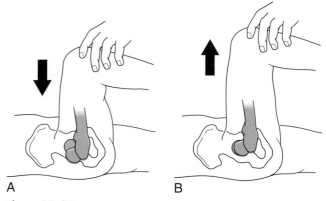

Figure 11–21
Telescoping of the hip. Because hip is not fixed in acetabulum, it moves down (A) and up (B).

Galeazzi Sign (Allis or Galeazzi Test). The Galeazzi test is good only for assessing unilateral congenital dislocation of the hip and may be used in children from 3 to 18 months of age. The child lies supine with the knees flexed and the hips flexed to 90°. A positive test is indicated if one knee is higher than the other (Fig. 11–20).

Telescoping Sign (Piston or Dupuytren's Test).[26] The telescoping sign is evident in a child with a dislocated hip. The child lies in the supine position. The examiner flexes the knee and hip to 90°. The femur is pushed down onto the examining table. The femur and leg are then lifted up and away from the table (Fig. 11–21). With the normal hip, little movement occurs with this action. With the dislocated hip, however, there is a lot of relative movement. This excessive movement is called telescoping, or **pistoning.**

Abduction Test (Harts' Sign).[26] If congenital dislocation of the hip is not diagnosed early, parents often note that when they change the child's diapers, one leg does not abduct as far as the other one. This is the basis for this test. The child lies supine with the hips and knees flexed to 90°. The examiner then passively abducts both legs, noting any asymmetry or limitation of movement. In addition, if one hip is dislocated, the child often demonstrates asymmetry of fat folds in the gluteal and upper leg area because of the "riding up" of the femur on the affected side.

Tests for Leg Length

There are two types of leg length discrepancy. One, called **true leg length discrepancy** or **true shortening,** is caused by an anatomic or structural change in the lower leg resulting from congenital maldevelopment (e.g., adolescent coxa vara, congenital hip dysplasia, bony abnormality) or trauma (e.g., fracture). Because an anatomic short leg results, the spine and pelvis are often affected, leading to lateral pelvic tilt and scoliosis.[27]

The second type of leg length discrepancy is called **functional leg length discrepancy** or **functional shortening** and is the result of compensation for a change that may have occurred because of positioning rather than

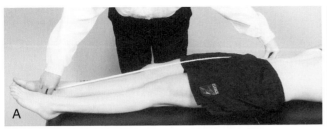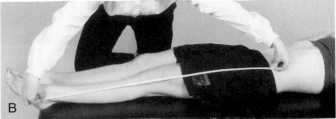

Figure 11–22
Measuring true leg length. (A) Measuring to the medial malleolus. (B) Measuring to the lateral malleolus.

structure. For example, a functional leg length discrepancy could occur because of unilateral foot pronation or spinal scoliosis.[27]

True Leg Length. Before any measuring is done, the examiner must set the pelvis square, level, or in balance with the lower limbs.[28-30] The legs should be 15 to 20 cm (4 to 8 inches) apart and parallel to each other (Fig. 11–22). If the legs are not placed in proper relation to the pelvis, **apparent shortening** of the limb may occur. The lower limbs must be placed in comparable positions relative to the pelvis, because abduction of the hip brings the medial malleolus closer to the ASIS on the same side and adduction of the hip takes the medial malleolus farther from the ASIS on the same side. If one hip is fixed in abduction or adduction as a result of contracture or some other cause, the normal hip should be adducted or abducted an equal amount to ensure accurate leg length measurement.

In North America, leg length measurement is usually taken from the ASIS to the medial malleolus; however, these values may be altered by muscle wasting or obesity. Measuring to the lateral malleolus is less likely to be affected by the muscle bulk. To obtain the leg length, the examiner measures from the ASIS to the lateral or medial malleolus. The flat metal end of the tape measure is placed immediately distal to the ASIS and pushed up against it. The thumb then presses the tape end firmly against the bone, rigidly fixing the tape measure against the bone. The index finger of the other hand is placed immediately distal to the lateral or medial malleolus and pushed against it. The thumbnail is brought down against the tip of the index finger so that the tape measure is pinched between them. A slight difference (as much as 1 to 1.5 cm) is considered normal; however, this difference can still cause symptoms.

The **Weber-Barstow maneuver** may also be used to measure leg length asymmetry. The patient lies supine with the hips and knees flexed (Fig. 11–23). The examiner stands at the patient's feet and palpates the distal aspect of the medial malleoli with the thumbs. The patient then

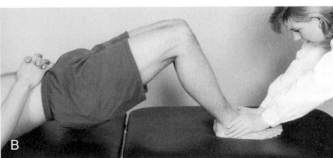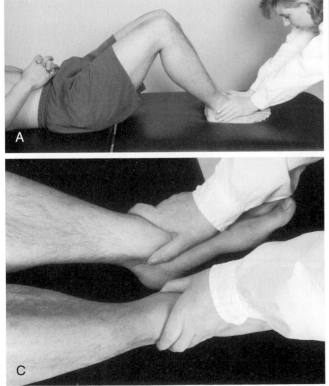

Figure 11–23
Weber-Barstow maneuver for leg length asymmetry. (A) Starting position. (B) Patient lifts hips off bed. (C) Comparing height of medial malleoli with the legs extended.

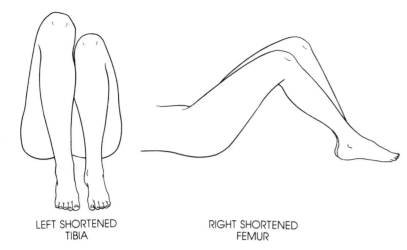

Figure 11–24
Leg length discrepancy.

LEFT SHORTENED
TIBIA

RIGHT SHORTENED
FEMUR

lifts the pelvis from the examining table and returns to the starting position. Next, the examiner passively extends the patient's legs and compares the positions of the malleoli using the borders of the thumbs. Different levels indicate asymmetry.[31]

If one leg is shorter than the other (Fig. 11–24), the examiner can determine where the difference is by measuring the following:

1. From the iliac crest to the greater trochanter of the femur (for coxa vara or coxa valga)
2. From the greater trochanter of the femur to the knee joint line on the lateral aspect (for femoral shaft shortening)
3. From the knee joint line on the medial side to the medial malleolus (for tibial shaft shortening)

The relative length of the tibia may also be examined with the patient lying prone. The examiner places the thumbs transversely across the soles of the feet just in front of the heels. The knees are flexed 90°, and the relative heights of the thumbs are noted. Care must be taken to ensure that the legs are perpendicular to the examining table (Fig. 11–25).[31]

Apparent or functional shortening (Fig. 11–26) of the leg is evident if the patient has a lateral pelvic tilt when the measurement is taken. Apparent or functional shortening of the limb is the result of adaptions the patient has made in response to pathology or contracture somewhere in the spine, pelvis, or lower limbs. In reality, there is no structural or anatomic difference in bone lengths. If there were, it would be called true shortening of the limb. When measuring the apparent leg length shortening, the examiner obtains the distance from the tip of the xiphisternum or umbilicus to the medial malleolus. Values obtained by these measurements may be affected by muscle wasting, obesity, asymmetric position of the xiphisternum or umbilicus, or asymmetric positioning of the lower limbs.

The neck-shaft angle of the femur (Fig. 11–27) is normally 150 to 160° at birth and decreases to between 120 and 135° in the adult (Fig. 11–28). If this angle is

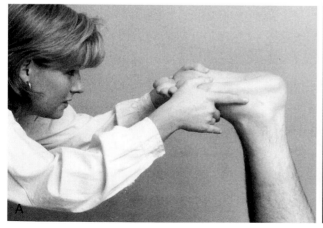

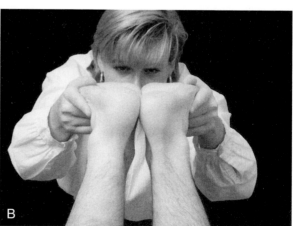

Figure 11–25
Prone knee flexion test for tibial shortening. The prone knee flexion test is completed as the examiner (A) passively flexes the patient's knees to 90° and (B) sights through the plane of the heel pads to see whether a difference in height is noticeable.

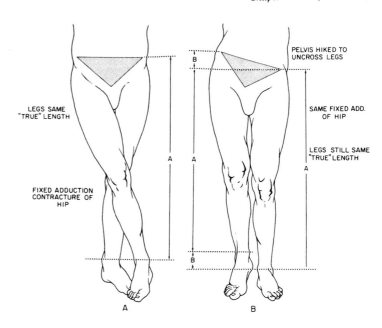

Figure 11–26

Functional shortening due to adduction contracture. (A) Legs crossed. (B) Legs uncrossed. Note that uncrossing causes pelvis to elevate on one side, but true leg length is equal on both sides. (From the American Orthopaedic Association: Manual of Orthopaedic Surgery. Chicago, 1972, p. 45.)

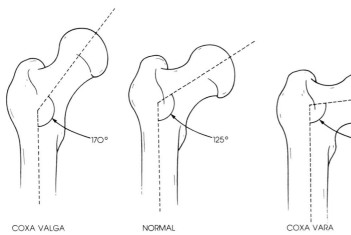

COXA VALGA   NORMAL   COXA VARA

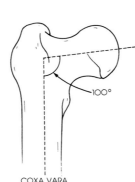

Figure 11–27
Neck-shaft angles of the femur in adults.

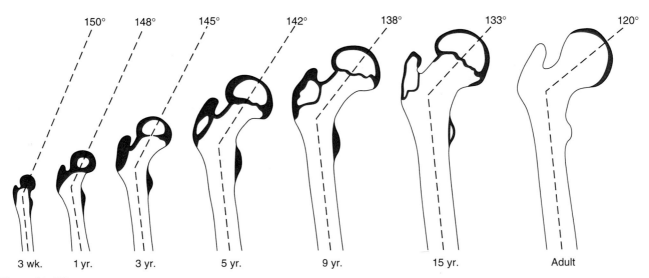

Figure 11–28
Mean angle of the femoral neck shaft in different age groups. Red area indicates cartilage. (Modified from von Lanz, T., and W. Wachsmuth: Praktische Anatomie. Berlin, Julius Springer, 1938, p. 143.)

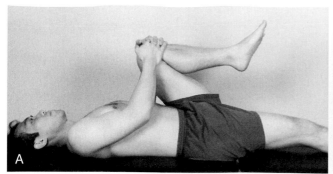
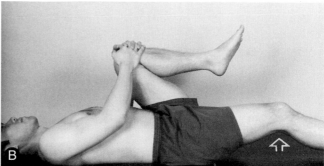

Figure 11–29
Thomas test. (A) Negative test. (B) Positive test.

less than 120° in an adult, it is known as **coxa vara**; if it is more than 135° in the adult, it is known as **coxa valga**.

Standing (Functional) Leg Length. The patient is first assessed while in a relaxed stance. In this position, the examiner palpates the ASIS and the PSIS, noting any asymmetry. The examiner then places the patient in a symmetric stance, ensuring that the subtalar joint is in neutral position (see Chapter 13), the toes are facing straight ahead, and the knees are extended. The ASIS and PSIS are again assessed for asymmetry. If differences are still noted, the examiner should check for structural leg length differences, sacroiliac joint dysfunction, or weak gluteus medius or quadratus lumborum muscles.

Tests for Muscle Tightness or Pathology

Sign of the Buttock. The patient lies supine and the examiner performs a straight leg raising test. If there is limitation on straight leg raising, the examiner flexes the patient's knee to see whether further hip flexion can be obtained. If hip flexion does not increase, the lesion is in the buttock and not in the hip, sciatic nerve, or hamstring muscles. There may also be some limited trunk flexion. Causes of a positive test include ischial bursitis, a neoplasm, or an abscess in the buttock.

Thomas Test. The Thomas test is used to assess a hip flexion contracture, the most common contracture of the hip. The patient lies supine while the examiner checks for excessive lordosis, which is usually present with tight hip flexors. The examiner flexes one of the patient's hips, bringing the knee to the chest to flatten out the lumbar spine, and the patient holds the flexed hip against the chest. If there is no flexion contracture, the hip being tested (the straight leg) remains on the examining table. If a contracture is present, the patient's straight leg rises off the table (Fig. 11–29). The angle of contracture can be measured. If the lower limb is pushed down onto the table, the patient may exhibit an increased lordosis; again, this result indicates a positive test. When doing the test, if measurements are taken, the examiner must be sure the restriction is in the hip and not the pelvis or lumbar spine.[32] If the leg does not lift off the table but abducts as the other leg is flexed to the chest, it is called the "J" **sign** and is indicative of a tight iliotibial band on the extended leg side.

Rectus Femoris Contracture Test (Method 1). The patient lies supine with the knees bent over the end or edge of the examining table. The patient flexes one knee onto the chest and holds it (Fig. 11–30). The angle of the test knee should remain at 90° when the opposite knee is flexed to the chest. If it does not (i.e., the test knee extends slightly), a contracture is probably present. The examiner may attempt to passively flex the knee to see whether it will remain at 90° of its own volition. The examiner should always palpate for muscle tightness when doing any contracture test. If there is no palpable tightness, the probable cause of restriction is tight joint structures (e.g., the capsule). The two sides should be tested and compared.

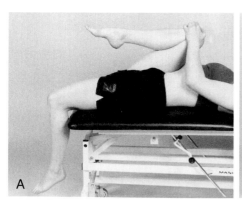
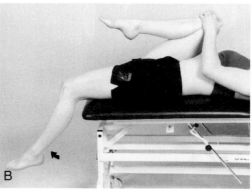

Figure 11–30
Rectus femoris contracture. (A) The movement leg is brought to the chest. The test leg remains bent over the end of the examining table, indicating a negative test. (B) The test knee extends, indicating a positive test.

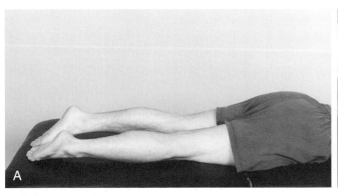
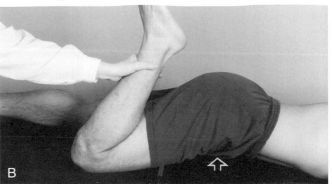

Figure 11–31

Ely's test for a tight rectus femoris. (A) Position for the test. (B) Posture test shown by hip flexion when the knee is flexed.

Ely's Test (Tight Rectus Femoris, Method 2). The patient lies prone, and the examiner passively flexes the patient's knee (Fig. 11–31).[33] On flexion of the knee, the patient's hip on the same side spontaneously flexes, indicating that the rectus femoris muscle is tight on that side and that the test is positive. The two sides should be tested and compared.

Ober's Test. Ober's test assesses the tensor fasciae latae (iliotibial band) for contracture (Fig. 11–32).[34] The patient is in the side lying position with the lower leg flexed at the hip and knee for stability. The examiner then passively abducts and extends the patient's upper leg with the knee straight or flexed to 90°. The examiner slowly lowers the upper limb; if a contracture is present, the leg remains abducted and does not fall to the table. When doing this test, it is important to extend the hip slightly so that the iliotibial band passes over the greater trochanter of the femur. To do this, the examiner stabilizes the pelvis at the same time to stop the pelvis from "falling backward." Ober originally described the test with the knee flexed.[34] However, the iliotibial band has

a greater stretch placed on it when the knee is extended. Also, when the knee is flexed during the test, greater stress is placed on the femoral nerve. If neurological signs (i.e., pain, paresthesia) occur during the test, the examiner should consider pathology affecting the femoral nerve. Likewise, tenderness over the greater trochanter should lead the examiner to consider trochanteric bursitis.

Adduction Contracture Test. The patient lies supine with the ASISs level. If a contracture is present, the affected leg forms an angle of less than 90° with the line joining the two ASISs. If the examiner then attempts to "balance" the lower limb with the pelvis, the pelvis shifts up on the affected side or down on the unaffected side, and balancing is not possible. This type of contracture can lead to **functional shortening** of the limb rather than true shortening (see Fig. 11–26).

In patients with **adductor spasticity,** especially children, abduction is performed quickly by the examiner. The patient is supine. If there is a "grab" or kicking in of the stretch reflex at less than 30°, the test for adductor

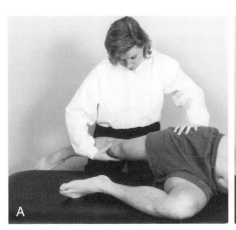
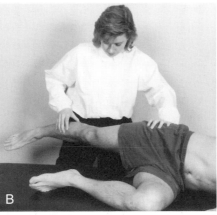
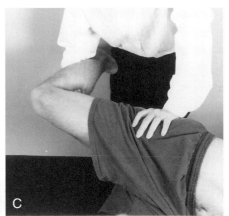

Figure 11–32

Ober's test. (A) Knee straight. (B) The hip is passively extended by the examiner to ensure that the tensor fasciae latae runs over the greater trochanter. A positive test is indicated when the leg remains abducted while the patient's muscles are relaxed. (C) Test done with the knee flexed.

spasticity is positive. The test should be repeated with the knee flexed to rule out medial hamstring contracture.[35]

Abduction Contracture Test. The patient lies supine with the ASISs level. If a contracture is present, the affected leg forms an angle of more than 90° with a line joining each ASIS. If the examiner then attempts to balance the lower limb with the pelvis, the pelvis shifts down on the affected side or up on the unaffected side, and balancing is not possible. This type of contracture can lead to **functional lengthening** of the limb rather than true lengthening.

Noble Compression Test. This test is used to determine whether iliotibial band friction syndrome exists near the knee (Fig. 11–33).[36] The patient lies supine and the knee is flexed to 90° accompanied by hip flexion. The examiner then applies pressure with the thumb to the lateral femoral epicondyle or 1 to 2 cm (0.4 to 0.8 inch) proximal to it. While the pressure is maintained, the patient slowly extends the knee. At approximately 30° of flexion (0° being a straight leg), if the patient complains of severe pain over the lateral femoral condyle, a positive test is indicated. The patient usually says it is the same pain that accompanies the patient's activity (e.g., running).

Piriformis Test. The patient is in the side lying position with the test leg uppermost. The patient flexes the test hip to 60° with the knee flexed. The examiner stabilizes the hip with one hand and applies a downward pressure to the knee (Fig. 11–34). If the piriformis muscle is tight, pain is elicited in the muscle. If the piriformis muscle is pinching the sciatic nerve, pain results in the buttock, and sciatica may be experienced by the patient.[4, 22] In about 15% of the population, the sciatic nerve, all or in part, passes through the piriformis muscle rather than below it.[3] It is these people who are more likely to suffer from **piriformis syndrome.** Resisted lateral rotation with the muscle on stretch (hip medially rotated) can cause the same sciatica.[37]

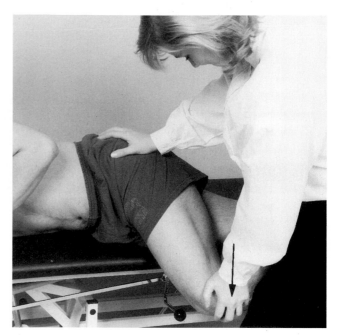

Figure 11–34
Piriformis test.

Hamstrings Contracture Test (Method 1). The patient is instructed to sit with one knee flexed against the chest to stabilize the pelvis and the other knee extended (Fig. 11–35). The patient then attempts to flex the trunk and touch the toes of the extended lower limb (test leg) with the fingers. The test is repeated on the other side. A comparison is made between the two sides. Normally, the patient should be able to at least touch the toes while keeping the knee extended. If he or she is unable to do so, it is an indication of tight hamstrings on the straight leg.

Tripod Sign (Hamstrings Contracture, Method 2). The patient is seated with both knees flexed to 90° over the edge of the examining table (Fig. 11–36).[38] The examiner then passively extends one knee. If the hamstring muscles on that side are tight, the patient extends the trunk to relieve the tension in the hamstring muscles. The leg is returned to its starting position, and the other leg is tested and compared with the first side. Extension of the spine is indicative of a positive test. The examiner must be aware that nerve root problems (stretching of the sciatic nerve) can cause a similar positive sign.

90-90 Straight Leg Raising Test (Hamstrings Contracture, Method 3). The supine patient flexes the hip to 90° while the knee is bent. The patient then grasps behind the knee with both hands to stabilize the hips at 90° of flexion. The patient actively extends each knee in turn as much as possible. For normal flexibility in the hamstrings, knee extension should be within 20° of full extension (Fig. 11–37).[4, 39] Nerve root symptoms may also result, as this positioning is similar to the slump test done in supine lying instead of sitting.

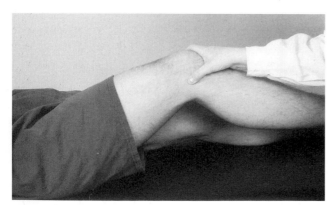

Figure 11–33
Noble compression test for iliotibial band friction syndrome. The patient extends the knee. The examiner is indicating where pain is felt at about 30° of flexion.

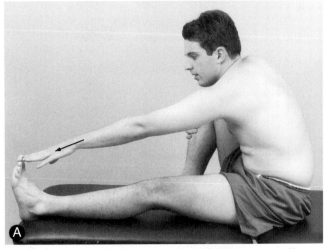

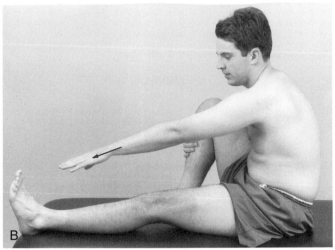

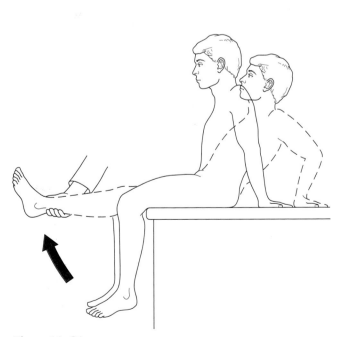

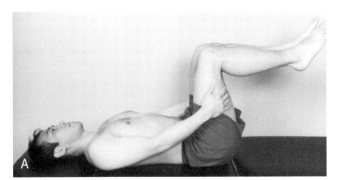

Figure 11–35
Test for hamstring tightness (method 1). (A) Negative test.
(B) Positive test. (C) Hypermobility of hamstrings.

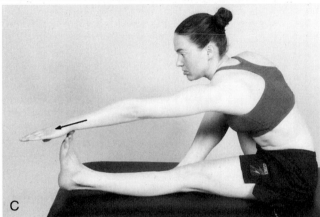

Figure 11–36
Tripod sign.

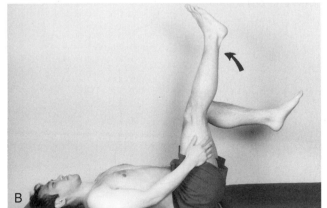

Figure 11–37
The 90-90 straight leg raising test.

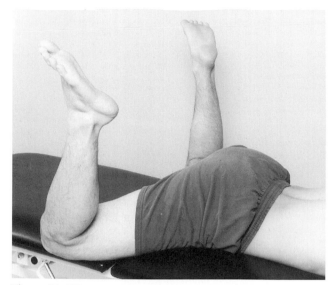

Figure 11–38
Phelps' test. Hips are abducted and knees are flexed to 90°. If abduction increases with knee flexion, test is positive.

Phelps' Test.[17] The patient lies prone with the knees extended. The examiner passively abducts both of the patient's legs as far as possible. The knees are then flexed to 90° (Fig. 11–38), and the examiner then tries to abduct the hips further. If abduction increases, the test is considered positive for contracture of the gracilis muscle.

Other Tests

Fulcrum Test. The fulcrum test[40] is used to assess for possible stress fracture of the femoral shaft. The patient sits with the knees bent over the end of bed with feet dangling. The examiner places an arm under the patient's thigh to act as a fulcrum (Fig. 11–39). The fulcrum arm

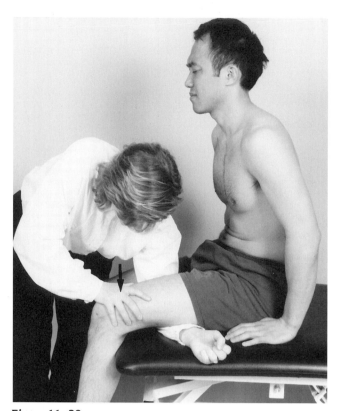

Figure 11–39
Fulcrum test. Examiner places arm under femur and carefully applies a downward force at the knee.

is moved from distal to proximal along the thigh as gentle pressure is applied to the dorsum of the knee with the examiner's opposite hand. If a stress fracture is present, the patient complains of a sharp pain and expresses apprehension when the fulcrum arm is under the fracture site. A bone scan confirms the diagnosis.

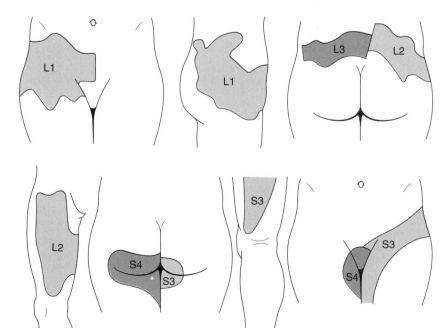

Figure 11–40
Dermatomes around the hip. Only one side is illustrated.

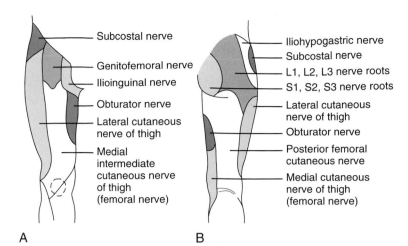

Figure 11-41
Sensory distribution of peripheral nerves around the hip. (A) Anterior view. (B) Posterior view.

Reflexes and Cutaneous Distribution

There are no reflexes around the hip that can easily be evaluated. However, the examiner should assess the normal dermatome patterns of the nerve roots (Fig. 11–40) as well as the cutaneous distribution of the peripheral nerves (Fig. 11–41). Because dermatomes vary from person to person, the accompanying diagrams are estimations only. Testing for altered sensation is performed by running the relaxed hands and fingers of the examiner over the pelvis and legs anteriorly, posteriorly, and laterally in a sensation scanning assessment. Any difference in sensation should be noted and can be mapped out more exactly using a pinwheel, pin, cotton batten, and/or brush.

True hip pain is usually referred to the groin, but it may also be referred to the ankle, knee, lumbar spine, and sacroiliac joints (Fig. 11–42). In children with hip problems (e.g., slipped capital femoral epiphysis, Legg-Calvé-Perthes disease), sensory symptoms may be manifested only in the knee. Similarly, the knee, sacroiliac joints, and lumbar spine may refer pain to the hip. Table 11–8 illustrates muscles of the hip and their referral pattern if injured.

Figure 11-42
Referred pain around the hip. Right side demonstrates referral to the hip. Left side shows referral from hip.

Table 11–8
Hip Muscles and Referral of Pain

Muscle	Referral Pattern
Iliopsoas	Lateral to lumbar spine, anterior thigh
Gluteus maximus	Sacral and gluteal area to lateral aspect of pelvis and posterosuperior thigh
Gluteus medius	Lumbar and sacral gluteal area to lateral aspect of pelvis and upper thigh
Gluteus minimus	Gluteal area to area below iliac crest down lateral aspect of thigh and leg
Piriformis	Sacrum, gluteal area down posterior aspect of thigh
Tensor fasciae latae	Lateral thigh
Sartorius	Anteromedial thigh (along course of muscle)
Pectineus	Groin to upper medial thigh
Rectus femoris	Anterior thigh to knee
Adductor longus and brevis	Anterior thigh to medial thigh to anterior knee to anteromedial leg to ankle
Adductor magnus	Groin along medial thigh to above knee
Gracilis	Anteromedial thigh to knee
Hamstrings	Gluteal area along posterior thigh to knee and posteromedial calf

Peripheral Nerve Injuries About the Hip

Sciatic Nerve (L4 *through* S3). The sciatic nerve (Fig. 11–43 and Table 11–9) may be injured anywhere along its path from the lumbosacral spine down the back of the leg to the knee. If it is injured, the hamstrings and all muscles below the knee will be affected. The result is a high steppage gait with an inability to stand on the heels or toes. There is sensory alteration in the entire foot except the instep and medial malleolus, along with muscle atrophy. In the hip region, the sciatic nerve may be compressed by the piriformis muscle **(piriformis syndrome)**.[41] In 15% of the population, the nerve passes through the muscle instead of below it. Usually, the symptoms are primarily in the common peroneal branch of the sciatic nerve. Burning pain and hyperesthesia may be felt in the sacral and/or gluteal region as well as in the sciatic nerve distribution. Medial rotation with extension of the hip accentuates the problem.

Superior Gluteal Nerve (L4 *through* S1). The superior gluteal nerve may be compressed as it passes between the piriformis and inferior border of the gluteus minimus muscle. The patient complains of acute gluteal pain that increases with ambulation. The hip is often medially rotated, and there is weakness of the hip abductors, resulting in a Trendelenburg's gait. Tenderness may be palpated just lateral to the greater sciatic notch.

Femoral Nerve (L2 *through* L4). The femoral nerve (Fig. 11–44), although not commonly injured, may be compressed during childbirth or with anterior dislocation of the femur or may be traumatized during hernia surgery, stripping of varicose veins, or fractures. The patient is not able to flex the thigh on the trunk or extend the knee. The deep tendon knee reflex is also lost. Wasting of the quadriceps is most evident. Sensory loss includes the medial aspect of the distal thigh **(anterior femoral cutaneous nerve)** and the medial aspect of the leg and foot **(saphenous nerve)**.

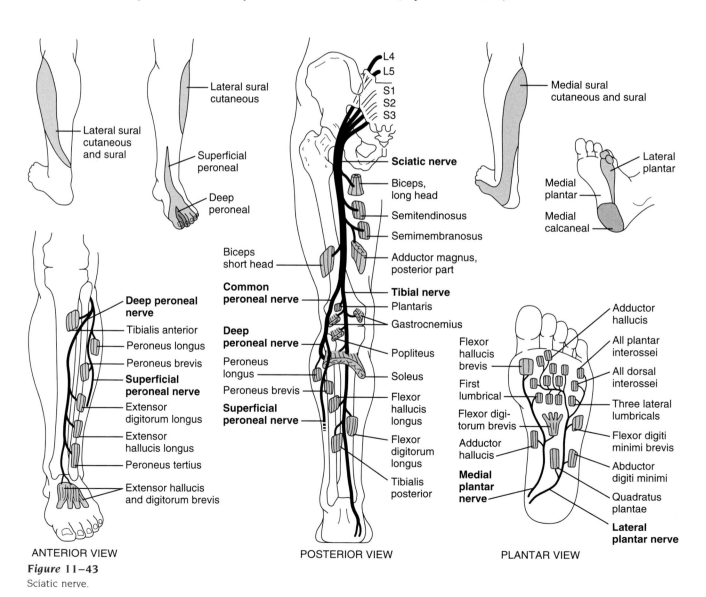

ANTERIOR VIEW   POSTERIOR VIEW   PLANTAR VIEW

Figure 11–43
Sciatic nerve.

Table 11–9
Peripheral Nerve Injuries (Neuropathy) About the Hip

	Muscle Weakness	Sensory Alteration	Reflexes Affected
Sciatic nerve (L4 through S3)	Hamstrings Tibialis anterior Extensor digitorum longus Extensor digitorum brevis Extensor hallucis longus Peroneus tertius Peroneus longus Peroneus brevis Gastrocnemius Soleus Plantaris Tibialis posterior Flexor digitorum longus Flexor hallucis longus Flexor accessorius (quadratus plantae) Abductor digiti minimi Flexor digiti minimi Lumbricales Interossei Adductor hallucis Abductor hallucis Flexor digitorum brevis Flexor hallucis brevis	Posterior thigh and leg Whole foot except instep and medial malleolus	Medial hamstrings (L5–S1) Lateral hamstrings (S1–S2) Achilles (S1–S2) Tibialis posterior (L4–L5)
Superior gluteal nerve	Gluteus medius Gluteus minimus Tensor fasciae latae	None	None
Femoral nerve (L2 through L4)	Iliacus Psoas Sartorius Pectineus Quadriceps	Medial side of thigh and leg	Patellar (L3–L4)
Obturator nerve (L2 through L4)	Adductor brevis Adductor magnus Adductor longus Obturator externus Gracilis	Middle thigh on anterior aspect	None

Obturator Nerve (L2 through L4). The obturator nerve (Fig. 11–45) may be compressed as it leaves the pelvis and enters the leg in the obturator tunnel. Injury to the nerve may be caused by pelvic or hip surgery, pregnancy **(obstetric palsy)**, fractures, or tumors.[41] Because the obturator nerve controls primarily the adductors, hip adduction is affected, as are knee flexion (gracilis) and lateral rotation (obturator externus). Sensory deficit is small, involving a small area in the middle medial part of the thigh, although the patient may complain of pain from the symphysis pubis to the medial aspect of the knee.

Joint Play Movements

The joint play movements (Fig. 11–46) are completed with the patient in the supine position. The examiner should attempt to compare the amounts of available

movement on the two sides. Small differences may be difficult to detect because of the large muscle bulk in the area.

> **Joint Play Movements of the Hip**
>
> - Caudal glide of the femur (long leg traction or long-axis extension)
> - Compression
> - Lateral distraction
> - Quadrant test

Caudal Glide. The examiner places both hands around the patient's leg, slightly above the ankle. The examiner then leans back, applying a long-axis extension to the entire lower limb. Part of the movement occurs in the

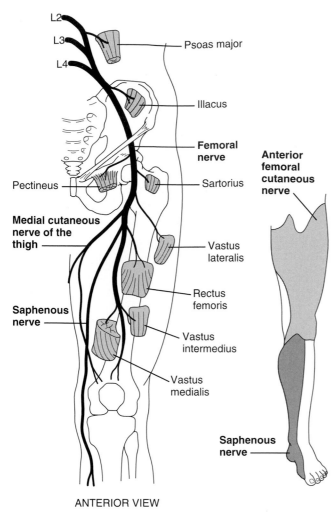

ANTERIOR VIEW

Figure 11–44
Femoral nerve.

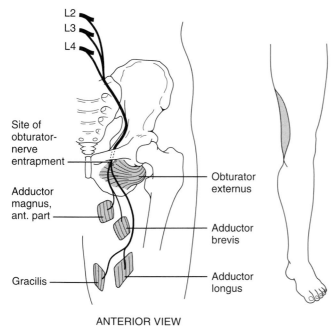

ANTERIOR VIEW

Figure 11–45
Obturator nerve.

knee. If one suspects some pathology in the knee or the knee is stiff, both hands should be placed around the thigh just proximal to the knee, and traction force should again be applied (see Fig. 11–46A). The first method enables the examiner to apply a greater force. During the movement, any telescoping or excessive movement occurring in the hip should be noted, as it may indicate an unstable joint.

Compression. The examiner places the patient's knee in the resting position and then applies a compressive force to the hip through the longitudinal axis of the femur by pushing through the femoral condyles (see Fig. 11–46B).

Lateral Distraction. The examiner applies a lateral distraction force to the hip by placing a wide strap around the leg as high up in the groin as possible. The strap is then wrapped around the examiner's buttocks. The examiner leans back, using the buttocks to apply the distraction force to the hip. The proximal hand is used to palpate the hip or greater trochanter movement, while the distal hand prevents abduction of the leg, and, hence, torque to the hip (see Fig. 11–46C).

Quadrant (Scouring) Test.[42] The examiner flexes and adducts the patient's hip so that the hip faces the patient's opposite shoulder and resistance to the movement is felt. As slight resistance is maintained, the patient's hip is taken into abduction while maintaining flexion in an arc of movement. As the movement is performed, the examiner should look for any irregularity in the movement (e.g., "bumps"), pain, or patient apprehension, which may give an indication of where the pathology is occurring in the hip (see Fig. 11–46D).[42]

Palpation

During palpation of the hip and associated muscles, the examiner should note any tenderness, temperature, muscle spasm, or other signs and symptoms that may indicate the source of pathology.

Anterior Aspect

The following structures should be palpated anteriorly, as shown in Figure 11–47.

Iliac Crest, Greater Trochanter, and Anterior Superior Iliac Spine. The iliac crests are easily palpated and should be level. The crest should be palpated for any tenderness, because several muscles insert into this structure. In athletes, a condition called a "hip pointer" may be located on the iliac crest. This occurs from a strain or contusion of the muscles that insert into the crest. The iliac tubercle is felt during palpation along the lateral aspect of the crest. The examiner then moves anteriorly to the ASIS. The greater trochanter, located approximately 10 cm (4 inches) distal to the iliac tubercle of the iliac crest, is palpated next. If the examiner's thumbs are placed over each ASIS, the fingers will naturally lie

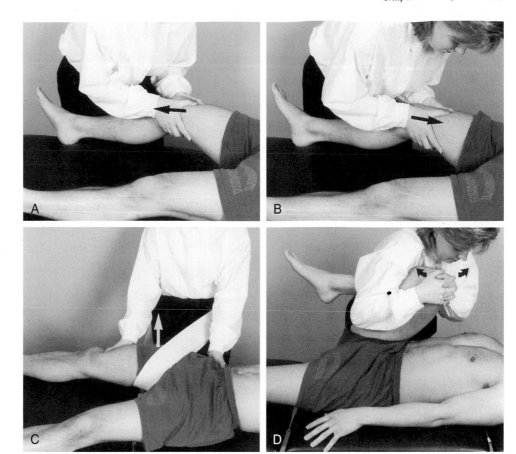

Figure 11-46

Joint play movements of the hip. (A) Long leg traction (applied above the knee). (B) Compression. (C) Lateral distraction. (D) Quadrant test.

along the lateral aspects of the thigh, and the greater trochanter can be felt with the fingers on each side. If the trochanteric bursa is swollen, it may also be palpated over the greater trochanter.

Inguinal Ligament, Femoral Triangle, Hip Joint, and Symphysis Pubis. The examiner's fingers are placed on the ASIS. Palpation gently continues along the inguinal liga-

ment to the pelvic tubercles (symphysis pubis), with the examiner noting any signs of pathology. The psoas bursa, if swollen, is usually palpable under the inguinal ligament at its midpoint. Moving distal to the inguinal ligament, the examiner palpates the femoral triangle, the boundaries of which are the inguinal ligament superiorly, the sartorius muscle laterally, and the adductor longus mus-

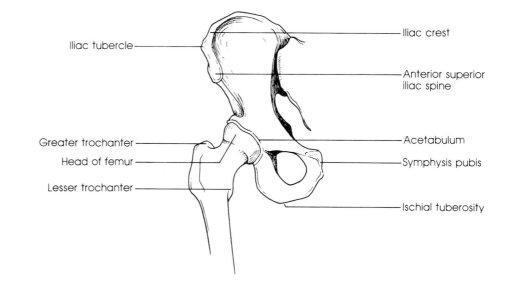

Figure 11-47

Landmarks of the hip (anterior view).

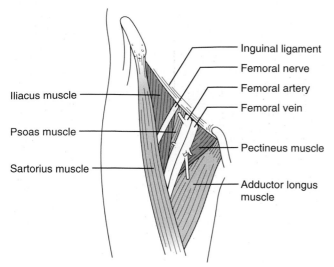

Figure 11–48
Femoral triangle containing the femoral artery, vein, and nerve. Note the inguinal ligament above, iliacus and psoas laterally, and adductors medially. The sartorius attaches to the anterosuperior spine, whereas the adductor muscles attach along the pubic ramus. (Modified from Anson, B.J.: Atlas of Human Anatomy. Philadelphia, W.B. Saunders Co., 1963, p. 583.)

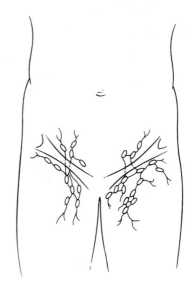

Figure 11–49
Lymph glands in the groin area.

cle medially (Fig. 11–48). Within the femoral triangle, the examiner may palpate swollen lymph glands (Fig. 11–49) and the femoral artery. The femoral nerve lies lateral to the artery and the femoral vein lies medial to it, but neither of these structures is easily palpated. At this stage, the examiner may decide to palpate for an inguinal hernia in the male. The head of the femur is then palpated. Although the hip joint is deep and not easily palpable, the surrounding structures may show signs of pathology. The head of the femur is 1 to 2 cm (0.4 to 0.8 inch) below the middle third of the inguinal ligament and is found on a horizontal line running halfway between the pubic tubercle and the greater trochanter.

The examiner concludes the anterior palpation by palpating the hip flexor, adductor, and abductor muscles for signs of pathology.

Posterior Aspect

The patient is then asked to lie in the prone position so that the following structures can be palpated posteriorly.

Iliac Crest, Posterior Superior Iliac Spine, Ischial Tuberosity, and Greater Trochanter. The examiner begins posterior palpation by following the iliac crests, which are easily palpable, posteriorly to the PSIS. On most patients, each PSIS is evident by the presence of overlying skin dimples. As the examiner moves caudally, the ischial tuberosities, which are approximately at the level of the gluteal folds, may be felt. If the ischial bursa is swollen, it is sometimes

palpable over the ischial tuberosities. The tuberosities should also be palpated for possible tenderness of the hamstring muscle insertions. Laterally, the posterior aspect of the greater trochanter is felt. If the distance between the ischial tuberosity and greater trochanter is divided in half, the fingers will lie over the sciatic nerve as it enters the lower limb. Normally, the nerve is not palpable. The examiner then palpates upward from the midpoint to determine whether there is any tenderness of the hip lateral rotators, especially the piriformis muscle. In addition, the gluteal and hamstring muscle bellies should be palpated for signs of pathology.

Sacroiliac, Lumbosacral, and Sacrococcygeal Joints. If the examiner suspects pathology in these joints, they should be palpated. Detailed descriptions of their palpation are given in Chapters 9 and 10.

Diagnostic Imaging

Plain Film Radiography

Normally, the standard views of the hip include anteroposterior views and axial or frog-leg views.

Anteroposterior View. The examiner should compare the two hips, noting the following features:

1. Joint spaces and pelvic lines (Fig. 11–50).
2. Presence of any bone disease (i.e., Legg-Calvé-Perthes disease, bony cysts, or tumors; Fig. 11–51).
3. Neck-shaft angle. The examiner should note whether the angle is normal or whether the patient exhibits a coxa vara or coxa valga (see Fig. 11–27).
4. Shape of the femoral head.
5. Presence of osteophytes or arthritis (Fig. 11–52).
6. Whether **Shenton's line** is normal. Normally, Shenton's line is curved, drawn along the medial curved edge of the femur and continuing upward in a smooth

Figure 11–50

Pelvic lines. The iliopubic (ip) and ilioischial (ii) lines help in assessing the anterior and posterior columns. The acetabular dome (D) and anterior (a) and posterior (p) lips (rims) of the acetabulum are seen. The teardrop figure (*arrows*) is a composite shadow made up laterally of the anterior aspect of the acetabular fossa and medially of the quadrilateral surface of the ilium. The more posterior aspect of the quadrilateral surface (represented by the ilioischial line) is superimposed on the teardrop in this nonrotated view. (From Weissman, B.N.W., and C.B. Sledge: Orthopedic Radiology. Philadelphia, W.B. Saunders Co., 1986, p. 343.)

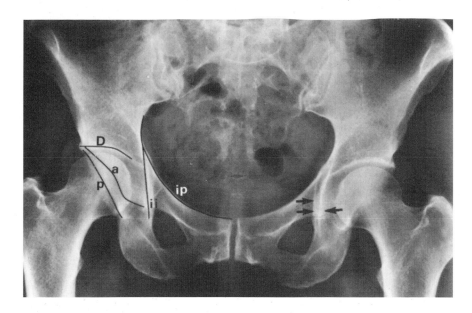

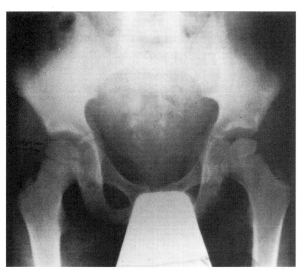

Figure 11–51

Legg-Calvé-Perthes disease of the left hip.

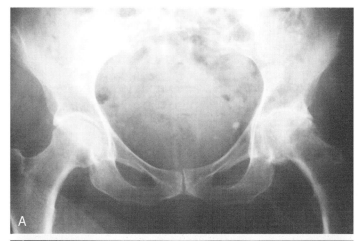

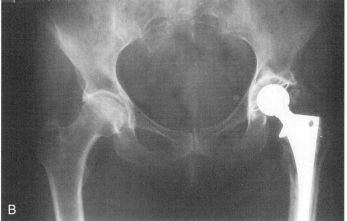

Figure 11–52

Arthritis of the left hip. (A) Before surgery. Note decreased joint space and unevenness of femoral head. (B) After total hip surgery.

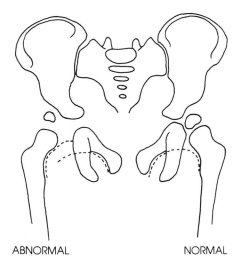

ABNORMAL   NORMAL

Figure 11–53
Shenton's line.

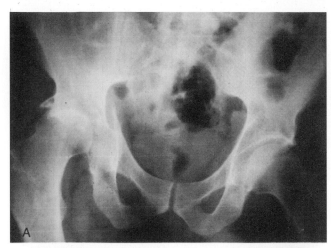

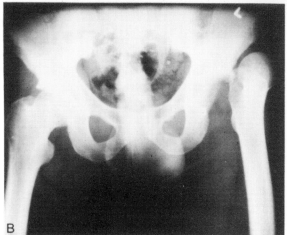

Figure 11–54
Trauma to the hip. (A) Fractured right acetabulum. (B) Dislocated left femur.

arc along the inferior edge of the pubis (Fig. 11–53). If the head of the femur is dislocated or fractured, two lines form two separate arcs, indicating a broken line. A broken Shenton's line is diagnostic.

7. Any evidence of fracture or dislocation (Fig. 11–54 and 11–55). Is the pelvic ring intact, or has it been disrupted? Disruption of the pelvic ring indicates severe injury.

8. Evidence of pelvic distortion.

9. Whether Hilgenreiner's and Perkins' lines are within normal limits.[43] **Hilgenreiner's line** is horizontal, drawn between the inferior parts of the ilium. **Perkins' line** is vertical, drawn through the upper outer point of

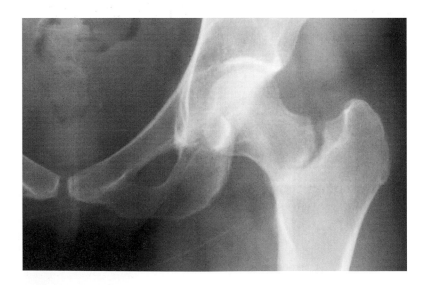

Figure 11–55
Stress fracture of the femoral neck.

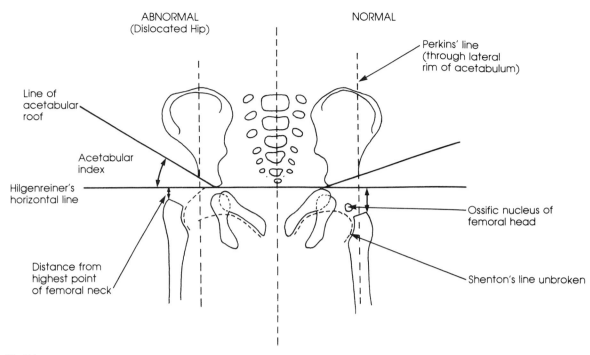

ABNORMAL
(Dislocated Hip)

NORMAL

Perkins' line
(through lateral
rim of acetabulum)

Line of
acetabular
roof

Acetabular
index

Hilgenreiner's
horizontal line

Ossific nucleus of
femoral head

Distance from
highest point
of femoral neck

Shenton's line unbroken

Figure 11–56
Radiological findings in congenital dislocation of the hip compared with normal findings in a 12- to 15-month-old child. Acetabular index: normal = 30°, in newborn = 27.5°. If the ossific nucleus of the femoral head is present, it should sit in the inner lower quadrant.

the acetabulum (Fig. 11–56). Normally, the developing femoral head or ossification center of the femoral head lies in the inner distal quadrant formed by the two lines. If the ossification center lies in the upper outer quadrant, the finding is indicative of a dislocation. In the newborn, the ossification center is not visible (Fig. 11–57).

10. Whether the femoral head and acetabulum are normal on both sides. In congenital dislocation of the hip, both structures may show dysplasia, and the **acetabular index** on the affected side may be more than the normal 30°. The acetabular index is determined by first drawing Hilgenreiner's line. An intersecting line is drawn from the lateral to the medial edge of the acetabulum, and the angle formed by the two lines is called the acetabular index, or **Hilgenreiner's angle** (Table 11–10). The greater the slope angle, the less stable the femoral head in the acetabulum.

11. **"Sagging rope" sign.** With Legg-Calvé-Perthes disease, only the head of the femur is affected. If avascular necrosis of a developing femoral head occurs, the sagging rope sign may be seen (Fig. 11–58). The sign

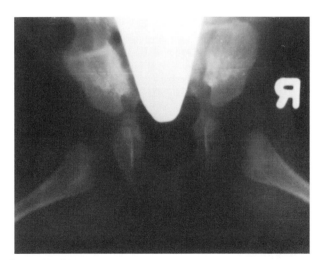

Figure 11–57
Radiograph of the hip in the newborn. Ossification of the femoral head has not yet developed.

Table 11–10
Average Values of Hilgenreiner's Angle (Acetabular Index)

	Newborn	**6 Months Old**	**1 Year Old**
Male	26°	20°	20°
Female	28°	22°	20°

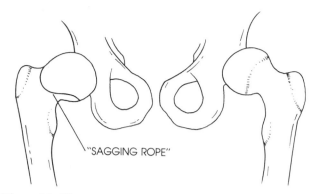

Figure 11–58
Sagging rope sign.

indicates damage to the growth plate with marked metaphyseal reaction. Its presence indicates a severe disease process.

12. "Teardrop" sign. Migration of the femoral head upward in relation to the pelvis, caused by degeneration as seen in osteoarthritis, may be detected by the teardrop sign (Fig. 11–59). The teardrop is visible at the base of the pubic bone, extending vertically downward to terminate in a round teardrop, or head. The x-ray beam must be centered relative to the pelvis. A line is drawn between the two teardrops and extended to the femoral heads

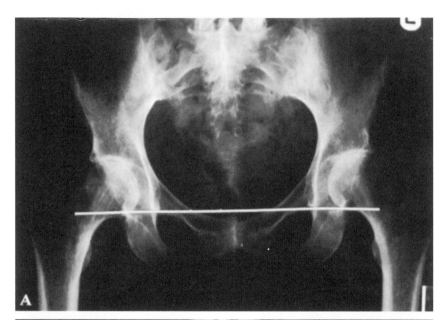

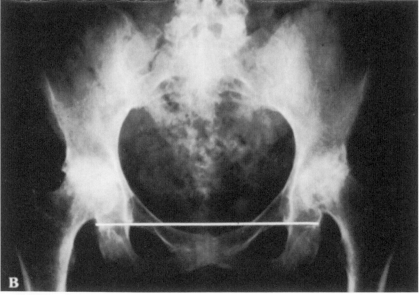

Figure 11–59

Teardrop sign. (A) A line has been drawn between the tips of the two "teardrops" and extended into the femoral neck. Osteoarthritis of both hip joints appears to be equal, with equivalent narrowing of the joint space, but the left hip is already at a slightly higher level than the right in relation to the line. (B) Later, both hips have gradually moved upward as a result of loss of the bone at the apex of each femoral head. The left hip is now at a higher level than the right, confirming the original observation that the process of destruction in the left hip was more advanced. (From Greubel-Lee, D.M.: Disorders of the Hip. Philadelphia, J.B. Lippincott, 1983, pp. 61, 146.)

on both sides. The examiner can then measure from the teardrop to the femoral head. A difference of more than 10 mm between the two sides indicates significant migration of the head of the femur. Serial films or films taken over time often show a progression of the migration.

13. **"Head-at-risk" signs.** With Legg-Calvé-Perthes disease, the examiner should note the following radiologic head-at-risk signs on an anteroposterior film:

   a. Cage's sign, a small osteoporotic segment on the lateral side of the epiphysis that appears to be translucent (Fig. 11–60)

   b. Calcification lateral to the epiphysis (if collapse is occurring)

   c. Lateral subluxation of the head (an increase in the inferomedial joint space)

   d. Angle of the epiphyseal line (horizontal, in this case)

   e. Metaphyseal reaction.

Patients who exhibit three or more head-at-risk signs have a poor prognosis, and surgery is usually performed.

14. Signs of a **slipped capital femoral epiphysis.** With a slipped capital femoral epiphysis (Fig. 11–61), the following x-ray signs may be noted:

   a. The epiphyseal line may widen.

   b. Lipping or stepping may be seen, as occurs on lateral films.

   c. The superior femoral neck line does not

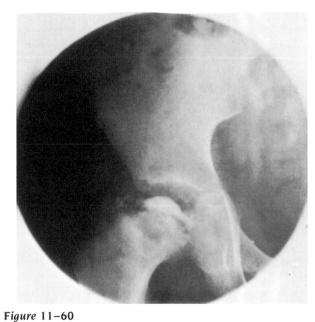

Figure 11–60

All of the signs of the "head-at-risk" are present: lateral subluxation, abnormal direction of the growth plates, Cage's sign, lateral calcification, and irregularity of the epiphysis. (From Greubel-Lee, D.M.: Disorders of the Hip. Philadelphia, J.B. Lippincott, 1983, p. 146.)

transect the overhanging ossified epiphysis as it does in the normal hip.

   d. Shenton's line does not describe a continuous arc. (The line is also broken if the hip is dislocated or subluxed.)

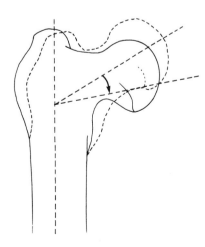 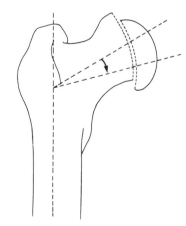

CONGENITAL   FRACTURE   SLIPPED CAPITAL FEMORAL EPIPHYSIS

Figure 11–61

Some causes of coxa vara.

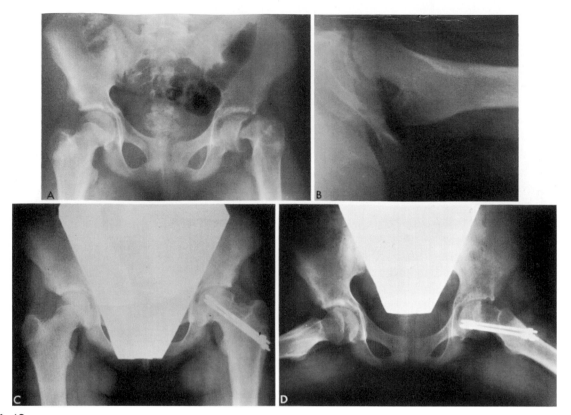

Figure 11–62

Acute slipped femoral epiphysis in a 14-year-old boy. After a fall, the patient complained of severe pain in the left groin and anterior thigh and was unable to bear weight on the left lower limb. (A and B) Preoperative radiographs show the severe slip on the left. The patient was placed in bilateral split Russell traction with medial rotation straps on the left thigh and leg. Gradually, within a period of 3 to 4 days, the slip was reduced. (C and D) Postoperative radiographs approximately 6 months later show closure of epiphyseal plate and normal position of femoral head. The hip had full range of motion. (From Tachdjian, M.O.: Pediatric Orthopedics. Philadelphia, W.B. Saunders Co., 1972, p. 470.)

In addition to a slipped capital femoral epiphysis causing a coxa vara, fractures or congenital malformations can lead to the same deformity (Figs. 11–62 and 11–63).

Lateral (Axial "Frog-Leg") View. For this view, the patient is supine with the hips in flexion, abduction, and lateral rotation. This view provides a true lateral view of the femoral head and neck.[44] The examiner looks for any pelvic distortion or any slipping of the femoral head, as may be seen in slipped capital femoral epiphysis. The lateral view is the first in which slipping may be seen.

Arthrography

Although arthrograms are not routinely done on the hip, they may be done if the hip cannot be reduced following a dislocation (Fig. 11–64). The arthrogram may indicate a possible inverted limbus (infolding of a meniscus-like structure) or an hourglass configuration from a contracted capsule. It is also useful in congenital dislocation of the hip to show where the unossified femoral head lies relative to the labrum. A normal hip arthrogram is shown in Figure 11–65.

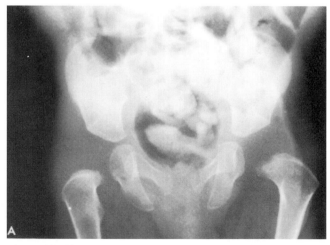

Figure 11–63

Congenital coxa vara of the left hip in an infant. (A) Anteroposterior radiographs of both hips at 3 months of age, taken because of limited abduction of left hip and suspicion of congenital hip dislocation. It was interpreted to be normal. (B and C) Radiographs of the hips of same patient at 1 year of age when he started walking with a painless gluteus medius lurch on the left. Varus deformity of the left hip is evident. (From Tachdjian, M.O.: Pediatric Orthopedics. Philadelphia, W.B. Saunders Co., 1972, p. 587.)

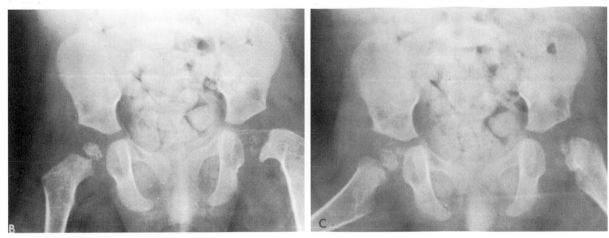

Figure 11–63 *Continued*

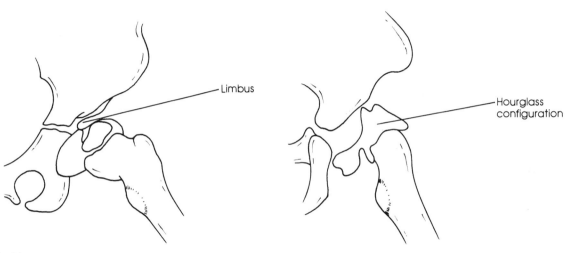

Limbus

Hourglass configuration

Figure 11–64
Drawings of arthrograms in congenital dislocation of the hip.

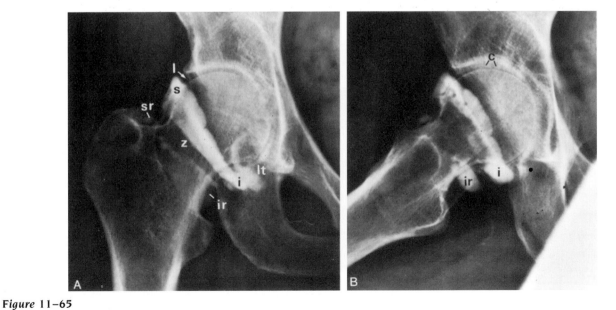

Figure 11–65
Normal hip arthrogram. Normal examination after intra-articular injection of approximately 6 ml of contrast medium. (A) Anteroposterior and (B) frog lateral views. c = contrast agent outlining articular cartilage (recess capitus); i = inferior articular recess; ir = recess colli inferior; l = acetabular labrum; lt = defect on contrast from transverse ligament; s = superior articular recess; sr = recess colli superior; z = zona orbicularis (impression on the intra-articular contrast by the iliofemoral ischiofemoral ligaments of the hip joint capsule). (From Weissman, B.N.W., and C.B. Sledge: Orthopedic Radiology. Philadelphia, W.B. Saunders Co., 1986, p. 396.)

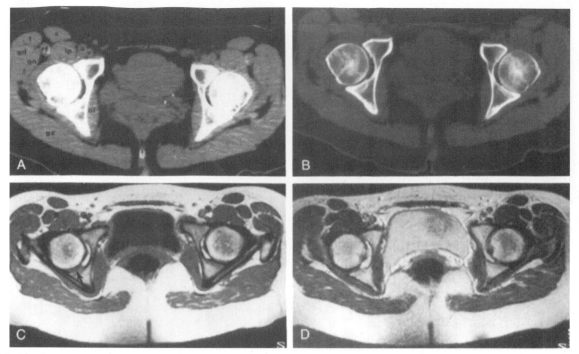

Figure 11–66

(A) Normal computed tomography (CT) image at the level of the midacetabulum obtained with soft-tissue window settings, showing the homogenous, intermediate signal of musculature. a = common femoral artery; gd = gluteus medius; gn = gluteus minimus; gx = gluteus maximus; ip = iliopsoas; oi = obturator internus; ra = rectus abdominis; rf = rectus femoris; s = sartorius; t = tensor fasciae latae; v = common femoral vein. (B) Axial CT at bone window settings reveals improved delineation of cortical and medullary osseous details. Note anterior and posterior semilunar acetabular articular surfaces and the central nonarticular acetabular fossa. (C) Normal midacetabular T1-weighted axial 0.4-T magnetic resonance image (TR, 600 msec; TE, 20 msec) of a different patient shows a normal, high-signal-intensity image of muscle and absence of signal in the cortical bone. The thin articular hyaline cartilage is of intermediate signal intensity (*arrow*). (D) T2-weighted magnetic resonance image (TR, 2,000 msec; TE, 80 msec) shows decreasing high-signal intensity in fatty marrow and subcutaneous tissue with increased signal intensity in the fluid-filled urinary bladder. (From Pitt, M.J., P.J. Lund, and D.P. Speer: Imaging of the pelvis and hip. Orthop. Clin. North Am. 21:553, 1990.)

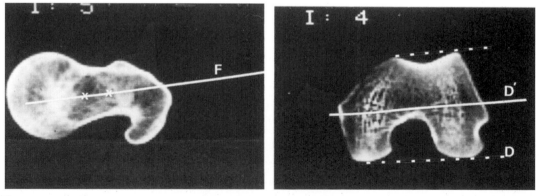

Figure 11–67

Computed tomography for determining femoral anteversion (using a femoral specimen). The diacondylar line (D) is drawn along the condyles, although Hernandez and coworkers construct it (D') midway between the anterior and posterior femoral surfaces (dashed lines). The axis of the femoral neck (F) is shown. The angle between the femoral neck axis (F) and the diacondylar line is the angle of anteversion. In this case, there is 2° of retroversion. (From Weissman, B.N.W., and C.B. Sledge: Orthopedic Radiology. Philadelphia, W.B. Saunders Co., 1986, p. 399.)

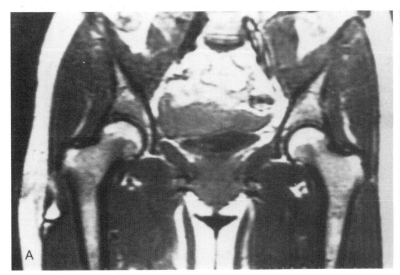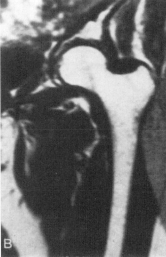

Figure 11–68

(A) Normal magnetic resonance imaging scan of a young adult. Spin-echo T1-weighted image (600/25). Note the bright signal of fat in the region of the femoral epiphysis and the greater trochanter. The intermediate signal intensity in the femoral neck represents hemopoietic marrow. (B) Normal elderly woman with same imaging sequence shows replacement of hemopoietic marrow in the femoral neck by fatty marrow. (From Dalinka, M.K., and L.M. Neustadter: Radiology of the hip. In Steinberg, M.E. [ed.]: The Hip and Its Disorders. Philadelphia, W.B. Saunders Co., 1991, p. 68.)

Computed Tomography

Computed tomography scanning is useful in assessing abnormalities of the hip. For example, it can be used to measure anteversion and retroversion, and it can show the size and shape of the acetabulum and femoral head as well as the congruity and position of the femoral head relative to the acetabulum (Figs. 11–66 and 11–67). In newborns, the lack of ossification limits its use.

Magnetic Resonance Imaging

Magnetic resonance imaging (Fig. 11–68) is a useful technique to study the hip because it is able to show soft tissue (e.g., bursitis, tendon lesions) as well as osseous tissue (e.g., osteonecrosis). This ability makes it an excellent technique to use for congenital abnormalities.

Scintigraphy (Bone Scan)

Bone scans may be used in the hip to help diagnose stress fractures (especially of femoral neck), necrosis, and tumors.

Ultrasonography

Ultrasonography is a nonirradiation technique that may be used to detect hip abnormalities and soft-tissue problems such as swelling.[45]

Précis of the Hip Assessment*

History
Observation
Examination
    Active movements (supine)
       Hip flexion
       Hip abduction
       Hip adduction
       Hip lateral rotation
       Hip medial rotation
    Passive movements (supine) as in active movements (if necessary)
    Resisted isometric movements (supine)
       Hip flexion
       Hip extension
       Hip adduction
       Hip abduction

       Hip medial rotation
       Hip lateral rotation
       Knee flexion
       Knee extension
    Special tests (supine)
    Reflexes and cutaneous sensation (supine)
       Reflexes
       Sensory scan
       Peripheral nerves
    Joint play movements (supine)
       Caudal glide
       Compression
       Lateral distraction
       Quadrant test
    Palpation (supine)

Active movement (prone)
 Hip extension
Passive movement (prone)
 Hip extension
Resisted isometric movements (prone)
 Hip medial rotation (if not previously done)
 Hip lateral rotation (if not previously done)
 Knee flexion (if not previously done)
 Knee extension (if not previously done)
Special tests (prone and side lying)

Reflexes and cutaneous sensation (prone)
Palpation (prone)
Diagnostic imaging

---

* The précis is shown in an order that limits the amount of moving the patient must do but ensures that all necessary structures are tested.

After the rest of the examination is completed, the examiner can ask the patient to perform the appropriate functional test.

After any examination, the patient should be warned of the possibility of exacerbation of symptoms as a result of the assessment.

Case Studies

When doing these case studies, the examiner should list the appropriate questions to be asked and why they are being asked, what to look for and why, and what things should be tested and why. Depending on the answers of the patient (and the examiner should consider different responses), several possible causes of the patient's problem may become evident (examples are given in parentheses). A differential diagnosis chart (Table 11–11) should be made up. The examiner can then decide how different diagnoses may affect the treatment plan.

1. A 14-year-old boy was well until he fell from a chair onto his buttocks. He did not appear hurt, but 1 week later his parents brought him in for assessment because of a limp and pain in his right thigh and knee. The teenager is a tall, thin boy who prefers to walk with the right foot laterally rotated. Design your assessment plan for this patient (slipped capital femoral epiphysis versus ischial bursitis).

2. A 71-year-old woman had an Austin Moore prosthesis inserted into the left hip 1 day ago. The prosthesis has relieved the pain she had in her hip. X-rays reveal that the prosthesis is solid. The surgeon has asked you to get the patient up and moving. Before doing this, however, you must do a bedside assessment. Outline how you would do the assessment.

3. A 7-year-old boy is brought by his parents for assessment. He walks with a limp and has done so during the past 5 weeks at irregular times, the limp becoming more pronounced when the boy becomes tired. The boy also complains of a painful left knee. Describe your assessment plan for this patient (Legg-Calvé-Perthes disease versus slipped capital femoral epiphysis).

4. A 3-week-old girl is referred to you to be fit with a Pavlik harness for congenital dislocation of the hip. Before you can fit the harness, you must do an assessment. Design your assessment plan for this patient.

5. A 55-year-old man presents complaining of hip and back pain. There is some sciatica with pain into the groin. The pain is especially bad when he walks. He has a desk job but has been very active throughout his life. Describe your assessment plan for this patient (piriformis syndrome versus lumbar spondylosis).

6. A 35-year-old woman presents complaining of lateral hip pain. She states she was in a motor vehicle accident 2 weeks ago in which she was hit from the passenger side (she was driving) and her car was pushed against a

---

Table 11–11
Differential Diagnosis of Slipped Capital Femoral Epiphysis and Ischial Bursitis

	Slipped Capital Femoral Epiphysis	**Ischial Bursitis**
History	Trauma may or may not be a factor Growth spurt may be involved More common on boys May be acute or chronic Pain into hip, groin, thigh to knee	Usually results from trauma (fall) Usually acute but can become chronic Pain over ischial tuberosity and sometimes into hamstrings
Observation	Lurching gait	Gait generally normal although may be antalgic
Active movement	Abduction, medial rotation, and flexion limited	Flexion limited
Passive movement	Capsular pattern	Noncapsular pattern
Resisted isometric movement	Normal but stress may cause pain	Hamstrings contraction sometimes painful
Special tests	True leg length difference Trendelenburg's test positive	Leg lengths equal Trendelenburg's test negative
Sensation	Normal	Normal
Reflexes	Normal	Normal
Joint play movements	May cause pain or relief	Normal
Diagnostic imaging	Diagnostic	Negative

telephone pole. She was wearing a seat belt. Describe your assessment plan for this patient (trochanteric bursitis versus muscle contusion).

7. An 18-year-old man was surfing when he was thrown by a wave and hurt his hip. The hip is medially rotated and shortened. He has some sciatic pain. Describe your

assessment plan for this patient (posterior hip dislocation versus trochanteric fracture).

8. A 23-year-old female diver comes to you complaining of hip pain. She says it bothers her when she does any quick flexion of the hip. Describe your assessment plan for this patient (psoas bursitis versus psoas strain).

References

Cited References

1. Reid, D.C.: Sports Injury Assessment and Rehabilitation. New York, Churchill Livingstone, 1992.
2. Allen, W.C.: Coxa saltans: The snapping hip revisited. J. Am. Acad. Orthop. Surg. 3:303–308, 1995.
3. Mellman, M.R., E.J. McPherson, L.D. Dorr, and P. Kwong: Differential diagnosis of back and lower extremity problems. In Watkins, R.G. (ed.): The Spine in Sport. St. Louis, C.V. Mosby Co., 1996.
4. Saudek, C.E.: The hip. In Gould, J.A. (ed.): Orthopedic and Sports Physical Therapy. St. Louis, C.V. Mosby, Co., 1990.
5. Brand, R.A., and R.D. Crowninshield: The effect of cane use on hip contact force. Clin. Orthop. 147:181–184, 1980.
6. Aspinall, W.: Clinical implications of iliopsoas dysfunction. J. Man. Manip. Ther. 1:41–46, 1993.
7. Ombregt, L., P. Bissehop, H.J. ter Veer, and T. Van de Velde: A System of Orthopedic Medicine. London, W.B. Saunders Co., 1995.
8. Klaue, K., C.W. Durnin, and R. Ganz: The acetabular rim syndrome: A clinical presentation of dysplasia of the hip. J. Bone Joint Surg. Br. 73:423–429, 1991.
9. Tis, L.L., D.H. Perrin, D.B. Snead, and A. Weltman: Isokinetic strength of the trunk and hip in female runners. Isok. Exerc. Sci. 1:22–25, 1991.
10. Donatelli, R., P.A. Catlin, G.S. Backer, D.L. Drane, and S.M. Slater: Isokinetic hip abductor to adductor torque ratio in normals. Isok. Exerc. Sci. 1:103–111, 1991.
11. D'Aubigné, R.M., and M. Postel: Functional results of hip arthroplasty with acrylic prosthesis. J. Bone Joint Surg. Am. 36:451–475, 1954.
12. Murray, D.: The hip. In Pynsent, P., J. Fairbank, and A. Carr (eds.): Outcome Measures in Orthopedics. Oxford, Butterworth Heinemann, 1994.
13. Harris, W.H.: Traumatic arthritis of the hip after dislocation and acetabular fractures: Treatment by mold arthroplasty. An end result study using a new method of result evaluation. J. Bone Joint Surg. Am. 51:737–755, 1969.
14. Kavanagh, B.F., and R.H. Fitzgerald: Clinical and roentgenographic assessment of total hip arthroplasty: A new hip score. Clin. Orthop. 193:133–140, 1985.
15. Johanson, N.A., M.E. Charlson, T.P. Szatrowski, and C.S. Ranawat: A self-administered hip-rating questionnaire for the assessment of outcome after total hip replacement. J. Bone Joint Surg. Am. 74:587–597, 1992.
16. Burton, K.E., V. Wright, and J. Richards: Patients' expectations in relation to outcome of total hip replacement surgery. Ann. Rheum. Dis. 38:471–474, 1979.
17. Evans, R.C.: Illustrated Essentials in Orthopedic Physical Assessment. St. Louis, C.V. Mosby Co., 1994.
18. Adams, M.C.: Outline of Orthopaedics. London, E & S Livingstone, 1968.
19. Tachdjian, M.O.: Pediatric Orthopedics. Philadelphia, W.B. Saunders Co., 1972.
20. Crane, L.: Femoral torsion and its relation to toeing-in and toeing-out. J. Bone Joint Surg. Am. 41:421–428, 1959.
21. Staheli, L.T.: Medial femoral torsion. Orthop. Clin. North Am. 11:39–50, 1980.
22. Lee, D.: The Pelvic Girdle. Edinburgh, Churchill Livingstone, 1989.
23. Callaghan, J.J.: Examination of the hip. In Clarke, C.R., and M. Bonfiglio (eds.): Orthopedics: Essentials of Diagnosis and Treatment. New York, Churchill Livingstone, 1994.
24. Darmonov, A.V.: Clinical screening for congenital dislocation of the hip. J. Bone Joint Surg. Am. 78:383–388, 1996.
25. Moore, F.H.: Examining infants' hips: Can it do harm? J. Bone Joint Surg. Br. 71:4–5, 1989.
26. LeVeau, B.: Hip. In Richardson, J.K., and Z.A. Iglarsh: Clinical Orthopedic Physical Therapy. Philadelphia, W.B. Saunders Co., 1994.
27. Bolz, S., and G.J. Davies: Leg length differences and correlation with total leg strength. J. Orthop. Sports Phys. Ther. 6:123–129, 1984.
28. Clarke, G.R.: Unequal leg length: An accurate method of detection and some clinical results. Rheumatol. Phys. Med. 11:385–390, 1972.
29. Fisk, J.W., and M.L. Balgent: Clinical and radiological assessment of leg length. N. Z. Med. J. 81:477–480, 1975.
30. Woerman, A.L., and S.A. Binder-Macleod: Leg-length discrepancy assessment: Accuracy and percision in five clinical methods of evaluation. J. Orthop. Sports Phys. Ther. 5:230–239, 1984.
31. Woerman, A.L.: Evaluation and treatment of dysfunction in the lumbar-pelvic-hip complex. In Donatelli, R., and M.J. Wooden (eds.): Orthopedic Physical Therapy. Edinburgh, Churchill Livingstone, 1989.
32. Thurston, A.: Assessment of fixed flexion deformity of the hip. Clin. Orthop. 169:186–189, 1982.
33. Gruebel-Lee, D.M.: Disorders of the Hip. Philadelphia, J.B. Lippincott Co., 1983.
34. Ober, F.B.: The role of the iliotibial and fascia lata as a factor in the causation of low-back disabilities and sciatica. J. Bone Joint Surg. 18:105–110, 1936.
35. Crawford, A.H.: Neurologic disorders. In Steinberg, M.E. (ed.): The Hip and Its Disorders. Philadelphia, W.B. Saunders Co., 1991.
36. Noble, H.B., M.R. Hajek, and M. Porter: Diagnosis and treatment of iliotibial band tightness in runners. Phys. Sportsmed. 10:67–68, 71–72, 74, 1982.
37. Garrick, J.G., and D.R. Webb: Sports Injuries: Diagnosis and Treatment. Philadelphia, W.B. Saunders, Co., 1990.
38. American Orthopaedic Association: Manual of Orthopaedic Surgery. Chicago, American Orthopaedic Association, 1972.
39. Palmar, M.L., and M. Epler: Clinical Assessment Procedures in Physical Therapy. Philadelphia, J.B. Lippincott, 1990.
40. Johnson, A.W., C.B. Weiss, and D.L. Wheeler: Stress fractures of the femoral shaft in athletes—more common than expected: A new clinical test. Am J. Sports Med. 22:248–256, 1994.
41. Pecina, M.M., J. Krmpotic-Nemanic, and A.D. Markiewitz: Tunnel Syndromes. Boca Raton, Florida, CRC Press, 1991.
42. Maitland, G.D.: The Peripheral Joints: Examination and Recording Guide. Adelaide, Australia, Virgo Press, 1973.
43. Perkins, G.: Signs by which to diagnose congenital dislocation of the hip. Clin. Orthop. 274:3–5, 1992.
44. Bigg-Wither, G., and P. Kelly: Diagnostic imaging in musculoskeletal physiotherapy. In Refshauge, K., and E. Gass (eds.): Musculoskeletal Physiotherapy. Oxford, Butterworth Heinemann, 1995.
45. Harke, H.T., and S.J. Kumar: The role of ultrasound in the diagnosis and management of congenital and dysplasia of the hip. J. Bone Joint Surg. Br. 73:622–628, 1991.

General References

Andersson, G.: Hip assessment: A comparison of nine different methods. J. Bone Joint Surg. Br. 54:621–625, 1972.

Bassett, L.W., R.H. Gold, and L.L. Seeger: MRI Atlas of the Musculoskeletal System. London, Martin Dunitz Ltd., 1989.

Beetham, W.P., H.F. Polley, C.H. Slocumb, and W.F. Weaver: Physical Examination of the Joints. Philadelphia, W.B. Saunders Co., 1965.

Bertol, P., M.F. Macnicol, and G.P. Mitchell: Radiographic features of neonatal congenital dislocation of the hip. J. Bone Joint Surg. Br. 64:176–179, 1982.

Bos, C.F.A., J.L. Bloem, W.R. Obermann, and P.M. Roging: Magnetic resonance imaging in congenital dislocation of the hip. J. Bone Joint Surg. Br. 70:174–178, 1988.

Brignall, C.G., and G.D. Stainky: The snapping hip. J. Bone Joint Surg. Br. 73:253–254, 1991.

Broughton, N.S., D.I. Brougham, W.G. Cole, and M.B. Menelaus: Reliability of radiological measurements in the assessment of the child's hip. J. Bone Joint Surg. Br. 71:6–8, 1989.

Bryant, M.J., W.G. Kernehan, J.R. Nixon, and R.A. Mellan: A statistical analysis of hip scores. J. Bone Joint Surg. Br. 75:705–709, 1993.

Caborn, D.N., L.J. Grollman, J.A. Nyland, and T. Brosky: Running. In Fu, F.H., and D.A. Stone (eds.): Sports Injuries: Mechanisms, Prevention, Treatment. Baltimore, Williams & Wilkins, 1994.

Callaghan, J.J., S.H. Dysart, C.F. Savory, and W.J. Hopkinson: Assessing the results of hip replacement: A comparison of five different rating systems. J. Bone Joint Surg. Br. 72:1008–1009, 1990.

Cameron, D.M., and R.W. Bohannon: Relationship between active knee extension and active straight leg raise test measurements. J. Orthop. Sports Phys. Ther. 17:257–259, 1993.

Campbell, J.D.: Injuries to the pelvis, hip, and thigh. In Orthopedic Knowledge Update: Sports Medicine. Rosemont, Illinois, American Academy of Orthopaedic Surgeons, 1994.

Chung, S.M.K.: Hip Disorders in Infants and Children. Philadelphia, Lea & Febiger, 1981.

Clarke, G.R.: Unequal leg length: An accurate method of detection and some clinical results. Rheumatol. Phys. Med. 11:385–390, 1972.

Clarkson, H.M., and G.B. Gilewich: Musculoskeletal Assessment: Joint Range of Motion and Manual Muscle Strength. Baltimore, Williams & Wilkins, 1989.

Crock, H.V.: An atlas of the arterial supply of the head and neck of the femur in man. Clin. Orthop. 152:17–27, 1980.

Crouch, J.E.: Functional Human Anatomy. Philadelphia, Lea & Febiger, 1973.

Cyriax, J.: Textbook of Orthopaedic Medicine, vol. 1: Diagnosis of Soft Tissue Lesions. London, Bailliere Tindall, 1975.

Dalinka, M.K., and L.M. Neustadter: Radiology of the hip. In Steinberg, M.E. (ed.): The Hip and Its Disorders. Philadelphia, W.B. Saunders Co., 1991.

Danbert, R.J.: Clinical assessment and treatment of leg length inequalities. J. Manip. Physiol. Ther. 11:290–295, 1988.

Debrunner, H.N.: Orthopaedic Diagnosis. London, E & S Longman Group Ltd., 1973.

Dorrell, J.H., and A. Catterall: The torn acetabular labrum. J. Bone Joint Surg. Br. 68:400–403, 1986.

D'Souza, L., D. Hynes, and F. McManus: Radiological screening for congenital hip dislocation in the infant 'at risk'. J. Bone Joint Surg. Br. 78:319–320, 1996.

Edelson, R., and P. Stevens: Meralgia paresthetica in children. J. Bone Joint Surg. Am. 76:993–999, 1994.

Ekstrand, J., M. Wiktorsson, P. Oberg, and J. Gillquist: Lower extremity goniometric measurements: A study to determine their reliability. Arch. Phys. Med. Rehabil. 663:171–175, 1982.

Fickel, T.E.: "Snapping hip" and sacroiliac sprain: Example of a cause-effect relationship. J. Manip. Physiol. Ther. 12:390–392, 1989.

Fisk, J.W., and M.L. Bargent: Clinical and radiological assessment of leg length. N. Z. Med. J. 81:477–480, 1975.

Forrester, D.M., and J.C. Brown: The Radiology of Joint Disease. Philadelphia, W.B. Saunders Co., 1987.

Friberg, O.: Clinical symptoms and biomechanics of lumbar spine and hip joint in leg length inequality. Spine 8:643–651, 1983.

Gajdosik, R.L., M.A. Rieck, D.K. Sullivan, and S.E. Wightman: Comparison of four clinical tests for assessing hamstring muscle length. J. Orthop. Sports Phys. Ther. 18:614–618, 1993.

Gelberman, R.H., M.S. Cohen, B.A. Shaw, J.R. Kasser, P.P. Griffin, and R.H. Wilkinson: The association of femoral retroversion with slipped capital femoral epiphysis. J. Bone Joint Surg. Am. 68:1000–1007, 1986.

Gerberg, L.F.: Nontraumatic hip pain in active children: A critical differential. Phys. Sportsmed. 24:69–74, 1996.

Goddard, N.J., and P.T. Gosling: Intra-articular fluid pressure and pain in osteoarthritis of the hip. J. Bone Joint Surg. Br. 70:52–55, 1988.

Gogia, P.P., and J.H. Braatz: Validity and reliability of leg length measurements. J. Orthop. Sports Phys. Ther. 8:185–188, 1986.

Grieve, G.P.: The hip. Physiotherapy 57:212–219, 1971.

Guidera, K.J., M.E. Einbecker, C.G. Berman, J.A. Ogden, J.A. Arrington, and R. Murtagh: Magnetic resonance imaging evaluation of congenital dislocation of the hips. Clin. Orthop. 261:96–101, 1990.

Harcke, H.T., and S.J. Kumar: The role of ultrasound in the diagnosis and management of congenital dislocation and dysplasia of the hip. J. Bone Joint Surg. Am. 73:622–628, 1991.

Hardcastle, P., and S. Nade: The significance of the Trendelenburg test. J. Bone Joint Surg. Br. 67:741–746, 1985.

Hernandez, R.J., and A.K. Poznanski: CT evaluation of pediatric hip disorders. Orthop. Clin. North Am. 16:513–541, 1985.

Hicklin, S.P., and M.C. DePretis: Lower extremity: Hip. In Myers, R.S. (ed.): Saunders Manual of Physical Therapy Practice. Philadelphia, W.B. Saunders Co., 1995.

Hoaglund, F.T., A.C. Yau, and W.L. Wong: Osteoarthritis of the hip and other joints in southern Chinese in Hong Kong. J. Bone Joint Surg. Am. 55:545–557, 1973.

Hoaglund, F.T., and W.D. Low: Anatomy of the femoral neck and head, with comparative data from Caucasians and Hong Kong Chinese. Clin. Orthop. 152:10–16, 1980.

Hollinshead, W.H., and D.B. Jenkins: Functional Anatomy of the Limbs and Back. Philadelphia, W.B. Saunders Co., 1981.

Hoppenfeld, S.: Physical Examination of the Spine and Extremities. New York, Appleton-Century-Crofts, 1976.

Hunt, G.C., W.A. Fromherz, J. Danoff, and T. Waggoner: Femoral transverse torque: An assessment method. J. Orthop. Sports Phys. Ther. 7:319–324, 1986.

Jones, D.A.: Neonatal hip stability and the Barlow test. J. Bone Joint Surg. Br. 73:216–218, 1991.

Judge, R.D., G.D. Zuidema, and F.T. Fitzgerald: Clinical Diagnosis: A Physiological Approach. Boston, Little, Brown and Co., 1982.

Kallio, P.E., E.T. Mah, B.K. Foster, D.C. Paterson, and G.W. LeQuesne: Slipped capital femoral epiphysis: Incidence and clinical assessment of physical instability. J. Bone Joint Surg. Br. 77:752–755, 1995.

Kaltenborn, F.M.: Mobilization of the Extremity. Oslo, Olaf Norlis Bokhandel, 1980.

Kane, T.J., G. Henry, and D. Furry: A simple roentgenographic measurement of femoral anteversion. J. Bone Joint Surg. Am. 74:1540–1542, 1992.

Kapandji, I.A.: The Physiology of the Joints, vol. 2: Lower Limb. New York, Churchill Livingstone, 1970.

Kernohan, W.G., G.E. Nugent, P.E. Haugh, B.P. Trainor, and R.A. Mollan: Sensitivity of manual palpation in testing the neonatal hip. Clin. Orthop. 294:211–215, 1993.

Kopell, H.P., and W.A. Thompson: Peripheral entrapment neuropathies of the lower extremity. New Engl. J. Med. 262:56–60, 1960.

Landon, G.C., and J.O. Galante: Physical examination of the hip joint. In Post, M. (ed.): Physical Examination of the Musculoskeletal System. Chicago, Year Book Medical Publishers, 1987.

Larson, C.B.: Rating scale for hip disabilities. Clin. Orthop. 31:85–93, 1963.

Lausten, G.S., F. Jorgensen, and J. Boesen: Measurement of anteversion of the femoral neck: Ultrasound and computerized tomography compared. J. Bone Joint Surg. Br. 71:237–239, 1989.

McGann, W.A.: History and physical examination. In Steinberg, M.E. (ed.): The Hip and Its Disorders. Philadelphia, W.B. Saunders Co., 1991.

McRae, R.: Clinical Orthopaedic Examination. New York, Churchill Livingstone, 1976.

Milch, H.: The measurement of hip motion in the sagittal and coronal planes. J. Bone Joint Surg. Am. 41:731–736, 1959.

Montgomery, W.H., M. Pink, and J. Perry: Electromyographic analysis of hip and knee musculature during running. Am. J. Sports Med. 22:272–278, 1994.

Morscher, E., and G. Figner: Measurement of leg length. Prog. Orthop. Surg. 1:21–27, 1977.

Moseley, C.F.: The biomechanics of the pediatric hip. Orthop. Clin. North Am. 11:3–16, 1980.

Murphy, S.B., S.R. Simon, P.K. Kijewski, R.H. Wilkinson, and N.T. Griscom: Femoral anteversion. J. Bone Joint Surg. Am. 69:1169–1176, 1987.

Nichols, P.J.R., and N.T.J. Bailey: The accuracy of measuring leg length difference: An "observer error" experiment. Br. Med. J. 2:1247–1248, 1955.

O'Donoghue, D.H.: Treatment of Injuries to Athletes, 4th ed. Philadelphia, W.B. Saunders Co., 1984.

Pavlov, H.: Roentgen examination of groin and hip pain in the athlete. Clin. Sports Med. 6:829–843, 1987.

Pearrsal, A.W.: Assessing acute hip injury: Examination, diagnosis and triage. Phys. Sportsmed. 23:36–48, 1995.

Pellecchia, G.L., N. Lugo-Larcheveque, and P.A. DeLuca: Differential diagnosis in physical therapy evaluation of thigh pain in an adolescent boy. J. Orthop. Sports Phys. Ther. 23:51–55, 1996.

Peterson, H.A., R.A. Klassen, R.A. McLeod, and A.D. Hoffman: The use of computerized tomography in dislocation of the hip and femoral neck anteversion in children. J. Bone Joint Surg. Br. 63:198–208, 1981.

Pitt, M.J., P.J. Lund, and D.P. Speer: Imaging of the pelvis and hip. Orthop. Clin. North Am. 21:545–559, 1990.

Poggi, J.J., J.J. Callahan, C.E. Spritzer, T. Roark, and R.D. Goldner: Changes on magnetic resonance images after traumatic hip dislocation. Clin. Orthop. 319:249–259, 1995.

Radin, E.L.: Biomechanics of the hip. Clin. Orthop. 152:28–34, 1980.

Rask, M.R.: Superior gluteal nerve entrapment syndrome. Muscle Nerve 3:304–307, 1980.

Reigger-Krugh, C., and J.J. Keysor: Skeletal malalignments of the lower quarter: Correlated and compensatory motions and postures. J. Orthop. Sports Phys. Ther. 23:164–170, 1996.

Roach, K.E., and T.P. Miles: Normal hip and knee active range of motion: The relationship to age. Phys. Ther. 71:656–665, 1991.

Rydell, N.: Biomechanics of the hip. Clin. Orthop. 92:6–15, 1973.

Sanders, B., and W.C. Nemeth: Hip and thigh injuries. In Zachazewski, J.E., D.J. Magee, and W.S. Quillen: Athletic Injuries and Rehabilitation. Philadelphia, W.B. Saunders Co., 1996.

Schaberg, J.E., M.C. Harper, and W.C. Allen: The snapping hip syndrome. Am. J. Sports Med. 12:361–365, 1984.

Schmalzried, T.P., H.C. Amstutz, and F.J. Dorey: Nerve palsy associated with total hip replacement. J. Bone Joint Surg. Am. 73:1074–1080, 1991.

Siffert, R.S.: Lower limb-length discrepancy. J. Bone Joint Surg. Am. 69:1100–1106, 1987.

Staheli, L.T.: Torsional deformity. Pediatr. Clin. North Am. 33:1373–1383, 1986.

Starkey, C., and J. Ryan: Evaluation of Orthopedic and Athletic Injuries. Philadelphia, F.A. Davis Co., 1996.

Swain, R., and S. Snodgrass: Managing groin pain: Even when the cause is not obvious. Phys. Sportsmed. 23:55–66, 1995.

Tomberlin, J.P., and H.D. Saunders: Evaluation, Treatment, and Prevention of Musculoskeletal Disorders. Chaska, Minnesota, The Saunders Group, 1994.

Wadsworth, C.T.: Manual Examination and Treatment of the Spine and Extremities. Baltimore, Williams & Wilkins, 1988.

Waters, P.M., and M.B. Mills: Hip and pelvic injuries in the young athlete. In Stanitski, C.L., J.C. DeLee, and D. Drez (eds.): Pediatric and Adolescent Sports Medicine. Philadelphia, W.B. Saunders Co., 1994.

Wiessman, B.N.W., and C.B. Sledge: Orthopedic Radiology. Philadelphia, W.B. Saunders Co., 1986.

Williams, P.L., and Warwick, P. (eds.): Gray's Anatomy, 36th British ed. Edinburgh, Churchill Livingstone, 1980.

Yoshioka, Y., and T.D. Cooke: Femoral anteversion: Assessment based on functional axes. J. Orthop. Res. 5:86–91, 1987.

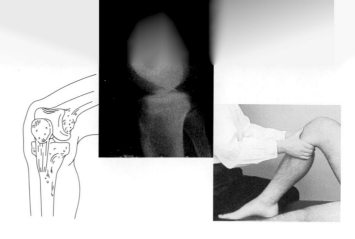

12

Knee

The knee joint is particularly susceptible to traumatic injury because it is located at the ends of two long lever arms, the tibia and the femur. In addition, because the joint connects one long bone "sitting" on another long bone, it depends on the ligaments and muscles that surround it for its strength and stability, not on its bony configuration.

Because the knee joint depends on its ligaments to such a great extent, it is imperative that the ligaments be tested during the examination of the knee. Therefore, the ligamentous tests are not included under Special Tests but instead are listed in a separate section to ensure that testing of the ligaments is always included in the examination of the knee.

Because of its anatomic arrangement, the knee is a complicated area to assess, and the examiner must take time to ensure that all of the relevant structures are tested. It must also be remembered that the lumbar spine, hip, and ankle may refer pain to the knee, and these joints must be assessed if it appears that joints other than the knee may be involved. For example, a slipped capital femoral epiphysis at the hip commonly refers pain to the knee, and this pain may predominate.

Applied Anatomy

The **tibiofemoral joint** is the largest joint in the body. It is a modified hinge joint having three degrees of freedom. The synovium around the joint is extensive; it communicates with many of the bursae and pouches around the knee joint. Although the synovial membrane "encapsulates" the entire knee joint, its distribution within the knee is such that the cruciate ligaments, which run from the middle of the tibial plateau to the intercondylar area of the femur, are extrasynovial. ("Cruciate" means that the ligaments cross each other.)

The articular surfaces of the tibia and femur are not congruent, which enables the two bones to move different amounts, guided by the muscles and ligaments. The two bones approach congruency in full extension, which is the close packed position. Kaltenborn[1] has stated that the close packed position includes full lateral rotation of the tibia. The lateral femoral condyle projects anteriorly more than the medial femoral condyle to help prevent lateral dislocation of the patella. In females, this enlargement is important because of the female's broader pelvis and increased inward angle of the femur, which allow the femoral condyles to be parallel with the ground (Fig. 12–1). The resting position of the joint is approximately 25° of flexion, and the capsular pattern is flexion more limited than extension.

Tibiofemoral Joint	
Resting position:	25° flexion
Close packed position:	Full extension, lateral rotation of tibia
Capsular pattern:	Flexion, extension

The space between the tibia and femur is partially filled by two menisci that are attached to the tibia to add congruency. The **medial meniscus** is a small part of a large circle (i.e., C-shaped) and is thicker posteriorly than anteriorly. The **lateral meniscus** is a large part of a small circle (i.e., O-shaped) and is generally of equal thickness throughout. Both menisci are thicker along the periphery and thinner along the inner margin.

During the movement from extension to flexion, both menisci move posteriorly, the lateral meniscus being displaced more than the medial meniscus. The menisci are avascular in their cartilaginous inner two thirds and are partly vascular and fibrous in their outer one

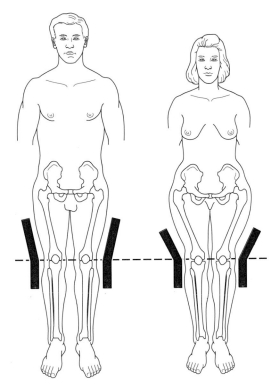

Figure 12–1
Q-angle differences in males and females. Because of the broader pelvis in the female, it is necessary for the femur to come inward at an increased angle to make the distal end of the condyles parallel with the ground. The quadriceps, patella, and patellar tendon form an angle centered at the patella. As the quadriceps contracts, the angle tends to straighten, which forces the patella laterally. (Redrawn from O'Donoghue, D.H.: Treatment of Injuries to Athletes, 4th ed. Philadelphia, W.B. Saunders Co., 1984, p. 522.)

third.[2] They are held in place by the coronary ligaments attaching to the tibia.

The menisci serve several functions in the knee. They aid in lubrication and nutrition of the joint and act as shock absorbers, spreading the stress over the articular cartilage and decreasing cartilage wear. They make the joint surfaces more congruent and improve weight distri-

bution by increasing the area of contact between the condyles. The menisci reduce friction during movement and aid the ligaments and capsule in preventing hyperextension. The menisci prevent the joint capsule from entering the joint and participate in the "locking" mechanism of the joint by directing the movement of the femoral articular condyles. Because more recent literature indicates that removal of the entire meniscus can lead to early degeneration of the joint,[3, 4] most surgeons today remove only the torn portion of the meniscus, or, if the tear is in the outer one third, the surgeon may attempt to surgically repair (suture) the meniscus.

Because the meniscus possesses minimal innervation, there is minimal or no pain when it is damaged unless the coronary ligaments have been damaged as well. Because the menisci are primarily avascular, especially in the inner two thirds, there is seldom bloody effusion in injury; however, there may be synovial effusion. Their poor blood supply, especially in the inner two thirds, gives them a low regeneration potential.

The lateral meniscus is not as firmly attached to the tibia as the medial meniscus and therefore is less prone to injury. The coronary ligaments, also referred to as the meniscotibial ligaments, tend to be longer on the lateral aspect, and the horns of the lateral meniscus are closer together. The lateral meniscus has an excursion of 10 mm, and the medial meniscus has an excursion of 2 mm.

The **patellofemoral joint** is a modified plane joint, the lateral articular surface of the patella being wider. The patella contains the thickest layer of cartilage in the body. It has five facets, or ridges: superior, inferior, lateral, medial, and odd. It is the odd facet that is most frequently the first part of the patella to be affected in chondromalacia patellae (i.e., premature degeneration of the patellar cartilage) or patellofemoral syndrome.

During the movement from flexion to extension, different parts of the patella articulate with the femoral condyles (Fig. 12–2).[5, 6] The odd facet does not come into contact with the femoral condyles until at least 135°

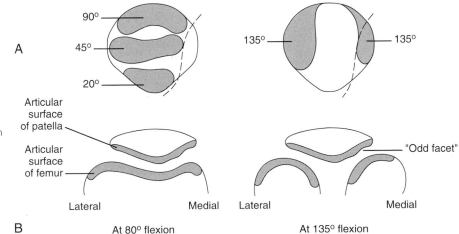

Figure 12–2
(A) Area of contact of the patella during different degrees of flexion. (B) Articulation between patella and femur.

of flexion is reached. Incorrect alignment or malalignment of the patellar movement over the femoral condyles can lead to patellofemoral arthralgia. The capsule of this joint is continuous with the capsule of the tibiofemoral joint.

The **patella** improves the efficiency of extension during the last 30° of extension (i.e., 30 to 0° of extension, with the straight leg being 0°), because it holds the quadriceps tendon away from the axis of movement. The patella also functions as a guide for the quadriceps tendon, decreases friction of the quadriceps mechanism, controls capsular tension in the knee, acts as a bony shield for the cartilage of the femoral condyles, and improves the aesthetic appearance of the knee.

Patellar Loading with Activity

Walking:	0.3 times the body weight
Climbing stairs:	2.5 times the body weight
Descending stairs:	3.5 times the body weight
Squatting:	7 times the body weight

The **superior tibiofibular joint** is a plane synovial joint between the tibia and the head of the fibula. Movement occurs in this joint with any activity involving the ankle. Hypomobility at this joint can lead to pain in the knee area on activity, because the fibula can bear up to one sixth of the body weight. In approximately 10% of the population, the capsule of this joint is continuous with that of the tibiofemoral joint.

Patient History

In addition to the questions listed under Patient History in Chapter 1, the examiner should obtain the following information from the patient:

1. How did the accident occur or what was the mechanism of injury? The primary mechanisms of injury in the knee are a valgus force (with or without rotation), hyperextension, flexion with posterior translation, and a varus force.[7] The first often results in injury to the medial collateral ligament, frequently accompanied by injury to the posteromedial capsule, medial meniscus, and anterior cruciate ("terrible triad"). The second leads to anterior cruciate injuries, often associated with meniscus tears. The third mechanism of injury often involves the posterior cruciate ligament, and the fourth mechanism involves the lateral collateral ligament, the posterolateral capsule, and the posterior cruciate ligament. Was the injury the result of trauma, such as a direct or an indirect blow? Was the patient bearing weight at the time of injury? From which direction did the injuring force come? For example, meniscal injuries, especially

those on the medial side, occur as a result of a torsion injury that combines compression and rotation. Slowly developing forces tend to cause bony avulsions, whereas rapidly developing forces tend to tear ligaments. Table 12–1 lists typical mechanisms of injury to the knee and the structures injured. The lower limb may be viewed as an open (foot off the ground) or a closed (foot on the ground) kinetic chain. There is less chance of injury when the lower limb is an open kinetic chain. As a closed kinetic chain, the lower limb is an encapsulated system in which all parts work in concert. Forces applied to one part of the chain must be absorbed by that part as well as by other parts of the closed chain. If the forces are too great, injury results.

2. Has the knee been injured before, or does it have any feeling of weakness?

3. What is the patient able or unable to do functionally? Is there disability on running, cutting, pivoting, twisting, climbing, or descending stairs? Positive responses to these questions should alert the examiner to instability or meniscus problems.[8]

4. Is there any "clicking," or was there a "pop" when the injury occurred? A distinct pop may indicate an anterior cruciate ligament tear or osteochondral fracture.

5. Did the injury occur during acceleration, during deceleration, or when the patient was moving at a constant speed? Acceleration and twisting injuries may involve the meniscus. Deceleration injuries often involve the cruciate ligaments. Constant speed with cutting may involve the anterior cruciate ligament.

6. Is there any pain? If so, where? What type is it? Is it diffuse? Aching? Retropatellar? Aching pain may indicate degenerative changes, whereas sharp, "catching" pain usually indicates a mechanical problem. Arthritic pain is more likely to be associated with stiffness in the morning and eases with activity. Pain at rest is not usually mechanical in origin. Pain during activity is usually seen in structural abnormalities such as subluxation or patellar tracking disorders. Pain after activity is characteristic of inflammatory disorders such as synovial plica irritation or early tendinitis. Generalized pain in the area of the knee is usually characteristic of contusions or partial tears of muscles or ligaments. Instability rather than pain tends to be the major presenting factor in complex ligament disruptions. Pain in the knee on ankle movements may implicate the superior tibiofibular joint.

7. Do certain positions or activities have an increased or decreased effect on the pain? Which activities produce pain? How much activity is needed to produce pain? Which positions or activities ease the pain? Does the pain go away when activity ceases? The examiner must take note of constant pain that is unrelated to activity, time, or posture, because it is usually indicative of serious pathology such as a tumor. Does the patient have confidence in the knee? Such a question gives the examiner some idea of the functional impairment from the patient's perspective.[9]

Table 12–1
Mechanisms of Injury to the Knee and Possible Structures Injured

Mechanism of Injury	Structure Possibly Injured
Varus or valgus contact without rotation	1. Collateral ligament 2. Epiphyseal fracture 3. Patellar dislocation or subluxation
Varus or valgus contact with rotation	1. Collateral and cruciate ligaments 2. Collateral ligaments and patellar dislocation or subluxation 3. Meniscus tear
Blow to patellofemoral joint, or fall on flexed knee, foot dorsiflexed	1. Patellar articular injury or osteochondral fracture
Blow to tibial tubercle, or fall on flexed knee, foot plantar flexed	1. Posterior cruciate ligament
Anterior blow to tibia, resulting in knee hyperextension	1. Anterior cruciate ligament 2. Anterior and posterior cruciate ligament
Noncontact hyperextension	1. Anterior cruciate ligament 2. Posterior capsule
Noncontact deceleration	1. Anterior cruciate ligament
Noncontact deceleration, with tibial medial rotation or femoral lateral rotation on fixed tibia	1. Anterior cruciate ligament
Noncontact, quickly turning one way with tibia rotated in opposite direction	1. Patellar dislocation or subluxation
Noncontact, rotation with varus or valgus loading	1. Meniscus injury
Noncontact, compressive rotation	1. Meniscus injury 2. Osteochondral fracture
Hyperflexion	1. Meniscus (posterior horn) 2. Anterior cruciate ligament
Forced medial rotation	1. Meniscus injury (lateral meniscus)
Forced lateral rotation	1. Meniscus injury (medial meniscus) 2. Medial collateral ligament and possibly anterior cruciate ligament 3. Patellar dislocation
Flexion-varus-medial rotation	1. Anterolateral instability
Flexion-varus-lateral rotation	1. Anteromedial instability
Dashboard injury	1. Isolated posterior cruciate ligament 2. Posterior cruciate ligament and posterior capsule 3. Posterolateral instability 4. Posteromedial instability 5. Patellar fracture 6. Tibial fracture (proximal) 7. Tibial plateau fracture 8. Acetabular and pelvic fracture

Adapted from Clancy, W.G.: Evaluation of acute knee injuries. American Association of Orthopaedic Surgeons, Symposium on Sports Medicine: The Knee. St. Louis, C.V. Mosby, 1985; and Strobel, M., and H.W. Stedtfeld: Diagnostic Evaluation of the Knee. Berlin, Springer-Verlag, 1990.

8. Does the knee "give way"?[9] This finding usually indicates instability in the knee, meniscus pathology, patellar subluxation (if present when rotation or stopping is involved), undisplaced osteochondritis dissecans, patellofemoral syndrome, plica, or loose body. Giving way when walking uphill or downhill is more likely the result of a retropatellar lesion.[8] If the patient complains that the patella "slips out of place," it may be because of patellar subluxation or a pathological plica.[10]

9. Has the knee ever locked? True locking of the knee is rare. Loose bodies may cause recurrent locking. Locking must be differentiated from catching, which is momentary locking or giving way as a result of reflex inhibition or pain.[10] **Locking** in the knee usually means that the knee cannot fully extend, and it is related to meniscus pathology. Hamstring muscle spasm may also limit extension and is sometimes referred to as **spasm locking.**

10. On movement, is there any grating or clicking in the knee? Grating or clicking may be caused by degeneration or by one structure's snapping over another.

11. Is the joint swollen? Does the swelling occur with activity or several hours after activity, or does the joint feel tight at rest? Swelling with activity may be caused by instability, and tightness at rest may be caused by arthritic changes or patellofemoral dysfunction. Is the

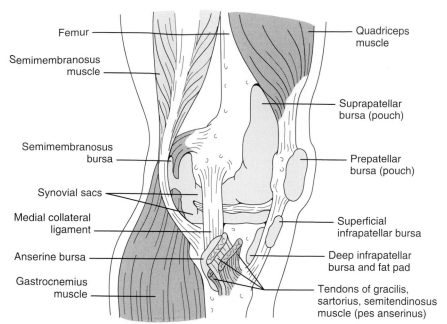

Figure 12–3
The bursae around the knee (medial aspect).

swelling recurrent? If so, what activity causes it? Swelling with pivoting or twisting may be a result of meniscus problems or instability at the tibiofemoral joint. Recurrent swelling caused by climbing or descending slopes or stairs may be related to patellofemoral dysfunction.[10] Often, there is no swelling in the knee after severe injury, because the fluid extravasates into the soft tissues surrounding the joint and because a number of structures around the knee joint are avascular and can be injured without bloody swelling occurring. Synovial swelling may occur 8 to 24 hours after the injury; swelling caused by blood begins to occur almost immediately. Localized swelling may be caused by an inflamed bursa (Fig. 12–3).

12. Is the gait normal? Does the patient put weight on the limb? Can the patient extend the knee while walking? Is the stride length altered on the affected limb? All these questions give an indication of the patient's functional disability and how much the knee is bothering the patient.

13. What type of shoes does the patient wear? Shoes with negative heels (e.g., "earth shoes") can increase the incidence of patellofemoral syndrome.

Observation

For a proper observation, the patient must be suitably undressed so that the examiner can observe the posture of the spine as well as the hips, knees, and ankles. Initially, the examiner should note whether the patient puts weight on the affected limb or stands with only a slight amount of weight on the affected side. In addition to the common observational items mentioned in Chapter 1, the examiner should look for the following alterations around the knee.

Anterior View, Standing

From the anterior aspect (Fig. 12–4), the examiner should note any malalignment, including **genu varum** (bowleg) or **genu valgum** (knock-knee) deformity (Fig. 12–5). Any observable malalignment may lead to or be the result of malalignment elsewhere (Table 12–2).[11]

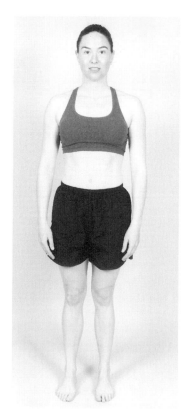

Figure 12–4
Anterior view of the lower limbs.

Figure 12–5

Genu varum and genu valgum. (A) Tibia vara of proximal third. Genu varum deformity located mainly in proximal tibia. Along with lateral tibial torsion and medial femoral torsion, this gives a "bandy-legged" appearance. (B) Genu varum of entire lower extremities. (C) Genu valgum deformity of both lower extremities. (From Hughston, J.C., W.M. Walsh, and G. Puddu: Patellar Subluxation and Dislocation. Philadelphia, W.B. Saunders Co., 1984, p. 221.)

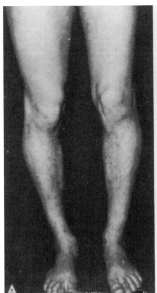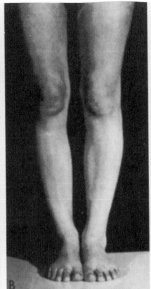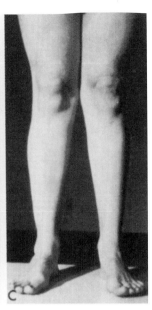

Table 12–2
Malalignment About the Knee and Possible Correlated and Compensatory Motions or Postures

Malalignment	Possible Correlated Motions or Postures	Possible Compensatory Motions or Postures
Genu valgum	Pes planus Excessive subtalar pronation Lateral tibial torsion Lateral patellar subluxation Excessive hip adduction Ipsilateral hip excessive medial rotation Lumbar spine contralateral rotation	Forefoot varus Excessive subtalar supination to allow the lateral heel to contact the ground In-toeing to decrease lateral pelvic sway during gait Ipsilateral pelvic lateral rotation
Genu varum	Excessive lateral angulation of the tibia in the frontal plane; tibial varum Medial tibial torsion Ipsilateral hip lateral rotation Excessive hip abduction	Forefoot valgus Excessive subtalar pronation to allow the medial heel to contact the ground Ipsilateral pelvic medial rotation
Genu recurvatum	Ankle plantar flexion Excessive anterior pelvic tilt	Posterior pelvic tilt Flexed trunk posture Excessive thoracic kyphosis
Lateral tibial torsion	Out-toeing Excessive subtalar supination with related rotation along the lower quarter	Functional forefoot varus Excessive subtalar pronation with relaxed rotation along the lower quarter
Medial tibial torsion	In-toeing Metatarsus adductus Excessive subtalar pronation with related rotation along the lower quarter	Functional forefoot valgus Excessive subtalar supination with relaxed rotation along the lower quarter
Excessive tibial retroversion (posterior slant of tibial plateaus)	Genu recurvatum	
Inadequate tibial retrotorsion (posterior deflection of proximal tibia due to hamstrings pull)	Flexed knee posture	
Inadequate tibial retroflexion (bowing of the tibia)	Altered alignment of Achilles tendon causing altered associated joint motion	
Bowleg deformity of the tibia (tibial varum)	Medial tibial torsion	Forefoot valgus Excessive subtalar pronation

From Riegger-Krugh, C., and J.J. Keysor: Skeletal malalignments of the lower quarter: Correlated and compensatory motions and postures. J. Orthop. Sports Phys. Ther. 23:166–167, 1996.

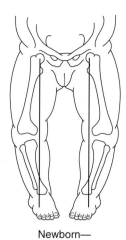

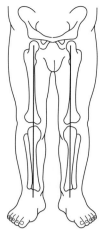

Newborn—
moderate genu varum

6 months—
minimal genu varum

1 year, 7 months—
legs straight

Figure 12-6

Physiological evolution of lower limb alignment at various ages in infancy and childhood. (Redrawn from Tachdjian, M.O.: Pediatric Orthopedics. Philadelphia, W.B. Saunders Co., 1972, p. 1463.)

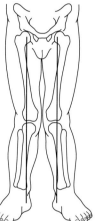

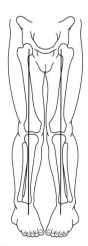

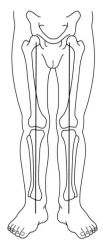

2 years, 6 months—
physiological genu valgum

Protective toeing-in

4 to 6 years—
legs straight with normal toeing-out

These deformities may be unilateral or bilateral. If two or more fingers fit between the knees when the ankles are together, the patient has a varus deformity.[12] Although in adults the legs should be relatively straight, in the child, the normal development of the knee is from genu varum to straight, to genu valgum, and then to straight. Initially, a child's lower limbs are in genu varum until 18 or 19 months, when they straighten. The knee then goes into genu valgum until about 3 to 4 years of age (Fig. 12–6). The limbs should be almost straight by age 6 and should remain that way. In the adult, the knee is normally in approximately 6° of valgus.

To observe genu varum and genu valgum, the patient is positioned so that the patellae face forward and the medial aspects of the knees and medial malleoli of both limbs are as close together as possible. If the knees touch and the ankles do not, the patient has a genu

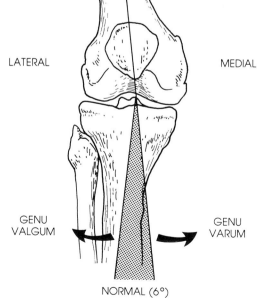

Figure 12-7

Normal tibiofemoral shaft angle.

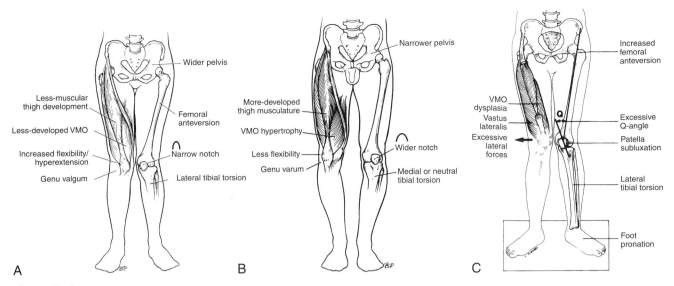

Figure 12–8

(A) Normal female alignment with wider pelvis, femoral anteversion, genu valgum, hyperflexibility, lateral tibial torsion, and narrow notch. (B) Normal male alignment demonstrates a narrower pelvis, more developed musculature, genu varum, medial or neutral tibial torsion, and wider notch. (C) Miserable malalignment syndrome is a term coined to describe patients who have increased femoral anteversion, genu valgum, vastus medialis obliquus (VMO) dysplasia, lateral tibial torsion, and forefoot pronation. These factors create excessive lateral forces and contribute to patellofemoral dysfunction. (From Griffin, L.Y. [ed.]: Rehabilitation of the Injured Knee. St. Louis, C.V. Mosby Co., 1995, pp. 298–299.)

valgum. A distance of 9 to 10 cm (3.5 to 4 inches) between the ankles is considered excessive. If the ankles touch and the knees do not, the patient has a genu varum. On x-ray studies, the normal **tibiofemoral shaft angle** is approximately 6° (Fig. 12–7).

Alignment is often different between males and females. Some of these misalignments, if excessive, can lead to patellofemoral symptoms. These excessive differences are sometimes referred to as **miserable malalignment syndrome** (Fig. 12–8).

The patient is asked to extend the knees to see whether the movement can be performed and what effect it has on the knee. Both knees should extend equally. If not, something must be limiting the movement (swelling, loose body, or meniscus). Normally, a person does not stand with the knees fully extended. If, however, the patient has an excessive lordosis, the knees are often hyperextended to maintain the center of gravity. This change can lead to posterior knee pain.

Is there any apparent swelling in the knees? If there is intracapsular swelling, or at least sufficient swelling, the knee assumes a position of 15 to 25° of flexion, which provides the synovial cavity with the maximum capacity to hold fluid. This position is also called the **resting position** of the knee.

Is the swelling intracapsular or extracapsular? Intracapsular swelling is evident over the entire joint; extracapsular swelling tends to be more localized. An example

of extracapsular swelling is shown in Figure 12–9, which illustrates **prepatellar bursitis**.

The examiner should ask the patient to contract the quadriceps muscles to see whether there is any visible wasting of the muscles, especially of the vastus medialis obliquus. The prominence of the vastus medialis results from the obliquity of the distal fibers, the inferior position of its insertion, and the thinness of the fascial covering compared with the other quadriceps muscles. Muscle defects (third-degree strain or rupture) should also be watched for when the patient contracts the muscles.

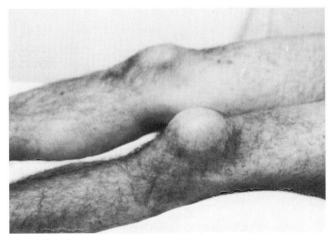

Figure 12–9

Prepatellar bursitis.

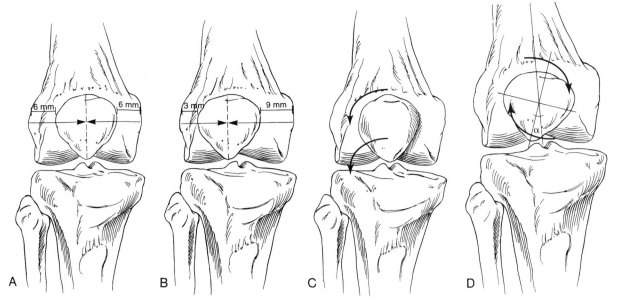

Figure 12–10

Assessment of the patellar glide component. Ideally, the patella should be centered on the superior portion of the femoral articular surface at 20° flexion. (A) Ideal alignment. (B) Lateral glide of the patella. (C) Lateral tilt of the patella. (D) Lateral rotation of inferior pole of patella. (From McConnell, J., and J. Fulkerson: The knee: Patellofemoral and soft tissue injuries. *In* Zachazewski, J.E., D.J. Magee, and W.S. Quillen [eds.]: Athletic Injuries and Rehabilitation. Philadelphia, W.B. Saunders Co., 1996, pp. 711–712.)

Third-degree strains may be indicated by muscle "bunching," abnormal mechanics (e.g., unilateral patella alta with patella tendon rupture), or a palpable defect.[10]

The position of the patella should be noted. When viewing the patellae, the examiner should note whether they face straight ahead, tilt outward ("grasshopper eyes" patellae), tilt inward ("squinting" patellae), or are rotated in or out (Fig. 12–10). Rotation and tilt may be caused by tight structures that alter the position of the patella. These tight structures may include muscles (e.g., rectus femoris, iliotibial band, gastrocnemius) or fascia (e.g., lateral retinaculum). Normally, the patellae should face straight ahead with no lateral tilt or rotation. If these deviations are seen in the observation phase, they are considered static problems, and the examiner should test patellar movement passively and watch the patellae during active movements to see whether it is a dynamic problem as well.[13] A squinting or rotated patella may be indicative of medial femoral or lateral tibial torsion (Fig. 12–11). Patients with abnormal torsion are prone to patellofemoral instability.

Any bruising or discoloration around the knee should also be noted, as well as any scars or signs indicating recent injury or surgery.

Lateral View, Standing

The examiner then views the patient from both sides for comparison. It should be noted whether **genu recurva-**

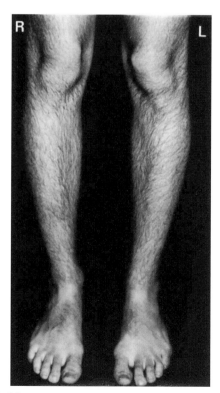

Figure 12–11

"Squinting" patellae, especially prominent on the patient's left knee. Both patellae point inward in a medial fashion, a sign of excessive femoral anteversion or increased medial femoral torsion. (From Carson, W.G., S.L. James, R.L. Larsen, et al.: Patellofemoral disorders: Physical and radiographic evaluation. Part I: Physical examination. Clin. Orthop. 185:169, 1984.)

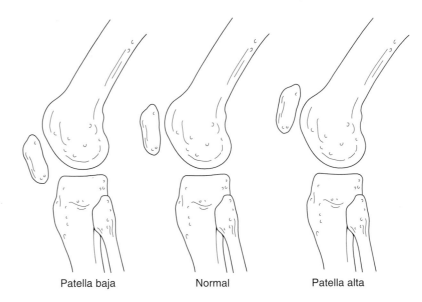

Figure 12–12

The normal patellar posture for exerting deceleration forces in the functional position of 45° of knee flexion places the patellar articular surface squarely against the anterior femur. A lower posture represents patella baja. A higher posture represents patella alta. Patella alta makes the patella less efficient in exerting normal forces. (Redrawn from Hughston, J.C., W.M. Walsh, and G. Puddu: Patellar Subluxation and Dislocation. Philadelphia, W.B. Saunders Co., 1984, p. 8.)

Patella baja   Normal   Patella alta

tum (hyperextended knee) is present and whether one or both patellae are higher **(patella alta)** or lower **(patella baja)** than normal (Fig. 12–12). With an abnormally high patella, a **"camel sign"** may be present (Fig. 12–13); because of the high patella (one "hump"), the infrapatellar fat pad (second hump) becomes more prominent. This finding is especially noticeable in females. In this position, the examiner should also note (Fig. 12–14) whether the inferior pole of the patella is tilted in (inferior tilt). Ideally, the plane of the patella and that of the femoral condyles should be the same. If the inferior pole tilts in, fat pad irritation may occur.[13] Habitual genu

recurvatum may make a patient prone to posterior cruciate tears because of the stretching of the posterior oblique ligament.[10] If one knee (normal) hyperextends and the other one (injured) does not, it may indicate meniscus pathology that is limiting extension. Osteoarthritic lipping (Fig. 12–15) or synovial hypertrophy (rheumatoid arthritis) may also limit movement.

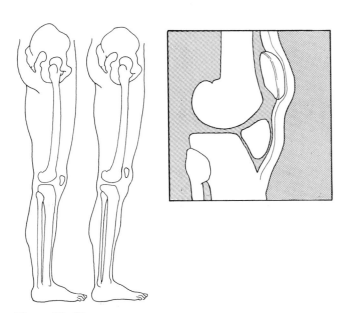

Figure 12–13

Camel sign. Double hump seen from side caused by high-riding patella and uncovered infrapatellar fat pad. (From Hughston, J.C., W.M. Walsh, and G. Puddu: Patellar Subluxation and Dislocation. Philadelphia, W.B. Saunders Co., 1984, p. 22.)

A   B

Figure 12–14

Assessment of the anteroposterior component of the patella. Ideally, the superior and inferior poles of the patella should be parallel in the sagittal plane of the knee (A). Commonly, in individuals with patella malalignment, the inferior patellar pole pushes posteriorly into the infrapatellar fat pad (B). This may irritate the fat pad. (From McConnell, J., and J. Fulkerson: The knee: Patellofemoral and soft tissue injuries. In Zachazewski, J.E., D.J. Magee, and W.S. Quillen [eds.]: Athletic Injuries and Rehabilitation. Philadelphia, W.B. Saunders Co., 1996, pp. 712.)

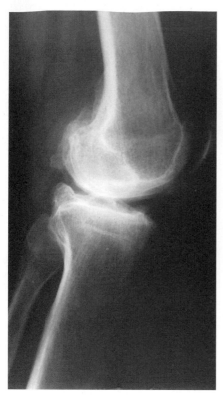

Figure 12–15
Osteophytic lipping in posterior knee limits flexion and produces a bone-to-bone end feel.

Posterior View, Standing

Next, the examiner views the patient from behind, looking for findings similar to those from the anterior aspect.

In addition, the examiner looks for abnormal swellings such as a popliteal (Baker's) cyst, which is caused by herniation of synovial tissue through a weakening in the posterior capsule wall (Fig. 12–16).

Anterior and Lateral Views, Sitting

For the final part of the observation, the patient sits with the knee flexed to 90° and the feet either not bearing weight (on a stool) or dangling free. The patient is observed from the front and from the side. In this position, the patella should face forward and should rest on the distal end of the femur. With patella alta, the patella becomes more aligned with the anterior surface of the femur. If the patella is laterally displaced or laterally displaced with a patella alta, the patellae take on the appearance of "frog eyes" or "grasshopper eyes" (Fig. 12–17), meaning that the patellae face upward and outward, away from each other. Patella alta sometimes causes a concavity proximal to the patella in thin patients.[10] Any bony enlargements such as those seen in Osgood-Schlatter disease (i.e., an enlarged tibial tubercle) should be noted (Fig. 12–18), as should abnormal swelling. Swelling of the pes anserine bursa is best visualized in the seated position.[10]

In the same position, any **tibial torsion** should be noted (Fig. 12–19).[14, 15] If there is tibial torsion, it is medial torsion that is associated with genu varum; genu valgum is associated with lateral tibial torsion. Normally, the forefoot points straight forward or slightly laterally. With medial tibial torsion, the feet point toward each other, resulting in a "pigeon-toed" foot deformity. These deformities can be exacerbated by habitual postures. The

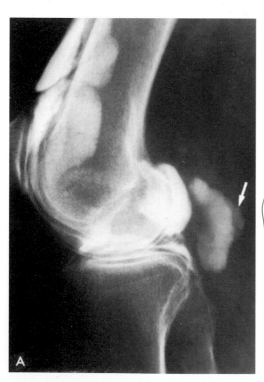

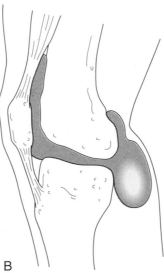

Figure 12–16
Popliteal (Baker's) cysts. (A) This 74-year-old man presented with the acute onset of calf pain and swelling without knee pain. The initial suspected diagnosis was popliteal thrombosis. A venogram was normal. The arthrogram revealed a collection of dye posterior to the joint space—a popliteal cyst (*arrow*). (From Reilly, B.M.: Practical Strategies in Outpatient Medicine. Philadelphia, W.B. Saunders Co., 1991, p. 1179.) (B) Schematic diagram of Baker's cyst.

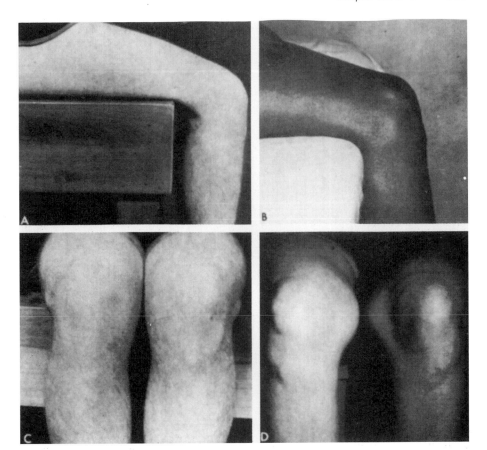

Figure 12–17

(A) Normal knee seen from side; patella faces straight ahead in line with femur. (B) Patella alta seen from side; patella points toward ceiling. (C) Normal patellae seen from front; patellae centered in outline of knees. (D) High and lateral posturing of patellae seen from front, giving "grasshopper eyes" or "frog eyes" appearance. (From Hughston, J.C., W.M. Walsh, and G. Puddu: Patellar Subluxation and Dislocation. Philadelphia, W.B. Saunders Co., 1984, p. 23.)

positions illustrated in Figures 12–20 and 12–21A cause problems only if they are used habitually. Excessive tibial torsion can contribute to conditions such as chondromalacia patellae, patellofemoral instability, and fat pad entrapment. When standing, most people exhibit a lateral tibial torsion, the Fick angle (see Fig. 13–9), which increases as the child grows. This angle is approximately 5° in babies and as much as 18° in adults. To test for

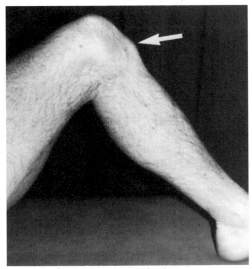

Figure 12–18

Osgood-Schlatter disease (enlarged tibial tuberosity).

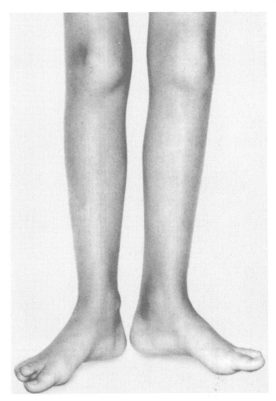

Figure 12–19

Exaggerated lateral tibial torsion. In stance, with the patellae facing straight forward, the feet point outward. (From Tachdjian, M.O.: Pediatric Orthopedics. Philadelphia, W.B. Saunders Co., 1990, p. 2816.)

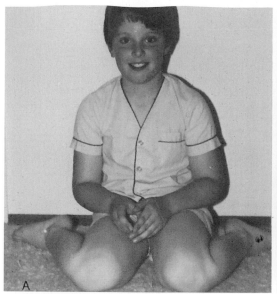
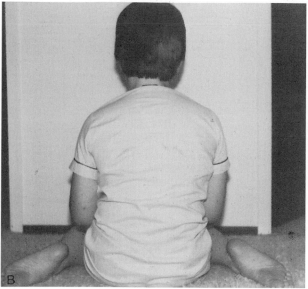

Figure 12–20
"Television" or "W" sitting position may lead to excessive lateral tibial torsion. (A) Anterior view.
(B) Posterior view.

tibial torsion, the examiner aligns the patient's straight legs (knees extended) so that the patellae face straight ahead. The examiner then looks at the feet to determine their angle relative to the shaft of the tibia.

Femoral torsion, or anteversion (discussed in Chapter 11), can also affect the position of the patella relative to the femur and tibia.

Gait

The examiner should also observe the patient's gait (see Chapter 14), noting any differences in stride length, walking speed, cadence, or linear and angular displacement.

In addition, the examiner should watch for abnormal patellar movement, indicating possible patellar tracking problems, and abnormal motion of the tibia relative to the femur, indicating possible instability problems.

Movement at the pelvis, hip, and ankle should also be observed. For example, weak hip abductors (positive Trendelenburg's sign) may lead to increased stress on the knee. If this is combined with medial tibial torsion, patellofemoral syndromes may result.[10, 16] Tight heel cords may result in gait with the knee flexed, which can put extra pressure on the patellofemoral joint. Similarly, pronation of the foot and lateral tibial torsion may lead to patellofemoral pathology or anteromedial joint pain.[10]

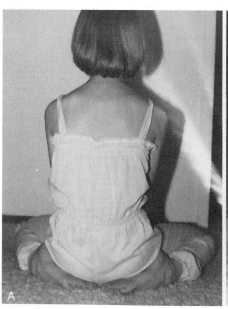
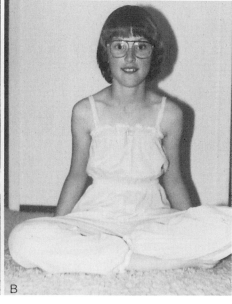

Figure 12–21
Medial tibial torsion. (A) Position to be avoided to prevent excessive medial tibial torsion. (B) Tailor position maintains normal medial tibial torsion.

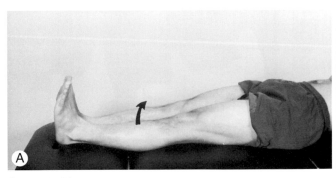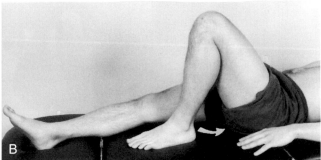

Figure 12-22
Active movements of the knee. (A) Extension. (B) Flexion.

Tight hamstrings result in increased knee flexion, which can lead to the need for more ankle dorsiflexion. If no further dorsiflexion is possible, the foot pronates to compensate, thus increasing the **dynamic Q-angle**.[17]

Examination

Active Movements

The examination is performed initially with the patient sitting and then with the patient in lying position. During the active movements, the examiner should observe (1) the excursion of the patella, to ensure that it tracks freely and smoothly; (2) the range of motion available; (3) whether pain occurs during the movement, and if so, where; and (4) what appears to be limiting the movement. The active movements may be done in the sitting or supine position, and, as always, the most painful movements should be done last (Fig. 12-22).

Active Movements of the Knee Complex

- Flexion (0 to 135°)
- Extension (0 to 15°)
- Medial rotation of the tibia on the femur (20 to 30°)
- Lateral rotation of the tibia on the femur (30 to 40°)
- Repetitive movements (if necessary)
- Sustained postures (if necessary)
- Combined movements (if necessary)

Full knee flexion is 135° (0° being straight knee). As the patient moves the knee through flexion and extension, the examiner should watch the movement of the patella as it "tracks" along the femoral trochlea. The examiner should note whether the movement is smooth from beginning to end or whether there is a lag or abrupt jump of the patella as it attempts to center in the groove.[18] It is important to realize that the patella does not follow a straight path as the knee moves from extension. Normally, it follows a curved pattern (Fig. 12-23). As in the observation phase, the examiner should note whether dynamic movement causes lateral tilt, anteroposterior tilt, or rotation of the patella during movement.[17]

Active knee extension is approximately 0° but may be −15°, especially in women, who are more likely to have hyperextended knees (genu recurvatum). The knee extensor muscles develop the greatest force about 60°, and the knee flexor muscles develop their greatest force at 45 to 10°. To complete the last 15° of knee extension, a 60% increase in force of the quadriceps muscles is required. The examiner should also watch for evidence of **quadriceps lag,** which results from loss of mechanical advantage, muscle atrophy, decreasing power of the muscle as it shortens, adhesion formation, effusion, or reflex inhibition. Active medial rotation of the tibia on

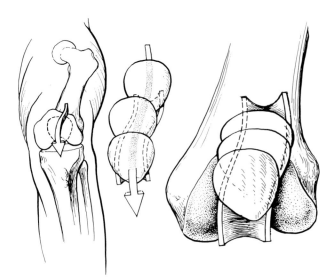

Figure 12-23
Multiplanar patellar path during knee flexion. (From Stanitski, C.L., J.C. DeLee, and D. Drez [ed.]: Pediatric and Adolescent Sports Medicine. Philadelphia, W.B. Saunders Co., 1994, p. 307.)

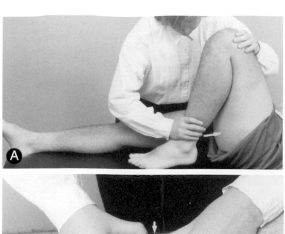

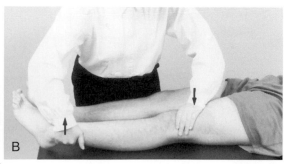

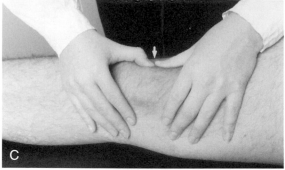

Figure 12–24
Passive movements of the knee. (A) Flexion. (B) Extension.
(C) Patella medial glide.

the femur should be 20 to 30°; active lateral rotation should be 30 to 40°.

If, during the history, the patient has complained that repetitive or combined movements or sustained postures have resulted in symptoms, these movements should also be tested.

Passive Movements

If, on active movements, the range of motion is full, overpressure may gently be applied to test the end feel of the various movements in the tibiofemoral joint. This action would preclude the need to do passive movements to the tibiofemoral joint. However, the examiner must do movements of the patella passively (Fig. 12–24).

At the tibiofemoral joint, the end feel of flexion is tissue approximation; the end feel of extension and of medial and lateral rotation of the tibia on the femur is

---

Passive Movements of the Knee Complex and Normal End Feel

- Flexion (tissue approximation)
- Extension (tissue stretch)
- Medial rotation of tibia on femur (tissue stretch)
- Lateral rotation of tibia on femur (tissue stretch)
- Patellar movement (tissue stretch—all directions)

---

tissue stretch. It must be remembered that during the passive movement, the examiner is also looking for a capsular pattern of the tibiofemoral joint. This pattern is more limitation of flexion than of extension. Passive medial rotation of the tibia on the femur should be approximately 30° when the knee is flexed to 90°. Passive lateral rotation of the tibia on the femur at 90° of knee flexion should be 40°.

Passive medial and lateral movement of the patella is also carried out to determine its mobility and to compare it with the unaffected side. Normally, the patella should move up to half its width medially and laterally in extension (Fig. 12–25). When the patella is pushed from side to side, the examiner should note whether it stays parallel to the femoral condyles or whether it tilts or rotates.[13] For example, if pushed medially when the medial structures are tight, the lateral border of the patella will tilt up. Likewise, tight lateral structures cause the medial border to tilt up. If the lateral structures are tight superiorly, the inferior pole of the patella medially rotates. These are examples of dynamic tilt and rotation problems of the patella. The side-to-side passive motion of the patella should also be tested in 45° of flexion, which is a more functional position and gives a better indication of functional instability of the patella.[19] The end feel of these movements is tissue stretch. Lateral displacement must be done with care, especially in patients who have experienced a dislocated patella.

The examiner must also ensure full and normal flexibility of the quadriceps, hamstring, iliotibial band, and abductor and adductor muscles of the thigh, as well as

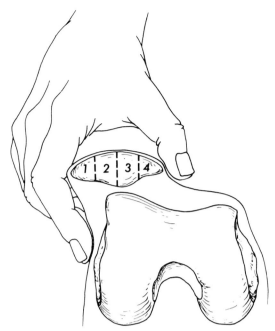

Figure 12–25

Passive lateral glide test demonstrating a patella being subluxed laterally to its second quadrant. Decreased patellar mobility (hypomobile) is manifested by less than one quadrant of medial and lateral glide; movement of more than two quadrants (one half of patellar width) is considered hypermobile. (From Jackson, D.W. [ed.]: The Anterior Cruciate Ligament: Current and Future Concepts. New York, Raven Press, 1993, p. 358.)

the gastrocnemius muscles (Fig. 12–26). Tightness of any of these structures or of the lateral retinaculum can alter gait and postural mechanics, which may lead to pathology. For example, tight hamstrings can contribute to patellofemoral pathology because of increased knee flexion at heel strike and during stance phase.[17] Limitation of hip rotation in extension can lead to patellofemoral pathology as well.[10] If the rectus femoris is tight, full excursion of the patella in the trochlea is not possible, especially if the hip is extended. A tight iliotibial band

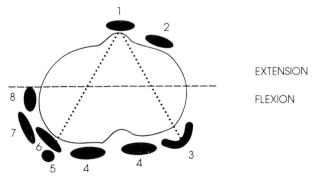

EXTENSION

FLEXION

Figure 12–26

Movement diagram of the knee showing quadriceps hamstrings tripod. 1 = Patellar tendon (quadriceps); 2 = iliotibial band; 3 = biceps femoris; 4 = gastrocnemius; 5 = semitendinosus; 6 = semimembranosus; 7 = gracilis; 8 = sartorius.

can lead to lateral tracking of the patella.[17, 20] Tests for the hamstring, abductor, adductor, and rectus femoris muscles have been described in Chapter 11. A functional test for the quadriceps (described under Special Tests in this chapter) is also a passive movement test (heel to buttock) for the femoral nerve. To test the gastrocnemius muscle, the examiner extends the patient's knee and, while holding it straight, dorsiflexes the patient's ankle. The examiner should be able to reach at least 90° (plantegrade), although 10 to 15° of dorsiflexion is more common.

Resisted Isometric Movements

For a proper test of the muscles, resisted isometric movements must be performed. The patient should be in the supine position (Fig. 12–27).

> **Resisted Isometric Movements of the Knee Complex**
>
> * Flexion of the knee
> * Extension of the knee
> * Ankle plantar flexion
> * Ankle dorsiflexion

Ideally, these resisted isometric movements are performed with the joint in its resting position. Segal and Jacob[21] suggest testing the quadriceps muscle at 0°, 30°, 60°, and 90° while observing any abnormal tibial movement (e.g., ligament instability) or excessive pain from patellar compression (e.g., patellofemoral syndrome). Table 12–3 lists the muscles acting at the knee.

Although these movements are tested with the patient in the supine lying position, the hamstrings are often tested with the patient prone. If the knee is flexed to 90° and the heel is turned out, the greatest stress is placed on the lateral hamstring muscle (biceps femoris) with resisted knee flexion. If the heel is turned in, the greatest stress is placed on the medial hamstring (semimembranosus and semitendinosus) muscles.

Ankle movements are tested because the gastrocnemius muscle crossing the posterior knee and both plantar and dorsiflexion movements cause movement of the fibula. Dorsiflexion causes the fibula to move up and increases the stress being applied to the ligaments supporting the superior tibiofibular joint. Plantar flexion decreases the stress on these ligaments and also brings the gastrocnemius into play, supporting the posterior knee and assisting knee flexion.

If the history has indicated concentric, eccentric, or econcentric movements have caused symptoms, these types of contractions should be tested as well, but only after isometric testing has been performed.

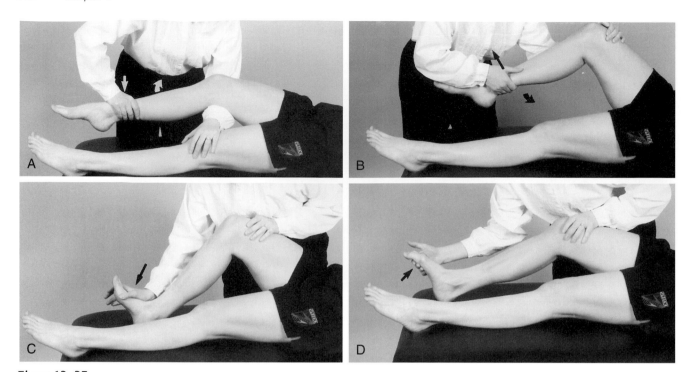

Figure 12–27
Resisted isometric movements of the knee. (A) Knee extension. (B) Knee flexion. (C) Ankle dorsiflexion.
(D) Ankle plantar flexion.

Table 12–3
Muscles of the Knee: Their Actions, Nerve Supply, and Nerve Root Derivation

Action	Muscles Acting	Nerve Supply	Nerve Root Derivation
Flexion of knee	1. Biceps femoris	Sciatic	L5, S1–S2
	2. Semimembranosus	Sciatic	L5, S1–S2
	3. Semitendinosus	Sciatic	L5, S1–S2
	4. Gracilis	Obturator	L2–L3
	5. Sartorius	Femoral	L2–L3
	6. Popliteus	Tibial	L4–L5, S1
	7. Gastrocnemius	Tibial	S1–S2
	8. Tensor fasciae latae (in 45 to 145° of flexion)	Superior gluteal	L4–L5
	9. Plantaris	Tibial	S1–S2
Extension of knee	1. Rectus femoris	Femoral	L2–L4
	2. Vastus medialis	Femoral	L2–L4
	3. Vastus intermedius	Femoral	L2–L4
	4. Vastus lateralis	Femoral	L2–L4
	5. Tensor fasciae latae (in 0 to 30° of flexion)	Superior gluteal	L4–L5
Medial rotation of flexed leg (non–weight bearing)	1. Popliteus	Tibial	L4–L5
	2. Semimembranosus	Sciatic	L5, S1–S2
	3. Semitendinosus	Sciatic	L5, S1–S2
	4. Sartorius	Femoral	L2–L3
	5. Gracilis	Obturator	L2–L3
Lateral rotation of flexed leg (non–weight bearing)	1. Biceps femoris	Sciatic	L5, S1–S2

Scoring Scale for Isokinetic and Isometric Strength Measurements of the Knee Joint

	Peak Torque		Difference		
	Uninjured	*Injured*	*Absolute*	*Percent*	*Score†*
Isokinetic					
Extension 60°/sec	————	————	————	————	————
Flexion 60°/sec	————	————	————	————	————
Extension 180°/sec	————	————	————	————	————
Flexion 180°/sec	————	————	————	————	————
Isometric					
Extension 60°	————	————	————	————	————
Flexion 60°	————	————	————	————	————
Total score (maximum 100 points)					————

†Scoring System
Isokinetic

17 points = per cent difference (uninjured − injured):	≤2%
15 points = per cent difference (uninjured − injured):	3 to 5%
13 points = per cent difference (uninjured − injured):	6 to 10%
9 points = per cent difference (uninjured − injured):	11 to 25%
5 points = per cent difference (uninjured − injured):	26 to 49%
0 points = per cent difference (uninjured − injured):	≥50%

Isometric

16 points = per cent difference (uninjured − injured):	≤2%
14 points = per cent difference (uninjured − injured):	3 to 5%
12 points = per cent difference (uninjured − injured):	6 to 10%
8 points = per cent difference (uninjured − injured):	11 to 25%
4 points = per cent difference (uninjured − injured):	26 to 49%
0 points = per cent difference (uninjured − injured):	≥50%

Figure 12–28
Scoring scale for isokinetic and isometric strength measurements of the knee joint. (Modified from Kannus, P., M. Jarvis, and K. Latvala: Knee strength evaluation. Scand. J. Sport Sci. 9:9, 1987.)

Kannus and colleagues[22] developed a scoring scale for measuring isokinetic and isometric strength (Fig. 12–28). The scale can be used to show improvement in strength over time. When using isokinetic values, different test parameters may be used. It is important to realize, however, that most knee isokinetic tests are not done with the knee in a functional position.

Isokinetic Test Parameters Commonly Used for the Knee

- Left-right peak torque ratio
- Left-right average (mean) torque ratio
- Ratio of peak torque to body weight
- Torque curve analysis
- Bilateral total work comparison
- Hamstrings-quadriceps ratio (left and right)
- Ratio of average power to body weight
- Time ratio to torque development
- Time to 50% peak torque
- Endurance (fatigue) ratio (first to last repetition)

Depending on the speed, the hamstring-quadriceps ratio is normally between 50 and 60%.[23] As the speed of isokinetic testing increases, however, the ratio approaches 100%.[24]

Functional Assessment

Instabilities produced on the examining table are easily produced functionally, especially in athletes who participate in activities such as vigorous cutting and jumping or rapid deceleration, which produce high physiological joint loads. Many numerical knee rating systems have been developed for the knee, many of them for specific populations (e.g., athletes) or to assess outcomes after surgery or for specific conditions. The examiner must pick the appropriate scale, realizing that each has advantages and disadvantages.[25]

Although full knee extension is usually preferable for everyday activities (e.g., standing, walking), full flexion (135°) is not necessary. However, approximately 117° of flexion is necessary for activities such as squatting to tie a shoelace or to pull on a sock. Sitting in a chair requires approximately 90° of flexion, and climbing stairs (average height) requires approximately 80° of flexion.

If the active, passive, and resisted isometric movements are performed with little difficulty, the examiner may put the patient through a series of **functional tests**

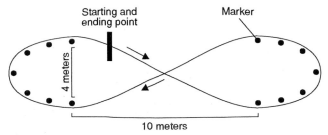

Figure 12–29

Figure-of-eight running track. (Redrawn from Fonseca, S.T., D.J. Magee, J. Wessel, and D.C. Reid: Validation of a performance test for outcome evaluation of knee function. Clin. J. Sport Med. 2:253, 1992.)

to see whether these sequential activities produce pain or other symptoms. These tests may be scored by the time taken to do the test or by the distance or height attained when doing the test. If the results are so measured, three measurements should be taken and averaged. In some cases, the results of different tests may be combined. Fonseca and coworkers[26] found that the time ratio of figure-of-eight running to straight running was one of the most effective ways of differentiating patients with anterior cruciate ligament deficiencies from normal patients (Fig. 12–29).

Sequential Functional Tests for the Knee

- Walking
- Ascending and descending stairs (walking → running)
- Squatting (both knees should flex symmetrically)
- Squatting and then bouncing at the end of the squat (again, the two knees should act symmetrically)
- Running straight ahead
- Running straight ahead and stopping on command
- Vertical jump
- Running and twisting (figure-of-eight running, carioca)
- Jumping and going into a full squat
- Hard cuts, twists, pivots

These functional activities, which are provided as examples, must be geared to the individual patient. Squatting reveals limitations of flexion and may cause impingement with meniscal lesions. Duck waddle, if attempted, can demonstrate increased symptoms in meniscal and ligamentous lesions. Older patients should not be expected to accomplish the last five movements unless they have been doing these or similar activities in the recent past. Daniel and coworkers[27] outlined

Table 12–4
Patient Activity Scale

Functional levels

Level I:	Activities of daily living (ADL)
Level II:	Straight running; sports that do not involve lower-limb agility activities; occupations involving heavy lifting
Level III:	Activities that require lower-limb agility but not involving jumping, hard cutting, or pivoting
Level IV:	Activities involving jumping, hard cutting, or pivoting

Intensity

W:	Work-related or occupational
LR:	Light recreational
VR:	Vigorous recreational
C:	Competitive

Exposure
Number of hours per year of participation at any given functional level and intensity

From Daniel, D., W. Akeson, and J. O'Conner (eds.): Knee Ligaments: Structure, Injury and Repair. New York, Raven Press, 1990, p. 522.

different functional and intensity levels that are useful especially for getting an indication of functional activities from a patient's perspective (Table 12–4). Functional strength tests for sedentary individuals are shown in Table 12–5.

Strobel and Stedtfeld[28] put forward the **one-leg hop test**. The patient stands and does a "long jump" hop on one leg while landing on the same leg. This is a **single-leg hop for distance** (Fig. 12–30A).[29, 30] Noyes and associates[29] considered symmetry of less than 85% between the legs to be abnormal. The test is repeated three times alternately with each leg. If instability is evident, the distance for the affected leg is less than that for the normal leg.

Table 12–5
Functional Testing of the Knee

Starting Position	Action	Functional Test
Standing	1. Walking backward 2. Running forward 20° (knee flexion)	6–8 m: Functional 3–6 m: Functionally fair 1–3 m: Functionally poor 0 m: Nonfunctional
Standing	1. Squat 20 to 30° 2. Jump, lifting body off floor	5 to 6 Repetitions: Functional 3 to 4 Repetitions: Functionally fair 1 to 2 Repetitions: Functionally poor 0 Repetitions: Nonfunctional

Data from Palmar, M.L., and M. Epler: Clinical Assessment Procedures in Physical Therapy. Philadelphia, J.B. Lippincott, 1990, pp. 275–276.

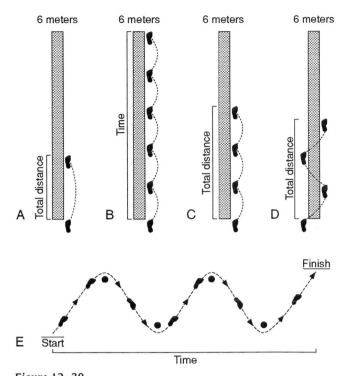

Figure 12–30

Hop tests. (A) Single hop for distance. (B) Timed hop. (C) Triple hop for distance. (D) Crossover hop for distance. (E) 30-m agility hop test.

Since the advent of the single-leg hop, modifications have been developed. Each test is usually repeated three times, and the average of the three scores is used as the measured value. These modifications include the following.

1. **Single-leg hop for time.** With this test, the patient is assessed for the time taken to hop 6 meters (20 ft) on one leg (Fig. 12–30B). The good leg is tested first, followed by the injured leg.[29–31]

2. **Triple hop.** With this test, the patient is asked to hop as far as possible, taking three hops. The distance for the good leg is compared with that for the injured leg (Fig. 12–30C).[29–31]

3. **Crossover hop.** A straight line is marked on the floor. The patient is asked to take three consecutive hops on one foot, crossing over the straight line each time (Fig. 12–30D). The good limb is tested, followed by the injured limb, and the average distances attained with each leg are compared.[29] Risberg and Ekeland[32] modified this test and called it the **side jump test.** For this test, two 6-m parallel lines are placed 30 cm (12 inches) apart on the floor. Outside one line, 10 marks are made at 60-cm (24-inch) intervals. Outside the other line, marks are made at 60-cm (24-inch) intervals but starting at 30 cm (12 inches), so that the marks are staggered from one side to the other. The good leg is timed, followed by the injured leg.

4. **Agility hop.** This hop test requires a space of 30 meters (100 ft). Cones are placed 6 m (20 ft) apart (Fig. 12–30E). The patient is then timed as he or she hops through the pylons. The good limb is tested, followed by the injured limb, and the average times attained with each leg are compared.[31]

5. **Stairs hop test.**[32] The patient is timed as he or she hops up and down several steps (20 to 25 steps recommended), first on the good leg and then on the injured leg.

These functional tests are for active persons and can be quite demanding. Losee[33] mentioned several additional tests. For example, in the **deceleration test,** the patient is asked to run at full speed and to stop suddenly on command.[9] The test is positive for rotary instability if the patient stops without using the quadriceps or decelerates in a crouched position (more than 30° flexion of the knee). The effect of the test can be accentuated by having the patient turn away from the affected leg just as he or she is about to stop.[34] As the patient does the test, the examiner should watch to ensure that the patient uses the affected leg to help stop. With instability problems, the patient uses only the good leg to stop, "hopping through" with the injured leg.

For the "disco test," the patient stands on one leg with the knee flexed 10 to 20°. The patient is asked to rotate or twist left and right while holding the flexed position (Fig. 12–31).[9] Apprehension during the test or refusal to do the test is a positive sign for rotary instabil-

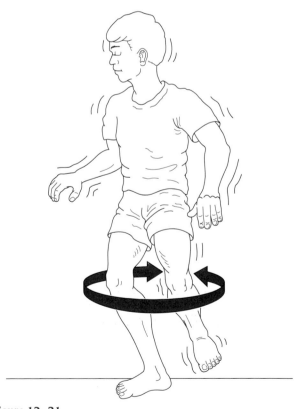

Figure 12–31

Losee disco test. Flexion, compression, and rotation may lead to shift of femur on tibia, causing rotary instability.

Cincinnati Knee Rating System

Symptoms (50 points):

Left	Right			Left	Right	
☐	☐	20	**1. Pain** No pain, normal knee, performs 100%.	☐	☐	*Location of pain:* Medial (inner side)
☐	☐	16	Occasional pain with strenuous sports or heavy work, knee not entirely normal, some limitations, but minor and tolerable.	☐	☐	Anterior-patellar (front/knee cap)
				☐	☐	Posterior (back of knee)
				☐	☐	Diffuse (all over)
☐	☐	12	Occasional pain with light recreational sports or moderate work activities, frequently brought on by vigorous activities, running, heavy labor, strenuous sports.	☐	☐	Diffuse (all over)
						Pain occurs on:
				☐	☐	Stairs
☐	☐	8	Pain, usually brought on by sports, light recreational activities, or moderate work. Occasionally occurs with walking, standing, or light work.	☐	☐	Sitting
				☐	☐	Kneeling
				☐	☐	Standing
☐	☐	4	Pain is a significant problem with activities as simple as walking. Relieved by rest. Unable to do sports.			*Type of pain:*
				☐	☐	Sharp
				☐	☐	Aching
☐	☐	0	Pain present all the time, occurs with walking, standing and at nighttime. Not relieved with rest.	☐	☐	Throbbing
				☐	☐	Burning
☐	☐		I do not know what my pain level is. I have not tested my knee.			

Intensity of pain:
☐ Mild ☐ Moderate ☐ Severe
Frequency: ☐ Intermittent ☐ Constant

Left	Right		
☐	☐	10	**2. Swelling** No swelling, normal knee, 100% activity.
☐	☐	8	Occasional swelling with strenuous sports or heavy work. Some limitations but minor and tolerable.
☐	☐	6	Occasional swelling with light recreational sports or moderate work activities, frequently brought on by vigorous activities, running, heavy labor, strenuous sports.
☐	☐	4	Swelling limits sports and moderate work. Occurs infrequently with simple walking activities or light work (about 3 times/year).
☐	☐	2	Swelling brought on by simple walking activities and light work. Relieved with rest.
☐	☐	0	Severe problem all of the time, with simple walking activities.
☐	☐		I do not know what my swelling level is. I have not tested my knee.

If swelling occurs it is: (check one box on each line)
Intensity: ☐ Mild ☐ Moderate ☐ Severe
Frequency: ☐ Intermittent ☐ Constant

Left	Right		
☐	☐	20	**3. Giving-way.** No giving-way, normal knee, performs 100%.
☐	☐	16	Occasional giving-way with strenuous sports or heavy work. Can participate in all sports but some guarding or limitations are still present.
☐	☐	12	Occasional giving-way with light recreational activities or moderate work. Able to compensate, limits vigorous activities; sports or heavy work; not able to cut or twist suddenly.
☐	☐	8	Giving-way limits sports and moderate work; occurs infrequently with walking or light work (about 3 times/year).
☐	☐	4	Giving-way with simple walking activities and light work. Occurs once per month. Requires guarding.
☐	☐	0	Severe problem with simple walking activities; cannot turn or twist while walking without giving-way.
☐	☐		I do not know my level of giving-way. I have not tested my knee.

4. Other Symptoms (unscored)

Left	Right	Knee stiffness	Left	Right	Kneecap grinding	Left	Right	Knee locking
☐	☐	None	☐	☐	None	☐	☐	None
☐	☐	Occasional	☐	☐	Mild	☐	☐	Occasional
☐	☐	Frequent	☐	☐	Moderate	☐	☐	Frequent
			☐	☐	Severe			

Figure 12–32

Cincinnati knee rating system. (From Noyes, F.R., G.H. McGinniss, and L.A. Mooar: Functional disability in the anterior cruciate insufficient knee syndrome. Sports Med. 1:287–288, 1984.)

Cincinnati Knee Rating System (*Continued*)

Function (50 points):

			5. Overall activity level
☐	☐	20	No limitation, normal knee, able to do everything including strenuous sports or heavy labor.
☐	☐	16	Perform sports including vigorous activities, but at a lower performance level, involves guarding or some limits to heavy labor.
☐	☐	12	Light recreational activities possible with rare symptoms, more strenuous activities cause problems. Active but in different sports, limited to moderate work.
☐	☐	8	No sports or recreational activities possible. Walking activities possible with rare symptoms, limited to light work.
☐	☐	4	Walking, activities of daily living cause moderate symptoms, frequent limitation.
☐	☐	0	Walking, activities of daily living cause severe problems, persistent symptoms.
☐	☐		I do not know what my real activity level is, I have not tested my knee, or I have given up strenuous sports.

			6. Walking
☐	☐	10	Normal, unlimited.
☐	☐	8	Slight/mild problem.
☐	☐	6	Moderate problem: smooth surface possible up to 800 m.
☐	☐	4	Severe problem: only 2–3 blocks possible.
☐	☐	2	Severe problem: requires cane, crutches.

			7. Stairs
☐	☐	10	Normal, unlimited.
☐	☐	8	Slight/mild problem.
☐	☐	6	Moderate problem: only 10–15 steps possible.
☐	☐	4	Severe problem: requires bannister, support.
☐	☐	2	Severe problem: only 1–5 steps possible.

			8. Running activity
☐	☐	5	Normal, unlimited: fully competitive, strenuous.
☐	☐	4	Slight/mild problem: run half-speed.
☐	☐	3	Moderate problem: only 2–4 km possible.
☐	☐	2	Severe problem: only 1–2 blocks possible.
☐	☐	1	Severe problem: only a few steps.

			9. Jumping or twisting activities
☐	☐	5	Normal, unlimited, fully competitive, strenuous.
☐	☐	4	Slight/mild problem: some guarding, but sports possible.
☐	☐	3	Moderate problem: gave up strenuous sports; recreational sports possible.
☐	☐	2	Severe problem: affects all sports, must constantly guard.
☐	☐	1	Severe problem: only light activity possible (golf, swimming).

Total: Left [ ] Right [ ] (Maximum: 100 points)

Figure 12–32 *Continued*

ity. If pain is felt on the joint line, it may be indicative of meniscus pathology, in which case it is called **Merke's sign.**[28] Pain on medial rotation along the joint line implies medial meniscus pathology, and pain on lateral rotation implies lateral meniscus pathology.

Larson[35] advocated the **leaning hop test.** For this test, the patient hops up and down on one leg while abducting the opposite leg. A positive test is apprehension during the test or refusal to do the test and is a positive sign for rotary instability.

Noyes and colleagues[36, 37] developed the Cincinnati Knee Rating System (Fig. 12–32), which deals with pain, swelling, stability, and activity level and is a good functional rating system for active persons. Irrgang and associates[38] make use of two scales, an Activities of Daily Living Scale and a Sports Activity Scale (Figs. 12–33 and 12–34), to detect clinically significant changes over time. The Knee Society[39] also has a rating scale (Fig. 12–35).

The Knee Society advocates keeping knee rating and functional assessment separate. This knee-rating scale deals first with pain, range of motion, and stability, giving positive points up to 100 and grouping deductions that can take away from the overall value. Function is dealt with separately on the scale.

Lysholm and Gillquist[40] developed a frequently used scale primarily designed to score clinical instability (Table 12–6). The most recent knee scale is the documentation form developed by the International Knee Documentation Committee (Fig. 12–36). Table 12–7 shows a patellofemoral joint evaluation scale that can be used to assess functional levels in patients with patellofemoral syndrome after surgery or nonsurgery.[41, 42] Each of these knee-rating scales is slightly different. The scale that works best for the examiner and the examiner's clientele should be used. Other knee-rating scales are also available.[40, 43–45]

Text continued on page 534

Activities of Daily Living Scale of the Knee Outcome Survey

Instructions:

The following questionnaire is designed to determine the symptoms and limitations that you experience because of your knee while you perform your usual *daily activities*. Please answer each question by ***checking the statement that best describes you over the last 1 to 2 days.*** For a given question, more than one of the statements may describe you, but please mark ONLY the statement which best describes you during your usual daily activities.

Symptoms

1. To what degree does pain in your knee affect your daily activity level?
   - ____ I never have pain in my knee.
   - ____ I have pain in my knee but it does not affect my daily activity.
   - ____ Pain affects my activity slightly.
   - ____ Pain affects my activity moderately.
   - ____ Pain affects my activity severely.
   - ____ Pain in my knee prevents me from performing all daily activities.

2. To what degree does grinding or grating of your knee affect your daily activity level?
   - ____ I never have grinding or grating in my knee.
   - ____ I have grinding or grating in my knee, but it does not affect my daily activity.
   - ____ Grinding or grating affects my activity slightly.
   - ____ Grinding or grating affects my activity moderately.
   - ____ Grinding or grating affects my activity severely.
   - ____ Grinding or grating in my knee prevents me from performing all daily activities.

3. To what degree does stiffness in your knee affect your daily activity level?
   - ____ I never have stiffness in my knee.
   - ____ I have stiffness in my knee, but it does not affect my daily activity.
   - ____ Stiffness affects my activity slightly.
   - ____ Stiffness affects my activity moderately.
   - ____ Stiffness affects my activity severely.
   - ____ Stiffness in my knee prevents me from performing all daily activities.

4. To what degree does swelling in your knee affect your daily activity level?
   - ____ I never have swelling in my knee.
   - ____ I have swelling in my knee, but it does not affect my daily activity.
   - ____ Swelling affects my activity slightly.
   - ____ Swelling affects my activity moderately.
   - ____ Swelling affects my activity severely.
   - ____ Swelling in my knee prevents me from performing all daily activities.

5. To what degree does slipping of your knee affect your daily activity level?
   - ____ I never have slipping of my knee.
   - ____ I have slipping of my knee, but it does not affect my daily activity.
   - ____ Slipping of my knee affects my activity slightly.
   - ____ Slipping of my knee affects my activity moderately.
   - ____ Slipping of my knee affects my activity severely.
   - ____ Slipping of my knee prevents me from performing all daily activities.

6. To what degree does buckling of your knee affect your daily activity level?
   - ____ I never have buckling of my knee.
   - ____ I have buckling of my knee, but it does not affect my daily activity level.
   - ____ Buckling of my knee affects my activity slightly.
   - ____ Buckling of my knee affects my activity moderately.
   - ____ Buckling of my knee affects my activity severely.
   - ____ Buckling of my knee prevents me from performing all daily activities.

7. To what degree does weakness or lack of strength of your leg affect your daily activity level?
   - ____ My leg never feels weak.
   - ____ My leg feels weak, but it does not affect my daily activity.
   - ____ Weakness affects my activity slightly.
   - ____ Weakness affects my activity moderately.
   - ____ Weakness affects my activity severely.
   - ____ Weakness of my leg prevents me from performing all daily activities.

Functional Disability with Activities of Daily Living

8. How does your knee affect your ability to walk?
   - ____ My knee does not affect my ability to walk.
   - ____ I have pain in my knee when walking, but it does not limit my ability to walk.
   - ____ My knee prevents me from walking more than 1 mile
   - ____ My knee prevents me from walking more than 1/2 mile.
   - ____ My knee prevents me from walking more than 1 block.
   - ____ My knee prevents me from walking.

9. Because of your knee, do you walk with crutches or a cane?
   - ____ I can walk without crutches or a cane.
   - ____ My knee causes me to walk with one crutch or a cane.
   - ____ My knee causes me to walk with two crutches.
   - ____ Because of my knee, I cannot walk, even with crutches.

10. Does your knee cause you to limp when you walk?
   - ____ I can walk without a limp.
   - ____ Sometimes my knee causes me to walk with a limp.
   - ____ Because of my knee, I cannot walk without a limp.

11. How does your knee affect your ability to go up stairs?
   - ____ My knee does not affect my ability to go up stairs.
   - ____ I have pain in my knee when going up stairs, but it does not limit my ability to go up stairs.
   - ____ I am able to go up stairs normally, but I need to rely on use of a railing.
   - ____ I am able to go up stairs one step at a time with the use of a railing.
   - ____ I have to use crutches or a cane to go up stairs.
   - ____ I cannot go up stairs.

Figure 12–33

Activities of daily living scale of the Knee Outcome Survey. (From Irrgang, J.J., M.R. Safran, and F.H. Fu: The knee: Ligamentous and meniscal injuries. *In* Zachazewski, J.E., D.J. Magee, and W.S. Quillen [eds.]: Athletic Injuries and Rehabilitation. Philadelphia, W.B. Saunders Co., 1996, pp. 683–684.)

Activities of Daily Living Scale of the Knee Outcome Survey (Continued)

12. How does your knee affect your ability to go down stairs?
    ___ My knee does not affect my ability to go down stairs.
    ___ I have pain in my knee when going down stairs, but it does not limit my ability to go down stairs.
    ___ I am able to go down stairs normally, but I need to rely on use of a railing.
    ___ I am able to go down stairs one step at a time with the use of a railing.
    ___ I have to use crutches or a cane to go down stairs.
    ___ I cannot go down stairs.

13. How does your knee affect your ability to stand?
    ___ My knee does not affect my ability to stand. I can stand for unlimited amounts of time.
    ___ I have pain in my knee when standing, but it does not limit my ability to stand.
    ___ Because of my knee, I cannot stand for more than 1 hour.
    ___ Because of my knee, I cannot stand for more than 1/2 hour.
    ___ Because of my knee, I cannot stand for more than 10 minutes.
    ___ I cannot stand because of my knee.

14. How does your knee affect your ability to kneel on the front of your knee?
    ___ My knee does not affect my ability to kneel on the front of my knee. I can kneel for unlimited amounts of time.
    ___ I have pain when kneeling on the front of my knee, but it does not limit my ability to kneel.
    ___ I cannot kneel on the front of my knee for more than 1 hour.
    ___ I cannot kneel on the front of my knee for more than 1/2 hour.
    ___ I cannot kneel on the front of my knee for more than 10 minutes.
    ___ I cannot kneel on the front of my knee.

15. How does your knee affect your ability to squat?
    ___ My knee does not affect my ability to squat. I can squat all the way down.
    ___ I have pain when squatting, but I can still squat all the way down.
    ___ I cannot squat more than 3/4 of the way down.
    ___ I cannot squat more than halfway down.
    ___ I cannot squat more than 1/4 of the way down.
    ___ I cannot squat at all.

16. How does your knee affect your ability to sit with your knee bent?
    ___ My knee does not affect my ability to sit with my knee bent. I can sit for unlimited amounts of time.
    ___ I have pain when sitting with my knee bent, but it does not limit my ability to sit.
    ___ I cannot sit with my knee bent for more than 1 hour.
    ___ I cannot sit with my knee bent for more than 1/2 hour.
    ___ I cannot sit with my knee bent for more than 10 minutes.
    ___ I cannot sit with my knee bent.

17. How does your knee affect your ability to rise from a chair?
    ___ My knee does not affect my ability to rise from a chair.
    ___ I have pain when rising from the seated position, but it does not affect my ability to rise from the seated position.
    ___ Because of my knee, I can only rise from a chair if I use my hands and arms to assist.
    ___ Because of my knee, I cannot rise from a chair.

18. How would you rate your current level of knee function during your *usual daily activities* on a scale from 0 to 100, with 100 being your level of knee function prior to your injury?

    _____

19. How would you rate the *overall function* of your knee during your *usual daily activities?*
    ___ normal
    ___ nearly normal
    ___ abnormal
    ___ severely abnormal

20. As a result of your knee injury, how would you rate your *current level of daily activity?*
    ___ normal
    ___ nearly normal
    ___ abnormal
    ___ severely abnormal

21. Since initiation of treatment for your knee, how would you describe your progress?
    ___ greatly improved
    ___ somewhat improved
    ___ neither improved/worsened
    ___ somewhat worse
    ___ greatly worse

Changes in Daily Activity Level

Please use the following scale to answer questions A–C below.

1 = I was able to perform *unlimited physical work,* which included lifting and climbing.
2 = I was able to perform *limited physical work,* which included lifting and climbing.
3 = I was able to perform *unlimited light activities,* which included walking on level surfaces and stairs.
4 = I was able to perform *limited light activities,* which included walking on level surfaces and stairs.
5 = I was *unable to perform light activities,* which included walking on level surfaces and stairs.

A. ___ *Prior to your knee injury,* how would you describe your usual daily activity? Please indicate only the **HIGHEST** level of activity that described you before your knee injury.

B. ___ *Prior to surgery or treatment* of your knee, how would you describe your usual daily activity? Please indicate only the **HIGHEST** level of activity that described you prior to surgery or treatment to your knee.

C. ___ How would you describe your *current level* of daily activity? Please indicate only the **HIGHEST** level of activity that describes you over the last 1 to 2 days.

Figure 12–33 *Continued*

Sports Activity Scale of the Knee Outcome Survey

Instructions:

The following questionnaire is designed to determine the symptoms and limitations that you experience because of your knee while you participate in sports activities. Please answer each question by checking the statement that best describes you over the last 1 to 2 days. For a given question, more than one of the statements may describe you, but please mark ONLY the statement which best describes you when you participate in sports activities.

Symptoms

1. To what degree does pain in your knee affect your sports activity level?
   - ___ I never have pain in my knee.
   - ___ Knee pain does not affect my activity.
   - ___ Slightly.
   - ___ Moderately.
   - ___ Severely.
   - ___ Prevents me from performing all sports activities.

2. To what degree does grinding or grating of your knee affect your sports activity level?
   - ___ I never have grinding or grating in my knee.
   - ___ Grinding/grating does not affect my activity.
   - ___ Slightly.
   - ___ Moderately.
   - ___ Severely.
   - ___ Prevents me from performing all sports activities.

3. To what degree does stiffness in your knee affect your sports activity level?
   - ___ I never have stiffness in my knee.
   - ___ Knee stiffness does not affect my activity.
   - ___ Slightly.
   - ___ Moderately.
   - ___ Severely.
   - ___ Prevents me from performing all sports activities.

4. To what degree does swelling in your knee affect your sports activity level?
   - ___ I never have swelling in my knee.
   - ___ Knee swelling does not affect my activity.
   - ___ Slightly.
   - ___ Moderately.
   - ___ Severely.
   - ___ Prevents me from performing all sports activities.

5. To what degree does partial giving way or slipping of your knee affect your sports activity level?
   - ___ I never have partial giving way or slipping of my knee.
   - ___ Partial giving way does not affect my activity.
   - ___ Slightly.
   - ___ Moderately.
   - ___ Severely.
   - ___ Prevents me from performing all sports activities.

6. To what degree does complete giving way or buckling of your knee affect your sports activity level?
   - ___ I never have complete giving way or buckling in my knee.
   - ___ Knee buckling does not affect my activity.
   - ___ Slightly.
   - ___ Moderately.
   - ___ Severely.
   - ___ Prevents me from performing all sports activities.

Functional Disability with Sports Activities

1. How does your knee affect your ability to run straight ahead?
   - ___ I am able to run straight ahead full speed without limitations.
   - ___ I have pain in my knee but it does not affect my ability.
   - ___ Slightly.
   - ___ Moderately.
   - ___ Severely.
   - ___ Prevents me from running.

2. How does your knee affect your ability to jump and land on your involved leg?
   - ___ I am able to jump and land on my involved leg without limitations.
   - ___ I have pain in my knee but it does not affect my ability.
   - ___ Slightly.
   - ___ Moderately.
   - ___ Severely.
   - ___ Prevents me from jumping and landing.

3. How does your knee affect your ability to stop and start quickly?
   - ___ I am able to start and stop quickly without limitations.
   - ___ I have pain in my knee but it does not affect my ability.
   - ___ Slightly.
   - ___ Moderately.
   - ___ Severely.
   - ___ Prevents me from stopping and starting quickly.

4. How does your knee affect your ability to cut and pivot on your involved leg?
   - ___ I am able to cut and pivot on my involved leg without limitations.
   - ___ I have pain in my knee but it does not affect my ability.
   - ___ Slightly.
   - ___ Moderately.
   - ___ Severely.
   - ___ Prevents me from jumping and landing.

Figure 12–34

Sports activity scale of the Knee Outcome Survey. (From Irrgang, J.J., M.R. Safran, and F.H. Fu: The knee: Ligamentous and meniscal injuries. *In* Zachazewski, J.E., D.J. Magee, and W.S. Quillen [eds.]: Athletic Injuries and Rehabilitation. Philadelphia, W.B. Saunders Co., 1996, p. 685.)

Knee Society Knee Score

Patient category
A. Unilateral or bilateral (opposite knee successfully replaced)
B. Unilateral, other knee symptomatic
C. Multiple arthritis or medical infirmity

Pain	Points	Function	Points
None	50	Walking	50
Mild or occasional	45	Unlimited	40
Stairs only	40	>10 blocks	30
Walking and stairs	30	5–10 blocks	20
Moderate		<5 blocks	10
Occasional	20	Housebound	0
Continual	10	Unable	
Severe	0	Stairs	
		Normal up and down	50
Range of Motion		Normal up; down with rail	40
(5° = 1 point)	25	Up and down with rail	30
		Up with rail; unable down	15
Stability (maximum		Unable	0
movement in any position)			
		Subtotal	
Anteroposterior			
<5 mm	10	Deductions (minus)	
5–10 mm	5	Cane	5
10 mm	0	Two canes	10
Mediolateral		Crutches or walker	20
<5°	15		
6°–9°	10	**Total deductions**	
10°–14°	5		
15°	0	**Function score**	

Subtotal

Deductions (minus)

Flexion contracture
5°–10°	2
10°–15°	5
16°–20°	10
>20°	15

Extension lag
<10°	5
10°–20°	10
>20°	15

Alignment
5°–10°	0
0°–4°	3 points each degree
11°–15°	3 points each degree
Other	20

Total deductions

Pain score
(if total is a minus number,
score is 0)

Figure 12–35

Knee Society Knee Score. (From Insall, J.N., L.D. Dorr, R.D. Scott, and W.N. Scott: Rationale of the Knee Society clinical rating system. Clin. Orthop. 248:14, 1989.)

Table 12–6
Lysholm Scoring Scale

	Points		Points
Limp (5 points)		**Walking, running and jumping (70 points)**	
None	5	Instability:	
Slight or periodic	3	Never giving way	30
Severe and constant	0	Rarely during athletic or other severe exertion	25
Support (5 points)		Frequently during athletic or other severe exertion (or unable to participate)	20
Full support	5	Occasionally in daily activities	10
Stick or crutch	3	Often in daily activities	5
Weight bearing impossible	0	Every step	0
Stair climbing (10 points)		Pain	
No problems	10	None	30
Slightly impaired	6	Inconstant and slight during severe exertion	25
One step at a time	2	Marked on giving way	20
Unable	0	Marked during severe exertion	15
Squatting (5 points)		Marked on or after walking more than 2 km	10
No problems	5	Marked on or after walking less than 2 km	5
Slightly impaired	4	Constant and severe	0
Not past 90°	2	Swelling	
Unable	0	None	10
		With giving way	7
		On severe exertion	5
		On ordinary exertion	2
		Constant	0
		Atrophy of thigh (5 points)	
		None	5
		1–2 cm	3
		More than 2 cm	0
		TOTAL SCORE	100

Modified from Lysholm, J., and J. Gillquist: Evaluation of knee ligament surgery results with special emphasis on use of a scoring scale. Am. J. Sports Med. 10:150–154, 1982.

Table 12–7
Patellofemoral Joint Evaluation Scale*

	Points		Points
Limp		**Inability, "giving way"**	
None	5	Never	20
Slight or episodic	3	Occasionally with vigorous activities	10
Severe	0	Frequently with vigorous activities	8
Assistive devices		Occasionally with daily activities	5
None	5	Frequently with daily activities	2
Cane or brace	3	Every day	0
Unable to bear weight	0	**Swelling**	
Stair climbing		None	10
No problem	20	After vigorous activities only	5
Slight impairment	15	After walking or mild activities	2
Very slowly	10	Constant	0
One step at a time, always same leg first	5	**Pain**	
Unable	0	None	35
Crepitation		Occasionally with vigorous activities	30
None	5	Marked with vigorous activities	20
Annoying	3	Marked after walking 1 mile or mild or moderate rest pain	15
Limits activities	2	Marked with walking <1 mile	10
Severe	0	Constant and severe	0

* Functional results were assessed according to the patellofemoral scoring scale. Excellent results equal 90–100 points, good 80–89, fair 60–79, and poor <60 points.

From Karlsson, J., R. Thomeé, and L. Sward: Eleven year follow up of patellofemoral pain syndromes. Clin. J. Sport Med. 6:23, 1996.

Guidelines for Evaluating Outcome of Knee Ligament Injury or Surgery

Name: _____ First name: _____ DOB: __/__/__ med. rec. #:_____

Examiner: _____ Date of examination: __/__/__ Date of injury/ies: __/__/__; __/__/__ Date of surgeries: __/__/__

Causes of injury: ☐ ADL*[2] ☐ traff. ☐ non-pivoting non-contact sports ☐ pivoting non-contact sp. ☐ contact sp. ☐ work

Time inj. to surg.: _____ (months) ☐ acute (0-2 weeks) ☐ subacute (2-8 weeks) ☐ chronic (>8 weeks)

Knee involved: ☐ r. ☐ l. opposite knee: ☐ norm. ☐ injured exam. under anesthes.: ☐ yes ☐ no

Postop. diagnosis: _____

Surgical proced.: _____

Status menisci: norm. ☐ med. ☐ lat. 1/3 removed: ☐ med. ☐ lat. 2/3 removed: ☐ med. ☐ lat. compl. rem. ☐ med. ☐ lat.

Morphotype: ☐ lax ☐ normal ☐ tight ☐ varus ☐ valgus

Activ. level*[3]: preinjury: ☐ I ☐ II ☐ III ☐ IV pretreatment: ☐ I ☐ II ☐ III ☐ IV

present: ☐ I ☐ II ☐ III ☐ IV Eventual change knee-related: ☐ yes ☐ no

GROUPS (PROBLEM AREA)	QUALIFICATION WITHIN GROUPS *[4]				GROUP QUALIFIC.			
	A: normal	B: nearly norm.	C: abnormal	D: sev. abnorm.	A	B	C	D*[4]
1. PATIENT SUBJECTIVE ASSESSMENT								
How does your knee function?	☐ normally	☐ nearly norm.	☐ abnormally	☐ sev. abnorm.				
On a scale of 0 to 3 how does your knee affect your activity level?	☐ 0	☐ 1	☐ 2	☐ 3	☐	☐	☐	☐
2. SYMPTOMS (absence of significant symptoms, at highest activity level known by patient) *[5]								
No pain at activity level *[3]	☐ I	☐ II	☐ III	☐ IV or worse				
No swelling at activity level *[3]	☐ I	☐ II	☐ III	☐ IV or worse				
No partial giving way at activity level *[3]	☐ I	☐ II	☐ III	☐ IV or worse				
No complete giving way at activity level *[3]	☐ I	☐ II	☐ III	☐ IV or worse	☐	☐	☐	☐
3. RANGE OF MOTION: Flex./ext.: documented side: __/__/__ opposite side: __/__/__ *[6]								
Lack of extension (from zero anatomic)	☐ <3°	☐ 3-5°	☐ 6-10°	☐ >10°				
△ *[7] lack of flexion	☐ 0-5°	☐ 6-15°	☐ 16-25°	☐ >25°	☐	☐	☐	☐
4. LIGAMENT EXAMINATION *[8]		3 to 5mm or	6 to 10mm					
△ *[7] Lachman (in 25°. flex.) *[9]	☐ −1 to 2mm	☐ −1 to −3mm[10]	☐ or <−3mm	☐ >10mm				
idem (alternative measurement, optional)	☐ −1 to 2mm	☐ 3-5/−1 to −3mm	☐ 6-10/<−3mm	☐ >10mm				
Endpoint: ☐ firm ☐ soft								
△ *[7] total a.p.transl. in 70° flex. *[9]	☐ 0 to 2mm	☐ 3 to 5mm	☐ 6 to 10mm	☐ >10mm				
idem (alternative measurement, optional)	☐ 0 to 2mm	☐ 3 to 5mm	☐ 6 to 10mm	☐ >10mm				
△ *[7] post. sag in 70° flex.	☐ 0 to 2mm	☐ 3 to 5mm	☐ 6 to 10mm	☐ >10mm				
△ *[7] med. joint opening (valgus rotation)	☐ 0 to 2mm	☐ 3 to 5mm	☐ 6 to 10mm	☐ >10mm				
△ *[7] lat. joint opening (varus rotation)	☐ 0 to 2mm	☐ 3 to 5mm	☐ 6 to 10mm	☐ >10mm				
Pivot shift *[11]	☐ neg.	☐ + (glide)	☐ ++ (clunk)	☐ +++ (gross)				
△ *[7] reversed pivot shift	☐ equal (neg.)	☐ slight	☐ marked	☐ gross				
	☐ equal (pos.)				☐	☐	☐	☐
5. COMPARTMENTAL FINDINGS *[12]								
△ *[7] Crepitus patellofemoral	☐ none/equal	☐ moderate	☐ painful	☐ severe				
△ *[7] Crepitus medial compartment	☐ none	☐ moderate	☐ painful	☐ severe				
△ *[7] Crepitus lateral compartment	☐ none	☐ moderate	☐ painful	☐ severe				
6. HARVEST SITE PATHOLOGY *[13]								
Tenderness, irritation, numbness	☐ none	☐ slight	☐ moderate	☐ severe				
7. X-RAY FINDINGS (DEGENERATIVE JOINT DISEASE) *[14]								
Patellofemoral cartilage space	☐ normal	☐ >4mm	☐ 2-4mm	☐ <2mm				
Medial compartment cartilage space	☐ normal	☐ >4mm	☐ 2-4mm	☐ <2mm				
Lateral compartment cartilage space	☐ normal	☐ >4mm	☐ 2-4mm	☐ <2mm				
8. FUNCTIONAL TEST *[15]								
△ One leg hop (percent of opposite side)	☐ 90-100%	☐ 76-90%	☐ 50-75%	☐ <50%				
FINAL EVALUATION					☐	☐	☐	☐

Figure 12–36

International Knee Documentation Committee guidelines for evaluating outcome after knee ligament injury and/or surgery. (From Hefti, F., W. Mullen, R.P. Jakob, and H.-U. Staubli: Evaluation of knee ligament injuries with the I KDC form. Knee Surg. Sports Traumatol. Arthrosc. 1:226–234, 1993. © Springer-Verlag.)

Ligament Stability

Because the knee, more than any other joint in the body, depends on its ligaments to maintain its integrity, it is imperative that the ligaments be tested. The ligaments of the knee joint act as primary stabilizers and guide the movement of the bones in proper relation to one another. Depending on the motion being tested, the ligaments act as primary or secondary restraints (Table 12–8). For example, the anterior cruciate ligament is the primary restraint to anterior tibial displacement and a secondary restraint to varus-valgus motion in full extension and rotation.[38, 46] If the primary restraint is injured, pathological motion occurs. If the secondary restraint is injured but the primary restraint is not, pathological motion in that direction does not occur. If both primary and secondary restraints are injured, the pathological motion is greater.[38] There are several ligaments around the knee, but four deserve special mention (Fig. 12–37).

Collateral and Cruciate Ligaments

Collateral Ligaments. The **medial (tibial) collateral ligament** lies more posteriorly than anteriorly on the medial aspect of the tibiofemoral joint. It is made up of two layers, one superficial and one deep. The deep layer is a thickening of the joint capsule that blends with the medial meniscus; it is sometimes called the medial capsular ligament. The superficial layer is a strong, broad triangular strap. It starts distal to the adductor tubercle and extends to the medial surface of the tibia, approximately 6 cm (2.4 inches) below the joint line. It blends with the posterior capsule and is separated from the capsule and the medial meniscus by a bursa.

The entire medial collateral ligament is tight throughout the full range of motion, although there is

Table 12–8
Primary and Secondary Restraints of the Knee

Tibial Motion	Primary Restraints	Secondary Restraints
Anterior translation	ACL	MCL, LCL; middle third of mediolateral capsule; popliteus corner, semimembranosus corner, iliotibial band
Posterior translation	PCL	MCL, LCL; posterior third of mediolateral capsule; popliteus tendon; anterior and posterior meniscofemoral ligaments
Valgus rotation	MCL	ACL, PCL; posterior capsule when knee fully extended, semimembranosus corner
Varus rotation	LCL	ACL, PCL; posterior capsule when knee fully extended, popliteus corner
Lateral rotation	MCL, LCL	Popliteus corner
Medial rotation	ACL, PCL	Anteroposterior meniscofemoral ligaments, semimembranosus corner

ACL = anterior cruciate ligament; LCL = lateral collateral ligament; MCL = medial collateral ligament; PCL = posterior cruciate ligament.

Modified from Zachazewski, J.E., D.J. Magee, and W.S. Quillen (eds.): Athletic Injuries and Rehabilitation. Philadelphia, W.B. Saunders Co., 1996, p. 627.

varying stress placed on different parts of the ligament as it moves through the full range because of the shape of the femoral condyles. All of its fibers are taut on full extension. In flexion, the anterior fibers are the most taut; in midrange, the posterior fibers are the most taut.[47]

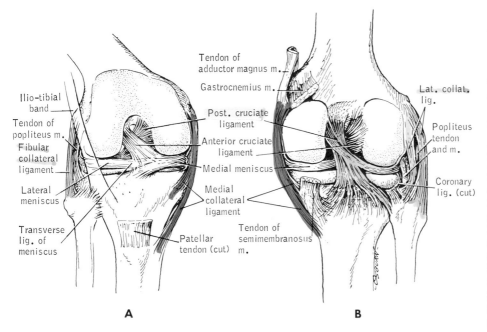

A   **B**

Figure 12–37
Anatomic drawings of knee. (A) Anterior view. The patellar tendon is sectioned, the patella is reflected upward, and the knee is flexed. Note that the cruciate ligament rises in front of the anterior tibial spine, not from it. Note also that the medial meniscus is firmly attached to the medial collateral ligament. (B) Posterior view with the knee extended. The posterior ligament has been removed. The two layers of the medial collateral ligament are shown, as is the tibial portion of the lateral collateral ligament. The posterior cruciate ligament rises behind the tibia, not on its upper surface. Observe the femoral attachment of the anterior cruciate ligament on the back of the notch. (From O'Donoghue, D.H.: Treatment of Injuries to Athletes, 4th ed. Philadelphia, W.B. Saunders Co., 1984, p. 477.)

The **lateral (fibular) collateral ligament** is round and lies under the tendon of the biceps femoris muscle. It runs from the lateral epicondyle of the femur to the fibular head. It also lies more posteriorly than anteriorly. This ligament is tight in extension and loosens in flexion, especially after 30° flexion. As the knee flexes, it provides protection to the lateral aspect of the knee. It is not attached to the lateral meniscus but rather is separated from it by a small fat pad.[47]

Cruciate Ligaments. The cruciate ligaments cross each other and are the primary rotary stabilizers of the knee.[48] These strong ligaments are named in relation to their attachment to the tibia and are intracapsular but extrasynovial. Each ligament has an anteromedial and a posterolateral portion. The anterior cruciate ligament has in addition an intermediate portion.

The **anterior cruciate ligament** extends superiorly, posteriorly, and laterally, twisting on itself as it extends from the tibia to the femur. Its main functions are to prevent anterior movement of the tibia on the femur, to check lateral rotation of the tibia in flexion, and, to a lesser extent, to check extension and hyperextension at the knee. It also helps to control the normal rolling and gliding movement of the knee. The anteromedial bundle is tight in both flexion and extension, whereas the posterolateral bundle is tight on extension only. As a whole, the ligament has the least amount of stress on it between 30 and 60° flexion.[47-50]

The **posterior cruciate ligament** extends superiorly, anteriorly, and medially from the tibia to the femur. This strong, fan-shaped ligament, the stoutest ligament in the knee, is a primary stabilizer of the knee against posterior movement of the tibia on the femur, and it checks exten-

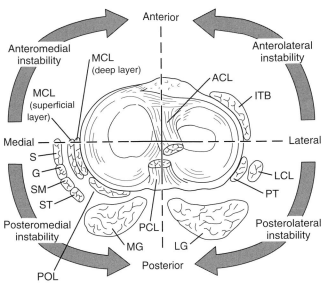

Figure 12–39

Instabilities about the knee. PCL = posterior cruciate ligament; POL = posterior oblique ligament; MCL = medial collateral ligament; ACL = anterior cruciate ligament; ITB = iliotibial band; LCL = lateral collateral ligament; PT = popliteal tendon, S = sartorius; G = gracilis; SM = semimembranosus; ST = semitendinosus; MG = medial gastrocnemius; LG = lateral gastrocnemius.

sion and hyperextension. In addition, the ligament helps to maintain rotary stability and functions as the knee's central axis of rotation. Along with the anterior cruciate ligament, it acts as a rotary guide to the "screwing home" mechanism of the knee.[47, 50] For the posterior cruciate ligament, the bulk of the fibers are tight at 30° flexion, but the posterolateral fibers are loose in early flexion.

With lateral rotation of the tibia, both collateral ligaments become more taut, and the cruciate ligaments become relaxed (Fig. 12–38). With medial rotation of the tibia, the reverse action occurs: the collateral ligaments become more relaxed, and the cruciate ligaments become tighter.[47, 51]

Testing of Ligaments

When testing the ligaments of the knee, the examiner must watch for four one-plane instabilities and four rotational instabilities (Table 12–9 and Fig. 12–39).

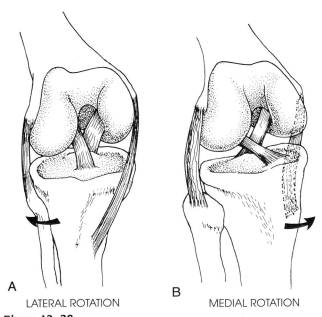

A LATERAL ROTATION   **B** MEDIAL ROTATION

Figure 12–38

Effect of tibial rotation on cruciate and collateral ligaments. (A) The collateral ligament is taut; the cruciate ligament is lax. (B) The collateral ligament is lax; the cruciate ligament is taut.

Instabilities About the Knee

- One-plane medial instability
- One-plane lateral instability
- One-plane anterior instability
- One-plane posterior instability
- Anteromedial rotary instability
- Anterolateral rotary instability
- Posteromedial rotary instability
- Posterolateral rotary instability

Table 12–9
Tests for Ligamentous Instability Around the Knee

Instability	Tests Used to Determine Instability	Structures Injured to Some Degree if Test Positive*	Notes
One-plane medial (straight medial)	1. Abduction (valgus) stress with knee in full extension	1. Medial collateral ligament (superficial and deep fibers) 2. Posterior oblique ligament 3. Posteromedial capsule 4. Anterior cruciate ligament 5. Posterior cruciate ligament 6. Medial quadriceps expansion 7. Semimembranosus muscle	1. If either cruciate ligament is torn (third-degree sprain) or stretched, rotary instability will also be evident 2. Order of injury is usually medial collateral ligament, then posteromedial corner, posterior capsule, anterior cruciate ligament, and finally posterior cruciate ligament
	2. Abduction (valgus) stress with knee slightly flexed (20 to 30°)	1. Medial collateral ligament (superficial and deep fibers) 2. Posterior oblique ligament 3. Posterior cruciate ligament	1. Depending on degree of pain, opening and end feel, primarily signifies medial collateral ligament sprain (first, second, or third degree) 2. If posterior cruciate ligament is torn (third-degree sprain), rotary instability will also be evident 3. Opening of 12 to 15° signifies injury to posterior cruciate ligament 4. If tibia is laterally rotated, stress is taken off posterior cruciate ligament 5. If tibia is medially rotated, stress is increased on cruciate ligaments while medial collateral ligament relaxes
One-plane lateral (straight lateral)	1. Adduction (varus) stress with knee in full extension	1. Lateral collateral ligament 2. Posterolateral capsule 3. Arcuate-popliteus complex 4. Biceps femoris tendon 5. Anterior cruciate ligament 6. Posterior cruciate ligament 7. Lateral gastrocnemius muscle	1. If either cruciate ligament is torn (third-degree sprain) or stretched, rotary instability will also be evident 2. Order of injury is lateral collateral ligament, arcuate-popliteus complex, anterior cruciate ligament, posterior cruciate ligament 3. With severe injury (third degree), common peroneal nerve and circulation may be affected
	2. Adduction (varus) stress with knee slightly flexed (20 to 30°) and tibia laterally rotated	1. Lateral collateral ligament 2. Posterolateral capsule 3. Arcuate-popliteus complex 4. Iliotibial band 5. Biceps femoris tendon	1. Depending on degree of pain, opening and end feel, primarily signifies lateral collateral ligament sprain (first, second, or third degree) 2. If tibia is not laterally rotated, maximum stress will not be placed on lateral collateral ligament

Table 12–9
Tests for Ligamentous Instability Around the Knee (Continued)

Instability	Tests Used to Determine Instability	Structures Injured to Some Degree if Test Positive*	Notes
One-plane lateral (straight lateral) *continued*			3. Lateral rotation of tibia results in relaxation of both cruciate ligaments 4. With flexion, the iliotibial band lies over the center of the lateral joint line 5. If tibia is medially rotated, stress is increased on both cruciate ligaments while lateral collateral ligament relaxes 6. Order of injury is lateral collateral ligament, arcuate-popliteus complex, and iliotibial band and/or biceps femoris
One-plane anterior	1. Lachman test (20 to 30° knee flexion)	1. Anterior cruciate ligament 2. Posterior oblique ligament 3. Arcuate-popliteus complex	1. Medial collateral ligament and iliotibial band lax in this position 2. Tests primarily posterolateral bundle of anterior cruciate ligament 3. Primarily tests anterior cruciate ligament but with severe injury (third-degree), structures in posteromedial and posterolateral corners may also be injured
	2. Anterior drawer sign (90° knee flexion) 3. Active drawer test	1. Anterior cruciate ligament 2. Posterolateral capsule 3. Posteromedial capsule 4. Medial collateral ligament 5. Iliotibial band 6. Posterior oblique ligament 7. Arcuate-popliteus complex	1. Tests primarily anteromedial bundle of anterior cruciate ligament 2. If anterior cruciate ligament and medial or lateral structures are torn (third-degree sprain) or stretched, rotary instability will also be evident 3. Be sure posterior cruciate has not been injured, giving possible false-positive test
One-plane posterior	1. Posterior drawer sign (90° knee flexion) 2. Posterior sag sign 3. Active drawer test 4. Reverse Lachman test 5. Godfrey test	1. Posterior cruciate ligament 2. Arcuate-popliteus complex 3. Posterior oblique ligament 4. Anterior cruciate ligament	1. If posterior cruciate ligament and medial or lateral structures are torn (third-degree sprain) or stretched, rotary instability will also be evident 2. With severe injury (third-degree), collateral ligaments may also be injured
Anteromedial rotary	1. Slocum test (foot laterally rotated 15°) 2. Lemaire's anteromedial jolt test 3. Dejour test	1. Medial collateral ligament (superficial and deep fibers) 2. Posterior oblique ligament 3. Posteromedial capsule 4. Anterior cruciate ligament	1. Test must not be done in extreme lateral rotation of tibia because passive stabilizing will result from "coiling" to maximum rotation

Table continued on following page

Table 12–9
Tests for Ligamentous Instability Around the Knee (*Continued*)

Instability	Tests Used to Determine Instability	Structures Injured to Some Degree if Test Positive*	Notes
Anterolateral rotary	1. Slocum test (foot medially rotated 30°) 2. Losee test 3. Jerk test of Hughston 4. Active pivot shift 5. Nakajima test	1. Anterior cruciate ligament 2. Posterolateral capsule 3. Arcuate-popliteus complex 4. Lateral collateral ligament 5. Iliotibial band	1. Tests bring about anterior *subluxation* of tibia on femur, causing patient to experience "giving way" sensation 2. Tests go from flexion to extension 3. Slocum test must not be done in extreme medial rotation of tibia because passive stabilization will result from "coiling" to maximum rotation 4. Shift may be "slip" (second degree) or "jerk" (third degree), depending on degree of sprain or injury
	1. Lateral pivot shift test of Macintosh 2. Slocum "ALRI" test 3. Crossover test 4. Flexion-rotation drawer test 5. Flexion-extension valgus test 6. Martens test	1. Anterior cruciate ligament 2. Posterolateral capsule 3. Arcuate-popliteus complex 4. Lateral collateral ligament 5. Iliotibial band	1. Tests cause *reduction* of subluxed tibia on femur 2. Tests go from extension to flexion 3. Shift may be "slip" (second degree) or "jerk" (third degree), depending on degree of sprain or injury
Posteromedial rotary	1. Hughston's posteromedial drawer sign 2. Posteromedial pivot shift test	1. Posterior cruciate ligament 2. Posterior oblique ligament 3. Medial collateral ligament (superficial and deep fibers) 4. Semimembranosus muscle 5. Posteromedial capsule 6. Anterior cruciate ligament	1. Watch for changing position of tibial tubercle relative to femoral condyles
Posterolateral rotary	1. Hughston's posterolateral drawer sign 2. Jakob test (reverse pivot shift maneuver) 3. External rotational recurvatum test 4. Dynamic posterior shift test 5. Loomer's test 6. Active posterolateral drawer sign	1. Posterior cruciate ligament 2. Arcuate-popliteus ligament 3. Lateral collateral ligament 4. Biceps femoris tendon 5. Posterolateral capsule 6. Anterior cruciate ligament	1. Watch for changing position of tibial tubercle relative to femoral condyles

* The amount of displacement gives an indication of how badly and how much of the structures are injured (i.e., first-, second-, or third-degree sprain).

There are a number of tests for each type of instability. The examiner should use the one or two tests that obtain the best results. It is not essential to do all of the tests discussed. The techniques chosen must be practiced diligently so that the examiner becomes proficient at doing them; only with practice will the examiner be able to determine which structures are injured. It is also important to understand that the direction of instability does not imply that only structures in that direction are injured. For example, with anterolateral rotary instability, it is not necessarily structures on the anterolateral side of the knee that are injured. In fact, posterior structures are often commonly injured as well. With anterolateral rotary instability, the posterolateral capsule, and arcuate-popliteal complex may also be injured.[9]

When testing for ligament stability of the knee, the examiner should keep the following points in mind.

1. The normal knee is tested first to establish a baseline and to show the patient what to expect. This action helps to gain the patient's confidence by showing what the test involves.

2. When one is comparing the normal and injured limbs, the test must be the same for both limbs. The examiner must use the same initial starting position and the same amount of force, apply the same force at the same point or throughout the range, and note the position at which the displacement occurs.[52]

3. The muscles must be relaxed if the tests are to be valid. Maximum laxity would be demonstrated with the patient under anesthesia.

4. The appropriate stress should be applied gently.

5. The stress is repeated several times and increased to the point of pain to demonstrate maximum laxity without causing muscle spasm.

6. It is not only the degree of opening but also the quality of the opening (i.e., the end feel) that is of concern. Left-right differences of 3 mm or more are classified as pathological.[52]

7. If the ligament is intact, there should be an abrupt stop or end feel when the ligament is stressed. A soft or indistinct end feel usually signifies ligamentous injury.[53]

8. Ligaments of the knee tend to act in concert to maintain stability, and individual ligaments are difficult to isolate in terms of their function. Therefore, more than one test may be found to be positive when assessing for the different instabilities. For example, a patient may exhibit a one-plane medial and one-plane anterior instability as well as an anteromedial and/or anterolateral rotary instability, depending on the severity of the injury to the various ligamentous structures.

9. Tests for ligament instability are more accurate for assessment of a chronic injury than for assessment of an acute injury in the unanesthetized knee because of the presence of muscle spasm and swelling in the acutely injured knee.

10. For the tests involving rotary instability in which the tibia is moved in relation to the femur, if the movement is into extension, subluxation of the tibia relative to the femur occurs in a positive test. If the movement is into flexion, reduction of the tibia relative to the femur occurs in a positive test.

11. Positive rotational tests should not be repeated too frequently because they may lead to articular cartilage damage, further meniscal tearing, or further damage to injured ligaments.

12. Because the ligamentous tests are subjective tests, the more experience the examiner has in doing them, the more accurate will be the interpretation of the test. The examiner should select only one or two from each group of tests and learn to do them well rather than learn all of the tests and risk doing them poorly.

Ligamentous Tests Commonly Performed on the Knee

One-plane medial instability:	Valgus stress at 0° and 30°
One-plane lateral instability:	Varus stress at 0° and 30°
One-plane anterior instability:	Lachman test Drawer test Active drawer test
One-plane posterior instability:	Posterior sag Drawer test Active drawer test Godfrey test
Anteromedial rotary instability:	Slocum test
Anterolateral rotary instability:	Pivot shift test Losee test Jerk test of Hughston Slocum ARLI test Crossover test Noyes flexion-rotation drawer test
Posteromedial rotary instability:	Hughston's posteromedial drawer test Posteromedial pivot shift test
Posterolateral rotary instability:	Hughston's posterolateral drawer test Jakob test External rotation recurvatum test Loomer's posterolateral rotary instability test

Tests for One-Plane Medial Instability

The **abduction (valgus stress) test** is an assessment for one-plane (straight) medial instability, which means that the tibia moves away from the femur (i.e., gaps) on the medial side (Fig. 12–40). The examiner applies a valgus stress (pushes the knee medially) at the knee while the ankle is stabilized in slight lateral rotation either with the hand or with the leg held between the examiner's arm and trunk. The knee is first in full extension and then it is slightly flexed so that it is "unlocked" (20 to 30°). It has been advocated that resting the test thigh on the examining table enables the patient to relax more and is easier for the examiner. The knee rests on the edge of the table; the lower leg is controlled by the

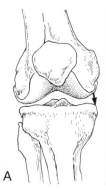

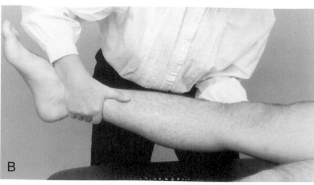

Figure 12–40
Abduction (valgus stress) test. (A) "Gapping" on the medial aspect of the knee. (B) Positioning for testing the medial collateral ligament (extended knee).

examiner's stabilizing the thigh on the table, and the lower leg is abducted, applying a valgus stress to the knee (Fig. 12–41).[10] Similarly, a varus stress may be applied to stress the lateral structures.

Hughston[10] advocates a third way to do this test. The patient is positioned as above, and the examiner faces the patient's foot, placing his or her body against the patient's thigh to help stabilize the upper leg in combination with one hand, which can also palpate the joint line. With the other hand, the examiner grasps the patient's big toe and applies a valgus stress, allowing any natural rotation of the tibia (Fig. 12–42). Similarly, a varus stress may be applied to test the lateral structures.

If the test is positive (i.e., the tibia moves away from the femur an excessive amount when a valgus stress is applied) when the knee is *in extension*, the following structures may have been injured to some degree:

1. Medial collateral ligament (superficial and deep fibers)
2. Posterior oblique ligament
3. Posteromedial capsule
4. Anterior cruciate ligament
5. Posterior cruciate ligament
6. Medial quadriceps expansion
7. Semimembranosus muscle.

A positive finding on full extension is classified as a major disruption of the knee. The examiner usually finds that one or more of the rotary tests are also positive. If the examiner applies lateral rotation to the foot when performing the test in extension and finds excessive lateral rotation on the affected side, it is a sign of possible anteromedial rotary instability.

If the test is positive when the knee *is flexed* to 20 to 30°, the following structures may have been injured to some degree:

1. Medial collateral ligament
2. Posterior oblique ligament
3. Posterior cruciate ligament
4. Posteromedial capsule.

This flexed part of the valgus stress test would be classified as the true test for one-plane medial instability.

If a stress radiograph is taken when the test is performed in full extension, a 5-mm opening is indicative of a grade 1 injury; up to 10 mm, a grade 2 injury; and more than 10 mm, a grade 3 injury.[47, 54]

Tests for One-Plane Lateral Instability

The **adduction (varus stress) test** is an assessment for one-plane lateral instability (i.e., the tibia moves away from the femur an excessive amount on the lateral aspect of the leg). The examiner applies a varus stress (pushes the knee laterally) at the knee while the ankle is stabilized (Fig. 12–43). The test is first done with the knee in full extension and then with the knee in 20 to 30° of flexion.

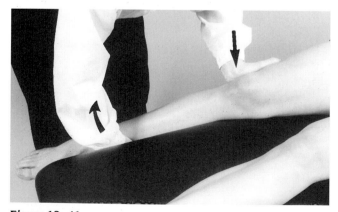

Figure 12–41
Applying a valgus stress with thigh supported on examining table.

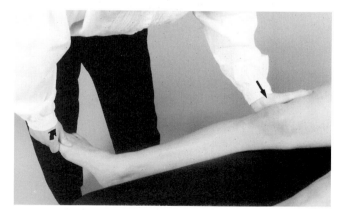

Figure 12–42
Hughston's valgus stress test.

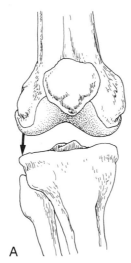
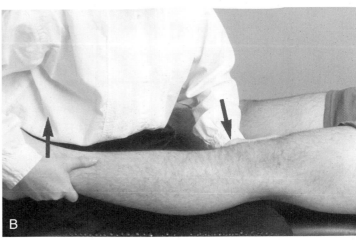

Figure 12–43
Adduction (varus stress) test.
(A) One-plane lateral instability "gapping" on the lateral aspect.
(B) Positioning for testing lateral collateral ligament in extension.

If the tibia is laterally rotated in full extension before the test, the cruciate ligaments will be uncoiled, and maximum stress will be placed on the collateral ligaments.

If the test is positive (i.e., the tibia moves away from the femur when a varus stress is applied) *in extension*, the following structures may have been injured to some degree:

1. Fibular or lateral collateral ligament
2. Posterolateral capsule
3. Arcuate-popliteus complex
4. Biceps femoris tendon
5. Posterior cruciate ligament
6. Anterior cruciate ligament
7. Lateral gastrocnemius muscle
8. Iliotibial band.

The examiner usually finds that one or more rotary instability tests are also positive. A positive test is indicative of major instability of the knee.

If the test is positive when the knee *is flexed* 20 to 30° with lateral rotation of the tibia, the following structures may have been injured to some degree:

1. Lateral collateral ligament
2. Posterolateral capsule
3. Arcuate-popliteus complex
4. Iliotibial band
5. Biceps femoris tendon.

This flexed part of the varus stress test is classified as the true test for one-plane lateral instability.

If a stress radiograph is taken when the test is performed in full extension, a 5-mm opening is indicative of a grade 1 injury; up to 8 mm, a grade 2 injury; and more than 8 mm, a grade 3 injury to the lateral ligaments of the knee.[47, 54]

Both varus and valgus stress testing **(varus-valgus test)** can be performed at the same time while the examiner palpates the joint line. The examiner holds the ankle between the examiner's waist and forearm while the patient lies supine with the knee extended and then flexed. At the same time, the examiner palpates the medial and lateral joint lines with the fingers. Varus and valgus stresses are applied with the heels of the hands (Fig. 12–44).[28]

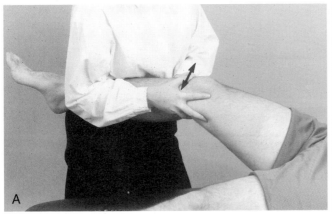
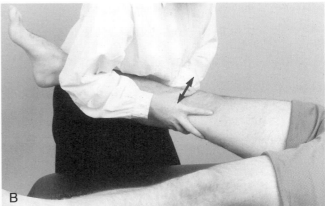

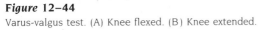

Figure 12–44
Varus-valgus test. (A) Knee flexed. (B) Knee extended.

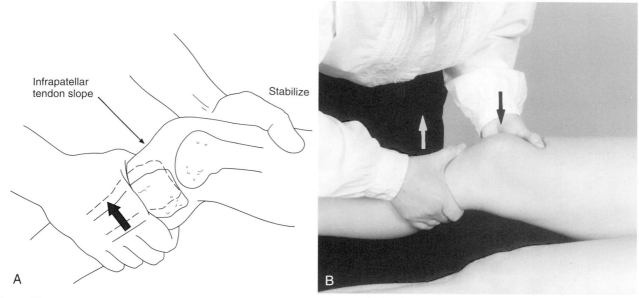

Figure 12–45
Hand position for classic Lachman test (A and B).

Tests for One-Plane Anterior Instability

Some clinicians[9, 10] believe that the posterior cruciate ligament should be tested (see Tests for One-Plane Posterior Instability) or observed for a posterior sag before the anterior cruciate ligament is tested to rule out false-positive tests for anterior translation. In either case, the examiner should be aware that a torn posterior cruciate can lead to a false-positive anterior translation test if the patient is tested in supine position with the knee flexed, because gravity causes the tibia to sag posteriorly.

Lachman Test. The Lachman test, which may also be referred to as the Ritchie, Trillat, or Lachman-Trillat test, is the best indicator of injury to the anterior cruciate ligament, especially the posterolateral band.[55–59] It is a test for one-plane anterior instability. The patient lies supine with the involved leg beside the examiner. The examiner holds the patient's knee between full extension and 30° of flexion. This position is close to the functional position of the knee, in which the anterior cruciate ligament plays a major role. The patient's femur is stabilized with one of the examiner's hands (the "outside" hand) while the proximal aspect of the tibia is moved forward with the other ("inside") hand (Fig. 12–45). Frank[60] reported that to achieve the best results, the tibia should be slightly laterally rotated and the anterior tibial translation force should be applied from the posteromedial aspect. Therefore, the hand on the tibia should apply the translation force. A positive sign is indicated by a "mushy" or soft end feel when the tibia is moved forward on the femur and disappearance of the infrapatellar tendon slope. A false-negative test may occur if the femur is not properly stabilized, if a meniscus lesion blocks translation, or if the tibia is medially rotated.[60] A positive sign indicates that the following structures may have been injured to some degree:

1. Anterior cruciate ligament (especially the posterolateral bundle)
2. Posterior oblique ligament
3. Arcuate-popliteus complex

Other ways of doing the Lachman test have also been advocated. The method that works for the examiner and that the examiner can use competently should be selected. Another method (modification 1) has the patient sitting with the leg over the edge of the examining table. The examiner sits facing the patient and supports the foot of the test leg on the examiner's thigh so that the patient's knee is flexed 30°. The examiner stabilizes the thigh with one hand and pulls the tibia forward with the other hand (Fig. 12–46). Abnormal forward motion is considered to be a positive test.[61]

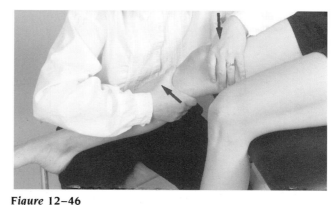

Figure 12–46
Lachman test (modification 1).

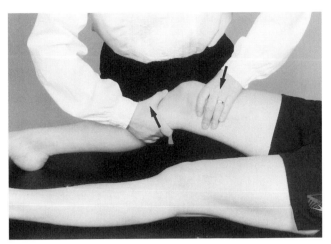

Figure 12–47
Stable Lachman test (modification 2).

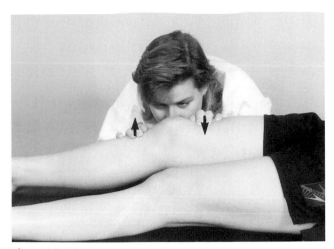

Figure 12–49
Lachman test (modification 4).

For examiners with small hands, the **stable Lachman test (modification 2)** is recommended. The patient lies supine with the knee resting on the examiner's knee (Fig. 12–47). One of the examiner's hands stabilizes the femur against the examiner's thigh, and the other hand applies an anterior stress.[28, 62]

Modification 3 has the patient lying supine while the examiner stabilizes the foot between the examiner's thorax and arm. Both hands are placed around the tibia, the knee is flexed 20 to 30°, and an anterior drawer movement is performed.[28] This technique allows gravity to control movement of the femur, which may not be sufficient to show a good positive test (Fig. 12–48).

Another way of doing the test (**modification 4**) is for the patient to lie supine while the examiner stands beside the leg to be tested with the eyes level with the knee. The examiner grasps the femur with one hand and the tibia with the other hand.[28] The tibia is pulled forward, and any abnormal motion is noted (Fig. 12–49). As with the regular Lachman test, the examiner may have diffi-culty stabilizing the femur if the examiner has small hands.

In the **prone Lachman Test (modification 5)**,[63, 64] the patient lies prone, and the examiner stabilizes the foot between the examiner's thorax and arm and places one hand around the tibia. The other hand stabilizes the femur (Fig. 12–50). Gravity assists anterior movement, but it is more difficult to determine the quality of the end feel.

In the **active (no touch) Lachman test (modification 6)**,[28, 65, 66] the patient lies supine with the knee over the examiner's forearm so that the knee is flexed approximately 30° (Fig. 12–51). The patient is asked to actively extend the knee, and the examiner watches for anterior displacement of the tibia relative to the unaffected side. The test may also be carried out with the foot held down on the table to increase the pull of the quadriceps. In this case, the test has been called the **maximum quadriceps test**.[28] The examiner must be certain that there is no posterior sag before performing the test.

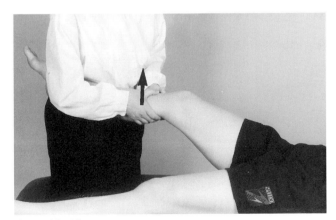

Figure 12–48
Lachman test (modification 3).

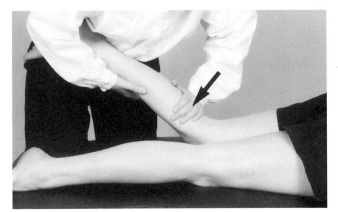

Figure 12–50
Prone Lachman test (modification 5).

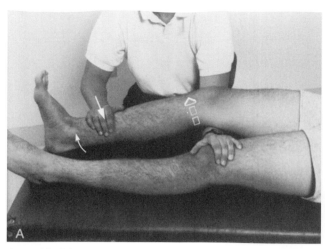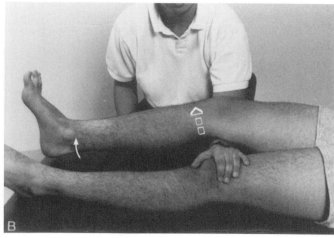

Figure 12–51

(A) Active Lachman (maximum quadriceps) test. (B) No-touch Lachman test (modification 6). Open arrow shows where the examiner watches for shift.

The Lachman test may be graded with a stress radiograph: a 3- to 6-mm opening is classified as a grade 1 injury; 6 to 9 mm, grade 2; 10 to 16 mm, grade 3; and 16 to 20 mm, grade 4.[28]

Drawer Sign. The drawer sign is a test for one-plane anterior and one-plane posterior instabilities.[67] The difficulty with this test is in determining the neutral starting position if the ligaments have been injured. The patient's knee is flexed to 90°, and the hip is flexed to 45°. In this position, the anterior cruciate ligament is almost parallel with the tibial plateau. The patient's foot is held on the table by the examiner's body with the examiner sitting on the patient's forefoot and the foot in neutral rotation. The examiner's hands are placed around the tibia to ensure that the hamstring muscles are relaxed (Figs. 12–52 and 12–53). The tibia is then drawn forward on the femur. The normal amount of movement that should be present is approximately 6 mm. This part of the test assesses one-plane anterior instability. If the test is posi-

tive (i.e., the tibia moves forward more than 6 mm on the femur), the following structures may have been injured to some degree:

1. Anterior cruciate ligament (especially the anteromedial bundle)
2. Posterolateral capsule
3. Posteromedial capsule
4. Medial collateral ligament (deep fibers)
5. Iliotibial band
6. Posterior oblique ligament
7. Arcuate-popliteus complex

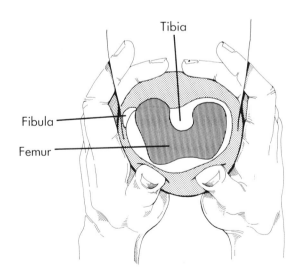

Figure 12–53

This view of the knee from above shows the inside of the knee joint during performance of the anterior drawer test in flexion. The hands are in place, and the overlay of the femur on the tibia demonstrates that the anterior and posterior motions are normal. The index fingers are ensuring that the hamstrings are relaxed. If, on pulling or pushing tibia, rotation of tibial plateau occurs, the examiner should check for rotary instabilities. (From Hughston, J.C.: Knee Ligaments: Injury and Repair. Mosby–Year Book Inc., 1993, p. 111.)

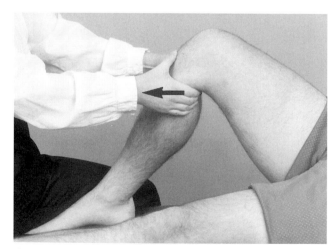

Figure 12–52

Position for drawer sign.

If only the anterior cruciate ligament is torn, the test is negative, because other structures (posterior capsule and posterolateral and posteromedial structures) limit movement. In addition, hemarthrosis, a torn medial meniscus (posterior horn) wedged against the medial femoral condyle, or hamstring spasm may result in a false-negative test. Hughston[10] points out that tearing of the coronary or meniscotibial ligament can allow the tibia to translate forward more than normal, even in the presence of an intact anterior cruciate ligament. In this case, when the anterior drawer test is performed, anteromedial rotation (subluxation) of the tibia occurs.

When performing this test, the examiner must ensure that the posterior cruciate ligament is not torn or injured. If it has been torn, it will allow the tibia to drop back on the femur, and when the examiner pulls the tibia forward, a large amount of movement will occur, giving a false-positive sign (see Posterior Sag Sign). Therefore, the test should be considered positive only if it is shown that the posterior sag is not present.

Weatherwax[68] described a modified way of testing the anterior drawer. The patient lies supine. The examiner flexes the patient's hip and knee to 90° and supports the lower leg between the examiner's trunk and forearm. The examiner places the hands around the tibia, as with the standard test, and applies sufficient force to slowly lift the patient's buttock off the table (Fig. 12–54).

If, when doing the anterior drawer test, there is an audible snap or palpable jerk (**Finochietto's jumping sign**) when the tibia is pulled forward and the tibia moves forward excessively, a meniscus lesion is probably accompanying the torn anterior cruciate ligament.[28]

After the anterior movement of the tibia on the fe-

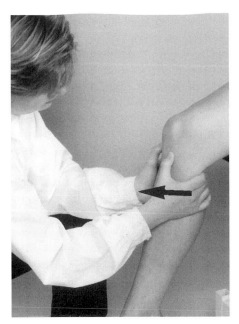

Figure 12–55
Anterior drawer test in sitting. Examiner feels anterior shift with thumbs.

mur, the posterior movement of the tibia on the femur should be completed. In this part of the test, the tibia is pushed back on the femur. This phase is a test for one-plane posterior instability. If the test is positive, the following structures may have been injured to some degree:

1. Posterior cruciate ligament
2. Arcuate-popliteus complex
3. Posterior oblique ligament
4. Anterior cruciate ligament

If the arcuate-popliteus complex remains intact, a positive posterior drawer sign may not be elicited.[69] If, when the tibia is pushed backward, the examiner forcefully rotates the tibia laterally and excessive movement occurs, the test is positive for posterolateral instability. Warren[70] calls this maneuver the **arcuate spin test.**

Feagin[63] advocated doing the drawer test with the patient sitting with the leg hanging relaxed over the end of the examining table. The examiner places the hands as with the standardized test and slowly draws the tibia first forward and then backward to test the anterior and posterior drawer (Fig. 12–55). The examiner uses the thumbs to palpate the tibia plateau movement relative to the femur. The examiner may also note any rotational deformity. The advantage of doing the test this way is that the posterior sag is eliminated because the effect of gravity is eliminated.

Active Drawer Test. The patient is positioned as for the normal drawer test. The examiner holds the patient's foot down. The patient is asked to try to straighten the leg, and the examiner prevents the patient from doing

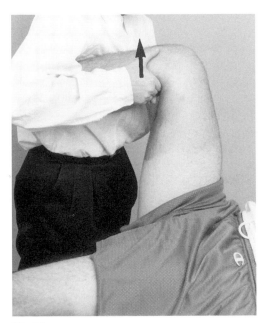

Figure 12–54
Anterior drawer test in 90° flexion with the hip flexed 90°.

so (isometric test). Muller[47] advocated allowing the foot to be free and noting when the foot is lifted off the table, which occurs only after the tibia has shifted forward and stabilized. If the anterior cruciate ligament or posterior cruciate ligament is torn, the anterior contour of the knee changes as the tibia is drawn forward. If the posterior cruciate ligament is torn, a posterior sag is evident before the patient contracts the quadriceps. Contraction of the quadriceps causes the tibia to shift foward to its normal position, indicating a positive test for a torn posterior cruciate ligament.[71] If there is no posterior sag present and if the tibia shifts forward more on the injured side than the noninjured side, it is a positive test for anterior cruciate ligament disruption (Fig. 12–56).[71] A second part of the test may be instituted by having the patient contract the hamstrings isometrically so that the tibial plateau moves posteriorly. This part of the test accentuates the posterior sag for posterior cruciate insufficiency, if present, and ensures maximum movement for anterior cruciate insufficiency if a quadriceps contraction is tried a second time.[28] The active drawer test is a better expression of posterior cruciate insufficiency than of anterior cruciate insufficiency.[72]

With the drawer sign or test, if the anterior or posterior cruciate ligament is torn (third-degree sprain), some rotary instability will be evident when the appropriate ligamentous tests are performed.

Tests for One-Plane Posterior Instability

Posterior Sag Sign (Gravity Drawer Test). The patient lies supine with the hip flexed to 45° and the knee flexed to 90°. In this position, the tibia "drops back," or sags back, on the femur if the posterior cruciate ligament is torn (Fig. 12–57). Posterior tibial displacement is more noticeable when the knee is flexed 90 to 110° than when the knee is only slightly flexed. It is a test for one-plane posterior instability. Normally, the medial tibial plateau extends 1 cm anteriorly beyond the femoral condyle when the knee is flexed 90°. If this "step" is lost, which is what occurs with a positive posterior sag due to a torn posterior cruciate ligament, this **step-off test** or **thumb sign** is considered positive.[12, 16, 72] The examiner must be careful because the position could result in a false-positive anterior drawer test for the anterior cruciate ligament if the sag remains unnoticed. If there is minimal or no swelling, the sag is evident because of an obvious concavity distal to the patella. If the posterior sag sign is present, the following structures may have been injured to some degree:

1. Posterior cruciate ligament
2. Arcuate-popliteus complex
3. Posterior oblique ligament
4. Anterior cruciate ligament

If it appears that the patient has a positive posterior sag sign, the patient should carefully extend the knee

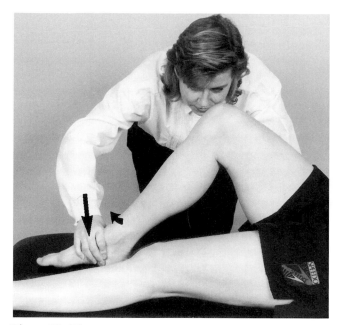

Figure 12–56
Active anterior drawer test. Examiner watches for anterior shift.

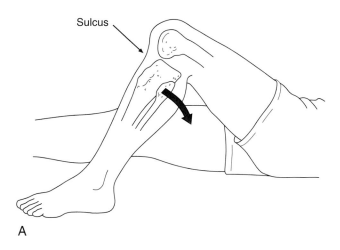

Sulcus

A

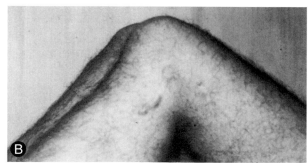

B

Figure 12–57
Sag sign. (A) Illustration of posterior sag sign. (B) Note profile of two knees; the left (nearer) sags backward compared with the normal right knee, indicating posterior cruciate defect. (A, Redrawn from and B, from O'Donoghue, D.H.: Treatment of Injuries to Athletes, 4th ed. Philadelphia, W.B. Saunders Co., 1984, p. 450.)

while the examiner holds the thigh in 90 to 100° of flexion. This action is sometimes called the **voluntary anterior drawer sign,** and the results are similar to those of the active anterior drawer test. As the patient does this slowly, the tibial plateau moves or shifts forward to its normal position, indicating that the tibia was previously posteriorly subluxed (posterior cruciate tear) on the femur.

Reverse Lachman Test.[28] The patient lies prone with the knee flexed to 30°, and the examiner grasps the tibia with one hand while fixing the femur with the other hand (Fig. 12–58). The examiner ensures that the hamstring muscles are relaxed. The examiner then pulls the tibia up (posteriorly), noting the amount of movement and the quality of the end feel. It is a test for the posterior cruciate ligament. The examiner should be wary of a false-positive test if the anterior cruciate ligament has been torn, because gravity may cause an anterior shift. This test is not as accurate for the posterior cruciate ligament as the posterior drawer test, because when the posterior cruciate ligament is torn, the greatest posterior displacement is at 90°.

Drawer Sign or Test. This test has been described previously.

Active Drawer Test. This test has been described previously.

Godfrey (Gravity) Test.[28] The patient lies supine, and the examiner holds both legs while flexing the patient's hips and knees to 90° (Fig. 12–59). If there is posterior instability, a posterior sag of the tibia is seen. If manual posterior pressure is applied to the tibia, posterior displacement may increase.

Tests for Anteromedial Rotary Instability

Slocum Test. The Slocum test assesses both anterior rotary instabilities.[73] The patient's knee is flexed to 80 or 90°, and the hip is flexed to 45°. The foot is first placed in 30° medial rotation (Fig. 12–60). The examiner then sits on the patient's forefoot to hold the foot in position and draws the tibia forward; if the test is positive, movement occurs primarily on the lateral side of the knee. This movement is excessive relative to the unaffected side and indicates anterolateral rotary instability. It also indicates that the following structures may have been injured to some degree:

1. Anterior cruciate ligament
2. Posterolateral capsule
3. Arcuate-popliteus complex
4. Lateral collateral ligament
5. Posterior cruciate ligament
6. Iliotibial band

If the examiner finds anterolateral instability during this first position of the Slocum test, the second part of the test, which assesses anteromedial rotary instability in this position, is of less value.[74]

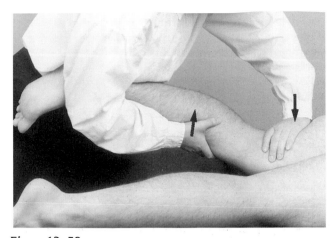

Figure 12–58
Reverse Lachman test.

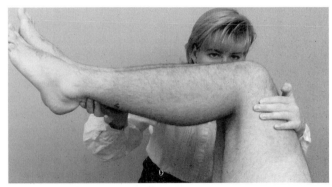

Figure 12–59
Godfrey test. Examiner watches for posterior shift, which is not evident in this case.

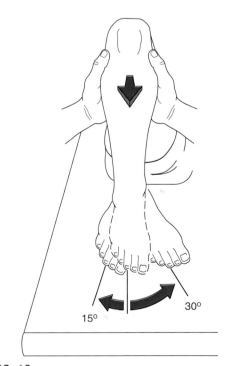

Figure 12–60
Slocum test.

In the second part of the test, the foot is placed in 15° of lateral rotation, and the tibia is drawn forward by the examiner. This part of the test is sometimes referred to as **Lemaire's T drawer test**. If the test is positive, the movement occurs primarily on the medial side of the knee. This movement is excessive relative to the unaffected side and indicates anteromedial rotary instability. It also indicates that the following structures may have been injured to some degree:

1. Medial collateral ligament (especially the superficial fibers, although the deep fibers may also be affected)
2. Posterior oblique ligament
3. Posteromedial capsule
4. Anterior cruciate ligament

For the Slocum test, it is imperative that the examiner medially or laterally rotate the foot to the degrees shown. If the examiner rotates the tibia as far as it will go, the test will be negative for movement, because this action tightens all of the remaining structures.

If a stress radiograph is taken during the test, minimal or no movement indicates a negative test; 1 mm or less, a grade 1 injury; 1 to 2 mm, a grade 2 injury; and more than 2 mm, a grade 3 injury.[54]

The test may also be performed with the patient sitting with the knees flexed over the edge of the examining table (Fig. 12–61).[47] The examiner applies an anterior or a posterior force while holding the foot medially or

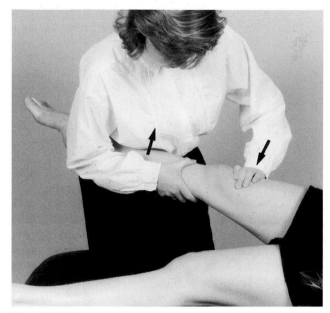

Figure 12–62
Dejour test.

laterally rotated. If this procedure is used, the examiner must remember that use of the anterior force tests for anterior rotary instability, whereas use of the posterior force tests for posterior rotary instability (see Hughston's Posteromedial and Posterolateral Drawer Sign in later sections). The examiner should note whether the movement is excessive on the medial or on the lateral side of the knee relative to the normal knee. Excessive movement indicates a positive test.

Dejour Test.[9] The patient lies supine. The examiner holds the patient's leg with one arm against the body and the hand under the calf to lift the tibia while applying a valgus stress. The other hand pushes the femur down (Fig. 12–62). In extension, this action causes anteromedial subluxation in the pathological knee. If the knee is then flexed, the tibial plateau reduces suddenly, indicating a positive test. If the jolt is painful, it indicates that the medial meniscus has been injured. If it is not painful, the posteromedial corner has been injured.

Tests for Anterolateral Rotary Instability

Slocum Test. This test has been described previously.

Lateral Pivot Shift Maneuver (Test of MacIntosh). This is the primary test used to assess anterolateral rotary instability of the knee and is an excellent test for ruptures of the anterior cruciate ligament.[75-78] It does have a disadvantage, however. In the apprehensive patient, because of the forces applied during the test, protective muscle contraction may lead to a false-negative test.[9] During this test, the tibia moves away from the femur on the lateral side (but rotates medially) and moves anteriorly in relation to the femur (Fig. 12–63).

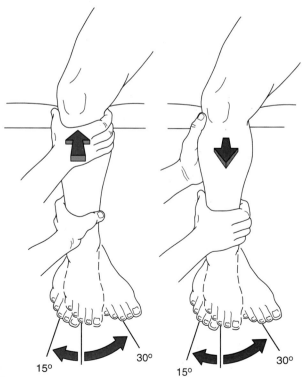

Figure 12–61
Slocum test with the patient in the sitting position.

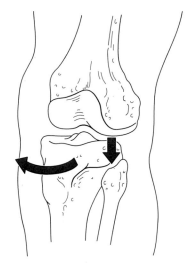

Figure 12–63
Anterolateral rotary instability.

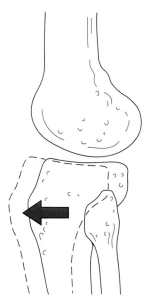

Figure 12–64
Anterior shift of the tibia during the lateral pivot shift test.

Normally, the knee's center of rotation changes constantly through its range of motion as a result of the shape of the femoral condyles, ligamentous restraint, and muscle tension. The path of movement of the tibia on the femur is described as a combination of rolling and sliding, with rolling predominating when the instant center is near the joint line and sliding predominating when the instant center shifts distally from the contact area. The MacIntosh test is a duplication of the anterior subluxation-reduction phenomenon that occurs during the normal gait cycle when the anterior cruciate ligament is torn. Therefore, it illustrates a **dynamic subluxation**. This shift occurs between 20 and 40° of flexion (0° being full extension). It is this phenomenon that gives the patient the clinical description of feeling the knee "give way" (Fig. 12–64).

The patient lies supine with the hip both flexed and abducted 30° and relaxed in slight medial rotation (20°). The examiner holds the patient's foot with one hand while the other hand is placed at the knee, holding the leg in slight medial rotation. This is done by placing the heel of the hand behind the fibula and over the lateral head of the gastrocnemius muscle with the tibia medially rotated, causing the tibia to sublux anteriorly as the knee is taken into extension (Fig. 12–65). Bach and colleagues[79] modified the position to slight lateral rotation, because they believed that lateral tibial rotation gives a more pronounced pivot shift when the test is positive. In slight flexion, the secondary restraints (i.e., hamstrings, lateral femoral condyle, and lateral meniscus) are less efficient than in full flexion. It is important to realize that in full extension subluxation does not occur, because of the "locking home" of the tibia on the femur.[9] With slight flexion, however, the secondary restraints are less restrictive, and subluxation occurs. The examiner then applies a valgus stress to the knee while maintaining a medial

rotation torque on the tibia at the ankle. The leg is then flexed, and at approximately 30 to 40° the tibia reduces or "jogs" backward. The patient says that that is what the "giving way" feels like, indicating a positive test. The reduction of the tibia on the femur is caused by the change in position of the iliotibial band when it switches from an extensor function to a flexor function, pulling

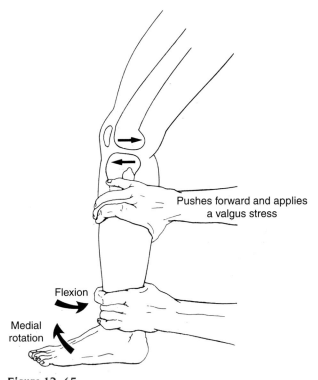

Pushes forward and applies
a valgus stress

Flexion

Medial
rotation

Figure 12–65
Lateral pivot shift test.

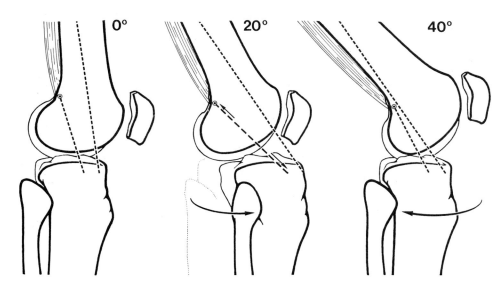

0° **20°** **40°**

Figure 12–66

Biomechanics of the pivot shift. Three phases occur during the pivot shift maneuver. Under load transmission in the lateral compartment, the tibia rolls from a reduced position in neutral rotation to anterior subluxation and some medial rotation. Under increasing flexion to 20°, the condyle becomes jammed behind the posterior slope of the lateral plateau. The iliotibial band, especially the femorotibial portion, becomes tight until, at 30 to 40°, it is gliding behind the flexion axis, initiating reduction in more flexion and some lateral rotation. (From Jakob, R.P.: Pathomechanical and clinical components of the pivot shift sign. Semin. Orthop. 2:12, 1987.)

the tibia back into its normal position (Fig. 12–66). The test involves two phases: first subluxation and then reduction. The iliotibial band must be intact for the test to work. In cases of anterolateral instability in which the iliotibial band has also been torn, the test does not work. In addition, if either meniscus has been torn, it may limit or prevent the subluxation reduction motion seen in the test.

If the patient is tense or apprehensive, the test can be modified; this is called the **soft pivot shift test** (Fig. 12–67). The patient lies supine and the examiner supports the test foot with one hand while placing the other hand over the calf muscle 10 to 20 cm (4 to 8 inches) distal to the knee joint. The examiner flexes and extends the knee slowly and gently. After three to five cycles, the examiner applies axial compression while the other hand over the calf exerts an anterior pressure. In a positive test, the tibia subluxes and reduces, but not with the same apprehensive, jerky feeling.[28] Kennedy[54] advocated pushing on the fibula with the thumb when performing

this maneuver. Because hip abduction and adduction has an effect on the iliotibial band, hip position plays an important role in the test. Subluxation is most obvious when the hip is abducted and least obvious when it is adducted. In addition, lateral rotation of the tibia allows greater subluxation because, like abduction, it decreases the stress on the iliotibial band.[28] If the test is positive, the following structures have probably been injured to some degree:

1. Anterior cruciate ligament
2. Posterolateral capsule
3. Arcuate-popliteus complex
4. Lateral collateral ligament
5. Iliotibial band

Active Pivot Shift Test.[80] The patient sits with the foot on the floor in neutral rotation and the knee flexed 80 to 90°. The patient is asked to isometrically contract the quadriceps while the examiner stabilizes the foot. A positive test is indicated by anterolateral subluxation of

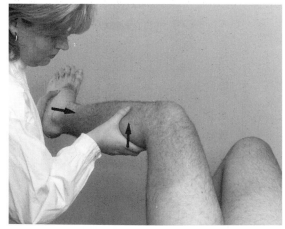

Figure 12–67
Soft pivot shift test. Examiner watches for anterior shift.

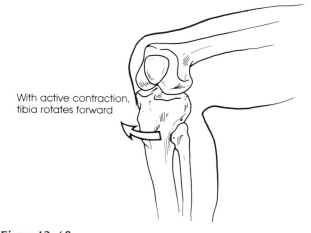

With active contraction, tibia rotates forward

Figure 12–68
Active pivot shift test.

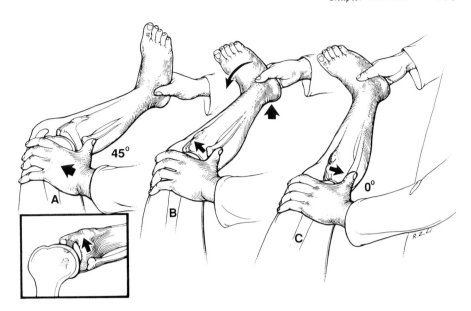

Figure 12–69
The Losee test begins with the knee in flexion and the tibia in lateral rotation and valgus stress. As the knee is extended, the foot is allowed to medially rotate, and the previously subluxed tibia reduces as the knee approaches full extension. A palpable "clunk" correlates with anterior cruciate ligament tear. (From Scott, W.N. [ed.]: Ligament and Extensor Mechanism Injuries of the Knee: Diagnosis and Treatment. St. Louis, Mosby–Year Book Inc., 1991, p. 96.)

the lateral tibial plateau and is indicative of anterolateral instability (Fig. 12–68).

Losee Test. This test is a clinical duplication of the anterolateral rotary instability mechanism of injury. The patient lies supine while relaxed.[81] The examiner holds the patient's ankle and foot so that the leg is laterally rotated and braced against the examiner's abdomen. The knee is then flexed to 30°, and the examiner ensures that the hamstring muscles are relaxed (Fig. 12–69). The lateral rotation ensures that the subluxation of the knee is reduced at the beginning of the test. With the examiner's other hand positioned so that the fingers lie over the patella and the thumb is hooked behind the fibular head, a valgus force is applied to the knee; the examiner uses the abdomen as a fulcrum while extending the patient's knee and applying forward pressure behind the fibular head with the thumb. The valgus stress compresses the structures in the lateral compartment and

makes the anterior subluxation, if present, more noticeable. At the same time, the foot and ankle are allowed to drift into medial rotation. If the foot and ankle are not allowed to rotate medially, the anterior subluxation of the lateral tibial plateau may be prevented. Just before full extension of the knee, there will be a "clunk" forward if the test is positive, and the patient must recognize the movement as the instability that was previously experienced. This clunk means that the tibia has subluxed anteriorly and indicates injury to the same structures as those indicated by a positive pivot shift maneuver.

Jerk Test of Hughston.[82] This test is similar to the pivot shift maneuver. The positioning of the patient and the examiner are the same, except that the patient's hip is flexed to 45°. With this test, the knee is first flexed to 90°. The leg is then extended, maintaining medial rotation and a valgus stress (Fig. 12–70). At approximately 20 to 30° of flexion, the tibia shifts forward, causing a

Figure 12–70
Jerk Test of Hughston. (A) The knee is flexed to 90°, and the heel of one hand is placed behind the fibular head to produce medial rotation of the tibia. (B) At 20 to 30°, the lateral tibial plateau subluxes anteriorly. (C) At full extension, the lateral tibial plateau is reduced. (From Irrgang, J.J., M.R. Safran, and F.H. Fu: The knee: Ligamentous and meniscal injuries. In Zachazewski, J.E., D.J. Magee, and W.S. Quillen [eds.]: Athletic Injuries and Rehabilitation. Philadelphia, W.B. Saunders Co., 1996, p. 644.)

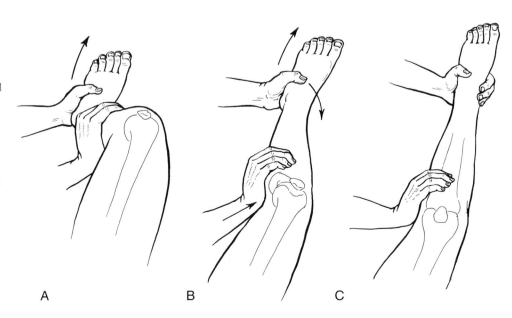

A   B   C

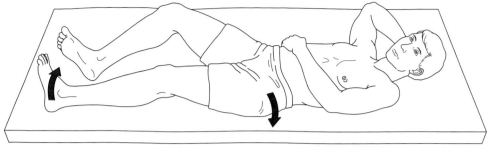
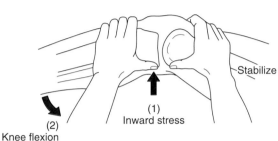

Figure 12–71
Slocum anterolateral rotary instability test.

subluxation of the lateral tibial plateau with a jerk if the test is positive. If the leg is carried into further extension, it spontaneously reduces. A positive jerk test indicates that the same structures are injured as indicated by a positive pivot shift maneuver and assesses anterolateral rotary instability. According to the literature,[47] this test is not as sensitive as the pivot shift test.

Slocum ALRI Test. Anterolateral rotary instability (ALRI) is also assessed by the Slocum ALRI test.[47, 74] The patient is in the side lying position (approximately 30° from supine). The bottom leg is the uninvolved leg. The knee of the uninvolved leg is flexed to add stability (Fig. 12–71). The foot of the involved leg rests and is stabilized on the examining table with the patient's foot in medial rotation and the knee in extension and valgus. This position helps to eliminate hip rotation during the test. The examiner applies a valgus stress to the knee while flexing the knee. The subluxation of the knee reduces at between 25 and 45° of flexion if the test is positive. A positive test indicates injury to the same structures as indicated in the pivot shift maneuver. The main advantage of this test is that it aids in relaxation of the patient's hamstring muscles and is easier to perform on heavy or tense patients.

Crossover Test of Arnold. The patient is asked to cross the uninvolved leg in front of the involved leg (Fig. 12–72). The examiner then carefully steps on the patient's involved foot to stabilize it and instructs the patient to rotate the upper torso away from the injured leg approximately 90° from the fixed foot. When this position is achieved, the patient contracts the quadriceps muscles, producing the same symptoms and testing the same structures as in the lateral pivot shift test.

Noyes Flexion-Rotation Drawer Test. Described by Noyes,[83] this test is a modification of the pivot shift

maneuver. It can be used in the acutely injured knee and is felt by some[7] to be more sensitive than the other anterolateral rotary instability tests. The patient lies supine, and the examiner holds the patient's ankle between the examiner's trunk and arm with the hands around the tibia (Fig. 12–73). The examiner flexes the patient's knee

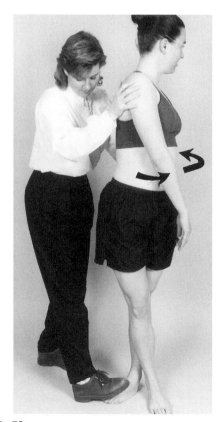

Figure 12–72
Crossover test.

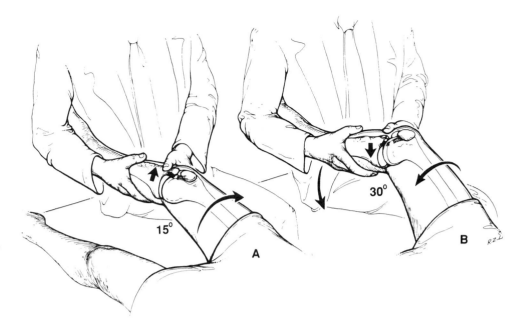

Figure 12–73

Flexion-rotation drawer test combines elements of Lachman test and lateral pivot shift. Flexion from (A) to (B) results in posterior reduction of subluxed tibia and medial rotation of femur. Positive test results correlate with anterior cruciate ligament disruption. (From Scott, W.N. [ed.]: Ligament and Extensor Mechanism Injuries of the Knee: Diagnosis and Treatment. St. Louis, Mosby–Year Book Inc., 1991, p. 94.)

to 20 to 30° while maintaining the tibia in neutral rotation. The tibia is then pushed posteriorly, as in a posterior drawer test. This posterior movement reduces the subluxation of the tibia, indicating a positive test for anterolateral rotary instability. If the tibia is alternately pushed posteriorly and released and the femur is allowed to rotate freely, the reduction and subluxation are seen and felt as the femur rotates medially and laterally.

Lemaire's Jolt Test.[9] The patient is in side lying position with the test leg uppermost. For the test to work, the patient must be relaxed. With one hand, the examiner medially rotates the tibia by grasping the foot and medially rotating it with the knee in extension. The back of the other hand pushes lightly against the biceps tendon and head of fibula while the hand on the foot flexes and extends the knee (Fig. 12–74). In a positive test, at about 15 to 20° of flexion, a "jolt" occurs with displacement of the tibia, indicating a positive test for anterolateral instability.

Flexion-Extension Valgus Test. The patient lies supine, and the examiner holds the patient's leg as in the Noyes test. The examiner palpates the joint line with the thumb and fingers of both hands, and a valgus stress and axial compression are applied while the knee is flexed and extended (Fig. 12–75). If the anterior cruciate ligament is torn, the examiner feels the reduction and subluxation. The tibia is not rotated, so the subluxation is easily felt.[84]

Figure 12–74

Lemaire's jolt test for anterolateral rotary instability.

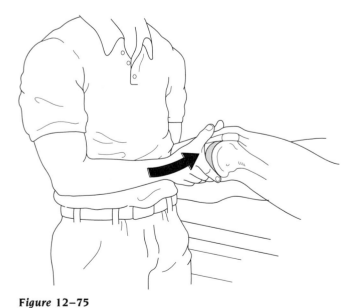

Figure 12–75

Flexion-extension valgus test. Arrow shows compression. (Redrawn from Hanks, G.A., D.M. Joyner, and A. Kalenak: Anterolateral instability of the knee. J. Sports Med. 9:226, 1981.)

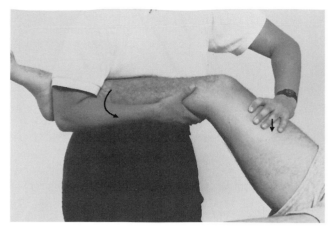

Figure 12–76
Martens test.

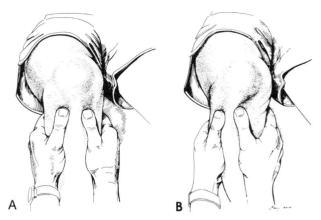

Figure 12–77
Posteromedial and posterolateral drawer test, anterior view.
(A) Starting position for posterolateral drawer test. (B) Positive posterolateral drawer test with posterior and lateral rotation of the lateral tibial condyle. (From Hughston, J.C., and L.A. Norwood: The posterolateral drawer test and external rotational recurvatum test for posterolateral rotary instability of the knee. Clin. Orthop. 147:83, 1980.)

Nakajima Test.[28] The patient lies supine, and the examiner stands on the side of the test leg. The patient's foot is held with one hand, which medially rotates the tibia. The knee is flexed to 90°. The examiner's other hand is placed over the lateral femoral condyle with the thumb behind the head of the fibula, pushing it forward. The examiner slowly extends the knee while pushing the head of the fibula forward, noting whether subluxation occurs, which indicates a positive test.

Martens Test.[28] The patient and examiner are positioned as for the Noyes test. The examiner grips the patient's leg distal to the knee joint with one hand and pushes the femur posteriorly with the other hand. A valgus stress is applied to the knee as the knee is flexed until the tibia reduces, indicating a positive test (Fig. 12–76).

Tests for Posteromedial Rotary Instability

Hughston's Posteromedial and Posterolateral Drawer Sign. The patient lies supine with the knee flexed to 80 to 90° and the hip flexed to 45° (Fig. 12–77).[85] The examiner medially rotates the patient's foot slightly and sits on the foot to stabilize it. The examiner then pushes the tibia posteriorly. If the tibia moves or rotates posteriorly

on the medial aspect an excessive amount relative to the normal knee, the test is positive and indicative of posteromedial rotary instability. A positive test indicates that the following structures have probably been injured to some degree:

1. Posterior cruciate ligament
2. Posterior oblique ligament
3. Medial collateral ligament (superficial and deep fibers)
4. Semimembranosus muscle
5. Posteromedial capsule
6. Anterior cruciate ligament

The medial tubercle rotates posteriorly around the posterior cruciate ligament when the tibia is in mild medial rotation. If the posterior cruciate ligament is also torn, the posteromedial movement is greater, and the tibia subluxes posteriorly (Fig. 12–78).

The test may also be done with the patient sitting with the knee flexed over the edge of the examining

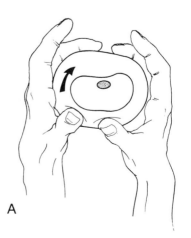
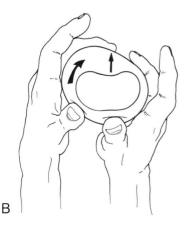

Figure 12–78
Posterolateral drawer test. (A) If the posterior cruciate ligament is intact, the tibia rotates posterolaterally. (B) If the posterior cruciate ligament is torn, the tibia rotates posterolaterally and subluxes posteriorly.

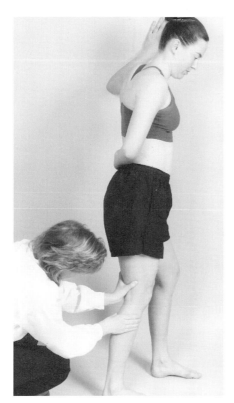

Figure 12–79
Jakob test (method 1, showing valgus stress and flexion).

table. The examiner pushes posteriorly while holding the patient's leg in medial rotation, watching for the same excessive movement.

Posterolateral rotary instability may be tested in a similar fashion.[85] The patient and examiner are in the same position, but the patient's foot is slightly laterally rotated. If the tibia rotates posteriorly on the lateral side an excessive amount relative to the uninvolved leg when the examiner pushes the tibia posteriorly, the test is positive for posterolateral rotary instability. The test is positive only if the posterior cruciate ligament is torn. The examiner may palpate the fibula while doing the movement to feel for excessive movement. The test indicates that the following structures have probably been injured to some degree:

1. Posterior cruciate ligament
2. Arcuate-popliteus complex
3. Lateral collateral ligament
4. Biceps femoris tendon
5. Posterolateral capsule
6. Anterior cruciate ligament

Posteromedial Pivot Shift Test.[86] The patient lies relaxed in the supine position. The examiner passively flexes the knee more than 45° while applying a varus stress, compression, and medial rotation of the tibia; in a "positive" knee, these movements cause subluxation of the medial tibial plateau posteriorly. The examiner then takes the knee into extension. At about 20 to 40° of

flexion, the tibia shifts into the reduced position. A positive test indicates that the following structures are injured:

1. Posterior cruciate ligament
2. Medial collateral ligament
3. Posterior oblique ligament

Tests for Posterolateral Rotary Instability

Hughston's Posteromedial and Posterolateral Drawer Sign. This test has been described previously.

Jakob Test (Reverse Pivot Shift Maneuver). This is a test for posterolateral rotary instability,[47, 87] and it can be performed in two ways. In the first method, the patient stands and leans against a wall with the uninjured side adjacent to the wall and the body weight distributed equally between the two feet (Fig. 12–79). The examiner's hands are placed above and below the involved knee, and a valgus stress is exerted while flexion of the patient's knee is initiated. If there is a jerk in the knee or the tibia shifts posteriorly and the "giving way" phenomenon occurs during this maneuver, it indicates injury to the same structures as indicated by a positive Hughston's posterolateral drawer sign.

In the second method, the patient lies in the supine position with the hamstring muscles relaxed. The examiner faces the patient, lifts the patient's leg, and supports the leg against the examiner's pelvis. The examiner's other hand supports the lateral side of the calf with the palm on the proximal fibula. The knee is flexed to 70 to 80° of flexion, and the foot is laterally rotated, causing the lateral tibial plateau to sublux posteriorly (Fig. 12–80A). The knee is taken into extension by its own weight

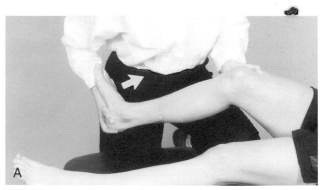

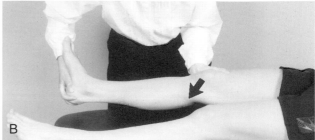

Figure 12–80
Reverse pivot shift test, method 2. (A) Flexed position with lateral rotation causes lateral tibial tubercle to sublux. (B) As the extended position is approached, the lateral tibial tubercle reduces.

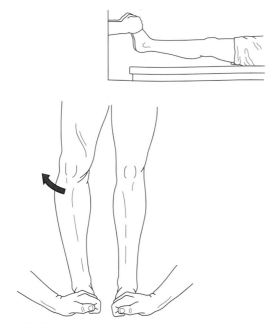

Figure 12–81
External rotational recurvatum test (method 1).

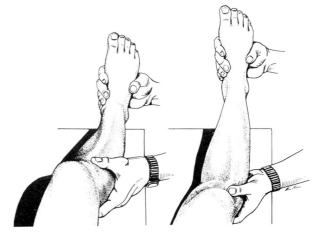

Figure 12–82
External recurvatum test (method 2). The test is begun by holding the knee in flexion (left). As the knee is slowly extended, the hand at the knee feels the lateral rotation and recurvatum at the posterolateral aspect of the knee. (From Hughston, J.C., and L.A. Norwood: The posterolateral drawer test and external rotational recurvatum test for posterolateral rotary instability of the knee. Clin. Orthop. 147:86, 1980.)

while the examiner leans on the foot to impart a valgus stress to the knee through the leg. As the knee approaches 20° of flexion, the lateral tibial tubercle shifts forward or anteriorly into the neutral rotation and reduces the subluxation, indicating a positive test (Fig. 12–80B). The leg is then flexed again, and the foot falls back into lateral rotation and posterior subluxation.

External Rotation Recurvatum Test. There are two methods for performing this test. In the first method, the patient lies in the supine position with the lower limbs relaxed. The examiner gently grasps the big toe of each foot and lifts both feet off the examining table (Fig. 12–81).[85, 88] The patient is told to keep the quadriceps muscles relaxed. While elevating the legs, the examiner watches the tibial tuberosities. With a positive test, the affected knee goes into relative hyperextension on the lateral aspect, with the tibia and tibial tuberosity rotating laterally. The affected knee has the appearance of a relative genu varum. It is a test for posterolateral rotary instability in extension and assesses the same structures previously mentioned.

In the second method, the patient lies supine and the examiner's hand holds the patient's heel or foot and flexes the knee to 30 to 40° (Fig. 12–82).[85] The examiner's other hand holds the posterolateral aspect of the patient's knee and slowly extends it. With the hand on the knee, the examiner feels the relative hyperextension and lateral rotation occurring in the injured limb compared with the uninjured limb. This is a test for posterolateral rotary instability and assesses the same structures as previously mentioned.

Loomer's Posterolateral Rotary Instability Test.[88, 89] The patient lies supine and flexes both hips and both knees

to 90°. The examiner then grasps the feet and maximally laterally rotates both tibias (Fig. 12–83). The test is considered positive if the injured tibia laterally rotates excessively and there is a posterior sag of the affected tibial tubercle; both signs must be present for a positive test. This test is similar to the **Bousquet external hypermobility test**[9] and is also called the **Dial test.**

Dynamic Posterior Shift Test.[90] The patient lies supine, and the examiner flexes the hip and knee of the test leg to 90° with the femur in neutral rotation. One hand of the examiner stabilizes the anterior thigh while the other hand extends the knee. If the test is positive, the tibia reduces anteriorly with a clunk as extension is reached.

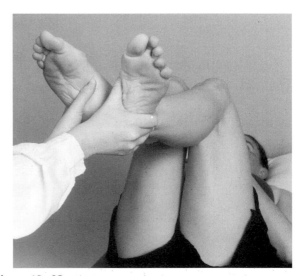

Figure 12–83
Loomer's test.

The test is positive for posterior and posterolateral instabilities. If the knee is painful before extension is accomplished, the hip flexion may be decreased, but the hamstrings must be kept tight (Fig. 12–84).

Active Posterolateral Drawer Sign.[91] The patient sits with the foot on the floor in neutral rotation. The knee is flexed to 80 to 90°. The patient is asked to isometrically contract the hamstrings, primarily the lateral one (biceps femoris), while the examiner stabilizes the foot. A positive test for posterolateral instability is posterior subluxation of the lateral tibial plateau (Fig. 12–85).

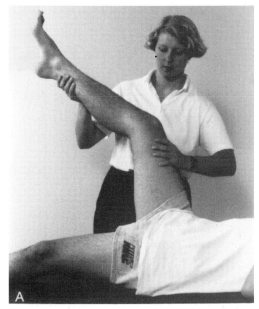

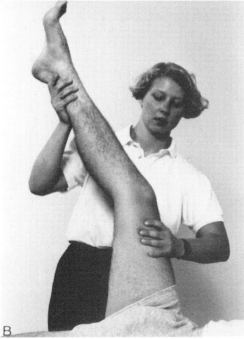

Figure 12–84
Dynamic posterior shift test. (A) Starting position in flexion. (B) Extended position in which posterior shift occurs.

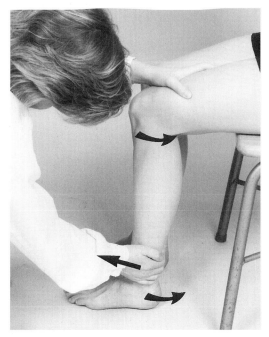

Figure 12–85
Active posterolateral drawer sign or test. Examiner watches for posterolateral shift.

Ligament Testing Devices

Ligament testing devices for the knee have been developed to help quantify the displacement occurring in the knee and how this displacement is modified when ligaments are injured. Most commonly, these devices test anteroposterior displacement, although more expensive ones may test other displacements. These devices are used primarily to assist in diagnosing ligament injuries (third-degree sprains) by detecting abnormal (pathological) motion, to provide a quantified measurement of motion, and to measure the amount of motion after surgery (e.g., whether normal motion limits were reestablished).[92–94]

The most commonly used ligament testing devices are the KT 1000 arthrometer, which measures anteriorposterior displacement; the Genucom, which measures anteroposterior, mediolateral, and rotation displacement; and the Stryker knee laxity tester. Of the three, the KT 1000 is most commonly used. Other units have been developed but are not commonly used.[9, 95–98] It is important to understand that these devices are adjuncts to clinical assessment and should be used primarily to confirm a clinical diagnosis.[10]

Each of these devices works on the principle of positioning the limb in a specific manner, applying a force that causes displacement, and subsequently measuring the amount of displacement or translation caused by the applied force.[92, 99, 100] The measurements obtained depend on the experience and ability of the examiner, the joint position, muscle activity or inactivity, the constraints present in the joint and those imposed by the testing systems, the amount of displacing force, and the measurement system used.[92] The greatest sources of error when using the arthrometer are the inability to stabilize the patellar sensor pad and lack of muscle relaxation.[101]

Because the KT 1000 arthrometer is the most commonly used testing device for anteroposterior displacement, it is briefly described here. More detailed descriptions of its use are found elsewhere[38, 99–101] and should be consulted if the examiner plans to use this device. The arthrometer is placed on the anterior aspect of the tibia and is held in place with two Velcro straps (Figs. 12–86 and 12–87). A thigh support and foot support help to hold the leg in proper alignment, with straps if necessary. There are two sensor pads, one on the tibial tubercle and one on the patella. These pads detect relative movement. Forces to translate the tibia are applied through a force-sensing handle.

After the device is properly positioned and the leg is properly relaxed, several tests may be performed, first on the good knee and then on the injured knee.

Quadriceps Neutral Test. The patient's knee is flexed to 90°, and the arthrometer is positioned on the leg. A 9-kg (20-lb) posterior force is applied through the apparatus to establish a reference position. The patient is then asked to perform an isolated quadriceps contraction. If the tibia shifts forward, the knee angle is altered until there is no movement of the tibia when the quadriceps contracts. This position is called the **quadriceps neutral angle** or **quadriceps active position,** and it is usually

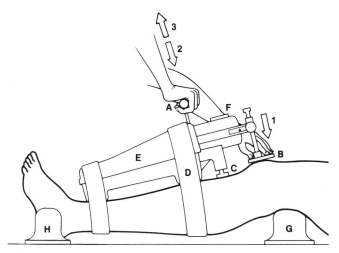

Figure 12–86
KT-1000 arthrometer. A posterior (2) or anterior (3) force is applied. A constant force (1) is applied to stabilize the patellar sensor pad. A = force handle; B = patellar sensor pad; C = tibial sensor pad; D = Velcro straps; E = arthrometer body; F = displacement dial; G = thigh support; H = foot support. (From Daniel, D., W. Akeson, and J. O'Conner [eds.]: Knee Ligaments: Structure, Injury and Repair. New York, Raven Press, 1990, p. 428.)

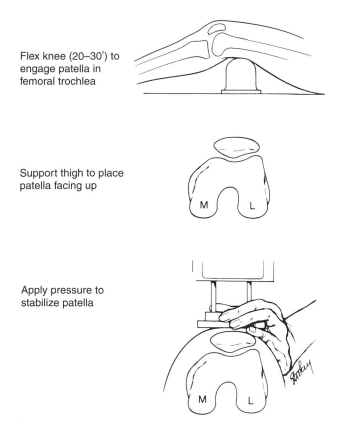

Flex knee (20–30°) to engage patella in femoral trochlea

Support thigh to place patella facing up

Apply pressure to stabilize patella

Figure 12–87
The knee is supported in a flexed position to engage the patella in the femoral trochlea. In some patients, the thigh support must be raised an additional 3 to 6 cm to provide sufficient knee flexion to engage the patella in the femoral trochlea. This may be done by placing a board under the thigh support. The thigh should be supported so that the patella is facing up. Occasionally, a thigh strap is used to accomplish this task. The examiner stabilizes the patellar sensor with manual pressure. The stabilizing hand should rest against the lateral thigh and should apply 1 to 2.25 kg (2 to 5 lb) of pressure on the patellar sensor pad. The hand position, patellar sensor position, and patellar sensor pressure must remain constant throughout the test. Variation of the pressure on the patellar sensor pad and rotation of the pad is a common cause of measurement error. (From Daniel, D., W. Akeson, and J. O'Conner [eds.]: Knee Ligaments: Structure, Injury and Repair. New York, Raven Press, 1990, p. 428.)

about 70° flexion (see Fig. 12–115). This position is found on the good knee and is used as a reference or starting position for the injured knee. If, when the injured knee is tested in this position, the anterior displacement is greater than 1 mm, the translation is abnormal and probably indicates a posterior cruciate ligament sprain.[92, 101]

Test in Quadriceps Active Position. With the patient's leg positioned at the quadriceps neutral angle, the examiner applies a 9-kg (20-lb) anterior force, followed by a 9-kg (20-lb) posterior force. The results for the good and injured knee are compared.[92, 101]

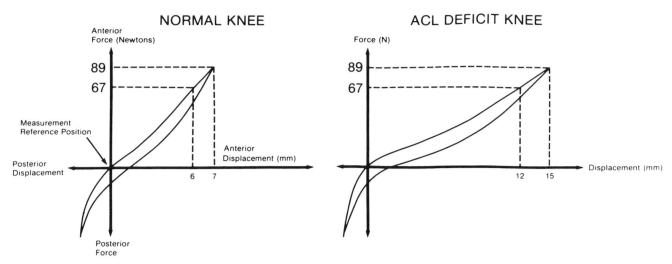

Figure 12-88

Force-displacement curves for normal knees and for knees with anterior cruciate ligament (ACL) deficit. The compliance index is obtained by measuring the displacement between the 67- and 89-N anterior-force levels. On this curve, the compliance index for the normal knee is 1 mm; for the knee with an ACL deficit, it is 3 mm. (From Daniel, D., W. Akeson, and J. O'Conner [eds.]: Knee Ligaments: Structure, Injury and Repair. New York, Raven Press, 1990, p. 433.)

Test in 30° Flexion. With the patient's leg positioned as shown in Figure 12–86, five tests are performed:

1. 9-kg (20-lb) posterior displacement
2. 7-kg (15-lb) anterior (Lachman) displacement
3. 9-kg (20-lb) anterior (Lachman) displacement
4. Maximum anterior (Lachman) displacement, usually 14 to 18 kg (30 to 40 lb)
5. Quadriceps active anterior displacement

The difference between the 7-kg and the 9-kg anterior displacement tests is called the **compliance index.** For the maximum anterior displacement test, the examiner manually pulls or translates the tibia forward on the femur, using a pull of approximately 14 to 18 kg (30 to 40 lb). For the quadriceps active test, the patient is asked to lift the heel slowly off the table; displacement as the heel leaves the table is noted. Differences of more than 3 mm between the good and injured legs are considered diagnostic for injury to the anterior cruciate or posterior cruciate.[92, 101] Force displacement curves (Fig. 12–88) and frequency distribution curves (Fig. 12–89) demonstrate differences between the normal and pathological knees. Tests involving larger translation forces have been found to be more responsive to translation differences.[102]

It is important to realize that the accuracy of the readings for these devices depends very much on positioning, muscle relaxation, and the experience of the operator. Reliability of any of these measuring devices may be greatly affected if these factors are not controlled.[92, 95, 96, 100, 103–109]

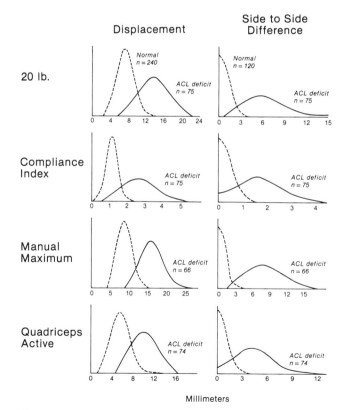

Figure 12-89

Frequency distribution curves of anterior laxity in normal knee in 30° of flexion and in knees with unilateral chronic anterior cruciate ligament disruption. (From Daniel, D.M., and M.L. Stone: Diagnosis of knee ligament injury: Test and measurements of joint laxity. In Feagin, J.A. [ed.]: The Crucial Ligaments. New York, Churchill Livingstone, 1988, pp. 287–300.)

Special Tests

Although most special tests on the knee are done only if the examiner suspects certain pathologies and wants to do a confirming test, tests for swelling should always be performed.

Special Tests Commonly Performed on the Knee

Meniscus lesions:	McMurray test
	Apley's test
	"Bounce home" test
Plica lesions:	Mediopatellar plica test
	Plica "stutter" test
	Hughston's plica test
Swelling:	Brush test
	Indentation test
	Patellar tap test
Patellofemoral syndrome:	Clarke's sign
	McConnell test
Quadriceps pull:	Q-angle
	Tubercle sulcus angle
Osteochondritis dissecans:	Wilson test
Patellar instability:	Apprehension test
Iliotibial band friction syndrome:	Noble compression test
Leg length:	Leg length tests

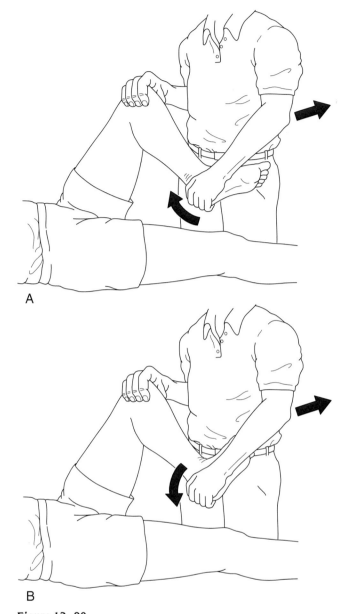

A

B

Figure 12–90
McMurray test. (A) Medial meniscus test. (B) Lateral meniscus test.

Tests for Meniscus Injury

Although there are several tests for a meniscus injury, none can be considered definitive without considerable experience on the part of the examiner. Because the menisci are avascular and have no nerve supply on their inner two thirds, an injury to the meniscus can result in little or no pain or swelling, making diagnosis even more difficult.

McMurray Test. The patient lies in the supine position with the knee completely flexed (the heel to the buttock).[110, 111] The examiner then medially rotates the tibia (Fig. 12–90). If there is a loose fragment of the lateral meniscus, this action causes a snap or click that is often accompanied by pain. By repeatedly changing the amount of flexion, the examiner can test the entire posterior aspect of the meniscus from the posterior horn to the middle segment. The anterior half of the meniscus is not as easily tested because the pressure on the meniscus is not as great. To test the medial meniscus, the examiner performs the same procedure with the knee laterally rotated. Kim and colleagues[112] reported that meniscus lesions may be found on the medial side with medial rotation and on the lateral side with lateral rotation.

The test may be modified by medially rotating the tibia, extending the knee, and moving through the full range of motion to test the lateral meniscus. The process is repeated several times. The tibia is then laterally rotated, and the process is repeated to test the medial mensicus. Both methods are described by McMurray.[110]

Apley's Test.[113] The patient lies in the prone position with the knee flexed to 90°. The patient's thigh is then anchored to the examining table with the examiner's knee (Fig. 12–91). The examiner medially and laterally rotates the tibia, combined first with distraction, while noting any restriction, excessive movement, or discomfort. Then the process is repeated using compression

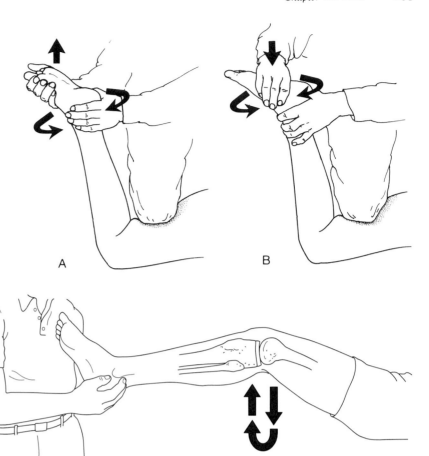

Figure 12–91
Apley's test. (A) Distraction. (B) Compression.

A   B

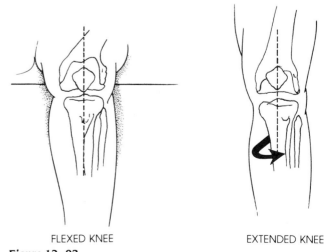

Figure 12–92
Bounce home test.

instead of distraction. If rotation plus distraction is more painful, the lesion is probably ligamentous. If the rotation plus compression is more painful, the lesion is probably a meniscus injury.

"Bounce Home" Test. The patient lies in the supine position, and the heel of the patient's foot is cupped in the examiner's hand (Fig. 12–92). The patient's knee is completely flexed, and the knee is passively allowed to extend. If extension is not complete or has a rubbery end feel ("springy block"), there is something blocking full extension. The most likely cause of a block is a torn meniscus. Oni[114] reported that if the knee is allowed to quickly extend in one movement or jerk and the patient experiences a sharp pain on the joint line, which may radiate up or down the leg, the test is positive for a meniscus lesion.

O'Donohue's Test. If a patient complains of pain along the joint line, the patient is asked to lie in the supine position. The examiner flexes the knee to 90°, rotates it medially and laterally twice, and then fully flexes and rotates it both ways again. A positive sign is indicated by increased pain on rotation in either or both positions and is indicative of capsular irritation or a meniscus tear.

Modified Helfet Test.[115] In the normal knee, the tibial tuberosity is in line with the midline of the patella when the knee is flexed to 90°. When the knee is extended, however, the tibial tubercle is in line with the lateral

border of the patella (Fig. 12–93). If this change does not occur with the change in movement, rotation is blocked, indicating that there is injury to the meniscus, there is a possible cruciate injury, or the quadriceps have insufficient strength to "screw home" the knee.

Test for Retreating or Retracting Meniscus. The patient sits on the edge of the examining table or lies in the supine position with the knee flexed to 90°.[115] The examiner places one finger over the joint line of the patient's

FLEXED KNEE   EXTENDED KNEE

Figure 12–93
Modified Helfet test (negative test shown).

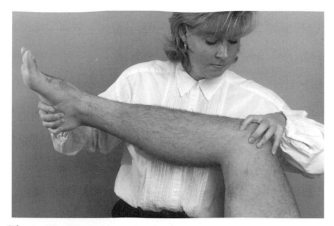

Figure 12-94
Test for a retreating meniscus.

knee anterior to the medial collateral ligament, where the curved margin of the medial femoral condyle approaches the tibial tuberosity (Fig. 12-94). The patient's leg and foot are then passively laterally rotated, and the meniscus normally disappears. The leg is medially and laterally rotated several times, with the meniscus appearing and disappearing. The knee must be flexed and the muscles relaxed to do the test. If the meniscus does not appear, a torn meniscus is indicated because rotation of the tibia is not occurring. The examiner must palpate carefully, because a distinct structure is difficult to palpate. If the examiner medially and laterally rotates the unaffected leg several times first, the meniscus can be felt pushing against the finger on medial rotation, and it disappears on lateral rotation.

Steinman's Tenderness Displacement Test. The Steinman's sign is indicated by point tenderness and pain on the joint line that appears to move anteriorly when the knee is extended and moves posteriorly when the knee is flexed. It is indicative of a possible meniscus tear. Medial pain is elicited on lateral rotation, and lateral pain is elicited on medial rotation.

Payr's Test. The patient lies supine with the test leg in the figure-four position (Fig. 12-95). If pain is elicited on the medial joint line, the test is considered positive for a meniscus lesion, primarily in the middle or posterior part of the meniscus.[28]

Bohler's Sign. The patient lies in the supine position, and the examiner applies varus and valgus stresses to the knee. Pain in the opposite joint line (valgus stress for lateral meniscus) on stress testing is a positive sign for meniscus pathology.[28]

Bragard's Sign. The patient lies supine and the examiner flexes the patient's knee. The examiner then laterally rotates the tibia and extends the knee (Fig. 12-96). Pain and tenderness on the medial joint line are indicative of medial meniscus pathology. If the examiner then medially rotates the tibia and flexes the knee, the pain and tenderness will decrease.[28] Both of these symptoms are indicative of medial meniscus pathology.

Kromer's Sign. This test is similar to Bohler's sign except that the knee is flexed and extended while the varus and valgus stresses are applied.[28] A positive test is indicated by the same pain on the opposite joint line.

Childress' Sign. The patient squats and performs a "duck walk."[28] Pain, snapping, or a click is considered positive for a posterior horn lesion of the meniscus.

Anderson Medial-Lateral Grind Test.[116] The patient lies supine. The examiner holds the test leg between the trunk and the arm while the index finger and thumb of the opposite hand are placed over the anterior joint line (Fig. 12-97). A valgus stress is applied to the knee as it is passively flexed to 45°; then, a varus stress is applied to the knee as it is passively extended, producing a circular motion to the knee. The motion is repeated, increasing the varus and valgus stresses with each rotation. A distinct grinding is felt on the joint line if there is meniscus pathology. The test may also show a pivot shift if the anterior cruciate ligament has been torn.

Passler Rotational Grind Test.[28] The patient sits with the test knee extended and held at the ankle between the examiner's legs proximal to the examiner's knees. The examiner places both thumbs over the medial joint line and moves the knee in a circular fashion, medially and laterally rotating the tibia while the knee is rotated through various flexion angles. Simultaneously, the examiner applies a varus or a valgus stress (Fig. 12-98). Pain elicited on the joint line is indicative of a meniscus lesion.

Cabot's Popliteal Sign.[28] The patient lies supine, and the examiner positions the test leg in the figure-four position. The examiner palpates the joint line with the thumb and forefinger of one hand and places the other hand proximal to the ankle of the test leg. The patient is asked to isometrically straighten the knee while the examiner resists the movement. A positive test, signifying a meniscus lesion, is indicated by pain on the joint (Fig. 12-99).

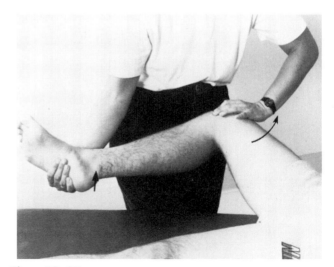

Figure 12-95
Payr's sign for a meniscus lesion.

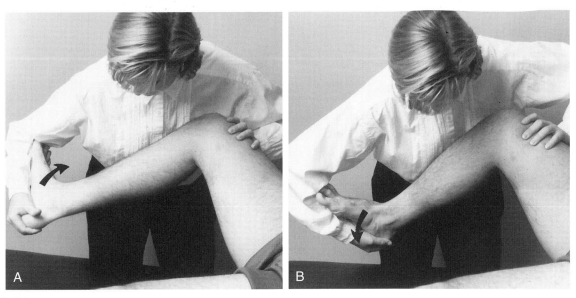

Figure 12–96
Bragard's sign for a meniscus lesion. (A) Medial meniscus test. (B) Lateral meniscus test.

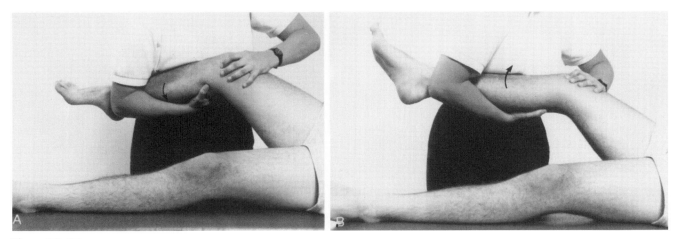

Figure 12–97
Anderson medial-lateral grind test. (A) Flexion and valgus stress. (B) Extension and varus stress.

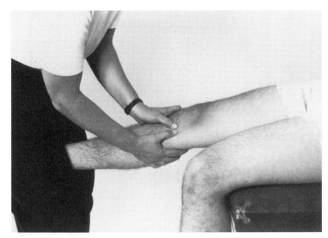

Figure 12–98
Passler rotational grind test for meniscus pathology.

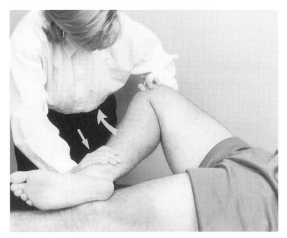

Figure 12–99
Cabot's popliteal sign for a meniscus lesion.

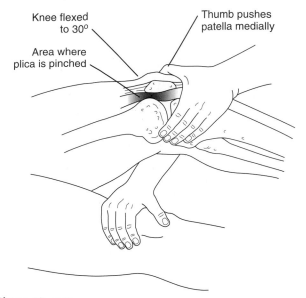

Knee flexed to 30°

Thumb pushes patella medially

Area where plica is pinched

Figure 12–100

Test for mediopatellar plica.

Plica Tests

Because an abnormal plica can mimic meniscus pathology, it is essential that the plica tests be performed as well as the meniscus tests if a meniscus injury is suspected.

Mediopatellar Plica Test. The patient lies in the supine position, and the examiner flexes the affected knee to 30° (Fig. 12–100). If the examiner then moves the patella medially, the patient complains of pain. This pain, indicating a positive test, is caused by pinching of the edge of the plica between the medial femoral condyle and the patella. The pain may be indicative of a mediopatellar plica.[117]

Plica "Stutter" Test. The patient is seated on the edge of the examining table with both knees flexed to 90°. The examiner places a finger over one patella to palpate during movement. The patient is then instructed to slowly extend the knee. If the test is positive, the patella stutters or jumps somewhere between 60° and 45° of flexion (0° being straight leg) during an otherwise smooth movement. The test is effective only if there is no joint swelling.

Hughston's Plica Test. The patient lies in the supine position, and the examiner flexes the knee and medially rotates the tibia with one arm and hand while pressing the patella medially with the heel of the other hand and palpating the medial femoral condyle with the fingers of the same hand (Fig. 12–101). The patient's knee is passively flexed and extended while the examiner feels for "popping" of the plical band under the fingers. The popping indicates a positive test.[82]

Tests for Swelling

When assessing swelling, the examiner must determine the type and amount of swelling that are present. Al-

though the tests for swelling are listed under Special Tests, the examiner should always be testing for swelling when examining the knee. In addition, the examiner must differentiate between swelling and synovial thickening. With swelling, the knee assumes its resting position of 15 to 25° of flexion, which allows the synovial cavity the maximum capacity for holding fluid. If the injury is sufficiently severe, the fluid extravasates into the soft tissue surrounding the joint as a result of torn structures (i.e., ligaments, capsule, synovium). Therefore, lack of effusion should not lull the examiner into thinking the injury is a minor one.

If the swelling consists of blood that results in a hemarthrosis, it may be caused by a ligament tear, osteochondral fracture, or peripheral meniscus tear. The swelling comes on very quickly (within 1 to 2 hours), and the skin becomes very taut. On palpation, it has a "doughy" feeling and is relatively hard to the touch. The joint surface feels warm. Usually, excess blood should be aspirated, or osteoarthritis may result from irritation of the cartilage.

Normally, synovial fluid swelling caused by joint irritation occurs in 8 to 24 hours. The feeling within the joint is a fluctuating or "boggy" feeling. The joint surface feels warm and tender. Swelling usually occurs with activity and disappears after a few days of inactivity.

The third type of swelling is purulent or pus swelling, in which the joint surface is hot to the touch. Often it is red, and the patient has general signs of infection or pyrexia.

Brush, Stroke, or Bulge Test. Also called the **wipe test,** this test assesses minimal effusion. The examiner com-

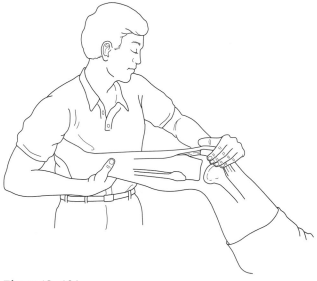

Figure 12–101

Examination for suprapatellar plica. The foot and tibia are held in medial rotation. The patella is displaced slightly medially with the fingers over the course of the plica. The knee is passively flexed and extended, eliciting a "pop" of the plica and associated tenderness. (Redrawn from Hughston, J.C., W.M. Walsh, and G. Puddu: Patellar Subluxation and Dislocation. Philadelphia, W.B. Saunders Co., 1984, p. 29.)

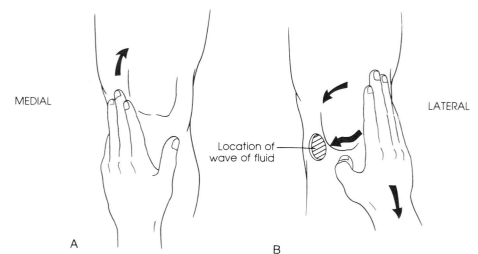

MEDIAL

LATERAL

Location of wave of fluid

Figure 12–102
Brush test for swelling. (A) Hand strokes up. (B) Hand strokes down.

A

B

mences just below the joint line on the medial side of the patella, stroking proximally toward the patient's hip as far as the suprapatellar pouch two or three times with the palm and fingers (Fig. 12–102). With the opposite hand, the examiner strokes down the lateral side of the patella. A wave of fluid passes to the medial side of the joint and bulges just below the medial distal portion or border of the patella. The wave of fluid may take up to 2 seconds to appear. Normally, the knee contains 1 to 7 ml of synovial fluid. This test shows as little as 4 to 8 ml of extra fluid within the knee.

Indentation Test.[118] The patient lies supine. The examiner passively flexes the good leg, noting an indentation on the lateral side of the patellar tendon (Fig. 12–103). The good knee is fully flexed, and the indentation remains. The injured knee is then slowly flexed while the examiner watches for the disappearance of the indentation. At that point, knee flexion is stopped. The disappearance of the indentation is caused by swelling and indicates a positive test. The angle at which the indentation disappears depends on the amount of swelling. The greater the swelling, the sooner the indentation disap-

pears. If the thumb and finger are placed on each side of the patellar tendon, the fluid can be made to fluctuate back and forth. This method, like the brush test, can detect minimal levels of swelling.

Peripatellar Swelling Test.[119] The patient lies supine with the knee extended. The examiner carefully milks fluid from the suprapatellar pouch distally. With the opposite hand, the examiner palpates adjacent to the patellar tendon (usually on the medial side) for fluid accumulation.

Fluctuation Test. The examiner places the palm of one hand over the suprapatellar pouch and the palm of the other hand anterior to the joint with the thumb and index finger just beyond the margins of the patella (Fig. 12–104). By pressing down with one hand and then the other, the examiner may feel the synovial fluid fluctuate under the hands and move from one hand to the other, indicating significant effusion.

Patellar Tap Test ("Ballotable Patella"). With the patient's knee extended or flexed to discomfort, the examiner applies a slight tap or pressure over the patella. When this is done, a floating of the patella should be

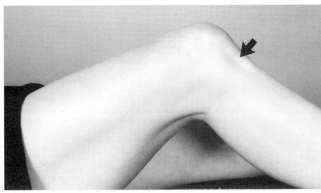

Figure 12–103
Indentation test. Arrow indicates where to watch for filling of indentation.

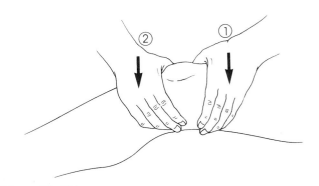

Figure 12–104
Hand positioning for fluctuation test. First one hand is pushed down (*arrow* 1); then the other hand is pushed down (*arrow* 2). The examiner will feel fluid shifting back and forth under one hand and then the other.

felt. This is sometimes called the "dancing patella" sign. A modification of this test calls for the examiner to apply the thumb and forefinger of one hand lightly on both sides of the patella. The examiner then strokes down on the suprapatellar pouch with the other hand.[28] A positive test is indicated by separation of the thumb and forefinger. This test can detect a large amount of swelling (40 to 50 ml) in the knee, which can also be noted by observation.

Tests for Patellofemoral Dysfunction

Clarke's Sign. This test assesses the presence of patellofemoral dysfunction. The examiner presses down slightly proximal to the upper pole or base of the patella with the web of the hand as the patient lies relaxed with the knee extended (Fig. 12–105). The patient is then asked to contract the quadriceps muscles while the examiner pushes down. If the patient can complete and maintain the contraction without pain, the test is considered negative. If the test causes retropatellar pain and the patient cannot hold a contraction, the test is considered positive. Because the examiner can achieve a positive test on anyone if sufficient pressure is applied to the patella, the amount of pressure that is applied must be controlled. The best way to do this is to repeat the procedure several times, increasing the pressure each time and comparing the results with those of the unaffected side. To test different parts of the patella, the knee should be tested in 30°, 60°, and 90° of flexion as well as in full extension.

McConnell Test for Chondromalacia Patellae. The patient is sitting with the femur laterally rotated. The patient performs isometric quadriceps contractions at 120°, 90°, 60°, 30°, and 0°, with each contraction held for 10 seconds. If pain is produced during any of the contractions, the patient's leg is passively returned to full extension by the examiner. The patient's leg is then fully supported on the examiner's knee, and the examiner pushes the patella medially. The medial glide is maintained while the knee is returned to the painful angle, and the patient performs an isometric contraction, again with the patella held medially. If the pain is decreased, the pain is patellofemoral in origin. Each angle is tested in a similar fashion.[120]

Waldron Test. This test also assesses the presence of patellofemoral syndrome.[15] The examiner palpates the patella while the patient performs several slow deep knee bends. As the patient goes through the range of motion, the examiner should note the amount of crepitus (significant only if accompanied by pain), where it occurs in the range of motion, the amount of pain, and whether there is "catching" or poor tracking of the patella throughout the movement. If pain and crepitus occur together during the movement, it is considered a positive sign.[15]

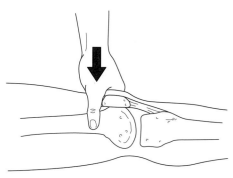

Figure 12–105
Clarke's sign.

Passive Patellar Tilt Test. The patient lies supine with the knee extended and the quadriceps relaxed. The examiner stands at the end of the examining table and lifts the lateral edge of the patella away from the lateral femoral condyle. The patella should not be pushed medially or laterally but rather should remain in the femoral trochlea.[121] The normal angle is 15°, although males may have an angle 5° less than that of females (Fig. 12–106). Patients with angles less than this are prone to patellofemoral syndrome.

Lateral Pull Test. The patient lies supine with the leg extended. The patient contracts the quadriceps while the examiner watches the movement of the patella.[121] Normally, the patella moves superiorly, or superiorly and laterally in equal proportions (Fig. 12–107). If lateral movement is excessive, the test is positive for lateral overpull of the quadriceps, resulting in a patellofemoral arthralgia.

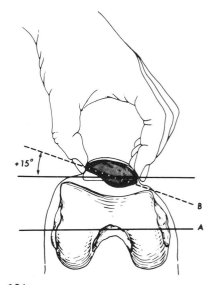

Figure 12–106
Passive patellar tilt test. (From Kolowich, P.A., L.E. Paulos, T.D. Rosenberg, and S. Farnsworth: Lateral release of the patella: Indications and contraindications. Am. J. Sports Med. 18:361, 1990.)

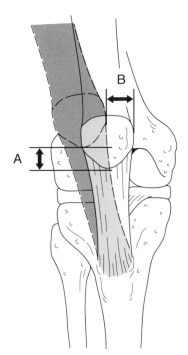

Figure 12–107

Lateral pull test. Normally, A > B or A = B; with lateral overpull of the quadriceps, B > A. (Redrawn from Kolowich, P.A., L.E. Paulos, T.D. Rosenberg, and S. Farnsworth. Lateral release of the patella: Indications and contraindications. Am. J. Sports Med. 18:361, 1990.)

Zohler's Sign.[28] The patient lies supine with the knees extended. The examiner pulls the patella distally and holds it in this position. The patient is asked to contract the quadriceps (Fig. 12–108). Pain is indicative of a positive test for chondromalacia patellae. However, the test may be positive in a large proportion of the normal population.

Frund's Sign. The patient is in the sitting position. The examiner percusses the patella in various positions of knee flexion. Pain is indicative of a positive test and may signify chondromalacia patellae.

Other Tests

Q-Angle or Patellofemoral Angle. The Q-angle (quadriceps angle) is defined as the angle between the quadriceps muscles (primarily the rectus femoris) and the patellar tendon (Fig. 12–109). The angle is obtained by first ensuring that the lower limbs are at a right angle to the line joining the two anterior superior iliac spines (ASISs). A line is then drawn from the ASIS to the midpoint of the patella on the same side and from the tibial tubercle to the midpoint of the patella. The angle formed by the crossing of these two lines is called the Q-angle. The foot should be placed in a neutral position in regard to supination and pronation and the hip in a neutral position in regard to medial and lateral rotation, because it has been found that different foot and hip positions alter the Q-angle.[122]

Normally, the Q-angle is 13° for males and 18° for females when the knee is straight (Fig. 12–110). Any angle less than 13° may be associated with chondromalacia patellae or patella alta. An angle greater than 18° is often associated with chondromalacia patellae, subluxing patella, increased femoral anteversion, genu valgum, lateral displacement of tibial tubercle, or increased lateral tibial torsion. During the test, which may be done either with radiographs or physically on the patient, the quadriceps should be relaxed. If measured with the patient in the sitting position, the Q-angle

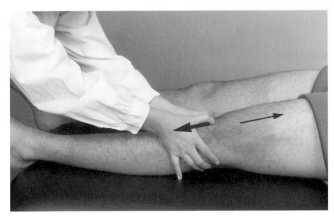

Figure 12–108

Zohler's sign for chondromalacia patellae.

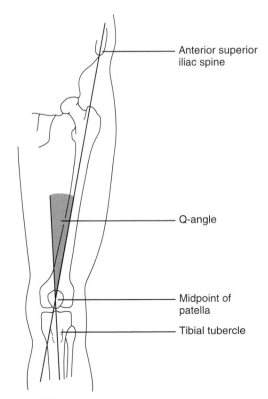

Figure 12–109

Quadriceps angle (Q-angle).

Anterior superior iliac spine

Q-angle

Midpoint of patella

Tibial tubercle

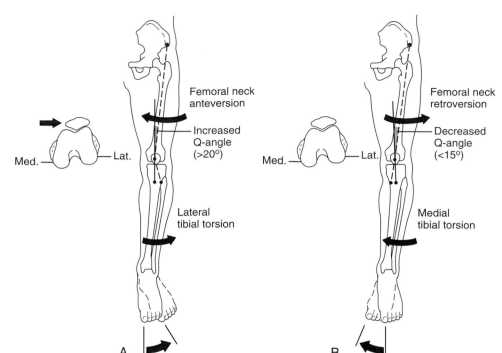

Figure 12–110

(A) Femoral neck anteversion and lateral tibial torsion increase the Q-angle and lead to lateral tracking of the patella on the femoral suicus. (B) Femoral neck retroversion and medial tibial torsion decrease the Q-angle and tend to centralize the tracking of the patella. (Redrawn from Tria, A.J., and R.C. Palumbo: Conservative treatment of patellofemoral pain. Semin. Orthop. 5:116–117, 1990.)

should be 0° (Fig. 12–111). While the patient is in a sitting position, the presence of the "**bayonet sign**," which indicates an abnormal alignment of the quadriceps musculature, patellar tendon, or tibial shaft, should be noted (Fig. 12–112).

Hughston advocates doing the test with the quadriceps contracted.[82] If measured with the quadriceps con-

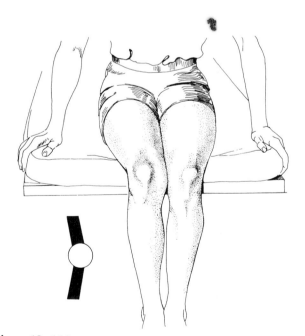

Figure 12–111

Q-angle in flexed position. Exaggerated Q-angle in the patient's right knee is seen as residual positive Q-angle with the knee flexed. Normally, the Q-angle in flexion should be 0°. (From Hughston, J.C., W.M. Walsh, and G. Puddu: Patellar Subluxation and Dislocation. Philadelphia, W.B. Saunders Co., 1984, p. 24.)

tracted and the knee fully extended, the Q-angle should be 8 to 10°. Any angle greater than 10° is considered abnormal. The examiner must ensure that a standardized measurement procedure is used to ensure consistent values.[123]

Tubercle Sulcus Angle (Q-Angle at 90°).[10, 120] This measurement is also used to measure the angle of quadriceps pull. A vertical line is drawn from the center of the patella to the center of the tibial tubercle. A second horizontal line is drawn through the femoral epicondyle (Fig. 12–113). Normally the lines are perpendicular. Angles greater than 10° from the perpendicular are considered abnormal. Lateral patellar subluxation may affect the results.

Another measurement, which is similar to the Q-angle, is the **A-angle,** which measures the relation of the patella to the tibial tubercle. This measurement, which is not as commonly used as the Q-angle, consists of a vertical line that divides the patella into two halves and a line drawn from the tibial tubercle to the apex of the inferior pole of the patella. The resulting angle is the A-angle (Fig. 12–114).[124, 125] Some have questioned the reliability of this measurement because of the difficulty in consistently finding appropriate landmarks.[126]

Daniel's Quadriceps Neutral Angle Test.[127] The patient lies supine, and the unaffected leg is tested first. The patient's hip is flexed to 45°, and the knee is flexed to 90° with the foot flat on the examining table. The patient is asked to extend the knee isometrically while the examiner holds down the foot. If tibial displacement is noted, knee flexion is decreased (posterior tibial displacement) or increased (anterior tibial displacement). The process is repeated until the angle at which there is no tibial

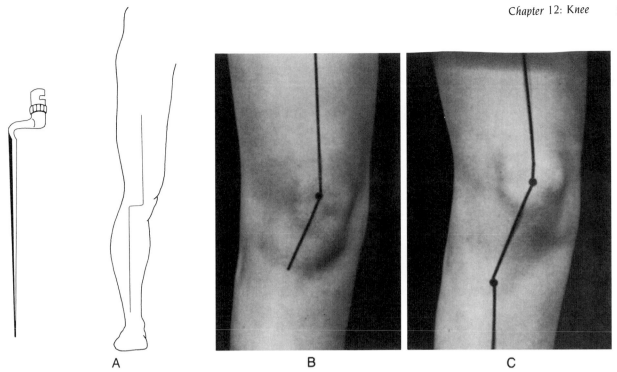

A   B   C

Figure 12-112

Increased Q-angle. (A) Bayonet sign. Tibia vara of proximal third causes a markedly increased Q-angle. Alignment of the quadriceps, patellar tendon, and tibial shaft resembles a French bayonet. (From Hughston, J.C., W.M. Walsh, and G. Puddu: Patellar Subluxation and Dislocation. Philadelphia, W.B. Saunders Co., 1984, p. 26.). (B) Q-angle with the knee in full extension is only slightly increased over normal. (C) However, with the knee flexed at 30°, there is failure of the tibia to derotate normally and failure of the patellar tendon to line up with the anterior crest of the tibia. This is not an infrequent finding in patients with patellofemoral arthralgia. (From Ficat, R.P., and D.S. Hungerford: Disorders of the Patello-Femoral Joint. Baltimore, Williams & Wilkins, 1977, p. 117.)

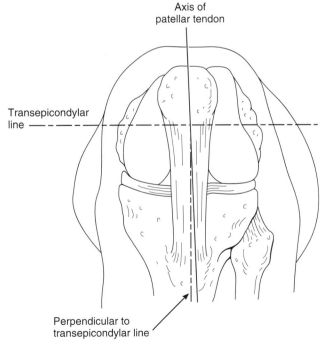

Figure 12-113

Tubercle sulcus angle of 90°. With the knee flexed to 90°, the transepicondylar line is assessed. The axis of the patellar tendon is compared with a perpendicular to the transepicondylar line. (Modified from Kolowich, P.A., L.E. Paulos, T.D. Rosenberg, and S. Farnsworth: Lateral release of the patella: Indications and contraindications. Am. J. Sports Med. 18:361, 1990.)

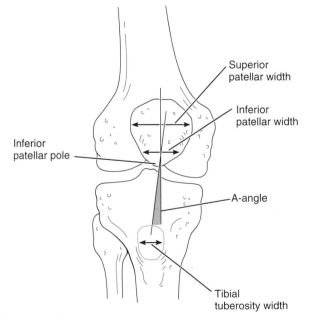

Figure 12-114

Location of landmarks of the A-angle. (Redrawn from Ehrat, M., J. Edwards, D. Hastings, and T. Worrell: Reliability of assessing patellar alignment. The A-angle. J. Orthop. Sports Phys. Ther. 19:23, 1994.)

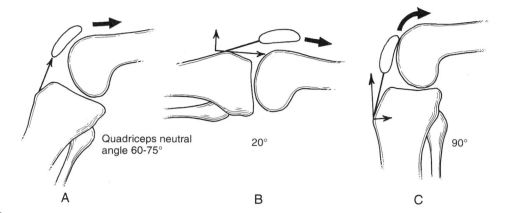

Quadriceps neutral
angle 60-75°

20°

90°

A

B

C

Figure 12–115

During open chain knee extension, tibial translation is a function of the shear force produced by the patellar tendon. (A) Quadriceps neutral position. The patellar tendon force is perpendicular to the tibial plateaus and results in compression of the joint surfaces without shear force. (B) At flexion angles less than the angle of the quadriceps neutral position, orientation of the patellar tendon produces anterior shear of the tibia. (C) At angles greater than the angle of the quadriceps neutral position, patellar tendon force causes a posterior shear of the tibia. (From Daniel, D.M., M.L. Stone, P. Barnett, and R. Sachs: Use of the quadriceps active test to diagnose posterior cruciate ligament disruption and measure posterior laxity of the knee. J. Bone Joint Surg. Am. 70:386–391, 1988.)

displacement is reached (Fig. 12–115). This angle, the quadriceps neutral angle, averages 70° (range, 60 to 90°). The injured knee is placed in the same neutral angle position, and the patient is asked to contract the quadriceps. Any anterior displacement is indicative of posterior cruciate ligament insufficiency. The quadriceps neutral angle is primarily used for machine testing of laxity (e.g., KT 1000 arthrometer, Stryker knee laxity test apparatus).

Wilson Test. This is a test for **osteochondritis dissecans.** The patient sits with the knee flexed over the examining table. The knee is then actively extended with the tibia medially rotated. At approximately 30° of flexion (0° being straight leg), the pain in the knee increases, and the patient is asked to stop the flexion movement.

The patient is then asked to rotate the tibia laterally, and the pain disappears. This finding indicates a positive test, which is indicative of osteochondritis dissecans of the femoral condyle. The test is positive only if the lesion is at the classic site for osteochondritis dissecans of the knee, namely, the medial femoral condyle near the intercondylar notch (Fig. 12–116).

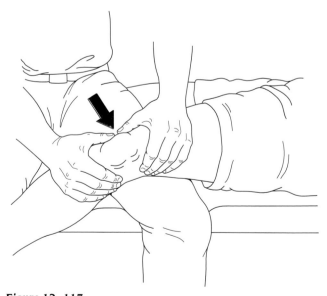

Figure 12–117

Apprehension test. (Redrawn from Hughston, J.C., W.M. Walsh, and G. Puddu: Patellar Subluxation and Dislocation. Philadelphia, W.B. Saunders Co., 1984, p. 29.)

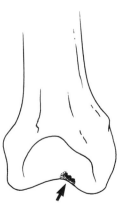

Figure 12–116

Classic site of osteochondritis dissecans.

Fairbank's Apprehension Test. This is a test for **dislocation of the patella.**[82, 128] The patient lies in the supine position with the quadriceps muscles relaxed and the knee flexed to 30° while the examiner carefully and slowly pushes the patella laterally (Fig. 12–117). If the patient feels as if the patella is going to dislocate, the patient will contract the quadriceps muscles to bring the patella back "into line." This action indicates a positive test. The patient will also have an apprehensive look.

Noble Compression Test. This is a test for **iliotibial band friction syndrome.**[129] The patient lies in the supine position, and the examiner flexes the patient's knee to 90°, accompanied by hip flexion (Fig. 12–118). Pressure is then applied to the lateral femoral epicondyle, or 1 to 2 cm (0.4 to 0.8 inch) proximal to it, with the thumb. While the pressure is maintained, the patient's knee is passively extended. At approximately 30° of flexion (0° being straight leg), the patient complains of severe pain over the lateral femoral condyle. Pain indicates a positive test. The patient states that it is the same pain that occurs with activity.

Functional Test for Quadriceps Contusion. The patient lies in the prone position while the examiner passively flexes the knee as much as possible. If passive knee flexion is 90° or more, it is only a mild contusion. If passive knee flexion is less than 90°, the contusion is moderate to severe, and the patient should not be allowed to bear weight. Normally, the heel-to-buttock distance should not exceed 10 cm (4 inches) in men and 5 cm (2 inches) in women.

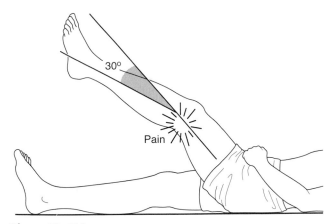

Figure 12–118
Noble compression test.

Test for Knee Extension Contracture (Heel Height Difference).[130] The patient lies prone with the thighs supported and the legs relaxed. The examiner measures the difference in heel height (Fig. 12–119). One centimeter of difference approximates 1°, depending on leg length. Swelling may also cause a positive test.

Tests for Hamstrings Tightness. These tests are described in Chapter 11.

Measurement of Leg Length. The patient lies in the supine position with the legs at a right angle to a line joining the two ASISs. With a tape measure, the examiner obtains the distance from one ASIS to the lateral or medial malleolus on that side, placing the metal end of

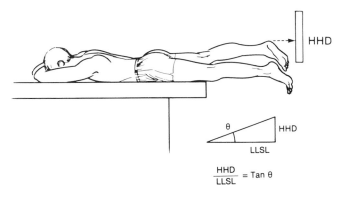

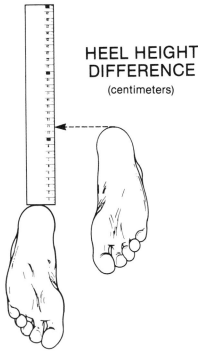

Figure 12–119
Heel height difference. The patient lies prone on the examining table with the lower limbs supported by the thighs. The difference in heel height is measured. The conversion of heel height difference to degrees of extension loss depends on the leg length. The tangent of angle θ is the heel height difference (HHD) divided by the lower-leg segment length (LLSL). The LLSL is proportional to patient height. (From Daniel, D., W. Akeson, and J. O'Conner [eds.]: Knee Ligaments: Structure, Injury and Repair. New York, Raven Press, 1990, p. 32.)

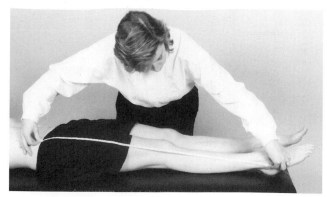

Figure 12–120
Measuring leg length (to the lateral malleolus).

the tape measure immediately distal to and up against the ASIS (Fig. 12–120). The tape is stretched so that the other hand pushes the tape against the distal aspect of the lateral (or medial) malleolus, and the reading on the tape measure is noted. The other side is tested similarly. A difference between the two sides of as much as 1.0 to 1.5 cm is considered normal. However, the examiner must remember that even this difference may result in pathological symptoms. If there is a difference, the examiner can determine its site of occurrence by measuring from the high point on the iliac crest to the greater trochanter (for coxa vara), from the greater trochanter to the lateral knee joint line (for femoral length), and from the medial knee joint line to the medial malleolus (for tibial length). The two legs are then compared. The examiner must also remember that torsion deformities to the femur or tibia can alter leg length.

Functional Leg Length. The patient stands in the normal relaxed stance. The examiner palpates the ASISs and then the posterior superior iliac spines (PSISs) and notes any differences. The examiner then positions the patient so that the patient's subtalar joints are in neutral while bearing weight (see Chapter 13). While the patient holds this position with the toes straight ahead and the knee straight, the examiner repalpates the ASISs and the

PSISs. If the previously noted differences remain, the pelvis and sacroiliac joints should be evaluated further. If the previously noted differences disappear, the examiner should suspect a functional leg length difference caused by hip, knee, ankle, or foot problems—primarily, ankle or foot problems.

Measurement of Muscle Bulk (Anthropometric Measurements for Effusion and Atrophy). The examiner selects areas where muscle bulk or swelling is greatest and measures the circumference of the leg. It is important to note on the patient's chart how far above or below the apex or base of the patella one is measuring and whether the tape measure is placed above or below that mark. The following are common measurement points:

1. 15 cm (6 inches) below the apex of the patella
2. Apex of the patella or joint line
3. 5 cm (2 inches) above the base of the patella
4. 10 cm (4 inches) above the base of the patella
5. 15 cm (6 inches) above the base of the patella
6. 23 cm (9 inches) above the base of the patella

Hughston[16] advocated using the lateral joint line rather than the patella for the beginning point of measurement; he believed that the joint line was more constant. The examiner must also note, if possible, whether swelling or muscle bulk is being measured and remember that there is no correlation between muscle bulk and strength.

Reflexes and Cutaneous Distribution

Having completed the ligamentous and other tests of the knee, if a scanning examination has not been carried out, the examiner next determines whether the reflexes around the knee joint are normal (Fig. 12–121). The patellar (L3–L4) and medial hamstring (L5–S1) reflexes should be checked for differences between the two sides.

The examiner must keep in mind the dermatome patterns of the various nerve roots (Fig. 12–122) as well as the cutaneous distribution of the peripheral nerves (Fig. 12–123). To test for altered sensation, a sensation

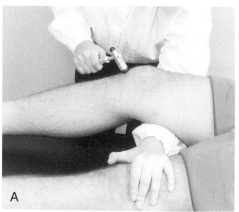
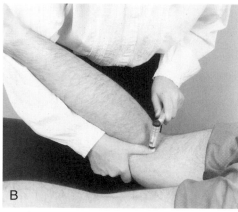

Figure 12–121
Reflexes of the knee. (A) Patellar (L3). (B) Medial hamstrings (L5).

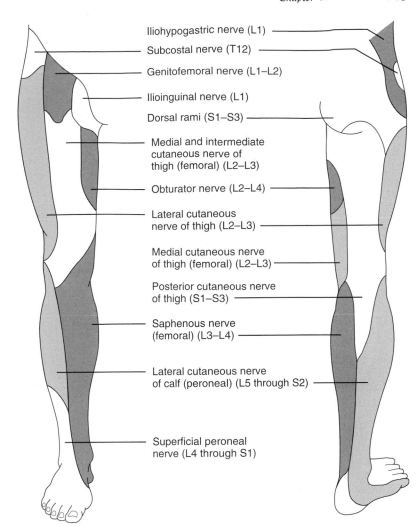

Iliohypogastric nerve (L1)
Subcostal nerve (T12)
Genitofemoral nerve (L1–L2)
Ilioinguinal nerve (L1)
Dorsal rami (S1–S3)
Medial and intermediate cutaneous nerve of thigh (femoral) (L2–L3)
Obturator nerve (L2–L4)
Lateral cutaneous nerve of thigh (L2–L3)
Medial cutaneous nerve of thigh (femoral) (L2–L3)
Posterior cutaneous nerve of thigh (S1–S3)
Saphenous nerve (femoral) (L3–L4)
Lateral cutaneous nerve of calf (peroneal) (L5 through S2)
Superficial peroneal nerve (L4 through S1)

Figure **12–122**
Peripheral nerve sensory distribution about the knee.

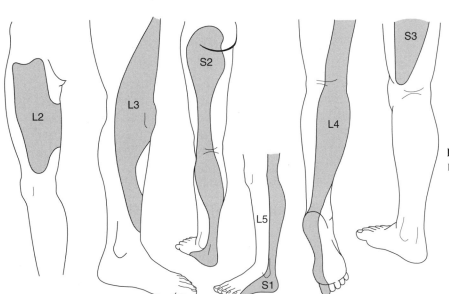

Figure **12–123**
Dermatomes about the knee.

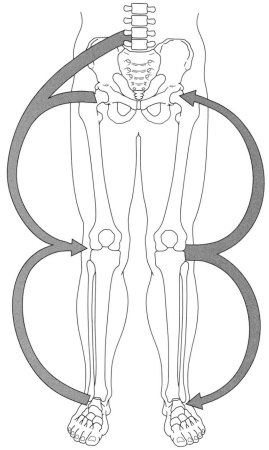

Figure 12-124
Patterns of referred pain to and from the knee.

Table 12-10
Knee Muscles and Referral of Pain

Muscle	Referral Pattern
Tensor fasciae latae	Lateral aspect of thigh
Sartorius	Over course of muscle (anterior thigh)
Quadriceps	Anterior thigh, patella, lateral thigh and knee (vastus lateralis)
Adductor longus and brevis	Superior anterolateral thigh, anterior thigh, proximal to patella and sometimes down anteromedial leg
Adductor magnus	Medial thigh from groin to adductor tubercle
Gracilis	Medial thigh (primarily the midportion)
Semimembranosus and semitendinosus	Ischial tuberosity, posterior thigh, and posteromedial calf
Biceps femoris	Posterior knee up posterior thigh
Popliteus	Posterior knee
Gastrocnemius	Posterior knee, posterolateral calf, and posteromedial calf to foot instep
Plantaris	Posterior knee and calf

True knee pain tends to be localized to the knee, but it may also be referred to the hip or ankle (Fig. 12–124). In a similar fashion, pain may be referred to the knee from the lumbar spine, hip (e.g., slipped capital femoral epiphysis in children), and ankle. Sometimes a lesion of the medial meniscus leads to irritation of the infrapatellar branch of the saphenous nerve. The result is a hyperaesthetic area the size of a quarter on the medial side of the knee. This finding is called **Turner's sign.**[28] Muscles about the knee and their pain referral pattern are shown in Table 12–10.

scanning examination should be performed using relaxed hands and fingers to cover all aspects of the thigh, knee, and leg. Any differences in sensation should be noted and can be mapped out further with the use of a pinwheel, pin, cotton batten, or brush.

Table 12-11
Peripheral Nerve Injuries (Neuropathy) About the Knee

Nerve	Muscle Weakness	Sensory Alteration	Reflexes Affected
Common peroneal nerve	Tibialis anterior (DP) Extensor digitorum brevis (DP) Extensor digitorum longus (DP) Extensor hallucis longus (DP) Peroneus tertius (DP) Peroneus longus (SP) Peroneus brevis (SP)	Area around head of fibula Web space between first and second toes (DP) Lateral aspect of leg and dorsum of foot (SP)	No common reflexes affected
Saphenous nerve	None	Medial side of knee, may extend down medial side of leg to medial malleolus	None

DP = deep peroneal branch; SP = superficial peroneal branch.

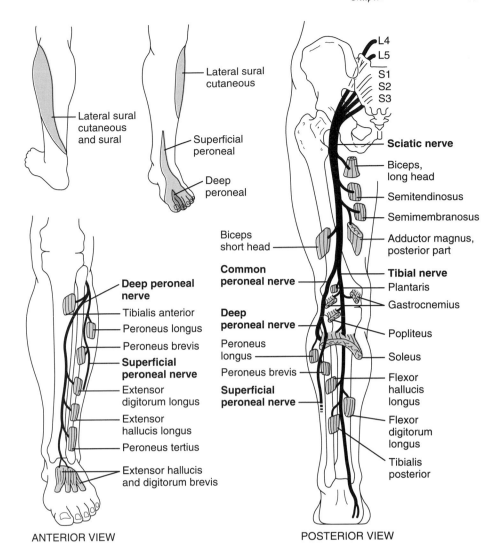

Figure 12–125
Common peroneal nerve.

ANTERIOR VIEW

POSTERIOR VIEW

Peripheral Nerve Injuries About the Knee

Common Peroneal Nerve (L4 *through* S2). This nerve is vulnerable to injury in the posterlateral knee and as it winds around the head of the fibula. It has also been reported that the nerve may be stretched as a result of pulling on the peroneus longus muscle in a lateral ankle sprain,[130–132] direct trauma, or a varus stress to the knee.[10] The result is weakness or paralysis of muscles supplied by the deep and superficial peroneal nerves, the two branches of the common peroneal nerve (Table 12–11). This causes an inability to dorsiflex the foot (drop foot), resulting in a steppage gait and an inability to evert the foot. Sensory loss is as shown in Figure 12–125.

Saphenous Nerve (L2 *through* L4). The saphenous nerve is a sensory branch of the femoral nerve that arises near the inguinal ligament and passes down the leg to supply the skin on the medial side of the knee and calf. The nerve is sometimes injured during surgery or trauma, or it may be entrapped as it passes between the vastus medialis and adductor magnus muscles. Entrapment may lead to medial knee pain (burning) that is aggravated by walking, standing, and quadriceps exercises.[133–135] Sensory loss after surgery or trauma is shown in Figure 11–41.

Joint Play Movements

For joint play movements on the knee, the patient is placed in the supine position (Fig. 12–126). The movement on the affected side is compared with that on the normal side.

Joint Play Movements of the Knee Complex

- Backward glide of tibia on femur
- Forward glide of tibia on femur
- Medial translation of tibia on femur
- Lateral translation of tibia on femur
- Medial displacement of patella
- Lateral displacement of patella
- Depression of patella
- Anteroposterior movement of fibula on tibia

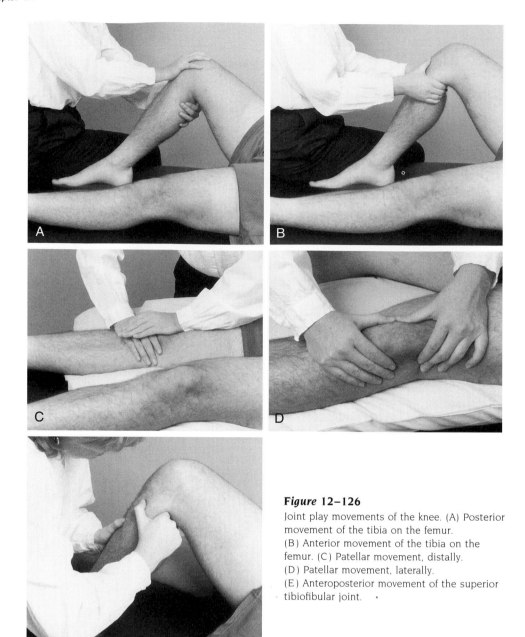

Figure 12–126
Joint play movements of the knee. (A) Posterior movement of the tibia on the femur.
(B) Anterior movement of the tibia on the femur. (C) Patellar movement, distally.
(D) Patellar movement, laterally.
(E) Anteroposterior movement of the superior tibiofibular joint.

Backward and Forward Movements of Tibia on Femur

The patient is asked to lie in the supine position with the test knee flexed to 90° and the hip flexed to 45°. The examiner then places the heel of the hand over the tibial tuberosity while stabilizing the patient's limb with the other hand and pushing backward with the heel of the hand. The end feel of the movement is normally tissue stretch. To perform the forward movement, the examiner places both hands around the posterior aspect of the tibia. Before performing the joint play movement, the examiner must ensure that the hamstrings and gastrocnemius muscles are relaxed. The tibia is then drawn forward on the femur. The examiner feels the quality of the movement, which normally is tissue stretch. These joint play movements are similar to those used in the anterior and posterior drawer tests for ligamentous stability.

Medial and Lateral Translation of Tibia on Femur

The patient lies supine, and the patient's leg is held between the examiner's trunk and arm. To test medial translation, the examiner puts one hand on the lateral side of the tibia and one hand on the medial side of the femur. The tibia is then pushed medially on the femur. Excessive movement may indicate a torn anterior cruciate ligament (Fig. 12–127). To test lateral translation,

Figure 12–127
Medial and lateral shift of tibia on femur. (A) Medial translation for anterior cruciate pathology. (B) Lateral translation for posterior cruciate pathology.

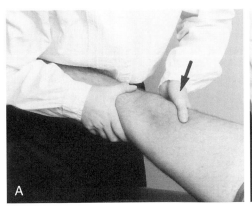
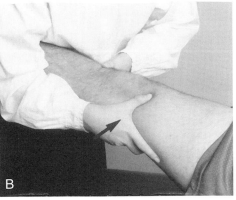

the examiner puts one hand on the medial side of the tibia and one hand on the lateral side of the femur. The tibia is then pushed laterally on the femur. Excessive movement may indicate a torn posterior cruciate ligament. The normal end feel of each movement is tissue stretch.[28] Liorzou[9] reports that Galway did a similar test with the knee flexed to 90° and the foot on the examining table. If the tibial plateau bulges laterally, the Wrisberg ligament or lateral meniscus may be injured.

Medial and Lateral Displacements of Patella

The patient is in the supine position with the knee slightly flexed on a pillow or over the examiner's knee (30° flexion). The examiner's thumbs are placed against the medial or lateral edge of the patella, and a force is applied to the side of the patella, with the fingers used for stabilization. The process is then repeated, with pressure applied to the other side of the patella. The other knee is tested as a comparison.

This joint play is similar to the passive movements of the patella; as in the passive test, the patella can be displaced by approximately half of its width medially and laterally. The examiner must do the movements slowly and carefully to ensure that the patella is not prone to dislocation.

Depression (Distal Movement) of Patella

The patient is in a supine position with the knee slightly flexed. The examiner then places one hand over the patient's patella so that the pisiform bone rests over the base of the patella. The other hand is placed so that the finger and thumb can grasp the medial and lateral edges of the patella to direct its movement. The examiner then rests the first hand over the second hand and applies a caudal force to the base of the patella, directing the caudal movement with the second hand so that the patella does not grind against the femoral condyles.

Anteroposterior Movement of Fibula on Tibia

The patient is supine with the knee flexed to 90° and the hip to 45°. The examiner then sits on the patient's foot and places one hand around the patient's knee to stabilize the knee and leg. The mobilizing hand is placed

around the head of the fibula. The fibula is drawn forward on the tibia, and the movement and end feel are tested. The fibula then slides back to its resting position of its own accord. The movement is tested several times and compared with that of the other side. Care must be taken when performing this technique because the common peroneal nerve, which winds around the head of the fibula, may be easily compressed, causing pain. If the superior tibiofibular joint is stiff or hypomobile, the test itself will cause discomfort.

Palpation

The patient lies supine with the knee slightly flexed. It is wise to put the knee in several positions during palpation. For example, meniscal cysts are best palpated at 45°, whereas the joint line is easiest to palpate at 90°. When palpating, the examiner looks for abnormal tenderness, swelling, nodules, or abnormal temperature. The following structures should be palpated (Fig. 12–128).

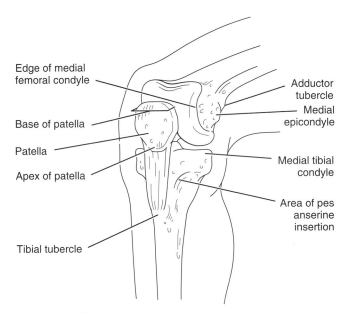

Edge of medial femoral condyle
Base of patella
Patella
Apex of patella
Tibial tubercle
Adductor tubercle
Medial epicondyle
Medial tibial condyle
Area of pes anserine insertion

Figure 12–128
Landmarks of the knee. (Adapted from Reilly, B.M.: Practical Strategies in Outpatient Medicine. Philadelphia, W.B. Saunders Co., 1991, p. 1175.)

Anterior Palpation With Knee Extended

Patella, Patellar Tendon, Patellar Retinaculum, Associated Bursa, Cartilaginous Surface of the Patella, and Plica. The patella can easily be palpated over the anterior aspect of the knee. The base of the patella lies superiorly, and the apex lies distally. After palpating the apex of the patella (for possible jumper's knee), the examiner moves distally, palpating the patellar tendon (for tendinitis) and the overlying infrapatellar bursa (for Parson's knee) as well as the fat pad that lies behind the tendon. When the knee is extended, the fat pad often extends beyond the sides of the tendon. Moving distally, the examiner comes to the tibial tuberosity, which should be palpated for enlargement (possible Osgood-Schlatter disease).

Returning to the patella, the examiner can palpate the skin lying over the patella for pathology (prepatellar bursitis or housemaid's knee) and then extend medially and laterally to palpate the patellar retinaculum on both sides of the patella. With the examiner pushing down on the lateral aspect of the patella, the medial retinaculum can be brought under tension and then palpated for tender areas. The lateral retinaculum can be palpated in a similar fashion, with the examiner pushing down on the medial aspect of the patella. By stressing the retinaculum, the examiner is separating the retinaculum from the underlying tissue.

With the quadriceps muscles relaxed, the articular facets of the patella are palpated for tenderness (possible chondromalacia patellae), as shown in Figure 12–129. This palpation is often facilitated by carefully pushing

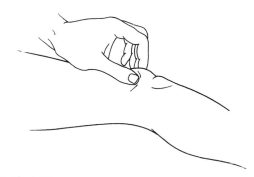

Figure 12–130
Palpation of the suprapatellar pouch.

the patella medially to palpate the medial facets and laterally to palpate the lateral facet.

As the medial edge of the patella is palpated, the examiner should carefully feel for the presence of a mediopatellar plica. The plica, if pathological, may be palpated as a thickened ridge medial to the patella. To help confirm the presence of the plica, the examiner flexes the patient's knee to 30° and pushes the patella medially. If the plica is present and pathological, this maneuver often causes pain.

Suprapatellar Pouch. Returning to the anterior surface of the patella and moving proximally beyond the base of the patella, the examiner's fingers will lie over the suprapatellar pouch. The examiner then lifts the skin and underlying tissue between the thumb and fingers (Fig. 12–130). In this way, the synovial membrane of the suprapatellar pouch, which is continuous with that of the knee joint, can be palpated. The examiner should feel for any thickness, tenderness, or nodules, the presence of which may indicate pathology.

Quadriceps Muscles (Vastus Medialis, Vastus Intermedius, Vastus Lateralis, and Rectus Femoris) and Sartorius. After palpating the suprapatellar pouch, the examiner palpates the quadriceps for tenderness (possible first- or second-degree strain), defects (third-degree strain), atonia, or hard masses (myositis ossificans).

Medial Collateral Ligament. If the examiner moves medially from the patella so that the fingers lie over the medial aspect of the tibiofemoral joint, the fingers will lie over the medial collateral ligament, which should be palpated along its entire length for tenderness (possible sprain) or other pathology (e.g., Pellegrini-Stieda syndrome).

Pes Anserinus. Medial and slightly distal to the tibial tuberosity, the examiner may palpate the pes anserinus (the common aponeurosis of the tendons of gracilis, semitendinosus, and sartorius muscles) for tenderness. Any associated swelling may indicate pes anserine bursitis.

Tensor Fasciae Latae (Iliotibial Band and Head of Fibula). As the examiner moves laterally from the tibial tuberosity, the head of the fibula can be palpated. Medial and

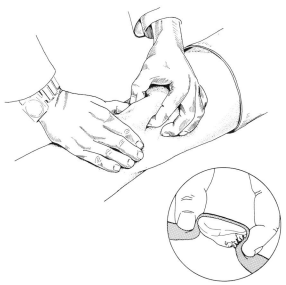

Figure 12–129
Checking for medial and lateral facet tenderness. Note that tenderness may be related to structures other than patellar surfaces beneath the examining finger. (From Hughston, J.C., W.M. Walsh, and G. Puddu: Patellar Subluxation and Dislocation. Philadelphia, W.B. Saunders Co., 1984, p. 28.)

slightly superior to the fibula, the examiner palpates the insertion of the iliotibial band into the lateral condyle of the tibia. When the knee is extended, it stands out as a strong, visible ridge anterolateral to the knee joint. As the examiner moves proximally, the iliotibial band is palpated along its entire length.

Anterior Palpation With Knee Flexed

Tibiofemoral Joint Line and Meniscal Cysts. The patient's knee is flexed at 45°, and the examiner palpates the joint line, especially on the lateral aspect, for any evidence of swelling (possible meniscal cyst), tenderness, or other pathology.

Tibiofemoral Joint Line, Tibial Plateau, Femoral Condyles, and Adductor Muscles. The patient's knee is flexed to 90°. If the examiner returns to the patella, palpates the apex of the patella, and moves medially or laterally, the fingers will lie on the tibiofemoral joint line, which should be palpated along its entire length. As the joint line is palpated, the examiner should also palpate the tibial plateau (for possible coronary ligament sprain) medially and laterally, as well as the femoral condyles.

Both condyles should be palpated carefully for any tenderness (e.g., osteochondritis dissecans). Beginning at the superior aspect of the femoral condyles, the examiner should note that the lateral condyle extends farther anteriorly (i.e., higher) than the medial condyle. The trochlear groove between the two condyles can then be palpated. As the medial condyle is palpated, a sharp edge appears on the condyle medially. If the edge is followed posteriorly, the adductor tubercle can be palpated on the posteromedial portion of the medial femoral condyle. After palpating the adductor tubercle, the examiner moves proximally, palpating the adductor muscles of the hip for tenderness or other signs of pathology.

Anterior Palpation With Foot of Test Leg Resting on Opposite Knee

Kennedy[54] has advocated palpation of the lateral collateral ligament by having the patient in the sitting or lying position (Fig. 12–131). The patient's knee is flexed to 90°, and the hip is laterally rotated so that the ankle of the test leg rests on the knee of the other leg. The examiner then places the knee into a varus position, and the ropelike ligament stands out if the ligament is intact.

Posterior Palpation With the Knee Slightly Flexed

Posterior Aspect of Knee Joint. The soft tissue on the posterior aspect of the knee should be palpated for tenderness or swelling (e.g., Baker's cyst). In some patients, the popliteal artery (pulse) may be palpated by running the hand down the center of the posterior knee.

Posterolateral Aspect of Knee Joint. The posterolateral corner of the knee is sometimes called the **popliteus corner**. The examiner should attempt to palpate the arcuate-popliteus complex, the lateral gastrocnemius muscle, the biceps femoris muscle, and possibly the lateral meniscus in this area. A sesamoid bone is sometimes found inserted in the tendon of the lateral head of the gastrocnemius muscle. This bone, referred to as the **fabella,** may be interpreted as a loose body in the posterolateral aspect of the knee by an unwary examiner.

Posteromedial Aspect of Knee Joint. The posteromedial corner of the knee joint is sometimes referred to as the **semimembranosus corner**. The examiner should attempt to palpate the posterior oblique ligament, the semimembranosus muscle, the medial gastrocnemius muscle, and possibly the medial mensicus in this area for tenderness or pathology.

Hamstring and Gastrocnemius Muscles. After the various parts of the posterior aspect of the knee have been palpated, the tendons and muscle bellies of the hamstring muscle group (biceps femoris, semitendinosus, and semimembranosus) proximally and of the gastrocnemius muscle distally should be palpated for tenderness, swelling, or other signs of pathology.

Diagnostic Imaging

Plain Film Radiography

For evaluation of knee injuries, anteroposterior and lateral views are most commonly obtained. Depending on the suspected pathology, other views may be taken as well. Usually, the anteroposterior view is taken with the patient bearing weight. Imaging should not be used indiscriminantly but should be considered an adjunct to examination; it is used primarily to confirm a diagnosis obtained by careful assessment.[136, 137]

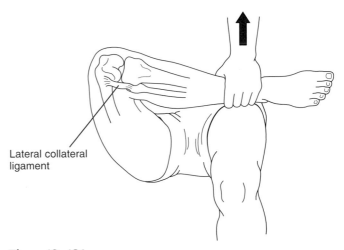

Lateral collateral ligament

Figure 12–131
Palpation of the lateral (fibular) collateral ligament.

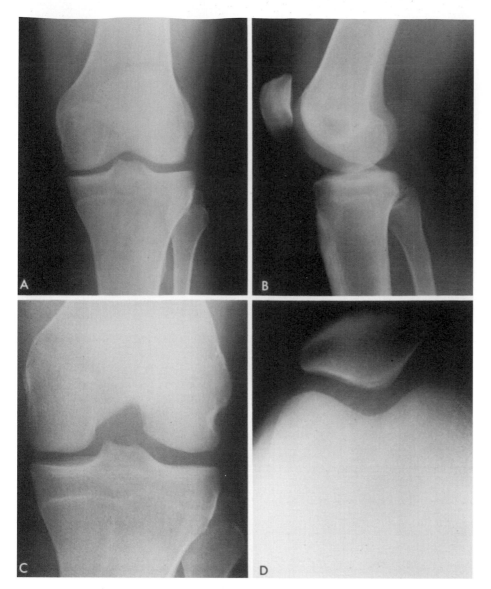

Figure 12–132

Normal radiographs of the knee. (A) Anteroposterior view. (B) Lateral view. (C) Tunnel view. (D) Skyline view. (From Reilly, B.M.: Practical Strategies in Outpatient Medicine. Philadelphia, W.B. Saunders Co., 1991, p. 1188.)

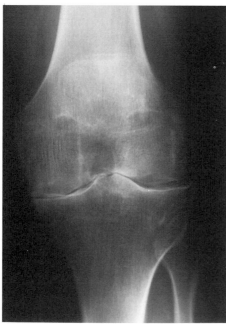

Figure 12–133

Anteroposterior x-ray showing degenerative arthritis of the knee. Note the loss of joint space caused by loss of cartilage (both sides) and meniscus (on medial side).

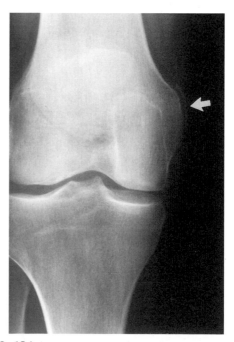

Figure 12–134

Pellegrini-Stieda syndrome. Note calcium formation within the substance of the medial collateral ligament (*arrow*).

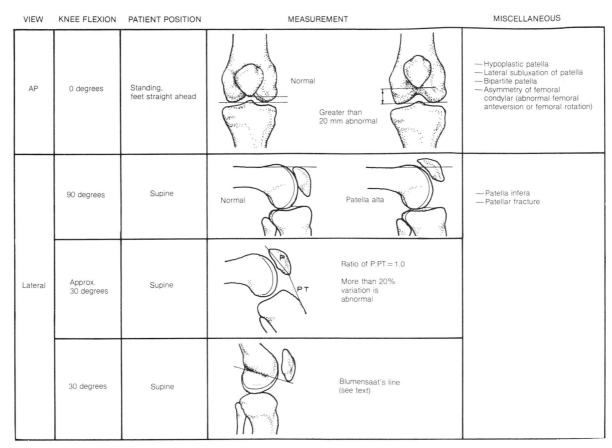

VIEW	KNEE FLEXION	PATIENT POSITION	MEASUREMENT	MISCELLANEOUS
AP	0 degrees	Standing, feet straight ahead	Normal / Greater than 20 mm abnormal	— Hypoplastic patella — Lateral subluxation of patella — Bipartite patella — Asymmetry of femoral condylar (abnormal femoral anteversion or femoral rotation)
Lateral	90 degrees	Supine	Normal / Patella alta	— Patella infera — Patellar fracture
	Approx. 30 degrees	Supine	Ratio of P:PT = 1.0 More than 20% variation is abnormal	
	30 degrees	Supine	Blumensaat's line (see text)	

Figure 12–135

Summary of radiographic findings in patella alta. (From Carson, W.G. Jr., S.L. James, R.L. Larsen, et al.: Patellofemoral disorders: Physical and radiographic evaluation: I: Physical examination. Clin. Orthop. 185:179, 1984.)

Anteroposterior View. When looking at radiographs of the knee (Fig. 12–132), the examiner should note any possible fractures (e.g., osteochondral), diminished joint space (possible osteoarthritis; Fig. 12–133), epiphyseal damage, lipping, loose bodies, alterations in bone texture, abnormal calcification, ossification (e.g., Pellegrini-Stieda syndrome; Fig. 12–134) or tumors, accessory ossification centers, varus or valgus deformity, patellar position, patella alta (Figs. 12–135 and 12–336) or baja, and asymmetry of femoral condyles.[138, 139] Stress, non–

Figure 12–136

Anteroposterior view of the knee. (A) Normal patellar position. (B) Patella alta. (C) Patella baja. (From Hughston, J.C., W.M. Walsh, and G. Puddu: Patellar Subluxation and Dislocation. Philadelphia, W.B. Saunders Co., 1984, p. 50.)

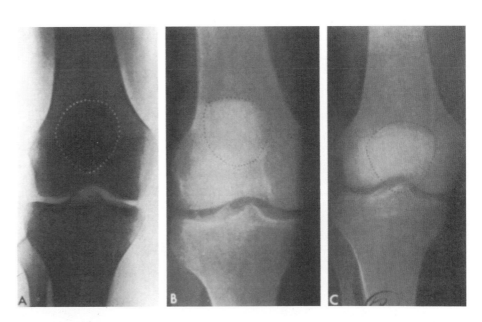

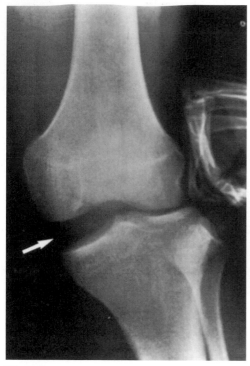

Figure 12–137

This valgus stress radiograph shows the patient's knee in full extension. Note the gapping on the medial side (*arrow*). (From Mital, M.A., and L.I. Karlin: Diagnostic arthroscopy in sports injuries. Orthop. Clin. North Am. 11:775, 1980.)

weight-bearing radiographs of this view illustrate excessive gapping medially or laterally, indicating ligamentous instablity (Fig. 12–137). The examiner should also remember the possible presence of the fabella, which is seen in 20% of the population. Epiphyseal fractures (Fig. 12–138) and osteochondritis dissecans (Fig. 12–139) may also be seen in this view. The presence of the Seg-

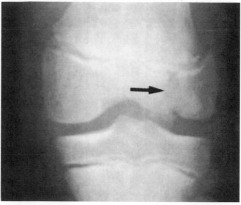

Figure 12–138

A Salter-Harris type III injury (*arrow*) of the growth plate and epiphysis. Main attention should be directed toward restitution of the joint surface. (From Ehrlich, M.G., and R.E. Strain: Epiphyseal injuries about the knee. Orthop. Clin. North Am. 10:93, 1979.)

und sign or **lateral capsular sign,** which is an avulsion fracture, often indicates severe lateral capsular injury and probably anterior cruciate ligament disruption (Fig. 12–140).[7, 140–142]

Lateral View. With this view,[82, 138, 143] the examiner should note the same structures as seen with the anteroposterior view (Figs. 12–141 and 12–142). This view is usually done in side lying with the knee flexed to 45°.[144] To determine the normal positioning of the patella, the standing, weight-bearing lateral view is used to determine the ratio of patellar length to patellar tendon length (Fig. 12–143); several methods are possible.[145–147] Berg and associates[148] reported that the Blackburne-Peel method was the most consistent. This view also illustrates Osgood-Schlatter disease (Fig. 12–144), the presence of the fabella (Fig. 12–145), and avulsion of the anterior cruciate insertion (Fig. 12–146).

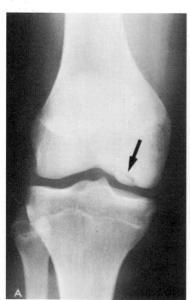
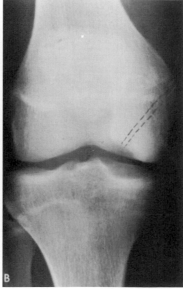

Figure 12–139

(A) Osteochondritis dissecans—actually an osteochondral fracture (*arrow*) of the femoral condyle—with almost the entire femoral attachment of the posterior cruciate ligament remaining attached to the fragment. (B) Three months after repair of posterior cruciate to femur. Excellent function is restored. Complete filling in of this defect is unlikely at this age. (From O'Donoghue, D.H.: Treatment of Injuries to Athletes, 4th ed. Philadelphia, W.B. Saunders Co., 1984, p. 575.)

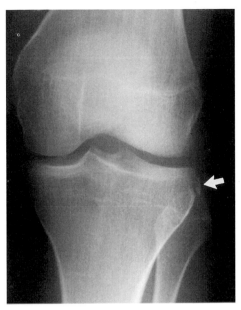

Figure 12–140

Segund sign. Note avulsion fracture adjacent to lateral tibial plateau (*arrow*). This lateral capsular injury often signifies an anterior cruciate ligament tear.

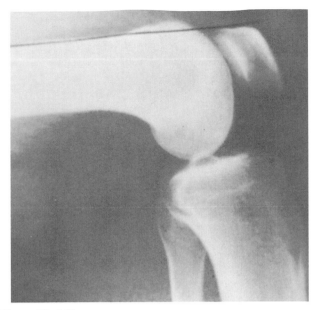

Figure 12–141

Lateral view at 90° shows the normal position of the patella. (From Hughston, J.C., W.M. Walsh, and G. Puddu: Patellar Subluxation and Dislocation. Philadelphia, W.B. Saunders Co., 1984, p. 52.)

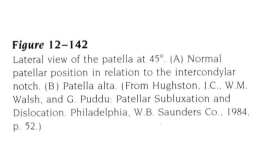

Figure 12–142

Lateral view of the patella at 45°. (A) Normal patellar position in relation to the intercondylar notch. (B) Patella alta. (From Hughston, J.C., W.M. Walsh, and G. Puddu: Patellar Subluxation and Dislocation. Philadelphia, W.B. Saunders Co., 1984, p. 52.)

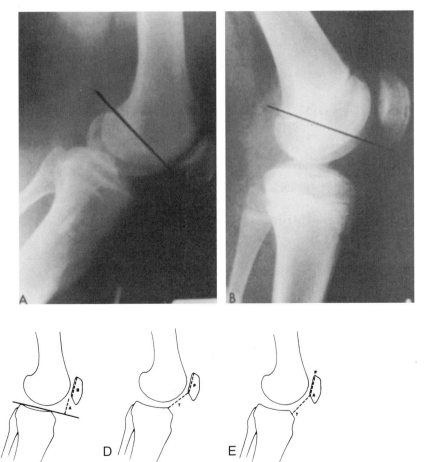

Figure 12–143

Indices for measurement of patellar height. (A) Insall-Salvati. (B) Modified Insall-Salvati. (C) Blackburne. (D) de Carvalho. (E) Caton. (From Grelsamer, R.P., and S. Meadows: The modified Insall-Salvati ratio for assessment of patellar height. Clin. Orthop. 282:172, 1992.)

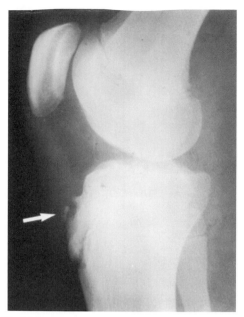

Figure 12–144

Osgood-Schlatter disease, showing epiphysitis of the entire epiphysis (*arrow*), with irregularity of the epiphyseal line. Because this epiphyseal cartilage is continuous with that of the upper tibia, it should not be disturbed. If surgery is used, exposure should be superficial to the epiphyseal cartilage. (From O'Donoghue, D.H.: Treatment of Injuries to Athletes, 4th ed. Philadelphia, W.B. Saunders Co., 1984, p. 574.)

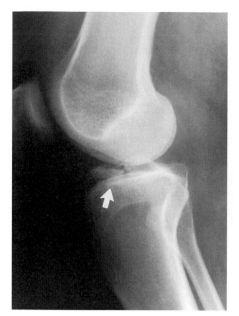

Figure 12–146

Avulsion fracture of the tibial insertion of the anterior cruciate ligament.

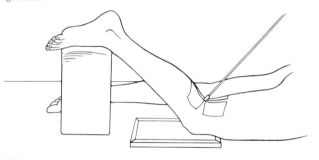

Figure 12–147

Position for intercondylar notch view. (From Larson, R.L., and W.A. Grana [eds.]: The Knee: Form, Function, Pathology and Treatment. Philadelphia, W.B. Saunders Co., 1993, p. 106.)

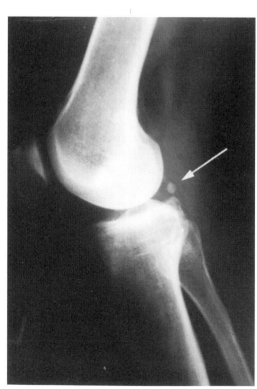

Figure 12–145

Sesamoid bone (fabella) in the gastrocnemius muscle.

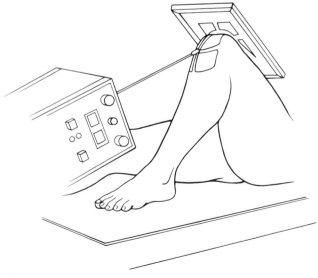

Figure 12–148

Positioning for the patellofemoral (skyline) view. (From Larson, R.L., and W.A. Grana [eds.]: The Knee: Form, Function, Pathology and Treatment. Philadelphia, W.B. Saunders Co., 1993, p. 107.)

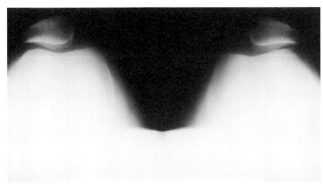

Figure 12–149

Skyline (sunrise) view of patellofemoral joints. Note the lateral displacement of both patellae, especially the one on the right. Note also the alpine hunter's cap shape of patella.

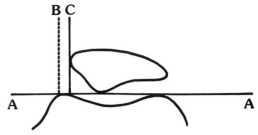

Figure 12–151

Lateral patellar displacement. A line is drawn through the highest points of the medial and lateral femoral condyles (AA). A perpendicular to that line, at the medial edge of the medial femoral condyle (B), normally lies 1 mm or less medial to the patella (line C). (From Laurin, C.A., R. Dussault, and H.P. Levesque: The tangential x-ray investigation of the patellofemoral joint. Clin. Orthop. 144:16, 1979.)

Intercondylar Notch (Tunnel View X-ray). With this view (patient prone, knee flexed to 90°), the tibia and intercondylar attachments of the cruciate ligaments can be examined (Fig. 12–147). Also, any loose bodies or possibility of osteochondritis dissecans, subluxation, patellar tilt (lateral or medial), or dislocation should be noted.

Axial (Skyline) View. This 30° tangential view (Fig. 12–148) is primarily used for suspected patellar problems such as patellar subluxation and dysplasia (Fig. 12–149).[139, 143, 149] It may be taken at different angles, as shown in Figures 12–150, 12–151, and 12–152, or it may be used to determine the type of patella present, as shown in Figure 12–153. Figure 12–154 illustrates abnormal patellar forms. Other patellofemoral measurements include lateral patellar displacement (see Fig. 12–151) and the lateral-to-medial trochlear ratio (see Fig. 12–152).[143]

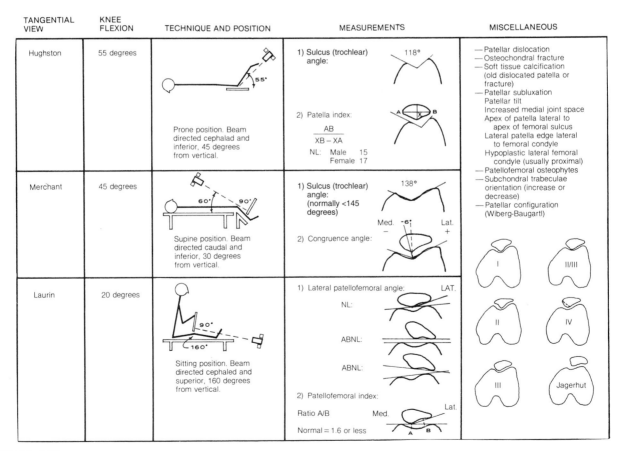

Figure 12–150

Summary of radiographic findings, tangential view. (From Carson, W.G. Jr., S.L. James, R.L. Larsen et al.: Patellofemoral disorders: Physical and radiographic evaluation: I: Physical examination. Clin. Orthop. 185:182, 1984.)

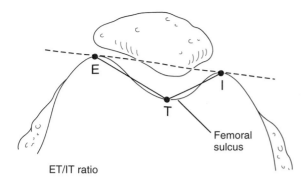

ET/IT ratio

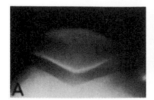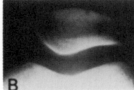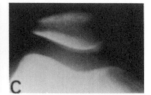

Figure 12–152

The lateral-medial trochlear ratio is the ratio between the external and internal segments (ET and IT) joining the highest points of the femoral condyles to the deepest point of the trochlear groove. It measures the dysplasia of the medial aspect of the trochlea. (Redrawn from Beaconsfield, T., E. Pintore, N. Maffulli, and G.J. Petri: Radiographic measurements in patellofemoral disorders. Clin. Orthop. 308:22, 1994.

Figure 12–153

Examples of patellar variations. (A) Wilberg type I. (B) Wilberg type II. (C) Wilberg type III. (From Ficat, R.P., and D.S. Hungerford. Disorders of the Patello-Femoral Joint. Baltimore, Williams & Wilkins, 1977, p. 53.)

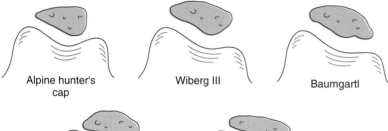

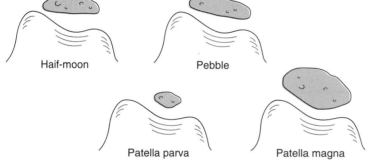

Alpine hunter's cap

Wiberg III

Baumgartl

Haif-moon

Pebble

Patella parva

Patella magna

Figure 12–154

Variations in patellar form that are considered dysplastic. (Redrawn from Ficat, R.P., and D.S. Hungerford. Disorders of the Patello-Femoral Joint. Baltimore, Williams & Wilkins, 1977, p. 55.)

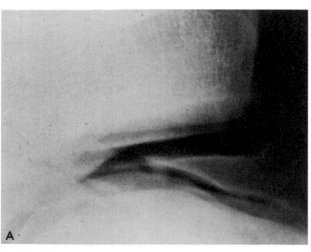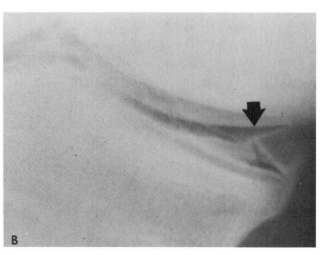

Figure 12–155

Arthrogram demonstrating a torn meniscus. The normal meniscus on the lateral side (A) is compared with the easily demonstrated tear in the medial meniscus (*arrow*) in the same patient (B). (From Reilly, B.M.: Practical Strategies in Outpatient Medicine. Philadelphia, W.B. Saunders Co., 1991, p. 1198.)

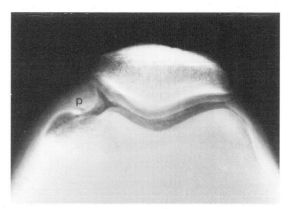

Figure 12–156
Tangential patellar view after arthrography, showing thinning and slight roughening of the patellar cartilage, especially medially. The mediopatellar plica (p) is markedly thickened. (From Weissman, B.N.W., and C.B. Sledge: Orthopedic Radiology. Philadelphia, W.B. Saunders Co., 1986, p. 536.)

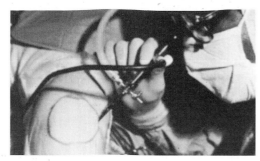

Figure 12–158
Arthroscopy of the knee. (From Patel, D.: Superior lateral-medial approach to arthroscopic meniscectomy. Orthop. Clin. North Am. 13:301, 1982.)

Arthrography

Arthrograms of the knee are used primarily to diagnose tears in the menisci (Fig. 12–155) and plica (Fig. 12–156). Double-contrast arthrograms are also used (Fig. 12–157). Arthrograms combined with computed tomography (CT) scans (CT arthrograms) are useful for assessing meniscus tears, articular cartilage, meniscal and popliteal cysts, and synovial plica.[150]

Arthroscopy

The arthroscope is being used increasingly to diagnose lesions of the knee and to repair many of them surgically.[151–153] By using various approaches to the knee, the surgeon is able to view all of the structures to determine whether they have been injured (Fig. 12–158).

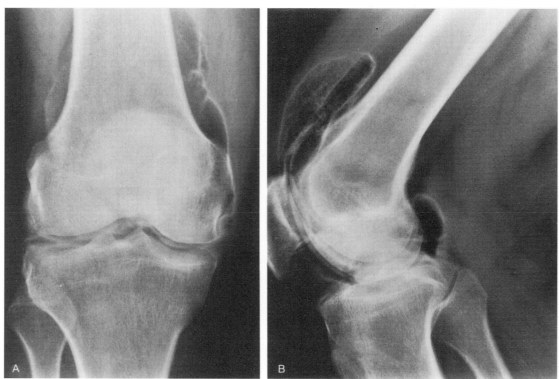

Figure 12–157
Double-contrast arthrogram. (A) The anteroposterior view demonstrates the menisci and articular cartilage. (B) The lateral projection illustrates the extent of the joint space. (From Forrester, D.M., and J.C. Brown: The Radiology of Joint Disease, 3rd ed. Philadelphia, W.B. Saunders Co., 1987, p. 200.)

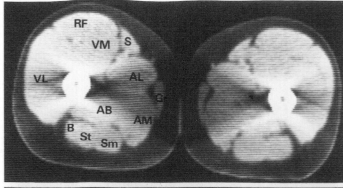

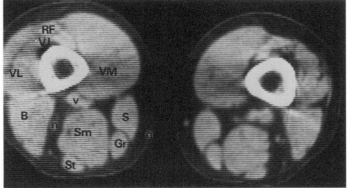

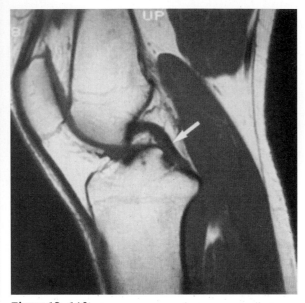

Figure 12–159

Muscular anatomy as shown on computed tomography scan; images through the upper femur (A) and lower third of femur (B) are shown. AB = adductor brevis; AL = adductor longus; AM = adductor magnus; B = biceps femoris; Gr = gracilis; n = tibial and common peroneal nerves; RF = rectus femoris; S = sartorius; Sm = semimembranosus; St = semitendinosus; V = deep femoral vein and artery; VI = vastus intermedius; VL = vastus lateralis; VM = vastus medialis. (From Weissman, B.N.W., and C.B. Sledge: Orthopedic Radiology. Philadelphia, W.B. Saunders Co., 1986, p. 504.)

Figure 12–160

Magnetic resonance image showing intact posterior cruciate ligament (*arrow*). (From Strobel, M., and H.W. Stedtfeld: Diagnostic Evaluation of the Knee. Berlin, Springer-Verlag, 1990, p. 243.)

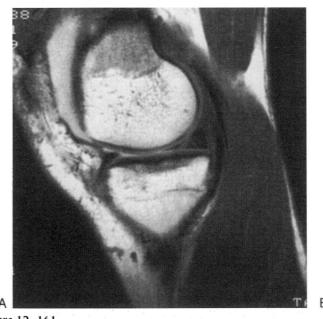

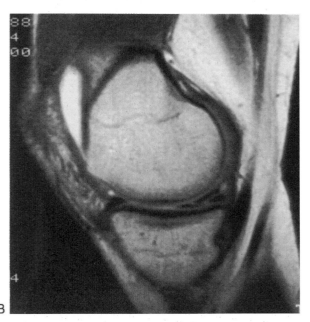

Figure 12–161

Magnetic resonance image showing lesion of the posterior horn of the medial meniscus (A). In some cases, contrast can be enhanced by the intra-articular injection of gadolinium diethylenetriamene penta-acetic acid (DTPA). (B) Inferior longitudinal tear with an associated horizontal tear. (From Strobel, M., and H.W. Stedtfeld: Diagnostic Evaluation of the Knee. Berlin, Springer-Verlag, 1990, p. 240.)

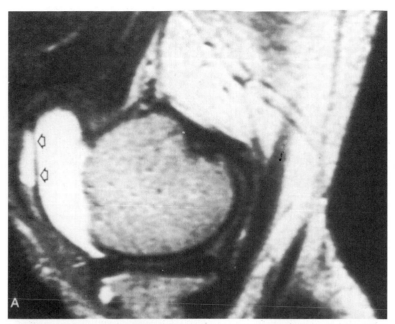

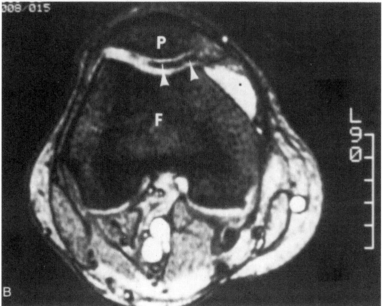

Figure 12–162

Magnetic resonance image of medial patellar plica. (A) Sagittal, T2-weighted image located medial to the patella demonstrates an effusion present within the knee joint that appears white. The vertical linear band seen within the joint (*open arrows*) represents the medial plica. (B) Transaxial STIR image through the patellofemoral joint again demonstrates the effusion (*arrowheads*), which appears bright and surrounds a tongue-like extension of tissue arising from the medial joint line and located between the patella (P) and the femur (F). This tissue represents a medial plica. In this location, plicae can become hypertrophied and lead to symptoms and signs of internal derangement. (From Kursunoglu-Brahme, S., and D. Resnick: Magnetic resonance imaging of the knee. Orthop. Clin. North Am. 21:571, 1990.)

Computed Tomography

CT scans are often used to view soft tissue as well as bone (Fig. 12–159).

Magnetic Resonance Imaging

Magnetic resonance imaging (MRI) is advantageous because of its ability to show soft tissue as well as bone tissue while providing no exposure to ionizing radiation.

MRI has been found to be useful in diagnosing lesions of the menisci and cruciate ligaments (Figs. 12–160, 12–161, 12–162, and 12–163), but it should be used only to confirm or clarify a clinical diagnosis.[34, 142, 154–156]

Xeroradiography

Xeroradiography may be used to delineate the edge of bone (Fig. 12–164).

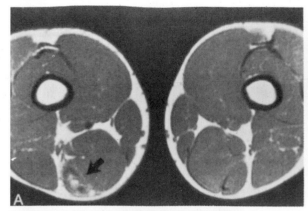

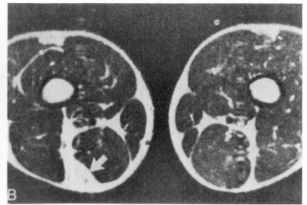

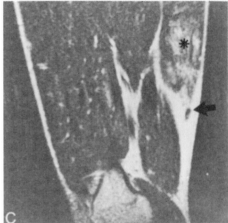

Figure 12–163

Magnetic resonance (MR) images showing tendon rupture in a 22-year-old athlete who pulled his hamstring on two occasions and was unable to run. Seven centimeters above the patella, (A) axial T1-weighted (TR, 600 msec; TE, 20 msec) and (B) T2-weighted (TR, 2,000 msec; TE, 85 msec) MR images show abnormally high signal intensity of the right semitendinosus muscle (*arrows*) compared with the normal left side. (C) Sagittal T2-weighted MR image (TR, 2,000 msec; TE, 85 msec) discloses that retracted semitendinosus muscle (*asterisk*) has an abnormally high signal intensity. The arrow indicates a torn musculotendinous junction. (From Bassett, L.W., and R.H. Gold: Magnetic resonance imaging of the musculoskeletal system: An overview. Clin. Orthop. 244:20, 1989.)

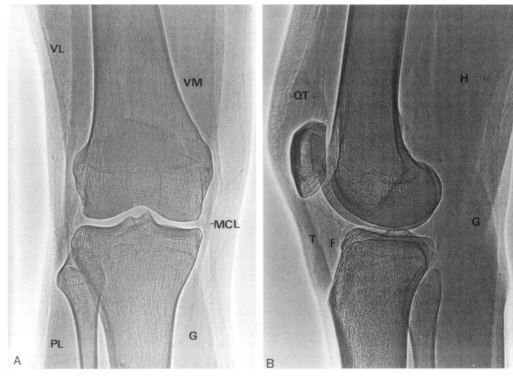

Figure 12–164

Xeroradiography of the knee. (A) Anteroposterior view. (B) Lateral view. F = infrapatellar fat pad; G = gastrocnemius; H = hamstrings; MCL = medial collateral ligament; PL = peroneus longus; QT = quadriceps tendon; T = patellar tendon; VL = vastus lateralis; VM = vastus medialis. (From Weissman, B.N.W., and C.B. Sledge: Orthopedic Radiology. Philadelphia, W.B. Saunders Co., 1986, p. 504.)

Précis of the Knee Assessment*

History
Observation
Examination
    Active movement
        Knee flexion
        Knee extension
        Medial rotation of the tibia on the femur
        Lateral rotation of the tibia on the femur
    Passive movements (as in active movements)
    Resisted isometric movements
        Knee flexion
        Knee extension
        Ankle plantar flexion
        Ankle dorsiflexion
    Tests for ligament stability
        Test for one-plane medial instability
        Test for one-plane lateral instability
        Tests for one-plane anterior and posterior
            instabilities
        Tests for anteromedial and anterolateral rotary
            instabilities
        Tests for posteromedial and posterolateral rotary
            instabilities
    Functional assessment
    Special tests
        Tests for meniscus injury

        Plica tests
        Tests for swelling
        Other tests
    Reflexes and cutaneous distribution
    Joint play movements
        Backward and forward movements of the tibia on the
            femur
        Medial and lateral translation of the tibia on the femur
        Medial and lateral displacements of the patella
        Depression of the patella
        Anteroposterior movement of the fibula on the tibia
    Palpation
    Diagnostic imaging

*Although examination of the knee may be carried out with the patient in the supine position, some of the tests may require the patient to move to other positions (e.g., standing, lying, prone, sitting). When these tests are used, the examination should be planned in such a way that the movement and, therefore, the discomfort experienced by the patient are kept to a minimum. The sequence should be from standing to sitting, to supine lying, to side lying, and finally, to prone lying.

After any examination, the patient should be warned of the possibility of exacerbation of symptoms as a result of the assessment.

Case Studies

When doing these case studies, the examiner should list the appropriate questions to be asked and why they are being asked, what to look for and why, and what things should be tested and why. Depending on the answers of the patient (and the examiner should consider different responses), several possible causes of the patient's problem may become evident (examples are given in parentheses). A differential diagnosis chart should be made. The examiner can then decide how different diagnoses may affect the treatment plan. For example, a 16-year old female volleyball player comes to you complaining of knee pain (Table 12–12). Her knee is painful when she plays, and she sometimes feels a clicking when going up and down stairs. Describe your assessment plan for this patient (meniscus pathology versus plica syndrome).

Table 12–12
Differential Diagnosis of Meniscus and Medial Patellar Plica Syndrome

	Medial Meniscus	**Medial Patellar Plica Syndrome**
History	Mechanism of injury: rotation, flexion, and valgus stress (may be acute or insidious)	Mechanism of injury; flexion, rotation (usually insidious onset)
Pain	Joint line	May be joint line but also superomedial to joint line
Swelling	May be present	May be present
Locking or giving way	Locking more likely	Giving way more likely
Active movement	May be limited	Usually full but extremes of motion may be painful, catching may occur on movement
Passive movement	Pain at extremes	Pain possible at extreme of flexion
Resisted isometric movement	Normal	Normal unless pinching causes pain and reflex inhibition
Ligament tests	Negative	Negative
Special tests	McMurray may be positive, Apley's test may be positive	Mediopatellar plica test positive, plica "stutter" test positive, Hughston plica test positive
Palpation	Joint line tenderness	Plica may demonstrate thickening and be bandlike

1. A 59-year-old man presents to you complaining of moderate pain and swelling of 4 months' duration in his right knee. There is no history of trauma. The pain and swelling have become worse during the past month. Describe your assessment plan for this patient (osteoarthritis versus meniscus pathology).

2. A 24-year-old male football player is referred to you for treatment after a surgical repair to the anterior cruciate and medial collateral ligaments of the right knee. He is still in a splint, but the surgeon says the splint can be removed for treatment. Describe your assessment plan for this patient.

3. A 54-year-old man comes to you for treatment. He complains of difficulty when walking and pain in the left hamstrings that is referred into the area of the gluteal fold. There is ecchymosis evident in the posterior knee and a small amount in the superior calf area. Describe your assessment plan for this patient (hamstring strain versus sciatica).

4. An 18-year-old woman presents to your clinic complaining of anterior knee pain. Design your assessment plan for this patient (chondromalacia patellae versus plica syndrome).

5. A 17-year-old male soccer player comes to you complaining that his knee feels unstable. He says he was playing soccer, twisted to challenge a player, and felt a pop in his knee. Describe your assessment plan for this patient (osteochondral fracture versus anterior cruciate sprain).

6. A 10-year-old boy is brought to you by his parents. He is complaining of anterior knee pain. Describe your assessment plan for this patient (Osgood-Schlatter syndrome versus chondromalacia patellae).

7. A 20-year-old female rugby player comes to you complaining of lateral knee pain that is sometimes referred down the leg. The knee hurts when she walks. She vaguely remembers being kicked in the knee while playing rugby 10 days earlier. Describe your assessment plan for this patient (superior tibiofibular joint subluxation versus common peroneal nerve neuropraxia).

8. An 18-year-old female swimmer presents to you complaining of medial knee pain. She has just increased her training to 10,000 m per day. Describe your assessment plan for this patient (medial collateral ligament sprain versus chondromalacia patellae).

References

Cited References

1. Kaltenborn, F.M.: Mobilization of the Extremity Joints. Oslo, Olaf Norles Bokhandel, 1980.
2. Arnoczsky, S.P.: The blood supply of the meniscus and its role in healing and repair. American Association of Orthopaedic Surgeons, Symposium on Sports Medicine: The Knee. St. Louis, C.V. Mosby, 1985.
3. Radin, E.L., R. de Lamotte, and P. Maquet: Role of the menisci in the distribution of stress in the knee. Clin. Orthop. 185:290–294, 1984.
4. Seedhom, B.B.: Loadbearing function of the menisci. Physiotherapy 62:223–226, 1976.
5. Ficat, R.P., and D.S. Hungerford: The Patello-Femoral Joint. Baltimore, Williams & Wilkins, 1977.
6. Goodfellow, J., D.S. Hungerford, and M. Zindel: Patellofemoral joint mechanics and pathology: Functional anatomy of the patellofemoral joint. J. Bone Joint Surg. Br. 58:287–290, 1976.
7. Tria, A.J., and T.M. Hosea: Diagnosis of knee ligament injuries: Clinical. In Scott, W.N. (ed.): Ligament and Extensor Mechanism Injuries of the Knee: Diagnosis and Treatment. St. Louis, Mosby–Year Book Inc., 1991.
8. Levy, M., and A.D. Smith: Diagnosing meniscus injuries: Focus on the office exam. Phys. Sportsmed. 22:47–54, 1994.
9. Liorzou, G.: Knee Ligaments: Clinical Examination. Berlin, Springer-Verlag, 1991.
10. Hughston, J.C.: Knee Ligaments: Injury and Repair. St. Louis, C.V. Mosby, 1993.
11. Riegger-Krugh, C., and J.J. Keysor: Skeletal malalignments of the lower quarter: Correlated and compensatory motions and postures. J. Orthop. Sports Phys. Ther. 23:164–170, 1996.
12. Hawkins, R.J.: Musculoskeletal Examination. St. Louis, C.V. Mosby Co., 1995.
13. McConnell, J.: Management of patellofemoral problems. Manual Therapy 1:60–66, 1996.
14. Staheli, L.T., and G.M. Engel: Tibial torsion: A method of assessment and a survey of normal children. Clin. Orthop. 86:183–186, 1972.
15. Waldron, V.D.: A test for chondromalacia patellae. Orthop. Rev. 12:103, 1983.
16. Hughston, J.C.: Extensor mechanism examination. In Fox, J.M., and W. Del Pizzo: The Patellofemoral Joint. New York, McGraw-Hill Inc., 1993.
17. McConnell, J., and J. Fulkerson: The knee: Patellofemoral and soft tissue injuries. In Zachazewski, J.E., D.J. Magee, and W.S. Quillen (eds.): Athletic Injuries and Rehabilitation. Philadelphia, W.B. Saunders Co., 1996.
18. Fulkerson, J.P.: Patellofemoral pain disorders: Evaluation and management. J. Am. Acad. Orthop. Surg. 2:124–132, 1994.
19. Jacobson, K.E., and F.C. Flandry: Diagnosis of anterior knee pain. Clin. Sports Med. 8:179–195, 1989.
20. Rouse, S.J.: The role of the iliotibial tract in patellofemoral pain and iliotibial band friction syndromes. Physiotherapy 82:199–202, 1996.
21. Segal, P., and M. Jacob: The Knee. Chicago, Year Book Medical Publishers, 1983.
22. Kannus, P., M. Jarvineaa, and K. Latvala: Knee strength evaluation. Scand. J. Sport Sci. 9:9, 1987.
23. Goslin, B.R., and J. Charteris: Isokinetic dynamometry: Normative data for clinical use in lower extremity (knee) cases. Scand. J. Rehab. Med. 11:105–109, 1979.
24. Stafford, M.G., and W.A. Grana: Hamstring/quadriceps ratios in college football players: A high velocity evaluation. Am. J. Sports Med. 12:209–211, 1984.
25. Sgaglione, N.A., W. Del Pizzo, J.M. Fox, and M.J. Friedman: Critical analysis of knee ligament rating systems. Am. J. Sports Med. 23:660–667, 1995.
26. Fonseca, S.T., D.J. Magee, J. Wessel, and D.C. Reid: Validation of a performance test for outcome evaluation of knee function. Clin. J. Sport Med. 2:251–256, 1992.
27. Daniel, D.M., M.L. Stone, and B. Riehl: Ligament surgery: The evaluation of results. In Daniel, D., W. Akeson, and J. O'Conner (eds.): Knee Ligaments: Structure, Injury and Repair. New York, Raven Press, 1990.
28. Strobel, M., and H.W. Stedtfeld: Diagnostic Evaluation of the Knee. Berlin, Springer-Verlag, 1990.
29. Noyes, F.R., S.D. Barber, and R.E. Mangine: Abnormal lower limb symmetry determined by functional hop tests after anterior cruciate rupture. Am. J. Sports Med. 19:513–518, 1991.
30. Barber, S.D., F.R. Noyes, R.E. Mangine, J.W. McCloskey, and W. Hartman: Quantitative assessment of functional limitations in normal and anterior cruciate ligament-deficient knees. Clin. Orthop. 255:204–214, 1990.
31. Booher, L.D., K.M. Hench, T.W. Worrell, and J. Stikeleather: Reliability of three single-leg hop tests. J. Sports Rehab. 2:165–170, 1993.

32. Risberg, M.A., and A. Ekeland: Assessment of functional tests after anterior cruciate ligament surgery. J. Orthop. Sports Phys. Ther. 19:212–217, 1994.

33. Losee, R.E.: Diagnosis of chronic injury to the anterior cruciate ligament. Orthop. Clin. North Am. 16:83–97, 1985.

34. Jackson, D.W., L.D. Jennings, R.M. Maywoods, and P.E. Berger: Magnetic resonance imaging of the knee. Am. J. Sports Med. 16:29–37, 1988.

35. Larson, R.L.: Physical examination in the diagnosis of rotary instability. Clin. Orthop. 172:38–44, 1983.

36. Noyes, F.R., G.H. McGinniss, and L.A. Mooar: Functional disability in the anterior cruciate insufficient knee syndrome: Review of knee rating systems and projected risk factors in determining treatment. Sports Med. 1:278–302, 1984.

37. Noyes, F.R., S.D. Barber, and L.A. Mooar: A rationale for assessing sports activity levels and limitations in knee disorders. Clin. Orthop. 246:238–249, 1989.

38. Irrgang, J.C., M.C. Safran, and F.H. Fu: The knee: ligamentous and meniscal injuries. In Zachazewski, J.E., D.J. Magee, and W.S. Quillen (eds.): Athletic Injuries and Rehabilitation. Philadelphia, W.B. Saunders Co., 1996.

39. Insall, J.N., L.D. Dorr, R.D. Scott, and W.N. Scott: Rationale of the Knee Society clinical rating system. Clin. Orthop. 248:13–14, 1989.

40. Lysholm, J., and J. Gillquist: Evaluation of knee ligament surgery results with special emphasis on use of a scoring scale. Am. J. Sports Med. 10:150–154, 1982.

41. Shea, K.P., and J.P. Fulkerson: Preoperative computed tomography scanning and arthroscopy in predicting outcome after lateral retinacular release. Arthroscopy 8:327–334, 1992.

42. Karlsson, J., R. Thomeé, and L. Sward: Eleven year follow up of patellofemoral pain syndromes. Clin. J. Sport Med. 6:22–26, 1996.

43. Kettlekamp, D.B., and C. Thompson: Development of a knee scoring scale. Clin. Orthop. 107:93–99, 1975.

44. Aichroth, P., M.A. Freeman, I.S. Smillie, and W.A. Souter: A knee function assessment chart. J. Bone Joint Surg. Br. 60:308–309, 1978.

45. Larson, R.: Rating sheet for knee function. In Smillie, I. (ed.): Diseases of the Knee Joint. Edinburgh, Churchill Livingstone, 1974.

46. Shoemaker, S.C., and D.M. Daniel: The limits of knee motion: In vitro studies. In Daniel, D., W. Akeson, and J. O'Conner (eds.): Knee Ligaments: Structure, Injury and Repair. New York, Raven Press, 1990.

47. Muller, W.: The Knee: Form, Function and Ligament Reconstruction. New York, Springer-Verlag, 1983.

48. Detenbeck, L.C.: Function of the cruciate ligaments in knee stability. Am. J. Sports Med. 2:217–221, 1974.

49. Furman, W., J.L. Marshall, and F.G. Girgis: The anterior cruciate ligament: A functional analysis based on postmortem studies. J. Bone Joint Surg. Am. 58:179–185, 1976.

50. Girgis, F.G., J.L. Marshall, and A.R.S. Al Monajem: The cruciate ligaments of the knee joint: Anatomical, functional and experimental analysis. Clin. Orthop. 106:216–231, 1975.

51. Baker, C.L., L.A. Norwood, and J.C. Hughston: Acute combined posterior and posterolateral instability of the knee. Am. J. Sports Med. 12:204–208, 1984.

52. Daniel, D.M.: Diagnosis of a ligament injury. In Daniel, D., W. Akeson, and J. O'Conner (eds.): Knee Ligaments: Structure, Injury and Repair. New York, Raven Press, 1990.

53. Marshall, J.L., and W.H. Baugher: Stability examination of the knee: A single anatomic approach. Clin. Orthop. 146:78–83, 1980.

54. Kennedy, J.C.: The Injured Adolescent Knee. Baltimore, Williams & Wilkins, 1979.

55. Jonsson, T., B. Althoff, L. Peterson, and P. Renstrom: Clinical diagnosis of ruptures of the anterior cruciate ligament: A comparative study of the Lachman test and the anterior drawer sign. Am. J. Sports Med. 10:100–102, 1982.

56. Paessler, H.H., and D. Michel: How new is the Lachman test? Am. J. Sports Med. 20:95–98, 1992.

57. Torg, J.S., W. Conrad, and V. Allen: Clinical diagnosis of anterior cruciate ligament instability in the athlete. Am. J. Sports Med. 4:84–93, 1976.

58. Jackson, R.W.: The torn ACL: Natural history of untreated lesions and rationale for selective treatment. In Feagin, J.A. (ed.): The Crucial Ligaments. Edinburgh, Churchill Livingstone, 1988.

59. Rosenberg, T.D., and G.L. Rasmussen: The function of the anterior cruciate ligament during anterior drawer and Lachman's testing. Am. J. Sports Med. 12:318–322, 1984.

60. Frank, C.: Accurate interpretation of the Lachman test. Clin. Orthop. 213:163–166, 1986.

61. Bechtel, S.L., B.R. Ellman, and J.L. Jordon: Skier's knee: The cruciate connection. Phys. Sports Med. 12:50–54, 1984.

62. Wroble, R.R., and T.N. Lindenfeld: The stabilized Lachman test. Clin. Orthop. 237:209–212, 1988.

63. Feagin, J.A.: The Crucial Ligaments. Edinburgh, Churchill Livingstone, 1988.

64. Rebman, L.W.: Lachman's test: An alternative method. J. Orthop. Sports Phys. Ther. 9:381–382, 1988.

65. Cross, M.J., and K.J. Crichton: Clinical Examination of the Injured Knee. Baltimore, Williams & Wilkins, 1987.

66. Cross, M.J., D.R. Schmidt, and I.G. Mackie: A no-touch test for the anterior cruciate ligament. J. Bone Joint Surg. Br. 69:300, 1987.

67. Butler, D.L., F.R. Noyes, and E.S. Grood: Ligamentous restraints to anterior-posterior drawer in the human knee. J. Bone Joint Surg. Am. 62:259–270, 1980.

68. Weatherwax, R.J.: Anterior drawer sign. Clin. Orthop. 154:318–319, 1981.

69. Hughston, J.C.: The absent posterior drawer test in some acute posterior cruciate ligament tears of the knee. Am. J. Sports Med. 16:39–43, 1988.

70. Warren, R.F.: Physical diagnosis of the knee. In Post, M. (ed.): Physical Examination of the Musculoskeletal System. Chicago, Year Book Medical Publishers, 1987.

71. Daniel, D.M., M.L. Stone, P. Barnett, and R. Sachs: Use of the quadriceps active test to diagnose posterior cruciate ligament disruption and measure posterior laxity of the knee. J. Bone Joint Surg. Am. 70:386–391, 1988.

72. De Lee, J.C.: Ligamentous injury of the knee. In Stanitski, C.L., J.C. DeLee, and D. Drez (eds.): Pediatric and Adolescent Sports Medicine. Philadelphia, W.B. Saunders Co., 1994.

73. Slocum, D.B., and R.L. Larson: Rotary instability of the knee. J. Bone Joint Surg. Am. 50:211–225, 1968.

74. Slocum, D.B., S.L. James, R.L. Larson, and K.M. Singer: A clinical test for anterolateral rotary instability of the knee. Clin. Orthop. 118:63–69, 1976.

75. Fetto, J.F., and J.L. Marshall: Injury to the anterior cruciate ligament producing the pivot shift sign: An experimental study on cadaver specimens. J. Bone Joint Surg. Am. 61:710–714, 1979.

76. Galway, H.R., and D.L. MacIntosh: The lateral pivot shift: A symptom and sign of anterior cruciate ligament insufficiency. Clin. Orthop. 147:45–50, 1980.

77. Tamea, C.D., and C.E. Henning: Pathomechanics of the pivot shift maneuver. Am. J. Sports Med. 9:31–37, 1981.

78. Katz, J.W., and R.F. Fingeroth: The diagnostic accuracy of ruptures of the anterior cruciate ligament comparing the Lachman test, the anterior drawer sign and the pivot shift test in acute and chronic knee injuries. Am. J. Sports Med. 14:88–91, 1986.

79. Bach, B.R., R.F. Warren, and T.L. Wickiewitz: The pivot shift phenomenon: Results and description of a modified clinical test for anterior cruciate ligament insufficiency. Am. J. Sports Med. 16:571–576, 1988.

80. Peterson, L., M.I. Pitman, and J. Gold: The active pivot shift: The role of the popliteus muscle. Am. J. Sports Med. 12:313–317, 1984.

81. Losee, R.E., T.R.J. Ennis, and W.O. Southwick: Anterior subluxation of the lateral tibial plateau: A diagnostic test and operative review. J. Bone Joint Surg. Am. 60:1015–1030, 1978.

82. Hughston, J.C., W.M. Walsh, and G. Puddu: Patellar Subluxation and Dislocation. Philadelphia, W.B. Saunders Co., 1984.

83. Noyes, F.R., D.L. Butler, E.S. Grood, et al: Clinical paradoxes of anterior cruciate instability and a new test to detect its instability. Orthop. Trans. 2:36, 1978.

84. Hanks, G.A., D.M. Joyner, and A. Kalenak: Anterolateral instability of the knee. Am. J. Sports Med. 9:225–231, 1981.

85. Hughston, J.C., and L.A. Norwood: The posterolateral drawer test and external rotational recurvatum test for posterolateral rotary instability of the knee. Clin. Orthop. 147:82–87, 1980.

86. Owens, T.C.: Posteromedial pivot shift of the knee: A new test for rupture of the posterior cruciate ligament. J. Bone Joint Surg. Am. 76:532–539, 1994.

87. Jakob, R.P., H. Hassler, and H.U. Staeubli: Observations on rotary instability of the lateral compartment of the knee. Acta Orthop. Scand. (Suppl. 191) 52:1–32, 1981.

88. Swain, R.A., and F.D. Wilson: Diagnosing posterolateral rotary knee instability: Two clinical tests hold key. Phys. Sportsmed. 21:95–102, 1993.

89. Loomer, R.L.: A test for knee posterolateral rotary instability. Clin. Orthop. 264:235–238, 1991.

90. Shelbourne, K.D., F. Benedict, J.R. McCarroll, and A.C. Rettig: Dynamic posterior shift test: An adjuvant in evaluation of posterior tibial subluxation. Am. J. Sports Med. 17:275–277, 1989.

91. Shino, K., S. Horibe, and K. Ono: The voluntary evoked posterolateral drawer sign in the knee with posterolateral instability. Clin. Orthop. 215:179–186, 1987.

92. Daniel, D.M., and M.L. Stone: Instrumented measurement of knee motion. In Daniel, D., W. Akeson, and J. O'Conner (eds.): Knee Ligaments: Structure, Function, Injury and Repair. New York, Raven Press, 1990.

93. Harter, R.A., L.R. Osternig, and K.M. Singer: Instrumented Lachman tests for the evaluation of anterior laxity after reconstruction of the anterior cruciate ligament. J. Bone Joint Surg. Am. 71:975–983, 1989.

94. Daniel, D.M., L.L. Malcolm, G. Losse, M.L. Stone, R. Sachs, and R. Burks: Instrumented measurement of anterior laxity of the knee. J. Bone Joint Surg. Am. 67:720–726, 1985.

95. Edixhoven, P., R. Huiskes, R. De Graff, T.J. van Reno, and T.J. Slooff: Accuracy and reproducibility of instrumented knee drawer tests. J. Orthop. Res. 5:378–387, 1987.

96. Andersson, C., and J. Gillquist: Instrumented testing for evaluation of sagittal knee laxity. Clin. Orthop. 256:178–184, 1990.

97. Markolf, K.L., and H.C. Amstutz: The clinical relevance of instrumented testing for ACL insufficiency: Experience with the UCLA clinical knee testing apparatus. Clin. Orthop. 223:198–207, 1987.

98. Anderson, A.F., R.B. Snyder, C.F. Federspiel, and A.B. Lipscomb: Instrumented evaluation of knee laxity: A comparison of five arthrometers. Am. J. Sports Med. 20:135–140, 1992.

99. Daniel, D.M., and M.L. Stone: Diagnosis of knee ligament injury: Tests and measurements of joint laxity. In Feagin, J.A. (ed.): The Crucial Ligaments. Edinburgh, Churchill Livingstone, 1988.

100. Bach, B.R., and J.C. Johnson: Ligament testing devices. In Scott, W.N. (ed.): Ligament and Extensor Mechanism Injuries of the Knee: Diagnosis and Treatment. St. Louis, Mosby–Year Book Inc., 1991.

101. Daniel, D.M., and M.L. Stone: KT-1000 anterior-posterior displacement measurements. In Daniel, D., W. Akeson, and J. O'Conner (eds.): Knee Ligaments: Structure, Function, Injury and Repair. New York, Raven Press, 1990.

102. Stratford, P.W., D. Miseferi, R. Ogilvie, J. Binkley, and J. Wuori: Assessing the responsiveness of five KT 1000 knee arthrometer measures used to evaluate anterior laxity at the knee joint. Clin. J. Sport Med. 1:225–228, 1991.

103. Wroble, R.R., E.S. Grood, F.R. Noyes, and D.J. Schmitt: Reproducibility of genucom knee analysis system testing. Am. J. Sports Med. 18:387–395, 1990.

104. Wroble, R.R., L.A. Van Ginkel, E.S. Grood, F.R. Noyes, and B.L. Shaffer: Repeatability of the KT-1000 arthrometer in a normal population. Am. J. Sports Med. 18:396–399, 1990.

105. Highgenboten, C.L., A. Jackson, N.B. Meske: Genucom, KT-1000 and Stryker knee laxity measuring device comparisons: Device reproducibility and interdevice comparison in asymptomatic subjects. Am. J. Sports Med. 17:743–746, 1989.

106. McQuade, K.J., J.A. Sidles, and K.V. Larson: Reliability of the genucom knee analysis system. Clin. Orthop. 245:216–219, 1989.

107. Highgenboten, C.L., A.W. Jackson, K.A. Jansson, and N.B. Meske: KT-1000 arthrometer: Conscious and unconscious test results using 15, 20 and 30 pounds of force. Am. J. Sports Med. 20:450–454, 1992.

108. Kowalk, D.L., E.M. Wojtys, J. Disher, and P. Loubert: Quantitative analysis of the measuring capabilities of the KT-1000 knee ligament arthrometer. Am. J. Sports Med. 21:744–747, 1993.

109. Forster, I.W., C.D. Warren-Smith, and M. Tew: Is the KT-1000 knee ligament arthrometer reliable? J. Bone Joint Surg. Br. 71:843–847, 1989.

110. McMurray, T.P.: The semilunar cartilages. Br. J. Surg. 29:407–414, 1942.

111. Evans, P.J., G.D. Bell, and C. Frank: Prospective evaluation of the McMurray test. Am. J. Sports Med. 21:604–608, 1993.

112. Kim, S.J., B.H. Min, and D.Y. Han: Paradoxical phenomena of the McMurray test: An arthroscopic examination. Am. J. Sports Med. 24:83–87, 1996.

113. Apley, A.G.: The diagnosis of meniscus injuries: Some new clinical methods. J. Bone Joint Surg. Br. 29:78–84, 1947.

114. Oni, O.O.: The knee jerk test for diagnosis of torn meniscus. Clin. Orthop. 193:309, 1985.

115. Helfet, A.: Disorders of the Knee. Philadelphia, J.B. Lippincott Co., 1974.

116. Anderson, A.F., and A.B. Lipscomb: Clinical diagnosis of meniscal tears: Description of a new manipulative test. Am. J. Sports Med. 14:291–293, 1988.

117. Mital, M.A., and J. Hayden: Pain in the knee in children: The medial plica shelf syndrome. Orthop. Clin. North Am. 10:713–722, 1979.

118. Mann, G., A. Finsterbush, U. Frankel, and Y. Maton: A method of diagnosing small amounts of fluid in the knee. J. Bone Joint Surg. Br. 73:346–347, 1991.

119. Sibley, M.B., and F.H. Fu: Knee injuries. In Fu, F.H., and D.A. Stone (eds.): Sports Injuries: Mechanisms, Prevention, Treatment. Baltimore, Williams & Wilkins, 1994.

120. McConnell, J.: The management of chondromalacia patellae: A long term solution. Aust. J. Physiother. 32:215–223, 1986.

121. Kolowich, P.A., L.E. Paulos, T.D. Rosenberg, and S. Farnsworth: Lateral release of the patella: Indications and contraindications. Am. J. Sports Med. 18:359–365, 1990.

122. Olerud, C., and P. Berg: The variation of the Q angle with different positions of the foot. Clin. Orthop. 191:162–165, 1984.

123. Guerra, J.P., M.J. Arnold, and R.L. Gajdosik: Q-angle: Effects of isometric quadriceps contraction and body position. J. Orthop. Sports Phys. Ther. 19:200–204, 1994.

124. Arno, S.: The A-angle: A quantitative measurement of patella alignment and realignment. J. Orthop. Sports Phys. Ther. 12:237–242, 1990.

125. DiVeta, J.A., and W.D. Vogelbach: The clinical efficacy of the A-angle in measuring patellar alignment. J. Orthop. Sports Phys. Ther. 16:136–139, 1992.

126. Ehrat, M., J. Edwards, D. Hastings, and T. Worrell: Reliability of assessing patellar alignment: The A-angle. J. Orthop. Sports Phys. Ther. 19:22–27, 1994.

127. Daniel, D.M., M.L. Stone, P. Barnett, and R. Sachs: Use of the quadriceps active test to diagnose posterior cruciate ligament disruption and measure posterior laxity of the knee. J. Bone Joint Surg. Am. 70:386–391, 1988.

128. Fairbank, H.A.T.: Internal derangement of the knee in children and adolescents. Proc. Roy. Soc. Med. 30:427–432, 1937.

129. Noble, H.B., M.R. Hajek, and M. Porter: Diagnosis and treatment of iliotibial band tightness in runners. Phys. Sportsmed. 10:67–74, 1982.

130. Daniel, D.M., and M.L. Stone: Case studies. In Daniel, D., W. Akeson, and J. O'Conner (eds.): Knee Ligaments: Structure, Injury and Repair. New York, Raven Press, 1990.

131. Hyslop, G.H.: Injuries of the deep and superficial peroneal nerves complicating ankle sprain. Am. J. Surg. 51:436–438, 1941.

132. Sidey, J.D.: Weak ankles: A study of common peroneal entrapment neuropathy. Br. Med. J. 56:623–626, 1969.

133. Pecina, M.M., J. Krmpotic-Nemanic, and A.D. Markiewitz: Tunnel Syndromes. Boca Raton, Florida, CRC Press, 1991.

134. Worth, R.M., D.B. Kettlekamp, R.J. Defalque, and K.U. Duane: Saphenous nerve entrapment: A cause of medial nerve pain. Am. J. Sports Med. 12:80–81, 1984.

135. Cox, J.S., and J.B. Blanda: Periarticular pathologies. In DeLee, J.C., and D. Drez (eds.): Orthopedic Sports Medicine. Philadelphia, W.B. Saunders Co., 1994.

136. O'Shea, K.J., K.P. Murphy, D. Heekin, and P.J. Herzwurm: The diagnostic accuracy of history, physical examination and radiographs in the evaluation of traumatic knee disorders. Am. J. Sports Med. 24:164–167, 1996.

137. Gelb, H.J., S.G. Glasgow, A.A. Sapega, and J.S. Torg: Magnetic resonance imaging of knee disorders: Clinical value and cost-effectiveness in a sports medicine practice. Am. J. Sports Med. 24:99–103, 1996.

138. Carson, W.G. Jr., S.L. James, R.L. Larson, et al.: Patellofemoral disorders: Physical and radiographic evaluation: I: Physical examination. Clin. Orthop. 185:178–186, 1984.

139. Merchant, A.C.: Extensor mechanism injuries: Classification and diagnosis. In Scott, W.N. (ed.): Ligament and Extensor Mechanism Injuries of the Knee: Diagnosis and Treatment. St. Louis, Mosby–Year Book Inc., 1991.

140. Woods, G.W., R.F. Stanley, and H.S. Tullos: Lateral capsular sign: X-ray clue to a significant knee instability. Am. J. Sports Med. 7:27–33, 1979.

141. Altchek, D.W.: Diagnosing acute knee injuries: The office exam. Phys. Sportsmed. 21:85–96, 1993.

142. Schils, J.P., D. Resnick, and D.J. Sartoris: Diagnostic imaging of ligamentous injuries of the knee. In Daniel, D., W. Akeson, and J. O'Conner (eds.): Knee Ligaments: Structure, Injury and Repair. New York, Raven Press, 1990.

143. Beaconsfield, T., E. Pintore, N. Maffulli, and G.J. Petri: Radiographic measurements in patellofemoral disorders. Clin. Orthop. 308:18–28, 1994.

144. Grana, W.A.: Diagnostic evaluation. In Larson, R.L., and W.A. Grana (eds.): The Knee: Form, Function, Pathology and Treatment. Philadelphia, W.B. Saunders Co., 1993.

145. Grelsamer, R.P., and S. Meadows: The modified Insall-Salvati ratio for assessment of patellar height. Clin. Orthop. 282:170–176, 1992.

146. Haas, S.B., and G.R. Scuderi: Examination and radiographic assessment of the patellofemoral joint. Semin. Orthop. 5:108–114, 1990.

147. Grelsamer, R.P., C.S. Proctor, and A.N. Brazos: Evaluation of patellar shape in the sagittal plane: A clinical analysis. Am. J. Sports Med. 22:61–66, 1994.

148. Berg, E.E., S.L. Mason, and M.J. Zucas: Patellar height ratios: A comparison of four measurement methods. Am. J. Sports Med. 24:218–221, 1996.

149. Speakman, H.B., and J. Weisberg: The vastus medialis controversy. Physiotherapy 63:249–254, 1977.

150. Ghelman, B., and S. Schraft: Arthrography of the knee. In Scott, W.N. (ed.): Ligament and Extensor Mechanism Injuries of the Knee: Diagnosis and Treatment. St. Louis, Mosby–Year Book Inc., 1991.

151. Mital, M.A., and L.I. Karlin: Diagnostic arthroscopy in sports injuries. Orthop. Clin. North Am. 11:771–785, 1980.

152. McClelland, C.J.: Arthroscopy and arthroscopic surgery of the knee. Physiotherapy 70:154–156, 1984.

153. Noyes, F.R., R.W. Bassett, E.S. Grood, and D.L. Butler: Arthroscopy in acute traumatic hemarthrosis of the knee. J. Bone Joint Surg. Am. 62:687–695, 757, 1980.

154. Glashow, J.L., and M.J. Friedman: Diagnosis of knee ligament injuries: Magnetic resonance imaging. In Scott, W.N. (ed.): Ligament and Extensor Mechanism Injuries of the Knee: Diagnosis and Treatment. St. Louis, Mosby–Year Book Inc., 1991.

155. Arendt, E.A.: Assessment of the athlete with an acutely injured knee. In Griffin, L.Y. (ed.): Rehabilitation of the Injured Knee. St. Louis, C.V. Mosby Co., 1995.

156. Gelb, H.J., S.G. Glasgow, A.A. Sapega, and J.S. Torg: Magnetic resonance imaging of knee disorders: Clinical value and cost effectiveness in a sports medicine practice. Am. J. Sports Med. 24:99–103, 1996.

General References

Adams, J.C.: Outline of Orthopedics. London, E & S Livingstone, Ltd., 1968.

Ahstrom, J.P.: Reliability of history and physical examination in diagnosis of meniscus pathology. Curr. Pract. Orthop. Surg., vol. 7. St. Louis, C.V. Mosby Co., 1977.

Aichroth, P., M.A.R. Freeman, I.S. Smillie, and W.A. Souter: A knee function assessment chart. J. Bone Joint Surg. Br. 60:308–309, 1978.

Ando, T., H. Hirose, M. Inoue, K. Shino, and T. Doi: A new method using computed tomographic scan to measure the rectus femoris–patellar tendon Q-angle comparison with conventional method. Clin. Orthop. 289:213–219, 1993.

Andriacchi, T.P., and D. Birac: Functional testing in the anterior cruciate ligament-deficient knee. Clin. Orthop. 288:40–47, 1993.

Aprin, H., J. Shapiro, and M. Gershwind: Arthrography (plica views): A noninvasive method for diagnosis and prognosis of plica syndrome. Clin. Orthop. 183:90–95, 1984.

Arnold, J.A., T.P. Coker, L.M. Heaton, et al.: Natural history of anterior cruciate tears. Am. J. Sports Med. 7:305–313, 1979.

Back, B.R., and R.F. Warren: Radiographic indicators of the anterior cruciate ligament injury. In Feagin, J.A. (ed.): The Crucial Ligaments. Edinburgh, Churchill Livingstone, 1988.

Bassett, L.W., and R.H. Gold: Magnetic resonance imaging of the musculoskeletal system: An overview. Clin. Orthop. 244:17–28, 1989.

Bassett, L.W., R.H. Gold, and L.L. Seeger: MRI Atlas of the Musculoskeletal System. London, Martin Dunitz, 1989.

Beetham, W.P., H.P. Polley, C.H. Slocumb, and W.F. Weaver: Physical Extremities of the Joint. Philadelphia, W.B. Saunders Co., 1965.

Bigg-Wither, G., and P. Kelly: Diagnostic imaging in musculoskeletal physiotherapy. In Refshauge, K., and E. Gass (eds.): Musculoskeletal Physiotherapy: Clinical Science and Practice. Oxford, Butterworth-Heinemann Ltd., 1995.

Booker, J.M., and G.A. Thibodeau: Athletic Injury Assessment. St. Louis, C.V. Mosby Co., 1989.

Brantigan, O.C., and A.F. Voshell: The mechanics of the ligaments and menisci of the knee joint. J. Bone Joint Surg. 23:44–66, 1941.

Bryant, J.T., and T.D. Cooke: A biomechanical function of the ACL: Prevention of medial translation of the tibia. In Feagin, J.A. (ed.): The Crucial Ligaments. Edinburgh, Churchill Livingstone, 1988.

Burk, D.L., M.K. Dalinka, E. Kinal, et al.: Meniscal and ganglion cysts of the knee: MR evaluation. Am. J. Roentgenol. 150:331–336, 1988.

Cabaud, H.E., and D.B. Slocum: The diagnosis of chronic anterolateral rotary instability of the knee. Am. J. Sports Med. 5:99–104, 1977.

Cailliet, R.: Knee Pain and Disability. Philadelphia, F.A. Davis Co., 1973.

Clancy, W.G.: Evaluation of acute knee injuries. American Association of Orthopaedic Surgeons, Symposium on Sports Medicine: The Knee. St. Louis, C.V. Mosby Co., 1985.

Clarkson, H.M., and G.B. Gilewich: Musculoskeletal Assessment: Joint Range of Motion and Manual Muscle Strength. Baltimore, Williams & Wilkins, 1989.

Collins, H.R.: Anterolateral rotary instability. American Association of Orthopaedic Surgeons, Symposium on the Athlete's Knee. St. Louis, C.V. Mosby Co., 1980.

Conlan, T., W.P. Garth, and J.E. Lemons: Evaluation of the medial soft tissue restraints of the extensor mechanism of the knee. J. Bone Joint Surg. Am. 75:682–693, 1993.

Cooper, D.E.: Tests for posterolateral instability of the knee in normal subjects: Results of examination under anaesthesia. J. Bone Joint Surg. Am. 73:30–36, 1991.

Crues, J.V., R. Ryu, and F.W. Morgan: Meniscal pathology: The expanding role of magnetic resonance imaging. Clin. Orthop. 252:80–87, 1990.

Cyriax, J.: Textbook of Orthopaedic Medicine, vol. 1: Diagnosis of Soft Tissue Lesions. London, Bailliere Tindall, 1975.

Danzig, L.A., J.D. Newell, J. Guerra, and D. Resnick: Osseous landmarks of the normal knee. Clin. Orthop. 156:201–206, 1981.

Davies, G.J.: Examining the knee. Phys. Sportsmed. 6:48–67, 1978.

De Haven, K.E., and H.R. Collins: Diagnosis of internal derangement of the knee: The role of arthroscopy. J. Bone Joint Surg. Am. 57:802–810, 1975.

Deutsch, A.L., F.G. Shellock, and J.H. Mink: Imaging of the patellofemoral joint: Emphasis on advanced techniques. In Fu, F.H., and D.A. Stone (eds.): Sports Injuries: Mechanisms, Prevention, Treatment. Baltimore, Williams & Wilkins, 1994.

Donaldson, W.F., R.F. Warren, and T. Wickiewicz: A comparison of acute anterior cruciate ligament examinations: Initial vs examination under anesthesia. Am. J. Sports Med. 13:5–9, 1985.

Dontigny, R.L.: Terminal extension exercises for the knee. Phys. Ther. 52:45–46, 1972.

Doppman, J.L.: Baker's cyst and the normal gastrocnemiosemimembranosus bursa. Am. J. Roentgenol. 94:646–652, 1965.

Dowd, G.S., and G. Bentley: Radiographic assessment of patellar instability and chondromalacia patellae. J. Bone Joint Surg. Br. 68:297–300, 1986.

Ehrlich, M.G., and R.E. Strain: Epiphyseal injuries about the knee. Orthop. Clin. North Am. 10:91–103, 1979.

Ellison, A.E.: The pathogenesis and treatment of anterolateral rotary instability. Clin. Orthop. 147:51–55, 1980.

Engle, R.P.: Examination of the knee. In Engle, R.P. (ed.): Knee Ligament Rehabilitation. New York, Churchill Livingstone, 1991.

Evans, R.C.: Illustrated Essentials in Orthopedic Physical Assessment. St. Louis, C.V. Mosby Co., 1994.

Ewald, F.C.: The knee society total knee arthroplasty roentgenographic evaluation and scoring system. Clin. Orthop. 248:9–12, 1989.

Feagin, J.A.: Introduction: principles of diagnosis and treatment. In Feagin, J.A. (ed.): The Crucial Ligaments. Edinburgh, Churchill Livingstone, 1988.

Feagin, J.A., H.E. Cabaud, and W.W. Curl: The anterior cruciate ligament: Radiographic and clinical signs of successful and unsuccessful repairs. Clin. Orthop. 164:54–58, 1982.

Fetto, J.F., and J.L. Marshall: The natural history and diagnosis of anterior cruciate ligament insufficiency. Clin. Orthop. 147:29–38, 1980.

Fleming, B.C., B.D. Beynnon, and R.J. Johnson: The use of knee laxity testers for the determination of anterior-posterior stability of the knee: Pitfalls in practice. In Jackson, D.W. (ed.): The Anterior Cruciate Ligament: Current and Future Concepts. New York, Raven Press, 1993.

Fowler, P.J.: The classification and early diagnosis of knee joint instability. Clin. Orthop. 147:15–21, 1980.

Francis, R.S., and D.E. Scott: Hypertrophy of the vastus medialis in knee extension. Phys. Ther. 54:1066–1070, 1974.

Frankel, V.H., A.H. Burstein, and D.B. Brooks: Biomechanics of internal derangement of the knee. J. Bone Joint Surg. Am. 53:945–962, 1971.

Franklin, J.L., T.D. Rosenberg, L.E. Paulos, and E.P. France: Radiographic assessment of instability of the knee due to rupture of the anterior cruciate ligament: A quadriceps contraction technique. J. Bone Joint Surg. Am. 73:365–372, 1991.

Fu, F.H., M.J. Seel, and R.A. Berger: Patellofemoral biomechanics. In Fox, J.M., and W. Del Pizzo (eds.): The Patellofemoral Joint. New York, McGraw-Hill Inc., 1993.

Fulkerson, J.P.: Evaluation of the peripatellar soft tissues and retinaculum in patients with patellofemoral pain. Clin. Sports Med. 8:197–202, 1989.

Fulkerson, J.P.: Awareness of the retinaculum in evaluating patellofemoral pain. Am. J. Sports Med. 10:147–149, 1982.

Fulkerson, J.P.: Patellofemoral pain disorders: Evaluation and management. J. Am. Acad. Orthop. Surg. 2:124–132, 1994.

Gartland, J.J.: Fundamentals of Orthopedics. Philadelphia, W.B. Saunders Co., 1979.

Gersoff, W.K., and W.G. Clancy: Diagnosis of acute and chronic anterior cruciate ligament tears. Clin. Sports Med. 7:727–738, 1988.

Gillquist, J.: Diagnosis and classification of the instability of the knee joint. Sem. Orthop. 2:18–22, 1987.

Ginsburg, J.H., and J.C. Ellsasser: Problem areas in the diagnosis and treatment of ligament injuries of the knee. Clin. Orthop. 132:201–205, 1978.

Goodfellow, J., D.S. Hungerford, and C. Woods: Patellofemoral joint mechanics and pathology: Chondromalacia patellae. J. Bone Joint Surg. Br. 58:291–299, 1976.

Gough, J.V., and G. Ladley: An investigation into the effectiveness of various forms of quadriceps exercises. Physiotherapy 57:356–361, 1971.

Greenmill, B.J.: The importance of the medial quadriceps expansion in medial ligament injury. Can. J. Surg. 10:312–317, 1967.

Grood, E.S., S.F. Stowers, and F.R. Noyes: Limits of movement in the human knee: Effect of sectioning the posterior cruciate ligament and posterolateral structures. J. Bone Joint Surg. Am. 70:88–97, 1988.

Gurtler, R.A., R. Stine, and J.S. Torg: Lachman test evaluated: Quantification of a clinical observation. Clin. Orthop. 216:141–150, 1987.

Guzzanti, V., A. Gigante, A. DiLazzaro, and C. Fabbriciani: Patellofemoral malalignment in adolescents: Computerized tomographic assessment with and without quadriceps contraction. Am. J. Sports Med. 22:55–60, 1994.

Hardaker, W.G., T.L. Shipple, and F.H. Bassett: Diagnosis and treatment of the plica syndrome of the knee. J. Bone Joint Surg. Am. 62:221–225, 1980.

Hilyard, A.: Recent developments in the management of patellofemoral pain: The McConnell programme. Physiotherapy 76:559–565, 1990.

Hollinshead, W.H., and D.B. Jenkins: Functional Anatomy of the Limbs and Back. Philadelphia, W.B. Saunders Co., 1981.

Hoppenfeld, S.: Physical Examination of the Spine and Extremities. New York, Appleton-Century-Crofts, 1976.

Hoppenfeld, S.: Physical examination of the knee joint by complaint. Orthop. Clin. North Am. 10:3–20, 1979.

Hughston, J.C., J.R. Andrews, M.J. Cross, and A. Moschi: Classification of knee ligament instabilities: Part I. The medial compartment and cruciate ligaments. J. Bone Joint Surg. Am. 58:159–172, 1976.

Hughston, J.C., J.A. Bowden, J.R. Andrews, and L.A. Norwood: Acute tears of the posterior cruciate ligament. J. Bone Joint Surg. Am. 62:438–450, 1980.

Insall, J., K.A. Falvo, and D.W. Wise: Chondromalacia patellae: A prospective study. J. Bone Joint Surg. Am. 58:1–8, 1976.

Jackson, J.P.: Internal derangement of the knee joint. Physiotherapy 52:229–232, 1966.

Jakob, R.P.: Pathomechanical and clinical components of the pivot shift sign. Sem. Orthop. 2:9–17, 1987.

Jakob, R.P., H.U. Staubli, and J.T. Deland: Grading the pivot shift: Objective tests with implications for treatment. J. Bone Joint Surg. Br. 69:294–299, 1987.

Jensen, K.: Manual laxity tests for anterior cruciate ligament injuries. J. Orthop. Sports Phys. Ther. 11:474–481, 1990.

Kapandji, L.A.: The Physiology of the Joints, vol. 2: Lower Limb. New York, Churchill Livingstone, 1970.

Kennedy, J.C., R. Stewart, and D.M. Walker: Anterolateral rotary instability of the knee joint: An early analysis of the Ellison repair. J. Bone Joint Surg. Am. 60:1031–1032, 1978.

Kramer, J.F., D. Nusca, P. Fowler, and S. Webster-Bogaert: Test-retest reliability of the one-leg hop test following ACL reconstruction. Clin. J. Sport Med. 2:240–243, 1992.

Kursunoglu-Brahme, S., and D. Resnick: Magnetic resonance imaging of the knee. Orthop. Clin. North Am. 21:561–572, 1990.

Larson, R.L.: Clinical evaluation. In Larson, R.L., and W.A. Grana (eds.): The Knee: Form, Function, Pathology and Treatment. Philadelphia, W.B. Saunders Co., 1993.

Leib, F.J., and J. Perry: Quadriceps function. J. Bone Joint Surg. Am. 50:1535–1548, 1968.

Liu, S.H., L. Osti, F. Dorey, and L. Yao: Anterior cruciate ligament tear: A new diagnostic index on magnetic resonance imaging. Clin. Orthop. Relat. Res. 302:147–150, 1994.

Logan, A.L.: The Knee: Clinical Applications. Gaithersburg, Maryland, Aspen Publishers, 1994.

Losee, R.E.: The pivot shift. In Feagin, J.A. (ed.): The Crucial Ligaments. Edinburgh, Churchill Livingstone, 1988.

Losee, R.E.: Concepts of the pivot shift. Clin. Orthop. 172:45–51, 1983.

Lucie, R.S., J.D. Wiedel, and D.G. Messner: The acute pivot shift: Clinical correlation. Am. J. Sports Med. 12:189–191, 1984.

Macnicol, M.F.: The Problem Knee: Diagnosis and Management in the Younger Patient. London, Wm. Heinemann Med. Books, 1986.

Malek, M.M., and R.E. Manjini: Patellofemoral pain syndrome: A comprehensive and conservative approach. J. Orthop. Sports Phys. Ther. 2:108–116, 1981.

Malone, T., and S.T. Kegerreis: Evaluation process. In Mangine, R.E. (ed.): Physical Therapy of the Knee. Edinburgh, Churchill Livingstone, 1988.

Mandelbaum, B.R., G.A. Finerman, M.A. Reicher, et al.: Magnetic resonance imaging as a tool for evaluation of traumatic knee injuries. Am. J. Sports Med. 14:361–370, 1986.

Mayor, D.: Anatomical and functional aspects of the knee joint. Physiotherapy 52:224–228, 1966.

McRae, R.: Clinical Orthopaedic Examination. New York, Churchill Livingstone, 1976.

Meislin, R.J.: Managing collateral ligament tears of the knee. Phys. Sportsmed. 24:67–80, 1996.

Merchant, A.C.: The lateral patellar compression syndrome. In Fu, F.H., and D.A. Stone (eds.): Sports Injuries: Mechanisms, Prevention, Treatment. Baltimore, Williams & Wilkins, 1994.

Moller, B.N., and S. Kadin: Entrapment of the common peroneal nerve. Am. J. Sports Med. 15:90–91, 1987.

Moran, D.J., and R.T. Floyd: The Lachman test: Alternative techniques and applications for anterior cruciate ligament evaluation. Sports Med. Update 5:3–5, 1990.

Muller, W., R. Biedert, F. Hefti, R.P. Jakob, U. Munzinger, and H.U. Staubli: OAK knee evaluation: A new way to assess knee ligament injuries. Clin. Orthop. 232:37–50, 1988.

Myer, J.W., S.S. Schulthies, and C.W. Fellingham: Relative and absolute reliability of the KT-1000 arthrometer for injured knees. Am. J. Sports Med. 24:104–108, 1992.

Norwood, L.A., and M.J. Cross: Anterior cruciate ligament: Functional anatomy of its bundles in rotary instabilities. Am. J. Sports Med. 7:23–26, 1979.

Norwood, L.A., and J.C. Hughston: Combined anterolateral-anteromedial rotary instability of the knee. Clin. Orthop. 147:62–67, 1980.

Noyes, F.R., and E.S. Grood: Diagnosis of knee ligament injuries: Clinical concepts. In Feagin, J.A. (ed.): The Crucial Ligaments. Edinburgh, Churchill Livingstone, 1988.

Noyes, F.R., E.S. Grood, and D.L. Butler: Clinical laxity tests and functional stability of the knee: Biomechanical concepts. Clin. Orthop. 146:84–89, 1980.

Nunn, K.D., and J.L. Mayhew: Comparison of three methods of assessing strength imbalances at the knee. J. Orthop. Sports Phys. Ther. 10:134–137, 1988.

Oberlander, M.A., R.M. Shalvoy, and J.C. Hughston: The accuracy of the clinical knee examination documented by arthroscopy: A prospective study. Am. J. Sports Med. 21:773–778, 1993.

O'Donoghue, D.H.: Treatment of Injuries to Athletes, 4th ed. Philadelphia, W.B. Saunders Co., 1984.

Ogata, K., J.A. McCarthy, J. Dunlap, and P.R. Manske: Pathomechanisms of posterior sag of the tibia in posterior cruciate deficient knees. Am. J. Sports Med. 16:630–636, 1988.

Ombregt, L., P. Bisschop, H.J. ter Veer, and T. Van de Velde: A System of Orthopedic Medicine. London, W.B. Saunders Co., 1995.

Palmer, M.L., and M. Epler: Clinical Assessment Procedures in Physical Therapy. Philadelphia, J.B. Lippincott Co., 1990.

Patel, D.: Superior lateral-medial approach to arthroscopic meniscectomy. Orthop. Clin. North Am. 13:299–305, 1982.

Percy, E.C., and R.T. Strother: Patellalgia. Phys. Sports Med. 13:43–59, 1985.

Perry, J.: Function of quadriceps. J. Can. Physiother. Assoc. 24:130–132, 1972.

Pickett, J.C., and E.L. Radin: Chondromalacia of the Patella. Baltimore, Williams & Wilkins, 1983.

Pipkin, G.: Knee injuries: The role of the suprapatellar plica and suprapatellar bursa in simulating internal derangements. Clin. Orthop. 74:161–176, 1971.

Pynsent, P., J. Fairbank, and A. Carr: Outcome Measures in Orthopedics. Oxford, Butterworth-Heinemann Ltd., 1993.

Reid, D.C.: Functional Anatomy and Joint Mobilization. Edmonton, University of Alberta Bookstore, 1980.

Reid, D.C.: Sports Injury Assessment and Rehabilitation. New York, Churchill Livingstone, 1992.

Reid, D.C.: The myth, mystic and frustration of anterior knee pain. Clin. J. Sport Med. 3:139–143, 1993.

Reider, B., and S.D. D'Agata: Factors predisposing to knee injury. In DeLee, J.C., and D. Drez (eds.): Orthopedic Sports Medicine. Philadelphia, W.B. Saunders Co., 1994.

Reider, B., J.L. Marshall, B. Koslin, B. Ring, and F.G. Girgis: The anterior aspect of the knee joint. J. Bone Joint Surg. Am. 63:351–356, 1981.

Reilly, B.M.: Practical Strategies in Outpatient Medicine. Philadelphia, W.B. Saunders Co., 1984.

Renstrom, P., and R.J. Johnson: Anatomy and biomechanics of the menisci. Clin. Sports Med. 9:523–538, 1990.

Rovere, G.D., and D.M. Adair: Anterior cruciate-deficient knees: A review of the literature. Am. J. Sports Med. 11:412–419, 1983.

Rubinstein, R.A., D. Shelbourne, J.R. McCarroll, C.D. Van Meter, and A.C. Rettig: The accuracy of the clinical examination in the setting of posterior cruciate ligament injuries. Am. J. Sports Med. 22:550–557, 1994.

Rusche, K., and R.E. Mangine: Pathomechanics of injury to the patellofemoral and tibiofemoral joint. In Mangine, R.E. (ed.): Physical Therapy of the Knee. Edinburgh, Churchill Livingstone, 1988.

Smillie, I.S.: Diseases of the knee joint. Physiotherapy 70:144–150, 1984.

Stanitski, C.L.: Patellofemoral mechanism. In Stanitski, C.L., J.C. DeLee, and D. Drez (eds.): Pediatric and Adolescent Sports Medicine. Philadelphia, W.B. Saunders Co., 1994.

Starkey, C., and J. Ryan: Evaluation of Orthopedic and Athletic Injuries. Philadelphia, F.A. Davis Co., 1996.

Tachdjian, M.O.: Pediatric Orthopedics. Philadelphia, W.B. Saunders Co., 1972.

Tegner, Y., and J. Lysholm: Rating systems in the evaluation of knee ligament injuries. Clin. Orthop. 198:43–49, 1985.

Teitge, R.A., W. Faerber, P. Des Madryl, and T.M. Matelic: Stress radiographs of the patellofemoral joint. J. Bone Joint Surg. Am. 78:193–203, 1996.

Travell, J.G., and D.G. Simons: Myofascial Pain and Dysfunction: The Trigger Point Manual. Baltimore, Williams & Wilkins, 1983.

Tria, A.J., and R.C. Palumbo: Conservative treatment of patellofemoral pain. Semin. Orthop. 5:115–121, 1990.

Trickey, E.L.: Injuries to the posterior cruciate ligament: Diagnosis and treatment of early injuries and reconstruction of late instability. Clin. Orthop. 147:76–81, 1980.

Turner, J.S., and I.S. Smillie: The effect of tibial torsion on the pathology of the knee. J. Bone Joint Surg. Br. 63:396–398, 1981.

Wallace, L.A., R.E. Mangine, and T.R. Malone: The knee. In Gould, J.A. (ed.): Orthopedic and Sports Physical Therapy. St. Louis, C.V. Mosby Co., 1990.

Walsh, W.M.: Patellofemoral joint. In DeLee, J.C., and D. Drez (eds.): Orthopedic Sports Medicine. Philadelphia, W.B. Saunders Co., 1994.

Warren, L.F., J. Marshall, and F. Girgis: The prime static stabilizer of the medial side of the knee. J. Bone Joint Surg. Am. 56:665–674, 1974.

Warren, L.F., and J. Marshall: The supporting structures and layers on the medial side of the knee. J. Bone Joint Surg. Am. 61:56–62, 1979.

Wechsler, L.R., and N.A. Busis: Sports neurology. In Fu, F.H., and D.A. Stone (eds.): Sports Injuries: Mechanisms, Prevention, Treatment. Baltimore, Williams & Wilkins, 1994.

Weiss, J.R., J.J. Irrgang, R. Sawhney, S. Dearwater, and F.H. Fu: A functional assessment of anterior cruciate ligament deficiency in an acute and clinical setting. J. Orthop. Sports Phys. Ther. 11:372–373, 1990.

Weissman, B.N.W., and C.B. Sledge: Orthopedic Radiology. Philadelphia, W.B. Saunders Co., 1986.

Welsh, R.P.: Knee joint structure and function. Clin. Orthop. 147:7–14, 1980.

Wiles, P., and R. Sweetnam: Essentials of Orthopedics. London, J & A Churchill, Ltd., 1965.

Wojtys, E.M. (ed.): The ACL Deficient Knee. Rosemont, Illinois, American Academy of Orthopedic Surgeons, 1994.

Lower Leg, Ankle, and Foot

13

At least 80% of the general population has foot problems, but these problems can often be corrected by proper assessment, treatment, and, above all, care of the feet. Lesions of the ankle and foot can alter the mechanics of gait and, as a result, cause stress on other lower limb joints, which in turn may lead to pathology in these joints.

The foot and ankle combine flexibility with stability because of the many bones, their shapes, and their attachments. The lower leg, ankle, and foot have two principal functions: propulsion and support. For propulsion, they act like a flexible lever; for support, they act like a rigid structure that holds up the entire body.

Functions of the Foot

- Acts as a support base that provides the necessary stability for upright posture with minimal muscle effort
- Provides a mechanism for rotation of the tibia and fibula during the stance phase of gait
- Provides flexibility to adapt to uneven terrain
- Provides flexibility for absorption of shock
- Acts as a lever during push-off

Although the joints of the lower leg, ankle, and foot are discussed separately, they act as functional groups, not as isolated joints. As the terminal part of the lower kinetic chain, the lower leg, ankle, and foot have the ability to distribute and dissipate the different forces (e.g., compressive, shearing, rotary, tensile) acting on the body through contact with the ground.[1] This is especially evident during gait. In the foot, the movement occurring at each individual joint is minimal. However, when combined, there normally is sufficient range of motion in all of the joints to allow functional mobility as well as

functional stability. For ease of understanding, the joints of the foot are divided into three sections—hindfoot (rearfoot), midfoot, and forefoot.

Applied Anatomy

Hindfoot (Rearfoot)

Tibiofibular Joint. The inferior (distal) tibiofibular joint is a fibrous or syndesmosis type of joint. It is supported by the anterior tibiofibular, posterior tibiofibular, and inferior transverse ligaments as well as the interosseous ligaments (Fig. 13–1). The movements at this joint are minimal but allow a small amount of "spread" (1 to 2 mm) at the ankle joint during dorsiflexion. This same action allows the fibula to move up and down during dorsiflexion and plantar flexion. Dorsiflexion at the ankle joint will cause the fibula to move superiorly, putting stress on both the inferior tibiofibular joint at the ankle and the superior tibiofibular joint at the knee. The joint is supplied by the deep peroneal and tibial nerves.

Talocrural (Ankle) Joint. The talocrural joint is a uniaxial, modified hinge, synovial joint located between the **talus**, the **medial malleolus** of the tibia, and the **lateral malleolus** of the fibula. The talus is shaped so that in dorsiflexion it is wedged between the malleoli, allowing little or no inversion or eversion at the ankle joint. The talus is approximately 2.4 mm (1 inch) wider anteriorly than posteriorly. The medial malleolus is shorter, extending halfway down the talus, whereas the lateral malleolus extends almost to the level of the subtalar joint.

The talocrural joint is designed for stability, especially in dorsiflexion. In plantar flexion, it is much more mobile. This joint is responsible for the anterior-poste-

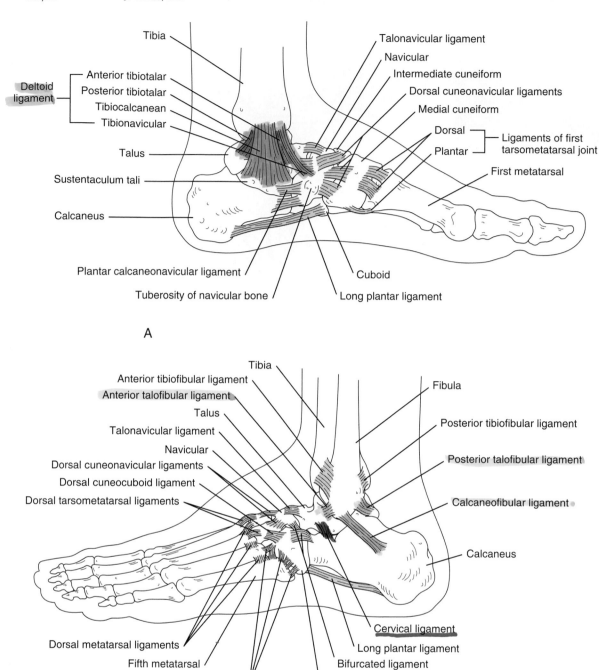

Figure 13-1
Ligaments of the hindfoot and midfoot. (A) Medial view. (B) Lateral view.

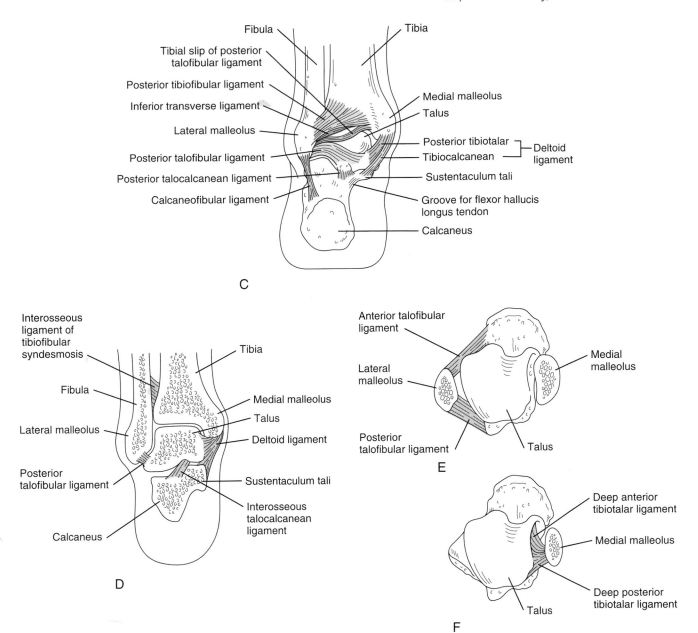

Figure 13-1 *Continued*
(C) Posterior view. (D) Coronal section through the left talocrural and talocalcanean joints.
(E) Superior view of ligaments on the lateral aspect. (F) Superior view of deep deltoid
ligament on the medial aspect.

rior (dorsiflexion–plantar flexion) movement that occurs in the ankle-foot complex. Its close packed position is maximum dorsiflexion, and its capsular pattern is more limitation of plantar flexion than of dorsiflexion. This joint is most stable in the dorsiflexed position. The resting position is 10° of plantar flexion, midway between maximum inversion and maximum eversion. The talocrural joint has one degree of freedom, and the movements possible at this joint are dorsiflexion and plantar flexion.

Joints of the Hindfoot

Tibiofibular joint	Resting position:	Plantar flexion
	Close packed position:	Maximum dorsiflexion
	Capsular pattern:	Pain on stress
Talocrural (ankle) joint	Resting position:	10° plantar flexion, midway between inversion and eversion
	Close packed position:	Maximum dorsiflexion
	Capsular pattern:	Plantar flexion, dorsiflexion
Subtalar joint	Resting position:	Midway between extremes of range of motion
	Close packed position:	Supination
	Capsular pattern:	Varus, valgus

On the medial side of the joint, the major ligament is the **deltoid** or **medial collateral ligament**, which consists of four separate ligaments: the tibionavicular, tibiocalcanean, and posterior tibiotalar ligaments superficially, all of which resist talar abduction, and the anterior tibiotalar ligament, which lies deep to the other three ligaments and resists lateral translation and lateral rotation of the talus.

On the lateral aspect, the talocrural joint is supported by the anterior talofibular ligament, which provides stability against excessive inversion of the talus; the posterior talofibular ligament, which resists ankle dorsiflexion, adduction ("tilt"), medial rotation, and medial translation of the talus; and the calcaneofibular ligament, which provides stability against maximum inversion at the ankle and subtalar joints. The anterior talofibular ligament is the ligament most commonly injured by a lateral ankle sprain, followed by the calcaneofibular ligament.

Subtalar (Talocalcanean) Joint. The subtalar joint is a

synovial joint having three degrees of freedom and a close packed position of supination. Supporting the subtalar joint are the lateral talocalcanean and medial talocalcanean ligaments. In addition, the interosseous talocalcanean and cervical ligaments limit eversion.

The movements possible at the subtalar joint are gliding and rotation. With injury to the area (e.g., sprain, fracture), this joint and the talocrural joint often become hypomobile, partially because the talus has no muscles attaching to it. Medial rotation of the leg causes a valgus (outward) movement of the calcaneus, whereas lateral rotation of the leg produces a varus (inward) movement of the calcaneus. The axis of the joint is at an angle of 40 to 45° inclined vertically and 15 to 18° to the sagittal plane.

Midfoot (Midtarsal Joints)

In isolation, the midtarsal joints allow only a minimal amount of movement. Taken together, however, they allow significant movement to enable the foot to adapt to many different positions without putting undue stress on the joints. **Chopart's joint** refers collectively to the midtarsal joints between the talus-calcaneus and the navicular-cuboid.

Talocalcaneonavicular Joint. The talocalcaneonavicular joint is a ball-and-socket synovial joint with three degrees of freedom. Its close packed position is supination, and the dorsal talonavicular ligament, bifurcated ligament, and plantar calcaneonavicular (spring) ligament support the joint (see Fig. 13–1; Fig. 13–2). Movements possible at this joint are gliding and rotation.

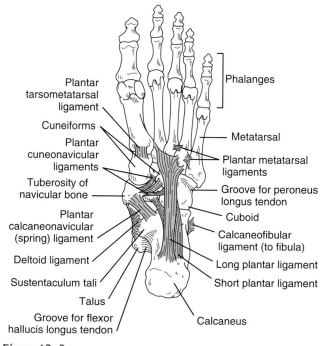

Figure 13–2

Ligaments on plantar aspect of foot.

Cuneonavicular Joint. The cuneonavicular joint is a plane synovial joint with a close packed position of supination. The movements possible at this joint are slight gliding and rotation.

Joints of the Midfoot (Midtarsal Joints)

Resting position:	Midway between extremes of range of motion
Close packed position:	Supination
Capsular pattern:	Dorsiflexion, plantar flexion, adduction, medial rotation

Cuboideonavicular Joint. The cuboideonavicular joint is fibrous, its close packed position being supination. The movements possible at this joint are slight gliding and rotation.

Intercuneiform Joints. The intercuneiform joints are plane synovial joints with a close packed position of supination. The movements possible at these joints are slight gliding and rotation.

Cuneocuboid Joint. The cuneocuboid joint is a plane synovial joint with a close packed position of supination. The movements of slight gliding and rotation are possible at this joint.

Calcaneocuboid Joint. The calcaneocuboid joint is saddle shaped with a close packed position of supination. Supporting this joint are the bifurcated ligament, the calcaneocuboid ligament, and the long plantar ligaments. The movement possible at this joint is gliding with conjunct rotation.

Forefoot

Tarsometatarsal Joints. The tarsometatarsal joints are plane synovial joints with a close packed position of supination. The movement possible at these joints is gliding. Taken together, these joints are referred to as Lisfranc's joint.[2]

Intermetatarsal Joints. The four intermetatarsal joints are plane synovial joints with a close packed position of supination. The movement possible at these joints is gliding.

Metatarsophalangeal Joints. The five metatarsophalangeal joints are condyloid synovial joints with two degrees of freedom. Their close packed position is full extension. Their capsular pattern is variable for the lateral four joints and more limitation of extension than flexion for the hallux (big toe); their resting position is 10° of extension. The movements possible at these joints are flexion, extension, abduction, and adduction.

Interphalangeal Joints. The interphalangeal joints are synovial hinge joints with one degree of freedom. The

Joints of the Forefoot

Tarsometa-tarsal joints	*Resting position:*	Midway between extremes of range of motion
	Close packed position:	Supination
	Capsular pattern:	None
Metatarso-phalangeal joints	*Resting position:*	Midway between extremes of range of motion (10° extension)
	Close packed position:	Full extension
	Capsular pattern:	Big toe: extension, flexion 2nd–5th toe: variable
Interpha-langeal joints	*Resting position:*	Slight flexion
	Close packed position:	Full extension
	Capsular pattern:	Flexion, extension

close packed position is full extension, and the capsular pattern is more limitation of flexion than of extension. The resting position of the distal and proximal interphalangeal joints is slight flexion. The movements possible at these joints are flexion and extension.

Patient History

It is important to take a detailed and complete history when assessing the lower leg, ankle, and foot. In addition to the questions listed under Patient History in Chapter 1, the examiner should obtain the following information from the patient:

1. What is the patient's occupation? Whether the patient stands a great deal and the types of surfaces on which the patient usually stands may have bearing on what is causing the problem.

2. What was the mechanism of injury? What was the position of the foot at the time of the injury? Ankle sprains occur most often when the foot is plantar flexed, inverted, and adducted, with injury to the anterior talofibular ligament.[3] This same mechanism can lead to a malleolar or talar dome fracture. Achilles tendinitis often arises as the result of overuse, increased activity, or change in a high-stress training program. A dorsiflexion injury, accompanied by a snapping and pain on the lateral aspect that rapidly diminishes, may indicate a tear

Table 13–1
Causes of Overuse Injuries to the Lower Limb

Prolonged training season

Impact force of activity

Training or competing on hard surfaces

Change of training surface

Downhill running

Lack of flexibility

Individual muscle weakness or poor reciprocal muscle
   strength

Overstriding

Poor posture

High mileage or sudden change in mileage

Too much, too soon

Overtraining

Anatomic factors (e.g., malalignment)

Wrong type of footwear

Road and/or sidewalk camber

From Taunton, J., C. Smith, and D.J. Magee: Leg, foot and ankle
injuries. In Zachazewski, J.E., D.J. Magee, and W.S. Quillen: Athletic
Injuries and Rehabilitation. Philadelphia, W.B. Saunders Co., 1996,
p. 730.

of the peroneal retinaculum.[4] Table 13–1 gives some
causes of overuse injuries in the lower limb.[5]

3. Did the patient notice a transient or fixed deformity of the foot or ankle at the time of injury? Was there
any transitory locking (e.g., loose body, muscle spasm)?
An affirmative answer may indicate a fracture causing
immediate swelling that decreased as it spread into the
surrounding tissue.

4. Was the patient able to continue the activity
after the injury? If so, the injury is probably not too
severe, provided there is no loss of stability. Inability to
bear weight, severe pain, and rapid swelling indicate a
severe injury.[4] Walking is compatible with a second-
degree sprain; pain with running usually indicates a first-
degree injury.[6]

5. Was there any swelling or bruising (ecchymosis)? How quickly and where did it develop? This question
can elicit some idea of the type of swelling (e.g., blood,
synovial, purulent) and whether it is intracapsular or extracapsular.

6. Are symptoms improving, becoming worse, or
staying the same? It is important to know the type of
onset and the duration and intensity of symptoms.

7. What are the sites and boundaries of pain or
abnormal sensation? The examiner should note whether
the pattern is one of a dermatome, a peripheral nerve,
or another painful structure.

8. What is the patient's usual activity or pastime?
Answers to this question should give some idea of the
stresses placed on the lower leg, ankle, and foot, how
frequently they are applied, and whether the patient is
suffering from a repetitive stress injury.

9. Does activity make a difference? Pain after activity suggests overuse. For example, with overuse injuries,
pain initially comes on after the activity. As the injury
progresses, pain or soreness is present at the beginning
of the activity, then goes away during the activity, only
to return afterward. In later stages of the problem, the
pain is constantly present. Pain during the activity suggests stress on the injured structure.

10. Where is the pain? Does the patient indicate a
specific location or area? For example, with shin splints
or a compartment syndrome, the patient usually indicates a diffuse area. With a stress fracture, the area of
pain tends to be more specific.

11. Does walking on various terrains make a difference in regard to the foot problem? If so, which terrains
cause the most obvious problem? For example, walking
on grass (an uneven surface) may bother the patient
more than walking on a sidewalk (a relatively even surface), or the patient may find walking on a relatively soft
surface (e.g., grass) easier than walking on a hard surface
(e.g., cement). Prepared surfaces such as sidewalks,
roads, and playing fields often have a camber to allow
water runoff. This camber can cause problems in some
cases of overuse.

12. What types of shoes does the patient wear? What
kind of heel do the shoes have? Are the shoes in good
condition? Does the patient make use of orthoses? If so,
are they still functional? When an appointment is being
made for an assessment, the patient should be told not
to wear new shoes, so the examiner can use the shoes
to determine the patient's usual shoe wear pattern. The
examiner should also note whether the shoes offer
proper support. Any orthoses used by the patient should
also be brought to the assessment.

13. Is there any history of previous injury or afflic-
tion? For example, poliomyelitis may lead to a pes cavus.
Systemic conditions such as diabetes, gout, psoriasis,
and collagen diseases may manifest themselves first in
the foot.

14. For active people, especially runners or joggers,
the following questions should also be considered[7]:

   a. How long has the patient been running or
      jogging?
   b. On what type of terrain and surface does
      the patient train?
   c. In what types of workouts does the patient
      participate? Have the workouts changed
      lately? How many workouts are done per
      week? How far does the patient run per
      week? (Joggers run approximately 2 to 30 km
      [1.2 to 18.6 miles] per week at a pace of
      5 to 10 minutes/km, and sports runners run
      30 to 65 km [18.6 to 40 miles] per week at
      a pace of 5 to 6 minutes/km. Long-distance
      runners run 60 to 180 km [37 to 112 miles]
      per week at a pace of 4 to 5 minutes/km.
      Elite runners run 100 to 270 km [62 to 168

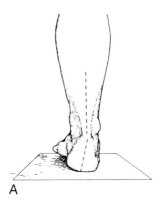
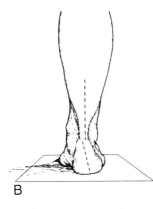

Figure 13–3

(A) Closed-chain (weight-bearing) supination of the subtalar joint (right foot). Supination of the subtalar joint in the weight-bearing foot results in motion of both the calcaneus and the talus. The calcaneus moves in the frontal plane, and the talus moves in the transverse and sagittal planes. The calcaneus inverts, and the talus simultaneously abducts and dorsiflexes relative to the calcaneus. The leg follows the motion of the talus in the transverse plane and laterally rotates. The leg also follows the sagittal plane motion of the talus to some degree. The dorsiflexion motion of the talus on the calcaneus, therefore, tends to impart a slight extension motion to the knee. (B) Closed-chain (weight-bearing) pronation of the subtalar joint (right foot). Pronation of the subtalar joint in the weight-bearing foot results in eversion of the calcaneus; the talus adducts and plantar flexes relative to the calcaneus. The leg follows the talus in a transverse plane and medially rotates. In a sagittal plane, the leg also moves to some extent with the talus. As the talus plantar flexes, the proximal aspect of the tibia moves forward to flex the knee slightly. (From Root, M.L., W.P. Orien, and J.H. Weed: Normal and Abnormal Function of the Foot. Los Angeles, Clinical Biomechanics Corp., 1977, p. 30.)

miles] per week at a pace of 3.3 to 4 minutes/km.)

    d. What types of warm-up, stretching, and postexercise routines does the patient do? The answers give the examiner some idea of whether the warm-up and stretching activities are static or ballistic and whether these activities could be detrimental.

    e. What types and styles of athletic shoes does the patient wear? (The patient should have the shoes at the examination.) Are they "control" or "cushioning" shoes? People with a cavus foot are more likely to need a cushioning shoe, whereas those with a planus foot are more likely to need a control shoe. The examiner should be able to tell if the shoes fit properly.

    f. Does the patient wear socks while training? If so, what kind (e.g., cotton, wool, nylon) and how many pairs?

    g. When was the patient's last race? How long was it? When is the patient's next race? The answers give the examiner some idea of how long the problem has been present and how long it will be until maximum stress is again placed on the joints.

Observation

Observation of the foot is extensive. Because of the stresses the foot is subjected to and because it, like the hand, can project signs of systemic problems and disease, the examiner should carry out a careful and meticulous inspection of the foot.

When performing the observation, one should remember to compare the weight-bearing (closed-chain) with the non–weight-bearing (open-chain) posture of the foot. During open-chain motion, the talus is considered fixed; during closed-chain motion, the talus moves to help the foot and leg adapt to the terrain and to the stresses that are applied to the foot. Even though the calcaneus is touching a surface in closed-chain movement, for descriptive purposes, it is still considered to be moving. The weight-bearing stance of the foot shows how the body compensates for structural abnormalities (Fig. 13–3). The non–weight-bearing posture shows functional and structural abilities without compensation (Fig. 13–4). The observation includes looking at the patient from the front, from the side, and from behind in the weight-bearing (standing) position and from the front, from the side, and from behind in the sitting position

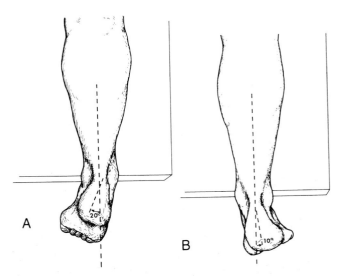

Figure 13–4

(A) Open-chain (non–weight-bearing) supination of the subtalar joint (right foot). When the non–weight-bearing foot is moved at the subtalar joint in the direction of supination, the talus is stable, and the calcaneus and foot move around the talus. The calcaneus and foot invert, plantar flex, and adduct. These positional changes, associated with subtalar joint supination, are readily visible when compared with the pronated position of the subtalar joint. (B) Open-chain (non–weight-bearing) pronation of the subtalar joint (right foot). When the subtalar joint is moved into a pronated position in the non–weight-bearing foot, the foot abducts, everts, and dorsiflexes around the stable talus. The positional variances can best be appreciated by comparing this illustration with the supinated position of the subtalar joint. (From Root, M.L., W.P. Orien, and J.H. Weed: Normal and Abnormal Function of the Foot. Los Angeles, Clinical Biomechanics Corp., 1977, p. 29.)

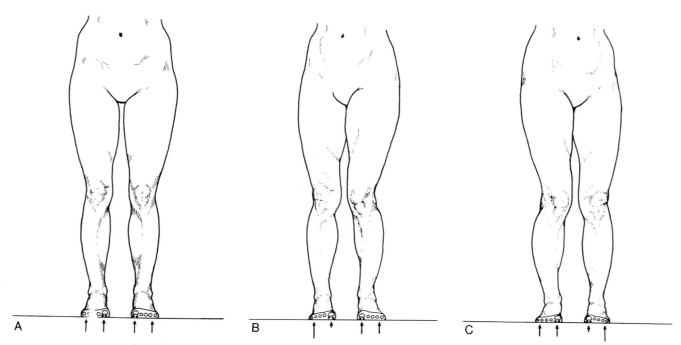

Figure 13–5

(A) During static stance, ground reaction forces (*arrows*) directed upward against the plantar aspects of both feet maintain the transverse plane equilibrium and stability of the lower extremities and pelvis. Equal ground reaction forces are exerted on the lateral and medial plantar surfaces of both feet. (B) When the trunk is rotated to the right, the right foot supinates and the left pronates. The right forefoot inverts from the ground; vertical ground reaction forces are greater against the lateral side of the forefoot (*large arrow*) and less against the medial side of the forefoot (*small arrow*). The left forefoot remains flat on the ground, and vertical ground reaction forces are distributed evenly against the forefoot (*equal arrows*). (C) When the trunk is rotated to the left, ground reaction exerts unequal forces against the left forefoot and equal forces against the right forefoot. (From Root, M.L., W.P. Orien, and J.H. Weed: Normal and Abnormal Function of the Foot. Los Angeles, Clinical Biomechanics Corp., 1977, p. 102.)

with the legs and feet not bearing weight. The examiner should note the patient's willingness and ability to use the feet. The bony and soft-tissue contours of the foot should be normal, and any deviation should be noted. Often, painful callosities may be found over abnormal bony prominences. Any scars or sinuses should also be noted.

Weight-Bearing Position, Anterior View

With the patient in a standing position, the examiner should observe whether the patient's hips and trunk are in normal position. Excessive lateral rotation of the hip or rotation of the trunk away from the opposite hip elevates the medial longitudinal arch of the foot, whereas

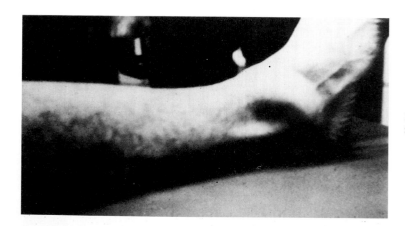

Figure 13–6
Swelling within the talocrural and subtalar joint capsule.

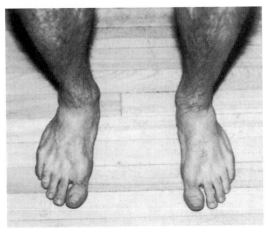

Figure 13–7
Anterosuperior view of the feet (weight-bearing position).

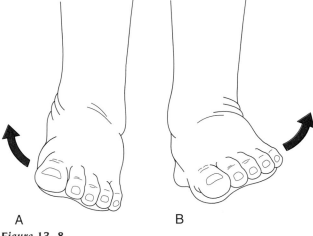

A   B

Figure 13–8
Supination (A) and pronation (B) of the foot (non–weight-bearing).

medial rotation of the hip or trunk rotation toward the opposite hip tends to flatten the arch (Fig. 13–5). Medial rotation of the hip can also cause **pigeon toes,** a condition more commonly associated with medial tibial torsion or rotation. If the iliotibial band is tight, the tightness may cause eversion and lateral rotation of the foot.

The examiner should also look at the tibia to note any local or general bone swelling (Fig. 13–6). Does the tibia have a normal shape, or is it bowed? Is there any torsional deformity? The medial malleolus usually lies anterior to the lateral malleolus. Pigeon toes, or toe-in deformity, is the result of a medial tibial torsion deformity; it does not constitute a foot deformity (Table 13–2).

Figure 13–7 shows the anterosuperior view of the feet in the weight-bearing stance. The examiner should note whether there is any asymmetry, any malalignment (Table 13–3), or any excessive supination or pronation of the foot. **Supination** of the foot involves inversion of

the heel, adduction of the forefoot, and plantar flexion at the subtalar joint and midtarsal joints so that the medial longitudinal arch is accentuated (Fig. 13–8A). In addition, there is lateral rotation of the leg in relation to the foot. Supination of the foot causes the proximal aspect of the tibia to move posteriorly. It is required during propulsion to give rigidity to the foot and requires less muscle work than pronation.

Pronation of the foot involves eversion of the heel, abduction of the forefoot, medial rotation of the leg in relation to the foot, and dorsiflexion of the subtalar and midtarsal joints (Fig. 13–8B), resulting in a decrease in the medial longitudinal arch. This movement causes the proximal aspect of the tibia to move anteriorly. The pronated foot has greater subtalar motion than the supinated foot and requires more muscle work to maintain stance stability than the supinated foot. The foot is much more mobile in this position.

Table 13–2
Causes of Toeing-In and Toeing-Out in Children

Level of Affection	Toe-In	Toe-Out
Feet-ankles	Pronated feet (protective toeing-in) Metatarsus varus Talipes varus and equinovarus	Pes valgus due to contracture of triceps surae muscle Talipes calcaneovalgus Congenital convex pes planovalgus
Leg-knee	Tibia vara (Blount's disease) and developmental genu varum Abnormal medial tibial torsion Genu valgum—developmental (protective toeing-in to shift body center of gravity medially)	Lateral tibial torsion Congenital absence of hypoplasia of the fibula
Femur-hip	Abnormal femoral antetorsion Spasticity of medial rotators of hip (cerebral palsy)	Abnormal femoral retroversion Flaccid paralysis of medial rotators of hip
Acetabulum	Maldirected—facing anteriorly	Maldirected—facing posteriorly

From Tachdjian, M.O.: Pediatric Orthopedics. Philadelphia, W.B. Saunders Co., 1990, p. 2817.

Table 13–3
Malalignment About the Foot and Ankle

Malalignment	Possible Correlated Motions or Postures	Possible Compensatory Motions or Postures
Ankle equinus	—	Hypermobile first ray Subtalar or midtarsal excessive pronation Hip or knee flexion Genu recurvatum
Rearfoot varus Excessive subtalar supination (calcaneal varus)	Tibial; tibial and femoral; or tibial, femoral, and pelvic lateral rotation	Excessive medial rotation along the lower quarter chain Hallux valgus Plantar flexed first ray Functional forefoot valgus Excessive or prolonged midtarsal pronation
Rearfoot valgus Excessive subtalar pronation (calcaneal valgus)	Tibial; tibial and femoral; or tibial, femoral, and pelvic medial rotation Hallux valgus	Excessive lateral rotation along the lower quarter chain Functional forefoot varus
Forefoot varus	Subtalar pronation and related rotation along the lower quarter	Plantar flexed first ray Hallux valgus Excessive midtarsal or subtalar pronation or prolonged pronation Excessive tibial; tibial and femoral; or tibial, femoral, and pelvic medial rotation, or all with contralateral lumbar spine rotation
Forefoot valgus	Hallux valgus Subtalar pronation and related rotation along the lower quarter	Excessive midtarsal or subtalar supination Excessive tibial; tibial and femoral; or tibial, femoral, and pelvic lateral rotation, or all with ipsilateral lumbar spine rotation
Metatarsus adductus	Hallux valgus Medial tibial torsion Flatfoot Toeing-in	—
Hallux valgus	Forefoot valgus Subtalar pronation and related rotation along the lower quarter	Excessive tibial; tibial and femoral; or tibial, femoral, and pelvic lateral rotation, or all with ipsilateral lumbar spine rotation

From Riegger-Krugh, C, and J.J. Keysor: Skeletal malalignment of the lower quarter: Correlated and compensatory motions and postures. J. Orthop. Sports Phys. Ther. 23:166, 1996.

The definitions used in this chapter are the ones preferred by orthopedists and podiatrists. Anatomists and kinesiologists such as Kapandji[8] refer to inversion as a combination of adduction and supination and to eversion as a combination of abduction and pronation. Lipscomb and Ibrahim[9] as well as Williams and Warwick[10] define supination and pronation as opposite the terms just mentioned. Because of the confusion in terminology concerning the terms supination and pronation, readers of books and articles on the foot must be careful to discern exactly what each author means.

In the infant, the foot is normally pronated. As the child matures, the foot begins to supinate, accompanied by development of the medial longitudinal arch. The foot also appears to be more pronated in the infant because of the fat pad in the medial longitudinal arch.

The examiner should note how the patient stands and walks. Normally, in standing, 50 to 60% of the weight is taken on the heel and 40 to 50% is taken by the metatarsal heads. The foot assumes a slight toe-out posi-tion. This angle (the **Fick angle**) is approximately 12 to 18° from the sagittal axis of the body, developing from 5° in children (Fig. 13–9).[11] During movement, the foot is subjected to high loading, and pathology may cause the gait to be altered. The cumulative force to which each foot is subjected during the day is the equivalent of 639 metric tons in a person who weighs approximately 90 kg, or the equivalent of walking 13 km per day.

Foot Loading During Gait

Walking:	1.2 times the body weight
Running:	2 times the body weight
Jumping (from height of 60 cm [2 feet]):	5 times the body weight

---

When weight bearing, if the relation of the foot to the ankle is normal, all of the metatarsal bones bear

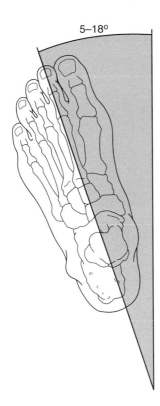

5–18°

Figure 13–9
Fick angle.

weight, and all of the metatarsal heads lie in the same transverse plane. The forefoot and hindfoot should be parallel to each other and to the floor. The midtarsal joints are in maximum pronation, and the subtalar joint is in neutral position. The subtalar and talocrural joints should be parallel to the floor. Finally, the posterior bisection of the calcaneus and distal one third of the leg should form two vertical, parallel lines.[12]

If the examiner has noted any asymmetry in standing, the examiner should place the talus (or foot) in neutral (see Special Tests) to see if the asymmetry disappears. If the asymmetry is present in normal standing, it is a **functional asymmetry**. If it is still present when the foot is in neutral, it is also an **anatomic asymmetry**, in which case a structural deformity is probably causing the asymmetry. Leg-heel and forefoot-heel alignment (see Special Tests) may also be checked, especially if asymmetry is present.

The examiner should note whether the patient uses a cane or other walking aid. Use of a cane in the opposite hand diminishes the stress on the ankle joint and foot by approximately one third.

Any prominent bumps or exostoses should be noted, as should any splaying (widening) of the forefoot. Splaying of the forefoot and metatarsus primus varus is more evident in weight bearing. There are three types of forefoot,[13] based on the length of the metatarsal bones (Fig. 13–10):

1. Index plus type. The first metatarsal (1) is longer than the second (2), with the others (3, 4, and 5) of progressively decreasing lengths, so that $1 > 2 > 3 > 4 > 5$.

2. Index plus-minus type. The first metatarsal is equal in length to the second metatarsal, with the others progressively diminishing in length, so that $1 = 2 > 3 > 4 > 5$.

3. Index minus type. The second metatarsal is longer than the first and third metatarsals. The fourth and fifth metatarsals are progressively shorter than the third, so that $1 < 2 > 3 > 4 > 5$.

The examiner should note whether the toenails appear normal. The examiner should look for warts, calluses, and corns. Warts are especially tender to the pinch (but not to direct pressure), but calluses are not. Plantar warts also tend to separate from the surrounding tissues, but calluses do not.

Any swelling or pitting edema within the ankle should be noted (Fig. 13–11). If there is any swelling, it should be noted whether it is intracapsular or extracapsular. Swelling above the lateral malleolus may be related to a fibular fracture or disruption of the syndesmosis. Peroneal retinacular injury may be indicated by swelling posterior to the lateral malleolus. Lateral ankle sprains initially swell distal to the lateral malleolus, but swelling may spread into the foot if the capsule has been torn (Table 13–4).[4] The examiner should also check the patient's gait for the position of the foot at heel strike, at foot flat, and at toe off. The gait cycle is described in greater detail in Chapter 14.

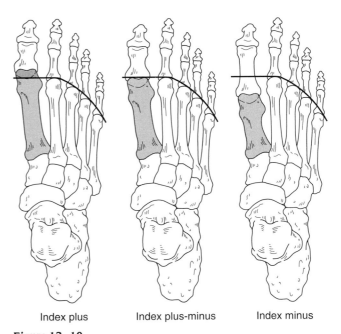

Index plus   Index plus-minus   Index minus

Figure 13–10
Metatarsal classifications.

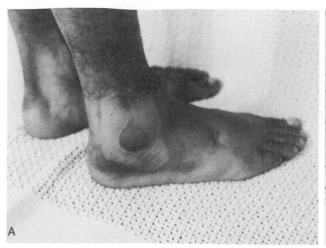
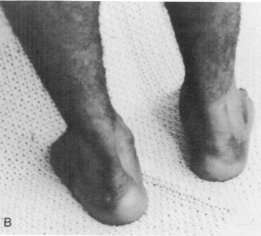

Figure 13–11
Ankle sprain. (A) Note pattern of pitting edema on top of the right foot. (B) The swelling is intracapsular, as indicated by swelling on both sides of the right Achilles tendon.

Any vasomotor changes should be recorded, including loss of hair on the foot, toenail changes, osteoporosis as seen on radiographs, and possible differences in temperature between the limbs. Systemic diseases such as diabetes can also lead to foot problems as a result of altered sensation, which facilitates injury.

The examiner should look for any circulatory impairment or presence of varicose veins. Brick-red color or cyanosis when the limb is dependent is an indication of impairment. Does this condition change to rapid blanching, or does it stay normal on elevation of the limbs? Change indicates circulatory impairment.

Weight-Bearing Position, Posterior View

From behind, the examiner compares the bulk of the calf muscles and notes any differences. Variation may be caused by peripheral nerve lesions, nerve root problems, or atrophy resulting from disuse after injury. The Achilles tendons on each side should be compared. If a tendon appears to curve out (Fig. 13–12), it may indicate a fallen medial longitudinal arch, resulting in a pes planus (flatfoot) condition **(Helbing's sign).**[14]

The examiner observes the calcaneus for normality of shape and position. Runners often build up bone and

Table 13–4
Classification of Ankle Sprains

Severity	Pathology	Signs and Symptoms	Disability
Grade I (mild) stable	Mild stretch No instability Single ligament involved (usually anterior talofibular ligament)	No hemorrhage Minimal swelling Point tenderness No anterior drawer sign No varus laxity	No or little limp Minimal functional loss Difficulty hopping Recovery 8 days (range, 2–10)
Grade II (moderate) stable	Large spectrum of injury Mild to moderate instability Complete tearing of anterior talofibular ligament, or partial tearing of anterior talofibular plus calcaneofibular ligaments	Some hemorrhage Localized swelling (margins of Achilles tendon less defined) Anterior drawer sign may be present No varus laxity	Limp with walking Unable to toe raise Unable to hop Unable to run Recovery 20 days (range, 10–30)
Grade III (severe) two-ligament, unstable	Significant instability Complete tear of anterior capsule, anterior talofibular and calcaneofibular ligaments	Diffuse swelling on both sides of Achilles tendon, early hemorrhage Possible tenderness medially and laterally Positive anterior drawer sign Positive varus laxity	Unable to bear weight fully Significant pain inhibition Initially almost complete loss of range of motion Recovery 40 days (range, 30–90)

From Reid, D.C.: Sports Injury Assessment and Rehabilitation. New York, Churchill Livingstone, 1992, p. 226.

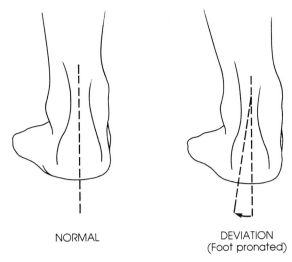

Figure 13-12
Normal and deviated Achilles tendon. The deviation is often seen with pes planus (flatfoot) and when the medial longitudinal arch is lower or has "dropped."

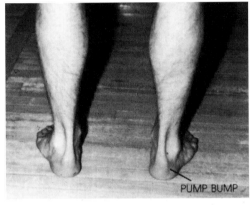

Figure 13-13
Posterior view of the leg and foot. Note "pump bumps."

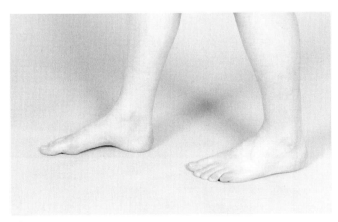

Figure 13-14
Lateral and medial views of the feet showing longitudinal arches.

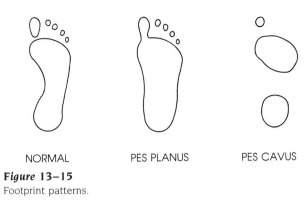

Figure 13-15
Footprint patterns.

a callus on the heel, producing a "pump bump" as a result of pressure on the heel (Fig. 13-13).

The malleoli are compared for positioning. Normally, the lateral malleolus extends farther distally than the medial malleolus; however, the medial malleolus extends farther anteriorly.

Weight-Bearing Position, Lateral View

With the side view, the examiner is primarily observing the longitudinal arches of the foot (Fig. 13-14). The examiner should note whether the medial arch is higher than the lateral arch (as would be expected). Differences in the arches may often be determined by looking at the footprint patterns (Fig. 13-15). The footprint pattern can be established by putting a light film of baby oil and then powder on the patient's foot and asking the patient to step down on a piece of colored paper.

The arches of the feet (Fig. 13-16) are maintained by three mechanisms[15]: (1) wedging of the interlocking tarsal and metatarsal bones; (2) tightening of the liga-

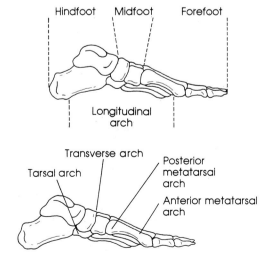

Figure 13-16
Divisions and arches of the foot (medial view).

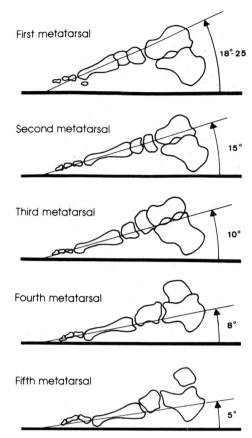

First metatarsal 18°-25

Second metatarsal 15°

Third metatarsal 10°

Fourth metatarsal 8°

Fifth metatarsal 5°

Figure 13–17
Angle formed by each metatarsal with the floor. (Modified from Jahss, M.H.: Disorders of the Foot. Philadelphia, W.B. Saunders Co., 1991, p. 1231.)

ments on the plantar aspect of the foot; and (3) the intrinsic and extrinsic muscles of the foot and their tendons, which help to support the arches. The longitudinal arches form a cone as a result of the angle of the metatar-

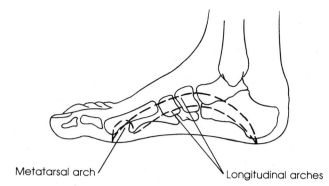

Metatarsal arch / Longitudinal arches

Figure 13–19
Arches of the foot (medial view).

sal bones in relation to the floor. With the medial longitudinal arch being more evident, this angle is greater on the medial side. The angle formed by each of the metatarsals with the floor is shown in Figure 13–17.

The **medial longitudinal arch** consists of the calcaneal tuberosity, the talus, the navicular, three cuneiforms, and the first, second, and third metatarsal bones (Figs. 13–18 and 13–19). This arch is maintained by the tibialis anterior, tibialis posterior, flexor digitorum longus, flexor hallucis longus, abductor hallucis, and flexor digitorum brevis muscles; the plantar fascia; and the plantar calcaneonavicular ligament.

The calcaneus, cuboid, and fourth and fifth metatarsal bones make up the **lateral longitudinal arch** (Fig. 13–20). This arch is more stable and less adjustable than the medial longitudinal arch. The arch is maintained by the peroneus longus, peroneus brevis, peroneus tertius, abductor digiti minimi, and flexor digitorum brevis muscles; the plantar fascia; the long plantar ligament; and the short plantar ligament.[15]

The **transverse arch** is maintained by the tibialis posterior, tibialis anterior, and peroneus longus muscles

Figure 13–18
Supports of the medial longitudinal arch of the foot.

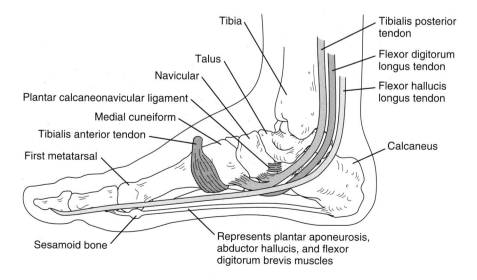

Tibia

Tibialis posterior tendon

Talus

Flexor digitorum longus tendon

Navicular

Flexor hallucis longus tendon

Plantar calcaneonavicular ligament

Medial cuneiform

Tibialis anterior tendon

First metatarsal

Calcaneus

Sesamoid bone

Represents plantar aponeurosis, abductor hallucis, and flexor digitorum brevis muscles

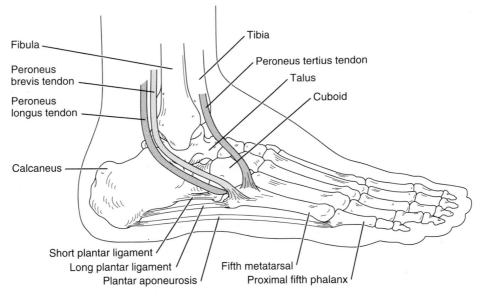

Figure 13–20

Supports of the lateral longitudinal arch of the foot: plantar aponeurosis (including the abductor digiti minimi and the flexor digitorum brevis IV and V); long plantar ligament; short plantar ligament.

and the plantar fascia (Fig. 13–21). This arch consists of the navicular, cuneiforms, cuboid, and metatarsal bones. The arch is sometimes divided into three parts: tarsal, posterior metatarsal, and anterior metatarsal. A loss of the anterior metatarsal arch results in callus formation under the heads of the metatarsal bones. The metatarsophalangeal joints are slightly extended when the patient is in the normal standing position because the longitudinal arches of the foot curve down toward the toes.[15]

Non–Weight-Bearing Position

With the patient in a supine, non–weight-bearing position, the examiner should look for abnormalities such as

callosities, plantar warts, scars, and sinuses or pressure sores on the soles of the feet. In addition, by looking at the foot from anterior to posterior, as shown in Fig. 13–22, the examiner can observe whether the patient has a "fallen" metatarsal arch. Normally, in the non–weight-bearing position, the arch can be seen. If it falls, callosities are often found over the metatarsal heads. The arch may be reversed, or it may fall because of an equinus forefoot, pes cavus, rheumatoid arthritis, short heel cord, or hammer toes. Abnormal width of one ankle in relation to the other **(Keen's sign)** may be caused by swelling, loss of integrity of the syndesmosis, or a malleolar fracture.

Young children should be assessed for clubfoot deformities, the most common of which is talipes equino-

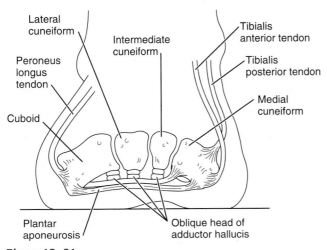

Figure 13–21

Supports of the transverse arch of the foot.

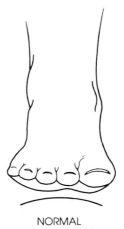 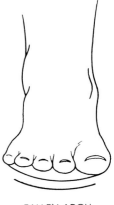

NORMAL   FALLEN ARCH

Figure 13–22

Fallen metatarsal arch.

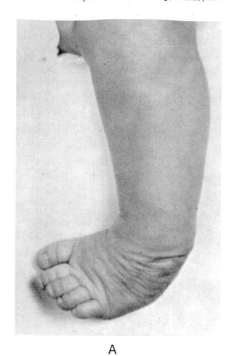
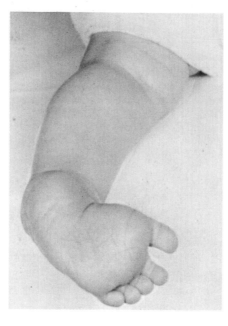

A   B

Figure 13–23

Talipes equinovarus (clubfoot) in a child aged 4 months. (A) Anterior view. (B) Posterior view. (From Klenerman, L.: The Foot and Its Disorders. Boston, Blackwell Scientific Publications, 1982, p. 64.)

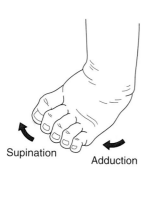
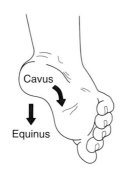

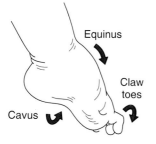
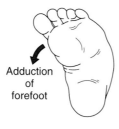

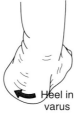

Figure 13–24

Components of talipes equinovarus.

varus (Figs. 13–23 and 13–24). These types of deformities are often associated with other anomalies, such as spina bifida.

Common Deformities, Deviations, and Injuries

Equinus Deformity (Talipes Equinus). This deformity is characterized by limited dorsiflexion (less than 10°) at the talocrural joint, usually as a result of contracture of the gastrocnemius or soleus muscles or Achilles tendon. It may also be caused by structural bone deformity (primarily in the talus), trauma, or inflammatory disease. The deformity causes increased stress to the forefoot, which may lead to a rocker-bottom foot and excessive pronation at the subtalar joint. This deviation can contribute to conditions such as plantar fasciitis, metatarsalgia, heel spurs, and talonavicular pain.[7]

Clubfoot. This congenital deformity is relatively common and can take many forms, the most common of which is **talipes equinovarus**. Its cause is unknown, but there are probably multifactorial genetic causes modified by environmental factors.[16] It sometimes coexists with other congenital deformities, such as spina bifida and cleft palate. The flexible form is easily treated, but the resistant type often requires surgery. On assessment, the range of motion is limited and the foot has abnormal form (see Fig. 13–24).

Hindfoot Varus (Subtalar Varus). This structural deviation involves inversion of the calcaneus when the subtalar joint is in the neutral position. The hindfoot is mildly rigid with calcaneal eversion; therefore, pronation is lim-

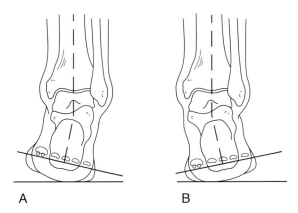

Figure 13–25
Hindfoot deformities (right foot). (A) Hindfoot varus. (B) Hindfoot valgus.

ited. It may contribute to the appearance of a pes cavus foot, making the medial longitudinal arch appear accentuated. It may be the result of tibia varus (genu varum), and, because of the extra subtalar pronation necessary at the beginning of stance, normal supination during early propulsion may be prevented. This deviation can contribute to conditions such as retrocalcaneal exostosis (pump bumps), shin splints, plantar fasciitis, hamstring strains, and knee and ankle pathology (Fig. 13–25).[7]

Hindfoot Valgus. This structural deformity involves eversion of the calcaneus when the subtalar joint is in the neutral position. The hindfoot is mobile, which may lead to excessive pronation and limited supination. It may result from genu valgum (knock knees) and may contribute to the appearance of a pes planus foot, with the medial longitudinal arch appearing flattened. Because of the increased mobility, it is less likely to cause problems than hindfoot varus. It is often associated with tibia valgus (see Fig. 13–25).

Forefoot Valgus. This structural midtarsal deviation involves eversion of the forefoot on the hindfoot when the subtalar joint is in the neutral position because the normal valgus tilt (35 to 45°) of the head and neck of the talus to its trochlea has been exceeded. With this deformity, during the weight-bearing phase of gait, the midtarsal joint is supinated so that the lateral aspect of the foot is brought into contact with the ground. Like hindfoot valgus, it contributes to increasing the medial longitudinal arch and therefore clinically resembles a cavus foot. The prolonged supination can contribute to conditions such as lateral ankle sprains, iliotibial band syndrome, plantar fasciitis, anterior tarsal tunnel syndrome, toe deformities, sesamoiditis, and leg and thigh pain (Fig. 13–26).[7, 17]

Forefoot Varus. This structural midtarsal joint deviation involves inversion of the forefoot on the hindfoot when the subtalar joint is in the neutral position. It occurs because the normal valgus tilt (35 to 45°) of the head and neck of the talus to its trochlea has not been

achieved.[7, 17, 18] Clinically, it contributes to decreasing the medial longitudinal arch and therefore resembles pes planus. With this deformity, during the weight-bearing phase of gait, the midtarsal joint is completely pronated in an attempt to bring the first metatarsal head in contact with the ground. The prolonged rotation that results can contribute to conditions such as tibialis posterior tendinitis, patellofemoral syndrome, toe deformities, ligamentous stress (medially), shin splints, plantar fasciitis, postural fatigue, and Morton's neuroma (see Fig. 13–26).

Metatarsus Adductus (Hooked Forefoot). This deformity is the most common foot deviation in children. It may be seen at birth but often is not noticed until the child begins to stand. The foot appears to be adducted and supinated, and the hindfoot may or may not be in valgus. It may be associated with hip dysplasia. Eighty-five to 90% of cases resolve spontaneously.[16]

Pes Cavus ("Hollow Foot" or Rigid Foot). A pes cavus may be caused by a congenital problem; a neurological problem such as spina bifida, poliomyelitis, or Charcot-Marie-Tooth disease; talipes equinovarus; or muscle imbalance. There may also be a genetic factor, because it tends to run in families.

The longitudinal arches are accentuated (Fig. 13–27), and the metatarsal heads are lower in relation to the hindfoot so that there is a "dropping" of the forefoot on the hindfoot at the tarsometatarsal joints. The soft tissues of the sole of the foot are abnormally short, which gives the foot a shortened appearance. If the deformity persists, the bones eventually alter their shape, perpetuating the deformity. The heel is normal, at least initially. Claw toes are often associated with the condition because of the dropping of the forefoot combined with the pull of the extensor tendons. The examiner often finds

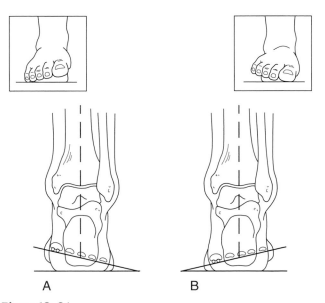

Figure 13–26
Forefoot deformities (right foot). (A) Forefoot varus. (B) Forefoot valgus.

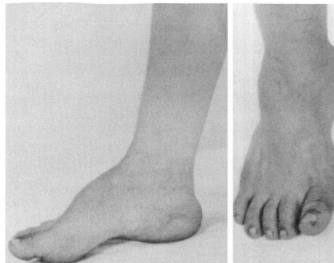
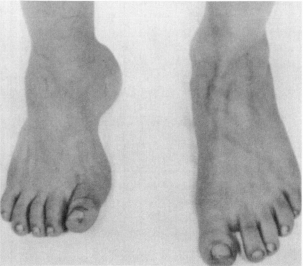

Figure 13–27
Pes cavus ("hollow foot"). Note the high medial longitudinal arch, early clawing of the big toe, and the heel in varus. (From Klenerman, L.: The Foot and Its Disorders. Boston, Blackwell Scientific Publications, 1982, p. 72.)

painful callosities beneath the metatarsal heads that are caused by the loss of the metatarsal arch and tenderness along the deformed toes. There is pain in the tarsal region after time because of osteoarthritic changes in these joints.

The longitudinal arches are high on both the medial and lateral aspects, so that a lateral longitudinal arch can in some severe cases be seen, and the forefoot is thickened and splayed (Table 13–5). The metatarsal heads are prominent on the sole of the foot, and the toes do not touch the ground, even on active or passive movement. This type of deformity leads to a rigid foot with very little ability to absorb shock and adapt to stress. People with this deformity have difficulty doing repetitive stress activity (e.g., long distance running, ballet) and

Table 13–5
Pes Cavus Classification

Classification	Features
1. Mild	Longitudinal arch appears high N.W.B.
	Longitudinal arch almost normal W.B.
	Toes clawed N.W.B.
	Toes may be normal W.B.
	May have hindfoot varus
2. Moderate	Longitudinal arch high N.W.B. and W.B.
	Claw toes evident N.W.B. and W.B.
	Calluses under prominent metatarsal heads
	Dorsiflexion may be limited
	Forefoot plantar flexed on hindfoot
3. Severe	Calcaneus cannot pronate past 5° varus
	Heel in varus, foot in valgus
	Decreased R.O.M. in foot

N.W.B. = non–weight bearing; W.B. = weight bearing; R.O.M. = range of motion.

require a cushioning shoe. In severe cases, the cavus foot is often associated with neurological disorders.[16]

Pes Planus (Flatfoot or Mobile Foot). Flatfoot may be congenital, or it may result from trauma, muscle weakness, ligament laxity, "dropping" of the talar head, paralysis, or a pronated foot. For example, a traumatic flatfoot may follow fracture of the calcaneus. It may also be caused by a postural deformity, such as medial rotation of the hips or medial tibial torsion. It is a relatively common foot deformity that often causes little or no problem. Therefore, the examiner should not necessarily assume that a flat, mobile foot needs to be treated. Because the foot is mobile, patients with flatfoot function very well without treatment and often need only a control shoe to avoid problems in prolonged stress situations.

It must be remembered that all infants have flat feet up to approximately 2 years of age. This appearance in part results from the fat pad in the longitudinal arch and in part from the incomplete formation of the arches. With pes planus, the medial longitudinal arch is reduced, so that on standing its borders are close to or in contact with the ground. If the condition persists into adulthood, it may become a permanent structural deformity, leading to a defect or alteration of the tarsal bones and the talonavicular joints.

There are two types of flatfoot deformities. The first type (**rigid** or **congenital flatfoot**) is relatively rare. The calcaneus is found in a valgus position, whereas the midtarsal region is in pronation. The talus faces medially and downward, and the navicular is displaced dorsally and laterally on the talus. There are accompanying soft-tissue contractures and bony changes. The second type is **acquired** or **flexible flatfoot** (Fig. 13–28). In this case,

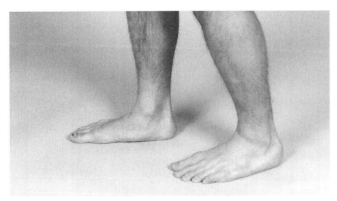

Figure 13–28
Pes planus (flatfoot).

the deformity is similar to the rigid flatfoot, but the foot is mobile (Table 13–6) and there are few, if any, soft-tissue contractures and bony changes. It is usually caused by hereditary factors and is sometimes called a **hypermobile flatfoot**. Flexible flatfoot may result from tibial or femoral torsion, coxa vara, or a defect in the subtalar joint. If the patient is asked to stand on tiptoes and the arch appears, it is an indication that the patient has a mobile flatfoot. This type of flatfoot seldom needs treatment.

Rocker-Bottom Foot. In the rocker-bottom foot deformity, the forefoot is dorsiflexed on the hindfoot. This results in a "broken midfoot," so that the medial and longitudinal arches are absent and the foot appears to be "bent" the wrong way (i.e., convex to the floor instead of the normal concave).

Splay Foot. This deformity, which is broadening of the forefoot, is often caused by weakness of the intrinsic muscles and associated weakness of the intermetatarsal ligament and dropping of the anterior metatarsal arch.

Morton's Metatarsalgia (Interdigital Neuroma). Morton's metatarsalgia refers to the formation of an interdigital neuroma as a result of injury to one of the digital nerves (Fig. 13–29). Usually, it is the digital nerve between the third and fourth toes, so the examiner must take care to differentially diagnose the condition from a stress fracture of one of the metatarsals in the same area (**march fracture**). While walking or running, the patient is sud-

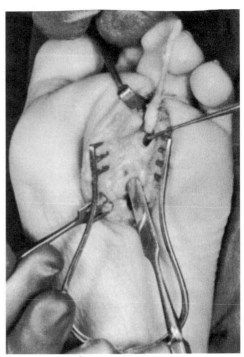

Figure 13–29
The applied anatomy of Morton's metatarsalgia. The interdigital nerve to the space between the third and fourth digits has been divided 2 cm above the neuroma and is reflected downward. The plantar digital vessels are seen entering the neuroma. The end of the flat dissector is on the upper margin of the transverse ligament. The end of the probe points to the intermetatarsophalangeal bursa. (From Klenerman, L.: The Foot and Its Disorders. Boston, Blackwell Scientific Publications, 1982, p. 143.)

denly seized with an agonizing pain on the outer border of the forefoot. The pain is often intermittent, like a cramp, shooting up the side and to the tip of the affected toe or the adjacent two toes. If the metatarsal bones are squeezed together, pain is elicited because of the pressure on the digital nerve. The condition tends to occur more frequently in women than in men.

Exostosis (Bony Spur). Exostosis is an abnormal bony outgrowth extending from the surface of the bone (Fig. 13–30). It is actually an increase in the bone mass at

Table 13–6
Pes Planus Classification

Classification	Features
1. Mild	4 to 6° hindfoot valgus 4 to 6° forefoot varus
2. Moderate	6 to 10° hindfoot valgus 6 to 10° forefoot varus Poor shock absorption at heel strike
3. Severe	10 to 15° hindfoot valgus 8 to 10° forefoot varus Equinus deformity may be present

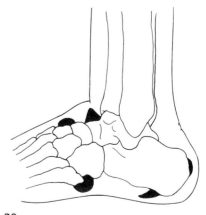

Figure 13–30
Common areas of exostosis formation in the foot.

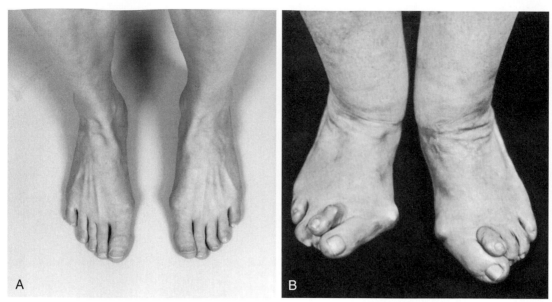

Figure 13–31

(A) An example of congruous hallux valgus. (B) Pathological hallux valgus with bilateral bunions and overlapped toes. Note how the deviating big toe (hallux) rotates and pushes under the second toe.
(B, From Gartland, J.J.: Fundamentals of Orthopedics. Philadelphia, W.B. Saunders Co., 1987, p. 401.)

the site of an irritative lesion in response to overuse, trauma, or excessive pressure. The common areas of occurrence in the foot are on the dorsal aspect of the tarsometatarsal joint, the head of the fifth metatarsal bone, the calcaneus (where it is often called a pump bump or runner's bump), the insertion of the plantar fascia, and the superior aspect of the navicular bone. Most often these exostoses are the result of poorly fitting footwear that leads to undue pressure on the bone.

Hallux Valgus. Hallux valgus is a relatively common condition in which there is medial deviation of the head of the first metatarsal bone in relation to the center of the body and lateral deviation of the head in relation to the center of the foot (Fig. 13–31). The cause of hallux valgus is varied. It may result from a hereditary factor and is often familial. Women tend to be affected more than men. Trying to keep up with fashion may be a contributing factor if the patient wears tight or pointed shoes, tight stockings, or high-heeled shoes.[19]

As the metatarsal bones move medially, the base of the proximal phalanx is carried with it, and the phalanx pivots around the adductor hallucis muscle that inserts into it, causing the distal end as well as the distal phalanx to deviate laterally in relation to the center of the body. The long flexor and extensor muscles then have a "bowstring" effect as they are displaced to the lateral side of the joint.

A callus develops over the medial side of the head of the metatarsal bone, and the bursa becomes thickened and inflamed; excessive bone (exostosis) forms, resulting in a **bunion** (Fig. 13–32).[5,20] These three changes—callus,

thickened bursa, and exostosis—make up the bunion, a condition separate from hallux valgus, although it is the result of hallux valgus.

In normal persons, the **metatarsophalangeal angle** (the angle between the longitudinal axis of the metatarsal bone and the proximal phalanx) is 8 to 20° (Fig. 13–33). This angle is increased to varying degrees in hallux valgus.

The first type (**congruous hallux valgus**) is a simple exaggeration of the normal relation of the metatarsal to

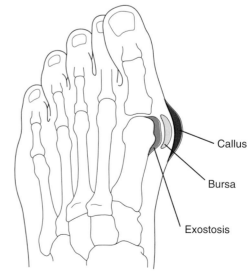

Figure 13–32
Bunion.

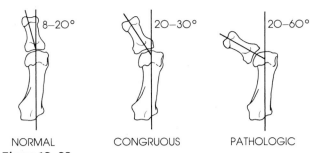

Figure 13-33

Metatarsophalangeal (hallux valgus) angle.

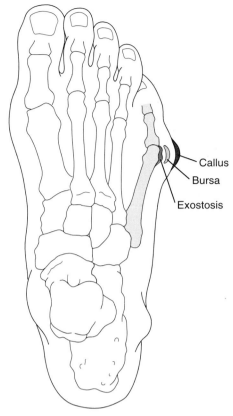

Figure 13-35

A bunionette or tailor's bunion.

the phalanx of the big toe. The deformity does not progress, and the valgus deformity is between 20° and 30°. The opposing joint surfaces are congruent. It requires little treatment, and often the biggest problem is cosmetic.

The second type (**pathological hallux valgus**) is a potentially progressive deformity, increasing from 20 to 60°. The joint surfaces are no longer congruent, and some may even go to subluxation. This type may occur in deviated (early) and subluxed (later) stages.

When looking at the foot, the examiner may find that there is a widening gap between the first and second metatarsal bones (increased **intermetatarsal angle**) and a lateral deflection of the phalanx at the metatarsophalangeal joint. The joint capsule lengthens on the medial aspect and is contracted on the lateral aspect. The toes rotate on the long axis so that the toenail faces medially because of the pull of the adductor hallucis muscle. Sometimes, the big toe deviates so far that it lies over or under the second toe.

Of all hallux valgus cases, 80% are caused by **metatarsus primus varus,** in which the intermetatarsal or

metatarsal angle is increased to more than 15° (Fig. 13–34).[21, 22] Metatarsus primus varus is an abduction deformity of the first metatarsal bone in relation to the tarsal and other metatarsal bones so that the medial border of the forefoot is curved. Normally, this angle is between 0 and 15°.

Bunionette (Tailor's Bunion). This deformity is characterized by prominence of the lateral aspect of the fifth toe metatarsal head (Fig. 13–35).[23] If associated with hallux valgus, it results in a splayed foot. It is often associated with a pronated foot.

Hallux Rigidus. Hallux rigidus is a condition in which dorsiflexion or extension of the big toe is limited because of osteoarthritis of the first metatarsophalangeal joint.[24] Hallux rigidus may also be caused by an anatomic abnormality of the foot, an abnormally long first metatarsal bone (index plus type forefoot; see Fig. 13–10), pronation of the forefoot, or trauma. There are two types: acute and chronic.

The acute, or adolescent, type is seen primarily in young people with long, narrow, pronated feet and occurs more frequently in boys than in girls. Pain and stiffness in the big toe come on quickly; the pain is described as constant, burning, throbbing, or aching. Tenderness may be palpated over the metatarsophalangeal joint, and the toe is initially held stiff because of muscle spasm. The first metatarsal head may be elevated, large, and tender.

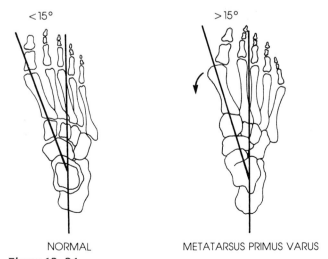

Figure 13-34

Normal foot and metatarsus primus varus. (Note increased intermetatarsal angle.)

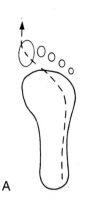
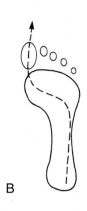
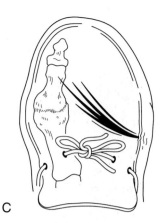

A   B   C

Figure 13–36

Weight-bearing patterns in hallux rigidus. (A) Hallux rigidus gait pattern. (B) Normal gait pattern. (C) Shoe develops oblique creases with hallux rigidus. (C redrawn from Jahss, M.H.: Disorders of the Foot. Philadelphia, W.B. Saunders Co., 1991, p. 60.)

The weight distribution pattern in the gait is shown in Figure 13–36.

The second (chronic) type of hallux rigidus is much more common and is seen primarily in adults—again, in men more frequently than in women. It is frequently bilateral and is usually the result of repeated minor trauma resulting in osteoarthritic changes to the metatarsophalangeal joint of the big toe. The toe stiffens gradually, and the pain, once established, persists. The patient complains primarily of pain at the base of the big toe on walking.

Plantar Flexed First Ray. This structural deformity occurs when the first ray (big toe) lies lower than the other four metatarsal bones, so that the forefoot is everted when the metatarsal bones are aligned. If present congenitally, it is indicative of a cavus foot. In its acquired form, it is seen as compensation for tibia varum (genu varum) with limited calcaneal eversion. This deformity can contribute to the same conditions seen with forefoot valgus.[7] The neutral position of the first ray is the position in which the first metatarsal head lies in the same transverse plane as the second through fourth metatarsal heads when they are maximally dorsiflexed.[25]

Turf Toe. Turf toe is a hyperextension injury (sprain) combined with compressive loading to the metatarsophalangeal joint of the hallux. It can cause a significant functional disability, especially in sports, where the hallux is put under high loads. It is often related to the use of flexible footwear and artificial turf.[26, 27]

Morton's (Atavistic or Grecian) Foot. With a Morton's foot, the second toe is longer than the first. Increased stress is put on this longer toe, and the big toe tends to be hypomobile. There is often hypertrophy of the second metatarsal bone because more stress is put through the second toe. In fact, the second metatarsal can become as large as the first metatarsal. People with this deformity often have difficulty putting on tight-fitting footwear (e.g., skates, ski boots) or dancing (e.g., en pointe in ballet). The different types of feet and their proportional representations in the population are shown in Figure 13–37.

Claw Toes. A claw-toe deformity results in hyperextension of the metatarsophalangeal joints and flexion of the proximal and distal interphalangeal joints (Fig. 13–38A). Claw toes usually result from the defective actions of lumbrical and interosseus muscles that cause the toes to become functionless. This condition may be unilateral or bilateral and is often associated with pes cavus, spina bifida, or other neurological problems.

Hammer Toes. A hammer-toe deformity consists of an extension contracture at the metatarsophalangeal joint and flexion contracture at the proximal interphalangeal joint; the distal interphalangeal joint may be flexed, straight, or hyperextended (Fig. 13–38B).[20, 28] The interosseus muscles are unable to hold the proximal phalanx in the neutral position and therefore lose their flexion effect. This results in clawing of the toe by the long flexors and extensors leading to and accentuating the deformity. The causes of hammer toe include an imbalance of the synergic muscles, hereditary factors, and mechanical factors such as poorly fitting shoes or hallux

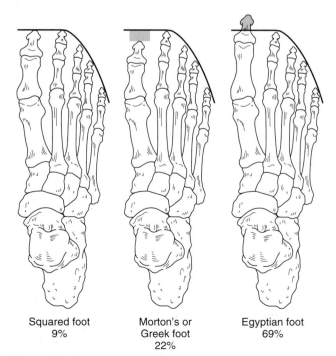

Squared foot
9%

Morton's or
Greek foot
22%

Egyptian foot
69%

Figure 13–37

Types of feet seen in the general population.

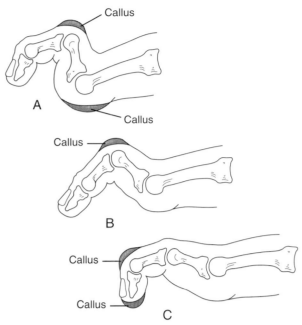

Callus
Callus
Callus
Callus
Callus

A

B

C

Figure 13–38

Toe deformities. (A) Claw toe. Note that the proximal and distal interphalangeal joints are hyperflexed and the metatarsophalangeal joint is dorsally subluxated. (B) Hammer toe. Note the flexion deformity of the proximal interphalangeal joints. The distal interphalangeal joint is in neutral position or slight flexion. (C) Mallet toe. There is flexion contracture of the distal interphalangeal joint. The proximal interphalangeal and metatarsophalangeal joints are in neutral position.

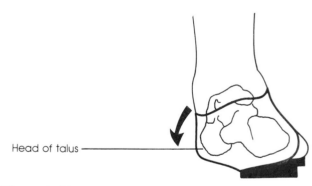

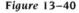
Head of talus

Figure 13–39

Pes planus (flatfoot) or calcaneus in valgus can lead to misshapen shoes. Note the prominence of the talar head.

valgus. It is usually seen only in one toe—the second toe. Often, there is a callus or corn over the dorsum of the flexed joint. The condition is often asymptomatic, especially if the hammer toe is flexible or semiflexible. The rigid type of hammer toe is likely to cause the greatest problems.

Mallet Toe. Mallet toe is associated with a flexion deformity of the distal interphalangeal joint (Fig. 13–38C).[20, 28] It can occur on any of the four lateral toes. Often, a corn or callus is present over the dorsum of the affected joint. The condition is usually asymptomatic. It is commonly seen with ill-fitting or poorly designed footwear.[23]

Polydactyly. This developmental anomaly is characterized by the presence of an extra digit or toe. It may be seen in isolation or with other anomalies such as polydactyly of the hands and **syndactyly** (webbing) of the toes. The primary problem with this anomaly is cosmesis.[29]

Shoes

The examiner looks at the patient's shoes, both inside and outside, for weight-bearing and wear patterns (Figs. 13–39 and 13–40). With the normal foot, the greatest wear on the shoe is beneath the ball of the foot and slightly to the lateral side. If shoes are too small or too narrow, they may pinch the feet, causing deformities and affecting normal growth. If shoes are worn out, they offer little support. If shoes are stiff, they limit proper movement of the foot.

Platform-type or high-heeled shoes often cause painful knees because the patient wearing these shoes usually walks with the knees flexed, which may increase the stress on the patella. Continuous wearing of high-heeled shoes may also lead to contracture of the calf muscles as well as sore knees and a painful back, because the lumbar spine goes into increased lordotic posture to maintain the center of gravity in its normal position. In addition, these shoes increase the potential for ankle sprains and fractures because a raised center of gravity puts the wearer off balance.

High-heeled and pointed shoes often contribute to hallux valgus, bunions, march fractures, and Morton's

Figure 13–40

Misshapen shoes caused by severely pronated feet. (From Gartland, J.J.: Fundamentals of Orthopedics. Philadelphia, W.B. Saunders Co., 1987, p. 398.)

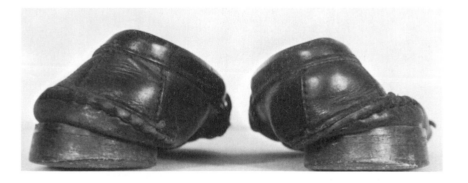

metatarsalgia as a result of the toes' being pushed together. Shoes with a negative heel (i.e., "earth shoes") may lead to hyperextension of the knees and patellofemoral syndrome. High-cut or high-top shoes that cover the medial and lateral malleoli offer more support than low-cut shoes or those that do not cover the malleoli.

Excessive bulging on the medial side of the shoe suggests a valgus or everted foot, whereas excessive bulging on the lateral side suggests an inverted foot. Drop foot resulting from musculature weakness scuffs the toe of the shoe. Oblique forefoot creases in the shoe indicate possible hallux rigidus; absence of forefoot creases indicates no toe-off action during gait.

Examination

As with any assessment, the examiner must compare one side with the other and note any asymmetry. This comparison is necessary because of individual differences among normal people.

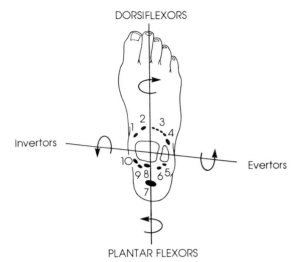

Figure 13–42

Motion diagram of the ankle. 1 = tibialis anterior; 2 = extensor hallucis longus; 3 = extensor digitorum longus; 4 = peroneus tertius; 5 = peroneus brevis; 6 = peroneus longus; 7 = Achilles tendon (soleus and gastrocnemius); 8 = flexor hallucis longus; 9 = flexor digitorum longus; 10 = tibialis posterior.

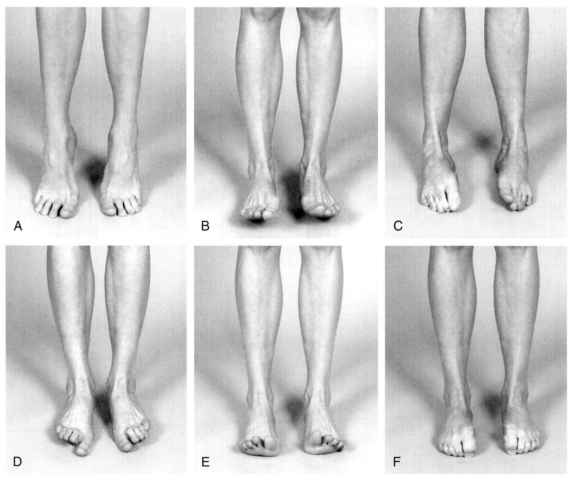

Figure 13–41

Active movements (weight-bearing posture). (A) Plantar flexion. (B) Dorsiflexion. (C) Supination. (D) Pronation. (E) Toe extension. (F) Toe flexion.

Active Movements

The first movements tested during the examination are active, with painful movements being done last. These movements should be done in both weight-bearing (Figs. 13–41 and 13–42) and non–weight-bearing (long leg sit-ting or supine lying; Fig. 13–43) positions, and any differences should be noted. Lindsjo and colleagues[30] advocated testing weight-bearing range of motion by putting the test foot on a 30-cm (12-inch) stool for ease of measurement and flexing the knee.

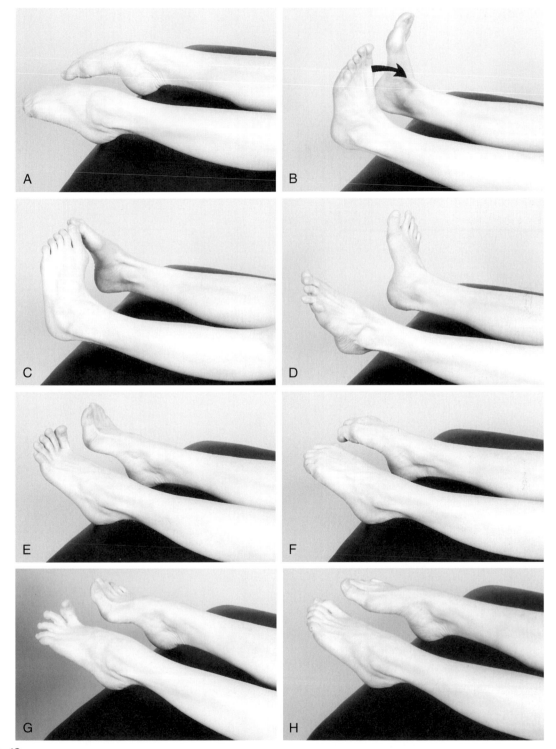

Figure 13–43

Active movements (non–weight-bearing posture). (A) Plantar flexion. (B) Dorsiflexion. (C) Supination. (D) Pronation. (E) Toe extension. (F) Toe flexion. (G) Toe abduction. (H) Toe adduction.

Weight-Bearing Active Movements of the Lower Leg, Ankle, and Foot

- Plantar flexion (flexion), standing on the toes
- Dorsiflexion (extension), standing on the heels
- Supination, standing on the lateral edge of the foot
- Pronation, standing on the medial edge of the foot
- Toe extension
- Toe flexion
- Combined movements (if necessary)
- Sustained positions (if necessary)
- Repetitive movements (if necessary)

Non–Weight-Bearing Active Movements of the Lower Leg, Ankle, and Foot

- Plantar flexion (flexion), 50°
- Dorsiflexion (extension), 20°
- Supination, 45 to 60°
- Pronation, 15 to 30°
- Toe extension, lateral four toes (MTP, 40°; PIP, 0°; DIP, 30°) and great toe (MTP, 70°; IP, 0°)
- Toe flexion, lateral four toes (MTP, 40°; PIP, 35°; DIP, 60°) and great toe (MTP, 45°; IP, 90°)
- Toe abduction
- Toe adduction
- Combined movements (if necessary)
- Sustained positions (if necessary)
- Repetitive movements (if necessary)

DIP = distal interphalangeal joint, MTP = metatarsophalangeal joint; PIP = proximal interphalangeal joint.

Plantar Flexion. Plantar flexion of the ankle is approximately 50° (see Fig. 13–43A), and the patient's heel normally inverts when the movement is performed in weight bearing (Fig. 13–44). If heel inversion does not occur, the foot is unstable.

Dorsiflexion. Dorsiflexion of the ankle is usually 20° past the anatomic position (plantegrade), which is with the foot at 90° to the bones of the leg (see Fig. 13–43B). For normal locomotion, 10° of dorsiflexion and 20 to 25° of plantar flexion at the ankle are required.

Supination and Pronation. Supination is 45 to 60° and pronation is 15 to 30°, although there is variability among individual patients (see Fig. 13–43C and D). It is more important to compare the movement with that of the patient's normal side (Figs. 13–45 and 13–46). Supination combines the movements of inversion, adduction,

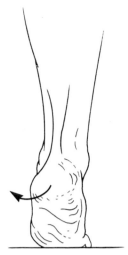

Figure 13–44
Inversion of heel while standing on toes (plantar flexion of ankle).

and plantar flexion; pronation combines the movements of eversion, abduction, and dorsiflexion of the foot and ankle. As the patient does the movement, the examiner should watch for the possibility of subluxation of various tendons. The peroneal tendons are especially prone to subluxation, and their subluxation is evident on eversion (Fig. 13–47).

Toe Extension and Flexion. Movement of the toes occurs at the metatarsophalangeal and proximal and distal interphalangeal joints (see Fig. 13–43E and F). Extension

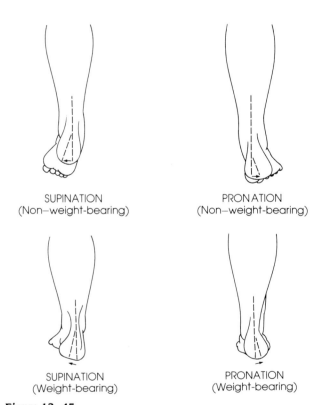

SUPINATION
(Non–weight-bearing)

PRONATION
(Non–weight-bearing)

SUPINATION
(Weight-bearing)

PRONATION
(Weight-bearing)

Figure 13–45
Supination and pronation of the foot in weight-bearing and non–weight-bearing postures (posterior views of the right limb).

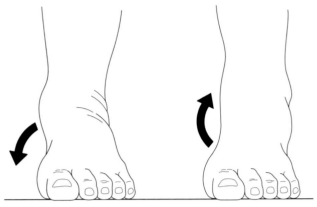

Figure 13–46

Anterior view of the foot in pronation and supination (weight-bearing stance).

Foot in pronation   Foot in supination

of the great toe occurs primarily at the metatarsophalangeal joint (70°); there is minimal or no extension at the interphalangeal joint. For the great toe, 45° flexion occurs at the metatarsophalangeal joint, and 90° occurs at the interphalangeal joint.

For the lateral four toes, extension occurs primarily at the metatarsophalangeal (40°) and distal interphalangeal joints (30°). Extension at the proximal interphalangeal joints is negligible. For the lateral four toes, 40° flexion occurs at the metatarsophalangeal joints, 35° occurs at the proximal interphalangeal joints, and 60° occurs at the distal interphalangeal joints.

Toe Abduction and Adduction. Abduction and adduction of the toes are measured with the second toe as midline.

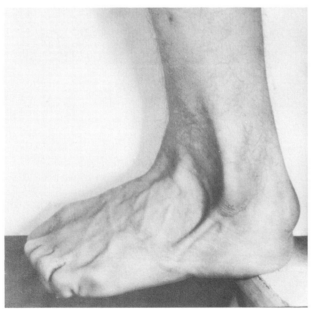

Figure 13–47

Habitual subluxation of the peroneal tendons. The peroneal tendons pass anterior to the retrofibular sulcus but not anterior to the distal fibula, in contradistinction to traumatic subluxation. (From Kelikian, H., and A.S. Kelikian: Disorders of the Ankle. Philadelphia, W.B. Saunders Co., 1985, p. 765.)

Although the range of motion of abduction can be measured, this is not usually done. The common practice is to ask the patient to spread the toes and then bring them back together (see Fig. 13–43G and H). The amount and quality of movement are compared with those of the unaffected side.

If the history has indicated that weight-bearing or non–weight-bearing combined or repetitive movements or sustained postures result in symptoms, these movements should also be tested. The patient should be asked to walk on the toes, heels, and outer and inner borders of the feet. These actions give an indication of the patient's muscle power and control and the functional range of motion. With a third-degree strain (rupture) of the Achilles tendon, the patient is not able to walk on the toes. Lack of dorsiflexion makes it difficult for the patient to walk on the heels. When the patient walks on the inner or outer borders of the feet, pain and difficulty are experienced in the presence of a subtalar lesion.

The examiner should also check the efficiency of the toes. Are the toes straight and parallel? Is the patient able to flex, extend, adduct, and abduct the toes? The toes have a primarily ambulatory function, although, with training, they can develop a prehensile function. The toes extend the weight-bearing area forward and, by so doing, reduce the load on the metatarsal heads. The great toe also has a primary function of "pushing off" during gait.

When assessing the active movements, the examiner must remember that peripheral nerve injuries may alter the pattern of movement. For example, the common peroneal nerve may be injured as it winds around the head of the fibula, resulting in altered nerve conduction to the peroneus longus and brevis muscles (superficial peroneal nerve) and/or the tibialis anterior, extensor digitorum longus, and extensor hallucis longus (deep peroneal nerve).[31] In such cases, the movements controlled by these muscles are altered. In addition, there are sensory changes that must be noted.

Passive Movements

The passive movements of the lower leg, ankle, and foot are performed with the patient in a non–weight-bearing position (Fig. 13–48). As with other joints, if the active range of motion is full, overpressure can be applied during the active, non–weight-bearing movements to negate the need to do passive movements. Each movement should be carefully checked, especially if deformities or asymmetries have been noticed during the observation. These deformities or asymmetries may cause problems in other areas of the lower kinetic chain. For example, limited dorsiflexion or tight heel cords may lead to anterior knee pain. Because the gastrocnemius is a two-joint muscle, dorsiflexion should be tested with the knee

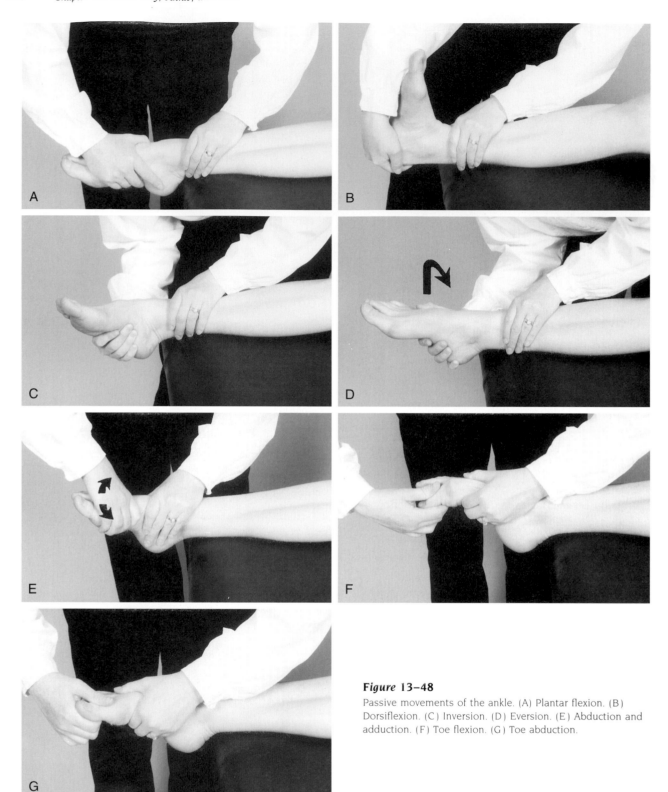

Figure 13–48
Passive movements of the ankle. (A) Plantar flexion. (B) Dorsiflexion. (C) Inversion. (D) Eversion. (E) Abduction and adduction. (F) Toe flexion. (G) Toe abduction.

straight. In a baby or young child, there is greater mobility and flexibility than in an adult. For example, in the newborn, the foot can readily be dorsiflexed passively, so that the toes and dorsum of the foot touch the skin over the tibia.

Some movements may be tested in combination to more closely approximate what occurs functionally. For example, instead of testing plantar flexion, adduction, and inversion separately, supination, as a combined movement, may be tested. Similarly, pronation may be tested as a combined movement, instead of dorsiflexion, abduction, and eversion.

Passive Movements of the Lower Leg, Ankle, and Foot and Normal End Feel

- Plantar flexion at the talocrural joint (tissue stretch)
- Dorsiflexion at the talocrural joint (tissue stretch)
- Inversion at the subtalar joint (tissue stretch)
- Eversion of the subtalar joint (tissue stretch)
- Adduction at the midtarsal joints (tissue stretch)
- Abduction at the midtarsal joints (tissue stretch)
- Flexion of the toes (tissue stretch)
- Extension of the toes (tissue stretch)
- Adduction of the toes (tissue stretch)
- Abduction of the toes (tissue stretch)

During passive movements of the ankle and foot, any capsular patterns should be noted. The capsular pattern of the talocrural joint is more limitation of plantar flexion than of dorsiflexion; the subtalar joint capsular pattern shows more limitation of varus range than of valgus range of motion. The midtarsal joint capsular pattern is dorsiflexion most limited, followed by plantar flexion, adduction, and medial rotation. The first metatarsophalangeal joint has a capsular pattern in which extension is most limited, followed by flexion. The pattern for the second through fifth metatarsophalangeal joints is variable. The capsular pattern of the interphalangeal joints is flexion most limited, followed by extension.

Resisted Isometric Movements

The resisted isometric movements are performed to test the contractile tissue around the foot, ankle, and lower leg. The patient is in the sitting or supine lying position, and the patient's foot is placed in the anatomic position (plantigrade or 90°; Fig. 13–49). Table 13–7 shows the muscles acting over the foot and ankle.

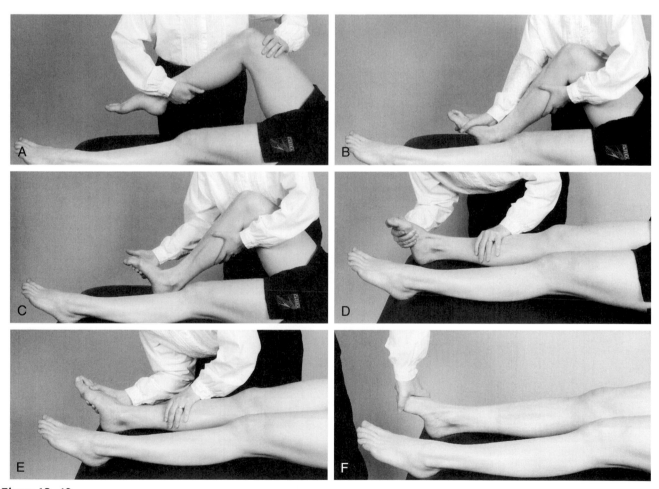

Figure 13–49
Resisted isometric movements of the lower leg, ankle, and foot. (A) Knee flexion. (B) Dorsiflexion. (C) Plantar flexion. (D) Supination. (E) Pronation. (F) Toe extension.

Table 13–7
Muscles of the Lower Limb, Ankle, and Foot: Their Actions, Nerve Supply, and Nerve Root Derivation
(Peripheral Nerves)

Action	Muscles Acting	Nerve Supply	Nerve Root Derivation
Plantar flexion (flexion) of ankle	1. Gastrocnemius*	Tibial	S1–S2
	2. Soleus*	Tibial	S1–S2
	3. Plantaris	Tibial	S1–S2
	4. Flexor digitorum longus	Tibial	S2–S3
	5. Peroneus longus	Superficial peroneal	L5, S1–S2
	6. Peroneus brevis	Superficial peroneal	L5, S1–S2
	7. Flexor hallucis longus	Tibial	S2–S3
	8. Tibialis posterior	Tibial	L4–L5
Dorsiflexion (extension) of ankle	1. Tibialis anterior	Deep peroneal	L4–L5
	2. Extensor digitorum longus	Deep peroneal	L5, S1
	3. Extensor hallucis longus	Deep peroneal	L5, S1
	4. Peroneus tertius	Deep peroneal	L5, S1
Inversion	1. Tibialis posterior	Tibial	L4–L5
	2. Flexor digitorum longus	Tibial	S2–S3
	3. Flexor hallucis longus	Tibial	S2–S3
	4. Tibialis anterior	Deep peroneal	L4–L5
	5. Extensor hallucis longus	Deep peroneal	L5, S1
Eversion	1. Peroneus longus	Superficial peroneal	L5, S1–S2
	2. Peroneus brevis	Superficial peroneal	L5, S1–S2
	3. Peroneus tertius	Deep peroneal	L5, S1
	4. Extensor digitorum longus	Deep peroneal	L5, S1
Flexion of toes	1. Flexor digitorum longus	Tibial	S2–S3
	2. Flexor hallucis longus	Tibial	S2–S3
	3. Flexor digitorum brevis	Tibial (medial plantar branch)	S2–S3
	4. Flexor hallucis brevis	Tibial (medial plantar branch)	S2–S3
	5. Flexor accessorius (Quadratus plantae)	Tibial (lateral plantar branch)	S2–S3
	6. Interossei	Tibial (lateral plantar branch)	S2–S3
	7. Flexor digiti minimi brevis	Tibial (lateral plantar branch)	S2–S3
	8. Lumbricals (metatarsophalangeal joints)	Tibial (1st by medial plantar branch; 2nd through 4th by lateral plantar branch)	S2–S3
Extension of toes	1. Extensor digitorum longus	Deep peroneal	L5, S1
	2. Extensor hallucis longus	Deep peroneal	L5, S1
	3. Extensor digitorum brevis	Deep peroneal (lateral terminal branch)	S1–S2
	4. Lumbricals (interphalangeal joints)	Tibial (1st by medial plantar branch; 2nd through 4th by lateral plantar branch)	S2–S3
Abduction of toes	1. Abductor hallucis	Tibial (medial plantar branch)	S2–S3
	2. Abductor digiti minimi	Tibial (lateral plantar branch)	S2–S3
	3. Dorsal interossei	Tibial (lateral plantar branch)	S2–S3
Adduction of toes	1. Adductor hallucis	Tibial (lateral plantar branch)	S2–S3
	2. Plantar interossei	Tibial (lateral plantar branch)	S2–S3

* The gastrocnemius and soleus muscles are sometimes grouped together as the triceps surae muscles.

Resisted Isometric Movements of the Lower Leg, Ankle, and Foot

- Knee flexion
- Plantar flexion
- Dorsiflexion
- Supination
- Pronation
- Toe extension
- Toe flexion

Dorsiflexion is sometimes tested with the patient's hip flexed to 45° and the knee flexed to 90°, as illustrated in Figure 13–49B. Testing with the patient in this position enables the examiner to exert a greater isometric force. Resisted isometric knee flexion must be performed, because the triceps surae (gastrocnemius and soleus muscles together) act on the knee as well as on the ankle and foot.

If the history has indicated that eccentric, concentric, or econcentric muscle action has caused symptoms, these movements should also be tested, but only after the isometric tests have been completed.

Functional Assessment

If the patient is able to do the movements already described with little difficulty, functional tests may be performed to see whether these sequential activities produce pain or other symptoms. Full range of motion is often not necessary for the patient to lead a functional life.

Functional Activities of the Lower Leg, Ankle, and Foot (in Sequential Order)

- Squatting (both ankles should dorsiflex symmetrically)
- Standing on toes (both ankles should plantar flex symmetrically)
- Squatting and bouncing at the end of a squat
- Standing on one foot at a time
- Standing on the toes, one foot at a time
- Going up and down stairs
- Walking on the toes
- Running straight ahead
- Running, twisting, and cutting
- Jumping
- Jumping and going into a full squat

These activities, which are examples only, must be geared to the individual patient. Older patients should not be expected to do some of the activities unless they have been doing these or similar ones in the recent past (Table 13–8). Because the functional tests place a stress on the other lower limb joints (e.g., knees, hip, sacroiliac, lumbar joints), the examiner must ensure that these joints exhibit no pathology before all of the tests are completed. On the other hand, functional tests for other joints in the lower limb (e.g., hop test for the knee) may not be sensitive enough to test ankle function.[32] As the patient completes the activities, the examiner must assess whether any symptoms (e.g., intermittent claudication or anterior compartment syndrome) occur within a specific time frame.[33, 34]

Range of Motion Necessary at the Foot and Ankle for Selected Locomotion Activities

Descending stairs:	Full dorsiflexion (20°)
Walking:	Dorsiflexion (10°); plantar flexion (20 to 25°)

Balance and proprioception are tested by asking the patient to stand on the unaffected leg and then on the affected leg, first with the eyes open, and then with the

Table 13–8
Functional Testing of the Foot and Ankle

Starting Position	Action	Functional Test
Standing on one leg*	Lift toes and forefeet off ground (dorsiflexion)	10 to 15 Repetitions: Functional 5 to 9 Repetitions: Functionally fair 1 to 4 Repetitions: Functionally poor 0 Repetitions: Nonfunctional
Standing on one leg*	Lift heels off ground (plantar flexion)	10 to 15 Repetitions: Functional 5 to 9 Repetitions: Functionally fair 1 to 4 Repetitions: Functionally poor 0 Repetitions: Nonfunctional
Standing on one leg*	Lift lateral aspect of foot off ground (ankle eversion)	5 to 6 Repetitions: Functional 3 to 4 Repetitions: Functionally fair 1 to 2 Repetitions: Functionally poor 0 Repetitions: Nonfunctional
Standing on one leg*	Lift medial aspect of foot off ground (ankle inversion)	5 to 6 Repetitions: Functional 3 to 4 Repetitions: Functionally fair 1 to 2 Repetitions: Functionally poor 0 Repetitions: Nonfunctional
Seated	Pull small towel up under toes or pick up and release small object (i.e., pencil, marble, cottonball) (toe flexion)	10 to 15 Repetitions: Functional 5 to 9 Repetitions: Functionally fair 1 to 4 Repetitions: Functionally poor 0 Repetitions: Nonfunctional
Seated	Lift toes off ground (toe extension)	10 to 15 Repetitions: Functional 5 to 9 Repetitions: Functionally fair 1 to 4 Repetitions: Functionally poor 0 Repetitions: Nonfunctional

* Hand may hold something for balance only.

Data from Palmer, M.L., and M. Epler: Clinical Assessment Procedures in Physical Therapy. Philadelphia, J.B. Lippincott Co., 1990, pp. 308–310.

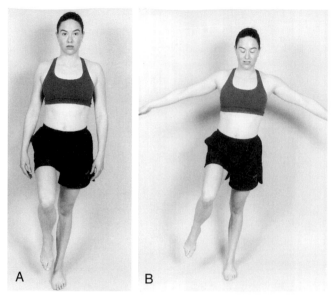

Figure 13–50
Balance and proprioception. (A) One leg, with eyes open. (B) One leg, with eyes closed.

Kaikkonen and colleagues[36] developed a numerical scoring system to evaluate functional outcome after ankle injury (Table 13–9). Other scales have been developed for specific pathologies (e.g., fractures) about the ankle.[37–40]

Special Tests

When assessing the lower leg, ankle, and foot, it is important to always assess the neutral position of the talus in both weight-bearing and non–weight-bearing situations. Other tests that should be carried out include

> **Special Tests Commonly Performed on the Lower Leg, Ankle, and Foot**
>
> * Neutral position of the talus (weight bearing and non–weight bearing)
> * Leg-heel alignment
> * Forefoot-heel alignment
> * Tests for tibial torsion
> * Anterior drawer sign of the ankle
> * Talar tilt
> * Leg length
> * Thompson test

eyes closed. Any differences in balance time or difficulty in balancing give an idea of proprioceptive ability, especially differences that occurred when the patient's eyes were closed (Fig. 13–50).[35]

Table 13–9
Scoring Scale for Subjective and Functional Follow-up Evaluation After Ankle Injury*

I	Subjective assessment of the injured ankle†		VI	Rising on toes with injured leg	
	No symptoms of any kind	15		More than 40 times	10
	Mild symptoms	10		30 to 39 times	5
	Moderate symptoms	5		Fewer than 30 times	0
	Severe symptoms	0	VII	Single-limbed stance with injured leg§	
II	Can you walk normally?			Longer than 55 seconds	10
	Yes	15		50 to 55 seconds	5
	No	0		Less than 50 seconds	0
III	Can you run normally?		VIII	Laxity of the ankle joint (ADS)	
	Yes	10		Stable (≤5 mm)	10
	No	0		Moderate instability (6–10 mm)	5
IV	Climbing down stairs‡			Severe instability (>10 mm)	0
	Less than 18 seconds	10	IX	Dorsiflexion range of motion, injured leg	
	18 to 20 seconds	5		≥10°	10
	Longer than 20 seconds	0		5°–9°	5
V	Rising on heels with injured leg			<5°	0
	More than 40 times	10			
	30 to 39 times	5			
	Fewer than 30 times	0			

* Total: Excellent, 85–100; good, 70–80; fair, 55–65; poor, ≤50.

† Pain, swelling, stiffness, tenderness, or giving way during activity (mild, only 1 of these symptoms is present; moderate, 2 to 3 of these symptoms are present; severe, 4 or more of these symptoms are present).

‡ Two levels of staircase (length, 12 m) with 44 steps (height, 18 cm; depth, 22 cm).

§ On square beam (10 cm × 10 cm × 30 cm).

ADS = anterior drawer sign.

From Kaikkonen, A., P. Kannus, and M. Jarvinen: A performance test protocol and scoring scale for the evaluation of ankle injuries. Am. J. Sports Med. 22:465, 1994.

alignment, functional leg length, and tibial torsion tests. Of the other tests, only those that the examiner wishes to use as confirming tests need be performed.

Tests for Neutral Position of the Talus

The neutral position of the talus is often referred to as the neutral or balanced position of the foot. This "neutral" position is an ideal position that, in reality, is not commonly found in people. For most patients, the subtalar joint is normally in slight valgus, with the forefoot in slight varus and the calcaneus in slight valgus. The tibia is in slight varus,[41] so each joint slightly compensates for the adjacent one. The neutral position is used as a starting position to determine foot and leg deviations. Functional asymmetry may be seen in the lower limb in normal standing; the examiner should then put the talus in the neutral position to see whether the asymmetry remains. If it does, there is **anatomic asymmetry** as well as **functional asymmetry**. If the asymmetry disappears, there is only functional asymmetry, which is often easier to treat.

Neutral Position of the Talus (Weight-Bearing Position). The patient stands with the feet in a relaxed standing position so that the base width and Fick angle are normal for the patient. Usually, only one foot is tested at a time. The examiner palpates the head of the talus on the dorsal aspect of the foot with the thumb and forefinger of one hand (Fig. 13–51). The patient is asked to slowly rotate the trunk to the right and then to the left, which causes the tibia to medially and laterally rotate so that the talus supinates and pronates. If the foot is positioned so that the talar head does not appear to bulge to either side, then the subtalar joint will be in its neutral position in weight bearing.[18]

Neutral Position of the Talus (Supine). The patient lies supine with the feet extending over the end of the exam-

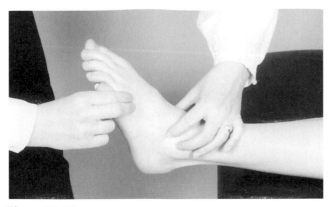

Figure 13–52
Determining the neutral position of the subtalar joint in supine position.

ining table. The examiner grasps the patient's foot over the fourth and fifth metatarsal heads, using the thumb and index finger of one hand. The examiner palpates both sides of the head of the talus on the dorsum of the foot with the thumb and index finger of the other hand (Fig. 13–52). The examiner then gently, passively dorsiflexes the foot until resistance is felt. While the examiner maintains the dorsiflexion, the foot is passively moved through an arc of supination (talar head bulges laterally) and pronation (talar head bulges medially). If the foot is positioned so that the talar head does not appear to bulge to either side, the subtalar joint will be in its neutral non–weight-bearing position.[12, 18, 25, 42]

Neutral Position of the Talus (Prone). The patient lies prone with the foot extended over the end of the examining table (Fig. 13–53). The examiner grasps the patient's

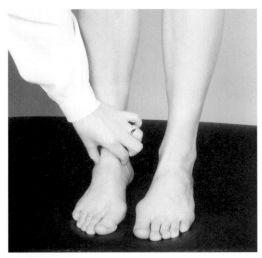

Figure 13–51
Determining the neutral position of the subtalar joint in standing (weight bearing).

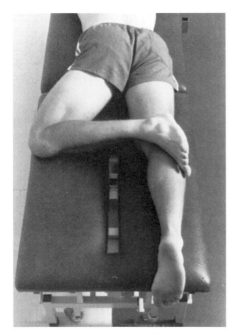

Figure 13–53
Prone lying with legs in figure-four position to assess neutral position of the subtalar joint.

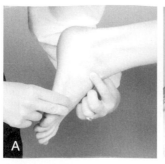
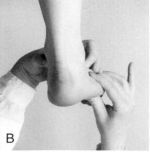

Figure 13–54
Determining the neutral position of the subtalar joints in the prone position. (A) Side view. (B) Superior view.

foot over the fourth and fifth metatarsal heads with the index finger and thumb of one hand. The examiner palpates both sides of the talus on the dorsum of the foot, using the thumb and index finger of the other hand. The examiner then passively and gently dorsiflexes the foot until resistance is felt (Fig. 13–54). While maintaining the dorsiflexed position, the examiner moves the foot back and forth through an arc of supination (talar head bulges laterally) and pronation (talar head bulges medially). As the arc of movement is performed, there is a point in the arc at which the foot appears to "fall off" to one side or the other more easily. This point is the neutral, non–weight-bearing position of the subtalar joint.[12, 18, 25, 42]

Tests for Alignment

Alignment tests are used to determine the relation of the leg to the hindfoot and the relation of the hindfoot to the forefoot. These tests are used to differentiate functional from anatomic (structural) deformities or asymmetries.

Leg-Heel Alignment. The patient lies in the prone position with the foot extending over the end of the examining table. The examiner then places a mark over the midline of the calcaneus at the insertion of the Achilles tendon. The examiner makes a second mark approximately 1 cm distal to the first mark and as close to the midline of the calcaneus as possible. A **calcaneal line** is then made to join the two marks. Next, the examiner makes two marks on the lower third of the leg in the midline. These two marks are joined, forming the **tibial line,** which represents the longitudinal axis of the tibia. The examiner then places the subtalar joint in the prone neutral position. While the subtalar joint is held in neutral, the examiner looks at the two lines. If the lines are parallel or in slight varus (2 to 8°), the leg-to-heel alignment is considered normal.[42] If the heel is inverted, the patient has hindfoot varus; if the heel is everted, the patient has hindfoot valgus (Fig. 13–55).

"Too Many Toes" Sign. The patient stands in a normal relaxed position while the examiner views the patient

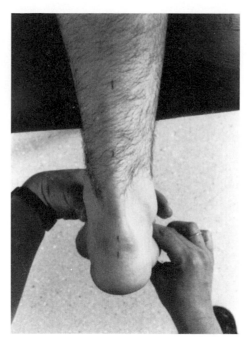

Figure 13–55
Alignment of leg and heel.

from behind. If the heel is in valgus, the forefoot abducted or the tibia laterally rotated more than normal, more toes can be seen on the affected side than on the normal side (Fig. 13–56).[43]

Forefoot-Heel Alignment. The patient lies supine with the feet extending over the end of the examining table. The examiner positions the subtalar joint in supine neutral position. While maintaining this position, the examiner pronates the midtarsal joints maximally and then observes the relation between the vertical axis of the heel and the plane of the second through fourth metatar-

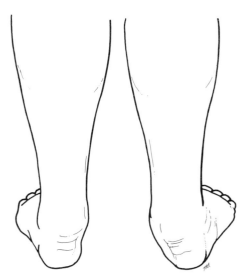

Figure 13–56
"Too-many-toes" sign signifying lateral foot or tibial rotation. Two and one-half toes seen on the left foot, four toes on the abnormal right foot. (From Baxter, D.E. [ed.]: The Foot and Ankle in Sport. St. Louis, C.V. Mosby, 1995, p. 45.)

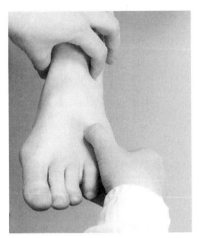

Figure 13-57
Alignment of forefoot and heel (superior view).

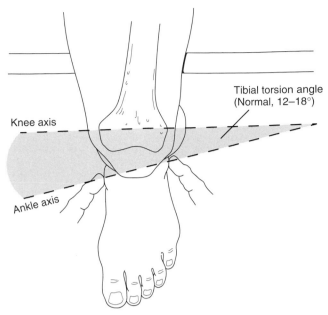

Figure 13-58
Determination of tibial torsion in sitting (superior view). The torsion angle determined by the intersection of the knee axis and the ankle axis. (Modified from Hunt, G.C. [ed]: Physical Therapy of the Foot and Ankle. Clinics in Physical Therapy. New York, Churchill Livingstone, 1988, p. 80.)

sal heads (Fig. 13–57). Normally, the plane is perpendicular to the vertical axis. If the medial side of the foot is raised, the patient has a forefoot varus; if the lateral side of the foot is raised, the patient has a forefoot valgus.[12, 42]

Tests for Tibial Torsion

When testing for tibial torsion, the examiner must realize that some lateral tibial torsion (13 to 18° in adults, less in children) is normally present.[44] If tibial torsion is more than 18°, it is referred to as a toe-out position. If tibial torsion is less than 13°, it is referred to as a toe-in position. Excessive toeing-in is sometimes referred to as pigeon toes and may be caused by medial tibial torsion, medial femoral torsion, or excessive femoral anteversion (see Table 13–2).

Tibial Torsion (Sitting). Tibial torsion is measured by having the patient sit with the knees over the edge of the examining table (Fig. 13–58). The examiner than places the thumb of one hand over the apex of one malleolus and the index finger of the same hand over the apex of the other malleolus. Next, the examiner visualizes the axes of the knee and of the ankle. The lines are not normally parallel but instead form an angle of 12 to 18° owing to lateral rotation of the tibia.[7]

Tibial Torsion (Supine). The patient lies supine. The examiner ensures that the femoral condyle lies in the frontal plane (patella facing straight up). The examiner palpates the apex of both malleoli with one hand and draws a line on the heel representing a line joining the two apices. A second line is drawn on the heel parallel to the floor. The angle formed by the intersection of the two lines indicates the amount of lateral tibial torsion.

Tibial Torsion (Prone). The patient lies prone with the knee flexed to 90°. The examiner views from above the angle formed by the foot and thigh (Fig. 13–59) after the subtalar joint has been placed in the neutral position, noting the angle the foot makes with the tibia.[45] This

method is most often used in children because it is easier to observe the feet from above.

Tests for Ligamentous Instability

Anterior Drawer Test of the Ankle. This test is designed primarily to test for injuries to the anterior talofibular ligament, the most frequently injured ligament in the

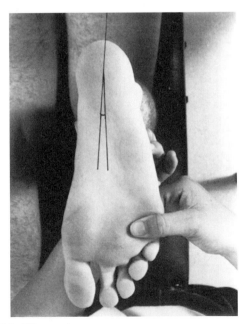

Figure 13-59
Measurement of tibial torsion in the prone position.

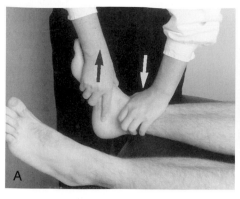
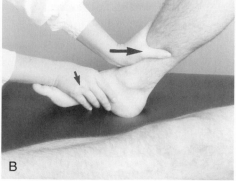

Figure 13–60
Anterior drawer test. (A) Method 1—drawing the foot forward. (B) Method 2—pushing the leg back.

ankle.[46, 47] The patient lies supine with the foot relaxed. The examiner stabilizes the tibia and fibula, holds the patient's foot in 20° of plantar flexion, and draws the talus forward in the ankle mortise (Fig. 13–60).[48, 49] Sometimes, a dimple appears over the area of the anterior

talofibular ligament on anterior translation (**dimple or suction sign**) if pain and muscle spasm are minimal.[50, 51] In the plantar-flexed position, the anterior talofibular ligament is perpendicular to the long axis of the tibia. By adding inversion, which gives an anterolateral stress, the examiner can increase the stress on the anterior talofibular ligament and the calcaneofibular ligament. A positive anterior drawer test may be obtained with a tear of only the anterior tibiofibular ligament, but anterior translation is greater if both ligaments are torn, especially if the foot is tested in dorsiflexion.[52] If straight

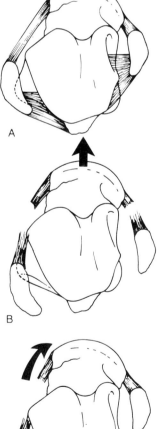

Figure 13–61
Anterior drawer test. (A) Normal relation between talus and malleoli. (B) Straight anterior translation (one-plane anterior instability). (C) Lateral rotary translation (anterolateral rotary instability).

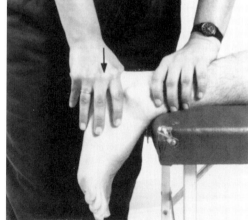

Figure 13–62
Prone anterior drawer test.

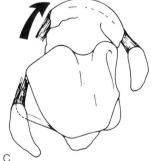

Figure 13–63
Talar tilt test.

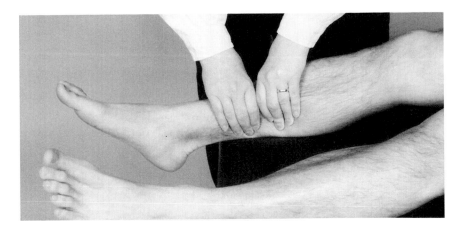

Figure 13–64
Squeeze test for stress fracture or ankle syndesmosis pathology.

anterior movement or translation occurs (Fig. 13–61B), the test indicates both medial and lateral ligament insufficiencies. This bilateral finding, which is often more evident in dorsiflexion, means that the superficial and deep deltoid ligaments, as well as the anterior talofibular ligament and anterolateral capsule, have been torn. If the tear is on only one side, only that side would translate forward. For example, with a lateral tear, the lateral side would translate forward, causing medial rotation of the talus and resulting in anterolateral rotary instability (Fig. 13–61C), which is increasingly evident with increasing plantar flexion of the foot.[11, 13, 53–55]

Ideally, the knee should be placed in 90° of flexion to alleviate tension on the Achilles tendon. The test should be performed in plantar flexion and in dorsiflexion to test for straight and rotational instabilities.

The test may also be performed by stabilizing the foot and talus and pushing the tibia and fibula posteriorly on the talus (see Fig. 13–60B). In this case, excessive posterior movement of the tibia and fibula on the talus indicates a positive test.

Prone Anterior Drawer Test.[56] The patient lies prone with the feet extending over the end of the examining table. With one hand, the examiner pushes the heel steadily forward (Fig. 13–62). A positive sign is indicated by excessive anterior movement and a "sucking in" of the skin on both sides of the Achilles tendon. The test, like the previous one, is indicative of ligamentous instability.

Talar Tilt. The patient lies in the supine or side lying position with the foot relaxed (Fig. 13–63).[11, 57] The patient's gastrocnemius muscle may be relaxed by flexion of the knee. This test is used to determine whether the calcaneofibular ligament is torn.[47, 52] The normal side is tested first for comparison. The foot is held in the anatomic position, which brings the calcaneofibular ligament perpendicular to the long axis of the talus. The talus is then tilted from side to side into adduction and abduction. Adduction tests the calcaneofibular ligament and, to some degree, the anterior talofibular ligament by increasing the stress on the ligament.[6] Abduction stresses the deltoid ligament, primarily the tibionavicular, tibiocalcaneal, and posterior tibiotalar ligaments. On

a radiograph, the talar tilt may be measured by obtaining the angle between the distal aspect of the tibia and the proximal surface of the talus (see later discussion of stress radiographs).

Squeeze Test of the Leg. The patient lies supine. The examiner grasps the lower leg at midcalf and squeezes the tibia and fibula together (Fig. 13–64). Pain in the lower leg may indicate a syndesmosis injury, provided that fracture, contusion, and compartment syndrome have been ruled out.[4, 58]

Kleiger Test. The patient sits with the knee flexed to 90° and the foot relaxed and not weight bearing. The examiner gently grasps the foot and rotates it laterally (Fig. 13–65).[3, 13] If the Kleiger test is positive, the patient

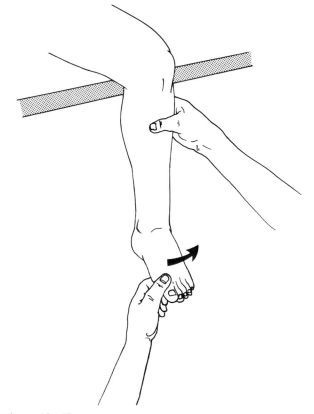

Figure 13–65
Kleiger test.

has pain medially and laterally, and the examiner may feel the talus displace from the medial malleolus, indicating a tear of the deltoid ligament. On a stress radiograph, the medial clear space is increased, suggesting rupture of the ligament (see later discussion) if the lateral malleolus is intact.

Other Tests

Functional Leg Length.[59] The patient stands in the normal relaxed stance (Fig. 13–66). The examiner palpates the anterior superior iliac spines and then the posterior superior iliac spines and notes any differences. The examiner then positions the patient so that the patient's subtalar joints are in neutral position while weight bearing. The patient maintains this position with the toes straight ahead and the knees straight, and the examiner repalpates the anterior and the posterior superior iliac spines. If the previously noted differences remain, the pelvis and sacroiliac joints should be evaluated further. If the previously noted differences disappear, the examiner should suspect a functional leg length difference resulting from hip, knee, or ankle and foot problems—primarily, ankle and foot problems (Tables 13–10 and 13–11). The examiner must then determine what is causing the difference. For example, foot pronation is often seen with forefoot or hindfoot varus, tibial varus, tight

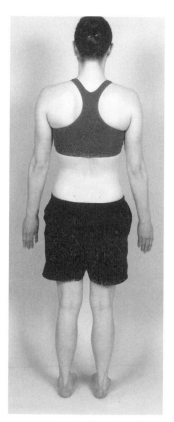

Figure 13–66
Functional leg length in standing position (subtalar joint in neutral). Dots on back indicate posterior superior iliac spines.

Table 13–10
Functional Limb Length Difference

Joint	Functional Lengthening	Functional Shortening
Foot	Supination	Pronation
Knee	Extension	Flexion
Hip	Lowering Extension Lateral rotation	Lifting Flexion Medial rotation
Sacroiliac	Anterior rotation	Posterior rotation

Modified from Wallace, L.A.: Lower quarter pain: Mechanical evaluation and treatment. *In* Grieve, G.P. (ed.): Modern Manual Therapy of the Vertebral Column. Edinburgh, Churchill Livingstone, 1986, p. 467.

muscles (e.g., calf, hamstrings, hip flexors), or weak muscles (e.g., ankle invertors, piriformis).

Thompson's (Simmonds') Test (Sign for Achilles Tendon Rupture). The patient lies prone or kneels on a chair with the feet over the edge of the table or chair (Fig. 13–67). While the patient is relaxed, the examiner squeezes the calf muscles. A positive test is indicated by the absence of plantar flexion when the muscle is squeezed and is indicative of a ruptured Achilles tendon (third-degree strain).[60–63] One should be careful not to assume that the Achilles tendon is not ruptured if the patient is able to plantar flex the foot while not bearing weight. The long flexor muscles can perform this function in the non–weight-bearing stance even with a rupture of the Achilles tendon.

Swing Test for Posterior Tibiotalar Subluxation.[64] The patient sits with feet dangling over the edge of the examining table (Fig. 13–68). The examiner holds the plantar aspect of the patient's feet and uses the fingers to keep the feet parallel to the floor. With the thumbs, the examiner palpates the anterior portion of the talus. The examiner then passively plantar flexes and dorsiflexes the foot and compares the quality and degree of movement between feet, especially into dorsiflexion. If resistance to normal dorsiflexion is felt in the injured ankle, it is indicative of a positive test for posterior tibiotalar subluxation.

Feiss Line.[12] The examiner marks the apex of the medial malleolus and the plantar aspect of the first metatarsophalangeal joint while the patient is not bearing weight. The examiner then palpates the navicular tuberosity on the lateral aspect of the foot, noting where it lies relative to a line joining the two previously made points. The patient then stands with the feet 8 to 15 cm (3 to 6 inches) apart. The two points are checked to ensure that they still represent the apex of the medial malleolus and the plantar aspect of the metatarsophalanageal joint. The navicular tuberosity is again palpated (Fig. 13–69). The navicular tuberosity normally lies on

Table 13–11
Dynamic Limb Length Evaluation

Asymmetric Shoe Wear	Asymmetric Callus	Asymmetric Posture	Asymmetric Alignment or Movement
Shoe upper	Medial first distal interphalangeal	Foot	Toe-out
Heel counter	Medial first metatarsal	Ankle	Toe grasp
Varus or valgus	Second and third metatarsal	Knee	Patellar alignment over foot
	heads	Hip	Knee flexion
Shoe sole	Fourth and fifth metatarsal heads	Pelvis	Hip drop
Posterior lateral heel	Calcaneus		Propulsion
Posterior central heel	Lateral		
Posterior medial heel	Central		
	Medial		

Modified from Wallace, L.A.: Limb length difference and back pain. In Grieve, G.P. (ed.): Modern Manual Therapy of the Vertebral Column. Edinburgh, Churchill Livingstone, 1986, p. 469.

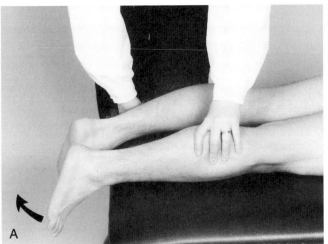
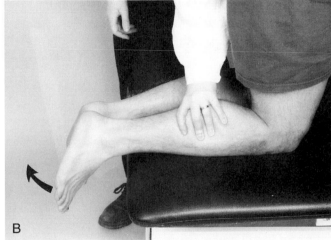

Figure 13–67
Thompson's test for Achilles tendon rupture. (A) Prone lying position. (B) Kneeling position. In each case, foot plantar flexes (*arrow*) if test result is negative.

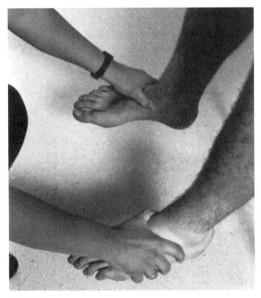

Figure 13–68
Swing test for posterior tibiotalar subluxation.

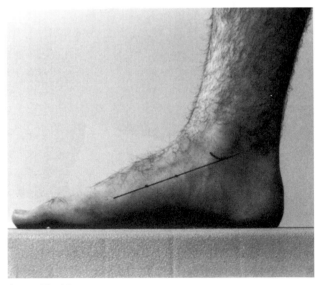

Figure 13–69
Feiss line in weight bearing. Navicular tuberosity is in normal position.

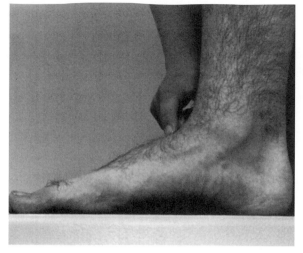

A

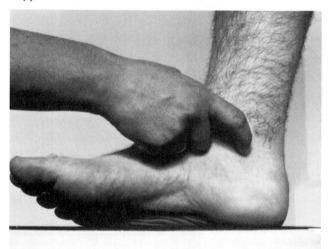

B

Figure 13–70

Tinel's sign. (A) Anterior tibial branch of deep peroneal nerve. (B) Posterior tibial nerve.

or very close to the line joining the two points. If the tuberosity falls one third of the distance to the floor, it represents a first-degree flatfoot; if it falls two thirds of the distance, it represents a second-degree flatfoot; and if it rests on the floor, it represents a third-degree flatfoot.

Hoffa's Test. The patient lies prone with the feet extended over the edge of the examining table. The examiner palpates the Achilles tendon while the patient plantar flexes and dorsiflexes the foot. If one Achilles tendon (the injured one) feels less taut than the other one, the test is considered positive for a calcaneal fracture. Passive dorsiflexion on the affected side is also greater.

Tinel's Sign at the Ankle (Percussion Sign). Tinel's sign may be elicited in two places around the ankle. The anterior tibial branch of the deep peroneal nerve may be percussed in front of the ankle (Fig. 13–70A). The posterior tibial nerve may be percussed as it passes behind the medial malleolus (Fig. 13–70B). In both cases, tingling or paresthesia felt distally is a positive sign.

Duchenne Test.[14] The patient lies supine with the legs straight. The examiner pushes up on the head of the first metatarsal through the sole, pushing the foot into dorsiflexion. The test is positive for a lesion of the superficial peroneal nerve or a lesion of L4, L5, or S1 if, when the patient is asked to plantar flex the foot, the medial border dorsiflexes and offers no resistance while the lateral border plantar flexes.

Morton's Test.[14] The patient lies supine. The examiner grasps the foot around the metatarsal heads and squeezes the heads together. Pain is a positive sign for stress fracture or neuroma.

Homans' Sign. The patient's foot is passively dorsiflexed with the knee extended. Pain in the calf indicates a positive Homans' sign for deep vein thrombophlebitis (Fig. 13–71). Tenderness is also elicited on palpation of the calf. In addition to these findings, the examiner may

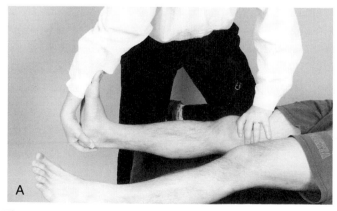

A

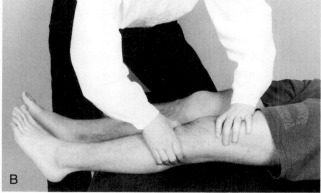

B

Figure 13–71

Homans' sign for thrombophlebitis. (A) Test. (B) Palpation for tenderness in thrombophlebitis.

find pallor and swelling in the leg and a loss of the dorsalis pedis pulse.

Buerger's Test. This test is designed to test the arterial blood supply to the lower limb.[14] The patient lies supine while the examiner elevates the patient's leg to 45° for at least 3 minutes. If the foot blanches or the prominent veins collapse shortly after elevation, the test is positive for poor arterial blood circulation. The patient is then asked to sit with the legs dangling over the edge of the bed. If it takes 1 to 2 minutes for the limb color to be restored and the veins to fill and become prominent, the test is confirmed positive.

Reflexes and Cutaneous Distribution

The examiner must be aware of the sensory distribution of the various peripheral nerves in the foot (especially the superficial peroneal, deep peroneal, and saphenous) and the branches of the tibial nerve (sural, medial calcaneal, medial plantar, and lateral plantar; Fig. 13–72).

The examiner must also differentiate between the peripheral nerve sensory distribution and the sensory nerve root distribution or dermatomes (Fig. 13–73). Although dermatomes vary among individuals, their pattern is never identical to the peripheral nerve distribution, which tends to be more consistent among patients.

The patient's sensation should be tested by the examiner's running his or her hands over the anterior, lateral, medial, and posterior surfaces of the patient's leg below the knee, foot, and toes (sensation scanning examination). Any difference in sensation should be noted and can be mapped out in more detail with a pinwheel, pin, cotton batten, and/or brush.

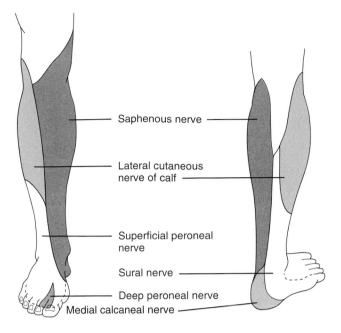

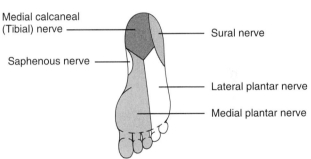

Figure 13–72
Peripheral nerve distribution in the lower leg, ankle, and foot.

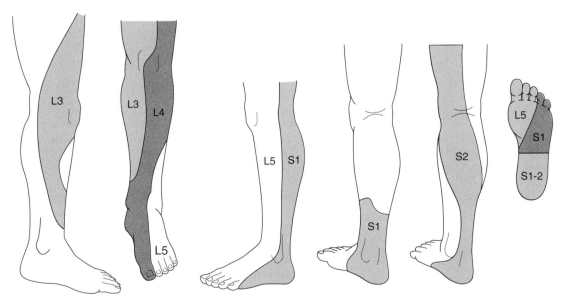

Figure 13–73
Dermatomes of the lower leg, ankle, and foot.

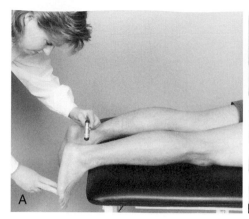
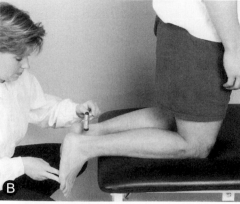

Figure 13–74
Test of Achilles reflex (S1–S2).
(A) Prone lying. (B) Kneeling.

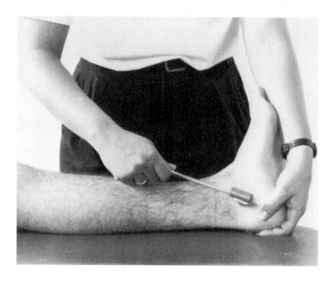

Figure 13–75
Tibialis posterior reflex.

The examiner must test the patient's reflexes. Commonly checked in this region is the Achilles reflex[65] (S1–S2; Fig. 13–74) and the posterior tibial reflex (L4–L5; Fig. 13–75). The examiner may also wish to test for pyramidal tract (upper motor neuron) disease. There are various methods for testing the pathological reflexes, including the Babinski, Chaddock, Oppenheim, and Gordon reflexes (Fig. 13–76). A positive sign in all of these tests is extension of the big toe. The Babinski reflex also causes

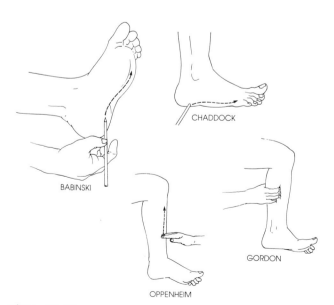

Figure 13–76
Pathological reflexes for pyramidal tract disease.

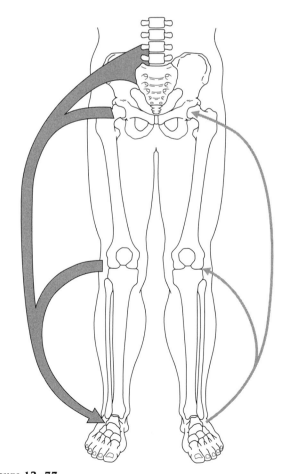

Figure 13–77
Pattern of referred pain to and from the ankle.

Table 13–12
Muscles of the Lower Leg, Ankle, and Foot and Referral of Pain

Muscle	Referral Pattern
Tibialis anterior	Anterior lower leg, medial dorsum of foot to hallux
Peroneus longus	Superolateral aspect of lower leg
Peroneus brevis	Lower lateral leg, over lateral malleolus and lateral aspect of foot
Peroneus tertius	Lower lateral leg, anterior to lateral malleolus and onto dorsum of foot, or behind lateral malleolus to lateral heel
Gastrocnemius	Behind knee, posterior leg to instep of foot
Soleus	Posterior leg to heel and sometimes to sole of foot
Plantaris	Posterior knee to upper half of posterior leg
Tibialis posterior	Posterior leg, Achilles tendon, heel and sole of foot
Extensor digitorum longus	Anterolateral leg to dorsum of foot
Extensor hallucis longus	Anterior leg to dorsomedial foot
Flexor digitorum longus	Posteromedial leg, over medial malleolus, distal sole of foot
Flexor hallucis longus	Plantar aspect of hallux
Extensor digitorum brevis and extensor hallucis brevis	Dorsum of foot
Abductor hallucis	Medial heel and instep
Abductor digiti minimi	Sole of foot over fifth metatarsal
Flexor digitorum brevis	Over metatarsal head
Quadratus plantae (flexor accessorius)	Plantar aspect of heel
Adductor hallucis	Sole of foot over metatarsals
Flexor hallucis brevis	Dorsal and plantar aspect of first metatarsal and hallux
Interossei	Dorsum and plantar aspect of equivalent metatarsal and toe

fanning of the second through fifth toes. The most common and reliable test is the Babinski test.[66]

The examiner must remember that pain may be referred to the lower leg, ankle, or foot from the lumbar spine, sacrum, hip, or knee (Fig. 13–77). Conversely, pain from a lesion in the lower leg, ankle, or foot may be transmitted to the hip or knee. Table 13–12 shows the muscles of the lower leg, ankle, and foot, and their patterns of pain referral.

Peripheral Nerve Injuries of the Lower Leg, Ankle, and Foot

Deep Peroneal Nerve (L4 through S2). The deep peroneal nerve, a branch of the common peroneal nerve, which is itself a branch of the sciatic nerve (Fig. 13–78), is most commonly injured (compressed) in **anterior compartment syndrome** in the leg, and where it passes under the extensor retinaculum (**anterior tarsal tunnel syndrome**).[67–72] Compression may be caused by trauma, tight shoelaces, a ganglion, or pes cavus.[69] Motor loss (Table 13–13) includes an inability to dorsiflex the foot (**drop foot**), which results in a steppage gait, and an inability to control ankle movement. Because the deep peroneal nerve is primarily motor, there is minimal sensory loss, but this loss can be aggravating, especially in anterior tarsal tunnel syndrome (see Fig. 13–78). The sensory loss is a small triangular area between the first and

second toes. Pain is often accentuated by plantar flexion.[69] With the tunnel syndrome, muscle weakness is minimal (extensor digitorum brevis); there is burning pain between the first and second toes that is sometimes referred to the dorsum of the foot.

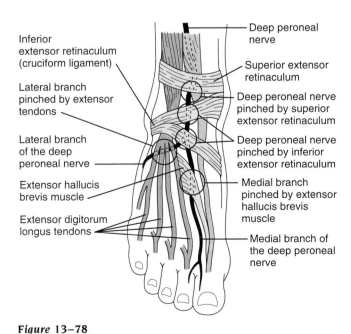

Figure 13–78
Compression of deep peroneal nerve by the extensor retinaculum or other structures.

Table 13–13
Peripheral Nerve Injuries (Neuropathy) of the Lower Leg, Ankle, and Foot

Nerve	Muscle Weakness	Sensory Alteration	Reflexes Affected
Deep peroneal nerve (L4 through S2)	Tibialis anterior Extensor digitorum longus Extensor digitorum brevis Extensor hallucis longus Peroneus tertius	Triangular area between the first and second toes	None
Superficial peroneal nerve (L4 through S2)	Peroneus longus Peroneus brevis	Lateral aspect of leg and dorsum of foot	None
Tibial nerve (L4 through S3)	Gastrocnemius Soleus Plantaris Tibialis posterior Flexor digitorum longus Flexor hallucis longus Flexor accessorius (quadratus plantae) Abductor digiti minimi Flexor digiti minimi Lumbricals Interossei Adductor hallucis Abductor hallucis Flexor digitorum brevis Flexor hallucis brevis	Sole of foot except medial border, plantar surface of toes	Achilles (S1–S2) Tibialis posterior (L4–L5)

Superficial Peroneal Nerve (L4 through S2). Injuries to the superficial peroneal nerve, a branch of the common peroneal nerve (Fig. 13–79), are rare but they have been reported to be associated with lateral ankle (inversion) sprains causing stretching of the nerve, or the nerve may be entrapped as it pierces the deep fascia to become subcutaneous about 10 to 13 cm (4 to 5 inches) above the lateral malleolus (Fig. 13–80).[31, 68, 71–76] Motor loss with the high lesion near the head of the fibula is primarily loss of foot eversion and loss of ankle stability. With both lesions, the sensory loss is the same. The superficial peroneal nerve has a greater sensory role than the deep

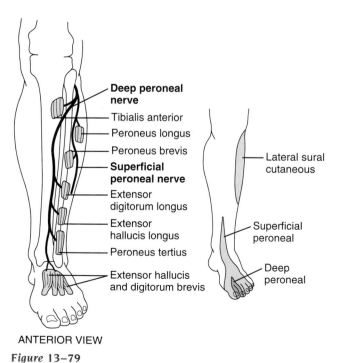

Deep peroneal nerve
— Tibialis anterior
— Peroneus longus
— Peroneus brevis
— **Superficial peroneal nerve**
— Extensor digitorum longus
— Extensor hallucis longus
— Peroneus tertius
— Extensor hallucis and digitorum brevis

— Lateral sural cutaneous
— Superficial peroneal
— Deep peroneal

ANTERIOR VIEW

Figure 13–79
Common peroneal nerve and its branches, the superficial and deep peroneal nerves.

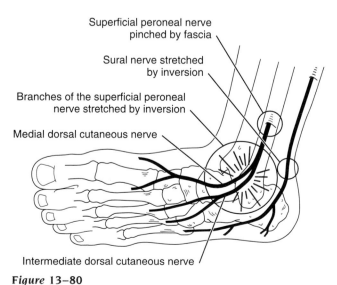

Superficial peroneal nerve pinched by fascia

Sural nerve stretched by inversion

Branches of the superficial peroneal nerve stretched by inversion

Medial dorsal cutaneous nerve

Intermediate dorsal cutaneous nerve

Figure 13–80
Stretching of the superficial peroneal nerve as a result of inversion of ankle.

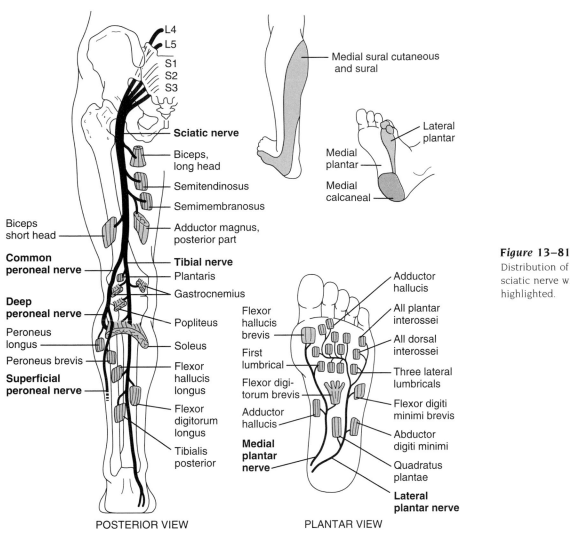

POSTERIOR VIEW   PLANTAR VIEW

Figure 13–81

Distribution of the branches of the sciatic nerve with tibial nerve highlighted.

branch; it supplies the lateral side of the leg and dorsum of the foot (see Fig. 13–79). This sensory alteration is often greater with activity. If the examiner plantar flexes and everts the foot while applying pressure over the distal site, symptoms usually result.[77]

Tibial Nerve (L4 through S3). The tibial nerve, a branch of the sciatic nerve (Fig. 13–81), has a major role to play in the lower leg, ankle, and foot because it supplies all the muscles in the posterior leg and on the sole of the foot. The nerve may be injured in the popliteal area at the knee from trauma (e.g., dislocation, blow) or from entrapment as it passes over the popliteus and under the soleus. **Popliteal entrapment syndrome** or injury may accompany an ankle sprain.[74] At the ankle, the nerve may be compressed as it passes through the tarsal tunnel, which is formed by the medial malleolus, calcaneus, and talus on one side and the deltoid ligament (primarily the tibiocalcanean ligament) on the other. This compression is referred to as **tarsal tunnel syndrome** (Fig. 13–82).[68]

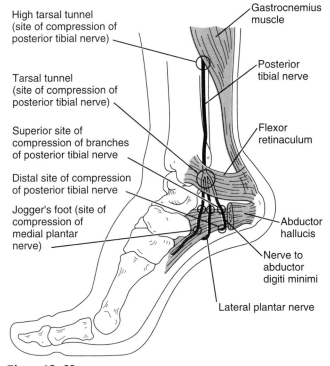

Figure 13–82

Tarsal tunnel syndrome.

Injury to the nerve at the knee causes a major functional disability. Functionally, the patient is unable to plantar flex and invert the foot, which has a major effect on gait. In addition, the patient is unable to flex, abduct, or adduct the toes. Sensory loss involves primarily the sole of the foot, lateral surface of the heel, and plantar surfaces of the toes. With popliteal entrapment syndrome, the popliteal artery is often compressed with the nerve, leading to vascular symptoms (e.g., numbness, tingling, intermittent cramping, weakened dorsalis pedis pulse) and neurological signs.

Compression in the tarsal tunnel may be caused by swelling after trauma, a space-occupying lesion (e.g., ganglion), inflammation (e.g., tendinitis), valgus deformity, or chronic inversion.[29, 70-72, 78-85] Sammarco and associates[86] reported the possibility of **double crush injury** in the lower limb involving the sciatic nerve (L4 through S3) and one of its branches. The examiner must always keep this possibility in mind when assessing for nerve pathology in the lower limb, especially in patients who do not appear to be recovering. Pain and paresthesia into the sole of the foot are often present and are worse after long periods of standing or walking or at night.[68] The pain may be localized or may radiate over the medial side of the ankle distal to the medial malleolus. The condition is sometimes misdiagnosed as plantar fasciitis (Table 13-14).[87] In long-standing cases, motor weakness may become evident in the muscles of the sole of the foot that are supplied by the terminal branches of the tibial nerve (i.e., the medial and lateral plantar nerves).

The **sural nerve** (L5 through S2) is a sensory branch of the tibial nerve supplying the skin on the posterolateral aspect of the lower one third of the leg and the lateral aspect of the foot. The **medial plantar nerve** (Fig. 13-83), another branch of the tibial nerve that is found

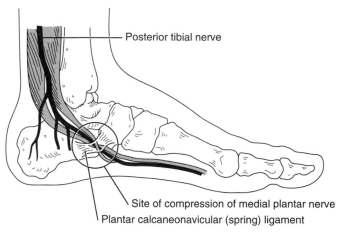

Figure 13–83
Jogger's foot (entrapment of the medial plantar nerve).

in the foot, may be entrapped in the longitudinal arch, causing aching in the arch, burning pain in the heel, and altered sensation in the sole of the foot behind the hallux. This condition is associated with hindfoot valgus and may be referred to as **jogger's foot**.[68, 72, 88, 89]

Similarly, the lateral plantar nerve may be entrapped between the deep fascia of the abductor hallucis and the quadratus plantae (flexor accessorius) muscles (Fig. 13-84).[68, 90] The patient complains of chronic, dull, aching heel pain that is accentuated by walking and running. There is no complaint of numbness. The condition is accentuated by excessive foot pronation.[90]

Sural Nerve. This nerve is a sensory branch of the tibial nerve supplying the lateral heel, foot, and posterolateral leg. Injury can result from a blow, trauma (e.g.,

Table 13–14
Differential Diagnosis of Plantar Fasciitis and Tarsal Tunnel Syndrome

	Plantar Fasciitis	**Tarsal Tunnel Syndrome**
Cause	Overuse	Trauma, space occupying lesion, inflammation, inversion, pronation, valgus deformity
Pain	Plantar aspect of foot, anterior calcaneus Worse with walking, running, and in the morning (sometimes improves with activity)	Medial heel and medial longitudinal arch Worse with standing, walking, and at night
Electrodiagnosis	Normal	Prolonged motor and sensory latencies
Active movements	Full range of motion	Full range of motion
Passive movements	Full range of motion	May have pain on pronation
Resisted isometric movements	Normal	Weakness of foot intrinsics may be present
Sensory deficits	No	Possible
Reflexes	Normal	Normal

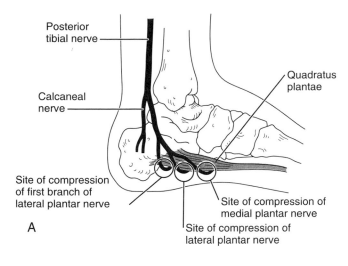

A

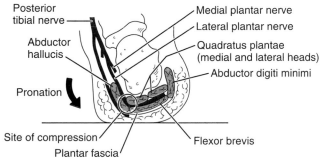

B

Figure 13–84

Entrapment of the lateral plantar nerve as it changes direction. (A) Medial view. (B) Posterior view.

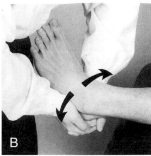

Figure 13–86

Joint play movements at the subtalar joint. (A) Talar rock with slight traction applied (*black arrow*). Talus is rocked anterior and posteriorly (*open arrows*). (B) Side tilt.

fracture), or stretching (e.g., accompanying an ankle sprain).[29, 71, 85] Shooting pain and paresthesia in its sensory distribution are diagnostic signs.[68]

Saphenous Nerve. This nerve is a sensory branch of the femoral nerve. If it is injured, sensation on the medial side of the leg and foot is affected.[91] More details are given in Chapter 12.

Joint Play Movements

The joint play movements (Figs. 13–85 through 13–88) are performed with the patient in the supine or side lying position, depending on which movement is being performed. A comparison of movement between the normal or unaffected side and the injured side should be made.

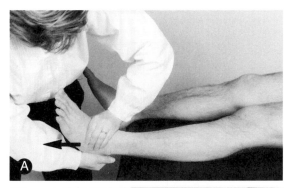

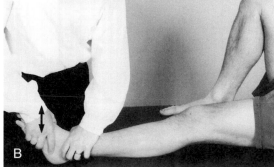

Figure 13–85

Joint play movements at the talocrural joint. (A) Long-axis extension. (B) Anteroposterior glide at the talocrural joint.

Joint Play Movements of the Lower Leg, Ankle, and Foot	
Talocrural (ankle joint)	• Long-axis extension (traction) • Anteroposterior glide
Subtalar joint	• Talar rock • Side tilt medially and laterally
Midtarsal joints	• Anteroposterior glide • Rotation
Tarsometatarsal joints	• Anteroposterior glide • Rotation
Metatarsophalangeal and interphalangeal joints	• Long-axis extension (traction) • Anteroposterior glide • Lateral or side glide • Rotation

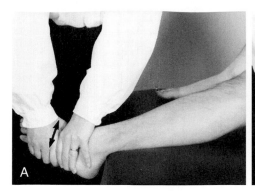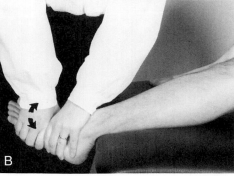

Figure 13–87
Joint play movements in the midtarsal and tarsometatarsal joints. (A) Anteroposterior glide. (B) Rotation.

Long-Axis Extension

Long-axis extension is performed by stabilizing the proximal segment and applying traction to the distal segment. For example, at the ankle, the examiner stabilizes the tibia and fibula by using a strap, or just allows the leg to relax. Both hands are then placed around the ankle, distal to the malleoli, and a distractive force is applied. At the metatarsophalangeal and interphalangeal joints, the examiner stabilizes the metatarsal bone or proximal phalanx and applies a distractive force to the proximal or distal phalanx, respectively.

Anteroposterior Glide

Anteroposterior glide at the ankle joint is performed by stabilizing the tibia and fibula and drawing the talus

and foot forward. To test the posterior movement, the examiner pushes the talus and foot back on the tibia and fibula. There is a difference in the arc of movement between the two actions in tests of joint play. During the anterior movement, the foot should move in an arc into plantar flexion; during the posterior movement, the foot should move in an arc into dorsiflexion. Although similar to the anterior drawer test, the movements are not the same.

Anteroposterior glide at the midtarsal and tarsometatarsal joints is performed in a fashion similar to that used to test the carpal bones at the wrist. For the midtarsal joints, the examiner stabilizes the navicular, talus, and calcaneus with one hand. The other hand is placed around the distal row of tarsal bones (cuneiforms and cuboid). If the hands are positioned properly, they should touch each other, as in Figure 13–87. An antero-

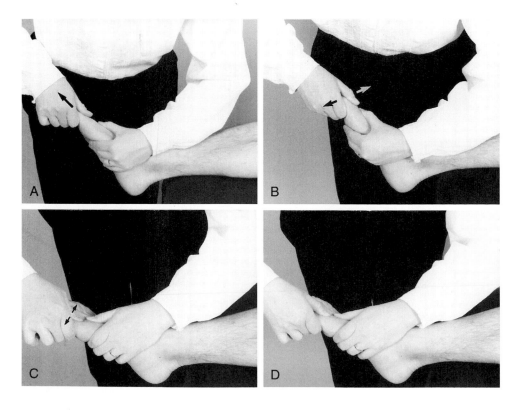

Figure 13–88
Joint play movements at the metatarsophalangeal and interphalangeal joints. (A) Long-axis extension. (B) Anteroposterior glide. (C) Side glide. (D) Rotation.

posterior gliding movement of the distal row of tarsal bones is applied while the proximal row of tarsal bones is stabilized. The examiner's hands are then moved distally so that the stabilizing hand rests over the distal row of tarsal bones and the mobilizing hand rests over the proximal aspect of the metatarsal bones. Again, the hands should be positioned so that they touch each other. An anteroposterior gliding movement of the metatarsal bones is applied while the distal row of tarsal bones is stabilized.

Anteroposterior glide of the metatarsophalangeal and interphalangeal joints is performed by stabilizing the proximal bone (metatarsal or phalanx) and moving the distal bone (phalanx) in an anteroposterior gliding motion in relation to the stabilized bone.

Talar Rock ~~sub talar~~

Talar rock is the only joint play movement performed with the patient in the side lying position.[57] Both the hip and knee are flexed. The examiner sits with his or her back to the patient, as illustrated in Figure 13–86A, and places both hands around the ankle just distal to the malleoli. A slight distractive force is applied to the ankle, and a rocking movement forward and backward (plantar flexion–dorsiflexion) is applied to the foot. Normally, the examiner should feel a "clunk" at the extreme of each movement. As with all joint play movements, the movement is compared with that of the unaffected side.

Side Tilt ~~subtalar~~

Side tilt at the subtalar joint is performed by placing both hands around the calcaneus (see Fig. 13–86B). The wrists are flexed and extended, tilting the calcaneus medially and laterally on the talus. The examiner keeps the patient's foot in the anatomic position while performing the movement. The movement is identical to that used to test the calcaneofibular ligament in the talar tilt test.

Rotation ~~midtarsal~~

Rotation at the midtarsal joints is performed in a similar fashion to the anteroposterior glide at these joints. The proximal row of tarsal bones (navicular, calcaneus, and talus) is stabilized, and the mobilizing hand is placed around the distal tarsal bones (cuneiforms and cuboid). The distal row of bones is then rotated on the proximal row of bones. Rotation at the tarsometatarsal joints is performed in a similar fashion.

Rotation at the metatarsophalangeal and interphalangeal joints is performed by stabilizing the proximal bone with one hand, applying slight traction, and rotating the distal bone with the other hand.

Side Glide

Side glide at the metatarsophalangeal and interphalangeal joints is performed by stabilizing the proximal bone with one hand. The examiner then uses the other hand to apply slight traction to the distal bone and moves the distal bone sideways (right and left) in relation to the stabilized bone without causing torsion motion at the joint.

Tests for Tarsal Bone Mobility

In addition to testing of the tarsal bones as a group, the bones should be tested individually, especially if symptoms resulted from group testing. The examiner may test these individual bones using whatever method is desired. An example of individual tarsal bone testing was put forward by Kaltenborn,[92] who advocates "10 tests" to determine the mobility of the tarsal bones.

Kaltenborn's 10 Tests for Tarsal Mobility

1. Fixate the second and third cuneiforms and mobilize the second metatarsal bone.
2. Fixate the second and third cuneiform bones and mobilize the third metatarsal bone.
3. Fixate the first cuneiform bone and mobilize the first metatarsal bone.
4. Fixate the navicular bone and mobilize the first, second, and third cuneiform bones.
5. Fixate the talus and mobilize the navicular bone.
6. Fixate the cuboid bone and mobilize the fourth and fifth metatarsal bones.
7. Fixate the navicular and third cuneiform bones and mobilize the cuboid bone.
8. Fixate the calcaneus and mobilize the cuboid bone.
9. Fixate the talus and mobilize the calcaneus.
10. Fixate the talus and mobilize the tibia and fibula.

Palpation

The examiner palpates for any swelling, noting whether it is intracapsular or extracapsular. Extracapsular swelling around the ankle is indicated by swelling on only one side of the Achilles tendon, whereas intracapsular swelling is indicated by swelling on both sides (see Fig. 13–11). Pitting edema, if present, should be noted. If swelling is present at the end of the day and absent after a night of recumbency, venous insufficiency, caused by a weakening or insufficiency of the action of the muscle pump of the lower leg muscles, may be implied. Swelling in the ankle may persist for many weeks after injury as a result of this insufficiency.

The examiner should also notice the texture of the skin and nails. It must be remembered that the skin of an ischemic foot shows a loss of hair and becomes thin and very inelastic. In addition, the nails become coarse, thickened, and irregular. Many of the nail changes seen in the hand in the presence of systemic disease are also seen in the foot (see Chapter 7). With poor circulation, the foot will also feel colder. The foot is palpated in the non–weight-bearing and long leg sitting or supine positions. The following structures, including the joints between them, should be palpated.

Palpation Anteriorly and Anteromedially

Toes and Metatarsal, Cuneiform, and Navicular Bones. Starting on the medial side, the great toe and its two phalanges are easily palpated. Moving proximally, the examiner comes to the first metatarsal bone (Fig. 13–89). The head of the first metatarsal should be palpated carefully. On the lateral aspect, the examiner palpates for any evidence of a bunion (exostosis, callus, and inflamed bursa), which is often associated with hallux valgus. On the plantar aspect, the two sesamoid bones just proximal to the head of the first metatarsal may be palpated. The examiner then palpates the first metatarsal bone along its length to the first cuneiform bone and notes any tenderness, swelling, or signs of pathology. As the examiner moves proximally past the first cuneiform on its medial aspect, a bony prominence is felt, the tubercle of the navicular bone. The examiner then returns to the first cuneiform bone and moves laterally on the dorsal and plantar surface, palpating the second and third cuneiforms (Fig. 13–90). Like the first cuneiform, the navicular and second and third cuneiform bones should be palpated on their dorsal and plantar aspects for signs of pathology such as fracture, exostosis, or **Köhler's bone disease** (osteochondritis of the navicular bone).

Moving laterally, the examiner palpates the three phalanges of each of the lateral four toes. Each of the lateral four metatarsals is palpated proximally to check for conditions such as **Freiberg's disease** (osteochondrosis of the second metatarsal head). Under the heads of the second and third metatarsals on the plantar aspect, the examiner should feel for any evidence of a callus, which may indicate a fallen metatarsal arch. Care must be taken to palpate the base of the fifth metatarsal (styloid process) and adjacent cuboid bone for signs of pathology. Also, the lateral aspect of the head of the fifth metatarsal may demonstrate a bunion similar to that seen on the first toe; this is called a tailor's bunion (see Fig. 13–35).

In addition to palpating the metatarsal bones, the examiner palpates between the bones for evidence of

pathology (e.g., interdigital neuroma) as well as the intrinsic muscles of the foot.

Medial Malleolus, Medial Tarsal Bones, and Posterior Tibial Artery. The examiner stabilizes the patient's heel by holding the calcaneus with one hand and palpates the distal edges of the medial malleolus for tenderness or swelling with the other hand. Moving from the distal extent of the medial malleolus along a line joining the navicular tubercle, the examiner moves along the talus until the head of the talus is reached. As the head of the talus is palpated, the examiner may evert and invert the foot, feeling the movement between the talar head and navicular bone. Eversion causes the head to become more prominent, as does the deformity pes planus. At the same time, the tibialis posterior tendon may be palpated where it inserts into the navicular and cuneiform bones. Rupture (third-degree strain) of this tendon leads to a valgus foot. The four ligaments that make up the deltoid ligament may also be palpated for signs of pathology.

Returning to the medial malleolus at its distal extent, the examiner moves farther distally (approximately one fingerwidth) until another bony prominence, the sustentaculum tali of the calcaneus, is felt. This bony prominence is often small and difficult to palpate. Moving farther posteriorly, the examiner palpates the medial aspect of the calcaneus for signs of pathology (e.g., sprain, fracture, tarsal tunnel syndrome). As the examiner moves to the plantar aspect of the calcaneus, the heel fat pad, intrinsic foot muscles, and plantar fascia are palpated for signs of pathology (e.g., heel bruise, plantar fasciitis, bone spur).

The examiner then returns to the medial malleolus and palpates along its posterior surface, noting the movement of the tibialis posterior and long flexor tendons (and checking for tendinitis) during plantar flexion and dorsiflexion and noting any swelling or crepitus. At the same time, the posterior tibial artery, which supplies blood to 75% of the foot, may be palpated as it runs posterior to the medial malleolus. This pulse is often difficult to palpate in individuals with "fat" ankles and in the presence of edema or synovial thickening.

Anterior Tibia, Neck of Talus, and Dorsalis Pedis Artery. The examiner moves to the anterior aspect of the medial malleolus and follows its course laterally onto the distal end of the tibia. As the examiner moves distally, the fingers will rest on the talus. If the foot is then plantar flexed and dorsiflexed, the anterior aspect of the articular surface of the talus can be palpated for signs of pathology (e.g., osteochondritis dissecans). As the examiner moves farther distally, the fingers can follow the course of the neck of the talus to the talar head. Moving distally from the tibia, the examiner should be able to palpate the long extensor tendons, the tibialis anterior tendon, and, with care, the extensor retinaculum (Fig. 13–91). If the examiner moves farther distally over the cuneiforms or

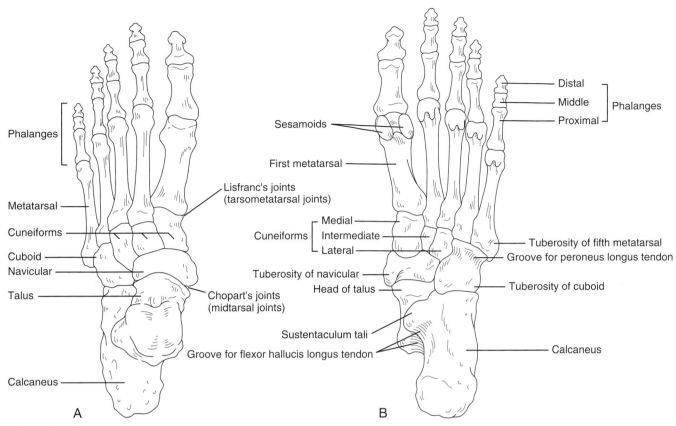

Figure 13-89

Bones of the ankle and foot. (A) Dorsal view. (B) Plantar view.

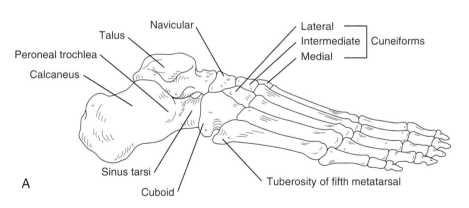

Figure 13-90

Bones of the foot from the lateral (A) and medial (B) sides.

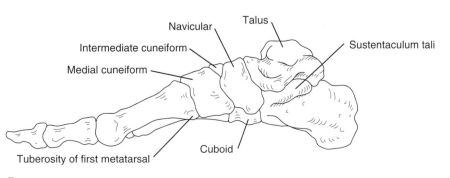

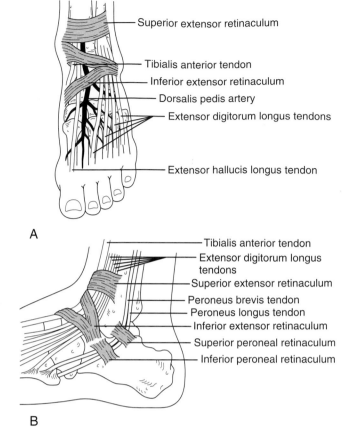

A

B

Figure 13–91
Retinaculum of the ankle. (A) Anterior view. (B) Lateral view.

between the first and second metatarsal bones, the dorsalis pedis pulse (branch of the anterior tibial artery) may be palpated. It may be found between the tendons of extensor digitorum longus and extensor hallucis longus over the junction of the first and second cuneiform bones. If an anterior compartment syndrome is suspected, this pulse should be palpated and compared with that of the opposite side. It should be remembered, however, that this pulse is normally absent in 10% of the population.

Palpation Anteriorly and Anterolaterally

Lateral Malleolus, Calcaneus, Sinus Tarsi, and Cuboid Bone. The lateral malleolus is palpated at the distal extent of the fibula. It should be noted that the lateral malleolus extends farther distally and lies more posterior than the medial malleolus. The examiner then stabilizes the calcaneus with one hand and palpates with the other hand, as done previously. As the examiner moves distally from the lateral malleolus, the fingers lie along the lateral edge of the calcaneus, which is palpated with care. At the same time, the peroneal tendons can be palpated as they angle around the lateral malleolus to their inser-

tion in the foot and up to their origin in the peroneal muscles of the leg. The peroneal retinaculum, which holds the peroneal tendons in place as they angle around the lateral malleolus, is also palpated for tenderness (see Fig. 13–91). While palpating the retinaculum, the examiner should ask the patient to invert and evert the foot. If the peroneal retinaculum is torn, the peroneal tendons will often slip out of their groove or dislocate on eversion (see Fig. 13–47). While the lateral malleolus is being palpated, the lateral ligaments (anterior talofibular, calcaneofibular, and posterior talofibular) should be palpated for tenderness and swelling (see Fig. 13–1).

Returning to the lateral malleolus, the examiner palpates its anterior surface and then moves anteriorly to the extensor digitorum brevis muscle, the only muscle on the dorsum of the foot. If the examiner palpates carefully and deeply through the muscle, a depression (the sinus tarsi) can be felt (Fig. 13–92). If the fingers are left in the depression and the foot is inverted, the neck of the talus will be felt and the fingers will be pushed deeper into the depression. Tenderness in this area may also be indicative of a sprain to the anterior talofibular ligament (see Fig. 13–92), the most frequently injured ligament in the lower leg, ankle, and foot.

The cuboid bone may be palpated in two ways. The examiner may move farther distally from the sinus tarsi (approximately one fingerwidth) so that the fingers lie over the cuboid bone. Or, the styloid process at the base of the fifth metatarsal bone may be palpated, and, as the examiner moves slightly proximally, the fingers will lie over the cuboid bone. In either case, the cuboid should be palpated on its dorsal, lateral, and plantar surfaces for signs of pathology.

Inferior Tibiofibular Joint, Tibia, and Muscles of the Leg. Starting at the lateral malleolus and following its anterior

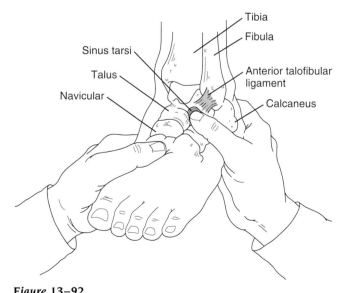

Figure 13–92
Palpation of the sinus tarsi and the anterior talofibular ligament.

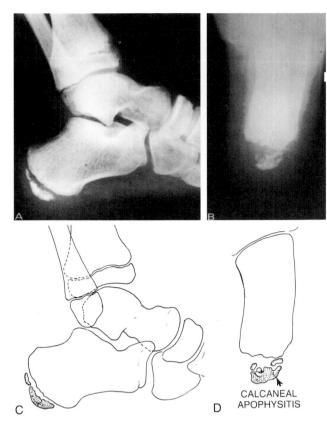

Figure 13–93

In Sever's disease (calcaneal apophysitis), there is fragmentation of the posterior apophysis off the calcaneus, causing achillodynia. (A) Lateral roentgenogram of a 10-year-old boy with pain around the insertion of the Achilles tendon. (B) Axial view of the calcaneus. (C and D) Representations of films A and B, respectively. (From Kelikian, H., and A.S. Kelikian: Disorders of the Ankle. Philadelphia, W.B. Saunders Co., 1985, p. 121.)

border, the examiner should note any signs of pathology. The inferior tibiofibular joint is almost impossible to feel; however, it lies between the tibia and fibula and just superior to the talus. The examiner then follows the "shin" or crest of the tibia superiorly, observing for signs of pathology (e.g., shin splints, anterior compartment syndrome, stress fracture). At the same time, the muscles of the lateral compartment (peronei) and anterior compartment (tibialis anterior and long extensors) should be carefully palpated for tenderness or swelling.

Palpation Posteriorly

The patient is then asked to lie in the prone position with the feet over the end of the examining table. The examiner palpates the following structures.

Calcaneus and Achilles Tendon. The examiner palpates the calcaneus and surrounding soft tissue for swelling (i.e., retrocalcaneal bursitis), exostosis (e.g., pump bump), or other signs of pathology. In children, care should be taken in palpating the calcaneal epiphysis for

evidence of **Sever's disease** (calcaneal apophysitis; Fig. 13–93). Moving proximally, the examiner palpates the Achilles tendon, noting any swelling or thickening (e.g., tendinitis, retro-Achilles bursitis) or crepitation on movement. Any swelling caused by an intracapsular sprain of the ankle would also be evident posteriorly. Proximal to the Achilles tendon, the dome or superior surface of the calcaneus may also be palpated.

Posterior Compartment Muscles of the Leg. Moving farther proximally, the examiner palpates the superficial (triceps surae) and deep (tibialis posterior and long flexors) posterior compartment muscles of the leg along their lengths for signs of pathology (e.g., strain, thrombosis).

Diagnostic Imaging

Plain Film Radiography

When viewing any radiograph, the examiner should look for changes and differences between the right and left lower legs, ankles, and feet, such as osteoporosis or alterations in soft tissue, joint space, and alignment. Both weight-bearing and non–weight-bearing views should be taken. Routinely, anteroposterior, lateral, and mortise views are taken.[4] However, x-rays should not be used indiscriminately. Stiell and colleagues[93–95] have developed rules for the proper use of x-rays after ankle or foot injuries (Fig. 13–94). To be viewed properly, indi-

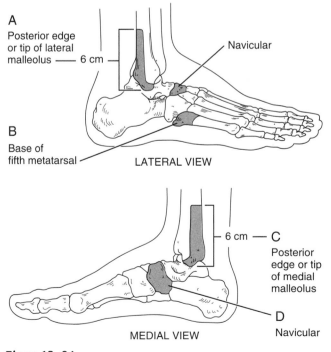

Figure 13–94

Ottawa rules for ankle and foot radiographic series in ankle injury patients. Radiographic series are needed only if there is bone tenderness at A, B, C, or D; inability to bear weight, and malleolar or midfoot pain.

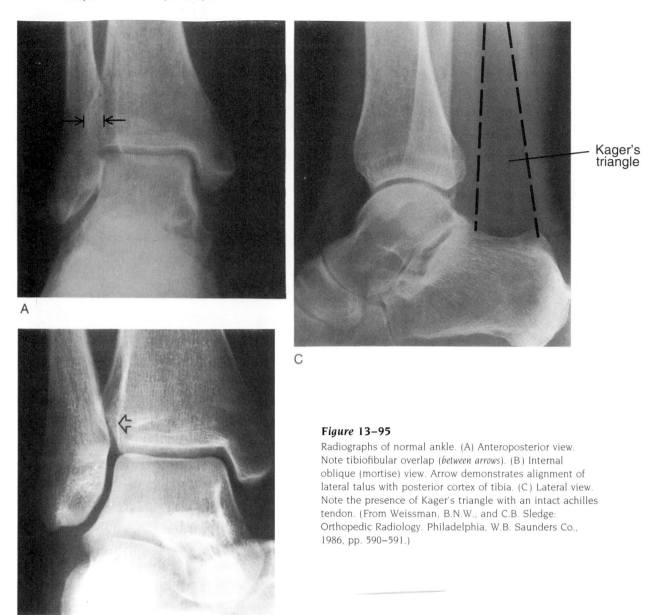

A

B

C

Kager's triangle

Figure 13-95

Radiographs of normal ankle. (A) Anteroposterior view. Note tibiofibular overlap (*between arrows*). (B) Internal oblique (mortise) view. Arrow demonstrates alignment of lateral talus with posterior cortex of tibia. (C) Lateral view. Note the presence of Kager's triangle with an intact achilles tendon. (From Weissman, B.N.W., and C.B. Sledge: Orthopedic Radiology. Philadelphia, W.B. Saunders Co., 1986, pp. 590–591.)

vidual radiographs must be made of the ankle, lower leg, and foot (Fig. 13–95).[4, 12, 96–99]

Anteroposterior View of the Ankle. The examiner notes the shape, position (whether the medial clear space is normal), and texture of the bones and determines whether there is any fractured or new subperiosteal bone. The medial clear space is the space between the talus and medial malleolus. It is normally 2 to 3 mm wide, and values greater than this indicate lateral talar shift with disruption of the ankle mortise and therefore of the tibiofibular syndesmosis.[4] The **tibiofibular overlap** (see Fig. 13–95A) should be at least 6 mm, and greater than 1 mm in the mortise view.[100] In addition, the configuration, congruity, and inclination of the talar dome in relation to the tibial vault above it should be noted, because it

may indicate osteochondritis dissecans (Fig. 13–96).[11] If there are epiphyseal plates present, the examiner should note whether they appear normal. Any increase or decrease in joint space, greater reduction of the tibial overlap, widening of the interosseus space, and greater visibility of the digital fossa should also be noted.

Mortise View of the Ankle. With this view, the ankle mortise and distal tibiofibular joint can be visualized. To obtain this view, which is a modification of the anteroposterior view, the foot and leg are medially rotated 15 to 30°.

Lateral View of Leg, Ankle, and Foot. With this view, the examiner notes the shape, position, and texture of bones, including the tibial tubercle (Fig. 13–97). Any fracture, new subperiosteal bone, or bone spurs should

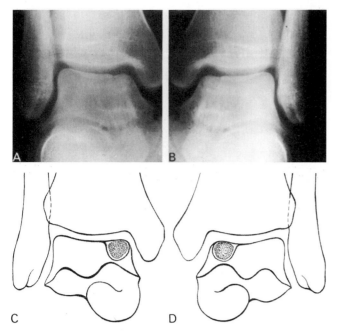

Figure 13-96

Bilateral osteochondritis dissecans of the talus. (A and B) Oblique anteroposterior films of the right and left ankles of a 29-year-old man without any antecedent trauma. (C and D) Illustrations of films A and B, respectively. (From Kelikian, H., and A.S. Kelikian: Disorders of the Ankle. Philadelphia, W.B. Saunders Co., 1985, p. 726.)

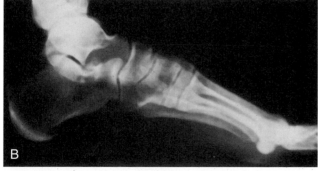

Figure 13-97

Lateral view of the foot. (A) Weight-bearing posture. The soft-tissue pads are flattened beneath the heel and in the forepart of the foot, and the first metatarsal head is elevated by the sesamoids beneath it. (B) Non–weight-bearing posture. The bony alignment and configuration are satisfactory, but the lack of resistance from the floor to the body weight permits variations, which make such views unsatisfactory for determining foot contours. (From Jahss, M.H.: Disorders of the Foot. Philadelphia, W.B. Saunders Co., 1991, pp. 68, 72.)

be noted (Fig. 13-98). The examiner must note whether the epiphyseal lines are normal and whether there is any increase or decrease in joint space. Although this view clearly shows the talus and calcaneus, there is overlap of the midtarsal, metatarsal, and phalangeal structures. On the lateral x-ray, the presence or absence of **Kager's triangle** (see Fig. 13-95C) may be used to diagnose a ruptured Achilles tendon.[101] When viewing lateral films, the examiner must also be aware of Sever's disease and Köhler's disease (Fig. 13-99).

Dorsoplanar View of the Foot. The dorsoplanar view is used primarily to project the forefoot. As with the previous views, the examiner should note the position, shape, and texture of the bones of the foot (Fig. 13-100). The presence of a metatarsus primus varus or a condition such as Köhler's disease should be noted.

Medial Oblique View of the Foot. This view is often taken because it gives the clearest picture of the tarsal bones and joints and the metatarsal shafts and bases (Fig. 13-101). The medial oblique view shows any pathology in the calcaneocuboid joint as well as the presence of a calcaneonavicular bar (Figs. 13-102 and 13-103).

Stress Oblique View. The examiner should note whether there is a calcaneonavicular bar or abnormality of the calcaneus or navicular bones.

Stress Film. The stress radiograph is used to compare the two ankles for integrity of the ligaments (Figs. 13-104 and 13-105).[53, 78, 102-106] With the application of an eversion or abduction stress, tilting of the talus by more than 10° is considered pathological.[107] An increase in the medial clear space (space between medial malleolus and talus) of more than 2 to 3 mm is considered pathological and usually indicates insufficiency of the deltoid ligament, especially the tibiotalar ligament. Instability may also be demonstrated by widening of the syndesmosis (the mortise between the tibia and fibula). An inversion or adduction stress causing 8 to 10° more movement on one side than the other is considered pathological and is indicative of torn lateral ligaments. If the talus has not moved, or if it is fixed but its distal end is unduly prominent, subtalar instability is suggested.

Measurements on Plain Radiographs. Plain radiographs may be used to measure different angles and axes. For example, Figure 13-106 shows the ankle joint axis, and Figure 13-107 shows the subtalar joint axis. Figures 13-108 and 13-109 show various angles measured in the ankle and foot. These angles may change during development, so in some cases serial radiographs may be of benefit.[108]

Abnormal Ossicles or Accessory Bones. The foot often exhibits abnormal ossicles, and their presence may lead to incorrect interpretation of films (Fig. 13-110). These bones are pieces of the prominences of various tarsal bones that for some reason (e.g., fracture, secondary ossification center) has separated from the normal bone.[109] A sesamoid bone, on the other hand, is incorpo-

Text continued on page 660

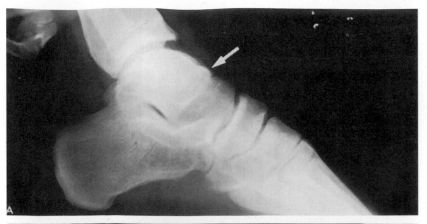

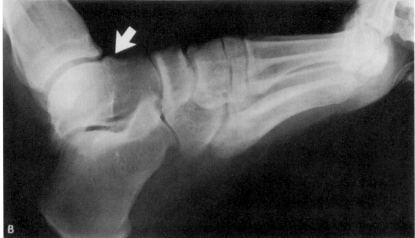

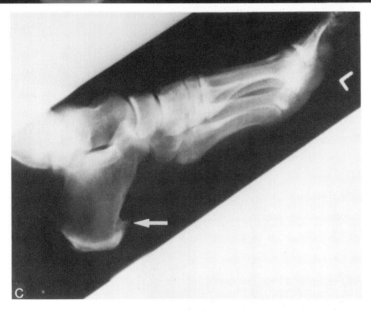

Figure 13–98

(A) Talotibial spurs. (B) Impingement occurs when foot is dorsiflexed. (C) Heel spur. (A and B from O'Donoghue, D.H.: Treatment of Injuries to Athletes, 4th ed. Philadelphia, W.B. Saunders Co., 1984, p. 627.)

Figure 13–99

Radiographs of the foot.
(A) Bilateral involvement with condensation in the early stage of Köhler's disease. (B) Same foot 2 years later shows restoration of contour on the way to completion. (From Jahss, M.H.: Disorders of the Foot. Philadelphia, W.B. Saunders Co., 1991, p. 608.)

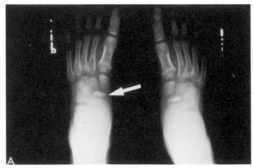

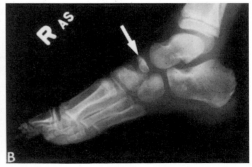

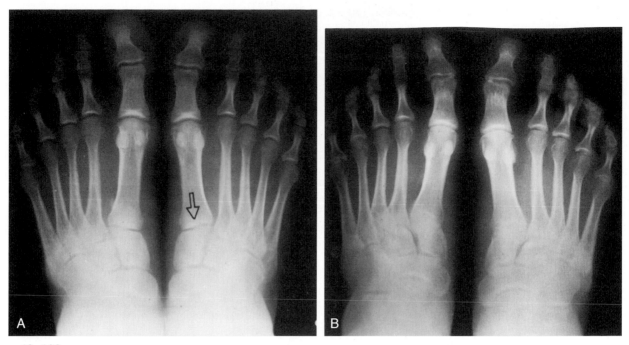

Figure 13–100

Dorsoplanar view of the foot. (A) Weight-bearing posture. The cuneiform–first metatarsal joint is clearly seen (*arrow*), as are the transverse intertarsal joints, in contrast to the non–weight-bearing radiographs. (B) Non–weight-bearing posture. The joint between the medial and middle cuneiforms is clearly seen; the other midtarsal joints are obscure. (From Jahss, M.H.: Disorders of the Foot. Philadelphia, W.B. Saunders Co., 1991, pp. 69, 71.)

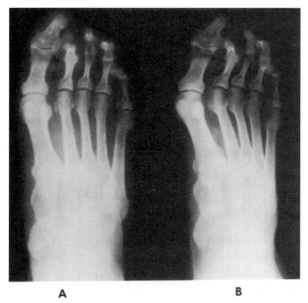

Figure 13–101

Metatarsals and phalanges. (A) With the beam centered directly over the foot, the metatarsal bases and adjacent tarsal bones are shown much more clearly than in B. (B) Both feet are examined with the beam centered between the feet (right foot shown). Marked overlap of metatarsal bases and adjacent tarsal bones is seen. The midtarsal joint can be seen as a continuous line or cyma. (From Klenerman, L.: The Foot and Its Disorders. Boston, Blackwell Scientific Publications, 1982, p. 306.)

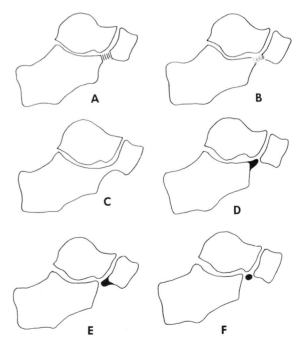

Figure 13–102

Diagrammatic representation of the types of union. (A) Fibrous. (B) Cartilaginous. (C) Osseous. (D) Prominent process on the calcaneus. (E) Prominent process on the navicular. (F) Separate calcaneonavicular ossicle (calcaneum secondarium). (From Klenerman, L.: The Foot and Its Disorders. Boston, Blackwell Scientific Publications, 1982, p. 336.)

Figure 13–103
Calcaneonavicular coalition or bar. (A) Total bony union, as well as bony breaks on the upper surfaces of the navicular and talus. The head of the talus may well be small. (B) Fibrous or cartilaginous, rather than osseous, union between the bones is seen with osteoarthritic changes of the opposing bone surfaces and an enlarged navicular. (From Klenerman, L.: The Foot and Its Disorders. Boston, Blackwell Scientific Publications, 1982, p. 340.)

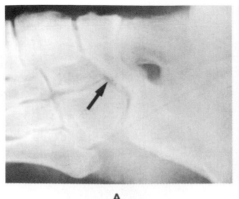
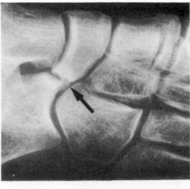

A   **B**

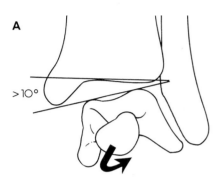
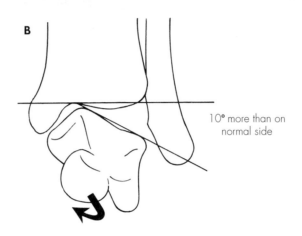

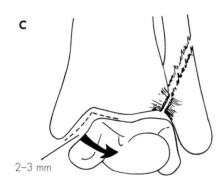

Figure 13–104
Positive findings on diagrammatic stress radiographs. (A) Abduction stress. (B) Adduction stress. (C) Increased (2 to 3 mm) medial clear space (lateral rotary stress).

Figure 13–105
Abnormal stress views: anterior talofibular and calcaneofibular ligament tears. Anteroposterior (A) and lateral (B) views of the right ankle showing hypertrophic lipping from the anterior tibia and talus. The syndesmosis is slightly wide. Comparison varus stress views of the right (C) and left (D) ankles show abnormal talar tilt on the right, particularly when compared with the normal left side. This is diagnostic of an anterior talofibular ligament tear on the right, with or without a calcaneofibular ligament tear. The anterior drawer test is abnormal on the right (E) compared with the left (F). Comparison can be made by noting the anterior shift of the midtalus in relation to the midtibia (*arrows*) on each side, the loss of parallelism of the subchondral cortices on the right, or the marked widening of the posterior joint space (*lines*) on the abnormal as compared with the normal side. This is consistent with an anterior talofibular ligament tear on the right. (From Weissman, B.N.W., and C.B. Sledge: Orthopedic Radiology. Philadelphia, W.B. Saunders Co., 1986, p. 600.)

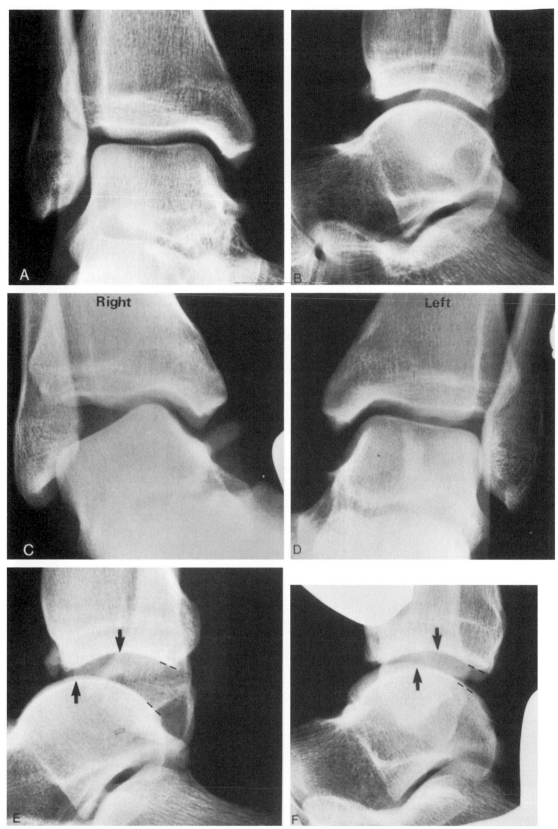

Figure 13–105

See legend on opposite page

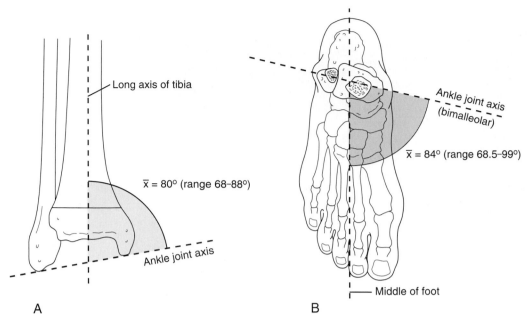

Figure 13–106

Orientation of the ankle joint axis. Mean values measure (A) 80° from a vertical reference and (B) 84° from the longitudinal reference of the foot. (Adapted from Hunt, G.C. [ed.]: Physical Therapy of the Foot and Ankle. New York, Churchill Livingstone, 1988; and Isman, R.E., and V.T. Inman: Anthropometric Studies of the Human Foot and Ankle: Technical Report No. 58. University of California, San Francisco, 1968.)

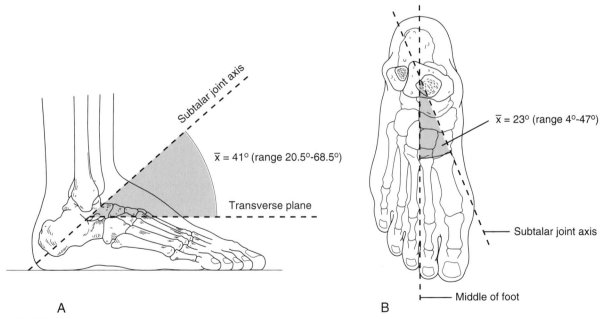

Figure 13–107

Orientation of the subtalar joint axis. Mean values measure (A) 41° from the transverse plane and (B) 23° medially from the longitudinal reference of the foot. (Adapted from G.C. Hunt [ed.]: Physical Therapy of the Foot and Ankle. New York, Churchill Livingstone, 1988; and Isman, R.E., and V.T. Inman: Anthropometric Studies of the Human Foot and Ankle: Technical Report No. 58. University of California, San Francisco, 1968.)

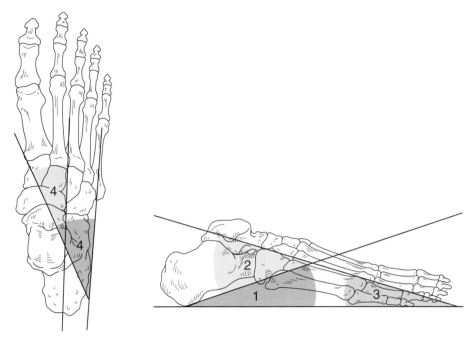

Figure 13–108

Angles of the foot. 1 = lateral talocalcaneal angle; 2 = calcaneal inclination angle; 3 = talar declination angle; 4 = talocalcaneal angle (2 methods).

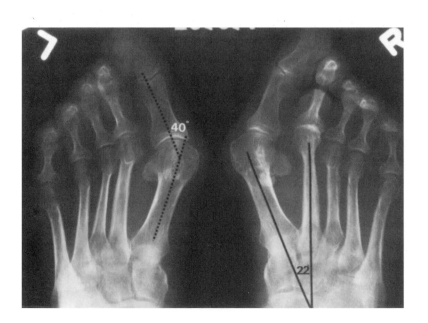

Figure 13–109

Measurement of hallux valgus deformity. On the left, the angle of intersection of the long axes of the proximal phalangeal and the first metatarsal shafts (*dotted lines*) is 40°. Normally, this angle is no greater than 10°. On the right, there is rotation of the great toe and lateral subluxation of the proximal phalanx, leaving about one half of the articular surface of the metacarpal uncovered. The angle of the first and second metatarsal shafts (*solid lines*) is 22°. On standing views, angles of greater than 10° indicate metatarsus primus varus. (From Weissman, B.N.W., and C.B. Sledge: Orthopedic Radiology. Philadelphia, W.B. Saunders Co., 1986, p. 657.)

rated into the substance of a tendon, with one surface articulating with the adjacent bones. A sesamoid bone moves with the tendon and is found over bony prominences or where the tendon makes a change in direction. In addition to the normal sesamoid bones under the big toe, sesamoid bones may also be found in the tendons of peroneus longus and tibialis posterior. Abnormal ossi-

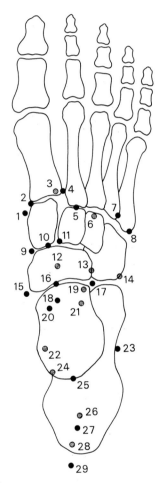

Figure 13–110

Accessory tarsal bones. 1 = os sesamoideum tibialis anterior; 2 = os cuneometatarsale I tibiale; 3 = os cuneometatarsale I plantare; 4 = os intermetatarsale I; 5 = os cuneometatarsale II dorsale; 6 = os unci; 7 = os intermetatarsale IV; 8 = os vesalianum; 9 = os paracuneiforme; 10 = os naviculocuneiforme I dorsale; 11 = os intercuneiforme; 12 = os sesamoideum tibialis posterior (according to Trolle, this may be the same as 15); 13 = os cuboideum secundarium; 14 = os peroneum; 15 = os tibiale (externum); 16 = os talonaviculare dorsale; 17 = os calcaneus secundarius; 18 = os supertalare; 19 = os trochleae; 20 = os talotibiale dorsale; 21 = os in sinu tarsi; 22 = os sustentaculi proprium; 23 = calcaneus accessorius; 24 = os talocalcaneare posterior; 25 = os trigonum; 26 = os aponeurosis plantaris; 27 = os supracalcaneum; 28 = os subcalcaneum; 29 = os tendinis Achilles. (From Klenerman, L.: The Foot and Its Disorders. Boston, Blackwell Scientific Publications, 1982, p. 361.)

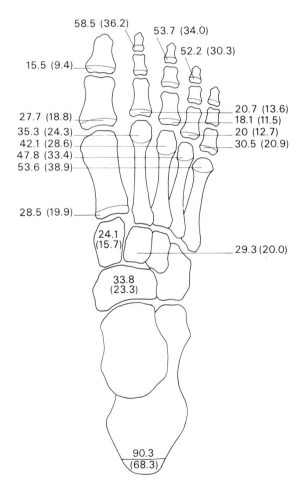

Figure 13–111

Anteroposterior diagram of the foot showing the times of appearance (in months) of the centers of ossification for boys (and for girls, in parentheses). (From Hoerr, N.L., S.I. Pyle, and C.C. Francis: Radiographic Atlas of Skeletal Development of the Foot and Ankle. Springfield, Illinois: Charles C Thomas, 1962, with kind permission of Charles C Thomas, Springfield, Illinois.)

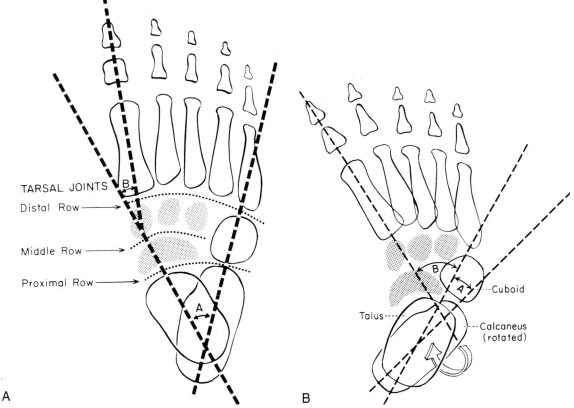

Figure 13–112

Representations of the foot as seen on radiographs. (A) Representation of the normal foot. The cuboid blocks medial movement of the foot at the middle row of tarsal joints because of its unique location. It alone occupies a position in both rows of tarsal joints. The talocalcaneal angle (angle A) is measured by drawing lines through the long axes of the talus and calcaneus. One should attempt to be as accurate as possible in making these measurements. The normal range for this measurement is 20 to 40° in the young child. The talus–first metatarsal angle (angle B) is measured by drawing lines through the long axis of the talus and along the long axis of the first metatarsal. The normal range is 0 to −20°. (B) Hindfoot varus, as manifested by a decreased talocalcaneal angle (angle A), and talonavicular subluxation, as manifested by a talocalcaneal angle of less than 15° and a talus–first metatarsal angle (angle B) of more than 15°. Talonavicular subluxation occurs through the medial movement of three bones, which move as a unit. The navicular, cuboid, and calcaneus move medially through the combined movements of medial translation and supination of the proximal tarsal bones, whereas the calcaneus inverts beneath the talus. (From Simons, G.W.: Analytical radiography and the progressive approach in talipes equinovarus. Orthop. Clin. North Am. 9:189, 1978.)

cles are more likely to occur in the foot than anywhere else in the body.

Films Showing Bone Development. Like the bones of the hand, the bones of the foot form within a certain time period (Fig. 13–111). However, because the foot is subjected to greater forces and environmental effects than the hand, it is not usually used to determine skeletal age. X-rays of the foot often show the developing bone deformities seen in clubfoot (Fig. 13–112). Although not all of the bones are present at birth, a series of films will show differences when compared with films of normal feet.

Arthrography

Arthrograms of the ankle are indicated whenever there is acute ligament injury, chronic ligament laxity, or indications of loose body or osteochondritis dissecans (Figs. 13–113 and 13–114).[4, 11, 110, 111] Leakage of the contrast

Text continued on page 665

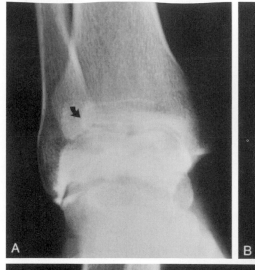

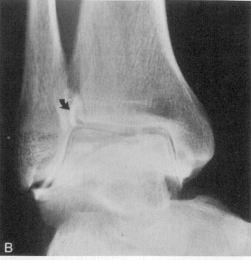

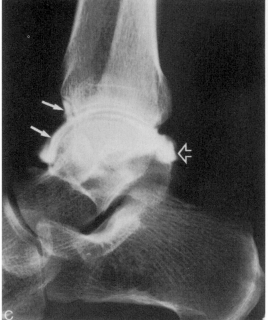

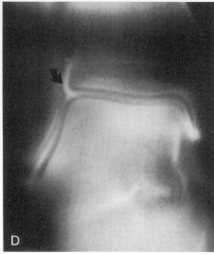

Figure 13–113

Normal positive-contrast ankle arthrogram. Anteroposterior (A), internal oblique or mortise (B) and lateral (C) views and a tomogram (D) in the internal oblique projection show contrast agent coating the articular surfaces and filling normally present anterior (*white arrows*), posterior (*open arrow*), and syndesmotic (*black arrows*) recesses. There is no extension of contrast medium into the soft tissue medially or laterally. (From Weissman, B.N.W., and C.B. Sledge: Orthopedic Radiology. Philadelphia, W.B. Saunders Co., 1986, p. 596.)

Figure 13–114

Contrast arthrography showing acute tear of the anterior tibiofibular ligament. (A) Anteroposterior arthrogram of the right ankle 14 hours after the injury showing extravasation of contrast medium in front and around the lateral aspect of the fibula. (B) Lateral view of the same. (C and D) Illustrations of arthrograms A and B, respectively. (Modified from Kelikian, H., and A.S. Kelikian: Disorders of the Ankle. Philadelphia, W.B. Saunders Co., 1985, p. 143.)

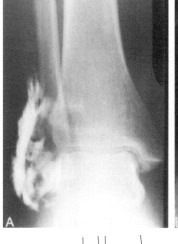

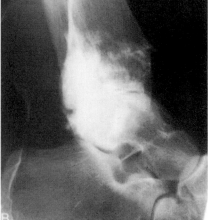

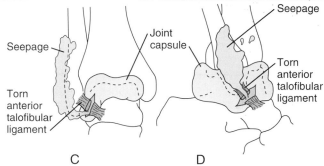

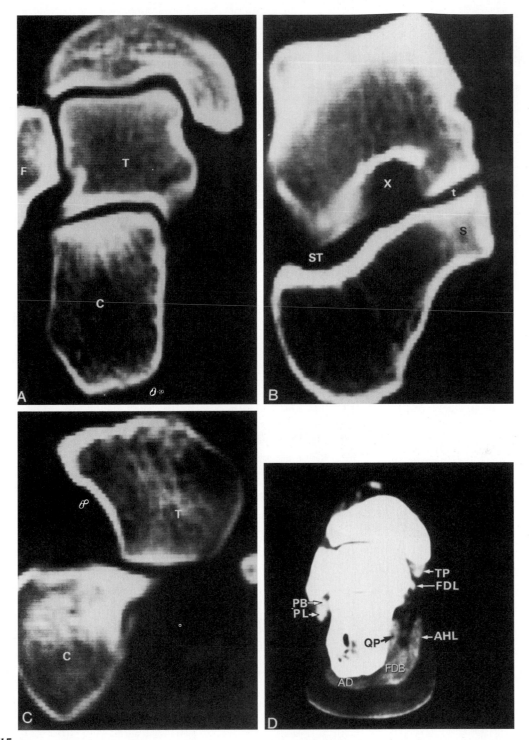

Figure 13–115

Normal anatomy of the ankle and foot as seen on computed tomography scans. (A) Coronal section through the ankle and subtalar joint. T = talus, C = calcaneus, F = fibula. (B) Farther anteriorly, the sustentaculum tali (S), the site of insertion of the talocalcaneal ligament (X), the subtalar joint (ST), and the mid-talocalcaneonavicular joint (t) are seen. (C) Anterior to the sustentaculum tali, the talus (T) and the calcaneus (C) are seen. (D) The peroneus brevis (PB), peroneus longus (PL), posterior tibial (TP), and flexor digitorum longus (FDL) muscles are seen. AHL = abductor hallucis longus, FDB = flexor digitorum brevis, QP = quadratus plantae, AD = abductor digiti quinti pedis. This scan is at the level of the posterior aspect of the sustentaculum tali. (From Weissman, B.N.W., and C.B. Sledge: Orthopedic Radiology. Philadelphia, W.B. Saunders Co., 1986, p. 632.)

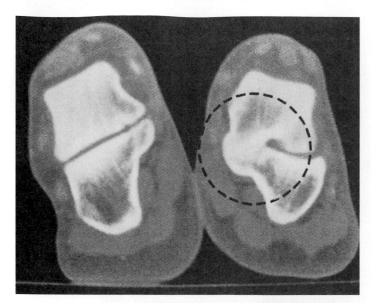

Figure 13–116

Coronal computed tomographic view showing talocalcaneal coalition on the right. (From Rettig, A.C., K.D. Shelbourne, H.F. Beltz, D.W. Robertson, and P. Arfken: Radiographic evaluation of foot and ankle injuries in the athlete. Clin. Sports Med. 6:914, 1987.)

Figure 13–117

Sagittal and coronal magnetic resonance images of the ankle. (A) Sagittal projection. Note the white bone marrow (BM) and subcutaneous fat (F), black tendons (T) and ligaments, grey muscles (M) and articular cartilage (C), and black cortical bone (B). (B) Coronal projection. Note the black appearance of the deltoid ligament (*white arrow*) and interosseous ligament (*black arrowhead*) between the talus and calcaneus. (From Kingston, S.: Magnetic resonance imaging of the ankle and foot. Clin. Sports Med. 7:19, 1988.)

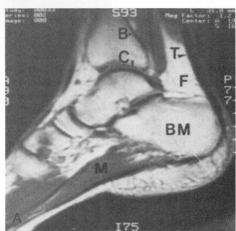

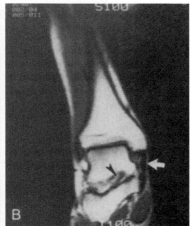

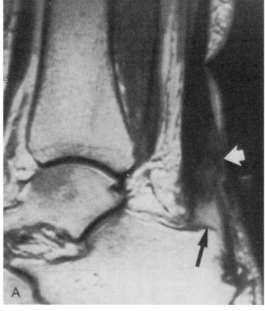

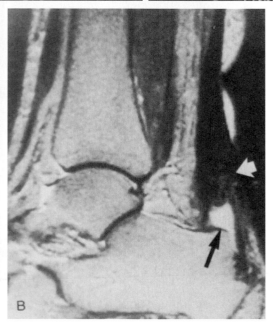

Figure 13–118

Magnetic resonance images showing partial Achilles tendon tear. (A) Sagittal, proton-density and (B) T2-weighted magnetic resonance images reveal a large tear at the Achilles insertion with intratendinous fluid (*long arrow*) and fraying and thickening of the distal tendon (*short arrow*).

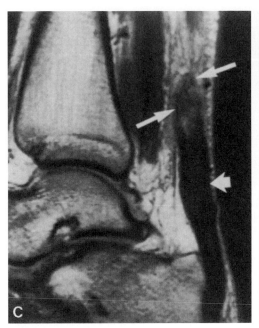
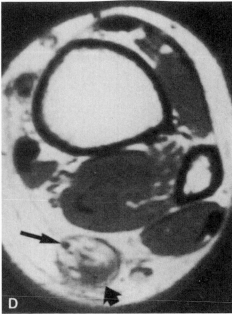

Figure 13–118 *Continued*

(C) Complete Achilles tendon tear. Sagittal, proton-density magnetic resonance image reveals disruption of the Achilles tendon (*long arrows*) and thickening of its distal portion (*short arrow*). (D) On an axial, T1-weighted magnetic resonance image, only gray granulation tissue is seen within the paratenon (*short arrow*). The intact plantaris tendon passes along the medial border of the paratenon (*long arrow*). (From Kerr, R., D.M. Forrester, and S. Kingston: Magnetic resonance imaging of foot and ankle trauma. Orthop. Clin. North Am. 21:593, 1990.)

medium indicates tearing of the joint capsule or capsular ligaments. Normally, the talocrural joint admits only about 6 ml of contrast medium.

Computed Tomography

Computed tomography scans are useful for determining the relation among the bones and for giving a view of the relation between bony and soft tissues (Figs. 13–115 and 13–116).

Magnetic Resonance Imaging

Magnetic resonance imaging (MRI) is an especially useful, although sometimes overused, technique for delineating bony and soft tissues around the ankle and foot (Figs. 13–117 and 13–118). MRI may be used to diagnose ruptured tendons (e.g., Achilles, peroneal), ligament tears, and fractures (e.g., osteochondral fractures, osteonecrosis).[112–114]

Bone Scans

Bone scans are used in the lower limb, ankle, and foot to diagnose stress fractures, primarily those of the tibia (Fig. 13–119) and metatarsal bones.

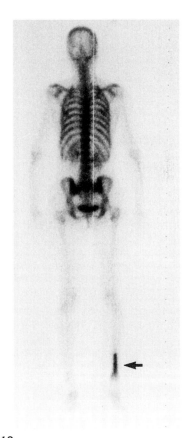

Figure 13–119

Bone scan of whole body. Arrow indicates area of increased isotope uptake ("hot spot") in the right tibia, which is consistent with a stress-related lesion.

Précis of the Lower Leg, Ankle, and Foot Assessment*

History
Observation
Examination
  Active movements, weight-bearing (standing)
    Plantar flexion
    Dorsiflexion
    Supination
    Pronation
    Toe extension
    Toe flexion
  Active movements, non–weight-bearing (sitting or supine lying)
    Plantar flexion
    Dorsiflexion
    Supination
    Pronation
    Toe extension
    Toe flexion
    Toe abduction
    Toe adduction
  Special tests (sitting)
    Tibial torsion
  Passive movements (supine lying)
    Plantar flexion at the talocrural (ankle) joint
    Dorsiflexion at the talocrural joint
    Inversion at the subtalar joint
    Eversion at the subtalar joint
    Adduction at the midtarsal joints
    Abduction at the midtarsal joints
    Flexion of the toes
    Extension of the toes
    Adduction of the toes
    Abduction of the toes
  Resisted isometric movements (supine lying)
    Knee flexion
    Plantar flexion
    Dorsiflexion

    Supination
    Pronation
    Toe extension
    Toe flexion
  Special tests (supine lying)
    Neutral position of talus
    Anterior drawer sign
    Talar tilt
    Leg length
  Reflexes and cutaneous distribution (supine lying)
  Joint play movements (supine and side lying)
    Long-axis extension
    Anteroposterior glide
    Talar rock
    Side tilt
    Rotation
    Side glide
    Tarsal bone mobility
  Palpation (supine lying and prone lying)
  Special tests (prone lying)
    Neutral position of talus
    Leg heel alignment
    Foot-heel alignment
    Tibial torsion
    Thompson test
  Functional assessment (standing)
  Special tests (standing)
    Neutral position of talus
  Diagnostic imaging

---

* The précis is shown in an order that limits the amount of moving that the patient has to do but ensures that all necessary structures are tested. It does not follow the order of the text.

After any examination, the patient should be warned of the possibility of exacerbation of symptoms as a result of the assessment.

Case Studies

When doing these case studies, the examiner should list the appropriate questions to be asked and why they are being asked, what to look for and why, and what things should be tested and why. Depending on the patient's answers (and the examiner should consider different responses), several possible causes of the patient's problem may become evident (examples are given in parentheses). A differential diagnosis chart should be made (see Table 13–15 as an example). The examiner can then decide how different diagnoses may affect the treatment plan.

1. A 38-year-old man ruptured his Achilles tendon 4 weeks earlier and had it surgically repaired. The cast has been removed. Describe your assessment plan for this patient.

2. A 24-year-old woman presents at your clinic with a painful left foot. There is no history of trauma; however, the pain has been present for approximately 6 years and has become worse in the last year. Describe your assessment plan for this patient (Morton's neuroma versus plantar fasciitis).

3. A 59-year-old man comes to you complaining of pain in his right calf and some numbness in his right foot. He also complains of some stiffness in his back. Describe your assessment plan for this patient (lumbar spondylosis versus tibial nerve palsy).

4. A 10-year-old boy recently had a triple arthrodesis for talipes equinovarus. The cast has now been removed. Describe your assessment plan for this patient.

5. A 16-year-old female volleyball player comes to you complaining of left ankle pain and difficulty walking after she stepped on another player's foot and went over on her ankle. The injury occurred 30 minutes ago and her ankle is swollen. Describe your assessment plan for this patient (malleolar fracture versus ligament sprain).

6. A 25-year-old woman tells you that she is training for a marathon but that every time she increases her mileage, her right foot hurts. Some time ago, someone told her she had a cavus foot. Describe your assessment plan for this patient.

7. Parents bring a 2-year-old boy to you and express concern that the child appears to have flat feet and "pigeon toes." Describe your assessment plan for this patient.

8. A 32-year-old woman comes to you complaining of ankle pain. She states that she sprained it 9 months earlier and thought it was better. However, she has now returned to training, and the ankle is bothering her. Describe your assessment plan for this patient (proprioceptive loss versus hypermobility).

Table 13–15
Differential Diagnosis of Lower Leg Compartment Syndrome

	Compartment Syndrome	Shin Splints	Stress Fracture	Tumor
Pain (type)	Severe cramping, diffuse pain, and tightness	Diffuse along medial two thirds of tibial border	Deep, nagging, localized with minimal radiation	Deep, nagging (bone) with some radiation
Pain with rest	Decreases or disappears	Decreases or disappears	Present, especially night pain	Present, often night pain
Pain with activity	Increases	Increases	Present (may increase)	Present
Pain with warm-up	May increase or become present	May disappear	Unilateral	Unaltered
Range of motion	Limited in acute phase	Limited	Normal	Normal
Onset	Gradual to sudden	Gradual	Gradual	?
Altered sensation	Sometimes	No	No	Sometimes
Muscle weakness or paralysis	Maybe	No	No	Not usually
Stretching	Increases pain	Increases pain	Minimal pain alteration	No increase in pain
Radiography	Normal	Normal	Early, negative; late, positive (?)	Usually positive
Bone scan	Negative	Periosteal uptake	Positive	Positive
Pulse	Affected sometimes	Normal	Normal	Normal
Palpation	Tender, tight compartment	Diffuse tenderness	Point tenderness	Point or diffuse tenderness
Cause	Muscle expansion	Overuse	Overuse	?
Duration and recovery	None without surgery	None without rest	Up to 3 months	None without treatment

From Magee, D.J.: Sports Physiotherapy Manual. Edmonton, University of Alberta Bookstore, 1988.

References

Cited References

1. Donatelli, R.: Abnormal biomechanics of the foot and ankle. J. Orthop. Sports Phys. Ther. 9:11–16, 1987.
2. Mantas, J.P.: Lisfranc injuries in the athlete. Clin. Sports Med. 13:719–730, 1994.
3. Kleiger, B.: Mechanisms of ankle injury. Orthop. Clin. North Am. 5:127–146, 1974.
4. Marder, R.A.: Current methods for the evaluation of ankle ligament injuries. J. Bone Joint Surg. Am. 76:1103–1111, 1994.
5. Taunton, J., C. Smith, and D.J. Magee: Leg, foot and ankle injuries. In Zachazewski, J.E., D.J. Magee, and W.S. Quillen: Athletic Injuries and Rehabilitation. Philadelphia, W.B. Saunders Co., 1996.
6. Reid, D.C.: Sports Injury Assessment and Rehabilitation. New York, Churchill Livingstone, 1992.
7. Hunt, G.C., and R.S. Brocato: Gait and foot pathomechanics. In Hunt, G.C. (ed.): Physical Therapy of the Foot and Ankle. Clinics in Physical Therapy. Edinburgh, Churchill Livingstone, 1988.
8. Kapandji, I.A.: The Physiology of the Joints, Vol. 2: Lower Limb. New York, Churchill Livingstone, 1970.
9. Lipscomb, A.B., and A.A. Ibrahim: Acute peroneal compartment syndrome in a well conditioned athlete: Report of a case. Am. J. Sports Med. 5:154–157, 1977.
10. Williams, P.L., and R. Warwick (eds.): Gray's Anatomy, 36th British ed. Philadelphia, W.B. Saunders Co., 1980.
11. Kelikian, H., and A.S. Kelikian: Disorders of the Ankle. Philadelphia, W.B. Saunders Co., 1985.
12. Palmer, M.L., and M. Epler: Clinical Assessment Procedures in Physical Therapy. Philadelphia, J.B. Lippincott Co., 1990.
13. Jahss, M.H.: Disorders of the Foot. Philadelphia, W.B. Saunders Co., 1982.
14. Evans, R.C.: Illustrated Essentials in Orthopedic Physical Assessment. St. Louis, C.V. Mosby Co., 1994.
15. Hamilton, J.J., and L.K. Ziemer: Functional Anatomy of the Human Ankle and Foot. American Association of Orthopaedic Surgeons, Symposium on the Foot and Ankle. St. Louis, C.V. Mosby Co., 1983.
16. Bowe, J.A.: The pediatric foot. In Lutter, L.D., M.S. Mizel, and G.B. Pfeffer (eds.): Orthopedic Knowledge Update: Foot and Ankle. Rosemont, Illinois, American Academy of Orthopaedic Surgeons, 1994.
17. Brown, L.P., and P. Yavorsky: Locomotor biomechanics and pathomechanics. A review. J. Orthop. Sports Phys. Ther. 9:3–10, 1987.
18. McPoil, T.G., and R.S. Brocato: The foot and ankle: Biomechanical evaluation and treatment. In Gould, J.A. (ed.): Orthopedic and Sports Physical Therapy. St. Louis, C.V. Mosby Co., 1990.
19. Pedowitz, W.J.: Deformities of the first ray. In Lutter, L.D., M.S. Mizel, and G.B.. Pfeffer (eds.): Orthopedic Knowledge Update: Foot and Ankle. Rosemont, Illinois, American Academy of Orthopaedic Surgeons, 1994.
20. Thompson, G.H.: Bunions and deformities of the toes in children and adolescents. J. Bone Joint Surg. Am. 77:1924–1936, 1995.
21. Durman, D.C.: Metatarsus primus varus and hallux valgus. Arch. Surg. 74:128–135, 1957.
22. Price, G.F.W.: Metatarsus primus varus, including various clinicoradiologic features of the female foot. Clin. Orthop. 145:217–223, 1979.

23. Romash, M.: Deformities of the lesser toes and bunionette. In Lutter, L.D., M.S. Mizel, and G.B. Pfeffer (eds.): Orthopedic Knowledge Update: Foot and Ankle. Rosemont, Illinois, American Academy of Orthopaedic Surgeons, 1994.

24. McMaster, M.J.: The pathogenesis of the hallux rigidus. J. Bone Joint Surg. Br. 60:82–87, 1978.

25. Root, M.L., W.P. Orien, and J.H. Weed: Normal and Abnormal Function of the Foot. Los Angeles, Clinical Biomechanics Corp., 1977.

26. Bowers, K.D., and R.B. Martin: Turf toe: A shoe related football injury. Med. Sci. Sports Exerc. 8:81–83, 1976.

27. Clanton, T.O., and J.J. Ford: Turf toe injury. Clin. Sports Med. 13:731–741, 1994.

28. Coughlin, M.J.: Conditions of the forefoot. In DeLee, J.C., and D. Drez (eds.): Orthopedic Sports Medicine: Principles and Practice. Philadelphia, W.B. Saunders Co., 1994.

29. Lian, G.: Nerve problems in the foot. In Lutter, L.D., M.S. Mizel, and G.B. Pfeffer (eds.): Orthopedic Knowledge Update: Foot and Ankle. Rosemont, Illinois, American Academy of Orthopaedic Surgeons, 1994.

30. Lindsjo, U., G. Danckwardt-Lilliestrom, and B. Sahlstedt: Measurement of the motion range in the loaded ankle. Clin. Orthop. 199:68–71, 1985.

31. Hyslop, G.H.: Injuries of the deep and superficial peroneal nerves complicating ankle sprain. Am. J. Surg. 51:436–438, 1941.

32. Worrell, T.W., L.D. Booher, and K.M. Hench: Closed kinetic chain assessment following inversion ankle sprain. J. Sports Rehab. 3:197–203, 1994.

33. Mubarak, S., and A. Hargens: Exertional compartment syndromes. American Association of Orthopaedic Surgeons, Symposium on the Foot and Leg in Running Sports. St. Louis, C.V. Mosby Co., 1982.

34. Reneman, R.S.: The anterior and the lateral compartmental syndrome of the leg due to intensive use of muscles. Clin. Orthop. 113:69–80, 1975.

35. Freeman, M.A.R., M.R.E. Dean, and I.W.F. Hanham: The etiology and prevention of functional instability of the foot. J. Bone Joint Surg. Br. 47:678–685, 1965.

36. Kaikkonen, A., P. Kannus, and M. Jarvinen: A performance test protocol and scoring scale for the evaluation of ankle injuries. Am. J. Sports Med. 22:462–469, 1994.

37. Seligson, D., J. Gassman, and M. Pope: Ankle Instability: Evaluation of the lateral ligaments. Am. J. Sports Med. 8:39–42, 1980.

38. Hildebrand, K.A., R.E. Buckley, N.G. Mohtadi, and P. Faris: Functional outcome measures after displaced intra-articular calcaneal fractures. J. Bone Joint Surg. Br. 75:119–123, 1996.

39. Merchant, T.C., and F.R. Dietz: Long-term follow up after fractures of the tibial and fibular shafts. J. Bone Joint Surg. Am. 71:599–606, 1989.

40. Olerud, C., and H. Molander: A scoring scale for symptom evaluation after ankle fracture. Arch. Orthop. Trauma Surg. 103:190–194, 1984.

41. Astrom, M., and T. Arvidson: Alignment and joint motion in the normal foot. J. Orthop. Sports Phys. Ther. 22:216–222, 1995.

42. Roy, S., and R. Irvin: Sports Medicine: Prevention, Evaluation, Management and Rehabilitation. Englewood Cliffs, New Jersey, Prentice-Hall, 1983.

43. Johnson, K.A.: Posterior tibial tendon. In Baxter, D.E. (ed.): The Foot and Ankle in Sport. St. Louis, C.V. Mosby Co., 1995.

44. Staheli, L.T., M. Corbett, C. Wyss, and H. King: Lower extremity rotational problems in children: Normal values to guide management. J. Bone Joint Surg. Am. 67:39–47, 1985.

45. Staheli, L.T.: Rotational problems of the lower extremities. Orthop. Clin. North Am. 18:503–512, 1987.

46. Lindstrand, A.: New aspects in the diagnosis of lateral ankle sprains. Orthop. Clin. North Am. 7:247–249, 1976.

47. Hollis, J.M., R.D. Blasier, and C.M. Flahiff: Simulated ankle ligamentous injury: Change in ankle stability. Am. J. Sports Med. 23:672–677, 1995.

48. Frost, H.M., and C.A. Hanson: Technique for testing the drawer sign in the ankle. Clin. Orthop. 123:49–51, 1977.

49. Birrer, R.B., T.J. Cartwright, and J.R. Denton: Immediate diagnosis of ankle trauma. Phys. Sportmed. 22:95–102, 1994.

50. Aradi, A.J., J. Wong, and M. Walsh: The dimple sign of a ruptured lateral ligament of the ankle: Brief report. J. Bone Joint Surg. Br. 70:327–328, 1988.

51. Davis, P.F., and S.G. Trevino: Ankle injuries. In Baxter, D.E. (ed.): The Foot and Ankle in Sport. St. Louis, C.V. Mosby Co., 1995.

52. Kjaersgaard-Andersen, P., L.H. Frich, F. Madsen, P. Helmig, P. Sogard, and J.O. Sojbjerg: Instability of the hindfoot after lesion of the lateral ankle ligaments: Investigations of the anterior drawer and adduction maneuvers in autopsy specimens. Clin. Orthop. 266:170–179, 1991.

53. Colter, J.M.: Lateral ligamentous injuries of the ankle. In Hamilton, W.C. (ed.): Traumatic Disorders of the Ankle. New York, Springer-Verlag, 1984.

54. Hamilton, W.C.: Anatomy. In Hamilton, W.C. (ed.): Traumatic Disorders of the Ankle. New York, Springer-Verlag, 1984.

55. Rasmussen, O., and I. Tovberg-Jensen: Anterolateral rotational instability in the ankle joint. Acta Orthop. Scand. 52:99–102, 1981.

56. Gungor, T.: A test for ankle instability: Brief report. J. Bone Joint Surg. Br. 70:487, 1988.

57. Mennell, J.M.: Foot Pain. Boston, Little, Brown & Co., 1969.

58. Hopkinson, W.J., P. St. Pierre, J.B. Ryan, and J.H. Wheeler: Syndesmosis sprains of the ankle. Foot Ankle 10:325–330, 1990.

59. Wallace, L.A.: Limb length difference and back pain. In Grieve, G.P. (ed.): Modern Manual Therapy of the Vertebral Column. Edinburgh, Churchill Livingstone, 1986.

60. Thompson, T., and J. Doherty: Spontaneous rupture of the tendon of Achilles: A new clinical diagnostic test. Anat. Res. 158:126–129, 1967.

61. Scott, B.W., and A. Al-Chalabi: How the Simmonds-Thompson test works. J. Bone Joint Surg. Br. 74:314–315, 1992.

62. Simmonds, F.A.: The diagnosis of a ruptured achilles tendon. Practitioner 179:56–58, 1957.

63. Thompson, T.C.: A test for rupture of the tendoachilles. Acta Orthop. Scand. 32:461–465, 1962.

64. Blood, S.D.: Treatment of the sprained ankle. J. Am. Osteopathic Assoc. 79:680–692, 1980.

65. Bowditch, M.G., P. Sanderson, and J.P. Livesey: The significance of an absent ankle reflex. J. Bone Joint Surg. Br. 78:276–279, 1996.

66. Bassetti, C.: Babinski and Babinski's sign. Spine 20:2591–2594, 1995.

67. Chusid, J.G., and J.J. McDonald: Correlative Neuroanatomy and Functional Neurology. Los Altos, Lange Medical Publications, 1967.

68. Schon, L.C., and D.E. Baxter: Neuropathies of the foot and ankle in athletes. Clin. Sports Med. 9:489–509, 1990.

69. Zengzhao, L., Z. Jiansheng, and Z. Li: Anterior tarsal tunnel syndrome. J. Bone Joint Surg. Br. 73:470–473, 1991.

70. Pecina, M.M., J. Krmpotic-Nemanic, and A.D. Markiewitz: Tunnel Syndromes. Boca Raton, Florida, CRC Press, 1991.

71. Wechsler, L.R., and N.A. Busis: Sports neurology. In Fu, F.H., and D.A. Stone (eds.): Sports Injuries: Mechanisms, Prevention, Treatment. Baltimore, Williams & Wilkins, 1994.

72. Baxter, D.E.: Functional nerve disorders. In Baxter, D.E. (ed.): The Foot and Ankle in Sport. St. Louis, C.V. Mosby Co., 1995.

73. Sidey, J.D.: Weak ankles: A study of common peroneal entrapment neuropathy. Br. Med. J. 3:623–626, 1969.

74. Nitz, A.J., J.J. Dobner, and D. Kersey: Nerve injury and grades II and III ankle sprains. Am. J. Sports Med. 13:177–182, 1985.

75. Kleinrensink, G.J., R. Stoeckart, J. Meulstee, et al.: Lowered motor conduction velocity of the peroneal nerve after inversion trauma. Med. Sci. Sports Exerc. 26:877–883, 1994.

76. Schon, L.C., and T.O. Clanton: Chronic leg pain. In Baxter, D.E. (ed.): The Foot and Ankle in Sport. St. Louis, C.V. Mosby Co., 1995.

77. Styf, J.: Entrapment of the superficial peroneal nerve: Diagnosis and results of decompression. J. Bone Joint Surg. Br. 71:131–135, 1989.

78. Kaplan, P.E., and W.T. Kernahan: Tarsal tunnel syndrome: An electrodiagnostic and surgical correlation. J. Bone Joint Surg. Am. 63:96–99, 1981.
79. Massey, E.W., and A.B. Plett: Neuropathy in joggers. Am. J. Sports Med. 6:209–211, 1978.
80. Murphy, P.C., and D.E. Baxter: Nerve entrapment of the foot and ankle in runners. Clin. Sports Med. 4:753–763, 1985.
81. Takakura, Y., C. Kitada, K. Sugimoto, Y. Tanaka, and S. Tamai: Tarsal tunnel syndrome: Causes and results of operative treatment. J. Bone Joint Surg. Br. 73:125–128, 1991.
82. Stefko, R.M., W.C. Lauerman, and J.D. Heckman: Tarsal tunnel syndrome caused by an unrecognized fracture of the posterior process of the talus (Cedell fracture). J. Bone Joint Surg. Am. 76:116–118, 1994.
83. Trepman, E.: Tarsal tunnel syndrome following Achilles tendon injury in dancers: Two cases. Clin. J. Sports Med. 3:192–194, 1993.
84. Jackson, D.L., and B.L. Haglund: Tarsal tunnel syndrome in runners. Sports Med. 13:146–149, 1992.
85. Mann, R.A.: Entrapment neuropathies of the foot. In DeLee, J.C., and D. Drez (eds.): Orthopedic Sports Medicine: Principles and Practice. Philadelphia, W.B. Saunders Co., 1994.
86. Sammarco, G.J., D.E. Chalk, and J.H. Feibel: Tarsal tunnel syndrome and additional nerve lesions in the same limb. Foot Ankle 14:71–77, 1993.
87. Jackson, D.L., and B. Haglund: Tarsal tunnel syndrome in athletes: Case reports and literature review. Am. J. Sports Med. 19:61–65, 1991.
88. Rask, M.R.: Medial plantar neuropraxia (jogger's foot): Report of three cases. Clin. Orthop. 134:193–195, 1978.
89. Pfeffer, G.B.: Plantar heel pain. In Baxter, D.E. (ed.): The Foot and Ankle in Sport. St. Louis, C.V. Mosby Co., 1995.
90. Johnson, E.R., K. Kirby, and J.S. Lieberman: Lateral plantar nerve entrapment: Foot pain in the power lifter. Am. J. Sports Med. 20:619–620, 1992.
91. House, J.A., and K. Ahmed: Entrapment neuropathy of the infrapatellar branch of the saphenous nerve. Am. J. Sports Med. 5:217–224, 1977.
92. Kaltenborn, F.M.: Mobilization of the Extremity Joints. Oslo, Olaf Norlis Bokhandel, 1980.
93. Stiell, I.G., G.H. Greenberg, R.D. McKnight, et al.: Decision rules for the use of radiography in acute ankle injuries: Refinement and prospective validation. JAMA. 269:1127–1132, 1993.
94. Stiell, I.G., R.D. McKnight, G.H. Greenberg, et al.: Implementation of the Ottawa ankle rules. JAMA. 271:827–832, 1994.
95. Stiell, I.G., G.H. Greenberg, R.D. McKnight, R.C. Nair, I. McDowell, and J.R. Worthington: A study to develop clinical decision rules for the use of radiography in acute ankle injuries. Ann. Emerg. Med. 21:384–390, 1992.
96. Black, H.: Roentgenographic considerations. Am. J. Sports Med. 5:238–240, 1977.
97. Hoffman, J.D.: Radiography of the ankle. In Hamilton, W.C. (ed.): Traumatic Disorders of the Ankle. New York, Springer-Verlag, 1984.
98. Renton, P., and W.J. Stripp: The radiology and radiography of the foot. In Klenerman, L. (ed.): The Foot and Its Disorders, 2nd ed. Boston, Blackwell Scientific Publications, 1982.
99. Rettig, A.C., K.D. Shelbourne, H.F. Beltz, D.W. Robertson, and P. Arfken: Radiographic evaluation of foot and ankle injuries in the athlete. Clin. Sports Med. 6:905–919, 1987.
100. Katcherian, D.: Soft-tissue injuries of the ankle. In Lutter, L.D., M.S. Mizel, and G.B. Pfeffer (eds.): Orthopedic Knowledge Update: Foot and Ankle. Rosemont, Illinois, American Academy of Orthopaedic Surgeons, 1994.
101. Cetti, R., and I. Andersen: Roentgenographic diagnosis of ruptured achilles tendon. Clin. Orthop. 286:215–221, 1993.
102. Rubin, G., and M. Witten: The talar-tilt angle and the fibular collateral ligaments: A method for the determination of talar-tilt. J. Bone Joint Surg. Am. 42:311–326, 1960.
103. Rijke, A.M., B. Jones, and P.A. Vierhout: Stress examination of traumatized lateral ligaments of the ankle. Clin. Orthop. 210:143–151, 1986.
104. Grace, D.L.: Lateral ankle ligament injuries: Inversion and anterior stress radiography. Clin. Orthop. 183:153–159, 1984.
105. Rijke, A.M.: Lateral ankle sprains: Graded stress radiography for accurate diagnosis. Phys. Sportsmed. 19:107–118, 1991.
106. Karlsson, J., T. Bergsten, L. Peterson, and B.E. Zachrisson: Radiographic evaluation of ankle joint stability. Clin. J. Sports Med. 1:166–175, 1991.
107. Cox, J.S., and T.F. Hewes: "Normal" talar tilt angle. Clin. Orthop. 140:37–41, 1979.
108. Vanderwilde, R., L.T. Staheli, D.E. Chew, and V. Malagon: Measurements on radiographs of the foot in normal infants and children. J. Bone Joint Surg. Am. 70:407–415, 1988.
109. Klenerman, L.: Examination of the foot. In Klenerman, L. (ed.): The Foot and Its Disorders, 2nd ed. Boston, Blackwell Scientific Publications, 1982.
110. Pavlov, H.: Ankle and subtalar arthrography. Clin. Sports Med. 1:47–49, 1982.
111. Raatikainen, T., M. Putkanen, and J. Puranen: Arthrography, clinical examination and stress radiograph in the diagnosis of acute injury to the lateral ligaments of the ankle. Am. J. Sports Med. 20:2–6, 1992.
112. Kerr, R., D.M. Forrester, and S. Kingston: Magnetic resonance imaging of foot and ankle trauma. Orthop. Clin. North Am. 21:591–601, 1990.
113. Terk, M.R., and P.K. Kwong: Magnetic resonance imaging of the foot and ankle. Clin. Sports Med. 13:883–908, 1994.
114. Rijke, A.M., H.T. Gietz, F.C. McCue, and P.M. Dee: Magnetic resonance imaging of injury to the lateral ankle ligaments. Am. J. Sports Med. 21:528–534, 1993.

General References

American Academy of Orthopaedic Surgeons: Athletic Training and Sports Medicine. Chicago, AAOS, 1984.
American Orthopedic Association: Manual of Orthopaedic Surgery. Chicago, 1972.
Anderson, K.J., J.F. Lecocq, and E.A. Lecocq: Recurrent anterior subluxation of the ankle joint: A report of two cases and an experimental study. J. Bone Joint Surg. Am. 34:853–860, 1952.
Basmajian, J.V., and G. Stecko: The role of muscles in arch support of the foot. J. Bone Joint Surg. Am. 45:1184–1190, 1964.
Baumhauer, J.F., D.N. Alosa, P.A. Renstrom, S. Trevino, and B. Beynnen: A prospective study of ankle injury risk factors. Am. J. Sports Med. 23:564–570, 1995.
Beetham, W.P., H.F. Polley, C.H. Slocumb, and W.F. Weaver: Physical Examination of the Joints. Philadelphia, W.B. Saunders Co., 1965.
Berridge, F.R., and J.G. Bonnin: The radiographic examination of the ankle joint including arthrography. Surg. Gynecol. Obstet. 79:383–389, 1944.
Bigg-Wither, G., and P. Kelly: Diagnostic imaging in musculoskeletal physiotherapy. In Refshauge, K., and E. Gass (eds.): Musculoskeletal Physiotherapy. Oxford, Butterworth-Heinemann, 1995.
Bloedel, P.K., and B. Hauger: The effects of limb length discrepancy on subtalar joint kinematics during running. J. Orthop. Sports Phys. Ther. 22:60–64, 1995.
Bojsen-Moller, F.: Anatomy of the forefoot: Normal and pathologic. Clin. Orthop. 142:10–18, 1979.
Bordelson, R.L.: Heel pain. In DeLee, J.C., and D. Drez (eds.): Orthopedic Sports Medicine: Principles and Practice. Philadelphia, W.B. Saunders Co., 1994.
Cailliet, R.: Foot and Ankle Pain. Philadelphia, F.A. Davis Co., 1968.
Campbell, D.G., A. Menz, and J. Isaacs: Dynamic ankle ultrasonography: A new imaging technique for acute ankle ligament injuries. Am. J. Sports Med. 22:855–858, 1994.
Campbell, J.W., and V.T. Inman: Treatment of plantar fasciitis and calcaneal spurs with the UC-BL shoe insert. Clin. Orthop. 103:57–62, 1974.

Carroll, N.C., R. McMurtry, and S.F. Leete: The pathoanatomy of congenital clubfoot. Orthop. Clin. North Am. 9:225–232, 1978.

Case, W.S.: Ankle injuries. In Sanders, B. (ed.): Sports Physical Therapy. Norwalk, Conn., Appleton & Lange, 1990.

Catterall, A.: A method of assessment of the clubfoot deformity. Clin. Orthop. 264:48–53, 1991.

Cawthorn, M., G. Cummings, J.R. Walker, and R. Donatelli: Isokinetic measurement of joint inversion and evertor force in three positions of plantar flexion and dorsiflexion. J. Orthop. Sports Phys. Ther. 14:75–81, 1991.

Chen, S.C.: Ankle injuries. In Helal, B., J.B. King, and W.J. Grange (eds.): Sports Injuries: Their Treatment. London, Chapman & Hall Medical, 1986.

Chew, J.T., S.B. Tan, C. Sivathasan, R. Pavanni, and S.K. Tan: Vascular assessment in the neuropathic diabetic foot. Clin. Orthop. 320:95–100, 1995.

Clarkson, H.M., and G.B. Gilewich: Musculoskeletal Assessment: Joint Range of Motion and Manual Muscle Strength. Baltimore, Williams & Wilkins, 1989.

Clement, D.B., J.E. Taunton, and G.W. Smart: Achilles tendinitis and peritendinitis: Etiology and treatment. Am. J. Sports Med. 12:179–184, 1984.

Close, J.R.: Some applications of the functional anatomy of the ankle joint. J. Bone Joint Surg. Am. 38:761–781, 1956.

Close, J.R., V.T. Inman, P.M. Poor, and F.N. Todd: The function of the subtalar joint. Clin. Orthop. 50:159–179, 1967.

Cohn, S.L., and W.C. Taylor: Vascular problems of the lower extremity in athletes. Clin. Sports Med. 9:449–470, 1990.

Coleman, S.S., and W.J. Chesnut: A simple test for hindfoot flexibility in the cavovarus foot. Clin. Orthop. 123:60–62, 1977.

Cooper, D.L., and J. Fair: Managing the pronated foot. Phys. Sportsmed. 7:131, 1979.

Cox, J.S., and R.L. Brand: Evaluation and treatment of lateral ankle sprains. Phys. Sportsmed. 5:51–55, 1977.

Cox, P.D.: Isokinetic strength testing of the ankle: A review. J. Orthop. Sports Phys. Ther. 47:97–106, 1985.

Cyriax, J.: Textbook of Orthopaedic Medicine: Diagnosis of Soft Tissue Lesions, vol. 1, 8th ed. London, Balliere Tindall, 1982.

Dahle, L.K., M. Mueller, A. Delitto, and J.E. Diamond: Visual assessment of foot type and relationship of foot type to lower extremity injury. J. Orthop. Sports Phys. Ther. 14:70–74, 1991.

DeBrunner, H.U.: Orthopaedic Diagnosis. London, E & S Livingstone, 1970.

DeCarlo, M.S., and R.W. Talbot: Evaluation of ankle joint proprioception following injection of the anterior talofibular ligament. J. Orthop. Sports Phys. Ther. 8:70–76, 1986.

DeValentine, S.: Evaluation and treatment of ankle fractures. Clin. Podiatr. 2:325–348, 1985.

Drecben, S.: Heel pain. In Lutter, L.D., M.S. Mizel, and G.B. Pfeffer (eds.): Orthopedic Knowledge Update: Foot and Ankle. Rosemont, Illinois, American Academy of Orthopaedic Surgeons, 1994.

Dreeben, S., P.B. Thomas, P.C. Noble, and H.S. Tallos: A new method for radiography of weight bearing metatarsal heads. Clin. Orthop. 224:260–267, 1987.

Ebbetts, J.: Manipulation of the foot. Physiotherapy 57:194–202, 1971.

Edgar, M.A.: Hallux valgus and associated conditions. In Klenerman, L. (ed.): The Foot and Its Disorders, 2nd ed. Boston, Blackwell Scientific Publications, 1982.

Engsberg, J.R.: A new method for quantifying pronation in overpronating and normal runners. Med. Sci. Sports Exerc. 28:299–304, 1996.

Faciszewski, T., R.T. Burks, and B.J. Manaster: Subtle injuries of the Lisfranc joint. J. Bone Joint Surg. Am. 72:1519–1522, 1990.

Fixsen, J.A.: The foot in childhood. In Klenerman, L. (ed.): The Foot and Its Disorders, 2nd ed. Boston, Blackwell Scientific Publications, 1982.

Forkin, D.M., C. Koczur, R. Battle, and R.A. Newton: Evaluation of kinesthetic deficits indicative of balance control in gymnasts with unilateral chronic ankle sprains. J. Orthop. Sports Phys. Ther. 23:245–250, 1996.

Fromherz, W.A.: Examination. In Hunt, G.C. (ed.): Physical Therapy of the Foot and Ankle. Clinics in Physical Therapy. Edinburgh, Churchill Livingstone, 1988.

Garbalosa, J.C., R. Donatelli, and M.J. Wooden: Dysfunction, evaluation and treatment of the foot and ankle. In Donatelli, R., and M.J. Wooden (eds.): Orthopedic Physical Therapy. Edinburgh, Churchill Livingstone, 1989.

Garrick, J.G.: The injured ankle: A sports medicine nemesis. Sports Med. Bull. 10:8–10, 1975.

Gartland, J.J.: Fundamentals of Orthopedics. Philadelphia, W.B. Saunders Co., 1979.

Gray, G.W.: Chain Reaction: Successful Strategies for Closed Chain Testing and Rehabilitation. Adrian, Michigan, Wynn Marketing Inc., 1989.

Gregg, J.R., and M. Das: Foot and ankle problems in the preadolescent and adolescent athlete. Clin. Sports Med. 1:131–147, 1982.

Gutrecht, J.A., R.E. Espinosa, and P.J. Dyck: Early descriptions of common neurological signs. Mayo Clin. Proc. 43:807–814, 1968.

Ha' Eri, G.B., V.L. Fornasier, and J. Schatzker: Morton's neuroma: Pathogenesis and ultrastructure. Clin. Orthop. 141:256–259, 1979.

Halpern, J.S.: Lower extremity peripheral nerve assessment. J. Emerg. Med. 15:333–337, 1989.

Hardy, A.E.: Assessment of foot movement. J. Bone Joint Surg. Br. 69:838–839, 1987.

Harter, R.A.: Clinical rationale for closed kinetic chain activities in functional testing and rehabilitation of ankle pathologies. J. Sports Med. 5:13–24, 1996.

Hartsell, H.D.: Isokinetics and muscle strength ratios of the ankle invertors/evertors: A pilot study. Isok. Exerc. Sci. 4:116–121, 1994.

Helfet, A.J., and D.M. Gruebel-Lee: Disorders of the Foot. Philadelphia, J.B. Lippincott Co., 1979.

Hlavac, H.F.: The Foot Book: Advice to Athletes. Mountain View, California, World Publications, 1977.

Hoerr, N.L., S.I. Pyle, and C.C. Francis: Radiographic Atlas of Skeletal Development of the Foot and Ankle. Springfield, Illinois, Charles C. Thomas, 1962.

Holden, C.E.A.: Compartmental syndromes following trauma. Clin. Orthop. 113:95–102, 1975.

Hollinshead, W.H., and D.B. Jenkins: Functional Anatomy of the Limbs and Back. Philadelphia, W.B. Saunders Co., 1981.

Hoppenfeld, S.: Physical Examination of the Spine and Extremities. New York, Appleton-Century-Crofts, 1976.

Hutton, W.C., J.R.R. Stott, and I.A.F. Stokes: The mechanics of the foot. In Klenerman, L. (ed.): The Foot and Its Disorders, 2nd ed. Boston, Blackwell Scientific Publications, 1982.

Inman, V.T.: The Joints of the Ankle. Baltimore, Williams & Wilkins, 1976.

Jones, D.C.: Tendon disorders of the foot and ankle. J. Am. Acad. Orthop. Surg. 1:87–94, 1993.

Judge, R.D., G.D. Zuidema, and F.T. Fitzgerald: Clinical Diagnosis: A Physiological Approach. Boston, Little, Brown & Co., 1982.

Kaumeyer, G., and T. Malone: Ankle injuries: Anatomical and biomechanical considerations necessary for the development of an injury prevention program. J. Orthop. Sports Phys. Ther. 1:171–177, 1980.

Kerr, R., D.M. Forrester, and S. Kingston: Magnetic resonance imaging of foot and ankle trauma. Orthop. Clin. North Am. 21:591–601, 1990.

Kibler, W.B., C. Goldbert, and T.J. Chandler: Functional biomechanical deficits in running athletes with plantar fasciitis. Am. J. Sports Med. 19:66–71, 1991.

Kingston, S.: Magnetic resonance imaging of the ankle and foot. Clin. Sports Med. 7:15–28, 1988.

Kiruchi, S., M. Hasue, and M. Watanabe: Ischemic contracture in the lower limb. Clin. Orthop. 134:185–192, 1978.

Kleiger, B.: The mechanism of ankle injuries. J. Bone Joint Surg. Am. 38:59–70, 1956.

Klenerman, L: Functional anatomy. In Klenerman, L. (ed.): The Foot and Its Disorders, 2nd ed. Boston, Blackwell Scientific Publications, 1982.

Konradsen, L., J.B. Ravn, and A.I. Sorensen: Proprioception at the ankle: The effect of anaesthetic blockade of ligament receptors. J. Bone Joint Surg. Br. 75:433–436, 1993.

Kopell, H.P., and W.A. Thompson: Peripheral entrapment neuropathies of the lower extremity. N. Engl. J. Med. 262:56–60, 1960.

Kotwick, J.E.: Biomechanics of the foot and ankle. Clin. Sports Med. 1:19–34, 1982.

Landeros, O., H.M. Frost, and C.C. Higgins: Post-traumatic anterior ankle instability. Clin. Orthop. 56:169–178, 1968.

Lassiter, T.E., T.R. Malone, and W.E. Garrett: Injury to the lateral ligaments of the ankle. Orthop. Clin. North Am. 20:629–640, 1989.

Lattanza, L., G.W. Gray, and R.M. Kantner: Closed vs open kinetic chain measurements of subtalar joint eversion: Implications for clinical practice. J. Orthop. Sports Phys. Ther. 9:310–314, 1987.

Leach, R.E., S. James, and S. Wasilewski: Achilles tendinitis. Am. J. Sports Med. 9:93–98, 1981.

Liu, S.H., and W.J. Jason: Lateral ankle sprains and instability problems. Clin. Sports Med. 13:793–809, 1994.

MacConaill, M.A., and J.V. Basmajian: Muscles and Movements: A Basis for Human Kinesiology. Baltimore, Williams & Wilkins, 1969.

Mack, R.P.: Ankle injuries in athletics. Clin. Sports Med. 1:71–84, 1982.

Maitland, G.D.: The Peripheral Joints: Examination and Recording Guide. Adelaide, Australia, Virgo Press, 1973.

Malekafzali, S., and M.B. Wood: Tibial torsion: A simple clinical apparatus for its measurement and its application to a normal adult population. Clin. Orthop. 145:154–157, 1979.

Mann, R.A.: Surgical implications of biomechanics of the foot and ankle. Clin. Orthop. 146:111–118, 1980.

Matsen, F.A.: Compartment syndrome: A unified concept. Clin. Orthop. 113:8–14, 1975.

McPoil, T.G., and G.C. Hunt: Evaluation and management of foot and ankle disorders: Present problems and future directions. J. Orthop. Sports Phys. Ther. 21:381–388, 1995.

McRae, R.: Clinical Orthopaedic Examination. New York, Churchill Livingstone, 1976.

Milbauer, D.L., and S. Patel: Roentgenographic techniques. In Nicholas, J.A., and E.B. Hershman (eds.): The Lower Extremity and Spine in Sports Medicine, vol 1. St. Louis, C.V. Mosby Co., 1986.

Morris, J.M.: Biomechanics of the foot and ankle. Clin. Orthop. 122:10–17, 1977.

Morton, D.J.: The Human Foot: Its Evolution, Physiology and Functional Disorders. Cambridge, Cambridge University Press, 1935.

Mubarak, S.J., and A.R. Hargens: Compartment Syndrome and Volkmann's Contracture. Philadelphia, W.B. Saunders Co., 1981.

Nigg, B.M.: The assessment of loads acting on the locomotor system in running and other sports activities. Semin. Orthop. 3:197–206, 1988.

Norfray, J.F., L. Schlachter, W.T. Kernaham, et al.: Early confirmation of stress fractures in joggers. JAMA. 243:1647–1649, 1980.

O'Doherty, D.: The foot and ankle. In Pynsent, P., J. Fairbank, and A. Carr (eds.): Outcome Measures in Orthopedics. Oxford, Butterworth-Heinemann, 1993.

O'Donoghue, D.H.: Treatment of Injuries to Athletes, 4th ed. Philadelphia, W.B. Saunders Co., 1984.

Ombregt, L., P. Bisschop, H.J. ter Veer, and T. Van de Velde: A System of Orthopedic Medicine. London, W.B. Saunders Co., 1995.

Parlasca, R., H. Shoji, and R.D. D'Ambrosia: Effects of ligamentous injury on ankle and subtalar joints: A kinematic study. Clin. Orthop. 140:266–272, 1979.

Picciano, A.M., M.S. Rowlando, and T. Worrell: Reliability of open and closed kinetic chain subtalar joint neutral positions and navicular drop test. J. Orthop. Sports Phys. Ther. 18:553–558, 1993.

Post, M.: Physical Examination of the Musculoskeletal System. Chicago, Year Book Medical Pub., 1987.

Regan, T.P., and J.C. Hughston: Chronic ankle "sprain" secondary to anomalous peroneal tendon. Clin. Orthop. 123:52–54, 1977.

Renstrom, P.A., and P. Kannus: Injuries of the foot and ankle. In DeLee, J.C., and D. Drez (eds.): Orthopedic Sports Medicine: Principles and Practice. Philadelphia, W.B. Saunders Co., 1994.

Richman, J.D., and P.S. Barre: The plantar ecchymosis sign in fractures of the calcaneus. Clin. Orthop. 207:122–125, 1986.

Riddle, D.L.: Foot and ankle. In Richardson, J.K., and Z.A. Iglarsh (eds.): Clinical Orthopedic Physical Therapy. Philadelphia, W.B. Saunders Co., 1994.

Riegger-Krugh, C., and J.J. Keysor: Skeletal malalignment of the lower quarter: Correlated and compensatory motions and postures. J. Orthop. Sports Phys. Ther. 23:164–170, 1996.

Root, M.L., W.P. Orien, and H.J. Weed: Normal and Abnormal Function of the Foot. Los Angeles, Clinical Biomechanics Corp., 1977.

Rorabeck, C.H., and I. Macnab: The pathophysiology of the anterior tibial compartment syndrome. Clin. Orthop. 113:52–57, 1975.

Rundle, E.: Foot and ankle. In Zuluaga, M., et al. (eds.): Sports Physiotherapy: Applied Science and Practice. Melbourne, Churchill Livingstone, 1995.

Samuelson, K.M.: Functional Anatomy. In Hamilton, W.C. (ed.): Traumatic Disorders of the Ankle. New York, Springer-Verlag, 1984.

Scheller, A.D., J.R. Kasser, and T.B. Quigley: Tendon injuries about the ankle. Orthop. Clin. North Am. 11:801–811, 1980.

Sell, K.E., T.M. Verity, T.W. Worrell, B.J. Pease, and J. Wigglesworth: Two measurement techniques for assessing subtalar joint position: A reliability study. J. Orthop. Sports Phys. Ther. 19:162–167, 1994.

Shea, M.P., and A. Manoli: Recognizing talar dome lesions. Phys. Sportsmed. 21:109–120, 1993.

Sheehan, G.: Medical Advice for Runners. Mountain View, California, World Publications, 1978.

Sidey, J.D.: Weak ankles: A study of common peroneal entrapment neuropathy. Br. Med. J. 3:623–626, 1969.

Simons, G.W.: Analytical radiography and the progressive approach in talipes equinovarus. Orthop. Clin. North Am. 9:187–206, 1978.

Soma, C.A., and B.R. Mandelbaum: Achilles tendon disorders. Clin. Sports Med. 13:811–823, 1994.

Spring, J.M., and G.W. Hyatt: Treatment of sprained ankles. Gen. Pract. 36:78–94, 1967.

Staheli, L.T., D.E. Chew, and M. Corbett: The longitudinal arch. J. Bone Joint Surg. Am. 69:426–428, 1987.

Starkey, C., and J. Ryan: Evaluation of Orthopedics and Athletic Injuries. Philadelphia, F.A. Davis Co., 1996.

Stuberg, W., J. Temme, P. Kaplan, A. Clarke, and R. Fuchs: Measurement of tibial torsion and thigh-foot angle using goniometry and computed tomography. Clin. Orthop. 272:208–212, 1991.

Subotnick, S.I.: History and physical examination. In Subotnick, S.I. (ed.): Sports Medicine of the Lower Extremity. Edinburgh, Churchill Livingstone, 1989.

Subotnick, S.I.: Podiatric Sports Medicine. Mount Kisco, New York, Futura Publishing Co., 1975.

Subotnick, S.I.: The Running Foot Doctor. Mountain View, California, World Publications, 1977.

Sweetman, R.: Pes cavus. Physiotherapy 49:204–208, 1963.

Tatro-Adams, D., S.F. McGann, and W. Carbone: Reliability of the figure of eight method of ankle measurement. J. Orthop. Sports Phys. Ther. 22:161–163, 1995.

Taylor, D.C., and F.H. Bassett: Syndesmosis ankle sprains: Diagnosing the injury and aiding recovery. Phys. Sportsmed. 21:39–46, 1993.

Testa, V.G., G. Capasso, and N. Maffulli: Paresthesia of the anterior aspect of the ankle: An early sign of lumbar spinal disorders in sportsmen. Physiother. 75:205–206, 1989.

Tomberlin, J.P., and H.D. Saunders: Evaluation, Treatment and Prevention of Musculoskeletal Disorders. Chaska, Minnesota, The Saunders Group, 1994.

Topp, R., and A. Mikesky: Reliability of isometric and isokinetic evaluations of ankle dorsi/plantar strength among older adults. Isok. Exerc. Sci. 4:157–163, 1994.

Travell, J.G., and D.G. Simons: Myofascial Pain and Dysfunction: The Trigger Point Manual (The Lower Extremities). Baltimore, Williams & Wilkins, 1992.

Vanderwilde, R.L., T. Stahei, D.E. Chew, and V. Malagon: Measurements on radiographs of the foot in normal infants and children. J. Bone Joint Surg. Am. 70:407–415, 1988.

Wadsworth, C.T.: Manual Examination and Treatment of the Spine and Extremities. Baltimore, Williams & Wilkins, 1988.

Walter, N.E., and M.D. Wolf: Stress fractures in young athletes. Am. J. Sports Med. 5:165–169, 1977.

Weissman, B.N.W., and C.B. Sledge: Orthopedic Radiology. Philadelphia, W.B. Saunders Co., 1986.

Wilkerson, G.B., and A.J. Nitz: Dynamic ankle stability: Mechanical and neuromuscular interrelationships. J. Sports Rehab. 3:43–57, 1994.

Williams, A., R. Evans, and P.D. Shirley: Imaging of Sports Injuries. London, Bailliere Tindall, 1989.

Yvars, M.F.: Osteochondral fractures of the dome of the talus. Clin. Orthop. 114:185–191, 1976.

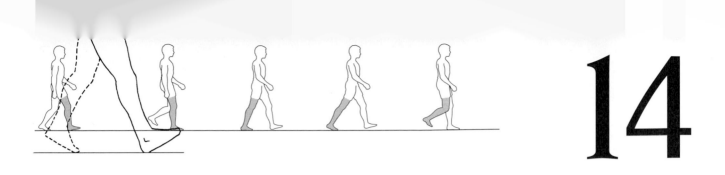

Gait Assessment

Walking is the simple act of falling forward and catching oneself. One foot is always in contact with the ground, and within a cycle there are two periods of single-leg support and two periods of double-leg support. With running, there is a period of time during which neither foot is in contact with the ground, a period called "double float."

The locomotion pattern tends to be variable and irregular until about the age of 7 years.[1] There are several functional tasks involved in gait, including forward progression, which is executed in a stepping movement in a wide range of rapid and comfortable walking speeds. Second, the body must be balanced alternately on one limb and then the other; this is accompanied by repeated adjustments of limb length. Finally, there is support of the upright body.

Gait assessment or analysis takes a great deal of time, practice, and technical skill combined with standardization for the clinician to develop the necessary skills.[2, 3] Most gait analysis today is performed with force platforms to measure ground reaction forces, electromyography to measure muscle activity, and high-speed video motion analysis systems to measure movement. Discussion of these techniques, however, is beyond the scope of this book. This chapter gives only a brief overview of a very complex task, assessment of normal and pathological gait; detailed assessment of gait is left to other authors.[4–12] The various terms commonly used to describe gait, the normal pattern of gait, the assessment of gait, and common abnormal gaits are reviewed.

Definitions[4–9]

Gait Cycle

The **gait cycle** is the time interval or sequence of motions occurring between two consecutive initial contacts of the same foot (Fig. 14–1). For example, if heel strike is the initial contact, the gait cycle for the right leg is from one heel strike to the next heel strike on the same foot. The gait cycle is a description of what happens in one leg. The same sequence of events is repeated with the other leg, but it is 180° out of phase.[6] Table 14–1 demonstrates the periods or phases of the gait cycle, the function of each phase, and what is happening in the opposite limb.[6] The gait cycle consists of two phases for each foot: **stance phase**, which makes up 60 to 65% of the walking cycle, and **swing phase**, which makes up 35 to 40% of the walking cycle. In addition, there are two periods of double support and one period of single-leg stance during the gait cycle.

As the velocity of the cycle increases, the cycle length or stride length decreases. For example, in jogging the gait cycle is 70% of the walking cycle, and in running the gait cycle is 60% that of walking.[13] In addition, as the speed of movement increases, the function of the muscles changes somewhat, and their electromyographic activity may increase or decrease.

Stance Phase

The stance phase of gait occurs when the foot is on the ground and bearing weight (Fig. 14–2). It allows the lower leg to support the weight of the body and, at the same time, allows for the advancement of the body over the supporting limb. Normally, this phase makes up 60% of the gait cycle and consists of five subphases, or instants.

Stages (Instants) of Stance Phase

- Initial contact (heel strike)
- Load response (foot flat)
- Midstance (single-leg stance)
- Terminal stance (heel off)
- Preswing (toe off)

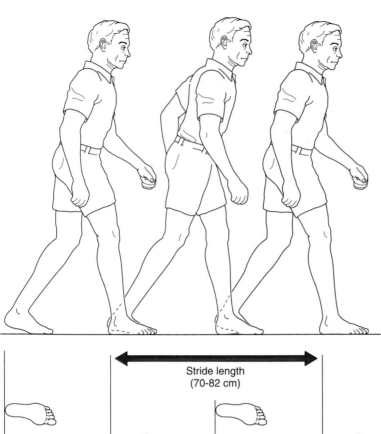

Figure 14–1
Gait cycle, stride length, and step length.

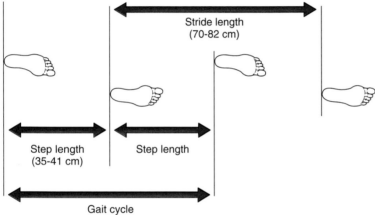

Table 14–1
Gait Cycle: Periods and Functions

Period	% of Cycle	Function	Contralateral Limb
Initial double limb support	0–12	Loading, weight transfer	Unloading and preparing for swing (preswing)
Single limb support	12–50	Support of entire body weight; center of mass moving forward	Swing
Second double limb support	50–62	Unloading and preparing for swing (preswing)	Loading, weight transfer
Initial swing	62–75	Foot clearance	Single limb support
Midswing	75–85	Limb advances in front of body	Single limb support
Terminal swing	85–100	Limb deceleration, preparation for weight transfer	Single limb support

From Sutherland, D.H., K.R. Kaufman, and J.R. Moitoza: Kinematics of normal human walking. *In* Rose, J., and J.G. Gamble (eds.): Human Locomotion. Baltimore, Williams & Wilkins, 1994, p. 27.

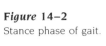

Figure 14-2
Stance phase of gait.

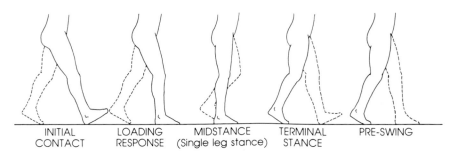

INITIAL   LOADING   MIDSTANCE   TERMINAL   PRE-SWING
CONTACT   RESPONSE (Single leg stance)   STANCE

The **initial contact** instant is the **weight-loading or weight acceptance period** of the stance leg, which accounts for the first 10% of the gait cycle. During this period, one foot is coming off the floor while the other foot is accepting body weight and absorbing the shock of initial contact. Because both feet are in contact with the floor, it is a period of **double support** or **double-leg stance**.

The **load response** and **midstance** instants consist of the **single support** or **single-leg stance**, which accounts for the next 40% of the gait cycle. During this period, one leg alone carries the body weight while the other leg goes through its swing phase. The stance leg must be able to hold the weight of the body, and the body must be able to balance on the one leg. In addition, lateral hip stability must be exhibited to maintain balance, and the tibia of the stance leg must advance over the stationary foot.

The **terminal stance** and **preswing** instants make up the **weight-unloading period,** which accounts for the next 10% of the gait cycle. During this period, the stance leg is unloading the body weight to the contralateral limb and preparing the leg for the swing phase. As with the first two instants, both feet are in contact, so double support occurs for the second time during the gait cycle.

Swing Phase

The swing phase of gait occurs when the foot is not bearing weight and is moving forward (Fig. 14–3). The swing phase allows the toes of the swing leg to clear the floor and allows for leg length adjustments. In addition, it allows the swing leg to advance forward. It makes

up approximately 40% of the gait cycle and consists of three subphases.

Acceleration occurs when the foot is lifted off the floor. During normal gait, rapid knee flexion and ankle dorsiflexion occur to allow the swing limb to accelerate forward. In some pathological conditions, loss or alteration of knee flexion and ankle dorsiflexion leads to alterations in gait.

The **midswing** instant occurs when the swing leg is adjacent to the weight-bearing leg, which is in midstance.

During the final instant (**terminal swing** or **deceleration**), the swinging leg slows down in preparation for initial contact with the floor. With normal gait, active quadriceps and hamstring muscle actions are required. The quadriceps muscles control knee extension, and the hamstrings control hip flexion.

During running or with increased velocity, the stance phase decreases and a **float phase** or **double unsupported phase** occurs while the double support phase disappears (Fig. 14–4).[13, 14] Although the single-leg stance phase decreases, the load increases two or three times.[13] The motion occurring at each of the joints (pelvis, hip, knee, ankle) is similar for walking and for running, but the required range of motion increases with the speed of the activity. For example, hip flexion in walking is about 40 to 45°, whereas in running it is to 60 to 75°.[15]

Subphases (Instants) of Swing Phase

- Initial swing (acceleration)
- Midswing
- Terminal swing (deceleration)

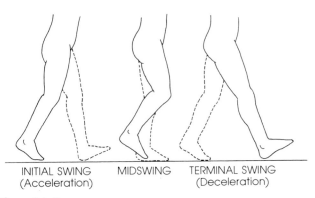

INITIAL SWING   MIDSWING   TERMINAL SWING
(Acceleration)   (Deceleration)

Figure 14-3
Swing phase of gait.

WALKING

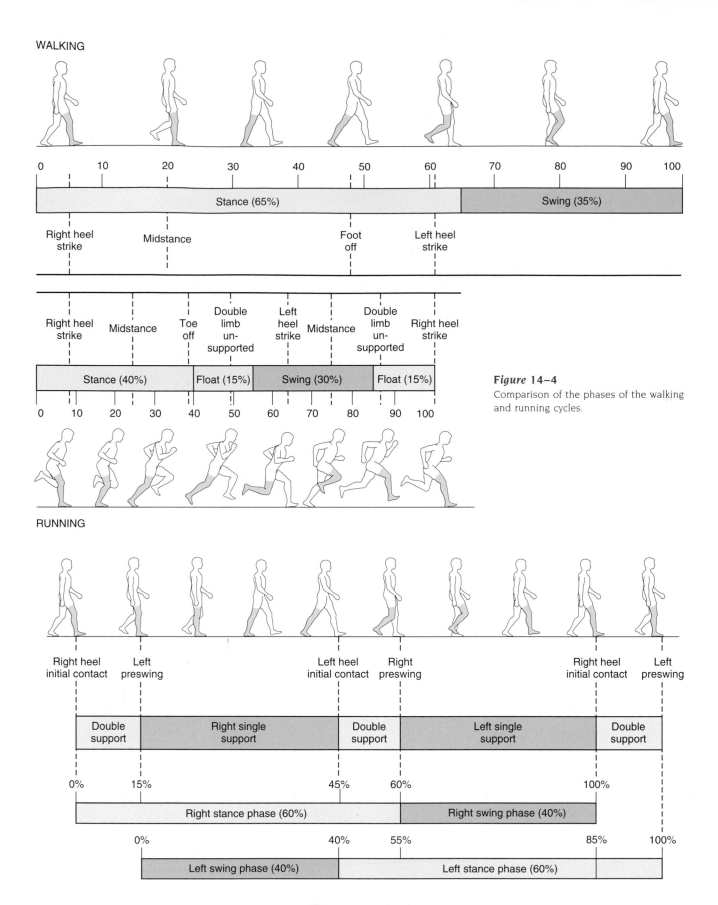

Stance (65%)   Swing (35%)

Right heel strike   Midstance   Foot off   Left heel strike

Right heel strike   Midstance   Toe off   Double limb un-supported   Left heel strike   Midstance   Double limb un-supported   Right heel strike

Stance (40%)   Float (15%)   Swing (30%)   Float (15%)

Figure 14–4
Comparison of the phases of the walking and running cycles.

RUNNING

Right heel initial contact   Left preswing   Left heel initial contact   Right preswing   Right heel initial contact   Left preswing

Double support   Right single support   Double support   Left single support   Double support

0%   15%   45%   60%   100%

Right stance phase (60%)   Right swing phase (40%)

0%   40%   55%   85%   100%

Left swing phase (40%)   Left stance phase (60%)

Time, percent of cycle

Figure 14–5
Time dimensions of the walking cycle. (Adapted from Inman, V.T., H.J. Ralston, and F. Todd: Human Walking. Baltimore, Williams & Wilkins, 1981, p. 26.)

Double-Leg Stance

Double-leg stance is that phase of gait in which parts of both feet are on the ground. In normal gait, it occurs twice during the gait cycle and represents about 25% of the cycle. This percentage increases the more slowly one walks; it becomes shorter as walking speed increases (Fig. 14–5) and disappears in running.

Single-Leg Stance

The single-leg stance phase of gait occurs when only one leg is on the ground; this occurs twice during the normal gait cycle and takes up approximately 30% of the cycle.

Normal Parameters of Gait[5–9, 16]

The parameters listed below and their values are what are considered normal for a population between the ages of 8 and 45 years. It should be pointed out, however, that a relatively normal gait pattern is seen in persons as young as 3 years of age.[1] There are, however, differences between individuals of the same sex and between men and women.[17] For the majority of the population outside of these ages, there are alterations caused by neurological development, balance control, aging, changes in limb length, and maturation.[1] For example, with maturity, walking velocity and step length increase, and cadence decreases.[18] It is also important to evaluate gait on the basis of normal gait of someone the same age. This is especially true for children.

> **Gait Parameters That Are Significantly Decreased in Women Compared With Men[17]**
>
> - Velocity
> - Stride and step length
> - Proportional distance of center of gravity from ground
> - Sagittal hip motion
> - Knee flexion in initial swing
> - Width of base of support
> - Vertical head excursion
> - Lateral head excursion
> - Shoulder sagittal motion
> - Elbow flexion

Base Width

The normal base width, which is the distance between the two feet, is 5 to 10 cm (2 to 4 inches; Fig. 14–6). If the base is wider, the examiner may suspect some pathology (e.g., cerebellar or inner ear problems) that

results in poor balance, a condition such as diabetes or peripheral neuropathy that may indicate a loss of sensation, or a musculoskeletal problem (e.g., tight hip abductors). In the first two cases, the patient tends to have a wider base to maintain balance. With increased speed, the base width normally decreases to zero, and in some cases, **crossover** occurs, in which one foot lands where the other should and vice versa. Such crossover can lead to gait alterations and other problems.[19]

Step Length

Step length, or gait length, is the distance between successive contact points on opposite feet (see Fig. 14–1). Normally, this distance is 35 to 41 cm (14 to 16 inches), and it should be equal for both legs. It varies with age and sex, with children taking smaller steps than adults and females taking smaller steps than males. Height also has an effect: a taller person takes larger steps. Step length tends to decrease with age, fatigue, pain, and

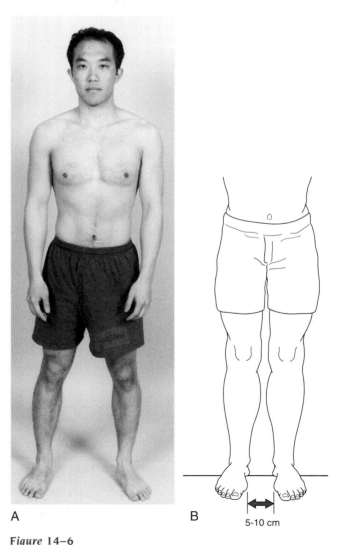

A   B   5-10 cm

Figure 14–6

(A) Wider-than-normal base width. (B) Normal base width.

disease. If step length is normal for both legs, the **rhythm of walking** will be smooth. If there is pain in one limb, the patient attempts to take weight off that limb as quickly as possible, altering the rhythm.

Stride Length

Stride length is the linear distance in the plane of progression between successive points of foot-to-floor contact of the same foot. The stride length is normally about 70 to 82 cm (27.5 to 32.3 inches) and in reality is one gait cycle. Stride length, like step length, decreases with age, pain, disease, and fatigue.[20] The age changes are often the result of decreased walking pace or speed.[20, 21]

Lateral Pelvic Shift (Pelvic List)

Lateral pelvic shift, or pelvic list, is the side-to-side movement of the pelvis during walking. It is necessary to center the weight of the body over the stance leg for balance (Fig. 14–7). The lateral pelvic shift is normally 2.5 to 5 cm (1 to 2 inches). It increases if the feet are farther apart. The pelvic list causes relative adduction of

the weight-bearing limb, facilitating the action of the hip adductors. If these muscles are weak, a Trendelenburg's gait results.

Vertical Pelvic Shift

Vertical pelvic shift keeps the center of gravity from moving up and down more than 5 cm (2 inches) during normal gait. By means of a vertical pelvic shift, the high point occurs during midstance and the low point during initial contact; the height of these points may increase during the swing phase if the knee is fused or does not bend because of protective spasm or swelling. The head is never higher during normal gait than it is when the person is standing on both feet. Therefore, if a person can stand in an opening, he or she should be able to move through the opening without hitting the head.[5] On the swing phase, the hip is lower on the swing side, and the patient must flex the knee and dorsiflex the foot to clear the toe. This action shortens the extremity length at midstance and decreases the center of gravity rise.

Pelvic Rotation

Pelvic rotation is necessary to lessen the angle of the femur with the floor, and, in so doing, it lengthens the femur (Fig. 14–8). It decreases the amplitude of displacement along the path traveled by the center of gravity

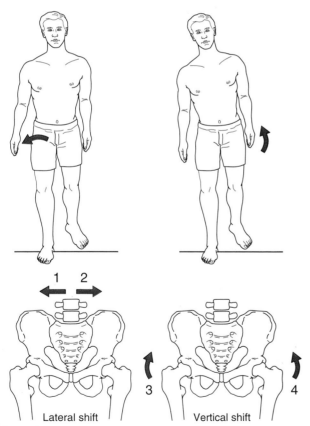

Figure 14–7
Pelvic shift. Numbers indicate that one lateral or vertical shift occurs, and then the other; they do not occur at the same time. 1 = right lateral shift; 2 = left lateral shift; 3 = right vertical shift; 4 = left vertical shift.

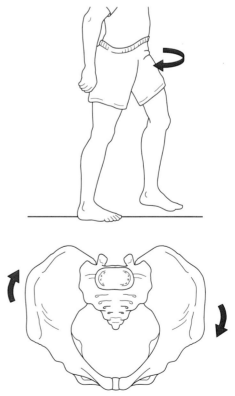

Figure 14–8
Pelvic rotation. Left forward pelvic rotation is illustrated.

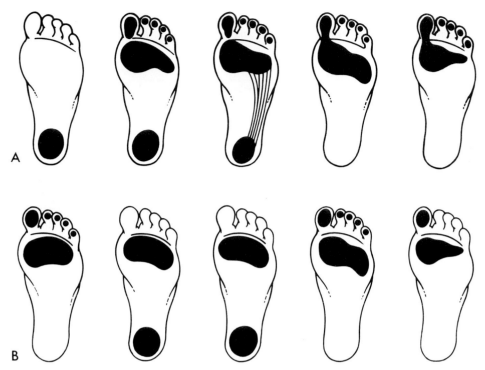

Figure 14–9
The cadence of gait. (A) Normal foot. (B) Cavus foot. (From Viladot, A.: Patologia del Antepié. Barcelona, Ediciones Toray, S.A., 1975.)

and thereby decreases the center-of-gravity dip. There is a total of 8° pelvic rotation, with 4° forward on the swing leg and 4° posteriorly on the stance leg. To maintain balance, the thorax rotates in the opposite direction. When the pelvis rotates clockwise, the thorax rotates counterclockwise, and vice versa. These concurrent rotations provide counterrotation forces and help regulate the speed of walking.

In the lower limb, rotation is evident at each joint. The farther the joint is from the trunk, the greater the amount of rotation. For example, rotation in the tibia is three times greater than rotation in the pelvis.[5]

Center of Gravity

Normally, in the standing position, the center of gravity is 5 cm (2 inches) anterior to the second sacral vertebra; it tends to be slightly higher in men than in women, because men tend to have a greater body mass in the shoulder area. The vertical and horizontal displacements of the center of gravity describe a figure-eight, occupying a 5-cm (2-inch) square within the pelvis during walking. The vertical displacement, which describes a smooth sinusoidal curve during walking, can be observed from the side. The patient's head descends during weight-loading and weight-unloading periods and rises during single-leg stance.

Normal Cadence

The normal cadence is between 90 and 120 steps per minute.[22, 23] The cadence of women is usually 6 to 9 steps per minute higher than that of men.[23] With age, the cadence decreases. Figure 14–9 illustrates the cadence of normal gait from heel strike to toe off. With pathology or deformity (e.g., a cavus foot), this pattern may be altered. As the pace of walking increases, the stride width increases, and the toeing-out angle decreases.

Normal Pattern of Gait[4–9, 24, 25]
Stance Phase

As previously mentioned, there are five instants involved during the stance phase of gait. These are now described in order of occurrence. This phase is the **closed kinetic chain** phase of gait. The action occurring at the various joints causes a "chain reaction" because of the stresses put on the joints and supporting structures with weight bearing. The foot becomes the fixed stable segment, and alterations occur from the foot up, with the joints of the foot adapting first, followed by those of the ankle, knee, hip, pelvis, spine, and finally the upper limb, which acts as a counterbalance to movement in the lower limb.[26] The relations between the joints are constantly changing.

Table 14–2
Summary of Joint Motions at the Hip, Knee, Tibia, Foot, and Ankle During the Stance Phase of Gait

		Hip	
		Kinetic Motion	
Phase	**Kinematic Motion**	*External Forces*	*Internal Forces*
Heel strike	20 to 40° of hip flexion moving toward extension Slight adduction and lateral rotation	Reaction force in front of joint; flexion moment moving toward extension; forward pelvic rotation	Gluteus maximus and hamstrings working eccentrically to resist flexion moment Erector spinae working eccentrically to resist forward bend
Foot flat	Hip moving into extension, adduction, medial rotation	Flexion moment	Gluteus maximus and hamstrings contracting concentrically to bring hip into extension Erector spinae resisting trunk flexion
Midstance	Moving through neutral position Pelvis rotating posteriorly	Reaction force posterior to hip joint; extension moment	Iliopsoas working eccentrically to resist extension Gluteus medius contracting in reverse action to stabilize opposite pelvis
Heel off	10 to 15° extension of hip abduction, lateral rotation	Extension moment decreasing after double-limb support begins	Iliopsoas activity continuing
Toe off	Moving toward 10° extension, abduction, lateral rotation	Decrease of extension moment	Adductor magnus working eccentrically to control or stabilize pelvis Iliopsoas activity continuing

	Knee and Tibia		
	Kinematic Motion		**Kinetic Motion**
Phase	*Knee*	*Tibia*	*External Forces*	*Internal Forces*

Phase	*Knee*	*Tibia*	*External Forces*	*Internal Forces*
Heel strike	In full extension before heel contact; flexing as heel strikes floor	Slight lateral rotation	Rapidly increasing reaction forces behind knee joint causing flexion moment	Quadriceps femoris contracting eccentrically to control rapid knee flexion and to prevent buckling
Foot flat	In 20° flexion moving toward extension	Medial rotation	Flexion moment	After foot is flat, quadriceps femoris activity becoming concentric to bring femur over tibia
Midstance	In 15° flexion moving toward extension	Neutral	Maximum flexion moment	Quadriceps femoris activity decreasing; gastrocnemius working eccentrically to control excessive knee extension
Heel off	In 4° flexion moving toward extension	Lateral rotation	Reaction forces moving anterior to joint; extension moment	Gastrocnemius beginning to work concentrically to start knee flexion
Toe off	Moving from near full extension to 40° flexion	Lateral rotation	Reaction forces moving posterior to joint as knee flexes; flexion moment	Quadriceps femoris contracting eccentrically

Table 14–2 summarizes the movement at the hip, knee, ankle, and foot during the stance phase.[27]

Initial Contact (Heel Strike)

Initial contact occurs when the limb first strikes the ground. Normally, this occurs when the heel strikes and the limb is being prepared to take weight. During the initial contact, the pelvis is level and medially rotated on the side of initial contact, whereas the trunk is aligned between the two lower limbs. The hip is flexed 30 to 49° and is medially rotated; the knee is slightly flexed or extended; the tibia is laterally rotated; the ankle is at 90° with the foot supinated; and the hindfoot is everted. At this instant, there is little force going through the limb.

If pain occurs in the heel at this time, it may be caused by a heel spur, bone bruise, heel fat-pad bruise,

Table 14–2
Summary of Joint Motions at the Hip, Knee, Tibia, Foot, and Ankle During the Stance Phase of Gait (Continued)

	Foot and Ankle			
	Kinematic Motion		Kinetic Motion	
Phase	Foot	Ankle	External Forces	Internal Forces
Heel strike	Supination (rigid) at heel contact	Moving into plantar flexion	Reaction forces behind joint axis; plantar flexion moment at heel strike	Dorsiflexors (tibialis anterior, extensor digitorum longus, and extensor hallucis longus) contracting eccentrically to slow plantar flexion
Foot flat	Pronation, adapting to support surface	Plantar flexion to dorsiflexion over a fixed foot	Maximum plantar flexion moment; reaction forces beginning to shift anterior, producing a dorsiflexion moment	Dorsiflexion activity decreasing; tibialis posterior, flexor hallucis longus, and flexor digitorum longus working eccentrically to control pronation
Midstance	Neutral	3° of dorsiflexion	Slight dorsiflexion moment	Plantar flexor muscles (gastrocsoleus and peroneal muscles), activated to control dorsiflexion of the tibia and fibula over a fixed foot, contracting eccentrically
Heel off	Supination as foot becomes rigid for push-off	15° dorsiflexion toward plantar flexion	Maximal dorsiflexion moment	Plantar flexor muscles beginning to contract concentrically to prepare for push-off
Toe off	Supination	20° plantar flexion	Dorsiflexion moment	Plantar flexor muscles at peak activity but becoming inactive as foot leaves ground

Modified from Giallonardo, L.M.: Gait. In Myers, R.S. (ed.): Saunders Manual of Physical Therapy Practice. Philadelphia, W.B. Saunders, Co., 1995, pp. 1108–1109.

or bursitis. This pain may cause increased flexion of the knee, with early plantar flexion to relieve the stress or pressure on the painful tissues. If the knee is weak, the patient may extend the knee by using the hand or may hit the heel hard on the ground to "whip" the knee into extension. A patient may do this because of weakness of the muscles (e.g., reflex inhibition, poliomyelitis, an internal derangement of the knee, a nerve root lesion [L2, L3, or L4], femoral neuropathy). In the past, this instant was referred to as "heel strike"; however, with some pathological gaits, heel strike may not be the first instant. Instead, the toes, the forefoot, or the entire foot may initially contact the ground. If the dorsiflexor muscles are weak, the foot "slaps" or "flops" down. The weakness may be caused by a peroneal neuropathy or nerve root lesion (L4). A knee flexion contracture or spasticity may cause the same alteration.

Load Response
(Weight Acceptance or Foot Flat)

Load response is a critical event in that the person subconsciously decides whether the limb is able to bear the weight of the body. The trunk is aligned with the stance leg. The pelvis drops slightly on the swing leg side and medially rotates on the same side. The flexed and later-

ally rotated hip moves into extension, and the knee flexes 15 to 25°. The tibia is medially rotated and begins to move forward over the fixed foot as the body swings over the foot. The ankle is plantar flexed, and the hindfoot is inverted. The foot moves into pronation, because this position unlocks the foot and enables it to adapt to different terrains and postures. The forefoot is pronated, unlocking the subtalar and metatarsal joints to enable them to absorb the shock more effectively, and the plantar aspect is in contact with the floor.

Abnormal responses include excessive or no knee motion as a result of weak quadriceps, plantar flexor contractures, or spasticity.[7]

Midstance (Single-Leg Support)

The midstance instant is a period of stationary foot support. Normally, the weight of the foot is evenly distributed over the entire foot. The trunk is aligned over the stance leg, and the pelvis shows a slight drop to the swing leg side.

During this stage, there is maximum extension of the hip (10 to 15°) with lateral rotation, and the greatest force is on the hip. Painful hip conditions cause this phase to be shortened as the patient "hurries through" the phase to decrease the pain. If the gluteus medius

(L5 nerve root) is weak, Trendelenburg's sign is present. The knee flexes, and the ankle is locked at 5 to 8° of dorsiflexion, rolling forward on the forefoot (roll-off). The foot is in contact with the floor; the forefoot is pronated, and the hindfoot is inverted. This instant is a critical event for the ankle. If pain is elicited during this period, the phase will be shortened and the heel may lift off early. This pain is commonly caused by conditions such as arthritis, rigid pes planus, fallen metatarsal or longitudinal arches, plantar fasciitis, or Morton's metatarsalgia. Therefore, pathology at the hip, ankle, or knee can modify the gait in this phase.

Terminal Stance (Heel Off)

In the final stages, the trunk is initially aligned over the lower limbs and moves toward the stance leg. The pelvis is initially level and posteriorly rotated and then dips to the swing leg side, remaining posteriorly rotated. The heel is in neutral and slight medial rotation; the knee is extended with the tibia laterally rotated. At the ankle, plantar flexion occurs as the critical event. This action helps to smooth the pathway of the center of gravity. The forefoot is initially in contact with the floor, and then the weight on the foot moves forward with plantar flexion so that only the big toe is in contact with the floor. At the same time, the forefoot moves from inversion to eversion.

Preswing (Toe Off)

The preswing phase is the acceleration phase as the toe pushes the leg forward. The trunk remains erect, the pelvis remains posteriorly rotated, and the hip is extended and slightly medially rotated. The knee flexes to 30 to 35° (critical event), and the ankle is plantar flexed. Because the center of gravity is anterior to the hip, the hip can be accelerated forward in initial swing.

If pain is elicited during this instant, it may be caused by a hallux rigidus, turf toe, or any other pathology involving the great toe (hallux), especially the metatarsophalangeal joint of the hallux. With injury to the joint, the patient is unable to push off on the medial aspect of the foot; instead, the patient pushes off on the lateral aspect of the foot to compensate for the painful metatarsophalangeal joint or, in some cases, a painful metatarsal arch resulting from increased pressure on the metatarsal heads. If the plantar flexors are weak (e.g., S1–S2 nerve root pathology), push-off may be absent. During this phase, the foot pronates so that there is a rigid base for better push-off.

Swing Phase

The swing phase of gait involves the lower limb in an **open kinetic chain**; the foot is not fixed on the ground, and the stresses on the limb are therefore less and easier to dissipate. During this phase, alterations occur from the spine down through the pelvis, hip, ankle, and foot. The pelvis and hip provide the most stability in the lower limb during the non–weight-bearing phase. Table 14–3 summarizes the motions occurring in the lower limb during the swing phase.

The three instants composing the swing phase of gait are now described in order of occurrence.

Initial Swing

During the first subphase of acceleration (Fig. 14–10), flexion and medial rotation of the hip and flexion of the

Table 14–3
Summary of Joint Motion and Forces During Swing Phase: Acceleration to Midswing and Midswing to Deceleration

	Acceleration to Midswing		Midswing to Deceleration	
Joint	*Kinematic Motion*	*Kinetic Motion*	*Kinematic Motion*	*Kinetic Motion*
Hip	Slight flexion (0 to 15°) moving to 30° flexion and lateral rotation to neutral	Hip flexors working concentrically to bring limb through; contralateral gluteus medius concentrically contracting to maintain pelvis position	Continued flexion at about 30 to 40°	Gluteus maximus contracting eccentrically to slow hip flexion
Knee	30 to 60° knee flexion and lateral rotation of tibia moving toward neutral	Hamstrings concentrically contracting	Moving to near full extension and slight lateral tibial rotation	Quadriceps femoris contracting concentrically and hamstrings contracting eccentrically
Ankle and foot	20° dorsiflexion and slight pronation	Dorsiflexors contracting concentrically	Ankle in neutral; foot in slight supination	Dorsiflexors contracting isometrically

From Giallonardo, L.M.: Gait. In Myers, R.S. (ed.): Saunders Manual of Physical Therapy Practice. Philadelphia, W.B. Saunders Co., 1995, p. 1110.

knee occur. The pelvis medially rotates and dips the swing leg side. The trunk is aligned with the stance leg. In addition, the ankle continues to plantar flex. The foot is not in contact with the floor. The forefoot continues supinating, and the hindfoot continues everting. The dorsiflexor muscles of the ankle contract to allow the foot to clear the ground, and the knee exhibits its maximum flexion of about 60°. If the quadriceps muscles are weak, the pelvis is thrust forward by the trunk muscles to provide forward momentum to the leg.

RANGE OF MOTION SUMMARY

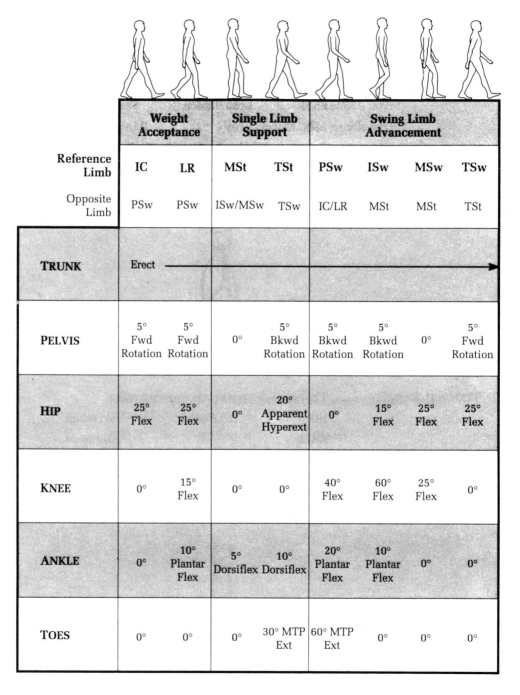

	Weight Acceptance		Single Limb Support		Swing Limb Advancement			
Reference Limb	IC	LR	MSt	TSt	PSw	ISw	MSw	TSw
Opposite Limb	PSw	PSw	ISw/MSw	TSw	IC/LR	MSt	MSt	TSt
TRUNK	Erect ———————————————————————————→							
PELVIS	5° Fwd Rotation	5° Fwd Rotation	0°	5° Bkwd Rotation	5° Bkwd Rotation	5° Bkwd Rotation	0°	5° Fwd Rotation
HIP	25° Flex	25° Flex	0°	20° Apparent Hyperext	0°	15° Flex	25° Flex	25° Flex
KNEE	0°	15° Flex	0°	0°	40° Flex	60° Flex	25° Flex	0°
ANKLE	0°	10° Plantar Flex	5° Dorsiflex	10° Dorsiflex	20° Plantar Flex	10° Plantar Flex	0°	0°
TOES	0°	0°	0°	30° MTP Ext	60° MTP Ext	0°	0°	0°

Figure 14–10

Normal range of motion during gait cycle. IC = initial contact; LR = load response; MSt = midstance; TSt = terminal stance; PSw = preswing; ISw = initial swing; MSw = midswing; TSw = terminal swing. (© 1991 LAREI, Rancho Los Amigos Medical Center, Downey, CA 90242; from The Pathokinesiology Service and The Physical Therapy Department, Rancho Los Amigos Medical Center: Observational Gait Analysis. Downey, California, Los Amigos Research and Educational Institute, Inc., 1996, p. 30.)

Midswing

During the midswing instant, the hip continues to flex and medially rotate, and the knee continues to flex. The ankle is in the anatomic position (90°) for the first 25% of the stance phase to permit the foot and midtarsal joints to unlock so that the foot can adapt to uneven terrain when it begins weight bearing. The forefoot is supinated, and the hindfoot is everted. The pelvis and trunk are in the same position as during the previous stage. If the ankle dorsiflexor muscles are weak (drop foot), the patient demonstrates a steppage gait. In such a gait, the hip flexes excessively so that the toes can clear the ground.

Terminal Swing (Deceleration)

During the final subphase, the hip continues to flex and medially rotate, and the knee reaches its maximum extension. At the ankle, dorsiflexion has occurred. The forefoot is supinated, and the hindfoot is everted. The trunk and pelvis maintain the same position as before. The hamstring muscles contract during the terminal phase to slow the swing; if the hamstrings are weak (e.g., S1–S2 nerve root lesion), heel strike may be excessively harsh to lock the knee in extension.

Joint Motion During Normal Gait

Although there is a tendency to talk about gait as action around joints, the examiner must not forget that muscles play a significant role in what happens at the joints.

Table 14–4 illustrates the actions of some of the muscles used during gait.[28]

Hip. The function of the hip is to extend the leg during the stance phase and flex the leg during the swing phase. The ligaments of the hip help to stabilize it in extension. The hip extensors help to initiate movement, as do the hip flexors; both groups of muscles work phasically. The hip flexors (primarily the iliopsoas muscles) fire to slow extension; the hip extensors (primarily the hamstring muscles) fire to slow flexion. In this way, they work eccentrically. The abductor muscles provide stability during single-leg support, a critical event for the hip.

If there is loss of movement of the hip, the compensatory mechanisms are increased mobility of the knee on the same side and increased mobility of the contralateral hip. In addition, the lumbar spine shows increased mobility.

Knee. When the knee is in flexion during the first three instants of the stance phase of gait, it acts as a shock absorber. Painful knees are not able to do this. One of the critical events of the knee is extension. The functions of the knee during gait are to bear weight, absorb shock, extend the stride length, and allow the foot to move through its swing. The quadriceps muscles use only 4 to 5% of their maximum voluntary contraction to extend the knee, but in so doing they help to control weight acceptance. The hamstring muscles flex the knee and slow the leg in the swing phase, working eccentrically.

If the knee has a flexion deformity, the hip is flexed and therefore loses its extension power, which is a critical event for the hip. Pathological conditions such as patel-

Table 14–4
Muscle Actions During Gait Cycle

Phase of Gait	Mechanical Goals	Active Muscle Groups	Examples
Stance Phase			
Initial contact	Position foot, begin deceleration	Ankle dorsiflexors, hip extensors, knee flexors	Anterior tibialis, gluteus maximus, hamstrings
Loading response	Accept weight, stabilize pelvis, decelerate mass	Knee extensors, hip abductors, ankle plantar flexors	Vasti, gluteus medius, gastrocnemius, soleus
Midstance	Stabilize knee, preserve momentum	Ankle plantar flexors (isometric)	Gastrocnemius, soleus
Terminal stance	Accelerate mass	Ankle plantar flexors (concentric)	Gastrocnemius, soleus
Swing Phase			
Preswing	Prepare for swing	Hip flexors	Iliopsoas, rectus femoris
Initial swing	Clear foot, vary cadence	Ankle dorsiflexors, hip flexors	Tibialis anterior, iliopsoas, rectus femoris
Midswing	Clear foot	Ankle dorsiflexors	Tibialis anterior
Terminal swing	Decelerate shank, decelerate leg, position foot, prepare for contact	Knee flexors, hip extensors, ankle dorsiflexors, knee extensors	Hamstrings, gluteus maximus, tibialis anterior, vasti

From Rab, G.T.: Muscle. *In* Rose, J., and J.G. Gamble (eds.): Human Locomotion. Baltimore, Williams & Wilkins, 1994, p. 113.

lofemoral syndrome also cause deviations from normal gait. For example, patients with patellofemoral syndrome show less knee flexion during the single-leg stance phase, combined with lateral femoral rotation during the swing phase.[29] On heel strike to foot flat, the femur then medially rotates, and if this compensating medial rotation is too great, it causes excessive pronation, which then stresses the medial aspect of the patellofemoral joint.

Gastrocnemius and Soleus. The gastrocnemius and soleus muscles are important in gait. They use 85% of their maximum voluntary contraction during normal walking. These muscles help to restrain the body's forward momentum during forward movement. They also contribute to knee and ankle stability, restrain forward rotation of the tibia on the talus during the stance phase, and minimize the vertical pelvic shift, thereby conserving energy.[30] To accomplish these functions during gait, the triceps surae work eccentrically and concentrically.

Foot and Ankle. The foot and ankle play major roles in gait in that the various joints allow the foot to accommodate to the ground. The joints of the foot and ankle work interdependently during normal gait. When the heel contacts the ground, the lower limb becomes a closed kinetic chain, and movements and stresses must be absorbed by the structures of the lower limb.

When looking at the ankle, the examiner should observe immediate plantar flexion at initial contact. Loss of this plantar flexion (e.g., tibial nerve neuropathy) results in inability to transfer weight to the anterior foot, increased ankle dorsiflexion, and increased knee flexion. In addition, the duration of single-leg stance on the affected side decreases, and the step length on the opposite side decreases. Furthermore, quadriceps action at the knee increases because of the lack of knee stability caused by the loss of the triceps surae, with the end result being that walking velocity decreases.[30] The foot then dorsiflexes through midstance or single-leg stance, with maximum dorsiflexion being reached just before heel off. The examiner should note whether there is sufficient plantar flexion during push-off.

Overview and Patient History

The assessment of a patient's gait should be included in any assessment of the lower limb. The examiner must keep in mind that the posture of the head, neck, thorax, and lumbar spine can affect gait even if no pathology is evident in the lower limb. The examiner must be able to identify the action of each body segment and note any deviation from normal during the individual phases of gait. For this reason, it is important to understand the normal parameters of gait and the mechanism of gait as it occurs. With this knowledge, the ways in which the gait is altered under pathological conditions can be better understood.

Musculoskeletal pathology tends to modify gait because of muscle weakness, pain, and/or altered range of motion, so the examiner should watch closely for these factors when observing gait. Many patients can adapt automatically to these changes, provided they have normal sensation and can develop selective control.[7] Patients with upper motor neuron lesions have greater alterations and cannot easily adapt because, in addition to the musculoskeletal problems, they also present with spasticity, control problems, and sensory disturbances.[7] It is important that the examiner read the patient's chart and take a history from the patient regarding any disease or injury, past or present, that may be causing gait problems.

Observation

The examiner should first perform a general overview of the patient's posture, looking for any asymmetry, and then observe the patient's gait, looking at stride length, step frequency, time of swing, speed of walking, and duration of the complete walking cycle. A steady gait pattern is usually established within three steps; it is initiated by the body's becoming unbalanced so that the patient can lift one foot off the ground to take the first step.[31] After this overview is completed, the examiner can look at specific parts of the gait in terms of phases and what happens at each joint during these phases.

Because gait constantly changes as one stops and starts, hurries, dawdles, and walks with others, it is important to remember whether the movements the patient is capable of are normal and whether the speeds, phases, strides, and durations of the cycles occur in normal combinations. In addition to observing walking at a normal speed, the patient's slow and fast gait speeds should be examined to see whether these changes affect the gait. The examiner must watch the lumbar spine, pelvis, hips, knees, feet, and ankles during these changes. Female patients should be in a bra and briefs, and male patients should be in shorts. The patient should walk barefoot. In this way, the motions of the toes, feet, legs, pelvis, trunk, and upper limbs can properly be observed.

The examiner should ask the patient to walk in the usual manner, using any aids necessary (e.g., parallel bars, crutches, walker, canes). While the patient is doing this, an initial general observation of any obvious limp or deformity should be made.

The examiner should observe the gait from the front, from behind, and from the side, in each instance observing from proximal to distal and watching the pelvis and lumbar spine down to the ankle and foot. In addition, the examiner should observe the movements in the trunk and upper limbs, which normally are in the opposite direction to those of the lower limbs. This method provides a sequential, thorough manner of assessment.

Rancho Los Amigos Medical Center has developed a very useful gait analysis chart (Fig. 14–11). By using the chart during observation, the examiner can determine deviations and their effect on gait in an easily used and easily retained method of recording. The dark gray boxes indicate what normally should occur; the lighter gray and white boxes indicate minor and major deviations from the normal, respectively. Minor deviations imply that the functional task of walking is not affected. Major deviations imply that the mechanics of walking are affected adversely.[32]

Anterior View

When observing from the front as the patient walks, the examiner should note whether any lateral tilt of the pelvis occurs, whether there is any sideways swaying of the trunk, whether the pelvis rotates on a horizontal plane,

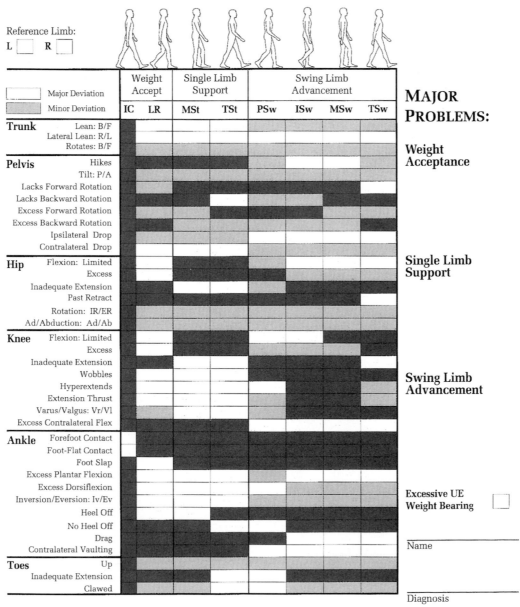

Figure 14–11

Gait analysis of the full body. (© 1996 LAREI, Rancho Los Amigos Medical Center, Downey, CA 90242; from The Pathokinesiology Service and The Physical Therapy Department, Rancho Los Amigos Medical Center: Observational Gait Analysis. Downey, California, Los Amigos Research and Educational Institute, Inc., 1996, p. 64.)

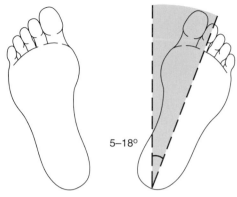

Figure 14–12
During stance and gait, the toes angle out 5 to 18° (Fick angle).

whether the trunk and upper extremity rotate in the opposite direction to the pelvis, and whether reciprocal arm swing is present. Usually, the trunk and upper extremity rotation is approximately 180° out of phase with the pelvis; that is, as the pelvis and lower limb rotate one way, the trunk and upper limb rotate in the opposite direction. This action helps provide a balancing effect and smooths the forward progression of the body. The examiner may also note movements at the hip (rotation and abduction-adduction), knee (rotation and abduction-adduction), and ankle and foot (amount of toe-out and toe-in, dorsiflexion–plantar flexion, supination-pronation). The examiner should note any bowing of the femur or the tibia, any medial or lateral rotation of the hips, and the position of the feet as the patient goes through the gait cycle (Fig. 14–12). This view is best used to examine the weight-loading period of the gait cycle. It should also be noted whether there is any abduction or circumduction of the swing leg, whether there is atrophy of the musculature of the anterior thigh and leg, and whether the base width is normal.

Lateral View

From the side, the examiner should observe rotation of the shoulder and thorax during the gait cycle, as well as reciprocal arm swing. Spinal posture (e.g., lordosis), pelvic rotation, and movements in the joints of the lower limbs should be noted. These movements include flexion-extension at the hip, flexion-extension at the knee, and dorsiflexion–plantar flexion at the ankle. From the lateral aspect, the examiner may also observe step length, stride length, cadence, and the other time dimensions of gait (see Fig. 14–5).[25] This view allows observation of the interactions between the walking surface and the various body parts.

The examiner must remember that there may be some compensation by the lumbar spine for limitation of movement in the hip. The patient should be observed to determine whether there is sufficient knee extension

at initial contact, followed almost immediately by slight flexion until the foot makes contact with the floor; whether there is control of the slightly flexed knee during load response and midstance; and whether there is sufficient flexion during preswing and initial swing. Also, any hyperextension of the knee during the gait cycle should be noted. Finally, the examiner should note whether there is coordination of movement among the hip, knee, and ankle; even or uneven gait length; and even or uneven duration of steps.

As the patient moves from initial contact to loading response, the foot flexes immediately, and the knee flexes until the foot is flat on the floor. During this period, the hip is also flexed. During midstance, the ankle dorsiflexes as the body pivots in an arc over the stationary foot. At the same time, the hip and knee extend, lengthening the leg. As the patient moves from terminal stance to preswing, the ankle plantar flexes to raise the heel, and the hip and knee flex as the weight is transferred to the opposite leg.

During the initial swing, the ankle is plantar flexed, and the hip and knee are maximally flexed. As the leg progresses to midswing, the ankle dorsiflexes, and the hip and knee begin to extend. As the patient moves from midswing to terminal swing, the ankle remains in the neutral position while the hip and knee continue extending. As the leg moves from terminal swing to initial contact, the knee reaches maximum extension; the ankle remains in neutral, and no further hip extension occurs at this stage.

Posterior View

When observing the gait cycle from behind, the examiner should notice the same structures that were viewed from the front. Rotation of the shoulders and thorax, reciprocal arm swing, and pelvic list and rotation may be noted posteriorly, as well as hip, knee, ankle, and subtalar joint movement. Heel rise and base of support (base width) are easier to view posteriorly. Any abnormal abduction or adduction movements or lateral displacement of the body segments should be noted. This view is best to examine the weight-unloading period of the gait cycle. The examiner can note whether heel rise is equal for both feet and whether the heels turn in or out. The observation should also include lateral movement of the spine and the musculature of the back, buttocks, posterior thigh, and calf.

Footwear

The patient should be asked to walk in normal footwear as well as in bare feet. The examiner should take time to observe the patient's footwear and observe any wearing down of the heels and/or socks, the condition of the shoe uppers, creases, and so on. The feet should also be examined for callus formations, blisters, corns, and bunions.

Different shoes can modify a patient's gait and the amount of energy necessary to perform gait. For example, high-heeled shoes alter movement, especially at the knee and ankle, which in turn increases the vertical loading.[33]

Locomotion Score

In addition to the detailed assessment of gait, locomotion scales or grading systems have been developed that include subjective and objective scores, which are combined for a total score. Figure 14–13 is a locomotion scoring scale that was developed for rheumatoid arthritis.[34] In addition to including all aspects of locomotion, it gives an overall estimation of functional disability for patients with rheumatoid arthritis.

Compensatory Mechanisms

The examiner must try to determine the primary cause of gait faults and the compensatory factors used to maintain an energy-saving gait. The patient tries to use the most energy-saving gait possible.[35] Speed of walking can also modify many of the normal parameters of gait.[36] Therefore, not only the gait pattern but also the speed of the activity and its effects must be noted. This type of assessment allows the examiner to set appropriate goals and plan a logical approach to treatment.

Abnormal Gait

Discussed next are some of the more common gait abnormalities; this list is by no means inclusive.

Detailed and Total Locomotion Score in Chronic Arthritis

UPPER EXTREMITIES

A.   Subjective score (max. 100 points)

1.   **Pain (max. 33 points)**
    33 None at ordinary activity   ____
    25 Mild, inconstant, unilaterally, not interfering with normal activity
    17 Mild bilateral or moderate unilateral, constant use of analgetics
    10 Severe pain despite large doses of analgesics, affecting activity
    5   Severe pain despite large doses of analgesics, affecting activity
    0   Severe bilateral, unable to work and use walking supports, prevents physical activity

2–4.   **Pain score reduction**   ____
    −10% Unilateral hand pain
    −25% Bilateral hand pain
    −25% Severe pain from both lower extremities or neck
                                            Sum: ____

ABILITY (max. 67 points)

Degree of disability

General (max. 20 points)	None	Mild	Moderate	Severe or unable
5–6. Manage work, household routines, shopping, child care (min. 3 of 4)	8 ☐	6 ☐	3 ☐	0 ☐ R 5 ☐ L 6
7–8. ADL (home and kitchen chore, personal care, dressing, etc.)	7 ☐	5 ☐	2 ☐	0 ☐ R 7 ☐ L 8
9–10. Drive a car or use public transportation	5 ☐		2 ☐	0 ☐ R 9 ☐ L 10

Special (max. 47 points)

	None	Mild	Moderate	Severe or unable
11–12. Feeding (hold knife, cup, open milk pack)	10 ☐	7 ☐	4 ☐	0 ☐ R 11 ☐ L 12
13–14. Carry 3 kg burden	5 ☐		2 ☐	0 ☐ R 13 ☐ L 14
15–18. Use telephone	5 ☐		2 ☐	0 ☐ R 15 ☐ L 16
17–18. Comb hair, brush teeth, shave	5 ☐		2 ☐	0 ☐ R 17 ☐ L 18

19–20. Wash the axillas	5 ☐		2 ☐	0 ☐ R 19 ☐ L 20
21–22. Reach things over shoulder level	5 ☐		2 ☐	0 ☐ R 21 ☐ L 22
23–24. Use of walking support(s)	12 ☐	7 ☐	4 ☐	0 ☐ R 23 ☐ L 24

Sum: right ____ left ____ Both (R/2 + L/2) ____

SUBJECTIVE SCORE: (pain: ____, ability: ____)   _____

B.   Objective score—physical signs (max. 100 points)

		Right	Left
Shoulder (max. 35 points)			
25–26. Flexion:	>90° = 10p, 45-90° = 5 p, <45° = 0p	☐25	☐26
27–28. Extension:	>20° = 5p, 0-20° = 3p, 0° = 0p	☐27	☐28
29–30. Abduction:	>90° = 10p, 45-90° = 5p, <45° = 0p	☐29	☐30
31–32. Medial rot.:	>15° = 5p, <15° = 0p	☐31	☐32
33–34. Lateral rot.:	>10° = 5p, <10° = 0p	☐33	☐34
Elbow (max. 35 points)			
35–36. Flexion (from 90°):	>120° = 10p, 100-120° = 7p, 90-100° = 4p, 0° = 0p	☐35	☐36
37–38. Extension defect:	0-30° = 10p, 30-60° = 7p, 60-90° = 4p, 90° = 0p	☐37	☐38
39–40. Deformity: none + stable = 5p, rigid deformity = 2p, laxid = 0p		☐39	☐40
41–42. Varus-valgus: <5° = 10p, 5-10° = 7p stressed varus-valgus >15° = 3p, >25° = 0p		☐41	☐42
Wrist (max. 15 points)			
43–44. Deformity (rigid, laxid): none = 15p, mild = 10p, moderate = 5p, severe = 0p		☐43	☐44
Hand (max. 15 points)			
45–46. Deformity (rigid, laxid): none = 15p, mild = 10p, moderate = 5p, severe = 0p		☐45	☐46

Sum: right ____ left ____ Both (R/2 + L/2) ____

OBJECTIVE SCORE: ____   **SUBJ. + OBJ. SCORE:** ☐ (a)
                                        (upper extremities)

Figure 14–13

Locomotion scoring scale. (Modified from Larsson, S.E., and B. Jonsson: Locomotion score in rheumatoid arthritis. Acta Orthop. Scand. 60:272, 1989 © Munksgaard International Publishers Ltd., Copenhagen, Denmark.)

Detailed and Total Locomotion Score in Chronic Arthritis (*Continued*)

LOWER EXTREMITIES

C. Subjective score (max. 100 points)

47. **Pain (max. 44 points)** ——
 44 None at ordinary activity
 40 Slight, occasional ache or awareness of pain, not influencing activity
 30 Mild bilateral or moderate unilateral, may take analgesics
 20 Moderate, affecting ordinary activities and work, consistent use of analgesics
 10 Severe pain in spite of optimal medication
 0 Severe, preventing most of activity or patient bedridden

48–50. **Pain score reduction** ——
 − 25% Moderate or severe pain from more than one ipsilateral joint
 − 50% Moderate or severe pain from more than one contralateral joint
 − 10% Severe pain from upper extremities or neck

           Sum: ——

   ABILITY (max. 56 points)

Walk (max. 36 points)
51. Limp: none = 12p, slight = 8p, moderate = 5p, severe = 0p ☐
52. Support: none = 12p, cane for long walks = 8p, cane most of time = 5p
    one crutch or can't use = 3p, two canes = 2p ☐
    two crutches or can't walk = 0p
53. Distance: unlimited = 12p, >400m = 8p, <400m = 5p ☐
    indoors only = 2p, bed or chair = 0p

Special (max. 20 points)
54. Climb stairs: without difficulty = 6p ☐
    with difficulty or by using banister = 3p
    with great difficulty or unable = 0p
55. Shoes and socks: without difficulty = 6p, with difficulty = 3p, unable = 0p ☐
56. Sitting: without difficulty = 6p, only short time or on high chair = 3p, unable to use any chair = 0p ☐

57. Transportation: can use public transportation = 2p, unable = 0p ☐

Sum: pain: ——, **ability:** —— (walk: ——, special: ——)

         SUBJECTIVE SCORE: ——

D.   **Objective score—physical signs (max. 100 points)**

              Right Left

Hip (max. 35 points)
58–59. Flexion: >90° = 10p, 60–90° = 5p, <60° = 0p ☐58 ☐59
60–61. Extension defect: 0-10° = 10p, 10–30° = 5p, >30° = 0p ☐60 ☐61
62–63. Abduction/adduction: >10° = 10p, −10–10° = 5p, <−10° = 0p ☐62 ☐63
64–65. Rotation: >0° = 5p, 0° = 0p ☐64 ☐65

Knee (max. 35 points)
66–67. Flexion: >100° = 10p, 80–100° = 8p, 60–80° = 5p ☐66 ☐67
68–69. Extension defect: 0° = 10p, 0–10° = 8p, 10–20° = 5p
    20-30° = 2p, >30° = 0p ☐68 ☐69
70–71. Varus-valgus: <7° = 10p, 7–15° = 8p
    stressed v/v 15–30° = 5p, >30° = 0p ☐70 ☐71
72–73. Deformity: none + stable = 5p, rigid = 2p, laxid = 0p ☐72 ☐73

Ankle (max. 15 points)
74–75. Deformity (rigid, laxid): none = 15p, mild = 10p, moderate = 5p, severe = 0p ☐74 ☐75

Feet (max. 15 points)
76–77. Deformity (rigid, laxid): None = 15p, mild = 10p, moderate = 5p, severe = 0p ☐76 ☐77

  SUM: right: —— **left:** —— **Both (R/2 + L/2):** ——
  OBJECTIVE SCORE: ——   **SUBJ. + OBJ. SCORE:** ☐ (b)
          (lower extremities)

    TOTAL LOCOMOTION SCORE: (a + b) ——

Figure 14–13 *Continued*

Antalgic (Painful) Gait

The antalgic or painful gait is self-protective and is the result of injury to the pelvis, hip, knee, ankle, or foot. The stance phase on the affected leg is shorter than that on the nonaffected leg, because the patient attempts to remove weight from the affected leg as quickly as possible; therefore, the amount of time on each leg should be noted. The swing phase of the uninvolved leg is decreased. The result is a shorter step length on the uninvolved side, decreased walking velocity, and decreased cadence.[25] In addition, the painful region is often supported by one hand, if it is within reach, and the other arm, acting as a counterbalance, is outstretched. If a painful hip is causing the problem, the patient also shifts the body weight over the painful hip. This shift decreases the pull of the abductor muscles, which decreases the pressure on the femoral head, from more than two times the body weight to approximately body weight, owing to vertical instead of angular placement of the load over the hip.

Arthrogenic (Stiff Hip or Knee) Gait

The arthrogenic gait results from stiffness, laxity, or deformity, and it may be painful or pain free. If the knee or hip is fused or the knee has recently been removed from a cylinder cast, the pelvis must be elevated by exaggerated plantar flexion of the opposite ankle and circumduction of the stiff leg (**circumducted gait**) to provide toe clearance. The patient with this gait lifts the entire leg higher than normal to clear the ground because of a stiff hip or knee (Fig. 14–14). The arc of movement helps to decrease the elevation needed to "clear" the affected leg. Because of the loss of flexibility in the hip, knee, or both, the gait lengths are different for the two legs. When the stiff limb is bearing weight, the gait length is usually smaller.

Ataxic Gait

If the patient has poor sensation or lacks muscle coordination, there is a tendency toward poor balance and a

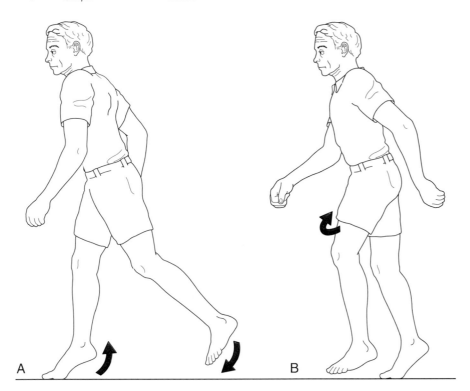

A   B

Figure 14–14
Arthrogenic (stiff knee or hip) gait.
(A) Excessive plantar flexion.
(B) Circumduction.

broad base (Fig. 14–15). The gait of a person with cerebellar ataxia includes a lurch or stagger, and all movements are exaggerated. The feet of an individual with sensory ataxia slap the ground because they cannot be felt. The patient also watches the feet while walking. The resulting gait is irregular, jerky, and weaving.

Contracture Gaits

Joints of the lower limb may exhibit contracture if immobilization has been prolonged or pathology to the joint has not been properly cared for. Hip flexion contracture often results in increased lumbar lordosis and extension of the trunk combined with knee flexion to get the foot on the ground. With a knee flexion contracture, the patient demonstrates excessive ankle dorsiflexion from late swing phase to early stance phase on the uninvolved leg and early heel rise on the involved side in terminal stance. Plantar flexion contracture at the ankle results in knee hyperextension (midstance of affected leg) and forward bending of the trunk with hip flexion (midstance to terminal stance of affected leg). Heel rise on the affected leg also occurs earlier.[25]

Equinus Gait

This childhood gait is seen with talipes equinovarus. Weight bearing is primarily on the dorsolateral or lateral edge of the foot, depending on the degree of deformity. The weight-bearing phase on the affected limb is decreased, and a limp is present. The pelvis and femur are laterally rotated to partially compensate for tibial and foot medial rotation.[1]

Gluteus Maximus Gait

If the gluteus maximus muscle, which is a primary hip extensor, is weak, the patient thrusts the thorax posteriorly at initial contact (heel strike) to maintain hip extension of the stance leg. The resulting gait involves a characteristic backward lurch of the trunk (Fig. 14–16).

Gluteus Medius (Trendelenburg's) Gait

If the hip abductor muscles (gluteus medius and minimus) are weak, the stabilizing effect of these muscles during stance phase is lost, and the patient exhibits an excessive lateral list in which the thorax is thrust laterally to keep the center of gravity over the stance leg (Fig. 14–17). A positive Trendelenburg's sign is also exhibited (i.e., the contralateral side droops because the ipsilateral hip abductors do not stabilize or prevent the droop). If there is bilateral weakness of the gluteus medius muscles, the gait shows accentuated side-to-side movement, resulting in a "wobbling" gait or "chorus girl swing." This gait may also be seen in patients with congenital dislocation of the hip and coxa vara.

Hemiplegic or Hemiparetic Gait

The patient with hemiplegic or hemiparetic gait swings the paraplegic leg outward and ahead in a circle (circumduction) or pushes it ahead (Fig. 14–18). In addition, the affected upper limb is carried across the trunk for

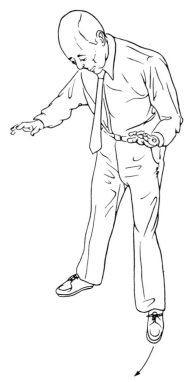

Figure 14–15

Ataxic gait. In cerebellar ataxia, the patient has poor balance and a broad base and therefore lurches, staggers, and exaggerates all movements. In sensory ataxia, the patient has a broad-based gait. Because the patient cannot feel the feet, the patient slaps them against the ground and looks down at them while walking. In both types of ataxia, the gait is irregular, jerky, and weaving. (From Judge, R.D., G.D. Zuidema, and F.T. Fitzgerald: Clinical Diagnosis: A Physiological Approach. Boston, Little, Brown & Co., 1982, p. 438.)

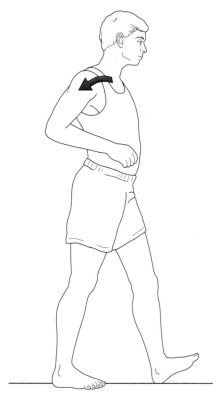

Figure 14–16

Gluteus maximus gait.

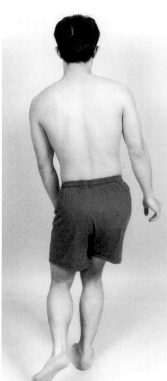

Figure 14–17

Gluteus medius (Trendelenburg's) gait.

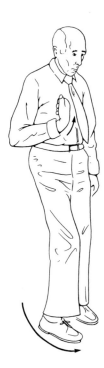

Figure 14–18

Hemiplegic (hemiparetic) gait. The arm is carried across the trunk, adducted at the shoulder. The forearm is rotated, the arm is flexed at the elbow and wrist, and the hand is flexed at the metacarpophalangeal joints. The leg is extended at the hip and knee. The patient either swings the affected leg outward in a circle (circumduction) or pushes it ahead. (From Judge, R.D., G.D. Zuidema, and F.T. Fitzgerald: Clinical Diagnosis: A Physiological Approach. Boston, Little, Brown & Co., 1982, p. 438.)

balance. This is sometimes referred to as a **neurogenic** or **flaccid gait**.

Parkinsonian Gait

The neck, trunk, and knees of a patient with parkinsonian gait are flexed. The gait is characterized by shuffling or short rapid steps (marche à petits pas) at times. The arms are held stiffly and do not have their normal associative movement (Fig. 14–19). During the gait, the patient may lean forward and walk progressively faster as though unable to stop (**festination**).

Plantar Flexor Gait

If the plantar flexor muscles are unable to perform their function, ankle and knee stability are greatly affected. Loss of the plantar flexors results in decrease or absence of push-off. The stance phase is less, and there is a shorter step length on the unaffected side.[25]

Psoatic Limp

The psoatic limp is seen in patients with conditions affecting the hip, such as Legg-Calvé-Perthes disease. The patient demonstrates a difficulty in swing-through, and the limp may be accompanied by exaggerated trunk and pelvic movement.[25] The limp may be caused by weak-

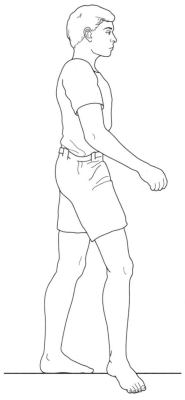

Figure 14–20
Psoatic limp. Note lateral rotation, flexion, and abduction of affected hip.

ness or reflex inhibition of the psoas major muscle. Classic manifestations of this limp are lateral rotation, flexion, and adduction of the hip (Fig. 14–20). The patient exaggerates movement of the pelvis and trunk to help move the thigh into flexion.

Quadriceps Gait

If the quadriceps muscles have been injured (e.g., femoral nerve neuropathy, reflex inhibition, trauma), the patient compensates in the trunk and lower leg. Forward flexion of the trunk combined with strong ankle plantar flexion causes the knee to extend (hyperextend). If the trunk, hip flexors, and ankle muscles cannot perform this movement, the patient may use a hand to extend the knee.[25]

Scissors Gait

This gait is the result of spastic paralysis of the hip adductor muscles, which causes the knees to be drawn together so that the legs can be swung forward only with great effort (Fig. 14–21). This is seen in spastic paraplegics and may be referred to as a **neurogenic** or **spastic gait**.

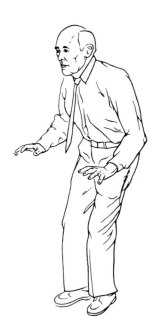

Figure 14–19
Parkinsonian gait. The head, trunk, and knees are flexed, and the arms are held rather stiffly with poor associative movement. The gait is shuffling or is characterized at times by short, rapid steps (marche à petits pas). The patient may lean forward and walk progressively faster, seemingly unable to stop (festination). (From Judge, R.D., G.D. Zuidema, and F.T. Fitzgerald: Clinical Diagnosis: A Physiological Approach. Boston, Little, Brown & Co., 1982, p. 496.)

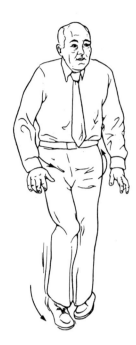

Figure 14–21
Scissors gait. Spasticity of thigh adduction, seen in spastic
paraplegics, draws the knees together. The legs are advanced (with
great effort) by swinging the hips. (From Judge, R.D., G.D. Zuidema,
and F.T. Fitzgerald: Clinical Diagnosis: A Physiological Approach.
Boston, Little, Brown & Co., 1982, p. 439.)

Short Leg Gait

If one leg is shorter than the other or there is a deformity
in one of the bones of the leg, the patient demonstrates
a lateral shift to the affected side, and the pelvis tilts
down on the affected side, creating a limp (Fig. 14–22).
The patient may also supinate the foot on the affected
side to try to "lengthen" the limb. The joints of the
unaffected limb may demonstrate exaggerated flexion,
or hip hiking may occur during the swing phase to allow
the foot to clear the ground.[25] The weight-bearing period
may be the same for the two legs. With proper footwear,
the gait may appear normal. This gait may also be termed
painless osteogenic gait.

Steppage or Drop Foot Gait

The patient with a steppage gait has weak or paralyzed
dorsiflexor muscles, resulting in a drop foot. To compensate and avoid dragging the toes against the ground, the
patient lifts the knee higher than normal (Fig. 14–23).
At initial contact, the foot slaps on the ground because
of loss of control of the dorsiflexor muscles.

Table 14–5 lists common gait pathologies that can
modify gait and the phase in which the deviation occurs.[27]

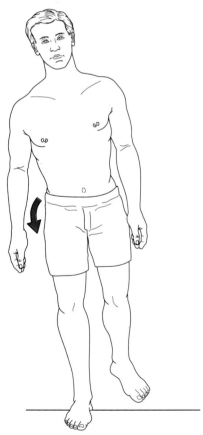

Figure 14–22
Short leg gait.

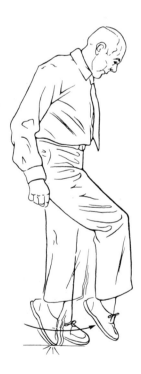

Figure 14–23
Steppage or drop foot gait. To avoid dragging the toes against the
ground (because the patient dorsiflexes the foot), the patient lifts
the knee high and slaps the foot to the ground on advancing. (From
Judge, R.D., G.D. Zuidema, and F.T. Fitzgerald: Clinical Diagnosis:
A Physiological Approach. Boston, Little, Brown & Co., 1982,
p. 438.)

Table 14–5
Common Gait Pathologies

Deviation	Phase	Cause
Excessive foot pronation	Midstance through toe off	Compensated forefoot or rearfoot varus deformity; uncompensated forefoot valgus deformity; pes planus; decreased ankle dorsiflexion; increased tibial varum; long limb; uncompensated medial rotation of tibia or femur; weak tibialis posterior
Excessive foot supination	Heel strike through midstance	Compensated forefoot valgus deformity; pes cavus; short limb; uncompensated lateral rotation of tibia or femur
Bouncing or exaggerated plantar flexion	Midstance through toe off	Heel cord contracture; increased tone of gastrocnemius and soleus
Insufficient push-off	Midstance through toe off	Gastrocnemius and soleus weakness; Achilles tendon rupture; metatarsalgia; hallux rigidus
Foot slap	Heel strike to foot flat	Dorsiflexor weakness
Steppage gait (hip and knee flex to clear foot)	Acceleration through deceleration	Dorsiflexor weakness
Excessive knee flexion	Heel strike through toe off	Hamstring contracture; decreased range of motion in ankle dorsiflexion; plantar flexor muscle weakness; lengthened limb; hip flexion contracture
Genu recurvatum (knee hyper-extension)	Heel strike through midstance	Quadriceps femoris weak or short; compensated hamstring weakness; Achilles tendon contracture; habit
Excessive medial or lateral femur rotation	Heel strike through toe off	Medial or lateral hamstrings tight, respectively; opposite muscle group weakness; anteversion or retroversion, respectively
Increased base of support (>4 inches)	Heel strike through toe off	Abductor muscle contracture; instability; genu valgum; leg length discrepancy
Decreased base of support (<2 inches)	Heel strike through toe off	Adductor muscle contracture; genu varum
Circumduction	Acceleration through deceleration	Increased limb length; abductor muscle shortening or overuse
Hip hiking	Acceleration through deceleration	Increased limb length; hamstring weakness; quadratus lumborum shortening
Inadequate hip flexion	Acceleration through heel strike	Hip flexor muscle weakness; hip extensor muscle shortening; increased limb length
Inadequate hip extension	Midstance through toe off	Hip flexion contracture; hip extensor muscle weakness
Excessive trunk back bending	Heel strike through midstance	Hip extensor of flexor muscle weakness; hip pain; decreased range of motion of knee
Excessive trunk forward bending	Deceleration through midstance	Quadriceps femoris and gluteus maximus weakness
Excessive trunk lateral flexion (compensated Trendelenburg's gait)	Foot flat through heel off	Gluteus medius weakness
Pelvic drop	Foot flat through heel off	Contralateral gluteus medius weakness

Modified from Giallonardo, L.M.: Gait. In Myers, R.S. (ed.): Saunders Manual of Physical Therapy Practice. Philadelphia, W.B. Saunders Co., 1995, p. 1112.

References

Cited References

1. Sutherland, D.H., and F. Valencia: Pediatric gait: Normal and abnormal development. *In* Drennan, J.C. (ed.): The Child's Foot and Ankle. New York, Raven Press, 1992.
2. Eastlack, M.E., J. Arvidson, L. Snyder-Mackler, J.V. Danoff, and C.L. McGarvey: Interrater reliability of videotaped observational gait-analysis assessments. Phys. Ther. 71:465–472, 1991.
3. Martin, P.E., G.D. Heise, and D.W. Morgan: Interrelationships between mechanical power, energy transfers, and walking and running economy. Med. Sci. Sports Exerc. 25:508–515, 1993.
4. Bowker, J.H., and C.B. Hall: Normal human gait. *In* Atlas of Orthotics: Biomechanical Principles and Applications. St. Louis, C.V. Mosby Co., 1975.
5. Inman, V.T., H.J. Ralston, and F. Todd: Human locomotion. *In* Rose, J., and J.G. Gamble (eds.): Human Locomotion. Baltimore, Williams & Wilkins, 1994.
6. Sutherland, D.H., K.R. Kaufman, and J.R. Moitoza: Kinematics of normal human walking. *In* Rose, J., and J.G. Gamble (eds.): Human Locomotion. Baltimore, Williams & Wilkins, 1994.
7. Adams, J.M., and J. Perry: Gait analysis: Clinical applications. *In* Rose, J., and J.G. Gamble (eds.): Human Locomotion. Baltimore, Williams & Wilkins, 1994.
8. Koerner, I.B.: Normal Human Locomotion and the Gait of the Amputee. Edmonton, University of Alberta Bookstore, 1979.
9. Koerner, I.: Observation of Human Gait [videotapes]. Health Sciences Audiovisual Education, University of Alberta, 1984.
10. Perry, J.: Gait Analysis: Normal and Pathological Function. Thorofare, New Jersey, Slack Inc., 1994.
11. Olsson, E.C.: Methods of studying gait. *In* Smidt, G.L. (ed.): Gait in Rehabilitation. New York, Churchill Livingstone, 1990.
12. Shiavi, R.: Electromyographic patterns in normal adult locomotion. *In* Smidt, G.L. (ed.): Gait in Rehabilitation. New York, Churchill Livingstone, 1990.
13. Adelaar, R.S.: The practical biomechanics of running. Am. J. Sports Med. 14:497–500, 1986.
14. Mann, R.A., G.T. Moran, and S.E. Dougherty: Comparative electromyography of the lower extremity in jogging, running, and sprinting. Am. J. Sports Med. 14:501–510, 1986.
15. Biden, E., J. O'Conner, and J.J. Collins: Gait analysis. *In* Daniel, D., W. Akeson, and J. O'Conner (eds.): Knee Ligaments: Structure, Function, Injury and Repair. New York, Raven Press, 1990.
16. Hoppenfeld, S.: Physical Examination of the Spine and Extremities. New York, Appleton-Century-Crofts, 1976.
17. Barry-Greb, T.L., and A.L. Harrison: Posture, gait, and functional abilities of the adolescent, pregnant and elderly female. Orthop. Phys. Ther. Clin. North Am. 5:1–21, 1996.
18. Sutherland, D.H., R. Olshen, L. Cooper, and S.L. Woo: The development of mature gait. J. Bone Joint Surg. Am. 62:336–353, 1980.
19. Subotnick, S.I.: Variations in angles of gait in running. Phys. Sportsmed. 7:110–114, 1979.
20. Ostrosky, K.M., J.M. Van Swearingen, R.G. Burdett, and Z. Gee: A comparison of gait characteristics in young and old subjects. Phys. Ther. 74:637–646, 1994.
21. Waters, R.L., H.J. Hislop, J. Perry, L. Thomas, and J. Campbell: Comparative cost of walking in young and old adults. J. Orthop. Res. 1:73–76, 1983.
22. Nuber, G.W.: Biomechanics of the foot and ankle during gait. Clin. Sports Med. 7:1–13, 1988.
23. Rodgers, M.M.: Dynamic foot mechanics. J. Orthop. Sports Phys. Ther. 21:306–316, 1995.
24. Perry, J., and H.J. Hislop: The mechanics of walking: A clinical interpretation. *In* Perry, J., and H.J. Hislop (eds.): Principles of Lower-Extremity Bracing. New York, American Physical Therapy Association, 1970.
25. Epler, M.: Gait. *In* Richardson, J.K., and Z.A. Iglarsh (eds.): Clinical Orthopedic Physical Therapy. Philadelphia, W.B. Saunders Co., 1994.
26. Krebs, D.E., D. Wong, D. Jevsevar, P.O. Riley, and W.A. Hodge: Trunk kinematics during locomotor activities. Phys. Ther. 72:505–514, 1992.
27. Giallonardo, L.M.: Gait. *In* Myers, R.S. (ed.): Saunders Manual of Physical Therapy Practice. Philadelphia, W.B. Saunders Co., 1995.
28. Rab, G.T.: Muscle. *In* Rose, J., and J.G. Gamble (eds.): Human Locomotion. Baltimore, Williams & Wilkins, 1994.
29. Dillon, P.Z., W.F. Updyke, and W.C. Allen: Gait analysis with reference to chondromalacia patella. J. Orthop. Sports Phys. Ther. 5:127–131, 1983.
30. Sutherland, D.H., L. Cooper, and D. Daniel: The role of the ankle plantar flexors in normal walking. J. Bone Joint Surg. Am. 62:354–363, 1980.
31. Mann, R.A., J.L. Hagy, V. White, and D. Liddell: The initiation of gait. J. Bone Joint Surg. Am. 61:232–239, 1979.
32. The Pathokinesiology Service and The Physical Therapy Department, Rancho Los Amigos Medical Center: Observational Gait Analysis. Downey, California, Los Amigos Research and Educational Institute, Inc., 1996.
33. Ebbeling, C.J., J. Hamill, and J.A. Crussemeyer: Lower extremity mechanics and energy cost of walking on high-heeled shoes. J. Orthop. Sports Phys. Ther. 19:190–196, 1994.
34. Larsson, S.E., and B. Jonsson: Locomotion score in rheumatoid arthritis. Acta Orthop. Scand. 60:271–277, 1989.
35. Gleim, G.W., N.S. Stachenfeld, and J.A. Nicholas: The influence of flexibility on the economy of walking and jogging. J. Orthop. Res. 8:814–823, 1990.
36. Murray, M.P., L.A. Mollinger, G.M. Gardner, and S.B. Sepic: Kinematic and EMG patterns during slow, free, and fast walking. J. Orthop. Res. 2:272–280, 1984.

General References

Andriacchi, T.P., G.B. Andersson, R.W. Fermier, D. Stern, and J.O. Galante: A study of lower-limb mechanics during stair climbing. J. Bone Joint Surg. Am. 62:749–757, 1980.

Brown, L.P., and P. Yavorsky: Locomotor biomechanics and pathomechanics: A review. J. Orthop. Sports Phys. Ther. 9:3–10, 1987.

Burdett, R.G., G.S. Skrinar, and S.R. Simon: Comparison of mechanical work and metabolic energy consumption during normal gait. J. Orthop. Res. 1:63–72, 1983.

Chondera, J.D.: Analysis of gait from footprints. Physiotherapy 60:179–181, 1974.

Crowinschield, R.D., R.A. Brand, and R.C. Johnson: The effects of walking velocity and age on hip kinematics and kinetics. Clin. Orthop. 132:140–144, 1978.

Eberhart, H.D., V.T. Inman, and B. Bresler: Principal elements in human locomotion. *In* Klopsteg, P.E., and P.D. Wilson (eds.): Human Limbs and Their Substitutes. New York, McGraw-Hill, 1954.

Engel, G.M., and L.T. Staheli: The natural history of torsion and other factors influencing gait in childhood. Clin. Orthop. 99:12–17, 1974.

Finley, F.R., K.A. Cody, and R.V. Finizie: Locomotion patterns in elderly women. Arch. Phys. Med. Rehabil. 50:140–146, 1969.

Gage, J.R., and S. Ounpuu: Gait analysis in clinical practice. Semin. Orthop. 4:72–87, 1989.

Garbalosa, J.C., R. Donatelli, and M.J. Wooden: Dysfunction, evaluation and treatment of the foot and ankle. *In* Donatelli, R., and M.J. Wooden (eds.): Orthopedic Physical Therapy. Edinburgh, Churchill Livingstone, 1989.

Gaudet, G., R. Goodman, M. Landry, G. Russell, and J.C. Wall: Measurement of step length and step width: A comparison of videotape and direct measurements. Physiother. Can. 42:12–15, 1990.

Gilbert, J.A., G.M. Maxwell, J.H. McElhaney, and F.W. Clippinger: A system to measure the forces and moments at the knee and hip during level walking. J. Orthop. Res. 2:281–288, 1984.

Gray, G.W.: Chain Reaction Successful Strategies for Closed Chain Testing and Rehabilitation. Adrian, Michigan, Wynn Marketing, 1989.

Grieve, D.W.: The assessment of gait. Physiotherapy 55:452–460, 1969.

Grieve, D.W.: Timing and placement of the feet. Semin. Orthop. 4:130–134, 1989.

Gruebel-Lee, D.M.: Disorders of Hip. Philadelphia, J.B. Lippincott Co., 1983.

Herzog, W., and P.J. Conway: Gait analysis of sacroiliac joint patients. J. Manip. Physiol. Ther. 17:124–127, 1994.

Hreljac, A.: Preferred and energetically optimal gait transition speeds in human locomotion. Med. Sci. Sports Exerc. 25:1158–1162, 1993.

Inman, V.T.: The Joints of the Ankle. Baltimore, Williams & Wilkins, 1976.

Inman, V.T.: Functional aspects of the abductor muscles of the hip. J. Bone Joint Surg. 29:607–619, 1947.

Inman, V.T.: Human locomotion: The classic. Clin. Orthop. 288:3–9, 1993.

Judge, R.D., G.D. Zuidema, and F.T. Fitzgerald: Clinical Diagnosis: A Physiological Approach. Boston, Little, Brown & Co., 1982.

Kadaba, M.P., H.K. Ramakrishnan, and M.E. Wootten: Measurement of lower extremity kinematics during level walking. J. Orthop. Res. 8:383–392, 1990.

Kadaba, M.P., H.K. Ramarkrishnan, M.E. Wootten, J. Gainey, G. Gordon, and G.V. Cochran: Repeatability of kinematic, kinetic, and electromyographic data in normal adult gait. J. Orthop. Res. 7:849–860, 1989.

Katoh, Y., E.Y. Chao, R.K. Laughman, E. Schneider, and B.F. Morrey: Biomechanical analysis of foot function during gait and clinical applications. Clin. Orthop. 2177:23–33, 1983.

Law, H.T.: Introduction: Techniques for the measurement of parameters related to human locomotion and their clinical applications. Semin. Orthop. 4:65–71, 1989.

Lehmann, J.F.: Push off and propulsion of the body in normal and abnormal gait. Clin. Orthop. 288:97–108, 1993.

Macleod, J.: Clinical Examination. New York, Churchill Livingstone, 1976.

Mann, R.A., and J.L. Hagy: The function of the toes in walking, jogging, and running [correction: 155:293]. Clin. Orthop. 142:24–29, 1979.

McCulloch, M.U., D. Brunt, and D. Van der Linden: The effect of foot orthotics and gait velocity on lower limb kinematics and temporal events of stance. J. Orthop. Sports Phys. Ther. 17:2–10, 1993.

McPoil, T.G., and M.W. Cornwall: Applied sports biomechanics in rehabilitation: Running. In Zachazewski, J.E., D.J. Magee, and W.S. Quillen (eds.): Athletic Injuries and Rehabilitation. Philadelphia, W.B. Saunders Co., 1996.

Minetti, A.E., C. Capelli, P. Zamparo, P.E. di Prampero, and F. Saibene: Effects of stride frequency on mechanical power and energy expenditure of walking. Med. Sci. Sports Exerc. 27:1194–1202, 1995.

Murray, M.P., A.B. Drought, and R.C. Kory: Walking patterns of normal men. J. Bone Joint Surg. Am. 46:335–360, 1964.

Murray, M.P.: Gait as a total pattern of movement. Am. J. Phys. Med. 46:290–333, 1967.

Murray, M.P., D.R. Gore, and B.H. Clarkson: Walking patterns of patients with unilateral pain due to osteoarthritis and avascular necrosis. J. Bone Joint Surg. Am. 53:259–274, 1971.

Olsson, E.: Gait analysis in orthopedics. Semin. Orthop. 4:111–119, 1989.

Perry, J.: Anatomy and biomechanics of the hindfoot. Clin. Orthop. 177:9–15, 1983.

Perry, J.: Pathological gait. In Atlas of Orthotics: Biomechanical Prinicples and Applications. St. Louis, C.V. Mosby Co., 1975.

Perry, J., and H. Hislop: Principles of Lower Extremity Bracing. Washington, American Physical Therapy Association, 1967.

Root, M.L., W.P. Orien, and J.H. Weed: Normal and Abnormal Function of the Foot. Los Angeles, Clinical Biomechanics Corp., 1977.

Saunders, J.B.M., V.T. Inman, and H.O. Eberhart: The major determinants in normal and pathological gait. J. Bone Joint Surg. Am. 35:543–558, 1953.

Schwab, G.H., D.R. Moynes, F.W. Jobe, and J. Perry: Lower extremity electromyographic analysis of running gait. Clin. Orthop. 176:166–170, 1983.

Simon, S.R., R.A. Mann, J.L. Hagy, and L.J. Larsen: Role of the posterior calf muscles in a normal gait. J. Bone Joint Surg. Am. 60:465–472, 1978.

Skinner, S.: Development of gait. In Rose, J., and J.G. Gamble (eds.): Human Locomotion. Baltimore, Williams & Wilkins, 1994.

Smidt, G.L.: Gait assessment and training in clinical practice. In Smidt, G.L. (ed.): Gait in Rehabilitation. New York, Churchill Livingstone, 1990.

Thurston, A.J., and J.D. Harris: Normal kinematics of the lumbar spine and pelvis. Spine 8:199–205, 1983.

Tiberio, D., and G.W. Gray: Kinematics and kinetics during gait. In Donatelli, R., and M.J. Wooden (eds.): Orthopedic Physical Therapy. Edinburgh, Churchill Livingstone, 1989.

Todd, F.N., L.W. Lamoreux, S.R. Skinner, et al.: Variations in the gait of normal children. J. Bone Joint Surg. Am. 71:196–204, 1989.

Tomaro, J., and R.G. Burdett: The effects of foot orthotics on the EMG activity of selected leg muscles during gait. J. Orthop. Sports Phys. Ther. 17:532–536, 1993.

Tomberlin, J.P., and H.D. Saunders: Evaluation, Treatment and Prevention of Musculoskeletal Disorders. Chaska, Minnesota, The Saunders Group, 1994.

Veicsteinas, A., P. Aghemo, R. Mrgaria, P. Cova, and M. Pozzolini: Energy cost of walking with lesions of the foot. J. Bone Joint Surg. Am. 61:1073–1076, 1979.

Wadsworth, C.T.: Manual Examination and Treatment of the Spine and Extremities. Baltimore, Williams & Wilkins, 1988.

Winter, D.A.: Energy assessment in pathological gait. Physiother. Can. 30:183–191, 1978.

Wooten, M.E., M.P. Kadaba, and G.V. Cochran: Dynamic electromyography: I. Numerical representation using principal component analysis. J. Orthop. Res. 8:247–258, 1990.

Wooten, M.E., M.P. Kadaba, and G.V. Cochran: Dynamic electromyography: II. Normal patterns during gait. J. Orthop. Res. 8:259–265, 1990.

Wright, D.G., S.M. Desai, and W.H. Henderson: Action of the subtalar and ankle joint complex during the stance phase of walking. J. Bone Joint Surg. Am. 46:361–382, 464, 1964.

Wyatt, M.P.: Gait in children. In Smidt, G.L. (ed.): Gait in Rehabilitation. New York, Churchill Livingstone, 1990.

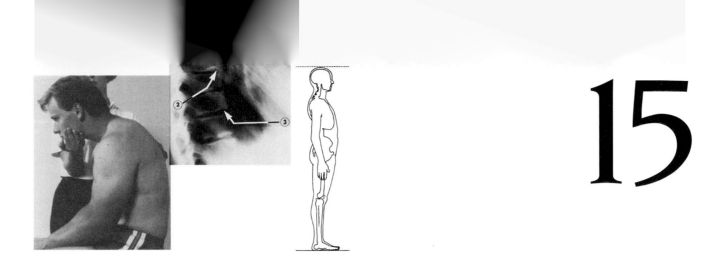

Assessment of Posture

Postural Development

Through evolution, human beings have assumed an upright erect or bipedal posture. The advantage of an erect posture is that it enables the hands to be free and the eyes to be farther from the ground so that the individual can see farther ahead. The disadvantages include an increased strain on the spine and lower limbs and comparative difficulties in respiration and transport of the blood to the brain.

Posture, which is the relative disposition of the body at any one moment, is a composite of the positions of the different joints of the body at that time. The position of each joint has an effect on the position of the other joints. Classically, ideal postural alignment (viewed from the side) is defined as a straight line (line of gravity) that passes through the ear lobe, the bodies of the cervical vertebrae, the tip of the shoulder, midway through the thorax, through the bodies of the lumbar vertebrae, slightly posterior to the hip joint, slightly anterior to the axis of the knee joint, and just anterior to the lateral malleolus.[1] **Correct posture** is the position in which minimum stress is applied to each joint. Upright posture is the normal standing posture for humans. If the upright posture is correct, minimal muscle activity is needed to maintain the position.

Any position that increases the stress to the joints may be called **faulty posture**. If a person has strong, flexible muscles, faulty postures may not affect the joints because he or she has the ability to change position readily so that the stresses do not become excessive. If the joints are stiff or too mobile, or the muscles are weak or shortened, however, the posture cannot be easily altered to the correct alignment, and the result can be some form of pathology. The pathology may be the result of the cumulative effect of repeated small stresses over a long period of time or of constant abnormal stresses over a short period of time. These chronic stresses can result in the same problems that are seen when a sudden (acute) severe stress is applied to the body. The abnormal stresses cause excessive wearing of the articular surfaces of joints and produce osteophytes and traction spurs, which represent the body's attempt to alter its structure to accommodate these repeated stresses. The soft tissue (e.g., muscles, ligaments) may become weakened, stretched, or traumatized by the increased stress. The application of an acute stress on the chronic stress may exacerbate the problem and produce the signs and symptoms that initially prompt the patient to seek aid.

At birth, the entire spine is concave forward, or flexed (Fig. 15–1). Curves of the spine found at birth are called **primary curves**. The curves that retain this position, those of the thoracic spine and sacrum, are therefore classified as primary curves of the spine. As the child grows (Fig. 15–2), **secondary curves** appear and are convex forward, or extended. At about the age of 3 months, when the child begins to lift the head, the cervical spine becomes convex forward, producing the cervical lordosis. In the lumbar spine, the secondary curve develops slightly later (6 to 8 months), when the child begins to sit up and walk. In old age, the secondary curves again begin to disappear as the spine starts to return to a flexed position as the result of disc degeneration, ligamentous calcification, osteoporosis, and vertebral wedging.

In the child, the center of gravity is at the level of the twelfth thoracic vertebra. As the child grows older, the center of gravity drops, eventually reaching the level of the second sacral vertebra in adults (slightly higher in males). The child stands with a wide base to maintain balance, and the knees are flexed. The knees are slightly bowed (genu varum) until about 18 months of age. The child then becomes slightly knock-kneed (genu valgum) until the age of 3 years. By the age of 6 years, the legs

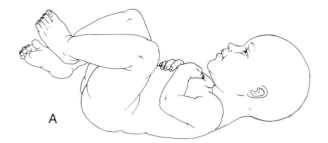

Figure 15–1
Postural development. (A) Flexed posture in a newborn. (B) Development of secondary cervical curve. (C) Development of secondary lumbar curve.

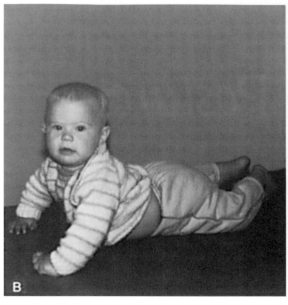

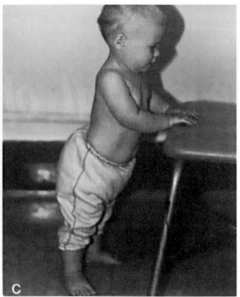

should naturally straighten (Fig. 15–3). The lumbar spine in the child has an exaggerated lumbar curve, or excessive lordosis. This accentuated curve is caused by the presence of large abdominal contents, weakness of the abdominal musculature, and the small pelvis characteristic of children at this age.

Initially, a child is flatfooted, or appears to be, as the result of the minimal development of the medial longitudinal arch and the fat pad that is found in the arch. As the child grows, the fat pad slowly decreases in size, making the medial arch more evident. In addition,

as the foot develops and the muscles strengthen, the arches of the feet develop normally and become more evident.

During adolescence, posture changes because of hormonal influence with the onset of puberty and musculoskeletal growth. Human beings go through two growth spurts, one when they are very young and a more obvious one when they are in adolescence. This second growth spurt lasts 2.5 to 4 years.[2] During this period, growth is accompanied by sexual maturation. Females develop quicker and sooner than males. Females enter puberty

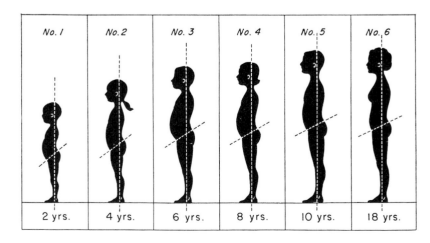

Figure 15–2
Postural changes with age. Apparent kyphosis at 6 and 8 years is caused by scapular winging. (From McMorris, R.O.: Faulty postures. Pediatr. Clin. North Am. 8:214, 1961.)

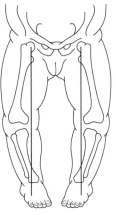
Newborn—
moderate genu varum

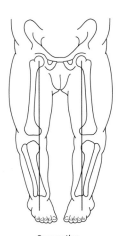
6 months—
minimal genu varum

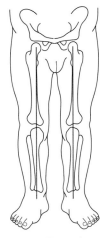
1 year, 7 months—
legs straight

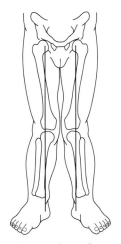
2 years, 6 months—
physiological genu valgum

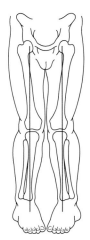
Protective toeing-in

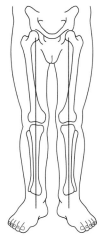
4 to 6 years—
legs straight with normal
toeing-out

Figure 15–3
Physiological evolution of lower limb alignment at various ages in infancy and childhood. (Redrawn from Tachdjian, M.O.: Pediatric Orthopedics. Philadelphia, W.B. Saunders Co., 1972, p. 1463.)

between 8 and 14 years of age, and puberty lasts about 3 years. Males enter puberty between 9.5 and 16 years of age, and it lasts up to 5 years.[2] It is during this period that body differences arise between males and females, with males tending toward longer leg and arm length, wider shoulders, smaller hip width, and greater overall skeletal size and height than females. Because of the rapid growth spurt, individuals, especially males, may appear ungainly, and poor postural habits and changes are more likely to occur at this age.

Factors Affecting Posture

Several anatomic features may affect correct posture. These factors may be enhanced or cause additional problems when combined with pathological or congenital states, such as Klippel-Feil syndrome, Scheuermann's disease (juvenile kyphosis), scoliosis, or disc disease.

Anatomic Factors Affecting Correct Posture

- Bony contours (e.g., hemivertebra)
- Laxity of ligamentous structures
- Fascial and musculotendinous tightness (e.g., tensor fasciae latae, pectorals, hip flexors)
- Muscle tonus (e.g., gluteus maximus, abdominals, erector spinae)
- Pelvic angle (normal is 30°)
- Joint position and mobility
- Neurogenic outflow and inflow

Causes of Poor Posture

There are many causes of poor posture (Fig. 15–4). Some of these causes are postural (positional), and some are structural.

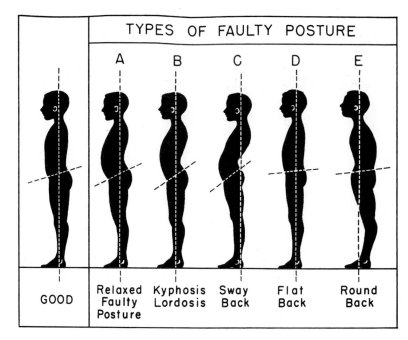

TYPES OF FAULTY POSTURE

A B C D E

GOOD | Relaxed Faulty Posture | Kyphosis Lordosis | Sway Back | Flat Back | Round Back

Figure 15–4

Examples of faulty posture. (From McMorris, R.O.: Faulty postures. Pediatr. Clin. North Am. 8:217, 1961.)

Postural (Positional) Factors

The most common postural problem is poor postural habit; that is, for whatever reason, the patient does not maintain a correct posture. This type of posture is often seen in the person who stands or sits for long periods and begins to slouch. Maintenance of correct posture requires muscles that are strong, flexible, and easily adaptable to environmental change. These muscles must continually work against gravity and in harmony with one another to maintain an upright posture.

Another cause of poor postural habits, especially in children, is not wanting to appear taller than one's peers. If a child has an early, rapid growth spurt there may be a tendency to slouch so as not to "stand out" and appear different. Such a spurt may also result in the unequal growth of the various structures, and this may lead to altered posture; for example, the growth of muscle may not keep up with the growth of bone. This process is sometimes evident in adolescents with tight hamstrings.

Another cause of poor posture is muscle imbalance or muscle contracture. For example, a tight iliopsoas muscle increases the lumbar lordosis in the lumbar spine.

Pain may also cause poor posture. Pressure on a nerve root in the lumbar spine can lead to pain in the back and result in a scoliosis as the body unconsciously adopts a posture that decreases the pain.

Respiratory conditions (e.g., emphysema), general weakness, excess weight, loss of proprioception, or muscle spasm (as seen in cerebral palsy) may also lead to poor posture.

The majority of postural nonstructural faults are relatively easy to correct after the problem has been identified. The treatment involves strengthening weak muscles, stretching tight structures, and teaching the patient

that it is his or her responsibility to maintain a correct upright posture in standing, sitting, and other activities of daily living.

Structural Factors

Structural deformities, which are the result of congenital anomalies, developmental problems, trauma, or disease, may cause an alteration of posture. For example, a significant difference in leg length or an anomaly of the spine such as a hemivertebra may alter the posture.

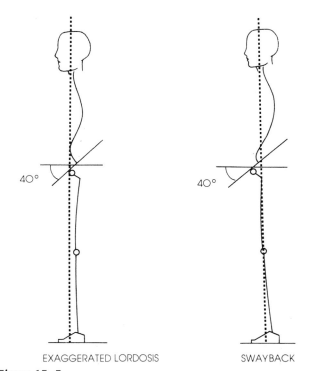

EXAGGERATED LORDOSIS   SWAYBACK

Figure 15–5

Examples of lordosis.

Structural deformities involve mainly changes in bone and therefore are not easily correctable without surgery. However, patients often can be relieved of symptoms by proper postural care instruction.

Common Spinal Deformities
Lordosis

Lordosis is an excessive anterior curvature of the spine (Fig. 15–5).[3–7] Pathologically, it is an exaggeration of the normal curves found in the cervical and lumbar spines. Causes of increased lordosis include (1) postural deformity; (2) lax muscles, especially the abdominal muscles; (3) a heavy abdomen, resulting from excess weight or pregnancy; (4) compensatory mechanisms that result from another deformity, such as kyphosis (Fig. 15–6); (5) hip flexion contracture; (6) spondylolisthesis; (7) congenital problems, such as bilateral congenital dislocation of the hip; (8) failure of segmentation of the neural arch of a facet joint segment; or (9) fashion (e.g., wearing high-heeled shoes). There are two types of exaggerated lordosis, pathological lordosis and swayback deformity.

Pathological Lordosis. In the patient with pathological lordosis, one may often observe sagging shoulders, medial rotation of the legs, and poking forward of the head so that it is in front of the center of gravity. This posture is adopted in an attempt to keep the center of gravity where it should be. Deviation in one part of the body often leads to deviation in another part of the body in an attempt to maintain the correct center of gravity and the correct visual plane. This type of exaggerated lordosis is the most common postural deviation seen.

The pelvic angle, normally approximately 30°, is increased with lordosis. With excessive or pathological lordosis, there is an increase in the pelvic angle to approximately 40°, accompanied by a mobile spine and an anterior pelvic tilt. Exaggerated lumbar lordosis is usually accompanied by tight hip flexors, tensor fasciae latae, and hip flexors, combined with weak abdominals.[8]

Swayback Deformity. With a swayback deformity, there is increased pelvic inclination to approximately 40°, and the thoracolumbar spine exhibits a kyphosis (Fig. 15–7).

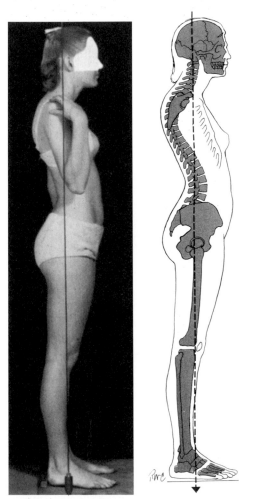

Figure 15–6
Faulty posture illustrating exaggerated lordosis and kyphosis. (From Kendall, F.P., and E.K. McCreary: Muscles: Testing and Function. Baltimore, Williams & Wilkins, 1983, p. 281.)

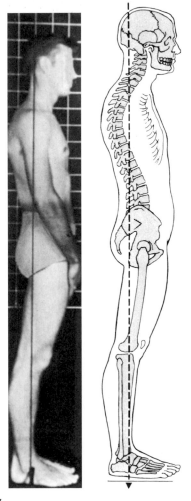

Figure 15–7
Faulty posture illustrating a swayback. (From Kendall, F.P., and E.K. McCreary: Muscles: Testing and Function. Baltimore, Williams & Wilkins, 1983, p. 284.)

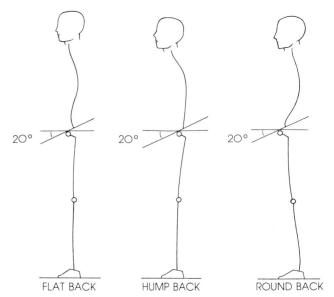

Figure 15-8
Examples of kyphosis.

A swayback deformity results in the spine's bending back rather sharply at the lumbosacral angle. With this postural deformity, the entire pelvis shifts anteriorly, causing the hips to move into extension. To maintain the center of gravity in its normal position, the thoracic spine flexes on the lumbar spine. The result is an increase in the lumbar and thoracic curves. Such a deformity may be associated with tight hip extensors, lower lumbar extensors, and upper abdominals, along with weak hip flexors, lower abdominals, and lower thoracic extensors.[1]

Kyphosis

Kyphosis is excessive posterior curvature of the spine (Figs. 15–8 and 15–9).[5, 7, 9–13] Pathologically, it is an exaggeration of the normal curve found in the thoracic spine. There are several causes of kyphosis, including tuberculosis, vertebral compression fractures, Scheuermann's disease, ankylosing spondylitis, senile osteoporosis, tumors, compensation in conjunction with lordosis, and congenital anomalies.[9] The congenital anomalies include a partial segmental defect, as seen in osseous metaplasia, or centrum hypoplasia and aplasia.[12, 14, 15] In addition, paralysis may lead to a kyphosis because of the loss of muscle action needed to maintain the correct posture combined with the forces of gravity.

Pathological conditions such as Scheuermann's vertebral osteochondritis may also result in a structural kyphosis (Fig. 15–10). In this condition, inflammation of the bone and cartilage occurs around the ring epiphysis of the vertebral body. The condition often leads to an

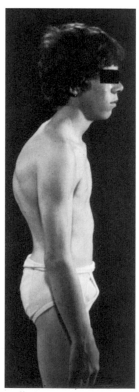

Figure 15-9
Faulty posture illustrating thoracic kyphosis. (From Moe, J.H., D.S. Bradford, R.B. Winter, and J.E. Lonstein: Scoliosis and Other Spinal Deformities. Philadelphia, W.B. Saunders Co., 1978, p. 152.)

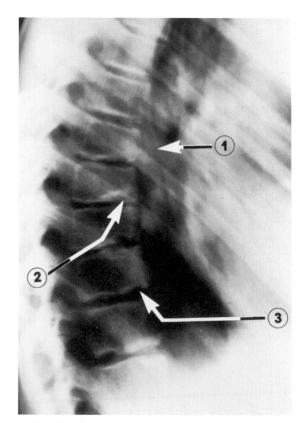

Figure 15-10
A classic x-ray appearance of the spine in a patient with Scheuermann's disease. Note the wedged vertebra (1), Schmorl's nodules (2), and marked irregularity of the vertebral end plates (3). (From Moe, J.H., D.S. Bradford, R.B. Winter, and J.E. Lonstein: Scoliosis and Other Spinal Deformities. Philadelphia, W.B. Saunders Co., 1978, p. 332.)

anterior wedging of the vertebra. It is a growth disorder that affects approximately 10% of the population, and in most cases several vertebrae are affected. The most common area for the disease to occur is between T10 and L2.

There are four types of kyphoses:

Round Back. The patient with a round back has a long, rounded curve with decreased pelvic inclination (<30°) and thoracolumbar kyphosis. The patient often presents with the trunk flexed forward and a decreased lumbar curve. On examination, there are tight hip extensors and trunk flexors with weak hip flexors and lumbar extensors.

Humpback or Gibbus. With humpback, there is a localized, sharp posterior angulation in the thoracic spine (Fig. 15–11).

Flat Back. A patient with flat back has decreased pelvic inclination to 20° and a mobile lumbar spine (Fig. 15–12).

Dowager's Hump. This is often seen in older patients, especially women. The deformity is caused by osteoporosis, in which the thoracic vertebral bodies begin to degenerate and wedge in an anterior direction, resulting in a kyphosis (Fig. 15–13).

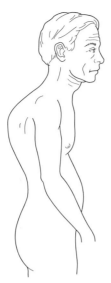

Figure 15–11
Humpback or gibbus deformity.

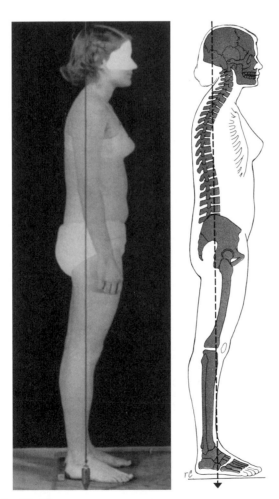

Figure 15–12
Faulty posture illustrating flat back. (From Kendall, F.P., and E.K. McCreary: Muscles: Testing and Function. Baltimore, Williams & Wilkins, 1983, p. 285.)

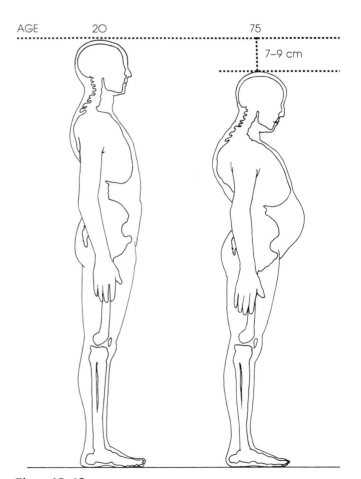

Figure 15–13
Loss of height resulting from osteoporosis leading to dowager's hump. Note the flexed head and protruding abdomen, which occur partially to maintain the center of gravity in its normal position.

Scoliosis

Scoliosis is a lateral curvature of the spine.[9, 11, 16–22] This type of deformity is often the most visible spinal deformity, especially in its severe forms. The most famous example of scoliosis is the "hunchback of Notre Dame." In the cervical spine, a scoliosis is called a **torticollis**. There are several types of scoliosis, some of which are nonstructural (Fig. 15–14) and some which are structural. **Nonstructural scoliosis** may be caused by postural problems, hysteria, nerve root irritation, inflammation, or compensation caused by leg length discrepancy or contracture (in the lumbar spine).[21] **Structural scoliosis** primarily involves bony deformity, which may be congenital or acquired. This type of scoliosis may be caused by wedge vertebra, hemivertebra (Fig. 15–15), or failure of segmentation. It may be idiopathic (genetic) (Fig. 15–16); neuromuscular, resulting from an upper or lower motor neuron lesion; or myopathic, resulting from muscular dystrophy. Or, it may be caused by arthrogryposis, resulting from persistent joint flexure or contracture,[15] or by conditions such as neurofibromatosis, mesenchymal disorders, or trauma. It is also seen in infection, tumors, and inflammatory conditions and in conjunction with malocclusion and ear problems (in the cervical spine).

With structural scoliosis, the patient lacks normal flexibility, and side bending becomes asymmetric. This type of scoliosis may be progressive, and the curve does not disappear on forward flexion. With nonstructural scoliosis, there is no bony deformity; this type of scoliosis is not progressive. The spine shows segmental limitation, and side bending is usually symmetric. The scoliotic

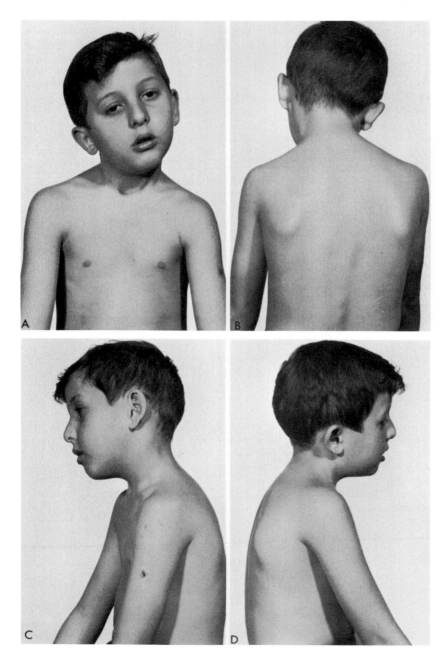

Figure 15–14

Congenital muscular torticollis on the right in a 10-year-old boy (A through D). Note the contracted sternocleidomastoid muscle. (From Tachdjian, M.O.: Pediatric Orthopedics. Philadelphia, W.B. Saunders Co., 1972, p. 74.)

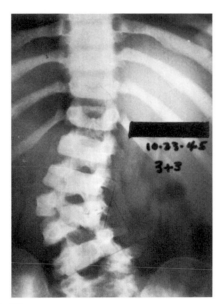

Figure 15–15
Scoliosis caused by hemivertebra. (From Moe, J.H., D.S. Bradford, R.B. Winter, and J.E. Lonstein: Scoliosis and Other Spinal Deformities. Philadelphia, W.B. Saunders Co., 1978, p. 134.)

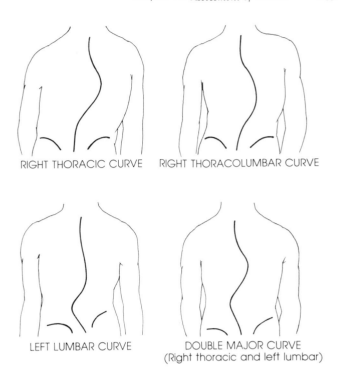

RIGHT THORACIC CURVE   RIGHT THORACOLUMBAR CURVE

LEFT LUMBAR CURVE   DOUBLE MAJOR CURVE
(Right thoracic and left lumbar)

Figure 15–17
Examples of scoliosis curve patterns.

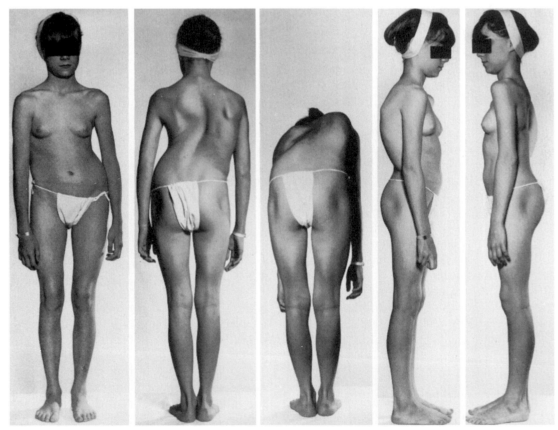

Figure 15–16
Idiopathic structural right thoracic scoliosis. (From Tachdjian, M.O.: Pediatric Orthopedics. Philadelphia, W.B. Saunders Co., 1972, p. 1200.)

Table 15–1
Types of Muscle Weakness or Tightness (Shortening) Associated With Postural Deviations

Postural Defect	Joints Commonly Affected	Muscles Commonly Shortened	Muscles Commonly Weakened
Forward head posture	Atlanto-occipital joint Cervical spine Temporomandibular joint Scapulothoracic joint Glenohumeral joint	Levator scapulae Sternocleidomastoid Scalenes Suboccipital muscles Upper trapezius Pectoralis major and minor	Hyoid muscles Lower cervical and thoracic erector spinae Middle and lower trapezius Rhomboids
Swayback posture	Thoracolumbar spine Pelvic joints Hip joint	Upper abdominals Internal intercostals Hip extensors Lower lumbar extensors	Lower abdominal muscles Lower thoracic extensors Hip flexor muscles
Lordotic posture	Thoracolumbar spine Pelvic joints Hip joint	Lumbar extensors Tight hip flexors	Abdominal muscles
Kyphotic posture	Thoracic spine	Intercostales Pectoralis major Serratus anterior Levator scapulae Upper trapezius	Thoracic erector spinae Rhomboids Middle and lower trapezius
Flat back posture	Lumbar spine Pelvic joints	Abdominals Hip extensors	Lumbar extensor muscles Hip flexor muscles
Flat upper back posture	Cervicothoracic spine Scapulothoracic joint	Thoracic erector spinae Scapula retractors	Scapula protractor muscles Anterior intercostal muscles
Scoliosis	Cervicothoracolumbar spine Pelvic joints Hip joint Foot joints	Muscles on the concave side Hip adductors Foot supinators on the short side	Muscles on the convex side Hip abductor muscles Foot pronator muscles on the long side

From Giallonardo, L.M.: Posture. In Myers, R.S. (ed.): Saunders Manual of Physical Therapy Practice. Philadelphia, W.B. Saunders Co., 1995, p. 1092.

curve disappears on forward flexion. This type of scoliosis is usually found in the cervical, lumbar, or thoracolumbar area.

Idiopathic scoliosis accounts for 75 to 85% of all cases of (structural) scoliosis. The vertebral bodies rotate into the convexity of the curve, with the spinous processes going toward the concavity of the curve. There is a fixed rotational prominence on the convex side, which is best seen on forward flexion from the skyline view. This prominence is sometimes called a "razorback spine." The disc spaces are narrowed on the concave side and widened on the convex side. There is distortion of the vertebral body, and vital capacity is considerably lowered if the lateral curvature exceeds 60°; compression and malposition of the organs within the rib cage also occur. Examples of scoliotic curves are shown in Figure 15–17.

Table 15–1 provides a summary of postural deviations and associated muscle dysfunction.[23]

Patient History

As with any history, the examiner must ensure that the information obtained is as complete as possible. By listening to the patient, the examiner can often comprehend the problem. The information should include a history of the problem, the patient's general condition and health, and family history. If a child is being examined, the examiner must also obtain prenatal and postnatal histories, including the health of the mother during pregnancy, any complications during pregnancy or delivery, and drugs taken by the mother during that period, especially during the first trimester, which is the period in which most of the congenital anomalies develop.

It should be remembered that it is unusual for a patient to present with just a postural problem. It is the symptoms produced by the pathology that are causing the postural abnormality that initiate the consultation. The examiner therefore must be cognizant of various underlying pathological conditions when assessing posture. The following questions should be asked:

1. Was there any history of injury? If so, what was the mechanism of injury? For example, lifting often causes lower spine problems, which may lead to altered posture.

2. If there is a history of injury, had the patient experienced any back injury or pain previously? If so, what caused that injury or pain? Was it a specific posture, sustained posture, or repetitive posture?

3. Are there any postures (e.g., standing with one foot on low stool, sitting with legs crossed) that give the patient relief or increase the patient's symptoms?[24] The

examiner can later test these postures to help determine the problem.

4. Does the family have any history of back problems or other special problems? Conditions such as hemivertebra, scoliosis, and Klippel-Feil syndrome may be congenital.

5. Has the patient had any previous illnesses, surgery, or severe injuries?

6. Is there a history of any other conditions, such as connective tissue diseases, that have a high incidence of associated spinal problems?

7. Does footwear make a difference to the patient's posture or symptoms? For example, high-heeled shoes often lead to excessive lordosis.[25]

8. How old is the patient? Many spinal problems begin in childhood or are the result of degeneration in the aged.

9. In the child, has there been a growth spurt? If so, when did it begin? Growth spurts often lead to tight muscles and altered posture.

10. For females, when did menarche begin? Does back pain appear to be associated with menses? Menarche indicates the point at which approximately two thirds of the female adolescent growth spurt has been completed.

11. For males, has there been a voice change? If so, when? This question also gives an indication of maturity or onset of puberty.

12. If a deformity is present, is it progressive or stationary?

13. Does the patient experience any neurological symptoms (e.g., a "pins and needles" feeling or numbness)?

14. What is the nature, extent, type, and duration of the pain?

15. What positions or activities increase the pain or discomfort?

16. What positions or activities decrease the pain or discomfort?

17. For children, is there difficulty in fitting clothes? For example, with scoliosis, the hem of a dress is usually uneven because of the spinal curvature.

18. Does the patient have any difficulty breathing? Structural deformities such as idiopathic scoliosis can lead to breathing problems in severe cases.

19. Which hand is the dominant one? Often, the dominant side shows a lower shoulder, with the hip slightly deviated to that side (Fig. 15–18). The spine may deviate slightly to the opposite side, and the opposite

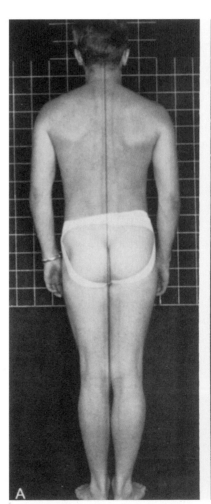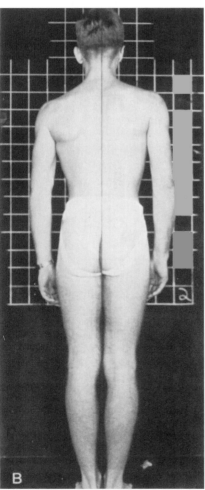

Figure 15–18
Effect of handedness on posture. (A) Right hand dominant. (B) Left hand dominant. (From Kendall, F.P., and E.K. McCreary: Muscles: Testing and Function. Baltimore, Williams & Wilkins, 1983, p. 294.)

foot is slightly more pronated.[5] The gluteus medius on the dominant side may also be weaker.

20. Has there been any previous treatment? If so, what was it? Was it successful?

Observation

To assess posture correctly, the patient must be adequately undressed. Male patients should be in shorts, and female patients should be in a bra and shorts. Ideally, the patient should not wear shoes or stockings. However, if the patient uses walking aids, braces, collars, or orthoses, they should be noted and may be used after the patient has been assessed in the "natural" state to determine the effect of the appliances.

The patient should be examined in the habitual, relaxed posture that is usually adopted. Often, it takes some time for the patient to adopt the usual posture because of tenseness or uncertainty.

In the standing and sitting positions, the assessment is the same as the observation for the upper and lower limb scanning examinations of the cervical and lumbar spines. Assessment of posture should be carried out with the patient in the standing, sitting, and lying (supine and prone) positions. After the patient has been examined in these positions, the examiner may decide to include other habitual, sustained, or repetitive postures assumed by the patient to see whether these postures increase or alter symptoms. The patient may also be assessed wearing different footwear to determine their effects on the posture and symptoms.

When observing a patient for abnormalities in posture, the examiner looks for asymmetry as a possible indication of what may be causing the postural fault. However, it is important for the examiner to realize that asymmetry between left and right sides is normal. The examiner must be able to differentiate normal deviations from asymmetry caused by pathology. It is also important to realize that postural deviations may not always cause symptoms, but they may do so with time.[26]

As the examiner is watching for asymmetry, he or she should also note potential causes of asymmetry. For example, the examiner should always watch for the presence of muscle wasting, soft tissue or bony swelling or enlargement, scars, and skin changes that may indicate present or past pathology.

Standing

The examiner should first determine the patient's body type (Fig. 15–19).[24] There are three body types: ectomorphic, mesomorphic, and endomorphic. The **ectomorph** is a person who has a thin body build characterized by a relative prominence of structures developed from the embryonic ectoderm. The **mesomorph** has a muscular or

sturdy body build characterized by relative prominence of structures developed by the embryonic mesoderm. The **endomorph** has a heavy or fat body build characterized by relative prominence of structures developed from the embryonic endoderm.

Body Types

- Ectomorph
- Mesomorph
- Endomorph

In addition to body type, the examiner should note the emotional attitude of the patient. Is the patient tense, bored, or lethargic? Does the patient appear to be healthy, emaciated, or overweight? Answers to these questions can help the examiner determine how much must be done to correct any problems. For example, if the patient is lethargic, it may take longer to correct the problem than if he or she appears truly interested in correcting the problem. The examiner must remember that posture is an expression of one's personality, sense of well-being, and self-esteem.

Anterior View

When observing the patient from the front (Fig. 15–20), the examiner should note whether the following conditions hold true:

1. The head is straight on the shoulders (in midline). The examiner should note whether the head is habitually tilted to one side or rotated (e.g., torticollis) (Fig. 15–21). The cause of altered head position must be established. For example, it may be the result of weak muscles, trauma, a hearing loss, temporomandibular joint problems, or the wearing of bifocal glasses.

2. The posture of the jaw is normal. In the resting position, normal jaw posture is when the lips are gently pressed together, the teeth are slightly apart (freeway space), and the tip of the tongue is behind the upper teeth in the roof of the mouth. This position maintains the mandible in a good posture (i.e., slight negative pressure in the mouth reduces the work of the muscles). It also enables respiration through the nose and diaphragmatic breathing.

3. The tip of the nose is in line with the manubrium sternum, xiphisternum, and umbilicus. This line is the **anterior line of reference** used to divide the body into right and left halves. If the umbilicus is used as a reference point, the examiner should remember that the umbilicus is almost always slightly off center.

4. The trapezius neck line is equal on both sides. The muscle bulk of the trapezius muscles should be equal, and the slope of the muscles should be approximately equal. Because the dominant arm usually shows

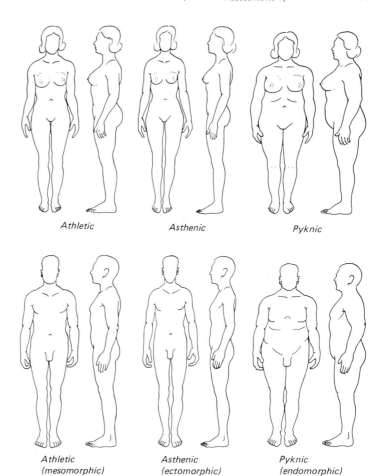

Figure 15–19

Male and female body types. (From Debrunner, H.U.: Orthopedic Diagnosis. London, E & S Livingstone, 1970, p. 86.)

Athletic   Asthenic   Pyknic

Athletic   Asthenic   Pyknic
(mesomorphic)   (ectomorphic)   (endomorphic)

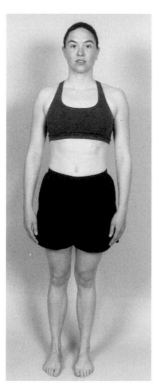

Figure 15–20

Posture in the standing position (anterior view).

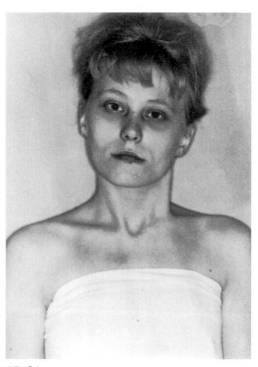

Figure 15–21

Congenital torticollis in 18-year-old girl. Note the asymmetry of the face. (From Tachdjian, M.O.: Pediatric Orthopedics. Philadelphia, W.B. Saunders Co., 1972, p. 68.)

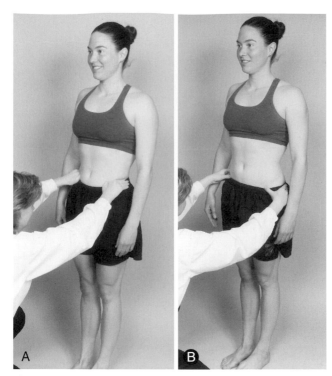

Figure 15–22
Viewing height equality. (A) Iliac crests. (B) Anterior superior iliac spines.

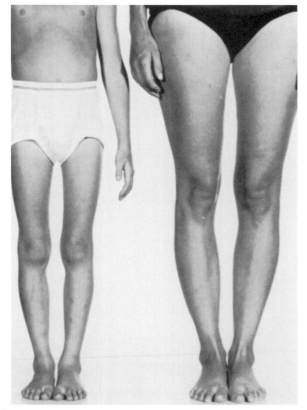

Figure 15–23
Bilateral genu varum in mother and son. Note the associated medial tibial torsion. (From Tachdjian, M.O.: Pediatric Orthopedics. Philadelphia, W.B. Saunders Co., 1972, p. 1462.)

greater laxity by being slightly lower, the slope on the dominant side may be slightly greater.

5. The shoulders are level. In most cases, the dominant side is slightly lower.

6. The clavicles and acromioclavicular joints are level and equal. They should be symmetric; any deviation should be noted. Deviations may be caused by subluxations or dislocations of the acromioclavicular or sternoclavicular joints, fractures, or clavicular rotation.

7. There is no protrusion, depression, or lateralization of the sternum, ribs, or costocartilage. If there are changes, they should be noted.

8. The waist angles are equal, and the arms are equidistant from the waist. If a scoliosis is present, one arm hangs closer to the body than the other arm. The examiner should also note whether the arms are equally rotated medially or laterally.

9. The carrying angle at each elbow is equal. Any deviation should be noted. The normal carrying angle varies from 5 to 15°.

10. The palms of both hands face the body in the relaxed standing position. Any differences should be noted and may give an indication of rotation in the upper limb.

11. The high points of the iliac crest are the same height on each side (Fig. 15–22). With a scoliosis, the patient may feel that one hip is "higher" than the other. This apparent high pelvis results from the lateral shift of the trunk; the pelvis is usually level. The same condition can cause the patient to feel that one leg is shorter than the other.

12. The anterior superior iliac spines (ASISs) are level. If one ASIS is higher than the other, there is a possibility that one leg is shorter than the other or that the pelvis is rotated more or shifted up or down more on one side.

13. The pubic bones are level at the symphysis pubis. Any deviation should be noted.

14. The patellae of the knees point straight ahead. Sometimes the patellae face outward ("frog eyes" patellae) or inward ("squinting" patellae). The position of the patella may also be altered by torsion of the femoral neck (anteversion-retroversion), femoral shaft, or tibial shaft.

15. The knees are straight. The knees may be in genu varum or genu valgum. If the ankles are together and the knees are more than two fingerwidths apart, the patient has some genu varum. If the knees are touching and the feet are apart, the patient has some genu valgum. Genu valgum is more likely to be seen in females. The examiner should note whether the deformity results from the femur, tibia, or both. In children, the knees go through a progression of being straight, going into genu varum (Fig. 15–23), being straight, going into genu valgum (Fig. 15–24), and finally being straight again during the first 6 years of life (see Fig. 15–3).[11]

16. The heads of the fibulae are level.

17. The medial and lateral malleoli of the ankles are

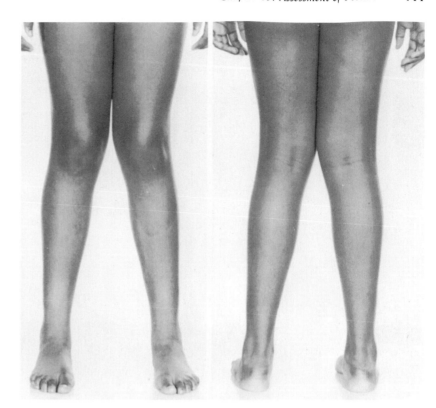

Figure 15-24

Bilateral genu valgum in an adolescent. (From Tachdjian, M.O.: Pediatric Orthopedics. Philadelphia, W.B. Saunders Co., 1972, p. 1467.)

level. Normally, the medial malleoli are slightly anterior to the lateral malleoli, but the lateral malleoli extend farther distally.

18. Two arches are present in the feet and equal on the two sides. In this position, only the medial longitudinal arch is visible. The examiner should note any pes planus (flatfoot), pes cavus ("hollow" foot), or other deformities.

19. The feet angle out equally (usually 5 to 18°; Fig. 15-25). This finding means that the tibias are normally slightly laterally rotated (lateral tibial torsion). The presence of pigeon toes usually indicates medial rotation of the tibias (medial tibial torsion).

20. There is no bowing of bone. Any bowing may indicate diseases such as osteomalacia or osteoporosis.

21. The bony and soft-tissue contours are equally symmetric on the two halves of the body. Any indication of muscle wasting, muscle hypertrophy on one side, or bony asymmetry should be noted. Such a finding may indicate muscle or nerve pathology, or it may simply be related to the patient's job or recreational pursuits. For example, a rodeo bull rider will show hypertrophy of the muscles and bones on one side (the arm that he uses to hang on!).

In addition, the patient's skin is observed for abnormalities such as hairy patches (e.g., diastematomyelia), pigmented lesions (e.g., café au lait spots, neurofibromatosis), subcutaneous tumors, and scars (e.g., Ehlers-Danlos syndrome), all of which may lead to or contribute to postural problems (Fig. 15-26).

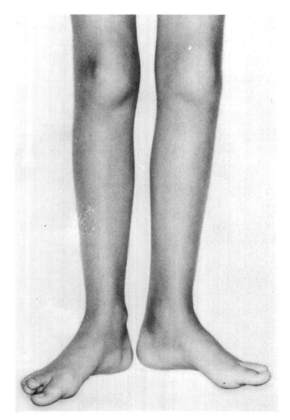

Figure 15-25

Exaggerated lateral tibial torsion. In stance, with the patellae facing straight forward, the feet point outward. (From Tachdjian, M.O.: Pediatric Orthopedics. Philadelphia, W.B. Saunders Co., 1972, p. 1461.)

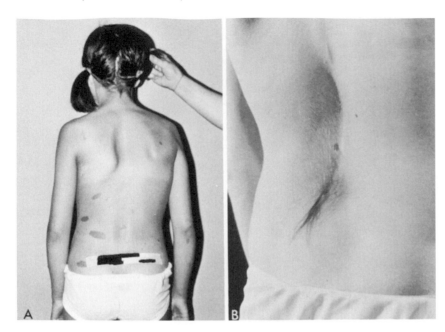

Figure 15–26
Abnormal skin markings. (A) Café au lait areas of pigmentation seen in neurofibromatosis. (B) Lumbar hair patch seen in diastematomyelia. (From Moe, J.H., D.S. Bradford, R.B. Winter, and J.E. Lonstein: Scoliosis and Other Spinal Deformities. Philadelphia, W.B. Saunders Co., 1978, p. 20.)

Lateral View

From the side, the examiner should note whether the following conditions hold true:

1. The ear lobe is in line with the tip of the shoulder (acromion process) and the high point of the iliac crest. This line is the **lateral line of reference** dividing the body into front and back halves (Fig. 15–27). If the chin pokes forward, an excessive lumbar lordosis may also be present. This compensatory change is caused by the body's

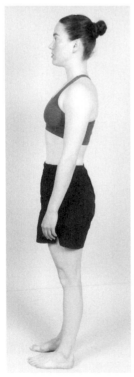

Figure 15–27
Posture in the standing position (side view).

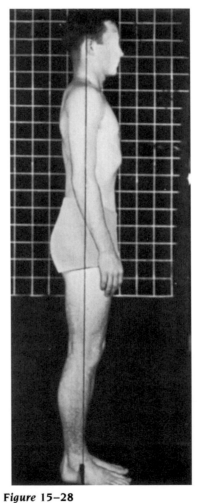

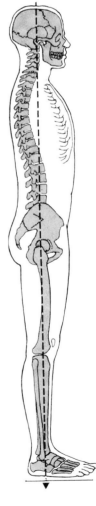

Figure 15–28
Correct postural alignment. (From Kendall, F.P., and E.K. McCreary: Muscles: Testing and Function. Baltimore, Williams & Wilkins, 1983, p. 280.)

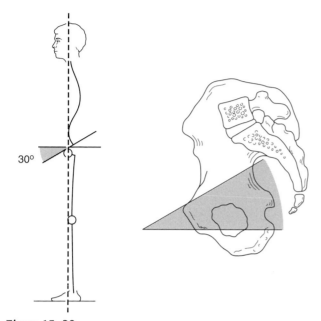

***Figure* 15–29**
Normal pelvic angle.

attempt to maintain the center of gravity in the normal position.

2. Each spinal segment has a normal curve (Fig. 15–28). Large gluteus maximus muscles or excessive fat may give the appearance of an exaggerated lordosis. The examiner should look at the spine in relation to the sacrum, not the gluteal muscles. Likewise, the scapulae may give the illusion of an increased kyphosis in the thoracic spine, especially if they are flat and the patient has rounded shoulders.

3. The shoulders are in proper alignment. If the shoulders droop forward, "rounded shoulders" are indicated. This improper alignment may be caused by habit or by tight pectoral muscles.

4. The chest, abdominal, and back muscles have proper tone. Weakness or spasm of any of these muscles can lead to postural alterations.

5. There are no chest deformities, such as pectus carinatum (undue prominence of the sternum) or pectus excavatum (undue depression of the sternum).

6. The pelvic angle is normal (30°; Fig. 15–29).

7. The knees are straight, flexed, or in recurvatum (hyperextended). Usually, in the normal standing position, the knees are slightly flexed (0 to 5°). Hyperextension of the knees may cause an increase in lordosis in the lumbar spine. Tight hamstrings or gastrocnemius muscles can also cause knee flexion.

Figure 15–30 illustrates normal posture and some of the abnormal deviations seen when viewing the patient from the side.

***Figure* 15–30**
Postural deviations obvious from the side view. (Redrawn from Reedco Research, Auburn, New York.)

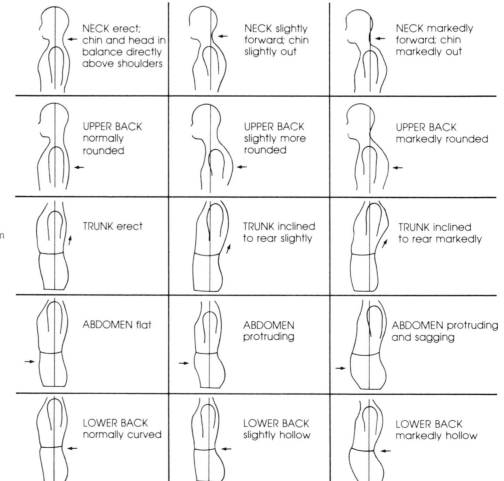

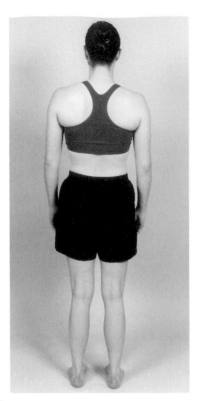

Figure 15–31
Posture in the standing position (posterior view).

Posterior View

When viewing from behind (Fig. 15–31), the examiner should note whether the following conditions hold true:

1. The shoulders are level, and the head is in midline. These findings should be compared with those from the anterior view.

2. The spines and inferior angles of the scapula are level (Fig. 15–32) and the medial borders of the scapulae are equidistant from the spine. If not, is there a rotational or winging deformity of one of the scapulae? Defects such as Sprengel's deformity should be noted (Fig. 15–33).

3. The spine is straight or curved laterally, indicating scoliosis. A plumbline may be dropped from the spinous process of the seventh cervical vertebra (Fig. 15–34). Normally, the line passes through the gluteal cleft. This line is the **posterior line of reference** used to divide the body into right and left halves. The distance from the vertical string to the gluteal cleft can be measured. This distance is sometimes used as a measurement of spinal imbalance, and it is noted whether the deviation is to the left or right. If a torticollis or cervicothoracic scoliosis is present, the plumbline should be dropped from the occipital protuberance.[9]

4. The ribs protrude or are symmetric on both sides.

5. The waist angles are level.

6. The arms are equidistant from the body and equally rotated.

7. The posterior superior iliac spines (PSISs) are level (Fig. 15–35). If one is higher than the other, one

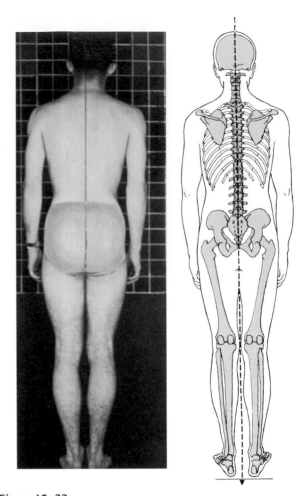

Figure 15–32
Correct postural alignment. (From Kendall, F.P., and E.K. McCreary: Muscles: Testing and Function. Baltimore, Williams & Wilkins, 1983, p. 290.)

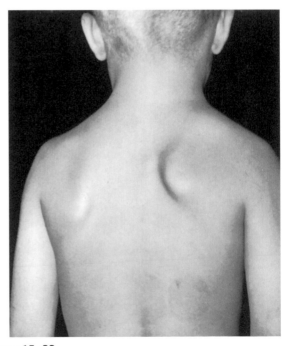

Figure 15–33
Sprengel's deformity. Note the small, high scapula on the right. (From Tachdjian, M.O.: Pediatric Orthopedics. Philadelphia, W.B. Saunders Co., 1972, p. 82.)

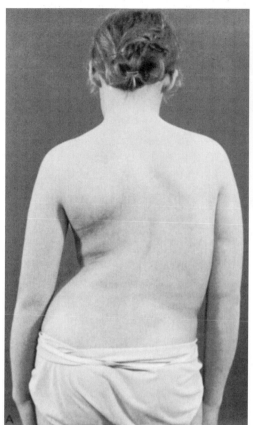
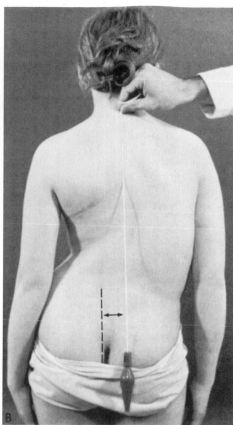

Figure 15–34

The patient is viewed from the back to evaluate the spine deformity. (A) A typical right thoracic curve is shown. The left shoulder is lower and the right scapula more prominent. Note the decreased distance between the right arm and the thorax, with the shift of the thorax to the right. The left iliac crest appears higher, but this is caused by the shift of the thorax, with fullness on the right and elimination of the waistline. The high hip is thus only apparent, not real. (B) Plumbline dropped from the prominent vertebra of C7 (vertebra prominens) measures the decompensation of the upper thorax over the pelvis. The distance from the vertical plumbline to the gluteal cleft is measured in centimeters and is recorded, noting the direction of fall from the occipital protuberance (inion). (From Moe, J.H., D.S. Bradford, R.B. Winter, and J.E. Lonstein: Scoliosis and Other Spinal Deformities. Philadelphia, W.B. Saunders Co., 1978, p. 14.)

Figure 15–35

Viewing height equality. (A) Posterior superior iliac spines. (B) Gluteal folds.

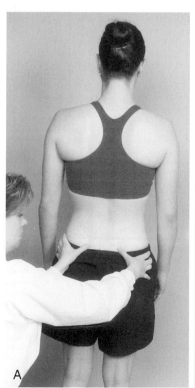
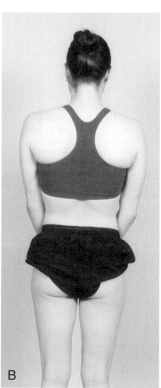

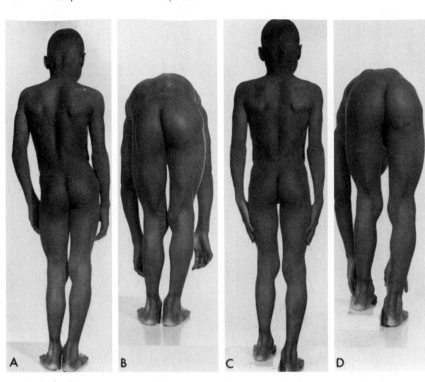

Figure 15–36
(A and B) Functional scoliosis resulting from short leg. (C and D) The spinal position with short leg is corrected. (From Tachdjian, M.O.: Pediatric Orthopedics. Philadelphia, W.B. Saunders Co., 1972, p. 1192.)

leg may be shorter or rotation of the pelvis may be present. The examiner should note how the PSISs relate to the ASISs. If the ASIS on one side and the PSIS on the other side are higher, there is a torsion deformity (anterior or posterior) at the sacroiliac joint. If the ASIS and PSIS on one side are higher than the ASIS and PSIS on the other side, there may be an upslip at the sacroiliac joint on the high side.

8. The gluteal folds are level. Muscle weakness, nerve root problems, or nerve palsy may lead to asymmetry.

9. The knee joints are level. If they are not, it may indicate that one leg is shorter than the other (Fig. 15–36).

10. Both of the Achilles tendons descend straight to the calcanei. If the tendons angle out, it may indicate a flatfoot deformity (pes planus).

11. The heels are straight or are angled in (varus) or out (valgus).

12. Bowing of femur or tibia is present or absent.

Figure 15–37 illustrates the normal posture and some of the abnormal deviations seen when viewing from behind.

When viewing posture, the examiner should remember that the pelvis is usually the key to proper back posture. The normal pelvic angle is 30°, and the pelvis

Table 15–2
Percentage of Mature Height Attained at Different Ages

Chronologic Age (Years)	Percentage of Eventual Height	
	Boys	Girls
1	42.2	44.7
2	49.5	52.8
3	53.8	57.0
4	58.0	61.8
5	61.8	66.2
6	65.2	70.3
7	69.0	74.0
8	72.0	77.5
9	75.0	80.7
10	78.0	84.4
11	81.1	88.4
12	84.2	92.9
13	87.3	96.5
14	91.5	98.3
15	96.1	99.1
16	98.3	99.6
17	99.3	100.0
18	99.8	100.0

From Bayley, N.: The accurate prediction of growth and adult height. Mod. Probl. Pediatr. 7:234–255, 1954.

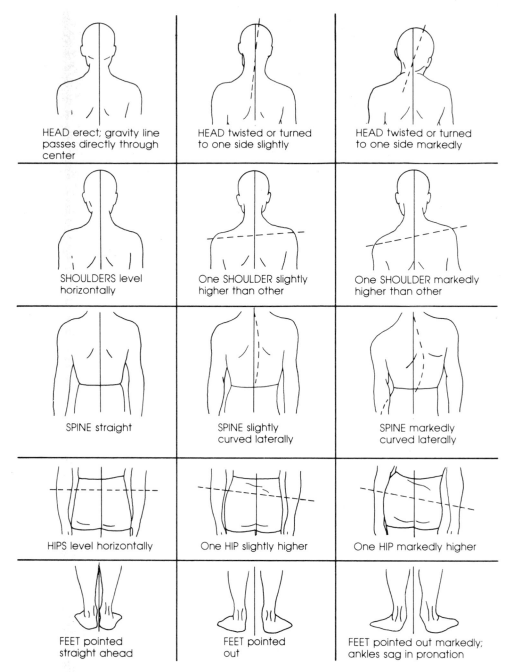

HEAD erect; gravity line passes directly through center

HEAD twisted or turned to one side slightly

HEAD twisted or turned to one side markedly

SHOULDERS level horizontally

One SHOULDER slightly higher than other

One SHOULDER markedly higher than other

SPINE straight

SPINE slightly curved laterally

SPINE markedly curved laterally

HIPS level horizontally

One HIP slightly higher

One HIP markedly higher

FEET pointed straight ahead

FEET pointed out

FEET pointed out markedly; ankles sag in pronation

Figure 15–37
Postural deviations obvious from the posterior view. (Redrawn from Reedco Research, Auburn, New York.)

is held or balanced in this position by muscles. For the pelvis to "sit properly" on the femur, the following muscles must be strong, supple (mobile), and balanced: abdominals, hip flexors, hip extensors, back extensors, hip rotators, and hip abductors and adductors.

If the height of the patient is measured, especially in a child, the focal height of the child may be estimated by the use of a chart such as the one shown in Table 15–2.[27]

After the standing posture has been assessed, the examiner may decide to assess some additional postures (e.g., positional, sustained, or repetitive), especially if the patient has complained in the history that these different positions have caused problems or symptoms.

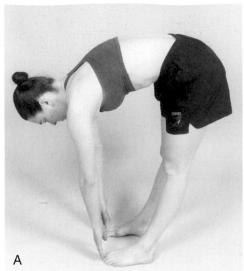
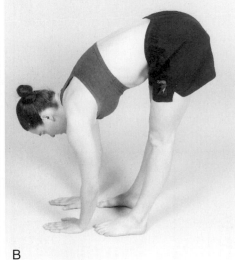

Figure 15-38
Posture in forward flexion.
(A) Normal range of motion. Note reversal of lumbar curve.
(B) Excessive range of motion due to excessive hip mobility.

Hump ———————
Hollow ———————

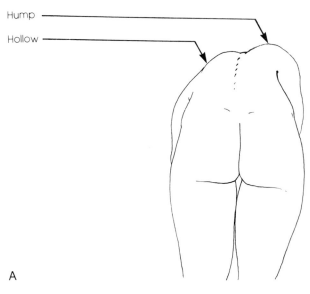

A

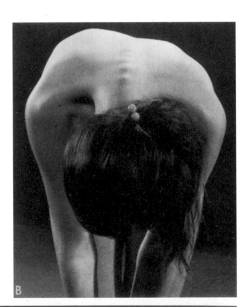

B

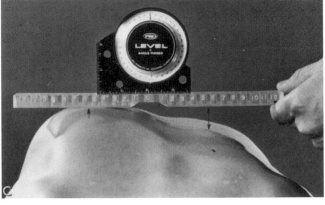

C

Figure 15-39
Rib hump in forward bending test.
(A) Posterior view. (B) Anterior view. The two sides are compared. Note the presence of a right thoracic prominence.
(C) Measurement of the prominence. The spirit level is positioned with the zero mark over the palpable spinous process in the area of maximal prominence. The level is made horizontal and the distance to the apex of the deformity (5 to 6 cm) noted. The perpendicular distance from the level to the hollow is measured at the same distance from the midline. A 2.4-cm right thoracic prominence is shown. (From Moe, J.H., D.S. Bradford, R.B. Winter, and J.E. Lonstein: Scoliosis and Other Spinal Deformities. Philadelphia, W.B. Saunders Co., 1978, p. 17.)

Forward Flexion

Having completed the assessment of normal standing, the examiner asks the patient to flex forward at the hips with the fingertips of both hands together so that the arms drop vertically (Fig. 15–38). The feet should be together, and both knees should be straight. Any alteration from this posture will cause the spine to rotate, giving a false view.

From this position, using the anterior and posterior skyline views, the examiner can note the following:

1. Whether there is any asymmetry of the rib cage (e.g., rib hump). If a hump is present, a level and tape measure may be used to obtain the perpendicular distance between the hump and hollow (Fig. 15–39).[9]

2. Whether there is any asymmetry in the spinal musculature.

3. Whether a kyphosis is present.

4. Whether lumbar spine straightens or flexes as it normally should.

5. Whether there is any restriction to forward bending such as spondylolisthesis or tight hamstrings (Figs. 15–40 and 15–41).

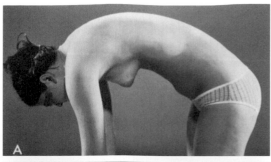
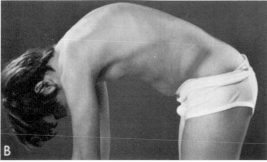

Figure 15–41
Forward bending position for viewing kyphosis (lateral view). (A) Normal thoracic roundness is demonstrated with a gentle curve to the whole spine. (B) An area of increased bending is seen in the thoracic spine, indicating structural changes, in a patient with Scheuermann's disease. (From Moe, J.H., D.S. Bradford, R.B. Winter, and J.E. Lonstein: Scoliosis and Other Spinal Deformities. Philadelphia, W.B. Saunders Co., 1978, p. 18.)

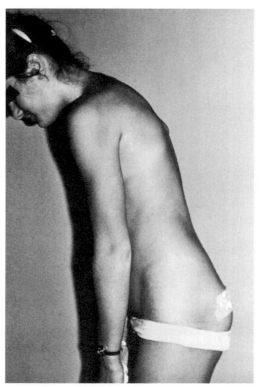

Figure 15–40
Abnormal forward bending resulting from tight hamstrings, in a patient with spondylolisthesis. (From Moe, J.H., D.S. Bradford, R.B. Winter, and J.E. Lonstein: Scoliosis and Other Spinal Deformities. Philadelphia, W.B. Saunders Co., 1978, p. 19.)

If, in the history, the patient complained that sustained forward flexion caused symptoms, the examiner should ask the patient to assume the symptom-causing posture and maintain it for 15 to 30 seconds to determine whether symptoms arise or increase. Flexion has been found to decrease the stress on the facet joints, but it can increase the pressure in the nucleus pulposus.[28, 29] Likewise, if repetitive forward flexion or combined movements (e.g., extension and rotation) have caused symptoms, the patient should be asked to do the repetitive or combined movements. Loading the spine by lifting an object may also cause symptoms and may be investigated if symptoms are not too great.

Sitting

With the patient seated on a stool so that the feet are on the ground and the back is unsupported, the examiner looks at the patient's posture (Fig. 15–42). Sitting without a back support causes the patient to support his or her own posture and increases the amount of muscle activity needed to maintain the posture.[28] This observation is carried out, as in the standing position, from the front, back, and side. If any anteroposterior or lateral

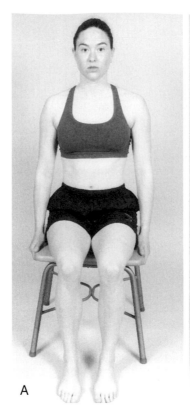
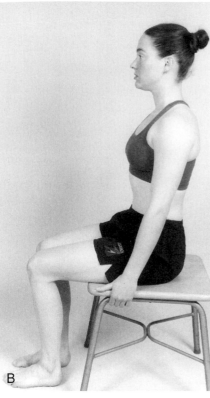

A   B

Figure 15–42
Posture in sitting position. (A) Anterior view. (B) Side view.

deviations of the spine are observed, the examiner should recall whether they were present when the patient was examined while standing. It should be noted whether the spinal curves increase or decrease when the patient is in the sitting position. From the front, it can be noted whether the knees are the same distance from the floor. If they are not, this may indicate a shortened tibia. From the side, it can be noted whether one knee protrudes farther than the other. If it does, this may indicate a shortened femur on the other side.

If the patient has complained in the history that going from standing to sitting or sitting to standing resulted in symptoms, the patient should be asked to repeat these maneuvers, provided the movements do not exacerbate the symptoms too much.

Supine Lying

With the patient in the supine lying position, the examiner notes the position of the head and cervical spine as well as the shoulder girdle. The chest area is observed for any protrusion (e.g., pectus carinatum) or sunken areas (e.g., pectus excavatum).

The abdominal musculature should be observed to see whether it is strong or flabby, and the waist angles should be noted to see whether they are equal. As in

the standing position, the ASISs should be viewed to see if they are level. Any extension in the lumbar spine should be noted. In addition, it should be noted whether bending the knees helps to decrease the lumbar curve; if it does, it may indicate tight hip flexors. The lower limbs should descend parallel from the pelvis. If they do not, or if they cannot be aligned parallel and at right angles to a line joining the ASISs, it may indicate an abduction or adduction contracture at the hip.

If, in the history, the patient has complained of symptoms on arising from supine lying or from going into the supine position, the examiner should ask the patient to repeat these movements, provided they do not exacerbate the symptoms.

Prone Lying

With the patient lying prone, the examiner notes the position of the head, neck, and shoulder girdle, as previously described. The head should be positioned so that it is not rotated, side flexed, or extended. Any condition such as Sprengel's deformity or rib hump should be noted, as should any spinal deviations. The examiner should determine whether the PSISs are level and should ensure that the musculature of the buttocks, posterior thighs, and calves is normal (Fig. 15–43).

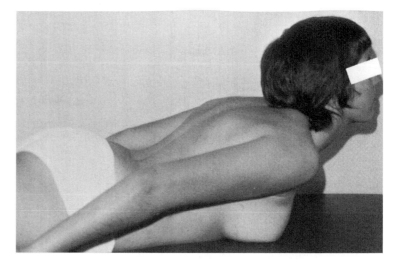

Figure 15–43

Structural kyphosis does not disappear on extension. (From Moe, J.H., D.S. Bradford, R.B. Winter, and J.E. Lonstein: Scoliosis and Other Spinal Deformities. Philadelphia, W.B. Saunders Co., 1978, p. 339.)

As with supine lying, if assuming the position or recovering from the position causes symptoms, the patient should be asked to repeat these movements, as long as symptoms are not made worse.

Examination

Assessment of posture primarily involves history and observation. If, on completing the history and observation, the examiner believes that a direct examination is necessary, the procedures outlined in this text for the various areas of the body should be followed. With every postural assessment, however, the examiner should perform two tests: the leg length measurement[30-33] and the slump test.

Leg Length Measurement. The patient lies supine with the pelvis set square or "balanced" on the legs (i.e., the legs at an angle of 90° to a line joining the ASISs). The legs should be 15 to 20 cm (6 to 8 inches) apart and parallel to each other (Fig. 15–44). The examiner then places one end of the tape measure against the distal aspect of the ASIS, holding it firmly against the bone. The index finger of the other hand is placed immediately distal to the medial or lateral malleolus and pushed against it. The thumbnail is brought down against the tip of the index fingers so that the tape measure is pinched between them. A reading is taken where the thumb and finger pinch together. A slight difference, up to 1.0 to 1.5 cm (0.4 to 0.6 inch), is considered normal but can still be relevant if pathology is present. Further information on measurement of true leg length may be found in Chapter 11.

Slump Test. The patient is seated on the edge of the examining table with the legs supported, the hips in neutral position (i.e., no rotation or abduction-adduction), and the hands behind the back (Fig. 15–45).

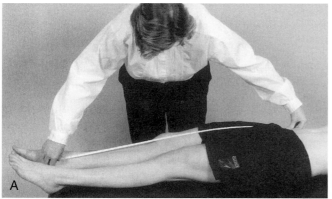
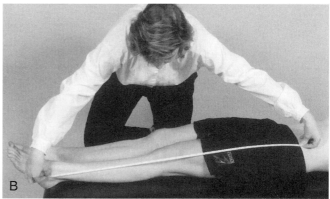

Figure 15–44

Measuring leg length (A) to medial malleolus; (B) to lateral malleolus.

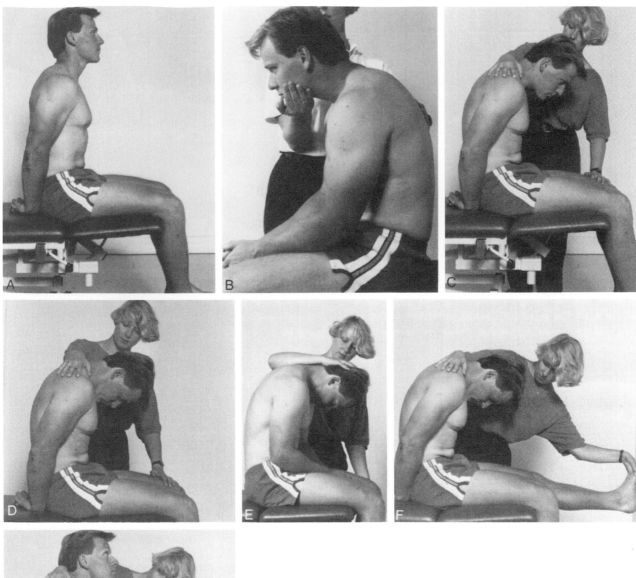

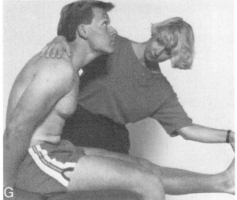

Figure 15–45
Sequence of subject postures in the slump test. (A) Patient sits erect. (B) Patient slumps lumbar and thoracic spine while examiner holds head in neutral.
(C) Examiner pushes down on shoulders while patient holds head in neutral.
(D) Patient flexes head. (E) Examiner carefully applies overpressure to cervical spine. (F) Examiner extends patient's knee and dorsiflexes foot. (G) Patient extends head.

The examination is performed in several steps. First, the patient is asked to "slump" the back into thoracic and lumbar flexion. The examiner maintains the patient's chin in the neutral position to prevent neck and head flexion. The examiner then uses one arm to apply overpressure across the shoulders to maintain flexion of the thoracic and lumbar spines. While this position is held, the patient is asked to actively flex the cervical spine and head as far as possible (i.e., chin to chest). The examiner then applies overpressure to maintain flexion of all three parts of the spine (cervical, thoracic, and lumbar), using the hand of the same arm to maintain overpressure in the cervical spine. With the other hand, the examiner then holds the patient's foot in maximum dorsiflexion. While the examiner holds these positions, the patient is asked to actively straighten the knee as much as possible. The test is repeated with the other leg and then with both legs at the same time. If the patient is unable to fully extend the knee because of pain, the examiner releases the overpressure to the cervical spine and the patient actively extends the neck. If the knee extends farther, the symptoms decrease with neck extension, or the positioning of the patient in-

creases the patient's symptoms, then the test is considered positive for increased tension in the neuromeningeal tract.[34-36] Further information on the slump test may be found in Chapter 9.

Additional Tests. Other tests may also be performed based on what the examiner has observed. For example, if the hip flexors appear tight, the Thomas test should be performed (see Chapter 11). Refer to Table 15–3 for a detailed presentation of good and faulty posture.

Table 15–3
Good and Faulty Posture: Summary Chart

Good Posture	Part	Faulty Posture
Head is held erect in a position of good balance.	Head	Chin up too high. Head protruding forward. Head tilted or rotated to one side.
Arms hang relaxed at the sides with palms of the hands facing toward the body. Elbows are slightly bent, so forearms hang slightly forward. Shoulders are level, and neither one is more forward or backward than the other when seen from the side. Scapulae lie flat against the rib cage. They are neither too close together nor too wide apart. In adults, a separation of approximately 10 cm (4 inches) is average.	Arms and shoulders	Holding the arms stiffly in any position forward, backward, or out from the body. Arms turned so that palms of hands face backward. One shoulder higher than the other. Both shoulders hiked up. One or both shoulders drooping forward or sloping. Shoulders rotated either clockwise or counterclockwise. Scapulae pulled back too hard. Scapulae too far apart. Scapulae too prominent, standing out from the rib cage ("winged scapulae").
A good position of the chest is one in which it is slightly up and slightly forward (while the back remains in good alignment). The chest appears to be in a position about halfway between that of a full inspiration and a forced expiration.	Chest	Depressed, or "hollow-chest" position. Lifted and held up too high, brought about by arching the back. Ribs more prominent on one side than on the other. Lower ribs flaring out or protruding.
In young children up to about the age of 10, the abdomen normally protrudes somewhat. In older children and adults, it should be flat.	Abdomen	Entire abdomen protrudes. Lower part of the abdomen protrudes while the upper part is pulled in.
The front of the pelvis and the thighs are in a straight line. The buttocks are not prominent in back but instead slope slightly downward. The spine has four natural curves. In the neck and lower back, the curve is forward, and in the upper back and lowest part of the spine (sacral region), it is backward. The sacral curve is a fixed curve, whereas the other three are flexible.	Spine and pelvis (side view)	The low back arches forward too much (lordosis). The pelvis tilts forward too much. The front of the thigh forms an angle with the pelvis when this tilt is present. The normal forward curve in the low back has straightened out. The pelvis tips backward and there is a slightly backward slant to the line of the pelvis in relation to the front of the hips (flat back). Increased backward curve in the upper back (kyphosis or round upper back). Increased forward curve in the neck. Almost always accompanied by round upper back and seen as a forward head. Lateral curve of the spine (scoliosis); toward one side (**C**-curve), toward both sides (**S**-curve).

Table continued on following page

Cyriax, J.: Textbook of Orthopaedic Medicine, Vol. 1: Diagnosis of Soft Tissue Lesions. London, Bailliere Tindall, 1982.

Dieck, G.S., J.L. Kelsey, V.K. Goel, M.M. Panjabi, S.D. Walter, and M.H. Laprade: An epidemiological study of the relationship between postural asymmetry in the teen years and subsequent back and neck pain. Spine 10:872–877, 1985.

During, J., H. Goudfrooij, W. Keessen, T.W. Beeker, and A. Crowe: Towards standards for posture-postural characteristics of the lower back system in normal and pathological conditions. Spine 10:83–87, 1985.

Itoi, E.: Roentgenographic analysis of posture in spinal osteoporotics. Spine 16:750–756, 1991.

Kapandji, I.A.: The Physiology of the Joints, Vol. 2: The Trunk and Vertebral Column. New York, Churchill Livingstone, 1974.

Kappler, R.: Postural balance and motion patterns. J. Am. Osteopath. Assoc. 81:598–606, 1982.

Littler, W.A.: Cardiorespiratory failure and scoliosis. Physiotherapy 60:69–70, 1974.

MacDougall, J.D., H.A. Wenger, and H.J. Green: Physiological Testing of the Elite Athlete. Ottawa, Canadian Association of Sports Sciences, 1982.

Matthews, D.K.: Measurement in Physical Education. Philadelphia, W.B. Saunders Co., 1973.

McKinnis, D.L.: The posture-movement dynamic. In Richardson, J.K., and Z.A. Iglarsh (eds.): Clinical Orthopedic Physical Therapy. Philadelphia, W.B. Saunders Co., 1994.

Mellin, G., and M. Poussa: Spinal mobility and posture in 8- to 16-year-old children. J. Orthop. Res. 10:211–216, 1992.

Mennell, J.: Back Pain: Diagnosis and Treatment Using Manipulative Techniques. Boston, Little, Brown & Co., 1960.

Murray, M.P., A. Seireg, and R.C. Scholz: Centre of gravity, center of pressure and supportive forces during human activities. J. Appl. Physiol. 23:831–838, 1967.

Nashner, L.M.: Sensory, neuromuscular and biomechanical contributions to human balance. In Duncan, P.W. (ed.): Balance: Proceedings of the American Physical Therapy Association Forum. Alexandria, American Physical Therapy Association, 1990.

Opila, K.A.: Gender and somatotype differences in postural alignment: Response to high-heeled shoes and simulated weight gain. Clin. Biomech. 3:145–152, 1988.

Pacelli, L.C.: Straight talk on posture. Phys. Sportsmed. 19:124–127, 1991.

Portnoy, H., and F. Morin: Electromyographic study of postural muscles in various positions and movements. Am. J. Physiol. 186:122–126, 1956.

Rothman, R.H., and F.A. Simeone: The Spine. Philadelphia, W.B. Saunders Co., 1982.

Torell, G., A. Nordwall, and A. Nachemson: The changing pattern of scoliosis treatment due to effective screening. J. Bone Joint Surg. Am. 63:337–341, 1981.

Tsai, L., and T. Wredmark: Spinal posture, sagittal mobility and subjective rating of back problems in former female elite gymnasts. Spine 18:872–875, 1993.

Vahos, J.P., A.J. Nitz, A.J. Threlkeld, R. Shapiro, and T. Horn: Electromyographic activity of selected trunk and hip muscles during a squat lift. Spine 19:687–695, 1994.

Walker, M.L., J.M. Rothstein, S.D. Finucane, and R.L. Lamb: Relationships between lumbar lordosis, pelvic tilt, and abdominal muscle performance. Phys. Ther. 67:512–516, 1987.

Williams, M.M., J.A. Hawley, R.A. McKenzie, and P.M. van Wijmen: A comparison of the effects of two sitting postures on back and referred pain. Spine 16:1185–1191, 1991.

Wolfson, L.I., R. Whipple, P. Amerman, and A. Kleinberg: Stressing the postural response: A quantitative method for testing balance. J. Am. Geriatr. Soc. 34:845–850, 1986.

Woollacott, M.: Postural control mechanisms in the young and old. In Duncan, P.W. (ed.): Balance: Proceedings of the American Physical Therapy Association Forum. Alexandria, American Physical Therapy Association, 1990.

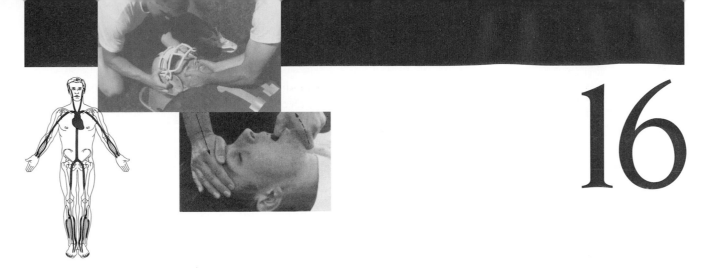

Emergency Sports Assessment

This chapter is provided to enable the health care professional to immediately assess a patient before application of first aid or transportation to the hospital. Such an assessment should be divided into two parts. The first part concerns the primary evaluation or survey, which is usually done at the location in which the patient is found to ensure that life-threatening situations are handled immediately. The secondary evaluation is performed when the examiner has more time and the patient is not under immediate threat of death or permanent disability.

Pre-event Preparation

Before any sporting event, the examiner should establish and practice **emergency protocols**. This preparation includes designating personnel for specific tasks and establishing emergency vehicle routes and entrances. The examiner and the assistants should know the location of additional medical assistance, emergency equipment (e.g., spinal board, neck supports, sandbags, stretchers, blankets, emergency first-aid kit), and a telephone. The equipment must be compatible with the needs, size, and age of the athletes, and with the equipment of other health professionals. Near the telephone, the examiner should post emergency telephone numbers (e.g., ambulance, physician, dentist), name and address of the sports facility, entrance to be used, and any obvious landmarks, because the person making the emergency call may forget information or give inappropriate information when under stress (Fig. 16–1). Included in the preparation is a communication plan for on-field or at-site injuries. This plan may involve pre-established hand signals (e.g., crossed arms: send physician out; hand on top of head: send ambulance or emergency medical services [EMS] personnel) or walkie-talkies to communicate with the sideline.[1]

Emergency Telephone Numbers

Ambulance _____ Fire/Inhalator _____

Acute Care Hospital (who will receive your athletes)

_____

Emergency Protocol

When you call the ambulance, state:

1. Your name

2. "There has been a suspected _____
   (*insert injury*)

   at _____ (*location*).

   Please send an ambulance to _____
   (*designated meeting spot*)

   I will meet the ambulance there."

3. Ask the estimated time of arrival (ETA).

4. Give them your phone number.

5. DO NOT HANG UP UNTIL THE OTHER PARTY DOES!

Note: If this information cannot be kept by the telephone it should be kept in your first-aid kit with a quarter ($0.25) in case you need to phone the ambulance from a pay phone.

Ambulance Route

Draw a map of the ambulance route to your facility and the designated meeting location.

Figure 16–1
Telephone emergency protocol (to be put near emergency telephones). (Modified from Sports Physiotherapy Division Newsletter, Canadian Physiotherapy Association, July/August 1991, p. 3.)

Emergency Protocol

- Designated personnel
- Emergency vehicle access routes
- Location of emergency equipment
- Location of telephone
- Communication plan

The examiner should take the time to give the facility a **safety check** by looking for potential hazards. Visiting teams should also be informed of emergency protocols. In addition, emergency situations and protocols must be practiced repeatedly to ensure that proper care will be given in an emergency.

Primary Assessment

After an injury occurs, the examiner must first take control of the situation and ensure that no additional harm comes to the patient. The primary survey, which takes 30 seconds to 2 minutes, with the maximum on-scene time being 10 minutes, is carried out with little or no movement of the patient.[2] With severe injuries, the longer the assessment takes, the higher the mortality rate is likely to be. If, at any time, a clinical finding indicates that a major injury has occurred (Table 16–1), the assessment process may be terminated to ensure the patient receives higher levels of care. This is done by calling for the ambulance or EMS. The examiner is designated as the **charge person,** or person in control.

Table 16–1

Priorities in the Management of Injuries: Beware of Injury to the Cervical Spine!

Highest priority
  1. Respiratory and cardiovascular impairment: facial, neck, and chest injuries
  2. Hemorrhage: external, severe

High priority
  3. Retroperitoneal injuries: shock, hemorrhage
  4. Intraperitoneal injuries: shock, hemorrhage
  5. Craniocerebral spinal cord injuries: open or closed, observation
  6. Severe burns: extensive soft-tissue wounds

Low priority
  7. Lower genitourinary tract: hemorrhage, extravasation
  8. Peripheral vascular, nerve, locomotor injuries: open or closed
  9. Facial and neck injuries: except priorities 1 and 2
  10. Cold exposure

Special
  11. Fractures, dislocations: splinting
  12. Tetanus prophylaxis

From Steichen, F.M.: The emergency management of the severely injured. J. Trauma 12:787, 1972.

The examiner takes control by not allowing the patient to be moved until some type of assessment is made, the spine is supported as much as possible, and, if required, assistance is obtained.

Emergency Evaluation

Airway evaluation (A):	5 to 7 seconds
Ventilation check (B):	5 to 8 seconds
Circulation/heart rate (C):	20 to 30 seconds
Blood loss:	20 to 30 seconds
Neurological injury:	10 to 20 seconds:
TOTAL TIME:	60 to 95 seconds

For the primary emergency assessment, the examiner should call at least one person to provide immediate assistance, relay messages, and obtain additional help, if necessary. This person is designated the **call person,** and he or she should know the location of the closest telephone and what telephone numbers to call in specific emergencies. This information can be posted on or by the telephone (see Fig. 16–1). When telephoning, the call person should state the caller's name, the number of the telephone being used, the exact emergency (type of injury), the degree of urgency, and the exact location of the facility; ask for an estimated time of arrival; and explain which is the best entrance to the facility for responding emergency personnel. Other individuals (as many as six or seven) may be called as necessary to act as transporters or help move the patient.

Emergency Telephone Information

- Caller's name
- Number of telephone being used
- Type of emergency
- Degree of urgency
- Exact location of facility
- Emergency vehicle access route
- Estimated time of arrival

While performing the initial assessment, the examiner must keep in mind that six situations can immediately threaten the life of a patient: airway obstruction, respiratory failure, cardiac arrest, severe heat injury, head (craniocerebral) injury, and cervical spine injury.[3] It is these situations along with control of severe bleeding that the examiner must practice repeatedly, because they are the most common emergency life-threatening situa-

Life-Threatening Emergency Situations

- Airway obstruction
- Respiratory failure
- Cardiac arrest
- Severe heat injury
- Head (craniocerebral) injury
- Cervical spine injury
- Severe bleeding

tions. Only practice can ensure proper care in an emergency.

Initially, the examiner **stabilizes and immobilizes the patient's head** and cervical spine in case the patient has suffered a cervical spine injury (Fig. 16–2).[4] If the patient has suffered trauma that is above the clavicles, he or she should be considered to have suffered a spinal injury to the cervical spine until proven otherwise.[5] Simultaneously, the examiner **talks to the patient.** If the patient replies in a normal voice and gives logical answers to questions, the examiner can assume that the airway is patent and the brain is receiving adequate perfusion. The examiner asks the patient what happened to determine how the injury occurred (mechanism of injury). The patient is asked to describe the symptoms (e.g., pain, numbness) and how severe he or she thinks the injury is. If the patient is unable to speak or is unconscious, witnesses are asked what happened. The examiner then explains to the patient what the examiner is going to do and reassures the patient.[6]

While the examiner is talking to the patient, he or she should be observing whether the patient moves, is still, or is having a seizure. If the patient moves, it means

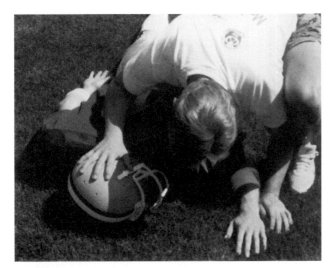

Figure 16–2
Stabilization of the patient's head and neck before initial assessment.

he or she is at least partially conscious, has no apparent neurological dysfunction, and has some cardiopulmonary function. If he or she is still, it means he or she is unconscious, has some neurological dysfunction, or has some other major system failure. A seizure indicates neurological, systemic, or psychological dysfunction. The examiner should also observe the position of the patient (e.g., normal, deformity) and look for altered joint alignment (e.g., fracture, dislocation), swelling, or discoloration.[1] In case there is a spinal cord injury, the patient should be left in the original position until the nature and severity of the injury have been determined, except in cases of respiratory or cardiac distress. A rapid assessment of **brain and spinal cord** can be accomplished by asking the patient to do simple movements such as sticking out the tongue[7] (see discussion of assessment for spinal cord injury).

Emergency On-Field Procedures

- Stabilize head and spine (do not move patient)
- Talk to patient and determine level of consciousness
- Move patient only if in respiratory or cardiac distress
- Check or establish airway
- Check heartbeat
- Check for bleeding, shock, cerebrospinal fluid
- Check pupils
- Check for spinal cord injury (neural watch)
- Position the patient
- Check for head injury
- Assess for heat injury
- Assess movement

Level of Consciousness

The examiner must quickly determine whether the patient is conscious. At no time during this initial assessment should ammonia inhalants be used to arouse the patient. Inhalants should be used only after the examiner is absolutely sure there is no spinal injury, because the fumes may cause a reflex head jerk, complicating the possible neck injury.[6] At this early stage, the examiner simply determines whether the patient is alert (fully conscious), confused (drowsy), in delirium, in obtundation (dulled sensations, especially pain and touch), in a stupor, or in a coma. A patient is classified as **alert** if he or she is able to carry on an appropriate conversation with no delays and is aware of time, place, and identity. A classification of **confused** implies that the patient is disoriented to time, place, and/or identity, has a short attention span, is easily bewildered, and has difficulty following commands. A patient in a **delirious** state is disoriented, restless, and irritable and may have hallucinations. An **obtunded** patient appears drowsy and lethargic but readily replies to verbal stimulation if the questions are simple. A patient is classified as **stuporous** if responses are elicited only in response to loud noises or painful stimulation. This type of patient is lethargic and does not respond to normal verbal communication. In a **comatose** state, the patient appears to be asleep and does not respond to verbal or painful stimuli, except in a rudimentary way (e.g., pulling away from a painful stimulus).

Levels of Consciousness

- Alertness
- Confusion (drowsiness)
- Delirium
- Obtundation
- Stupor
- Coma

The level of consciousness or arousal should be determined by talking to the patient, not by moving the patient. This stage is sometimes referred to as the "shake and shout" stage, in which the examiner tries to arouse the unconscious individual by gentle shaking (without allowing movement of the head and neck) and by shouting into each ear. If the patient does not respond to this verbal stimulus, the examiner can, at least initially, assume that the patient is unconscious or not fully conscious and proceed under that assumption. Further neurological assessment is left until the examiner is sure that the patient has a patent airway, is breathing normally, and has a heartbeat. If the patient is conscious, the examiner should reassure the patient that help has arrived. The patient should be informed of what the examiner is doing and proposes to do in terms of examining and moving the patient. Regardless of the patient's state of consciousness, the patient should not move or be moved until the examiner has had an opportunity to examine the patient.

Establishing the Airway

While waiting for assistance, the examiner can immediately begin to check for abnormal or arrested breathing, abnormal or arrested pulse, internal and external bleeding, and shock. This initial assessment is called the **ABCs (airway, breathing, and circulation)** of cardiopulmonary resuscitation (CPR). The first priority is to maintain an adequate airway, normal ventilation, and hemodynamic stability (see Table 16–1).[8, 9] Also, obvious bleeding should be controlled by compression.

While the cervical spine is protected and immobilized, the airway is quickly assessed for patency by looking, listening, and feeling for spontaneous respirations.[2, 5] Respirations can be determined by watching for movement of the chest, feeling the breath on the cheek, or hearing the air move in and out (Fig. 16–3). The normal resting ranges of respirations are 10 to 25 breaths per minute for adults and 20 to 25 breaths per minute for children. If a patient is not breathing and has no heartbeat, clinical death will occur between 0 and 4 minutes (Fig. 16–4). If breathing and heartbeat are not restored within 4 to 6 minutes, brain damage is probable. If there is no breathing and no heartbeat for 6 to 10 minutes, biological death occurs, and brain damage is very likely.[10]

If the patient is breathing with no difficulty, the rate and rhythm of the respirations and their characteristics should be noted. Cheyne-Stokes and ataxic respirations are often associated with head injuries.[11] Table 16–2 indicates some of the abnormal breathing patterns that may be seen in a patient in an emergency situation.

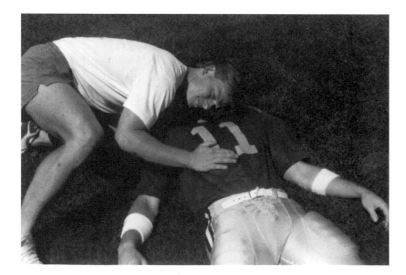

Figure 16–3

Examiner positioning to determine respiration of the patient. The examiner can feel the breath on the cheek, hear the breath, and watch the chest move.

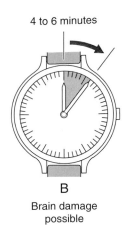
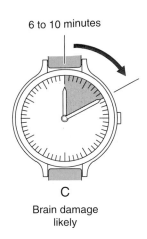

0 to 4 minutes   4 to 6 minutes   6 to 10 minutes

A   B   C

Brain damage unlikely   Brain damage possible   Brain damage likely

Figure 16–4
If the brain is deprived of oxygen for 4 to 6 minutes, brain damage is possible. After 6 minutes, brain damage is extremely likely.

If the conscious patient exhibits abnormal or arrested breathing (asphyxia), the examiner should look for possible causes.[12] Causes include compression of the trachea; tongue falling back, blocking the airway; foreign bodies (e.g., mouthguard, gum, chewing tobacco); swelling of the tissues (e.g., anaphylactic shock after a bee sting); fluid in the air passages; presence of harmful gases or fumes; and suffocation.

Causes of Asphyxia

- Compression of trachea
- Tongue blocking airway
- Foreign bodies
- Tissue swelling
- Fluid in air passages
- Harmful gases or fumes
- Suffocation

Falling back of the tongue is the most common cause of airway obstruction after a sport injury, especially in the unconscious patient. Normally, the tone of the muscles of the tongue ensures airway patency. However, in the unconscious person, especially one in the supine position, muscle tone is lost and the tongue falls back, potentially leading to an obstruction. If the tongue is the cause of obstruction, the examiner can simply pull the chin forward in a **chin lift** (Fig. 16–5A) or **jaw thrust** (Fig. 16–5B) **maneuver** to restore the airway, being careful to keep movement of the cervical spine to a minimum. The chin lift maneuver is less likely to compromise the cervical spine.[13, 14] Either maneuver pulls the retropharyngeal musculature forward, thus opening the airway.[12]

If the examiner can see an object obstructing the airway, an oral screw and tongue forceps can be used to remove the object (Fig. 16–6). The mouth should be held open with the oral screw or something similar, and the examiner can use a finger to sweep the mouth clear of debris (e.g., broken teeth, dentures, mouthguard,

Table 16–2
Abnormal Breathing Patterns

Term	Description	Location of Possible Neurological Lesions
Hyperpnea	Abnormal increase in the depth and rate of the respiratory movements	
Apnea	Periods of nonbreathing	Pons
Ataxic breathing (Biot's respiration)	Irregular breathing pattern, with deep and shallow breaths occurring randomly	Medulla
Hyperventilation	Prolonged, rapid hyperpnea, resulting in decreased carbon dioxide blood levels	Midbrain, pons
Cheyne-Stokes respirations	Periods of hyperpnea regularly alternating with periods of apnea, characterized by regular acceleration and deceleration in depth	Cerebrum, cerebellum, midbrain, pons
Cluster breathing	Breaths follow each other in disorderly sequence, with irregular pauses between them	Pons, medulla

Adapted from Hickey, J.V.: The Clinical Practice of Neurological and Neurosurgical Nursing. Philadelphia, J.B. Lippincott Co., 1986, p. 138.

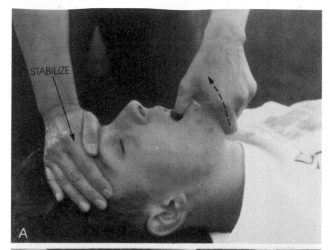

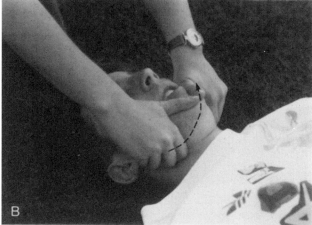

Figure 16–5

Chin lift (A) and jaw thrust (B) maneuvers. In both cases, the head should not be tilted if a cervical injury is suspected.

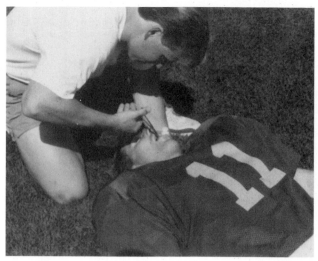

Figure 16–6

Use of tongue forceps and oral screw to maintain patent airway.

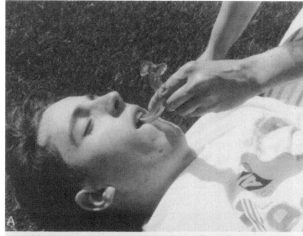

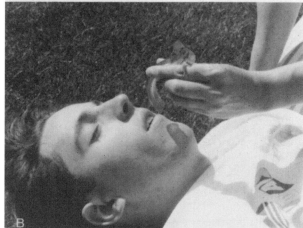

Figure 16–7

Inserting an oropharyngeal airway to establish a patent airway for a patient. (A) Inserting the oral airway; insert the airway wrong way up and gently rotate once in the mouth. (B) The airway as it would look when positioned in the mouth.

chewing gum, tobacco). If the jaw is not held open and blocked from closing, the examiner should put fingers in the patient's mouth only with caution. If the cause of the blockage is something other than the tongue (e.g., foreign body), the patient, if conscious, should be asked to cough. If this does not expel the object, the Heimlich maneuver should be performed until the patient expels the object. If the patient loses consciousness, he or she should be placed supine and ventilation attempted. If it is unsuccessful, 6 to 10 subdiaphragmatic abdominal thrusts are applied. This sequence of ventilation and subdiaphragmatic abdominal thrusts is repeated until a physician or EMS personnel arrive to perform a laryngoscopy.[15] Other causes of asphyxia may be treated by epinephrine (anaphylaxis) or intubation.[15] If the examiner is concerned about maintaining a patent airway, an oropharyngeal airway may be used (Fig. 16–7). As a last resort, a wide-bore needle (18-gauge or larger) may be inserted into the trachea to ensure an airway.

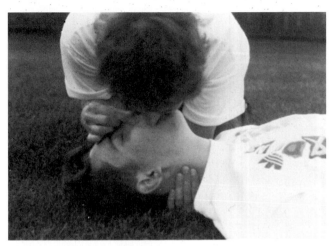

Figure 16–8
Mouth-to-mouth resuscitation.

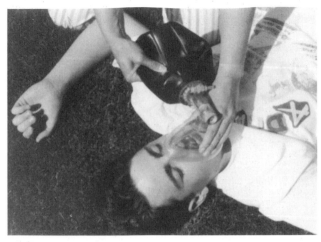

Figure 16–9
Use of a "bagger" to maintain air supply to a patient.

If the patient is not breathing, artificial ventilation (mouth-to-mouth resuscitation) must be initiated immediately, by using the breathing portion of the CPR techniques (Fig. 16–8), by "bagging" the patient (Fig. 16–9), or by using a combination of these methods.

If the patient is conscious but obviously in respiratory and/or cardiac distress, the examiner must deal with the presenting situation immediately (Table 16–3). If the

Table 16–3
Airway Obstruction

Conscious Athlete	*Unconscious Athlete*
1. If patient is breathing or coughing, leave alone but continue to watch	1. Head tilt if no cervical spine injury is suspected
2. If no air is going in and out of lungs, administer: Four abdominal thrusts (Heimlich maneuver); some people also administer four back blows	2. No response—try to ventilate
	3. No success—reposition head and try to ventilate again
3. Repeat until: Patient can breathe independently or patient becomes unconscious	4. If unsuccessful, follow with four abdominal thrusts (Heimlich maneuver); some people also administer four back blows
	5. Quick sweep of the mouth
	6. If unsuccessful, repeat steps 1 through 5 until: There is no longer obstruction, or qualified help arrives; a tracheotomy may follow if obstruction continues

Adapted from American Academy of Orthopaedic Surgeons: Athletic Training and Sports Medicine. Park Ridge, Illinois, AAOS, 1984, p. 454.

patient does not have a patent airway, an airway must be established, as has been described. If the patient is moving in an attempt to "get air," the examiner may assume that a severe cervical injury is less likely to have occurred. However, movement of the head in relation to the cervical spine should be kept to a minimum. Keeping in mind the possibility of a cervical injury, the examiner should position the patient so that airway clearance and resuscitation can easily be accomplished. This change in position must be performed very carefully to ensure that movement of the cervical spine is kept to a minimum. If the patient is reasonably comfortable in the side lying or prone position and there is no problem with cardiac function or breathing, it is not necessary to move the patient to the supine position.

After the airway has been established, whether by the use of an airway device (see Fig. 16–7), by proper head or jaw positioning (see Fig. 16–5), by the use of tongue forceps (see Fig. 16–6), or by a tracheotomy, the examiner must ensure that the airway is maintained and that the patient continues breathing. If respiration is not spontaneous, assisted ventilation (e.g., mouth-to-mouth, bagging) should be instituted. Ventilation can be compromised by a flail chest or pneumothorax (tension or open).[5] Endotracheal intubation is necessary if nasopharangeal bleeding, secretions, or aspirations prevent maintenance of an adequate airway or end-ventilation.[8] Transtracheal ventilation is the treatment of choice for patients with breathing problems caused by brain, cervical spine, or maxillofacial injuries. An endotracheal tube may cause straining and venous hypertension, leading to increased brain edema, and extension of the head and neck to open upper airways may aggravate cervical spine injuries. Also, hemorrhage in maxillofacial injuries prevents the effective use of a breathing mask and does not allow adequate visualization.[9]

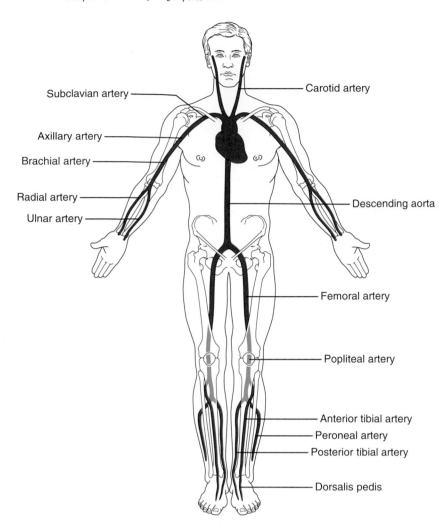

Subclavian artery

Axillary artery

Brachial artery

Radial artery

Ulnar artery

Carotid artery

Descending aorta

Femoral artery

Popliteal artery

Anterior tibial artery

Peroneal artery

Posterior tibial artery

Dorsalis pedis

Figure 16–10
Major arteries in the body. Pressure applied to any of the arteries (pressure points) can decrease bleeding if applied proximal to the bleeding.

Establishing Circulation

While the examiner is determining whether breathing is normal, the circulation should be checked for 10 or 15 seconds using the carotid (preferred), brachial, radial, or femoral pulse (Fig. 16–10). For a sedentary adult, the normal heart rate is 60 to 90 beats per minute. For children, it is 80 to 100 beats per minute. In the highly trained athlete of either sex, the rate may be as low as 40 beats per minute. With activity, the heart rate will be above these levels, and the examiner should take this fact into account when taking the pulse. In the fit person, depending on the type and level of activity, heart rate should decrease to slightly above normal values within 5 minutes. The examiner should note whether the pulse is absent, rapid and rebounding, or weak and diminishing.

The pulse is most often checked at the carotid artery because this artery is large and easy to locate. Therefore, the examiner has less chance of missing the pulse and does not have to move from the area of the patient's head to perform palpation. If a pulse cannot be detected, it should be assumed that the patient does not have a heartbeat, and CPR should be initiated. When the pulse

is assessed, the examiner should estimate its rate, strength, and rhythm to obtain an indication of the cardiac output. Circulatory sufficiency may also be determined by squeezing the nail bed or hypothenar eminence. **Capillary refill** is delayed if the pink color does not return to the nail bed or hypothenar eminence within 2 seconds after release of the pressure.[16] Squeezing the hypothenar eminence is a better indicator if the patient is hypothermic.

The pulse may also be used to determine the patient's blood pressure. If a carotid pulse can be palpated (Table 16–4), systolic blood pressure is 60 mm Hg or

Table 16–4
Rapid Assessment Criteria for Circulation

1. Skin color
2. Carotid pulse palpable (systolic blood pressure, ≥ 60 mm Hg)
   Femoral pulse palpable (systolic blood pressure, ≥ 70 mm Hg)
   Radial pulse palpable (systolic blood pressure, ≥ 80 mm Hg)

Modified from Driscoll, P., and D. Skinner: Initial assessment and management: I. Primary survey. Br. Med. J. 300:1266, 1990.

higher. If the femoral pulse is palpable, systolic blood pressure is 70 mm Hg or higher. If the radial pulse can be palpated, the systolic blood pressure is 80 mm Hg or higher.[7, 11, 16] Like heart rate, blood pressure should drop to almost normal levels within 5 minutes following termination of exercise.

A **weak or rapid pulse** usually indicates shock, heat exhaustion, hyoglycemia, fainting, or hyperventilation. A **slowing pulse** is sometimes seen when there is a large increase in intracranial pressure, which usually indicates a severe lower brain stem compression.[17] A pulse that is **rebounding and rapid** is often the result of hypertension, fright, heat stroke, or hyperglycemia.

If the pulse rate is beginning to weaken, the patient may be going into **shock** (Fig. 16–11). Shock is characterized by signs and symptoms that occur when the cardiac output is insufficient to fill the arterial tree and the blood is under insufficient pressure to provide organs and tissues with adequate blood flow. It should be noted, however, that patients who maintain pink skin, especially in the face and extremities, are seldom hypovolemic after injury. If the skin of the face or extremities turns ashgray or white, it usually indicates blood loss of at least 30%.[5] Common types of shock and their causes are shown in Table 16–5. A patient going into shock becomes restless and anxious. The pulse slowly becomes weak and rapid, and the skin becomes cold and wet, often clammy. Sweating may be profuse, and the face is initially pale and later cyanotic (blue) around the mouth. Respirations may be shallow, labored, rapid, or possibly irregular and gasping, especially if a chest injury has occurred. The eyes usually become dull and lusterless, and the pupils become increasingly dilated. The patient may complain

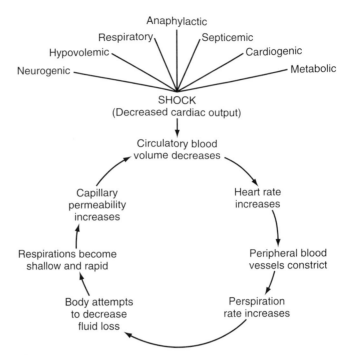

Figure 16–11
The shock cycle.

system injury, or pericardial tamponade (heart compression resulting from blood in the pericardium)—all emergency conditions that require physician intervention.[18] By the time hypovolemic shock becomes evident, blood loss may be as high as 20 to 25%. The normal range of blood pressure is 100 to 120 mm Hg for systolic pressure and 60 to 80 mm Hg for diastolic pressure. With shock, the blood pressure gradually decreases. If the blood pressure can be measured, it is best to assume that shock is developing in any injured adult whose systolic blood pressure is 100 mm Hg or less.

If the examiner is caring for a dark-skinned person, it may be difficult to determine from observation whether the patient is going into shock. A healthy person with dark skin usually has a red undertone and shows a

---

Signs and Symptoms of Shock

- Increased and weak heart rate
- Cold, clammy, pale skin
- Increased and shallow respiratory rate
- Profuse sweating
- Increased thirst
- Restlessness and anxiousness
- Altered level of consciousness
- Dilated pupils
- Nausea or vomiting

---

of thirst and feel nauseated or vomit. If shock develops quickly, the patient may lose consciousness. To prevent or delay the onset of shock, the examiner may cover the patient, elevate the patient's legs, or attempt to eliminate the cause of the problem.

Circulatory collapse in trauma patients is caused primarily by blood loss or **hypovolemic shock,** but the examiner must remember that shock in trauma may also be caused by tension pneumothorax, central nervous

Table 16–5
Types of Shock and Their Causes

Type	Cause
Hemorrhagic (hypovolemic)	Blood loss
Respiratory	Inadequate blood supply
Neurogenic	Loss of vascular control by nervous system
Psychogenic	Common fainting
Cardiogenic	Insufficient pumping of blood by the heart
Septic	Severe infection and blood vessel damage
Anaphylactic	Allergic reaction
Metabolic	Loss of body fluid

healthy pink color in the nail beds, lips, and mucous membranes of the mouth and tongue. A dark-skinned patient in shock, however, has a gray cast to the skin around the nose and mouth, especially if respiratory shock is being experienced. The mucous membranes of the mouth and tongue, the lips, and the nail beds have a blue tinge. If the shock is caused by hypovolemia, the mucous membranes of the mouth and tongue will not be blue, but rather they will have a pale, graying, waxy pallor.[19]

If no pulse is present, then the cardiac portion of CPR techniques should be initiated (Fig. 16–12C). Equipment such as shoulder pads or rib pads should be removed, at least anteriorly, to give the examiner clear access to the anterior chest wall. It should be remembered that CPR provides only approximately 25% of normal cardiac output, so it is imperative that it is performed properly by knowledgeable persons.[20] CPR is maintained until the patient recovers or EMS personnel arrive. If the patient is suspected of having a cervical spine injury, CPR must be done with care, because compression to the heart can cause repeated flexion-extension of the cervical spine.[9]

Assessment for Bleeding, Fluid Loss, and Shock

The examiner should look for any signs of external bleeding or **hemorrhage** (Table 16–6). The types of wounds in which external bleeding or hemorrhage may be seen are incisions, which are clean cuts, or lacerations, which have jagged edges. A contusion may produce internal bleeding, whereas a puncture or abrasion may also show bleeding or oozing on the surface. Major traumatic injuries such as fractures (e.g., pelvis, femur) can cause a great deal of internal bleeding. Of the five types of wounds, the puncture wound is probably the most difficult to treat because it has the highest probability of infection. The examiner should watch for bleeding from the lungs, which is indicated by bright, red, frothy blood appearing in the mouth. If there is bleeding from the stomach, it

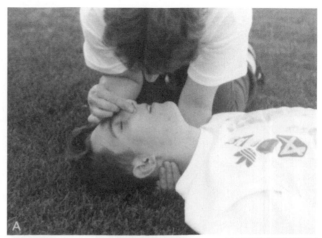
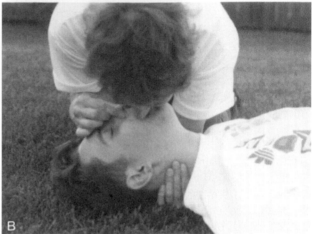
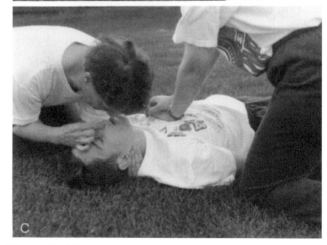

Figure 16–12
The ABCs of cardiopulmonary resuscitation. (A) Checking airway. (B) Applying breath to patient. (C) Cardiac compressions for circulation.

Table 16–6
Bleeding Characteristics and Their Source

Source	Bleeding Characteristics
Artery	Bright red, spurting or pulsating flow
Vein	Dark red, steady flow
Capillary	Slow, even flow
Lungs	Bright red, frothy
Stomach	"Coffee grounds" vomitus
Upper bowel	Tarry black stools
Kidneys	Smoky, red urine
Bladder	Red urine, difficulty urinating
Abdomen	Not seen; abdominal rigidity, pain, difficulty breathing

usually appears with vomitus and looks like coffee grounds. Bleeding from the upper bowel produces tarry-black stools. If the bleeding is from the lower bowel, the blood appears normal when it accompanies the stools. If bleeding is from the kidneys, it causes the urine to have a smoky, red appearance. If bleeding occurs in the bladder, the urine has a redder appearance, and the

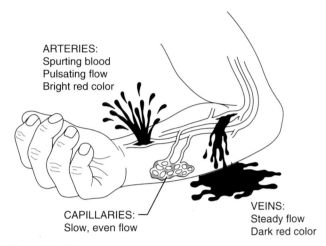

Figure 16–13
Bleeding characteristics.

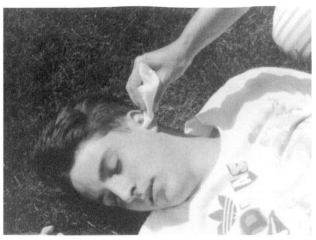

Figure 16–14
Checking the ear for blood and/or cerebrospinal fluid.

patient may have difficulty urinating. If the liver, spleen, or kidney is injured, serious internal bleeding may result; the blood will not be visible because it is contained within the abdominal cavity. In this case, the patient may experience abdominal rigidity, pain, and difficulty in breathing.

When inspecting a bleeding structure, the examiner should note the type of vessel affected. For example, an artery spurts blood, whereas a vein provides an even flow. Capillaries tend to ooze bright blood (Fig. 16–13).[10] Because arterial bleeding is of greatest concern, the examiner must be aware of the pressure points in the body (see Fig. 16–10) to apply proper treatment. The examiner chooses the pressure point closest to the area of bleeding and applies pressure to the artery to slow or stop the bleeding. Tourniquets should be used only with extreme caution and in selected instances (e.g., accidental amputation of a limb, very severe bleeding from a major artery, or the need to apply CPR with no assistance available). If a tourniquet is used, the time of tourniquet application should be noted carefully. Hemodynamic stability is best maintained by applying direct pressure to an open wound, keeping the patient in a recumbent position, and minimizing the number of times the patient is moved.[8]

If signs and symptoms of shock are present but visible bleeding is minimal, the examiner should suspect hidden bleeding within the abdomen, chest, or extremities.[11, 21] If bleeding is suspected in the abdomen, the examiner should check the abdominal wall for shape and distention. To check for bleeding in the chest or extremities, the examiner should look for deformities (e.g., fractures). The fingers may be used to percuss the chest area, noting any loss of hollow sounds, to help locate the presence of fluid or blood. Hyporesonance may indicate a solid organ or the presence of fluid or blood; hyperresonance usually indicates air- or gas-filled spaces.[11]

After the airway and the pulmonary and circulatory systems (ABCs) have been assessed and controlled, the examiner can proceed to the remainder of the primary assessment. The examiner should check the ears and nose for the presence of cerebrospinal fluid. If blood or cerebrospinal fluid leaks from the ear, it may be indicative of a skull fracture. The examiner should incline the head toward the affected side to facilitate drainage, unless a cervical injury is suspected. The examiner can place a gauze pad over the ear or nose where the bleeding is occurring to collect the fluid on the gauze (Fig. 16–14). The examiner should look for an "orange halo" forming on the pad (see Fig. 2–36). The halo is cerebrospinal fluid, the presence of which is a good indication of a skull fracture.[22]

Pupil Check

The examiner checks the pupils for shape and for response to light by using a penlight or by covering the eye with one hand and then taking it away. The pupil normally reacts to the intensity of light or focal distance. The pupils dilate in a dark environment or with a long focal distance, and they constrict in a light environment or with a short focal distance. Normally, the pupils are equally or almost equally dilated (diameter range, 2 to 6 mm; mean of 3.5 mm), but injury to the central nervous system (e.g., head injury) may cause the pupils to dilate unevenly. Some people normally have unequal pupil sizes, and the health care professional must be aware of this possibility. In a fully conscious, alert person who has sustained a blow near the eye, a dilated, fixed pupil is most likely the result of trauma to the short ciliary nerves of that eye rather than the result of third cranial nerve compression caused by brain herniation.[8] Drugs may also affect the pupillary size. For example, opiate drugs cause pinpoint pupils, whereas amphetamines may cause dilated pupils.[11]

To test pupil reaction, the examiner holds one hand over one eye and then moves the hand away quickly, or shines the light from a penlight into the eye, and ob-

Table 16–7
Some Common Causes of Unconsciousness in Patients

Category	Problem	Cause	Pathophysiology	Management
General	Loss of consciousness	Injury or disease	Shock, head injury, other injuries, diabetes, arteriosclerosis	Need for CPR, triage
Disease	Diabetic coma	Hyperglycemia and acidosis	Inadequate use of sugar, acidosis	Complex treatment for acidosis
	Insulin shock	Hypoglycemia	Excess insulin	Sugar
	Myocardial infarct	Damaged myocardium	Insufficient cardiac output	Oxygen, CPR, transport
	Stroke	Damaged brain	Loss of arterial supply to brain or hemorrhage within brain	Support, gentle transport
Injury	Hemorrhagic shock	Bleeding	Hypovolemia	Control external bleeding, recognize internal bleeding, CPR, transport
	Respiratory shock	Insufficient oxygen	Paralysis, chest damage, airway obstruction	Clear airway, supplemental oxygen, CPR, transport
	Anaphylactic shock	Acute contact with agent to which patient is sensitive	Allergic reaction	Intramuscular epinephrine, support, CPR, transport
	Cerebral contusion, concussion, or hematoma	Blunt head injury	Bleeding into or around brain, concussive effect	Airway, supplemental oxygen, CPR, careful monitoring, transport
Emotions	Psychogenic shock	Emotional reaction	Sudden drop in cerebral blood flow	Place supine, make comfortable, observe for injuries
Environment	Heatstroke	Excessive heat, inability to sweat	Brain damage from heat	Immediate cooling, support, CPR, transport
	Electric shock	Contact with electric current	Cardiac abnormalities, fibrillation	CPR, transport; do not treat until current controlled
	Systemic hypothermia	Prolonged exposure to cold	Diminished cerebral function, cardiac arrhythmias	CPR, rapid transport, warming at hospital
	Drowning	Oxygen, carbon dioxide, breath holding, water	Cerebral damage	CPR, transport
	Air embolism	Intravascular air	Obstruction to arterial blood flow by nitrogen bubbles	CPR, recompression
	Decompression sickness ("bends")	Intravascular nitrogen	Obstruction to arterial blood flow by nitrogen bubbles	CPR, recompression
Injected or ingested agents	Alcohol	Excess intake	Cerebral depression	Support, CPR, transport
	Drugs	Excess intake	Cerebral depression	Support, CPR, transport (bring drug)
	Plant poisons	Contact, ingestion	Direct cerebral or other toxic effect	Support, recognition, CPR, identify plant, local wound care, transport
	Animal poisons	Contact, ingestion, injection	Direct cerebral or other toxic effect	Recognition, support, CPR, identify agent, local wound care, transport
Neurological	Epilepsy	Brain injury, scar, genetic predisposition, disease	Excitable focus of motor activity in brain	Support, protect patient, transport in status epilepticus

From the American Academy of Orthopaedic Surgeons: Athletic Training and Sports Medicine, 2nd ed. Park Ridge, Illinois, AAOS, 1991, pp. 618–619.

serves the pupil's reaction when the light is shone on the eye (normal reaction: constriction) or when the light source is removed (normal reaction: dilation). The examiner tests the other eye in a similar fashion and compares the results. The **pupillary reaction** is classified as brisk (normal), sluggish, nonreactive, or fixed. An ovoid or slightly oval pupil or a fixed and dilated pupil indicates increasing intracranial pressure.[11] If both pupils are midsize, midposition, and nonreactive, midbrain damage is usually indicated. The fixation and dilation of both pupils is a terminal sign of anoxia and ischemia to the brain.[11, 23]

Assessment for Spinal Cord Injury

A spinal cord injury should be suspected, at least initially, if the patient has neck pain; the patient's head position is asymmetric or abnormal; the patient is having respiratory difficulty, especially if the chest is not moving (absence of abdominal or diaphragmatic breathing); the patient is demonstrating priapism (erection of the penis); or the patient is unconscious after a fall or other contact activity. Other indications of neurological injuries in the conscious patient include numbness, tingling, or burning, especially below the clavicles; muscle weakness; twitching; or paralysis of the arms and/or legs, especially bilaterally (flaccid paralysis).[11]

The examiner may ask the patient to "stick out the tongue," "wiggle the toes," "move the feet or arms," or "squeeze the (examiner's) fingers."[7] This quick test provides a rapid assessment of the brain and spinal cord by showing whether the patient can follow instructions and can do the activity.

> ### Situations in Which Cervical Spine Injury Must Be Suspected Until Proven Otherwise
>
> - Neck pain or stiffness
> - Cervical muscle spasm
> - Asymmetric or abnormal head position
> - Respiratory difficulty (chest not moving)
> - Priapism
> - Unconsciousness
> - Numbness, tingling, or burning
> - Muscle weakness or paralysis
> - Loss of bowel or bladder control

If the patient is unconscious (Table 16–7), the examiner should reassess the level of unconsciousness and treat the patient as though a spinal injury has occurred. In the unconscious patient, the examiner should watch for spontaneous limb movement, especially after the application of a painful stimulus, because movement indicates that the patient is less likely to have suffered a severe cervical injury.[11] In addition, the examiner should look for posturing that indicates a severe head injury.

Decerebrate rigidity is evidenced by all four extremities being in extension. With **decorticate rigidity,** the lower limbs are in extension and the upper limbs are in flexion (see Fig. 2–29).

Assessment for Head Injury (Neural Watch)

The patient's level of consciousness is then reassessed. The examiner should now institute a neural watch (Fig. 16–15) or a similar observation scheme to note any changes in the patient over time. The neural watch

Neural Watch Chart

Unit		Time 1 ( )	Time 2 ( )	Time 3 ( )
I. Vital signs	Blood pressure Pulse Respirations Temperature			
II. Conscious and	Oriented Disoriented Restless Combative			
	Unconscious			
III. Speech	Clear Rambling Garbled None			
IV. Will awaken to	Name Shaking Light pain Strong pain			
V. Nonverbal reaction to pain	Appropriate Inappropriate "Decerebrate" None			
VI. Pupils	Size on right Size on left Reacts on right Reacts on left			
VII. Ability to move	Right arm Left arm Right leg Left leg			
VIII. Sensation	Right side (normal/abnormal) Left side (normal/abnormal) Dermatome affected (specify) Peripheral nerve affected (specify)			

Figure 16–15

Neural watch chart. (Modified from American Academy of Orthopaedic Surgeons: Athletic Training and Sports Medicine. Park Ridge, Illinois, AAOS, 1984, p. 399.)

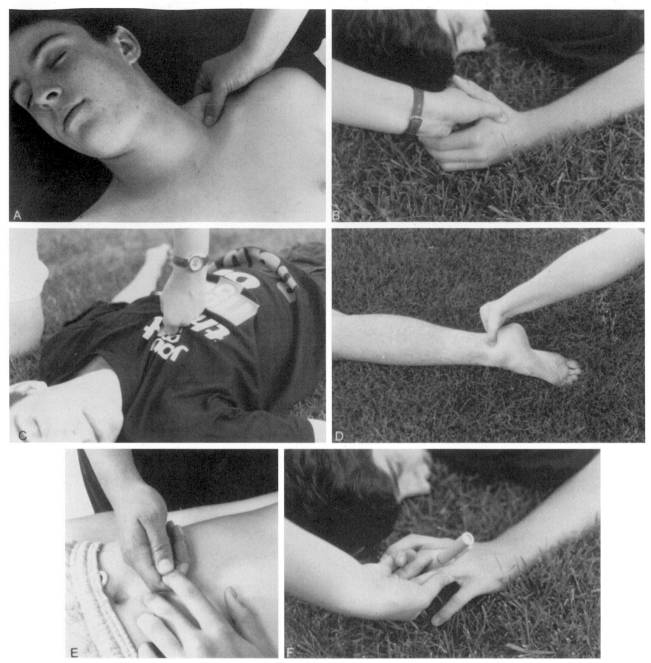

Figure 16–16
Use of physical stimuli to determine level of consciousness. (A) Squeezing trapezius. (B) Squeezing the soft tissue between thumb and index finger. (C) Knuckle to sternum. (D) Squeezing the Achilles tendon. (E) Squeezing a fingertip. (F) Squeezing a pen between the fingers.

should initially be performed **every 5 to 15 minutes,** because it also facilitates monitoring of the patient's vital signs.[11] After the patient has stabilized, neural watch recordings may be made **every 15 to 30 minutes.**[17] If possible, reassessment by the same examiner allows the detection of subtle changes.

The examination should include evaluation of the patient's facial expression; determination of the patient's orientation to time, place, and person; and presence of both posttraumatic amnesia and retrograde amnesia. Signs and symptoms that demand emergency action in a patient who has sustained a blow to the head are increased headache, nausea and vomiting, inequality of pupils, disorientation, progressive or sudden impairment of consciousness, gradual increase in blood pressure, and diminution of pulse rate.

Emergency Signs and Symptoms of Head Injury

- Increased headache
- Nausea and vomiting
- Inequality of pupils
- Disorientation
- Altered level of consciousness
- Increased blood pressure
- Decreased pulse rate
- Decreased reaction to pain
- Decreased or altered values on neural watch chart or Glasgow Coma Scale

---

Reaction to pain and the level of consciousness can be determined by the use of physical and verbal stimuli. If there is no cervical injury, the verbal stimuli may include calling the patient's name and shaking and shouting at the patient. Physical stimuli (Fig. 16–16) include squeezing the Achilles tendon, squeezing the trapezius muscle, squeezing the soft tissue between the patient's thumb and index finger, squeezing an object (pen or pencil) between the patient's fingers, squeezing a fingertip, or applying a knuckle to the sternum (this must be done with caution because it may cause bruising). In comatose patients, a motor response to a painful stimulus to an extremity may indicate intact pain appreciation from that site, especially if it is accompanied by a more remote response such as a grimace or a change in respiration or pulse.[8]

The level of consciousness can best be determined with the use of the **Glasgow Coma Scale** (GCS)[24] (Fig. 16–17). The sooner the patient is tested with the scale, the better, because the initial assessment can be used as a baseline for improvement or deterioration in the patient. The GCS is often performed in conjunction with the neural watch.

The first test of the GCS relates to eye opening. Eye opening may be spontaneous, in response to speech, or in response to pain, or there may be no response at all. Each of these responses is given a score. For example, spontaneous eye opening is given a value of 4, response to speech is given a value of 3, response to pain is given a value of 2, and no response at all is given a value of

Glasgow Coma Scale

				Time 1 (___)	Time 2 (___)
Eyes	Open	Spontaneously	4		
		To verbal command	3		
		To pain	2		
		No response	1	_____	_____
Best motor response	To verbal command	Obeys	6		
	To painful stimulus*	Localizes pain	5		
		Flexion-withdrawal	4		
		Flexion-abnormal (decorticate rigidity)	3		
		Extension (decerebrate rigidity)	2		
		No response	1	_____	_____
Best verbal response†		Oriented and converses	5		
		Disoriented and converses	4		
		Inappropriate words	3		
		Incomprehensible sounds	2		
		No response	1	_____	_____
Total			3–15	_____	_____

* Apply knuckles to sternum; observe arms.

† Arouse patient with painful stimulus if necessary.

Figure 16–17

The Glasgow Coma Scale, which is based on eye opening and verbal and motor responses, is a practical means of monitoring changes in level of consciousness. If responses on the scale are given numerical grades, the overall responsiveness of the patient can be expressed in a score that is the summation of the grades. The lowest score is 3, and the highest is 15.

1. Spontaneous opening of the eyes indicates functioning of the ascending reticular activating system. This finding does not necessarily mean that the patient is aware of the surroundings or of what is happening, but it does imply that the patient is in a state of arousal. A patient who opens the eyes in response to the examiner's voice is probably responding to the stimulus of sound, not necessarily to the command to do something, such as opening the eyes. If unsure, the examiner may try different sound-making objects (e.g., bell, horn, whistle) to elicit an appropriate response.

Motor response is given a value of 6 if the patient responds to a verbal command. Otherwise, the patient is scored on a 5-point scale depending on the motor response to a painful stimulus. When scoring motor responses, it is the ease with which the motor responses are elicited that constitutes the criteria for the best response. Commands given to the patient should be simple, such as "Move your arm." The patient should not be asked to squeeze the examiner's hand, nor should the examiner place something in the patient's hand and then ask the patient to grasp it. This action may cause a reflex grasp rather than a response to a command.[25]

If the patient does not give a motor response to a verbal command, the examiner should attempt to elicit a motor response to a painful stimulus. It is the type and quality of the patient's reaction to the painful stimulus that constitute the scoring criterion. The stimulus should not be applied to the face, because painful stimulus in the facial area may cause the eyes to close tightly as a protective reaction. Examples of application of a painful stimulus are shown in Figure 16–16. The painful stimulus should be applied to an area in which no injury has occurred and only in an amount sufficient to evoke a response. If the patient moves a limb when the painful stimulus is applied to more than one point, or if the patient tries to remove the hand that is applying the painful stimulus, the patient is localizing, and a value of 5 should be given. If the patient withdraws rapidly from the painful stimulus, a normal reflex withdrawal is being shown, and a value of 4 should be assigned. However, if application of a painful stimulus creates a decorticate or decerebrate posture (see Fig. 2–29), an abnormal response is being demonstrated, and a value of 3 or 2 is given, respectively. With **decorticate posturing,** the arms, wrists, and fingers are flexed, the upper limbs are adducted, and the legs are extended, medially rotated, and plantar flexed. **Decerebrate posturing,** which has a poorer prognosis, involves extension, adduction, and hyperpronation of the arms, with the lower limbs being in the same position as for decorticate posturing.[26] Decerebrate rigidity is usually bilateral. If the patient exhibits no reaction to the painful stimulus, a value of 1 is assigned. It is important to be sure that the "no" response is caused by a head injury and not by a spinal cord injury (i.e., flaccid paralysis), which involves lack of feeling or sensation. Any difference in reaction between limbs should be carefully noted, because this finding may be indicative of a specific focal injury.[27]

Verbal response is graded on a 5-point scale and measures the person's speech in response to simple questions such as "Where are you?" or "Are you winning the game?"[26] For verbal responses, the patient who converses appropriately shows proper orientation and awareness of self and environment and is given a grade of 5. The patient who is confused is disoriented and unable to completely interface with the environment. The patient is able to converse with the appropriate words and is given a grade of 4. The patient exhibiting inappropriate speech is unable to sustain a conversation with the examiner. This person is given a grade of 3. The term "vocalizing patient" implies that the patient only groans or makes incomprehensible sounds; this finding is assigned a grade of 2. Again, the examiner should make note of any possible mechanical reason for the inability to verbalize. If the patient makes no sounds and therefore has no verbal response, a grade of 1 is assigned.

It is vital that the initial scores on the GCS and the neural watch be obtained as soon as possible after the onset of injury, because amnesia may occur 10 to 20 minutes after a blow to the head, or there may be an expanding intracranial lesion.[25] With the GCS, the initial score is used as a basis for determining the severity of the patient's head injury. Patients who maintain a score of 8 or less on the GCS for 6 hours or longer are considered to have a serious head injury. A patient who scores from 9 to 11 is considered to have a moderate head injury, and one who scores 12 or more is considered to have a mild head injury.[27]

Deterioration of consciousness may result from many conditions, such as increased intracranial pressure caused by an expanding intracranial lesion, hypoxia (which can aggravate cerebral edema and increase the intracranial pressure), epilepsy, meningitis, or fat embolism. The examiner should always look for signs of expanding intracranial lesions, especially if the patient is conscious. These lesions are emergency conditions that

Head Injury and Glasgow Coma Scale Score (at 6 Hours After Injury)	
Normal:	15
Mild head injury:	12–14
Moderate head injury:	9–11
Severe head injury:	<8

must be attended to immediately because of their potentially high mortality rate (up to 50%). An expanding intracranial lesion is indicated by an altered state of consciousness, development of inequality of the pupils, unusual slowing of the heart rate (which primarily occurs after a lucid interval), irregular eye movements, and eyes that no longer track properly. There is also a tendency for the patient to demonstrate increased body temperature and irregular respiration.

Signs and Symptoms of an
Expanding Intracranial Lesion

- Severe headache
- Nausea and vomiting (projectile)
- Altered state of consciousness
- Inequality of pupils
- Irregular eye movements and tracking
- Decreased heart rate
- Increased body temperature
- Irregular respiration

Normal intracranial pressure ranges from 4 to 15 mm Hg, and intracranial pressure of more than 20 mm Hg is considered abnormal. Intracranial pressure of 40 mm Hg causes neurological dysfunction and impairment. Although the examiner in the emergency care setting has no way of determining the intracranial pressure, the signs and symptoms previously mentioned provide an indication that the pressure is increasing. Most patients who experience an increase in intracranial pressure complain of severe headache followed by vomiting (possibly projectile vomiting).

Signs and symptoms that indicate a good possibility of recovery for a head-injured patient, especially after unconsciousness, include response to noxious stimuli, eye opening, pupil activity, spontaneous eye movement, intact oculovestibular reflexes, and appropriate motor function responses. Neurological signs indicating a poor prognosis after a head injury include nonreactive pupils, absence of oculovestibular reflexes, severe extension patterns or no motor response at all, and increased intracranial pressure.[27]

If the patient experiences loss of consciousness or appears to have disturbed senses, is seeing stars or colors, is dizzy, or has auditory hallucinations or a severe headache, the patient should not be left alone or allowed to return to activity (Table 16–8). In addition, nausea, vomiting, lethargy, increasing blood pressure, disturbed sensation of smell, or a diminished pulse should lead the examiner to the same conclusion. Amnesia, hyperirritability, an open wound, unequal pupils, or leaking of cerebrospinal fluid or blood from the ears or nose also

Table 16–8
Indications for Immediate Removal From Activity

Area of Injury	Indications for Immediate Removal From Activity
Eye	Blunt trauma, visual difficulty, pain, laceration, obvious deformity
Head	Loss of consciousness, disturbed sensorium, stars or colors being seen, dizziness, auditory hallucinations, nausea, vomiting, lethargy, severe headache, rising blood pressure, disturbed smell, diminishing pulse, amnesia, hyperirritability, large contusion, open wounds, unequal pupils, leakage of cerebrospinal fluid or blood from ears or nose, numbness of one side of body
Spine	Obvious deformity, restricted motion, weakness of extremity, pain on movement, localized tenderness, numbness of extremity (pinched nerve), paresthesias
Extremities	Obvious deformity, crepitus, loss of range of motion, loss of sensation, effusion, pain on use, unstable joint, open wounds, significant tenderness, significant swelling
Abdomen	Dizziness or syncope, nausea, persisting pallor, vomiting, history of infectious mononucleosis, abnormal thirst, muscle guarding, localized tenderness, shoulder pain, distension, rapid pulse, clamminess and sweating

Reprinted by permission from the *New York State Journal of Medicine,* copyright by the Medical Society of the State of New York. Adapted from Greensher, J., H.C. Mofenson, and N.J. Merlis: First aid for school athletic emergencies. N.Y. State J. Med. 79:1058, 1979.

indicates an emergency condition. Numbness on one side of the body or a large contusion in the head area should likewise lead the examiner to handle the patient with care. If the frontal area of the brain is affected, the patient may experience lapses of memory, personality changes, or impairment of judgment. If the temporal lobe has been affected, the patient may experience feelings of unreality, déjà vu, or hallucinations involving odors, sounds, or visual disturbances such as macropsia (seeing objects as larger than they really are) or micropsia. The literature indicates that head injury depends not only on the magnitude and direction of impact and the structural features and physical reactions of the skull but also on the state of the head/brain at the moment of impact.[3, 26, 28]

If the patient has received a head injury and has been checked by a physician and it has been determined that it is not necessary to send the patient to the hospital, the clinician should ensure that the patient and whoever lives with the patient understands what to look for in terms of signs and symptoms that may indicate increasing severity of head injury. Figure 16–18 demonstrates typical home health care guidelines.

**Home Health Care Guidelines:
Head Injury Care**

The person you have been asked to watch has suffered a head injury, which at this time does *not* appear to be severe. However, to ensure proper care, please ensure that the following guidelines are followed for the next 24 hours.

1. Limited physical activity for at least 24 hours.

2. Liquid diet only for the next 8 to 24 hours.

3. Apply ice to the head for approximately 15 minutes every hour to relieve discomfort and swelling.

4. Tylenol may be given as needed but NO aspirin. No other medication for 24 hours without doctor's approval.

5. Awaken the patient every 2 hours during the next _____ hours and be aware of any symptoms in #6.

6. Appearance of any of the following signs and symptoms means that you should consult a doctor or go to an emergency room at a hospital **immediately:**

   - Nausea and/or vomiting
   - Weakness or numbness in arm, leg, or any other body part
   - Any visual difficulties or dizziness
   - Ringing in the ears
   - Mental confusion or disorientation, irritability, forgetfulness
   - Loss of coordination
   - Unusual sleepiness or difficulty in awakening
   - Progressively worsening headache
   - Persistent intense headache after 48 hours
   - Unequal pupil size; slow or no pupil reaction to light
   - Difficulty breathing
   - Irregular heartbeat
   - Convulsions or tremors

7. Call to arrange an appointment with your doctor or the team physician/therapist* for a follow-up visit. If unable to contact your doctor, go to an emergency room as soon as possible for an evaluation.

   *Consult: _____ at _____
   phone number

   or: _____ at _____
   phone number

SPECIAL INSTRUCTIONS, APPOINTMENTS:

Figure 16–18

Home health care guidelines for patients with head injuries. (Modified from Allman, F.L., and R.W. Crow: On-field evaluation of sports injuries. In Griffin, L.Y. [ed.]: Orthopedic Knowledge Update: Sports Medicine. Rosemont, Illinois, American Academy of Orthopaedic Surgeons, 1994, p. 144.)

Assessment for Heat Injury

If the examiner suspects a heat-type injury with no cervical injury, only heat exhaustion and heat stroke need be considered as life-threatening. **Heat fatigue or exhaustion** occurs when a person is exposed to high environmental temperature and/or humidity and perspires excessively without salt or fluid replacement. **Heat stroke** can occur when a nonacclimatized person is suddenly exposed to high environmental temperature and/or humidity. The thermal regulatory mechanism fails, perspiration stops, and the body temperature increases. Above 42°C oral body temperature, brain damage occurs, and death follows if emergency measures are not instituted. The diagnostic key in this situation are the **high body temperature** and the **absence of sweating**. Initial signs of heat injury include muscle cramps, excessive fatigue and/or weakness, loss of coordination, decreased reaction time, headache, decreased comprehension, dizziness, and nausea and vomiting.

Signs of Heat Injury

- Muscle cramps
- Excessive fatigue and/or weakness
- Loss of coordination
- Headache
- Decreased comprehension
- Dizziness
- Nausea and vomiting
- Decreased reaction time

The body temperature varies according to the site at which the measurement is taken. The oral body temperature is 37°C (98.6°F). Taken in the armpit or axilla, the temperature is 36.4 to 36.7°C (97.5 to 98.1°F) , and in the rectum, it is 37.3 to 37.6°C (99.1 to 99.7°F).

The examiner may palpate the skin to get some idea of the external temperature of the body and possible

Table 16–9
Skin Changes and Their Cause

Skin Change	Cause
Hot and dry	Heat stroke, high fever, hyperglycemia
Cold and clammy	Fainting, hypoglycemia, hyperventilation, shock
Cool and moist	Heat exhaustion
Cool and dry	Cold
White pallor	Decreased circulation
Cyanosis (blue pallor)	Respiratory distress
Red pallor	Fever, heat stroke, inflammation, exercise

pathology (Table 16–9). Hot and dry skin is often caused by heat stroke, high fever, or hyperglycemia. Cold and clammy skin is caused by hypoglycemia, shock, fainting, or hyperventilation. Cool and moist skin is often caused by heat exhaustion, whereas cool and dry skin is caused by exposure to cold.

Skin color can also play a significant role. Pallor, or "white" skin, indicates circulatory disturbance or decreased circulation and is most often associated with trauma and shock. Cyanosis, or a blue tint to the skin, indicates respiratory distress, as does a gray tint. Redness indicates an increase in blood flow as a result of fever, heat stroke, or exercise.

Assessment for Movement

If the patient has not already done so, the examiner asks the patient to move the limbs to reassess for a cervical spine injury and look for major trauma (e.g., fractures, dislocations, third-degree strains, third-degree sprains). At the same time, the examiner may palpate the areas of potential injury, noting any pain, abnormal bone or joint alignment, swelling, hypersensitive or hyposensitive areas, or palpable defect (third-degree strain).[1] If movement is relatively normal, the examiner quickly checks the myotomes of the upper or lower body for any possible motor involvement or motor impairment. Changes in limb power may be caused by a contractile tissue injury, a neurological injury, or an expanding intracranial lesion, which will be displayed as progressive weakness in the contralateral arm or leg.[17] Decreased limb power can also be caused by reflex inhibition as a result of previously unrecognized limb injury. In these cases, contractions are weak and painful. These types of injuries are placed in the low priority group (see Table 16–1) because they represent a threat to the limb rather than to the life of the patient.[9]

Positioning the Patient

Normally, a patient is left in the position in which he or she is found until the primary assessment is completed. However, if the patient is having difficulty breathing or there is no pulse, the patient must be positioned to do CPR. If the conscious patient is prone and in respiratory difficulty, the examiner, with assistance, should **log-roll** the patient (Fig. 16–19) onto a spinal board so that an attempt can be made to restore the airway. During any movement of the patient, traction of about 4.5 kg (10 lbs) should be applied to the cervical spine by the examiner to maintain stability. The patient should be reassured that others are going to carefully move the patient while he or she remains still. Before any movement is attempted, the patient and those who are going to assist the examiner should know what the examiner plans to do and what their jobs are. This requires **frequent practicing of emergency procedures.** The sequence of movement and positioning of the extremities and body of the patient should be thought out beforehand so that everyone is aware of what is going to happen. The proper procedure for moving the patient should be practiced often to ensure competency.

To roll the patient, at least three assistants are needed. There should be two-way communication between the examiner and the patient at all times to continually evaluate the patient's comfort level and neurological signs. The assistants should place the spinal board beside the patient and then kneel beside the spinal board and patient (see Fig. 16–19A). They should reach over the patient and hold the patient's shoulder, hip, and knees (see Fig. 16–19B). On command from the examiner, the assistants roll the patient toward them while the examiner stabilizes the head (see Fig. 16–19C and D), until the patient is lying supine on the spinal board (see Fig. 16–19E). Only rolling—not lifting—should occur. With the patient in the supine position, proper CPR techniques may be applied, or the patient may be transported. The patient may also be covered with a blanket to provide warmth.

If a spinal injury is suspected and the conscious patient is in the prone position but having no difficulty in breathing, the patient is log-rolled halfway toward the assistants while another assistant slides the spinal board as close as possible to the patient's side. The patient is then rolled directly onto the spinal board in the prone position. Similarly, if a spinal injury is suspected and the patient is in the supine position and breathing normally, the patient is rolled toward the assistants while another assistant slides the spinal board under the patient as far as possible. The patient is then rolled back onto the spinal board in the supine position. If a spinal injury is suspected and the patient is in side lying, the patient is log-rolled directly onto the spinal board and into the supine position. In each of these cases, the examiner controls the head, applies traction, and gives instructions to the assistants. The patient's head is then stabilized and immobilized with sandbags, a head immobilizer, or triangular bandages, and the patient is strapped to the spinal board with restraining belts. If a collar is used to stabilize the spine, it must do so during movement as well as when the patient is stationary; it must not hinder access to the carotid pulse, airway, or performance of CPR; it must be easy to assemble and apply; it must be adaptable to patients of all ages and sizes; and it must allow radiological examination without removal.[29, 30] Any major injury such as a head injury, a spinal injury, or a fracture requires appropriate handling, slow and deliberate management, and proper transportation to provide a satisfactory outcome. These techniques must be practiced repeatedly.

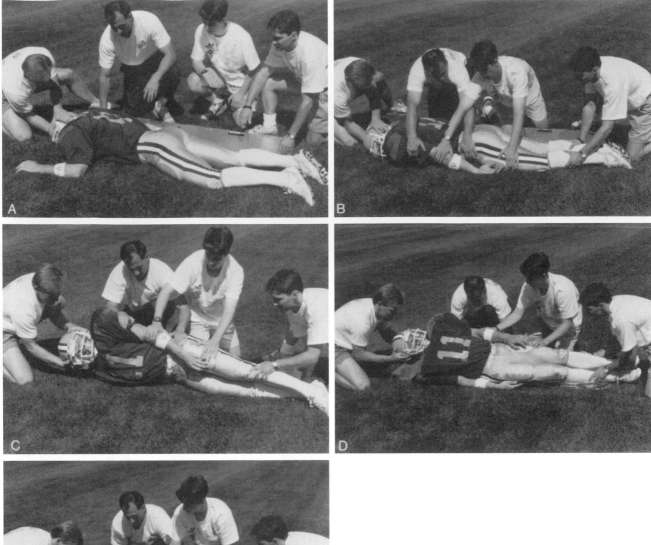

Figure 16–19

Moving a patient to the supine position after injury. Note that the head and neck are stabilized throughout the movement. (A) Patient prone, examiner stabilizes head and gives instruction to helpers. (B) through (E) Patient is log-rolled onto spinal board.

If possible and time permits, especially if the assistants are not used to working together, a simulated roll and transport using an uninjured person should be attempted before moving the patient to ensure that all involved know what they are doing in terms of patient positioning, movement sequence, and specific handling (e.g., head, hands, feet), so that any transfer or movement of the patient is effective and organized.

During the emergency assessment, if the patient is nauseated, is vomiting, or has fluid draining from the mouth, and if breathing and circulation are normal, the patient should be placed in the **recovery position** (Fig. 16–20) provided that there is no suspicion of a spinal injury. This side lying position enables the patient to be continually monitored (ABCs) and allows any change in condition to be observed easily while waiting for emergency personnel. The head should be positioned to keep the airway open and to allow drainage from the throat and mouth. If the blood flow to the heart and brain has diminished, circulation can be improved by elevating the lower limbs, provided that the position change can be accomplished without causing further pain, breathing problems, or aggravation of an injury. If the patient has breathing difficulties or a chest injury or has experienced a heart attack or stroke, it may be desirable to lower blood pressure in the injured parts by elevating the upper part of the body slightly, if the position change can be accomplished without causing further pain or breathing problems.

If the patient is unconscious and the cardiac and circulatory functions are not compromised, the patient should be left in the original position until consciousness is regained. However, if the patient is unconscious and lying supine, the examiner should always watch for the possibility that the patient may "swallow" the tongue and obstruct the airway. Also, an unconscious patient loses the cough reflex, and if vomiting or bleeding occurs, vomitus, mucus, or blood may enter and obstruct the airway. Therefore, the examiner may elect to put the patient in the recovery position.

If the patient is unconscious and in respiratory or cardiac distress, the examiner must quickly assess the patient and attempt to restore respiratory and cardiac function. This patient is then treated the same as the conscious patient.

If the patient's spine is twisted or flexed and the patient is reasonably comfortable, the patient should be stabilized in that position until a spinal injury is ruled out. If there has been a loss of breathing or cardiac function, the examiner must carefully correct the deformity, place the patient in the supine lying position, and perform the appropriate measures to deal with the problem.

If a cervical spine injury has occurred to a child of 7 years of age or younger, the examiner should realize that in these children, the head is normally larger in proportion to the rest of the body. If the child is positioned on a spinal board without modification, the neck will be forced into some flexion. To alleviate this prob-

lem, the spinal board should have a cutout for the head, or a pad for the chest or rest of the body should be added to elevate it in relation to the head.[31]

If the patient is in the water and unconscious, the patient must be reached as quickly as possible. The rescuer should not jump into the water, because this action creates waves that may rock the victim's head and could cause severe consequences if a neck injury has occurred. The examiner should approach the patient head-on and place an extended arm down the middle of the patient's back with the patient's head in the examiner's axilla. The examiner then grasps the patient's biceps with the forearm around the patient's forehead, slowly lifts the arm, and turns the patient face-up. The examiner's forearm locks the patient's head in the examiner's axilla during the turn. Once the patient is supine, both of the examiner's arms support the patient's head and spine in the water. An assistant then slides the spinal board under the patient in the water and blocks the patient's head with towels. The patient is next strapped to the spinal board with restraining straps and is lifted out of the water.[32] If a spinal board is not available and a cervical injury is suspected, the patient should be supported in the water until emergency personnel arrive.

In some sports (e.g., hockey, motor car or motorcycle racing, football), helmets are worn. Whether the helmet should be removed to institute emergency procedures is a controversial issue and often depends on the type of training (EMS versus sports therapy) and experience of the health care professional.[33] Generally, if the patient is unconscious, the helmet should not be removed unless the examiner is absolutely certain that there has not been a neck injury. In the patient who wears both helmet and shoulder pads, both should be left on the patient because they help to maintain the cervical sagittal alignment close to normal. Ideally, the helmet and shoulder pads should be removed in a controlled setting such as the emergency department.[34] Helmets should be removed only if the facemask or visor interferes with adequate ventilation[34, 35]; if the facemask interferes with the clinician's ability to restore an adequate airway[34, 35];

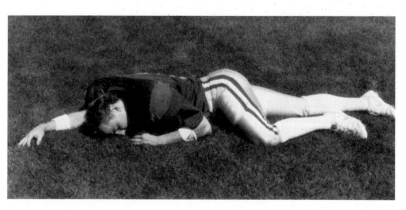

Figure 16–20
Recovery position.

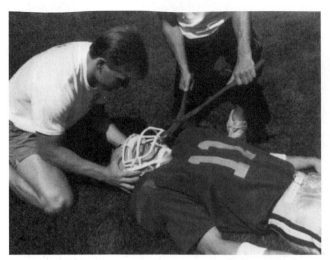

***Figure* 16–21**
Use of bolt cutters to remove mask.

if the helmet is so loose that it does not provide adequate immobilization of the head when secured to the spinal board[34, 35]; if life-threatening hemorrhage under the helmet cannot be controlled[34, 35]; if, in children, the helmet is too large and causes flexion of the neck when used as part of the immobilization[31, 34, 35]; or if it is necessary to defibrillate the patient. In the last case, the shoulder pads must be removed, so the helmet should be removed to maintain spinal position.[1] If the patient is in respiratory distress, facemasks can easily be removed with the use of bolt cutters or an X-Acto knife to cut the restraining straps while holding the mask in place (Fig. 16–21 and Fig. 16–22).

If, for whatever reason, the decision is made to remove the head gear, the neck and head must be held as rigid as possible. Therefore, at least two people

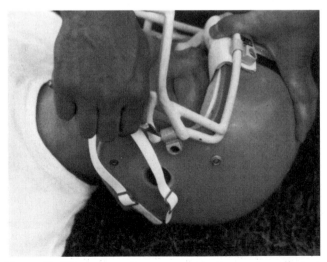

***Figure* 16–22**
Use of X-Acto knife to cut mask restraining straps.

are needed—one to stabilize the head and neck and one to remove the facemask. In-line traction is first applied to the helmet by one person, usually the assistant, to ensure initial stability. A second person, usually the examiner, then stands at the side of the patient and applies in-line traction by applying a traction force through the patient's chin and occiput (Fig. 16–23). The assistant stops applying traction and, if the helmet is a football helmet, first removes the cheek pads by sliding a flat object (e.g., scissors handle) between the cheek pad and helmet, twisting the object to cause the pads to unsnap. After the pads are removed, the assistant applies bilateral expansion to the helmet so that the ears are cleared as the helmet is removed.[1] After the helmet has been removed, the assistant reapplies in-line traction from the head, and the examiner then releases the traction and continues the primary examination.[28] If desired, the examiner may apply a cervical collar such as the Stifneck collar, but this should be done with caution, because cervical collars do not completely eliminate movement in the cervical spine.[36]

If the helmet is removed and the patient is wearing shoulder pads, the person holding the head must ensure that the head does not fall back into extension, and a modification must be made to the spinal board. The shoulder pads should be removed only if it is impossible to do this or if defibrillation is necessary.

If the patient is conscious and there appears to be no cervical injury or other severe injury, the patient may be moved to another area for a more appropriate and complete secondary assessment. If the injury is in the upper limb and the injured part is immobilized, the patient may first be moved from a supine to a sitting or kneeling position, then from sitting or kneeling to supported standing, to unsupported standing, and finally may walk off the field. During these changes in position, the examiner or assistants are positioned to provide support and assistance if the patient feels dizzy or un-

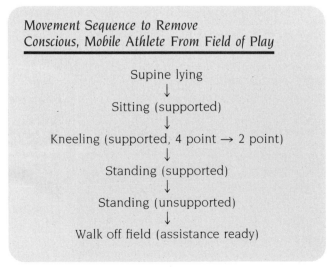

Movement Sequence to Remove
Conscious, Mobile Athlete From Field of Play

Supine lying
↓
Sitting (supported)
↓
Kneeling (supported, 4 point → 2 point)
↓
Standing (supported)
↓
Standing (unsupported)
↓
Walk off field (assistance ready)

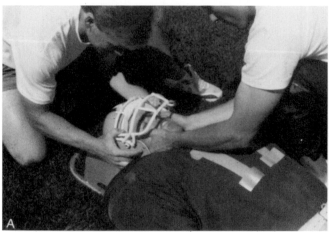

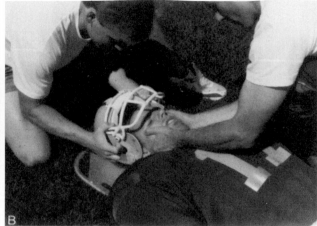

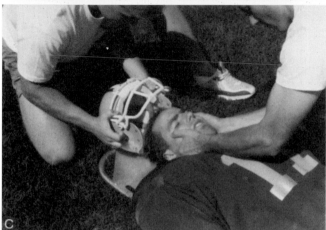

Figure 16–23
Removal of helmet. (A) Stabilize neck. (B) and (C) Remove helmet.

steady. If the injury is in the lower limb, the athlete may be helped off the field by teammates, stretcher, or pull cart. Spinal injuries require greater care and the use of a spinal board and cervical collar with support. Again, assistance may be required, and everyone, including the patient and assistants, should be aware of the movement sequence before it is attempted.

Injury Severity

During the primary assessment, the examiner must use some method of determining the severity of injury. There are several scales that may be used to test the severity of injury or to triage the patient, including the Galveston Orientation and Amnesia Test,[37] which tests for posttraumatic amnesia; the Abbreviated Injury Scale[38]; the Injury Severity Score[38-40]; the Trauma Score[41]; the Triage Index[42, 43]; the Circulation, Respiration, Abdomen, Motor, and Speech (CRAMS) Scale[44, 45]; and the Trauma Index.[46] Of these, the Trauma Score illustrates the ease of scoring (Fig. 16–24) and the survival probabilities (Table 16–10) that can be expected in trauma patients. This tool provides a dynamic score that monitors changes in the patient's condition and is useful in making triage decisions.

Table 16–10
Trauma Score and Probability of Survival Based on the Score

Trauma Score	Probability
16	0.99
15	0.98
14	0.95
13	0.91
12	0.83
11	0.71
10	0.55
9	0.37
8	0.22
7	0.12
6	0.07
5	0.04
4	0.02
3	0.01
2	0
1	0

From Champion, H.R., W.J. Sacco, A.J. Carnazzo, W. Copes, and W.J. Fouty: Trauma score. Crit. Care Med. 9:674, 1981.

Trauma Score

Trauma Score	Value	Points	Score
A. Respiratory rate	10–24	4	
Number of respirations in 15 sec, multiply by four	25–35	3	
	>35	2	
	<10	1	
	0	0	A. _____
B. Respiratory effort	Normal	1	
Shallow—markedly decreased chest movement or air exchange	Shallow, or retractive	0	
Retractive—use of accessory muscles or intercostal retraction			B. _____
C. Systolic blood pressure	>90	4	C. _____
Systolic cuff pressure—either arm; auscultate or palpate	70–90	3	
	50–69	2	
	<50	1	
No carotid pulse	0	0	
D. Capillary refill			
Normal—forehead, lip mucosa or nail bed color refill in 2 sec	Normal	2	
Delay—more than 2 sec of capillary refill	Delayed	1	
None—no capillary refill	None	0	D. _____

E. Glasgow Coma Scale (GCS)

			Total GCS Points	Score
1. Eye opening			14–15	5
Spontaneous	_____	4	11–13	4
To voice	_____	3	8–10	3
To pain	_____	2	5–7	2
None	_____	1	3–4	1 E. _____

2. Verbal response
Oriented _____ 5
Confused _____ 4
Inappropriate words _____ 3
Incomprehensible words _____ 2
None _____ 1

3. Motor response
Obeys command _____ 6
Purposeful movement (pain) _____ 5
Withdraw (pain) _____ 4
Flexion (pain) _____ 3
Extension (pain) _____ 2
None _____ 1

**Trauma Score
(Total points A + B + C + D + E):** _____

Total GCS points (1 + 2 + 3) _____

Figure 16–24

Trauma score. (From Champion, H.R., W.J. Sacco, A.J. Carnazzo, W. Copes, and W.J. Fouty: Trauma score. Crit. Care Med. 9:673, 1981.)

The CRAMS scale illustrates a similar scoring pattern (Table 16–11).

Secondary Assessment

The examiner can proceed to the secondary assessment if the patient is conscious, is able to respond by talking coherently, shows minimal or no distress in terms of breathing, and displays normal circulation. However, the examiner must keep in mind that the patient may still have suffered a catastrophic injury (e.g., cervical spine injury) that, although not life-threatening at the present time, could lead to problems. For the most part, the secondary survey is predicated on the patient's being clinically stable.[5]

If the patient is conscious, the examiner must constantly reassure the patient to reduce potential anxieties. By the time the secondary assessment begins, the examiner should have eliminated any possible life-threatening situations and can then complete the injury assessment. In the case of a sudden injury, the examiner should remember that the patient has had no time to prepare psychologically or practically for the injury. Therefore, the injury represents a sudden and frightening change

Table 16–11
CRAMS Scale

Circulation
2: Normal capillary refill and BP over 100 mm Hg systolic
1: Delayed capillary refill or BP 85–99 systolic
0: No capillary refill or BP less than 85 systolic _____

Respiration
2: Normal
1: Abnormal (labored, shallow, or rate over 35)
0: Absent _____

Abdomen
2: Abdomen and thorax not tender
1: Abdomen or thorax tender
0: Abdomen rigid, thorax flail, or deep penetrating injury to either abdomen or thorax _____

Motor
2: Normal (obeys commands)
1: Responds only to pain—no posturing
0: Posturing or no response _____

Speech
2: Normal (oriented)
1: Confused or inappropriate
0: No sounds or unintelligible sounds _____

(Score of 6 or less indicates referral to trauma center should be
initiated)   TOTAL   ══════════

CRAMS = Circulation, Respiration, Abdomen, Motor, and Speech.

From Hawkins, M.L., R.C. Treat, and A.R. Mansberger: Trauma victims: Field triage guidelines. South. Med. J. 80:564, 1987. Reprinted by permission from the Southern Medical Journal.

in the patient's physical state. Other concerns experienced by the patient may be related to the patient's job, financial situation, family, or prognosis, and these concerns, suddenly magnified, may affect the patient's behavior, especially in later secondary or "sideline" assessments.

The secondary assessment is a head-to-toe rapid physical examination[23] and can be performed after the examiner has ascertained that there is no threat to the patient's life. The patient must be conscious for the examiner to perform the secondary assessment properly. The secondary survey involves a complete body survey to detect other injuries that may cause serious complications or lead to a patient's not being allowed to return to activity. The patient should be instructed not to move unless requested by the examiner, who should also explain to the patient what is being done while the examination is being performed. It is important to maintain communication with the patient throughout the examination. During this time, the examiner is testing for pos-

sible spinal injuries, fractures, dislocations, or soft-tissue injuries.

While performing the assessment, the examiner is considering whether the patient should be allowed to return to activity (Table 16–12). The examiner must decide whether further evaluation is required on-site or whether the patient should be taken to some other venue (e.g., dressing room, hospital). In addition, the examiner should keep in mind that home monitoring may be necessary and therefore should determine whether a responsible person is at home to watch for changing signs and symptoms in the patient (see Fig. 16–18).

When progressing to the secondary assessment, the examiner must continue to do the neural watch or GCS and watch for signs of an expanding intracranial lesion or other complications. Advanced cerebral edema may further reduce the perfusion of an already damaged hemisphere, and compression of the descending motor tracts may decrease limb power. Also, the patient's level of consciousness can reveal a deficit previously overshadowed by other evidence of severe brain injury.

During the secondary assessment, there is time to carry out a more thorough assessment for head injury or perform other tests in addition to the neural watch and GCS. The patient's abilities to assimilate information and act with split-second timing are more likely to be impaired after concussion than are strength and endurance.

If a head injury is suspected, it is important to determine the patient's reasoning and processing ability. Questions such as "What day is it?", "Who is the opposition?", "Who is winning?", and "What is your telephone

Table 16–12
Emergency Care Levels of Decision

1. Is the injury life-threatening?
2. What care (first aid) must be given on-site or "on the field"?
3. Can and should the patient be moved?
4. If the patient is to be moved, what is the best way to do it?
5. What steps are to be taken before the patient is moved? Spinal board? Splinting? Instruction?
6. If the patient is to be moved, where to? Sidelines? Locker room? Training room? Hospital?
7. How is the patient to be transported? Ambulance? Parent's vehicle?
8. If the injury is not severe enough to require transportation to the hospital, what protocols are to be followed for return to activity?
9. If the patient is not allowed to return to activity, what protocols are to be followed?

Adapted from Haines, A.: Principles of emergency care. Athletic J. 26:66–67, 1984.

number and address?" test the patient's static memory ability. The examiner should also test for **retrograde amnesia** (loss of memory of events before the injury), **posttraumatic amnesia** (loss of memory of events after the injury), and injury severity (trauma scales). Immediate recall, another form of memory, is best tested by saying a series of single digits and asking the patient to repeat them. Normally, a person can repeat at least six digits, and many people can repeat eight or nine. Recent memory can be tested by giving the patient two to five common objects or names (e.g., the color "blue," the number "10," the word "ball," and the name "Mrs. Jones") to remember and then asking the patient to repeat these names 5 to 15 minutes later during the next neural watch. The patient can be asked to repeat the words two or three times when the examiner initially says them to test immediate recall or to ensure that the patient can say or remember the words. Short-term memory may be assessed by questions pertaining to the individual's assignments or "game plan" and events that

---

Common Head Injury Tests

- Static memory (What day is it? Who's winning?)
- Immediate recall (repeat series of single digits)
- Recent memory (recall three common objects or names after 15 minutes)
- Short term memory (What is the game plan?)
- Processing and concentration ability (minus-7 test, multiplying)
- Abstract relationships
- Coordination (eye-hand tests)
- Balance (Romberg test)
- Myotomes
- Eye coordination
- Visual disturbance tests

---

followed the injury.[47] For example, the examiner may ask one of the other players, such as a spare quarterback, to call out the number of a play and have the patient respond quickly with what the patient's assignment was during that play. Questions about the injury, preceding events, and posttraumatic events may also be asked. The correct answer to such questions must be known by the examiner or by someone present at the time of the examination.

Questions about names, places, spelling, and digital recall do not necessarily test the capacity for processing

information. To determine processing ability, the patient is asked to do the minus-7 test (e.g., $100 - 7 = 93$; $93 - 7 = 86$; $86 - 7 = 79$, and so on). This test provides the examiner with some idea of the calculating ability and concentration skills of the patient. Arithmetic ability (adding, subtracting, multiplying, and dividing) may also be evaluated to test processing ability. Similarly, the patient can be asked to name several important people from the present backward (e.g., the last three presidents of the United States), name the months of the year backward, or give the names of some familiar capital cities.

Finally, the patient should be tested to determine whether abstract relationships can be comprehended. For example, the examiner may quote a common proverb, such as "A bird in the hand is worth two in the bush," and then ask the patient to explain what it means. Patients with actual brain damage may give a concrete answer and fail to recognize the abstract principle involved.[27]

The examiner also checks coordination or motor neurological function. When testing for proper neurological function, the examiner should palpate the neck and back for any pain or tenderness.[25] There are a number of tests for eye-hand coordination, such as touching the finger to the nose, touching the finger to another finger at arm's length in front of the eyes, touching the examiner's palm and then touching the patient's own nose, touching the examiner's palm or finger at arm's length away from various positions, touching the thumb with the fingers, the hand flip test, the finger drumming test, and, finally, moving the heel of one leg down the shin of the other leg. These tests are described in greater detail in Chapter 2. Balance and motor coordination can be tested by determining whether the patient can maintain balance through unsupported standing, the Rhomberg test, standing with eyes closed, being pushed from side to side, balancing on one leg, or normal walking. Motor neurological function is tested by checking the patient's grip strength or the various myotomes.

Eye coordination and peripheral vision can be checked by asking the patient to follow the examiner's fingers up and down, side to side, diagonally, and in circles, noting any wandering eye movements. To test visual disturbance, the patient is asked to read or observe something from a short distance (e.g., eye chart, how many fingers the examiner is holding up). To test for vision at distance, the patient can be asked to read the score clock, as an example.

After brain function has been tested, the remainder of the secondary assessment is similar to the "clearing," or scanning, assessments performed for the cervical or lumbar spine. The examiner clears the different areas of the body so that a detailed assessment of the specifically injured joints or structures can be performed. At this stage, the assessment follows the same basic protocol as in the detailed assessment of specific joints; that is, a more detailed history of the injury is taken, the patient is observed for obvious or potential problems, and the entire body is quickly scanned for injury. This is followed by a detailed examination of the specifically injured structures, including active, passive, and resisted isometric movements, special tests, testing of reflexes and cutaneous sensory distribution, joint play movement tests (if applicable), and, finally, palpation and other diagnostic tests such as imaging and laboratory tests (see Chapters 3 to 13).

Because the examiner is one of the first persons to talk to the patient, the examiner will probably obtain the most accurate history. Simple nonleading questions should be asked, and information should be clarified in an attempt to find out what happened and what injury or injuries the patient believes have occurred. Appropriate questions related to specific joints or areas of the body can be found elsewhere in this text. The patient often can provide the examiner with the diagnosis if the examiner listens carefully. After the patient has been thoroughly questioned, others who witnessed the accident or injury may also be questioned to complete the history. Informed conversation with other persons sometimes helps to detect abnormal behavior that may not be noticed initially. If the patient has a previous medical file, it may also prove beneficial to review the contents for information regarding preexisting conditions, previous trauma, and medications.

As the patient history is obtained, the examiner continues to observe the patient and notes levels of consciousness, developing symptoms, pain patterns, and altered functional abilities. In addition, the examiner should carefully watch for developing signs and symptoms of an expanding intracranial lesion by noting changes in facial expression, the pupils, and the level of consciousness and performing the neural watch and GCS several times. The basic observation is the same as that performed during joint assessment and includes observation of bony and soft-tissue contours, scars, deformities, the ability to move, and body alignment.

The next part of the secondary assessment is the scanning examination, in which the examiner quickly scans the entire body through observation, by asking the patient to make particular movements (depending on where the suspected injury has occurred), and by testing myotomes, dermatomes, and reflexes. During this phase, the examiner should explain what is being done and why, not only to reassure the patient but also to ensure

cooperation and relaxation. This part of the examination may be done without removing the patient's clothes, although it is better to do so because clothing may obstruct the view of the injured area. However, if the examination is being performed in the presence of other people, clothing removal should be left to a later time, or the patient should be moved to a more appropriate location. If the clothes need to be removed, the patient should be warned, especially if in a public place, and every effort should be made to maintain the patient's dignity.

After the specific area or areas of injury have been narrowed down through the scanning examination, the examiner can perform a detailed assessment of the appropriate parts of the body, as specified in other chapters. Failure to perform a proper examination may lead to a missed assessment and more problems than originally anticipated.

The patient must be immediately sent to a hospital or trauma center if at any time during the primary or secondary evaluation the following signs are exhibited: pupillary or extraocular movement abnormality, facial or extremity weakness, amnesia, confusion or lethargy, sensory or cranial nerve abnormality, Babinski sign, deep tendon reflex asymmetry, or posttraumatic seizures.[23, 48] Proper care for the patient must always be uppermost in the mind of the examiner. Table 16–12 helps to outline the levels of decision making required of the examiner in the emergency sports assessment.

> ### Signs Indicating Need for Immediate Transport to Hospital
>
> - Abnormal pupil or extraocular movement
> - Increasing facial or extremity weakness or flaccid paralysis
> - Amnesia, confusion, or lethargy
> - Sensory or cranial nerve abnormality
> - Decreasing value in Glasgow Coma Scale
> - Positive Babinski sign
> - Deep tendon reflex asymmetry
> - Posttraumatic seizures

After the assessment has been completed and the patient has been stabilized, has returned to competition, or has been referred for further medical care by ambulance, the examiner should be sure to document what happened and the subsequent care that was given, noting any potential difficulties. These notes, if taken at the sideline, should be transferred to the patient's medical record as soon as possible.

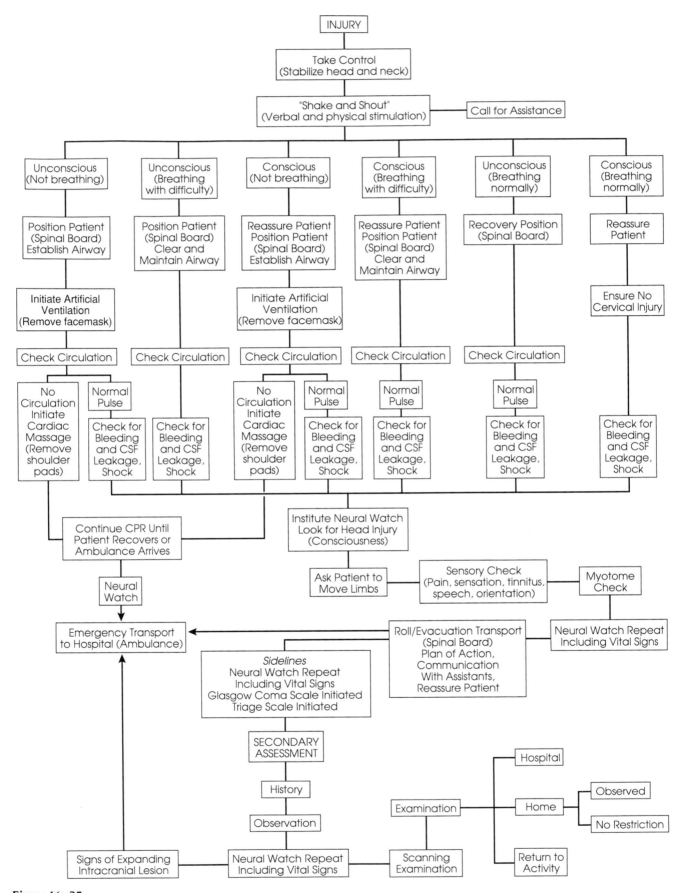

Figure 16–25
Assessment sequence following acute injury.

Précis of the Emergency Sports Assessment

The sequence to be followed for assessment of acute injury is shown in Figure 16–25.

Case Studies

When reviewing or practicing these case studies, the examiner should outline the necessary protocol for dealing with the described situations. The examiner can develop different scenarios depending on the degree of severity of the injury. These scenarios, including assessment and movement of the patient, should be practiced often so that the examiner is fully aware of what to do and how to handle emergency situations.

1. A diver misjudges his take-off from the 10-m board, hits his head on the concrete platform, and falls unconscious into the pool, displaying decorticate rigidity as he falls. Describe your emergency protocol for this patient.
2. A squash player is playing a squash game and is struck near the eye by her opponent's squash racquet. Describe your emergency protocol for this patient.
3. A 22-year-old professional basketball player is playing in a game. He is under his own net and suddenly collapses and lapses into unconsciousness. Describe your emergency protocol for this patient.
4. During a race on a hot, humid day, a 10,000-m runner collapses on the track during the event and lies motionless. Describe your emergency protocol for this patient.
5. During a baseball game, a batter is hit on the chest by a pitched ball and collapses at home plate. Describe your emergency protocol for this patient.

6. A defensive back tackles a runner and makes the tackle but does not move when the other players get up, even though he is conscious. He is having difficulty breathing. Describe your emergency protocol for this patient.
7. A rugby player hits his head during a collapsing scrum. He is knocked unconscious, is not breathing, and has no pulse. Describe your emergency protocol for this patient.
8. A hockey player receives a deep cut to the neck when another player's skate accidentally cuts him. He is bleeding profusely. Describe your emergency protocol for this patient.
9. A gymnast on the balance beam misses her dismount and lands on her head, neck, and shoulders and is knocked unconscious. Describe your emergency protocol for this patient.
10. A wrestler is thrown to the mat near the end of the first round. He lands hard on the side of his face with his neck twisted. He is lying prone and unconscious. Describe your emergency protocol for this patient.
11. While playing soccer, an athlete is stung by a bee and develops anaphylactic shock. Describe your emergency protocol for this patient.
12. A hockey player is "checked" into the boards from behind. He falls to the ice and has difficulty breathing; he had been chewing gum. Describe your emergency protocol for this patient.

References

Cited References

1. Starkey, C., and J. Ryan: Evaluation of Orthopedics and Athletic Injuries. Philadelphia, F.A. Davis Co., 1996.
2. Beaver, B.M.: Care of the multiple trauma victim: The first hour. Nurs. Clin. North Am. 25:11–21, 1990.
3. Torg, J.S., T.C. Quedenfeld, and W. Newell: When the athlete's life is threatened. Phys. Sportsmed. 3:54–60, 1975.
4. Fourré, M.: On-site management of cervical spine injuries. Phys. Sportsmed. 19:53–56, 1991.
5. Dick, B.H., and J.M. Anderson: Emergency care of the injured athlete. In Zachazewski, J.E., D.J. Magee, and W.S. Quillen (eds.): Athletic Injuries and Rehabilitation. Philadelphia, W.B. Saunders Co., 1996.
6. Allman, F.L., and R.W. Crow: On-field evaluation of sports injuries. In Griffin, L.Y. (ed.): Orthopedic Knowledge Update: Sports Medicine. Rosemont, Illinois, American Academy of Orthopaedic Surgeons, 1994.
7. Driscoll, P., and D. Skinner: Initial assessment and management: I. Primary survey. Br. Med. J. 300:1265–1266, 1990.
8. Hugenholtz, H., and M.T. Richard: The on-site management of athletes with head injuries. Phys. Sportsmed. 11:71–78, 1983.
9. Steichen, F.M.: The emergency management of the severely injured. J. Trauma 12:786–790, 1972.
10. American Academy of Orthopaedic Surgeons: Emergency Care and Transportation of the Sick and Injured. Chicago, AAOS, 1981.
11. Ward, R.: Emergency nursing priorities of the head injured patient. AXON 11:9–12, 1989.
12. Veenema, K.R., and J. Swenson: Laryngeal trauma: Securing the airway on the field. Phys. Sportsmed. 23:71–75, 1995.
13. Hochbaum, S.R.: Emergency airway management. Emerg. Med. Clin. North Am. 4:411–425, 1986.
14. Vegso, J.J., and R.C. Lehman: Field evaluation and management of head and neck injuries. Clin. Sports Med. 6:1–15, 1987.
15. Profera, L.M., and P. Paris: Managing airway obstruction. Phys. Sportsmed. 19:35–40, 1991.
16. Keitz, J.E.: Emergent assessment of the multiple trauma patient. Orthop. Nurs. 8:29–32, 1989.
17. Hayward, R.: Management of Acute Head Injuries. Oxford, Blackwell Scientific Pub., 1980.
18. Erickson, S.M., and B.S. Rich: Pulmonary and chest wall emergencies: On-site treatment of potentially fatal conditions. Phys. Sportsmed. 23:95–104, 1995.
19. Hafen, B.Q., and K.J. Karren: First Aid and Emergency Care Skills Manual. Englewood, California, Morton Pub. Co., 1982.
20. Jackson, R.E., and S.B. Freeman: Hemodynamics of cardiac massage. Emerg. Med. Clin. North Am. 1:501–513, 1983.
21. Rose, C.C.: Radiologic triage of the multiply-injured patient. Emerg. Med. Clin. North Am. 3:425–436, 1985.

22. Booher, J.M., and G.A. Thibodeau: Athletic Injury Assessment. St. Louis, C.V. Mosby Co., 1989.

23. Mahoney, B.D., and E. Ruiz: Acute resuscitation of the patient with head and spinal cord injuries. Emerg. Med. Clin. North Am. 1:583–594, 1983.

24. Teasdale, G., and B. Jennett: Assessment of coma and impaired consciousness: A practical scale. Lancet 2:81–83, 1974.

25. Topel, J.L.: Examination of the comotose patient. In Weiner, W.J., and C.G. Goetz (eds.): Neurology for the Non-neurologist. Philadelphia, J.B. Lippincott, 1989.

26. Gerberich, S.G., J.D. Priest, J. Grafft, and R.C. Siebert: Injuries to the brain and spinal cord: Assessment, emergency care and prevention. Minnesota Medicine Nov:691–696, 1982.

27. Manzi, D.B., and P.A. Weaver: Head Injury: The Acute Care Phase. Thorofare, New Jersey, Slack Inc., 1987.

28. Vegso, J.J., M.H. Bryant, and J.S. Torg: Field evaluation of head and neck injuries. In Torg, J.S. (ed.): Athletic Injuries to the Head, Neck and Face. Philadelphia, Lea & Febiger, 1982.

29. Karbi, O.A., D.A. Caspari, and C.H. Tator: Extrication, immobilization and radiologic investigation of patients with cervical spine injuries. Can. Med. Assoc. J. 139:617–621, 1988.

30. Chandler, D.R., C. Nemejc, R.H. Adkins, and R.L. Waters: Emergency cervical spine immobilization. Ann. Emerg. Med. 21:1185–1188, 1992.

31. Herzenberg, J.E., R.N. Hensinger, D.K. Dedrick, and W.A. Phillips: Emergency transport and positioning of young children who have an injury of the cervical spine. J. Bone Joint Surg. Am. 71:15–22, 1989.

32. Richards, R.N.: Rescuing the spine-injured diver. Phys. Sportsmed. 3:67–71, 1975.

33. Patel, M.N., and D.A. Rund: Emergency removal of football helmets. Phys. Sportsmed. 22:57–59, 1994.

34. Zachazewski, J.E., G. Geissler, and D. Hangen: Traumatic injuries to the cervical spine. In Zachazewski, J.E., D.J. Magee, and W.S. Quillen (eds.): Athletic Injuries and Rehabilitation. Philadelphia, W.B. Saunders Co., 1996.

35. Heckman, J.D.: Emergency Care and Transport of the Sick and Injured. Rosemont, Illinois, American Academy of Orthopaedic Surgeons, 1993.

36. Aprahamian, C., B.M. Thompson, W.A. Finger, and J.C. Darin: Experimental cervical spine injury model: Evaluation of airway management and splinting techniques. Ann. Emerg. Med. 13:584–587, 1984.

37. Davidoff, G., M. Jakubowski, D. Thomas, and M. Alpert: The spectrum of closed-head injuries in facial trauma victims: Incidence and impact. Ann. Emerg. Med. 17:27–30, 1988.

38. Baker, S.P., B. O'Neill, W. Haddon, and W.B. Long: The injury severity score: A method for describing patients with multiple injuries and evaluating emergency care. J. Trauma 14:187–196, 1974.

39. Baker, S.P., and B. O'Neill: The injury severity score: An update. J. Trauma 16:882–885, 1976.

40. Greenspan, L., B.A. McLellan, and H. Greig: Abbreviated injury scale and injury severity score: A scoring chart. J. Trauma 25:60–64, 1985.

41. Champion, H.R., W.J. Sacco, A.J. Carnazzo, W. Copes, and W.J. Fouty: Trauma score. Crit. Care Med. 9:672–676, 1981.

42. Champion, H.R., W.J. Sacco, D.S. Hannon, et al.: Assessment of injury severity: The triage index. Crit. Care Med. 8:201–208, 1980.

43. Lindsey, D.: Teaching the initial management of major multiple system trauma. J. Trauma 20:160–162, 1980.

44. Hawkins, M.L., R.C. Treat, and A.R. Mansberger: Trauma victims: Field triage guidelines. South. Med. J. 80:562–565, 1987.

45. Clemmer, T.P., J.F. Orme, F. Thomas, and K.A. Brooks: Prospective evaluation of the CRAMS scale for triaging major trauma. J. Trauma 25:188–191, 1985.

46. Kirkpatrick, J.R., and R.L. Youmans: Trauma index: An aid in the evaluation of injury victims: J. Trauma 11:711–714, 1971.

47. Hugenholtz, H., and M.T. Richard: Return to athletic competition following concussion. Can. Med. Assoc. J. 127:827–829, 1982.

48. Jones, R.K.: Assessment of minimal head injuries: indications for in-hospital care. Surg. Neurol. 2:101–104, 1974.

General References

Adelman, D.C., and S.L. Spector: Acute respiratory emergencies in emergency treatment of the injured athlete. Clin. Sports Med. 8:71–79, 1989.

American Academy of Orthopaedic Surgeons: Athletic Training and Sports Medicine. Park Ridge, Illinois, AAOS, 1984.

Andrews, J.: Difficult diagnoses in blunt thoracoabdominal trauma. J. Emerg. Nurs. 15:399–404, 1989.

Arnheim, D.D.: Modern Principles of Athletic Training. St. Louis, C.V. Mosby Co., 1985.

Axe, M.J.: Limb-threatening injuries in sport. Clin. Sports Med 8:101–109, 1989.

Bailes, J.E., and J.C. Maroon: Management of cervical spine injuries in athletes. Clin. Sports Med. 8:43–58, 1989.

Baker, J.H.: The first aid management of spinal cord injury. Semin. Orthop. 4:2–14, 1989.

Bernardo, L.M., A. Comway, and M. Bove: The ABC method of emotional assessment and intervention: A new approach in pediatric emergency care. J. Emerg. Nurs. 16:70–76, 1990.

Blanchard, B.M., and C.R. Castaldi: Injuries in youth hockey: On-ice emergency care. Phys. Sportsmed. 19:54–71, 1991.

Brukner, P., and K. Khan: Sporting emergencies. In Zuluaga, M., C. Briggs, J. Carlisle, et al. (eds.): Sports Physiotherapy: Applied Science and Practice. Melbourne, Australia: Churchill Livingstone, 1995.

Champion, H.R., W.J. Sacco, R.L. Lepper, E.N. Atzinger, W.S. Copes, and R.H. Prall: An anatomic index of injury severity. J. Trauma 20:197–202, 1980.

Coady, C., and W.D. Stanish: Emergencies in sports: The young athlete. Clin. Sports Med. 7:625–640, 1988.

Dailey, R.H.: Acute upper airway obstruction. Emerg. Med. Clin. North Am. 1:261–277, 1983.

Davies, G.J., and C.Y. Anast: The fractured femur: Acute emergency care treatment. J. Orthop. Sports Phys. Ther. 1:53–58, 1979.

De Podesta, M.: A practical and effective approach in dealing with emergency situations. Can. Athletic Ther. Assoc. J. 9:5–8, 1982.

Diamond, D.L.: Sports-related abdominal trauma. Clin. Sports Med. 8:91–99, 1989.

Fahey, T.D.: Athletic Training: Principles and Practice. Palo Alto, California, Mayfield Pub. Co., 1986.

Frasier, J.E.: Acute cardiac emergencies in the injured athlete. Clin. Sports Med. 8:81–90, 1989.

Gansche, M., D.P. Henderson, and J.S. Seidel: Vital signs as part of the prehospital assessment of the pediatric patient: A survey of paramedics. Ann. Emerg. Med. 19:173–178, 1990.

Greensher, J., H.C. Mofenson, and N.J. Merlis: First aid for school athletic emergencies. N.Y. State J. Med. 79:1058–1062, 1979.

Haines, A.: Principles of emergency care. Athletic Journal 26:8–10+, 1984.

Halpern, J.S.: Clinical notebook: Upper extremity peripheral nerve assessment. J. Emerg. Nurs. 15:261–265, 1989.

Halpern, J.S.: Clinical notebook: Lower extremity peripheral nerve assessment. J. Emerg. Nurs. 15:333–337, 1989.

Hawkins, M.L., R.C. Treat, and A.R. Mansberger: The trauma score: A simple method to evaluate quality of care. Am. Surg. 54:204–206, 1988.

Hickey, J.V.: The Clinical Practice of Neurological and Neurosurgical Nursing. Philadelphia, J.B. Lippincott Co., 1986.

Jacobs, L.M., A. Sinclair, A. Beisner, and R.B. D'Agostino: Prehospital advanced life support: Benefits in trauma. J. Trauma 24:8–13, 1984.

Kane, G., R. Engelhardt, J. Celentino, et al.: Empirical development and evaluation of prehospital trauma triage instruments. J. Trauma 25:482–489, 1985.

Levin, H.S., V.M. O'Donnell, and R.G. Grossman: The Galveston orientation and amnesia test (GOAT): A practical scale to assess cognition after head injury. J. Nerv. Ment. Dis. 167:675–684, 1979.

Long, S.E., S.E. Reid, H.J. Sweeney, and W.W. Johnson: Removing football helmets safely. Phys. Sportsmed. 8:119, 1980.

Lowery, D.W.: Soft tissue trauma of the head and neck. Phys. Sportsmed. 19:21–24, 1991.

Martinez, R.: Catastrophes at sporting events: A team physician's pivotal role. Phys. Sportsmed. 19:42–44, 1991.

McKnight, W.: Understanding the patient in emergency. Canadian Nurse July:20–23, 1976.

Meislen, H.W., K.V. Iserson, K.R. Kaback, M. Kobernick, A.B. Sanders, and S. Seifert: Airway trauma. Emerg. Med. Clin. North Am. 1:295–312, 1983.

Moore, S.: Airway maintenance: A primary consideration in the unconscious athlete. Athletic Training Spring:48–49, 1981.

Patterson, D.: Legal aspects of athletic injuries to the head and cervical spine. Clin. J. Sports Med. 6:197–210, 1987.

Round Table: Guidelines to help you in giving on-field care. Phys. Sportsmed. 3:51–63, 1975.

Roy, S., and R. Irvin: Sports Medicine: Prevention, Evaluation, Management, and Rehabilitation. Englewood Cliffs, New Jersey, Prentice Hall, 1983.

Ryan, A.J.: On-field diagnosis of head injuries. Phys. Sportsmed. 4:82–84, 1976.

San Diego Sports Medicine Center: Athletic Injury Disaster Plan. San Diego, Valhalla High School, 1987.

Schneider, R.C., and F.C. Kiss. First aid and diagnosis: The treatment of head injuries. In Schneider, R.C. (ed.): Head and Neck Injuries in Football. Baltimore, Williams & Wilkins Co., 1973.

Schneider, R.C.: The treatment of the athlete with neck, cervical spine and cervical cord trauma. In Schneider, R.C., J.C.

Kennedy, and M.L. Plant (eds.): Sports Injuries: Mechanisms, Prevention and Treatment. Baltimore, Williams & Wilkins, 1985.

Shatney, C.H.: Initial resuscitation and assessment of patients with multisystem blunt trauma. South. Med. J. 81:501–506, 1988.

Shires, G.T.: Initial management of the severely injured patient. JAMA 213:1872–1878, 1970.

Swaine, B.R., and S.J. Sullivan: Reliability of the scores for the finger-to-nose test in adults with traumatic brain injury. Phys. Ther. 73:71–78, 1993.

Teasdale, G., and B. Jennett: Assessment of coma and impaired consciousness: A practical scale. Lancet 2:81–83, 1974.

Torg, J.S.: Management guidelines for athletic injuries to the cervical spine. Clin. Sports Med. 6:53–60, 1987.

Waecherle, J.F.: Planning for emergencies. Phys. Sportsmed. 19:35–38, 1991.

Walters, B.C., and I. McNeill: Improving the record of patient assessment in the trauma room. J. Trauma 30:398–409, 1990.

Watkins, R.G., and W.M. Dillin: Cervical spine and spinal cord injuries. In Fu, F.H., and D.A. Stone (eds.): Sports Injuries: Mechanisms, Prevention, Treatment. Baltimore, Williams & Wilkins, 1994.

Weigelt, J.A.: Initial management of the trauma patient. Crit. Care Clin. 2:705–716, 1986.

Werman, H.A., R.N. Nelson, J.E. Campbell, R.L. Fowler, and P. Gandy: Basic trauma life support. Ann. Emerg. Med. 16:1240–1243, 1987.

West, J.G., M.A. Murdock, L.C. Baldwin, and E. Whalen: A method for evaluating field triage criteria. J. Trauma 26:655–659, 1986.

Wilberger, J.E., and J.C. Maroon: Head injuries in athletes. Clin. Sports Med. 8:1–9, 1989.

Yarnell, P.R., and S. Lynch: The "ding": Amnesic states in football trauma. Neurology 23:196–197, 1973.

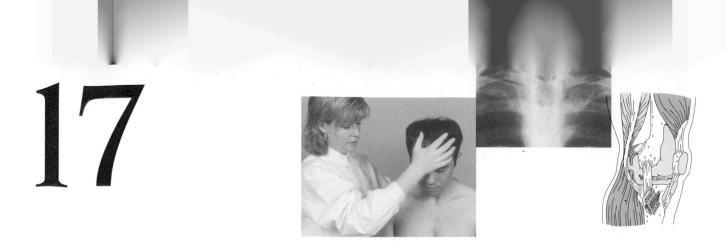

17

Preparticipation Evaluation

Preactivity evaluations, although they may be generic in some sense, are also usually designed to be specific for a given job, activity, sport, or age group.[1-3] For example, different occupations, activities, and sports have particular concerns, and participants are more prone to certain injuries when participating, for example, in football (trauma) compared with running (overuse). Similarly, each activity, job, or sport has different concerns regarding the population, age, or sex of participants.[3-5] The level or intensity of the examination may vary from a minimal medical examination or "physical" to a very extensive examination involving stress testing, profiling, x-rays, and other special protocols in addition to the medical examination.[6] It may also vary with the type of job or sport, the more strenuous activities and those involving contact or collision (Table 17–1) requiring a more detailed examination.[7]

Ideally, the preparticipation evaluation should be done at least 6 weeks before the activity begins.[8, 9] This allows time for consultation with specialists, if necessary, and time to correct minor defects such as skin disorders, muscle weaknesses, minor infections, and similar minor medical problems.[6]

Preparticipation evaluations are usually done by a family physician who is familiar with the athlete's and the family's history; he or she should be aware of any congenital or developmental problems, the patient's immunization status, and any recent injuries or illnesses and therefore can provide continuity of care.[8-10] Many people, however, do not have a family physician, and such a physician may not be interested or understand the demands of the proposed activity. A second method, especially in the case of a specific sport, is to use the team physician, who is familiar with the requirements and demands of the sport. This type of examination is often a group effort, with different health care professionals performing different parts of the assessment. This method, provided it is properly organized, enables a large number of people to be seen in a short time, but it can be impersonal, confusing, and noisy.[10-11] The third and least desirable method is to have the preparticipation examination done by the local health department. Although these agencies are efficient and effective, people working for local health departments are less likely to have an awareness of the activity's requirements or the patient's individual or family history.

Commonly, the preparticipation examination is done yearly, although it may not be as extensive after the first year with an organization.[9, 12, 13] Some locations require annual examinations.[14] In subsequent years with the same organization, the preparticipation evaluation may involve only those parts of the evaluation that could have been affected in the past season.[8] For example, strength testing may be performed only on those joints that suffered an injury in the past season to ensure that the patient is ready to participate again.

McKeag[15] has outlined five specific populations in which special areas of possible concern should be included in the examination. In the prepubescent patient (6 to 10 years of age), assessments should include examination for congenital abnormalities that may not have been diagnosed previously. In the pubescent patient (11 to 15 years of age), the examination should center on evaluation of physical maturity and good health practices to allow safe participation. The postpubescent or young adult group (16 to 30 years of age) has the widest variety of skills, levels, and motivation. For this group, the history of previous injuries and sport-specific examinations is particularly important. For the adult population (30 to 65 years of age), injury prevention (e.g., overuse), previous injury patterns, and conditioning should be included in the examination. The final group consists of elderly patients (65 years of age or older), who require an examination based on individual requirements, because many of these people take up exercising or increased physical activity after a medical illness.

Table 17–1
Classification of Sports

| | | Noncontact | | |
Contact/Collision	Limited Contact/Impact	Strenuous	Moderately Strenuous	Nonstrenuous
Boxing	Baseball	Aerobic dancing	Badminton	Archery
Field hockey	Basketball	Fencing	Curling	Golf
Football	Bicycling	Field	Table tennis	Riflery
Ice hockey	Diving	Discus		
Lacrosse	Field	Javelin		
Martial arts	High jump	Shot put		
Rodeo	Pole vault	Running		
Soccer	Gymnastics	Swimming		
Wrestling	Horseback riding	Tennis		
	Skating	Track		
	Ice	Weight lifting		
	Roller			
	Skiing			
	Cross-country			
	Downhill			
	Water			
	Softball			
	Squash, handball			
	Volleyball			

From Committee on Sports Medicine: Recommendations for participation in competitive sports. Pediatrics 81:737, 1988. Reproduced by permission of Pediatrics.

Objectives of the Evaluation

Preparticipation evaluations have many useful purposes.[6, 8, 16, 17] However, it is important to remember that the purpose of the examination is not to disqualify the patient but to **ensure the patient's health and safety.**[8] Therefore, a patient who is disqualified for any reason should be encouraged to find other activities, exercises, or sports that would not be precluded by the results of the examination. Most organizations require preparticipation evaluations for legal and insurance reasons. Such examinations can provide some protection in case of litigation, and many insurance companies require them as **a prerequisite for issuing an insurance policy.**[6] Usually, the evaluations are carried out to uncover any preexisting conditions that could rule out participation for reasons of safety and health. These conditions range from simple immaturity to loss of an organ or the presence of specific disease processes (e.g., rheumatic fever).

The preparticipation evaluation helps the examiner **develop a musculoskeletal profile**, which is used to determine whether the patient has the physical attributes for the activity. Patients who have had an injury or operation must be evaluated both physically and psychologically to ensure that they can withstand the forces normally encountered in the activity, exercise, or sport.[8]

By developing a physical fitness profile, the examiner can **establish baseline or normal values** for the patient so that future injury may be properly assessed. These values may be compared if an injury occurs or during the rehabilitation process. In other words, the assessment should not consist of simple "yes-no" questions. Instead, it must be very thorough and establish proper fitness

Objectives of Preparticipation Evaluation

- Meet legal and insurance requirements
- Uncover preexisting conditions
- Develop musculoskeletal profile
- Determine health status
- Prevent injuries
- Determine unsuspected correctable conditions
- Avoid misinterpretation of findings
- Establish baseline values
- Ensure that previous treatments have occurred
- Act as a screening process
- Foster good health practices
- Keep immunizations current
- Develop rapport with the patient
- Establish guidelines
- Counsel the patient
- Classify the patient

levels for the activity, both to decrease the incidence of injury and to ensure that the patient can take part at the level desired.

The preparticipation evaluation may also be used to determine the health status of the patient before he or she is exposed to participation or competition. It also helps to **prevent injuries** through identification of any abnormalities, physical inadequacies, or poor conditioning that may put the patient at risk.

The examination may **identify previously unsuspected conditions** that are amenable to correction or that preclude participation in the desired activity. Similarly, the evaluation helps to avoid misinterpretation of findings that appear to be new but existed previously. For this reason, a review of previous health records is also part of the preparticipation evaluation.

The preparticipation assessment is also worthwhile to **ensure that treatments are carried out** and that conditions previously diagnosed have been properly cared for. In this way, it acts as a screening process to ensure that treatment of potentially serious medical and surgical conditions has taken place. It also helps to rule out potentially serious or threatening conditions that may temporarily preclude the patient from participation. For example, with infectious mononucleosis, contact sports may be precluded for a time because the patient's spleen is enlarged and is more easily injured or ruptured. The preparticipation assessment also ensures that an injury that occurred at the end of the previous season has been properly cared for and rehabilitated. Often athletes do not go for treatment or put off treatment at the end of the season because they believe that the injury will heal with time. The preparticipation examination can ensure that proper treatment has taken place.

The assessment also gives the medical team a chance to **foster good health practices** and to promote optimum health and fitness. The assessment enables the health care providers to give proper health guidance and to determine the general state of health of the patient. For example, the examiner can ensure reasonable and proper weight for weight class athletes such as wrestlers and weightlifters. At the same time, the health team can explain the dangers involved in crash dieting and excessive dehydration.

The preparticipation evaluation also enables the health team to **bring immunizations up to date** and to rule out contagious diseases. Booster shots should be available during the examination for such diseases as tetanus, polio, diphtheria, smallpox, and hepatitis.

The assessment also gives the health care team, and especially the physician, a chance to **develop a rapport** with the patient. The examiner can learn what motivates the patient and, at the same time, help establish the patient's confidence in the health care staff. Any institution or team has a moral and legal obligation to ensure safety and health care if it sponsors particular programs

or activities. Meeting this obligation helps protect the organization from litigation and helps to fulfill insurance requirements.

The examination may also be used to establish guidelines for the patient, health care team, coaches, and administrators on questions of health, safety, and care. As well, it provides an opportunity to counsel the atypical athlete as to which sports or modifications of sports would provide suitable activity. It also enables a restriction from participation for those whose physical limitations present undue risk. Finally, it helps to classify the patient according to stature, qualifications, and abilities.

Setting Up the Examination

Preparticipation evaluations may be set up in different ways. In some cases, they may just involve a visit to a physician to obtain medical clearance to participate in an activity. In other cases, the evaluation may be more detailed and extensive. These extensive group evaluations are more likely to occur in higher level sporting activities where there is greater chance of injury if the patient is not healthy and fit. In the more detailed evaluation, individual stations may be set up in either a space-available format or a straight-line format (Fig. 17–1).[8, 18] With the first method, the patient checks in and then goes to whatever station is available until all are completed and then checks out. With the second method, the patient checks in and then goes to each station in a predetermined order and finally checks out.

Each station is set up to evaluate one or more particular aspects of the examination. Not every station has to be staffed with a physician. Often administrators, teachers, or therapists can staff the check-in and check-out stations. The check-in station enables the person or organization responsible for the preparticipation examination to ensure that the patient completes the legal requirements of the organization (e.g., informed consent, permission to participate), and the patients can be told how to proceed through the stations. A therapist, nurse, or some other suitably trained person can take the vital signs and perform the eye examination and profiling, whereas a dentist would do the dental examination. The maturation and medical examinations are done by physicians. At the check-out station, the patient's complete file is reviewed to ensure that all areas of the examination have been covered and that the patient has passed the examination, or to arrange for any additional tests, corrective exercises, or follow-up plans.[8] The patient is not told at the check-out whether he or she has passed or failed the preparticipation evaluation. This decision is the physician's, and the patient may be asked to wait to discuss the final decision with the physician.

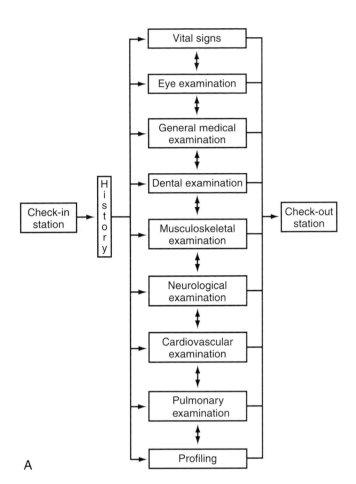

A

Station Examples for Examination

- Check-in
- Patient history
- Vital signs
    Blood pressure
    Heart rate
    Weight
- Eye examination
- Musculoskeletal examination
- Neurological examination
- Cardiovascular and pulmonary examination
- Additional medical examination
    Gastrointestinal examination
    Urogenital examination
    Dermatological examination
    Heat illness examination
    Laboratory examination
- Dental examination
- Musculoskeletal profile
    Body composition
    Maturity index
    Flexibility
    Strength, endurance, and power
    Agility, balance, and reaction time
    Cardiovascular fitness

Check-in

History

Vital signs

Eye examination

General medical examination

Dental examination

Musculoskeletal examination

Neurological examination

Cardiovascular examination

Pulmonary examination

Profiling

Check-out

B

Figure 17–1

Examples of traffic patterns for preparticipation screenings. (A) Space-available station method. (B) Straight-line station method.

Preparticipation History

In a preparticipation examination, the history plays a predominant role. A complete history can usually identify 60 to 75% of the problems affecting a patient.[6] For the young person, both the patient and his or her parent or guardian should provide the history to ensure completeness. The rest of the assessment proceeds from the information determined in the history. The history provides details regarding health problems and injuries and enables examiners to focus on any abnormalities that it brings out.[6] Generally, the history is completed by the patient's answering questions in a "yes-no" format. The "yes" answers then are investigated further in other parts of the assessment. It is important, however, that the "no" answers also be checked for accuracy. Ideally, oral histories are more accurate, but usually, because of time constraints, this is not possible. The history should include the patient's medical history as well as the family's to rule out any possible congenital, hereditary, or injury problems. It is important that a complete health history be obtained, because often the patient wants to leave out or hide information that may preclude the patient from taking part in the desired activity.

Some of the general questions can be used to

cross-reference questions asked in specific areas of assessment[6]:

1. Have you ever been a patient in a hospital, emergency room, or clinic?
2. Have you ever seen a physician for an injury or illness?
3. Have you ever had x-rays?
4. Have you ever had an operation?
5. Are you presently taking any medication or pills?
6. Do you have any allergies (to medications, insects, food, or other things)?
7. What was your last vaccination?
8. Have you ever been unable to participate in exercise or sport?

These general questions cover wide areas, and the specific parts of the assessmet should collaborate with the answers given to them. The following assessment sections outline questions pertaining to specific body systems that may lead to further examination or testing and possible concerns or issues that must be dealt with if the patient is going to take part in a particular activity.

Examination

The medical examination must be thorough and must be applicable to the activity, exercise, or sport in which the person hopes to participate. Health care professionals should always be alert for concealment, denial, or invention of problems. Depending on the particular activity, certain sites and structures must be emphasized (e.g., the ears in swimmers; the upper extremity in racquet sports; the spine, knees, and ankles in football players).

The initial part of the examination is done to establish the patient's baseline physiological parameters and vital statistics. This part of the examination may be performed by any health care professional who has knowledge or an understanding of the techniques.

Vital Statistics

Height:
Weight:
Pulse (heart rate):
    Males: 60–100 bpm
    Females: 60–100 bpm (may increase 10–15 bpm with pregnancy)
    Children: 120–140 bpm
    Well-conditioned athlete: 50+ bpm
Blood pressure:
    Adult: 120/80 mm Hg
    Children: 105/70 mm Hg (age: 10 years)

Table 17–2
Guidelines for Measurement of Blood Pressure

Posture	Blood pressure obtained in the sitting position is recommended. The subject should sit quietly for 5 minutes, with the back supported and the arm supported at the level of the heart, before blood pressure is recorded.
Circumstances	No caffeine during the hour preceding the reading. No smoking during the 30 minutes preceding the reading. A quiet, warm setting.
Equipment	Cuff size: the bladder should encircle and cover two thirds of the length of the arm; if it does not, place the bladder over the brachial artery. If bladder is too short, misleading high readings may result. Manometer: aneroid gauges should be calibrated every 6 months against a mercury manometer.

Technique	Number of readings:
	  On each occasion, take at least two readings, separated by as much time as is practical. If readings vary by more than 5 mm Hg, take additional readings until two consecutive readings are close.
	  If the initial values are elevated, obtain two other sets of readings at least 1 week apart.
	  Initially, take pressure in both arms; if the pressures differ, use the arm with the higher pressure.
	  If the arm pressure is elevated, take the pressure in one leg (particularly in patients younger than 30 years of age).
	Performance:
	  Inflate the bladder quickly to a pressure 20 mm Hg above the systolic pressure, as recognized by disappearance of the radial pulse.
	  Deflate the bladder by 3 mm Hg every second.
	  Record the Korotkoff phase V (disappearance), except in children, in whom use of phase IV (muffling) may be preferable if disappearance of the sounds is not perceived.
	  If the Korotkoff sounds are weak, have the patient raise the arm and open and close the hand 5 to 10 times, and then reinflate the bladder quickly.

Recordings	Blood pressure, patient position, arm and cuff size.

From Kaplan, N.M., R.B. Deveraux, and H.S. Miller: Systemic hyperextension. Med. Sci. Sports Exerc. 26:S269, 1994.

Table 17–3
Classification of Hypertension by Age in Children and Adolescents

	Magnitude of Hypertension*			
	Mild Stage 1	Moderate Stage 2	Severe Stage 3	Very Severe Stage 4
Child (6 to 9 years)†				
Systolic	120–124	125–129	130–139	≥140
Diastolic	75–79	80–84	85–89	≥90
Child (10 to 12 years)†				
Systolic	125–129	130–134	135–144	≥145
Diastolic	80–84	85–89	90–94	≥95
Child (13 to 15 years)†				
Systolic	135–139	140–149	150–159	≥160
Diastolic	85–89	90–94	95–99	≥100
Adolescent (16 to 18 years)†				
Systolic	140–149	150–159	160–179	≥180
Diastolic	90–94	95–99	100–109	≥110
Adult (>18 years)‡				
Systolic	140–159	160–179	180–209	≥210
Diastolic	90–99	100–109	110–119	≥120

* These definitions apply to persons who are not taking antihypertensive drugs and are not acutely ill. If the systolic and diastolic blood pressures fall into different categories, the higher category should be selected. In adults, isolated systolic hypertension is defined as a systolic blood pressure of 140 mm Hg or more and a diastolic blood pressure of less than 90 mm Hg and staged appropriately. Blood pressure values are based on the average of three or more readings taken at each of two or more visits after the initial screening.

† These levels are adapted from the recommendations of the Second Task Force on Blood Pressure Control in Children (Pediatrics 79:1–25, 1987) to be consistent with the classification in adults.

‡ From the Fifth Report of the Joint National Committee on Detection, Evaluation, and Treatment of High Blood Pressure (JNC V). Arch. Intern. Med. 153:154–183, 1993.

From Kaplan, N.M., R.B. Deveraux, and H.S. Miller: Systemic hyperextension. Med. Sci. Sports Exerc. 26:S269, 1994.

Table 17–2 outlines guidelines for blood pressure measurement.[19] High blood pressure values should be checked several times at 15- to 30-minute intervals, with the patient resting in between to determine whether a high reading is accurate or is being caused by anxiety ("white coat syndrome") or some similar reason. If three consecutive readings are high, the patient is said to have high blood pressure (hypertension). If the readings remain high, further investigation may be warranted (Table 17–3).[8, 19, 20]

Eye Examination

Visual acuity is usually examined with the use of a Snellon or common eye chart. For sports activities, peripheral vision and depth of perception may also be tested. Questions related to the eye examination include the following[6, 21]:

1. Have you had any problems with vision or your eyes?
2. Have you ever injured your eyes?
3. Do you wear glasses, contact lenses, or protective eyewear?
4. Are you color blind?
5. Do you have a peripheral vision problem?

Any abnormalities found or positive answers may require further examination. Uncorrected vision of less than 20/40 should be checked further.[16] Visual loss of 20/50 means that the patient can read at 20 feet what the average person can read at 50 feet. The health care professional should watch for problems that may preclude participation in the chosen activity or sport. Vision in only one eye results in lack of depth perception, which can be detrimental in certain activities. Patients with sight in only one eye should participate in physical activities only if they have an understanding of the dangers of participating and accept the risks.

Such patients should not participate in sports for which there is no adequate eye protection (e.g., boxing,

---

Examples of Eye Conditions or Signs and Symptoms Requiring Further Examination

- Visual loss greater than 20/40
- Vision in one eye only
- Severe myopia
- Retinal detachment
- Retinal tear

wrestling, martial arts). A special consent form should be obtained from the patient outlining the risks and his or her acceptance of them.[6, 22]

If the patient wears glasses, the health care professional should ensure that the lenses are plastic, polycarbonate, or heat-treated (safety) glass to prevent them from shattering during activity. Contact lenses should be of the soft type; the hard type may shatter.

Myopia or near-sightedness should be noted on the chart; such patients tend to have retinal degeneration, which increases the possiblity of retinal detachment. Patients who have retinal detachment are sometimes excluded from contact sports. People who have a retinal tear should be allowed to compete in strenuous activities only if cleared by a physician or specialist, and they should have a qualifying letter allowing them to participate.

Pupil size should also be evaluated. In some patients, the pupils are of obvious different size (anisocoria). This difference should be noted in case the patient has to be evaluated for a head injury at a later date.[23]

Musculoskeletal Examination

Like the neurological examination to be discussed later, the musculoskeletal examination is a very important part of a preparticipation evaluation. Questions in the history related to this examination include the following:

1. Have you ever pulled (strained) or hurt a muscle?
2. Have you ever torn (sprained) or stretched a ligament?
3. Have you ever subluxed or dislocated a joint or had a bone come out of joint?
4. Have you ever broken (fractured) a bone?
5. Have any of your joints ever swollen?
6. Have you ever had pain in the muscles or joints during or after activity, exercise, or sport?

A positive response to any of these questions requires further investigation.

The musculoskeletal examination begins with observation of the patient's posture (Chapter 15), looking for any asymmetry. Asymmetry, combined with the history, may lead the examiner to do a detailed assessment of a specific joint (see Chapters 3 through 13). If no problems are noted, the examiner can do a quick **upper and lower scanning examination** to check for potential problems and abnormal movement (e.g., hypomobility, hypermobility, capsular patterns, weakness, abnormal movement patterns, cheating movements). Depending on the proposed activity, emphasis may be placed on specific joints (Table 17–4).[15]

Table 17–4
Areas of Sport-Specific Emphasis

Sport	Physical Examination Emphasis
Ballet	Feet, ankles, knees, hips, spine
Baseball	Arms, elbows, shoulders
Basketball	Feet, ankles, knees, shoulders
Football	Ankles, knees, back, head, neck
Gymnastics	Ankles, knees, spine, shoulders, elbows, wrists
Hockey	Ankles, knees, back, shoulders, head, neck
Ice skating	Feet, ankles, shins, spine
Racquet sports	Feet, ankles, knees, shoulders, elbows, wrists
Rowing	Achilles tendons, knees, spine, shoulders, elbows, wrists, hands
Running	Feet, ankles, knees, hips, back
Soccer	Feet, ankles, shins, knees, thighs, pelvis, hips, neck
Softball	Ankles, knees, shoulders, elbows
Swimming	Shoulders, throat, ears
Synchronized swimming	Shoulders, back, knees, throat, ears
Track/cross-country	Feet, ankles, shins, knees, thighs, hips, shoulders
Volleyball	Ankles, knees, shoulders, hands
Wrestling	Shoulders, skin, % body fat

Adapted from Johnson, M.D.: Tailoring the preparticipation exam to female athletes. Phys. Sportsmed. 20:71, 1992; and McKeag, D.B.: Preparticipation screening of the potential athlete. Clin. Sports Med. 8:386, 1989.

Upper and Lower Scanning Examination

- Cervical spine: flexion, extension, side flexion, rotation
- Shoulder shrug (resistance may be added)
- Shoulder: elevation through abduction, forward flexion and the plane of the scapula; medial and lateral rotation (resistance may be added)
- Elbow: flexion, extension, supination, pronation
- Wrist: flexion, extension, radial and ulnar deviation
- Fingers and thumb: open hands wide, make a tight fist
- Thoracic and lumbar spine: flexion (touch toes, knees straight), extension, side flexion, rotation
- Tighten quadriceps
- Hip, knee, ankle, and foot: squat and bounce, heel-toe walking

If any deviation, weakness, or abnormality is found, or if the patient has reported a previous injury to a joint, a more detailed examination may be performed to assess active movements, passive movements, resisted isometric movements, special tests, functional tests, reflexes, sensation, myotomes, joint play, and palpation.

When looking for musculoskeletal problems, it is important to consider whether the proposed activity will

---

Examples of Musculoskeletal Conditions or Signs and Symptoms Requiring Further Examination

- Joint or spinal instability (static and dynamic)
- Unhealed muscle or ligament injury
- Unhealed or healing fracture
- Degenerative diseases
- Inflammatory diseases
- Unusual hypermobility or hypomobility
- Muscle weakness
- Growth or maturation disorders
- Repetitive stress disorders

---

exacerbate an existing disease, increase an existing deformity, or cause further bone or joint damage. When looking for orthopedic problems, the examiner may, depending on the activity or sport, look at the patient's flexibility as well as static and dynamic stability. Spinal instability (especially instability of the cervical or lumbar spine) or spondylolisthesis may preclude the patient from taking part in contact, collision, or impact activities. Maturation may also have to be considered when dealing with patients who are still growing, as may previous injuries, congenital problems, and growth abnormalities.

Neurological Examination and Convulsive Disorders

The neurological examination is very important, especially in contact or collision activities. Some of the more common questions asked in the neurological examination include the following[6]:

1. Have you ever been knocked out or been unconscious?
2. Have you ever had a head injury?
3. Have you ever had a seizure?
4. Have you ever had a stinger or burner?
5. Have you ever had a time when one or more of your limbs went numb or "to sleep" during activity?
6. Have you ever been in a motor vehicle accident or fallen and hit your head?

A positive answer to any of these questions could have a significant impact on whether the patient is allowed to participate in contact or collision activities.

In the neurological examination, the examiner may assess the status of a head injury (Chapter 2), perform a cranial nerve assessment (Chapter 2) or sensation scan, and evaluate the different reflexes (Chapter 1) if problems are suspected. The health care team must check for concussions and nerve palsies. Any positive neurological signs and symptoms uncovered in the examination should preclude strenuous activity until investigated further. Recurrent concussions or nerve palsies should be investigated further by a specialist before clearance to participate is given.

Examples of Neurological Conditions or Signs and Symptoms Requiring Further Examination

- More than one concussion
- Any history of head injury
- Any history of seizure
- Any history of stinger, burner, or neurapraxia
- Any history of transient quadriplegia
- Any history of nerve palsy

With convulsive disorders, the health care team needs to know about the frequency of the episodes, how or whether control has been achieved, the use of routine medication, any activating circumstances, and whether the patient understands the disorder, its hazards, and its predisposing factors. Patients with epilepsy should be discouraged from activities such as skiing, scuba diving, parachuting, and climbing because of their inherent dangers.[6] If the event involves water sports (e.g., swimming alone, scuba diving), auto racing, or any activity in which recurrent head trauma or unexpected falls may cause serious injury (e.g., mountain climbing, working at heights), then the patient with convulsive disorders should be discouraged from taking part. Patients whose activities should be restricted include those who experience daily or weekly seizures, those who display bizzare forms of psychomotor epilepsy, and those whose postconvalescent state is prolonged or typically includes marked abnormal behavior. It is important to have an understanding of whether the medication taken can maintain good control of the patient's condition in stress situations. For example, hyperventilation may precipitate an epileptic seizure, and seizures tends to occur after exercise, not during the event. In addition, it is important to understand whether the extent or intensity of the participation poses a significant threat to the patient's physical condition.

Cardiovascular Examination

The cardiovascular examination should be performed in a quiet area because of the need to auscultate. In this part of the evaluation, the examiner looks for subtle but significant cardiac abnormalities so as to reduce the incidence of unexpected sudden death in sport.[9, 24, 25] More than 90% of sudden deaths in exercise and sports among participants younger than 30 years of age involve the cardiovascular system.

The following questions should be asked in the history concerning the cardiovascular system[6]:

1. Have you ever experienced dizziness during or after activity, exercise, or sport?
2. Have you ever experienced chest pain during or after activity, exercise, or sport?
3. When doing an activity, exercise, or sport, do you

tire more quickly than others doing the same things?
4. Have you ever had high blood pressure?
5. Has your heart ever "raced" or skipped beats?
6. Have you ever been told you have a heart murmur?
7. Has anyone in your family ever had or died from heart problems?
8. Has anyone in your family died suddenly before the age of 50?

Examples of Cardiovascular Conditions or Signs and Symptoms Requiring Further Examination

* Chest pain
* Dizziness with activity
* Abnormal heartbeat (rate, rhythm)
* Abnormal hypertension (labile or organic)
* Heart murmur
* Family history of heart problems
* Hypertrophic cardiomegaly
* Conduction abnormalities
* Arrhythmias
* Valvular problems
* Coronary artery defects
* Aortic coarctation
* Marfan's syndrome
* Atrial septal defects
* Dextrocardia
* Enlarged (athlete's) heart
* Atherosclerotic disease
* Mitral insufficiency
* Anemia
* Enlarged spleen

If the answer to any of these questions is yes, the examiner must consider the possibility of cardiomegaly, conduction abnormalities, arrhythmias, valvular problems, coronary artery defects, and lung or related problems.[26] If cardiovascular problems are suspected, the examiner may organize further tests (e.g., electrocardiogram, treadmill stress tests) to detect cardiac abnormalities.

When looking for cardiovascular problems, the examiner should be alert for the following unusual or abnormal findings:

1. Heart rate faster than 120 bpm or inappropriate tachycardia for a specific activity
2. Arrhythmias or irregular beats
3. Midsystolic clicks, indicating a leaky valve or mitral valve prolapse
4. Murmurs that are grade 3 or louder.

The loudness of **systolic murmurs** is graded from 1 to 6, with grade 1 being a very faint murmur requiring concentration to be heard. A grade 2 murmur is a faint murmur but one that is heard immediately after the stethoscope is placed on the chest. Grade 3 is an intermediate murmur louder than grade 2. Most human dynamically significant murmurs are at least grade 3. Grade 4 is a loud murmur, frequently associated with palpable sensation, known as a thrill. A grade 5 murmur is a very loud murmur still requiring at least the edge of the stethoscope to remain in contact with the chest. The grade 6 murmur is a murmur audible with the stethoscope just breaking contact with the chest.[27] **Diastolic murmurs** are graded from 1 to 4, 1 representing the faintest and 4 the loudest murmur. Benign functional murmur or systemic mitral valve prolapse does not preclude exercise or sport but must be evaluated on an individual basis.

The health care team must be aware of congenital heart abnormalities such as aortic coarctation (stenosis of the artery), which may be revealed by a difference in the femoral and brachial pulses. In such a case, strenuous activity is contraindicated. As another example, 90% of patients with Marfan's syndrome (an autosomal dominant condition) have cardiac abnormalities. The health care team must be aware of atrial septal defects (an abnormal communication between the chambers of the heart), dextrocardia (the heart is moved within the thoracic cavity), and paroxysmal auricular tachycardia (an abnormal increase in heartbeat for short periods). Patients with these conditions are disqualified from all competitive sports because of the possibility of fainting in a stressful situation. The examiner must also be aware of heart enlargement (athlete's heart). This condition does not necessarily preclude activity or sport but should be investigated further if found. If any of these abnormalities have been surgically corrected, they should be evaluated by a specialist on an individual basis to determine whether the patient can take part in the proposed activity.

Hypertrophic cardiomyelopathy is the most common cause of sudden death in athletes, followed by aortic rupture associated with Marfan's syndrome, congenital coronary artery anomalies, and atherosclerotic coronary artery disease.[6, 28] If any of these conditions is present, strenuous activity is precluded.

Other cardiovascular problems include thromboembolic disease, pulse irregularities, valvular problems such as mitral insufficiency or mitral valve prolapse, and abnormally high blood pressure (hypertension). Systolic pressure of 140 mm Hg on repeated measurements is considered abnormal. Also, patients with labile hypertension (an unstable condition of free and rapid change in tension) or organic hypertension caused by structural problems should be investigated further. These patients should have a complete comprehensive coronary risk factor work-up (Tables 17–5 and 17–6). Mild hypertension does not preclude exercise or sports, but this slight abnormality should be noted and evaluated on an individual basis.[6] When taking blood pressure, it is important that a proper cuff size be used to ensure an accurate reading. If the initial reading is high, the reading should

Table 17–5

Detecting Cardiac Risks in Preparticipation Examinations: Key Physical Findings of Cardiac Evaluation by Physician

Heart rate faster than 120 beats per minute
- If repeated tests on second occasion are high, suggest monitoring and recording of pulse at home by a trained parent or nurse friend.
- Pulse recovery tests after jumping or hopping exercises are useless routines except for multiple extrasystoles or arrhythmias.

Multiple extrasystoles or arrhythmias. Check after jumping or hopping 20 times to ascertain if arrhythmias appear or disappear.

Resting blood pressure higher than 130/80 mm Hg for students aged 6 to 11 years, 140/90 mm Hg for students aged 12 to 18 years.
- For validity, be certain that the pressure cuff covers at least two thirds of the upper arm, from elbow to shoulder (adult cuff = 30 × 13 cm; pediatric cuff = 22 × 10 cm; obese cuff = 39 × 15 cm).
- If high, repeat test three times and take average.

All systolic murmurs grade 3 to 6 or louder at any location; all diastolic murmurs of any intensity at any location; or any continuous murmur. Heart should be auscultated at four chest locations:
- Pulmonic area (second intercostal space at left sternal border).
- Aortic area (second intercostal space at right sternal border).
- Tricuspid area (fourth intercostal space at left sternal border).
- Mitral area (fourth intercostal space at left midclavicular line).

Routinely palpate femoral and brachial pulses. Note if absent or if large discrepancy exists between them.

Modified from Schell, N.B.: Cardiac evaluation of school sports participants: Guidelines approved by the Medical Society of New York. N.Y. State J. Med. 78:942–943, 1978.

Table 17–6

Detecting Cardiac Risks in Preparticipation Examinations: Key Historical Facts Obtained From Students, Parents, and School Health Records

Cyanotic heart disease early in life

Murmur early in life based on anatomic diagnosis of left-to-right shunt or pulmonic or aortic stenosis

Rheumatic heart disease

Fainting spells (syncope)

Chest or abdominal pains (not otherwise diagnosed)

Dyspnea on exertion

Cardiac surgery

Enlarged heart

Cardiac rhythm disturbances

Familial heart disease* or rhythm disturbances

Functional or innocent murmur of 4 or more years' duration

* Hypertension, early stroke (before 50 years), or early coronary (before 50 years) in close relatives.

Modified from Schell, N.B.: Cardiac evaluation of school sports participants: Guidelines approved by the Medical Society of New York. N.Y. State J. Med. 78:942–943, 1978.

be repeated two or three times after the patient has been lying supine for 20 to 30 minutes. Only if the blood pressure is elevated after the third reading should the patient be considered hypertensive.

Another condition the examiner should be aware of is anemia. If anemia is suspected, the level of hemoglobin (the oxygen-carrying pigment in human blood) is tested. Anemia is more likely to be seen in women during menstruation, and sickle cell anemia is more common in black individuals. In some cases, anemia is caused by an increase in blood volume, which decreases the concentration of red blood cells. In this case, the individual has normal red blood cells but appears to be anemic.

If cardiovascular or cardiopulmonary disease is suspected, an exercise stress test is often recommended.[16] Figure 17–2 outlines a flow chart for considerations before doing such a test. Twenty to 35% of those with heart

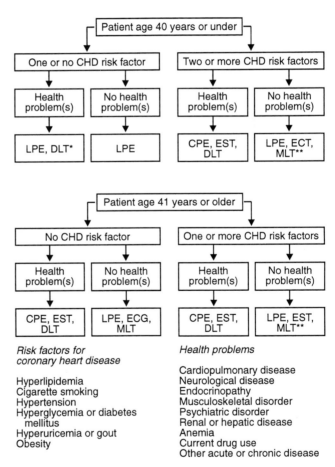

Risk factors for coronary heart disease

Hyperlipidemia
Cigarette smoking
Hypertension
Hyperglycemia or diabetes mellitus
Hyperuricemia or gout
Obesity

Health problems

Cardiopulmonary disease
Neurological disease
Endocrinopathy
Musculoskeletal disorder
Psychiatric disorder
Renal or hepatic disease
Anemia
Current drug use
Other acute or chronic disease

* Exercise stress testing is recommended if patient has cardiopulmonary disease

**Diagnostic laboratory testing is indicated if CDH risk factors include hyperlipidemia, hyperglycemia, or hyperuricemia

Figure 17–2

Preexercise evaluation flow sheet. CDH = coronary heart disease; CPE = comprehensive physical examination; DLT = diagnostic laboratory testing; ECG = resting electrocardiogram; EST = exercise stress test; LPE = limited physical examination; MLT = minimal laboratory testing. (Redrawn from Taylor, R.B.: Pre-exercise evaluation: Which procedures are really needed? Consultant April:94–101, 1983.)

Table 17–7
Classification of Sports Based on Peak Dynamic and Static Components During Competition

	Low Dynamic	Moderate Dynamic	High Dynamic
Low static	Billiards Bowling Cricket Curling Golf Riflery	Baseball Softball Table tennis Tennis (doubles) Volleyball	Badminton Cross-country skiing (classic technique) Field hockey* Orienteering Race walking Racquetball Running (long-distance) Soccer* Squash Tennis (singles)
Moderate static	Archery Auto racing*† Diving*† Equestrian*† Motorcycling*†	Fencing Field events (jumping) Figure skating* Football (American) Rodeo*† Rugby* Running (sprint) Surfing*† Synchronized swimming†	Basketball* Ice hockey* Cross-country skiing (skating technique) Football (Australian rules)* Lacrosse* Running (middle-distance) Swimming Team handball
High static	Bobsledding*† Field events (throwing) Gymnastics*† Karate/Judo* Luge*† Sailing Rock climbing*† Water skiing*† Weight lifting*† Wind surfing*†	Body building*† Downhill skiing*† Wrestling*	Boxing* Canoeing/kayaking Cycling*† Decathlon Rowing Speed skating

* Danger of bodily collision.

† Increased risk if syncope occurs.

From Mitchell, J.H., W.L. Hashell, and P.B. Raven: Classification of sports. Med. Sci. Sports Exerc. 26:S244, 1994.

disease will have a normal stress test, so it is important to remember that any stress test is only valid to the load at which the heart has been stressed when doing the test. Forty-five percent of runners older than 40 years of age have irregular results on electrocardiograms. Furthermore, different types of activity (e.g., static or dynamic) lead to different stresses on the heart. Table 17–7 outlines a sports classification based on peak dynamic and static components during competition.[29]

Pulmonary Examination

The pulmonary examination is often done in conjunction with the cardiovascular examination in a quiet area. Questions related to the pulmonary system may include the following:

1. Have you ever experienced long periods of intermittent coughing?
2. Have you ever experienced coughing during or after activity, exercise, or sport?
3. Have you ever experienced shortness of breath or wheezing during or after activity, exercise, or sport?

The examiner auscultates for clear breath sounds and watches for symmetric diaphragm excursion.[6] Any required controlling medications should be noted and recorded. The ears, nose, and mouth may also be checked

Examples of Pulmonary Conditions or Signs and Symptoms Requiring Further Examination

- Abnormal coughing
- Abnormal shortness of breath
- Abnormal breath sounds (e.g., wheezing, rhonchi, rales)
- Asthma (uncontrolled or exertional)
- Exercise-induced bronchospasm
- Pulmonary insufficiency
- Severe allergies

during this examination. If abnormalities are found, appropriate lung function tests may be ordered.[30] If there is concern about an active disease process, a chest x-ray may be in order.

Respiratory problems such as tuberculosis, uncontrolled asthma, exertional asthma, exercise-induced bronchospasm, pulmonary insufficiency resulting from a collapsed lung, or bronchial asthma should be checked and discussed with the patient.[16]

Urogenital Examination

Depending on whether the athlete is male or female, the examination is modified to meet the individual needs. For example, females may be asked about their menstrual history (e.g., when did it begin? when was the last period? are there any abnormalities?) or gynecologic problems. Males may be given a genital examination looking for abnormalities, hernias, or absence of a testicle.[6] Common history questions asked in the urogenital examination (males and females) include the following:

1. Have you ever had any problems with your kidneys or genitourinary organs?
2. Have you ever been diagnosed as having sugar, albumin, or blood in your urine?

The medical team must check for hernias, kidney problems, albuminuria (excessive protein in the urine), and venereal disease. Generally, athletes with one kidney should be warned of the danger of contact sports, especially if the kidney is abnormally positioned or is diseased.[22] In males, the examiner should be aware of an undescended or atrophied testicle or testicular torsion. A urinalysis should be carried out if diabetes or kidney disease is suspected. These conditions do not preclude activity, exercise, or sport, but they may be amenable to treatment, and the patient and the sponsoring organization must be made aware of potential dangers caused by these conditions.

> **Examples of Urogenital Conditions or Signs and Symptoms Requiring Further Examination**
>
> - Hernia (femoral or inguinal)
> - Absent or undescended testicle
> - One kidney or diseased kidney
> - Albuminuria
> - Hemoglobinuria
> - Nephroptosis
> - Hematuria
> - Exercise amenorrhea

Dehydration, athletic pseudonephritis, hemoglobinuria, nephroptosis, and hematuria are all possible problems of the urogenital system. For females, it is important to determine whether they have a regular period and their menstrual pattern because of concern about exercise amenorrhea and its relation to bone density and osteoporosis.[16, 31]

Gastrointestinal Examination

The gastrointestinal examination involves evaluation of the digestive system, eating habits, and nutrition. Some of the questions that may be asked include the following[32]:

1. Do you feel you eat regularly and have a well-balanced diet?
2. Are there certain food groups you will not eat?
3. Have you ever been on a diet?
4. Do you view yourself as too thin, too fat, or just right?
5. Have you ever tried to control your weight? If so, how?
6. Have you ever had excessive heartburn or indigestion?

A positive answer to any of these questions requires further investigation.

> **Examples of Gastrointestinal Conditions or Signs and Symptoms Requiring Further Examination**
>
> - Organomegaly (e.g., enlarged liver, spleen)
> - Anorexia
> - Bulimia

The examiner should palpate the abdomen for masses or organomegaly.[8] The health care team has to ensure that there is no inflammation of the liver (hepatitis, enlarged liver, or enlarged spleen), especially for contact sports.

In some cases and for some sports, notably the esthetic or weight-conscious sports (e.g., gymnastics, ballet, synchronized swimming, wrestling), it is advisable to check the patient's nutritional status, especially if there appears to be a tendency toward anorexia or bulimia.[33] This is best done by having the patient record his or her food intake for at least 3 days and having the record analyzed by a nutritionist, who can then calculate dietary intake in relation to the activity level of the patient. It also provides an opportunity to determine what supplements the patient is using, in case they contain banned substances.

Dermatological Examination

The preparticipation examination is a good time to catch any developing skin conditions and those that may be amenable to treatment. Generally, the questions that relate to the dermatological examination would be the following:

1. Have you had any problems with acne?
2. Have you had any problems with rashes or itching, especially in areas covered by clothes, equipment, or footwear?

The answers to such questions give the examiner some idea of skin conditions, most of which are easily dealt with by treatment.

> *Examples of Dermatological Conditions or Signs and Symptoms Requiring Further Examination*
>
> - Severe acne
> - Dermatitis (e.g., contact, clothes)
> - Herpes (e.g., simplex, gladiatorum)
> - Boils
> - Warts
> - Fungal infection
> - Impetigo
> - Tinea capitis or corporis
> - Molluscum contagiosum
> - Psoriasis

The examiner must ensure that the athlete has any dermatological problems under control, because many of these conditions are contagious, including infection or viral infection, such as herpes simplex, herpes gladiatorum, boils, impetigo, or warts; fungal infection; and contact dermatitis.

Examination for Heat Disorders

Examination for heat disorders should be included if the activity, exercise, or sport is going to take place where there is high temperature, high humidity, or a combination of the two (e.g., moderate temperature and high humidity). These are often the conditions that lead to heat disorders. Questions in the history related to heat disorders may include the following:

1. Have you ever suffered from a heat disorder?
2. Have you ever suffered muscle cramps?
3. Have you ever participated in an activity, exercise, or sport in a high-temperature, high-humidity environment?
4. Have you ever passed out or become dizzy in the heat?
5. Have you been on medication or do you drink a lot of caffeinated beverages?

Intake of antihistamines or excessive caffeine, as well as lack of fluid and/or metabolites, can increase the risk of heat disorders. If a patient has a history of heat-related

disorders, the condition should be thoroughly investigated, because it could lead to life-threatening situations.

> *Examples of Heat Disorders or Heat-Related Signs and Symptoms Requiring Further Examination*
>
> - Heat exhaustion
> - Heat stroke
> - Excessive muscle cramps in heat

General Medical Problems

In addition to the problems previously described, there are general systemic problems that the medical team must be aware of. Some of the general medical questions include the following:

1. Have you ever been diagnosed with a systemic disease (e.g., diabetes)?
2. Have you ever been diagnosed with a progressive disease (e.g., muscular dystrophy, multiple sclerosis)?
3. Have you ever been told you have cancer?

The presence of diabetes does not rule out activity, but the examiner must ensure that there is good control by the use of medication, and it must be determined whether the extent or intensity of the activity poses a significant threat to the patient's physical condition.[34] The examiner also has to be concerned about problems such as acute infection, malignancy, and progressive diseases such as multiple sclerosis.

Acute illnesses tend to be self limiting and usually require only that the patient be temporarily withdrawn from activity, often to prevent spread to other participants.[6] Dehydration is enhanced by febrile illness, which could, in certain circumstances, lead to heat disorders.

Dental Examination

Questions to be asked concerning the patient's dental record include the following[21]:

1. When did you last see a dentist?
2. Have you ever had any problems with your teeth or gums?
3. Have you ever had any teeth knocked out, damaged, or extracted?
4. Do you wear a mouthguard?
5. Do you smoke or chew tobacco?
6. Have you ever had an injury to your face or jaws?

When looking for dental problems, which is usually done by a dentist, it is important to determine how many teeth the patient has and the last time he or she saw a dentist. This becomes important because of the potential for liability if teeth are avulsed (knocked out). It also provides an opportunity for mouthguards to be fitted and for any dental appliance work to be checked to be sure it is in good condition.

Laboratory Tests

Laboratory tests are not usually included in the preparticipation assessment. However, if the examiner suspects problems for which laboratory tests are diagnostic, then they may be ordered. For example, if heart disease is suspected or an older population is being examined, serum cholesterol, triglyceride, or high-density lipoprotein tests may be ordered.

The incidence of iron deficiency anemia in postmenarche female athletes is as high as 15%. Plasma ferritin is used to measure iron status. In males, anemia may occur during a growth spurt, with inadequate diet, or with peptic ulcer. Sickle cell anemia is common in blacks. Hemoglobin is often checked if sickle cell anemia is suspected. The prepubertal level of hemoglobin is about 11.5 g/dl of blood, and the postpubertal value is 14.5 g/dl of blood for males and 12.0 g/dl or higher for females.

In some sports and at some levels of competition, drug screening must be performed, and the preparticipation examination is a place where such a screen may be included.

Physical Fitness Profile

It is important for the health care team to establish a physical fitness profile for each participant, especially in highly organized sports. Basically, profiling is the gathering of information about the physical attributes of the participant.[35] Such profiling helps to determine whether the person possesses the attributes, skills, and abilities necessary for participation and to meet the demands of the activity, and it should be geared to the specific activity, exercise, or sport (Table 17–8).[14, 35–40] It should be designed to stress the body so that any weakness or pathology that exists will be apparent. In this way, it may be used as a **screening device** to prevent injury.[35, 41] The profile also provides a **baseline** in the event of injury or to demonstrate the need for, or effect of, conditioning necessary to take part in the activity. A physical fitness profile can involve many parameters or aspects, including strength, endurance, flexibility, cardiovascular fitness, and maturation. To be effective, the program or test must exhibit several characteristics.[42]

Characteristics of Physical Fitness Profile

- The variables being tested must be relevant to the activity, exercise, or sport
- The test must be reliable and valid
- Test protocols must be as specific to the activity, exercise, or sport as possible
- The test must be standardized and controlled
- The rights of the patient and confidentiality must be respected
- Testing may be repeated at regular intervals if the purpose is to show effectiveness of a training program
- Results must be conveyed to the patient in a meaningful way that the patient can understand.

Strength

Strength is one of the attributes that is commonly examined in a physical fitness profile. The way in which the health care team determines strength depends on the activity, exercise, or sport, the equipment available, and the demands of the activity. The strength measures may involve isometric, isotonic, or isokinetic testing, functional activities, lifting of free weights, or, in some cases, simply a hand grip test.[43, 44] In some cases, it may involve muscle fiber typing. If a general indication of strength is desired, a hand grip is relatively easy, and standard tests can be used (see Chapter 7). Functional strength tests are often used because they are easy and provide comparable results.[8] However, the examiner should make these tests as activity-specific as possible.

Examples of Functional Strength Tests

- Bench press, leg press
- Sit-ups
- Push-ups
- Pull-ups

More sophisticated methods may be used, especially if the patient has a history of injury to specific muscles or joints (see the sections on functional testing in Chapters 3 through 13).

Isokinetic testing (i.e., Cybex, KinCom, Biodex) is more likely to be used to test specific joints, looking for potential discrepancies between left and right sides, agonist versus antagonist, and differences in strength and endurance. However, it is important to realize that many of these tests are not done in functional, activity-specific positions.

Table 17–8
Tests Used to Determine Athletic Fitness for Specific Sports*

	Speed	Strength	Muscle Endurance	Power	Quickness and Agility	Reaction Time	Flexibility	Cardiores-piratory Endurance	Balance	Anaerobic Endurance	Body Composition	Kinesthetic Perception
Football	X	X	—	X	X	X	X	—	X	X	X	X
Basketball	X	—	X	X	X	—	X	X	X	X	X	X
Baseball	X	—	—	X	—	X	X	—	—	X	—	—
Track and field												
Sprinters	X	X	—	X	—	X	X	—	—	X	X	—
Throwers	—	X	—	X	X	—	X	—	X	X	X	X
Jumpers	X	X	—	X	—	—	X	—	X	X	X	X
Distance	—	—	X	—	—	—	X	X	—	—	X	—
Volleyball	—	—	X	X	X	X	X	X	X	X	X	X
Soccer	X	—	X	—	X	—	X	X	X	—	X	X
Rodeo	—	X	—	X	X	X	X	—	X	—	—	X
Tennis	—	—	X	X	X	X	X	X	—	X	X	X
Golf	—	—	X	—	—	—	X	X	X	—	X	X
Skiing	—	X	X	X	X	—	X	X	X	—	X	X
Wrestling	—	X	X	X	X	—	X	X	X	—	X	X
Gymnastics	X	X	X	X	X	—	X	—	X	—	X	X

Test examples:

Speed: 20-, 40-, 100-yard dashes
Strength: 1 repetition max
Muscle endurance: 225-lb or 285-lb bench test, sit-up, pull-up, dip, push-up
Power: vertical jump, standing broad jump, two-hand medicine ball put
Agility: 20-yard shuttle run, Semo agility test, T-test
Reaction time: Dekan Auto Performance Analyzer
Flexibility: sit and reach test, shoulder rotation test
Cardiorespiratory endurance: 1.5-mile run, 12-minute run
Balance: Nelson balance test
Anaerobic endurance: Margaria-Kalamen leg power test, 40-yard repeated sprint test
Body composition: skinfold measurements
Kinesthetic perception: distance perception jump

* Xs denote areas of physical fitness that are most needed in each sport.

From Bridgman, R.: A coach's guide to testing for athletic attributes. National Strength and Conditioning Assoc. J. 13:35, 1991.

Power

Power is the ability to move a weight over a distance. This weight may be an object or the human body. Depending on the activity, exercise, or sport, power may be included as part of the physical fitness profile. As with all profile parameters, power measurements should be related to the activity, exercise, or sport in which the patient will be participating.

Examples of Power Activities

- Throwing a medicine ball
- Jump for height
- Two-legged hop
- Single-leg hop for distance
- Stair climbing

Flexibility and Range of Motion

Flexibility is a very important consideration when profiling a patient for a specific activity.[45, 46] In some cases, less flexibility is better than too much, but in some activities, excessive flexibility is necessary to succeed. Therefore, flexibility testing must be specific to the activity in which the patient wishes to take part, or it may be position-specific. For example, in running sports, lower limb flexibility (especially hip flexors, hamstrings, rectus femoris, iliotibial band, and gastrocnemius) is of greatest importance, whereas in swimming, upper limb flexibility (especially shoulder abduction and medial and lateral rotation) is more important. In some activities, such as ballet, gymnastics, and synchronized swimming, overall flexibility is essential. In baseball, pitchers often require greater shoulder, hip, and trunk flexibility than other players.[3] Flexibility may be measured with the use of a goniometer, flexometer, or tape measure.[46]

Determinants of Range of Motion[47]

- Shape of the bone and cartilage
- Muscle power and tone
- Muscle bulk
- Ligaments and joint capsule laxity
- Extensibility of the skin and subcutaneous tissue
- Race (Indians are more mobile than blacks, who are more mobile than Caucasians)
- Sex (women are more mobile than men)
- Age (range of motion decreases with age)
- Genetic makeup
- The dominant limb tends to be less mobile than the nondominant limb
- Day-to-day stresses on joints

When considering range of motion, it is important to realize that hypermobility or laxity in one joint or in one direction of joint movement does not necessarily mean hypermobility in all joints or in all directions. Similarly, normal range of motion charts are often not valid when dealing with persons who, by virtue of their activities (e.g., ballet, gymnastics, synchronized swimming), are hypermobile. Values that are considered normal for these types of activities would be considered hypermobile or abnormal for the general population. It is also important to realize that hypermobility (laxity) and hypomobility are not necessarily pathological states. In pathological states, hypermobility is referred to as mechanical or clinical instability (see Chapter 1). The range of motion available may be the result of genetic makeup or the stresses placed on individual joints. Tight-jointed people tend to be more susceptible to muscle strains, nerve pinch syndromes, and overstress tendinitis. Hypermobile or loose-jointed people are more susceptible to ligament sprains, chronic back pain, disc prolapse, spondylolisthesis, pes planus, joint effusion, and tendinitis caused by lack of control. In the hypermobile athlete, if strength and endurance are not at the appropriate level to support the joints, the joints are often unstable or are subjected to potentially injuring loads. These athletes tend to do very poorly in strength events.

Various criteria can be used to determine a patient's generalized joint laxity. However, the points previously mentioned must be kept in mind when looking at these generalized values. Carter and Wilkinson[48] have developed a 5-point system. If the patient meets all criteria, he or she is said to exhibit general joint hypermobility.

Carter and Wilkinson's Criteria for Generalized Joint Laxity (Hypermobility)

- Passive apposition of the thumb to the flexor aspect of the forearm
- Passive hyperextension of the fingers so they lie parallel with the extensor aspect of the forearm
- Ability to hyperextend elbows at least 10°
- Ability to hyperextend knees at least 10°
- Excessive passive dorsiflexion of the ankle and eversion of the foot

---

Nicholas[49] established criteria for determining whether a patient is tight jointed (hypomobile). It should be realized, however, that under these criteria, the majority of the North American population today would be classed as hypomobile!

It is important to understand the principles of hypermobility and hypomobility. If a person is hypermobile, then he or she must avoid further stretching and support the joint through strengthening programs. The patient must be taught proper positioning, and if there are hyper-

- Patient is unable to touch the floor with the palms, bending at the knees with the waist straight
- Patient is unable to sit comfortably in the lotus position
- Patient demonstrates less than 20° hyperextension at the knees when lying prone with the legs hanging over the end of the table
- Patient is unable to position the feet at 180° while standing with the knees flexed at 15 to 30°
- Patient has no upper limb laxity on shoulder flexion, elbow hyperextension, or forearm hypersupination

mobile joints, there are probably hypomobile joints nearby that need to be mobilized. It is essential to make sure that these patients have improved strength, endurance, muscular speed of reaction, and balanced activities to help support the hypermobile joints.

If the person is hypomobile, he or she may be treated by mobilization or manipulation of the affected joint in the direction of tightness. Tight supporting structures also must be stretched, and active exercises must be given to maintain the restored range of motion. It is important with these patients to retrain their kinesthetic sense so that they can maintain the acquired range of motion.

Speed

Speed is often considered an important component of a physical fitness profile, depending on the activity, exercise, or sport. It is a function of distance covered per unit time.[8]

Examples of Functional Speed Tests

- Timed 40-yard (40-m) run
- Timed 100-yard (100-m) run
- Timed 440-yard (400-m) run

Cardiovascular Fitness and Endurance

Because almost every activity involves stresses on the heart and vascular system, it is important to know the level of the stresses produced and whether the cardiovascular system can respond to those stresses. Therefore, the cardiovascular system must be evaluated to determine how it responds to these or equivalent loads.[50]

There are many methods that can be used to determine cardiovascular (aerobic) fitness, but the method chosen must be related to the specific activity or population.[51,52] As an example, ice hockey players who are tested

on a bicycle may show very good cardiovascular fitness; however, when they get on the ice and skate, their cardiovascular fitness may not be as evident because they are being tested in a different type of activity.

Examples of Common Endurance Tests

- Harvard step test
- 12-minute walk-run
- 1.5-mile (2.4-km) run
- Submaximal ergometer test
- Treadmill test

The Harvard step test is one of the most common general cardiovascular fitness tests done for a physical fitness profile. It is relatively simple, is easy to set up, and takes a minimal amount of time to do. To set up the test, an 18-inch platform is used. The patient is instructed to step with both feet onto the platform at a rate of about 30 times per minute (a metronome is used for cadence). The patient is made to step for 3.5 minutes at a pace of 2 seconds per step and then sprint as fast as possible for 30 seconds (total time: 4 minutes). The patient then immediately sits down in a chair and relaxes for 3 minutes while the pulse is determined. The pulse is taken at 30, 60, 120, and 180 seconds after the exercise. The index formula for the pulse is

$$\text{Index} = \frac{\text{duration of exercise (in seconds)} \times 100}{2 \times \text{the sum of any three pulse counts}}$$

The higher the index, the better the person's fitness. If the index is less than 65, the patient is not ready for sports activity. Cooper[53,54] developed an indirect method for measuring fitness using a 12-minute walk-run test. From the distance covered in 12 minutes, he developed tables for men and women that showed the patient's fitness category. He later went on to use a similar method for activities such as swimming and cycling.

Other, more detailed tests may be done, including a respiratory quotient test (direct method), the Astrand nomogram (indirect method), and the Sjostrad PWC$_{170}$ test (indirect method).[55]

Although not commonly done except in high-level sports, maximum tests are necessary to get the most complete diagnostic data on a patient's response to exercise. This is important because half the abnormalities are missed if the test stops at 85% of predicted maximum heart rate, which the simplest tests tend to do.[56] Even if a maximum test is performed, 10 to 15% of the normal population may show an abnormal response.[56] It must be remembered that cardiovascular tests clear the subject only up to the heart rate at which he or she has been tested. In most cases, maximum testing is not done, but if a person is showing abnormalities, such a test may be done as a second diagnostic procedure. These tests must, however, be performed under very controlled conditions, where there are proper facilities to handle cardiac emergencies.

Although anaerobic fitness is not directly related to the cardiovascular system, it is tested through its effects on the cardiovascular system. If the proposed activity, exercise, or sport is primarily anaerobic, consideration must be given to including this measurement as part of the profile.[57]

Agility, Balance, and Reaction Time

For activities requiring agility, balance, and reaction time, the physical fitness profile should include these items. Ideally, testing should be related to the specific activity. Agility is defined as the ability to change directions rapidly when moving at a high rate of speed.[8] Agility and balance tests are often measured by time or accuracy (e.g., correct two out of three).[8, 58]

Maturation and Growth

Maturation assessment is a method of determining how far a patient has progressed toward physical maturity; it can be used as an injury prevention measure by matching athletes for contact sports. It also helps to identify periods of rapid growth.[59–61] Maturation profiling should not be used to push children into specific activities unless chosen by the child, and it should not be used to exclude a child unless documented evidence demonstrates unacceptable risk for the child.[62] In adolescents, growth patterns can have an effect on participation in activities, exercise, and sport and may have a role in affecting injury

> **Agility and Balance Tests**
> ***
> - Carioca
> - Run-and-cut drills
> - Back-pedal and throw at stationary or moving target
> - Kick at stationary or moving target (different distances)
> - One-arm spin
> - Shuttle drills
> - Pivoting drills
> - Blocking drills
> - Figure-of-eight running
> - Front-to-back and side-to-side hops
> - Sidestep tests
> - Beam-walking tests

patterns. For example, a growth spurt for a gymnast may adversely affect balance and flexibility. Pubertal growth accounts for 20 to 25% of final adult height, and pubertal weight gain accounts for 50% of ideal adult weight.[32]

Skeletal development is usually measured by wrist x-rays, using the *Radiographic Atlas of Skeletal Development of the Wrist and Hand*, by W.W. Greulich and S.U. Pyle,[63] for interpretation.

The most common method of measuring maturation in males and females is the Tanner scale.[15, 59, 64] The five stages of the Tanner scale are based on pictoral standards of genitalia and pubic hair for males and breast development and pubic hair for females (Figs. 17–3,

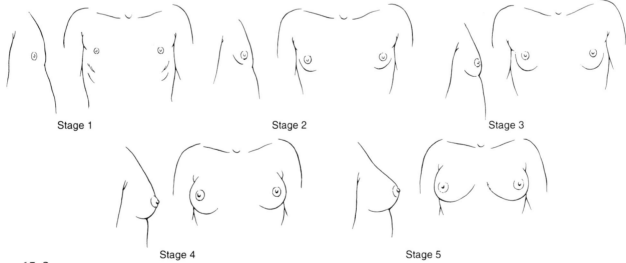

Stage 1   Stage 2   Stage 3

Stage 4   Stage 5

Figure 17–3

Breast development in girls. The development of the mammae can be divided into five stages: In *stage 1*, only the nipple is raised above the level of the breast (as in the child). In *stage 2*, the budding stage, there is bud-shaped elevation of the areola. On palpation, a fairly hard button can be felt that is disk- or cherry-shaped. The aerola is increased in diameter, and the surrounding area is slightly elevated. In *stage 3*, there is further elevation of the mammae; the areolar diameter is further increased, and the shape of mammae is visibly feminine. In *stage 4*, fat deposits increase, and the areola forms a secondary elevation above that of the breast. This secondary mound occurs in approximately half of all girls and in some cases persists in adulthood. In *stage 5*, the adult stage, the areola usually subsides to the level of the breast and is strongly pigmented. (From Halpern, B., T. Blackburn, B. Incremona, and S. Weintraub: Preparticipation sports physicals. In Zachazewski, J.E., D.J. Magee, and W.S. Quillen [eds.]: Athletic Injuries and Rehabilitation. Philadelphia, W.B. Saunders Co., 1996, p. 855.)

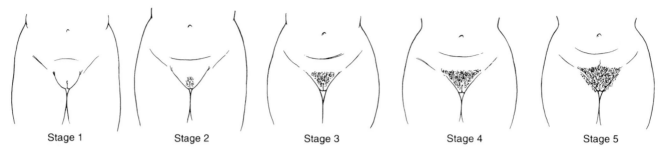

| Stage 1 | Stage 2 | Stage 3 | Stage 4 | Stage 5 |

Figure 17–4

Pubic hair development in females. In the development of pubic hair, five stages can be distinguished. In *stage* 1, there is no growth of pubic hair. In *stage* 2, initial, scarcely pigmented hair is present, especially along the labia (not visible on black-and-white photograph). In *stage* 3, sparse dark, visibly pigmented, curly pubic hair is present on the labia. In *stage* 4, hair that is adult in type but not in extent is present. In *stage* 5, there is lateral spreading (type and spread of hair are adult). (From Halpern, B., T. Blackburn, B. Incremona, and S. Weintraub: Preparticipation sports physicals. In Zachazewski, J.E., D.J. Magee, and W.S. Quillen [eds.]: Athletic Injuries and Rehabilitation. Philadelphia, W.B. Saunders Co., 1996, p. 855.)

17–4, 17–5, and Table 17–9). Some people have recommended that collision sports not be allowed for boys until they reach the level 5 of development. For females, onset of menstruation is another suitable index of maturity and maturation.

Body Composition and Anthropometry

Body composition profiling is designed to provide a relatively detailed analysis of muscle, fat, and bone mass.[61, 65] Anthropometry may be used to determine the patient's body type (mesomorphic, endomorphic, and ectomorphic) to see whether he or she is properly suited for the desired activity, exercise, sport, or position played in sport.

Anthropometry also involves body fat measurements, such as skinfold measurements or underwater weighing.[66] Of the two, skinfold measurement is more common because it is easier and faster. Seven skinfold sites are most commonly used (Fig. 17–6), although some people believe that measurement at three sites is sufficient (i.e., a different three for males and females).[66] Most males should fall below 12 to 15% body fat. Endurance athletes (gymnasts, wrestlers) are often below 7%. Football, baseball, and soccer players average 10 to 12%.[67] No one should be below 5% body fat. Generally, if the percentage of body fat is greater than the upper normal limit of 14% for males and 17% for females, the patient should be put on a weight loss program or weight

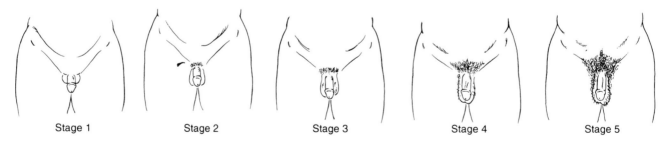

| Stage 1 | Stage 2 | Stage 3 | Stage 4 | Stage 5 |

Figure 17–5

Genital and pubic hair development in males. The development of external genitalia and pubic hair can be divided into five stages. In *stage* 1, the testes, scrotum, and penis are the same size and shape as in the young child, and there is no growth of pubic hair (hair in pubic area is no different from that on the rest of the abdomen). In *stage* 2, there is enlargement of the scrotum and testes. The skin of scrotum becomes redder, thinner, and wrinkled. The penis is no longer (or is scarcely so). Pubic hair is slightly pigmented. In *stage* 3, there is enlargement of the penis, especially in length, further enlargement of testes, and descent of scrotum. Dark, definitely pigmented, curly pubic hair is present around the base of penis. Stage 3 can be photographed. In *stage* 4, there is continued enlargement of the penis and sculpturing of the glans, with increased pigmentation of the scrotum. This stage is sometimes best described as not quite adult. Pubic hair is definitely adult in type but not in extent (no further than the inguinal fold). In *stage* 5, the adult stage, the scrotum is ample, and the penis reaches almost to the bottom of the scrotum. Pubic hair spreads to the medial surface of the thighs but not upward. In 80% of men, hair spreads along the linea alba. (From Halpern, B., T. Blackburn, B. Incremona, and S. Weintraub: Preparticipation sports physicals. In Zachazewski, J.E., D.J. Magee, and W.S. Quillen [eds.]: Athletic Injuries and Rehabilitation. Philadelphia, W.B. Saunders Co., 1996, p. 855.)

Table 17-9
Maturity Staging Guidelines

Boys Stage	Pubic Hair	Penis	Testis	Girls Stage	Pubic Hair	Breasts
1	None	Preadolescent (infantile)	—	1	Preadolescent (none)	Preadolescent (no germinal button)
2	Slight, long, slight pigmentation	Slight enlargement	Enlarged scrotum, pink slight rugae	2	Sparse, lightly pigmented, straight medial border of labia	Breast and papilla elevated as small mound; areolar diameter increased
3	Darker, starts to curl, small amount	Longer	Larger	3	Darker, beginning to curl, increased	Breast and areola enlarged; no contour separation
4	Coarse, curly, adult type, but less quantity	Increase in glans size and breadth of penis	Larger, darker scrotum	4	Coarse, curly, abundant, but less than adult	Areola and papilla form secondary mound
5	Adult, spread to inner thighs	Adult	Adult	5	Adult female triangle and spread to medial surface	Mature, nipple projects, areola part of general breast contour

From Tanner, J.M.: Growth and Adolescence. Oxford, Blackwell Scientific Pub., 1962.

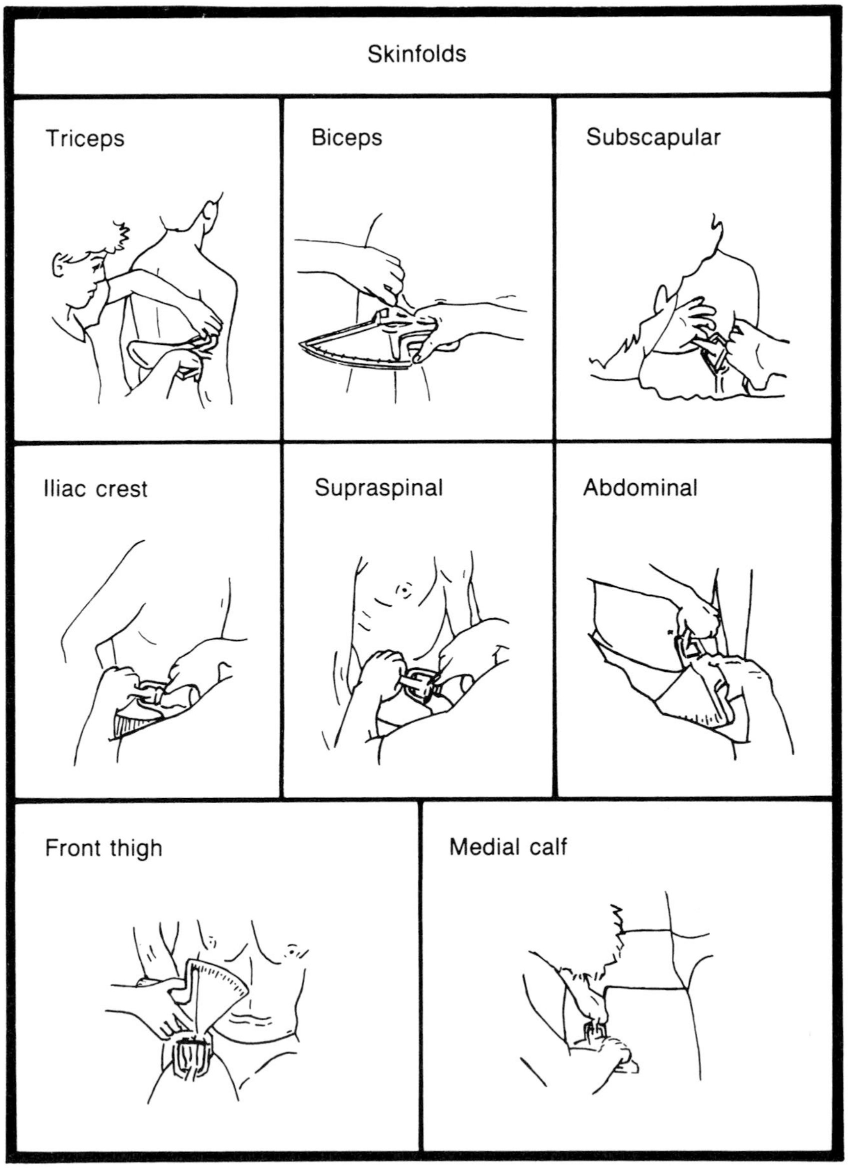

Figure 17-6
Skinfold sites from measuring body fat. (Reprinted, by permission, from Ross, W.D., and M.J. Marfell-Jones: Kinanthropometry. In MacDougal, J.D., H.A. Wenger, and H.J. Green [eds.]: Physiological Testing of the High Performance Athlete, 2nd ed. Champaign, Illinois, Human Kinetics, 1991, p. 238.)

training to increase lean body mass; but again, this depends on the activity in which the patient wishes to participate.

Other methods of body composition measurement include girth measurements, bone diameter measurements, ultrasound measurement, and arm radiograph measurements.[65]

Should the Individual Be Allowed to Participate?

For any preparticipation evaluation, the physician is the final arbitrator. The physician can decide that no participation is allowed; that the patient failed with conditions (i.e., if the conditions are corrected, the decision will be reconsidered); that limited participation (in specific sports or activities) is allowed; that clearance is withheld until additional tests, rehabilitation, or other clearances are completed; or that full, unlimited participation is allowed.[9, 68] In making the decision about participation in an activity, health care professionals must realize that virtually everyone is suited for some activity, exercise, or sport, and each person should be matched as nearly as possible to the activities that are appropriate in terms of ability, physical makeup and maturity, and emotional maturity.

Any decision as to whether someone should be allowed to participate in an activity must be based on accurate diagnosis of the condition, knowledge of the disease process for the condition, knowledge of the sport, knowledge of the physical needs of the patient and the activity, and direct evaluation of the individual. The examiner must also keep in mind the rights of the handicapped and the limits of informed consent. Although standards are given for participation, in the end, the health care team must make their final decision on an individual basis, being primarily concerned with the health and safety of the patient. If necessary, a clearance form may be completed for the patient's file, outlining the physician's decisions.

Any athlete with a solitary paired organ, such as an eye, kidney, or testicle, should not take part in contact sports, especially if the organ is abnormal. Children should be channeled into noncontact sports. High-caliber or older athletes know the rules and should make their own decision. Table 17–10 provides a list of conditions that are contraindications to specific types of activity.[10, 15]

Conditions of Passing or Failing Preparticipation Evaluation[9]

Passed (91 to 95%)
- Unconditional
- No reservations
- Cleared for all sports and all levels of exertion
- No preexisting or current medical problems
- No contraindications for collision or contact sports

Passed With Conditions
- Has a medical problem needing follow-up
- Can participate in sports at present
- Follow-up must be made before sports participation

Passed With Reservations
- No collision sports (hockey, rugby, lacrosse)
- No contact sports (football, basketball, wrestling)

Failed With Reservations
- Not cleared for REQUESTED sport (other sports can be considered)
- Collision not permitted, contact to be limited
- Contact not permitted, noncontact sports allowed

Failed With Conditions
- Can be reconsidered after medical problem is addressed

Failed (<1%)
- Unconditional
- No reservations
- Cannot be cleared for any sport or any level of competition

Table 17–10
Conditions Commonly Disqualifying an Athlete From Participation in Sports

Conditions	Type of Sport			
	Collision*	Contact†	Noncontact‡	Others§
Eyes				
Absence of one eye	??	??	—	—
Congenital glaucoma	X	X	—	—
Retinal detachment	X	X	—	—
Severe myopia	?	?	—	—
Musculoskeletal				
Acute inflammatory conditions	X	X	X	X
Spinal instability	X	X	?	?
Congenital or growth abnormalities that are incompatible with demands of sport	X	X	X	—
Chronic or unhealed conditions (unless cleared by physician)	X	X	X	X
Neurological				
Uncontrolled convulsive disorder	X	X	X	?
Controlled convulsive disorder	?	?	?	?
Repeated concussions	X	X	—	—
Serious head trauma	X	X	—	—
Previous head surgery	X	X	—	—
Transient quadriplegia (unless cleared by physician)	X	X	—	—
Cardiovascular				
Acute infection	X	X	X	X
Cardiomegaly	X	X	X	X
Enlarged spleen	X	X	—	—
Hemorrhage (bleeding) disorders	X	X	X	—
Heart abnormalities (unless cleared by cardiologist)	X	X	X	X
Organic hypertension	X	X	X	X
Previous heart surgery (unless cleared by cardiologist)	X	X	X	X
Pulmonary				
Acute infection	X	X	X	X
Pulmonary insufficiency	X	X	X	X
Uncontrolled asthma (unless cleared by pulmonary physician)	X	X	X	X
Urogenital				
Absence of one kidney	??	??	—	—
Acute infection	X	X	X	X
Enlarged liver	X	X	—	—
Hernia (inguinal or femoral, unless cleared by physician)	X	X	X	—
Renal disease	X	X	X	X
Absent or undescended testicle (unless cleared by physician)	??	??	—	—
Gastrointestinal				
Jaundice	X	X	X	X
Dermatological				
Acute infection (e.g., boils, herpes simplex, impetigo)	X	X	?	?
General or systemic disease				
Acute systemic infection or illness	?	?	?	?
Uncontrolled diabetes	X	X	X	X
Physical immaturity (relative to level of competition)	X	X	—	—

* Examples include boxing, football, hockey (ice and field), rugby.

† Examples include baseball, basketball, lacrosse, martial arts, rodeo, soccer, volleyball, wrestling.

‡ Examples include dance, rowing, skiing, squash, swimming, tennis, track/cross-country.

§ Examples include archery, bowling, golf, shooting, track and field events.

? = Depends on individual case and clearance by physician; ?? = Athlete may compete if athlete knows risks and informed consent form is completed (protective equipment may be necessary); X = Participation prohibited; — = Participation permitted.

Adapted from the American Medical Association Committee on Medical Aspects of Sports: Medical Evaluation of the Athlete: A Guide. Chicago, American Medical Association, 1966, pp. 7–8.

References

Cited References

1. Superko, H.R., E. Bernauer, and J. Voss: Effects of a mandatory health screening and physical maintenance program for law enforcement officers. Phys. Sportsmed. 16:99–109, 1988.
2. Binda, C.: Precamp physical exams: Their value may be greater than you think. Phys. Sportsmed. 17:167–169, 1989.
3. Gurry, M., A. Pappas, J. Michaels, et al.: A comprehensive preseason fitness evaluation for professional baseball players. Phys. Sportsmed. 13:63–74, 1985.
4. Tanji, T.L.: The preparticipation exam: Special concerns for the Special Olympics. Phys. Sportsmed. 19:61–68, 1991.
5. Hudson, P.B.: Preparticipation screening of Special Olympics athletes. Phys. Sportsmed. 16:97–104, 1988.
6. Hunter, S.C.: Preparticipation physical examination. In Griffin, L.Y. (ed.): Orthopedic Knowledge Update: Sports Medicine. Rosemont, Illinois, American Academy of Orthopaedic Surgeons, 1994.
7. Committee on Sports Medicine: Recommendations for participation in competitive sports. Pediatrics 81:737–739, 1988.
8. Sanders, B., and W.C. Nemeth: Preparticipation physical examination. J. Orthop. Sports Phys. Ther. 23:144–163, 1996.
9. American Academy of Orthopaedic Surgeons: Athletic Training and Sports Medicine. Rosemont, Illinois, A.A.O.S., 1991.
10. Harvey, J.: The preparticipation examination of the child athlete. Clin. Sports Med. 1:353–369, 1982.
11. DuRaaut, R.H., C. Seymore, C.W. Linder, et al.: The preparticipation examination of athletes: Comparison of single and multiple examiners. Am. J. Dis. Child. 139:657–666, 1985.
12. Sampler, P.: Preparticipation exams: Are they worth the time and trouble. Phys. Sportsmed. 14:180–187, 1986.
13. St. Rauss, R.H., M.D. Johnson, W.B. Kibler, and D. Smith: Keys to successful preparticipation exams. Phys. Sportsmed. 21:109–123, 1993.
14. Feinstein, R.A., E.J. Soileau, and W.A. Daniel: A national survey of preparticipation physical examination requirements. Phys. Sportsmed. 16:51–59, 1988.
15. McKeag, D.B.: Preparticipation screening of the potential athlete. Clin. Sports Med. 8:373–397, 1989.
16. Stanley, K.: Preparticipation evaluation of the young athlete. In Stanitski, C.L., J.C. DeLee, and D. Drez (eds.): Pediatric and Adolescent Sports Medicine. Philadelphia, W.B. Saunders Co., 1994.
17. Smilkstein, G.: Health evaluation of high school athletes. Phys. Sportsmed. 9:73–80, 1981.
18. McKeag, D.B.: Preseason physical examination for the prevention of sports injuries. Sports Med. 2:413–431, 1985.
19. Kaplan, N.M., R.B. Deveraux, and H.S. Miller: Systemic hyperextension. Med. Sci. Sports Exerc. 26:S268–S270, 1994.
20. Zabetakis, P.M.: Profiling the hypertensive patient in sports. Clin. Sports Med. 3:137–152, 1984.
21. Bonci, C.M., and R. Ryan: Preparticipation screening in intercollegiate athletics. Postgraduate Advances in Sports Medicine. Philadelphia, University of Pennsylvania Medical School and Forum Medicum, Inc., 1988.
22. Dorsen, P.J.: Should athletes with one eye, kidney or testicle play contact sports? Phys. Sportsmed. 14:130–138, 1986.
23. Halpern, B., T. Blackburn, B. Incremona, and S. Weintraub: Preparticipation sports physicals. In Zachazewski, J.E., D.J. Magee, and W.S. Quillen (eds.): Athletic Injuries and Rehabilitation. Philadelphia, W.B. Saunders Co., 1996.
24. Strong, W.B., and D. Steed: Cardiovascular evaluation of the young athlete. Pediatr. Clin. North Am. 29:1325–1339, 1982.
25. Huston, T.P., J.C. Puffer, and W.M. Rodney: The athletic heart syndrome. New. Engl. J. Med. 313:24–32, 1985.
26. Salem, D.N., and J.M. Isner: Cardiac screening in athletes. Orthop. Clin. North Am. 11:687–695, 1980.
27. Pflieger, K.L., and W.B. Strong: Screening for heart murmurs: What's normal and what's not. Phys. Sportsmed. 20:71–81, 1992.
28. Braden, D.S., and W.B. Strong: Preparticipation screening for sudden cardiac death in high school and college athletes. Phys. Sportsmed. 16:128–144, 1988.
29. Mitchell, J.H., W.L. Hashell, and P.B. Raven: Classification of sports. Med. Sci. Sports Exerc. 26:S242–S245, 1994.
30. Belman, M.J., and R.R. King: Pulmonary profiling in exercise. Clin. Sports Med. 3:119–136, 1984.
31. Lombardo, J.A.: Preparticipation physical evaluation. Prim. Care 11:3–21, 1984.
32. Johnson, M.D.: Tailoring the preparticipation exam to female athletes. Phys. Sportsmed. 20:61–72, 1992.
33. Slavin, J.L.: Assessing athletes' nutritional status: Making it part of the sports medicine physical. Phys. Sportsmed. 19:79–94, 1991.
34. Nelson, M.A.: The child athlete with chronic disease. In Stanitski, C.L., J.C. DeLee, and D. Drez (eds.): Pediatric and Adolescent Sports Medicine. Philadelphia, W.B. Saunders Co., 1994.
35. Nicholas, J.A.: The value of sports profiling. Clin. Sports Med. 3:3–10, 1984.
36. Marino, M.: Profiling swimmers. Clin. Sports Med. 3:211–229, 1984.
37. Sapega, A.A., J. Minkoff, M. Valsamis, and J.A. Nicholas: Musculoskeletal performance testing and profiling of elite competitive fencers. Clin. Sports Med. 3:231–244, 1984.
38. Bridgman, R.: A coach's guide to testing for athletic attributes. National Strength and Conditioning Assoc. J. 13:34–37, 1991.
39. Gleim, G.W.: The profiling of professional football players. Clin. Sports Med. 3:185–197, 1984.
40. Skinner, J.S.: Exercise Testing and Exercise Prescription for Special Cases: Theoretical Basis and Clinical Application. Philadelphia, Lea & Febiger, 1993.
41. Hershman, E.: The profile for prevention of musculoskeletal injury. Clin. Sports Med. 3:65–84, 1984.
42. MacDougal, J.D., and H.A. Wenger: The purpose of physiological testing. In MacDougal, J.D., H.A. Wenger, and H.J. Green (eds.): Physiological Testing of the High Performance Athlete. Champaign, Illinois, Human Kinetics, 1991.
43. Marino, M., and G.W. Gleim: Muscle strength and fiber typing. Clin. Sports Med. 3:85–100, 1984.
44. Sale, D.G.: Testing strength and power. In MacDougal, J.D., H.A. Wenger, and H.J. Green (eds.): Physiological Testing of the High Performance Athlete. Champaign, Illinois, Human Kinetics, 1991.
45. Corbin, C.B.: Flexibility. Clin. Sports Med. 3:101–117, 1994.
46. Hubley-Kozey, C.L.: Testing flexibility. In MacDougal, J.D., H.A. Wenger, and H.J. Green (eds.): Physiological Testing of the High Performance Athlete. Champaign, Illinois, Human Kinetics, 1991.
47. Kibler, W.B., T.J. Chandler, T. Uhl, and R.E. Maddux: A musculoskeletal approach to the preparticipation physical examination: Preventing injury and improving performance. Am. J. Sports Med. 17:525–531, 1989.
48. Carter, C., and J. Wilkinson: Persistent joint laxity and congenital dislocation of the hip. J. Bone Joint Surg. Br. 46:40–45, 1969.
49. Nicholas, J.A.: Risk factors, sports medicine and the orthopedic system: An overview. J. Sports Med. 3:243–259, 1975.
50. Squires, R.W., and A.A. Bove: Cardiovascular profiling. Clin. Sports Med. 3:11–29, 1984.
51. Wasserman, K., J.E. Hansen, D.Y. Sue, B.J. Whipp, and R. Casaburi: Principles of Exercise Testing and Interpretation. Philadelphia, Lea & Febiger, 1994.

52. Thoden, J.S.: Testing aerobic power. *In* MacDougal, J.D., H.A. Wenger, and H.J. Green (eds.): Physiological Testing of the High Performance Athlete. Champaign, Illinois, Human Kinetics, 1991.

53. Cooper, K.H.: The New Aerobics. New York, Bantam Books., 1970.

54. Cooper, K.M.: A means of assessing maximal oxygen intake. JAMA 203:201–204, 1968.

55. Astrand, P.D., and K. Rodahl: Textbook of Work Physiology. Toronto, McGraw-Hill Book Co., 1977.

56. Kowal, D.M., and W.L. Daniels: Recommendations for the screening of military personnel over 35 years of age for physical training programs. Am. J. Sports Med. 7:186–190, 1979.

57. Bouchard, C., A.W. Taylor, J.A. Simoneau, and S. Dulac: Testing anaerobic power and capacity. *In* MacDougal, J.D., H.A. Wenger, and H.J. Green (eds.): Physiological Testing of the High Performance Athlete. Champaign, Illinois, Human Kinetics, 1991.

58. Tippett, S.R., and M.L. Voight: Functional Progressions for Sports Rehabilitation. Champaign, Illinois, Human Kinetics, 1995.

59. Caine, D.J., and J. Broekhoff: Maturity assessment: A viable preventive measure against physical and psychological insult to the young athlete. Phys. Sportsmed. 15:67–80, 1987.

60. Whieldon, D.: Maturity sorting: New balance for young athletes. Phys. Sportsmed. 6:127–132, 1978.

61. Ross, W.D., and M.J. Marfell-Jones: Kinanthropometry. *In* MacDougal, J.D., H A. Wenger, and H.J. Green (eds.): Physiological Testing of the High Performance Athlete. Champaign, Illinois, Human Kinetics, 1991.

62. Goldberg, B., and R. Boiardo: Profiling children for sports participation. Clin. Sports Med. 3:153–169, 1984.

63. Greulich, W.W., and S.U. Pyle: Radiographic Atlas of Skeletal Development of the Wrist and Hand. Stanford, California, Stanford University Press, 1959.

64. Tanner, J.M.: Growth and Adolescence. Oxford, Blackwell Scientific Pub., 1962.

65. Katch, F.I., and V.L. Katch: The body composition profile: Techniques of measurement and applications. Clin. Sports Med. 3:31–63, 1984.

66. Jackson, A.S., and M.L. Pollock: Practical assessment of body composition. Phys. Sportsmed. 13:772–90, 1985.

67. Coleman, A.E.: Skinfold estimates of body fat in major league baseball players. Phys. Sportsmed. 9:77–82, 1981.

68. Magnes, S.A., J.M. Henderson, and S.C. Hunter: What conditions limit sports participation: Experience with 10,540 athletes. Phys. Sportsmed. 20:143–160, 1992.

General References

Abdenour, T.E., and N.J. Weir: Medical assessment of the prospective student athlete. Athletic Training, Summer: 122–123, 1986.

Armstrong, C.: Preseason medical examinations and an injury recording profile. Can. Athl. Ther. Assoc. J. Fall:13–14, 1981.

Boissonnault, W.G., and C. Bass: Medical screening examination: Not optional for physical therapists. J. Orthop. Sports Phys. Ther. 14:241–242, 1991.

Brown, R.T.: Targeting teen health problems: Maximizing the preparticipation exam. Phys. Sportsmed. 21:77–80, 1993.

Cahill, B.R., and E.H. Griffith: Effect of preseason conditioning on the incidence and severity of high school football knee injuries. Am. J. Sports Med. 6:180–184, 1978.

Cheitlen, M.D., P.S. Douglas, and W.W. Parmley: Acquired valvular heart disease. Med. Sci. Sports Exerc. 26:S254–S260, 1994.

Clement, J.D., R.A. Graves, R.M. Lane, and J. Weisz: Minimum standards of physical fitness required of candidates for collision sports at the University of Maine. J. Maine Med. Assoc. 58:121–123, 1967.

Dyment, P.G.: New guidelines for sports participation. Phys. Sportsmed. 16:45–46, 1988.

Eggart, J.S., D. Leigh, and G. Vargamini: Preseason athletic physical examination. *In* Gould, J.A. (ed.): Orthopedic and Sports Physical Therapy. St. Louis, C.V. Mosby Co., 1990.

Feinstein, R.A., E. Colvin, and M.K. Oh: Echo cardiographic screening as part of a preparticipation examination. Clin. J. Sports Med. 3:149–152, 1993.

Feiring, D.C., and G.L. Derscheid: The role of preseason conditioning in preventing athletic injuries. Clin. Sports Med. 8:361–372, 1989.

Gettman, L.R., T.W. Storer, and R.D. Ward: Fitness changes in professional football players during preseason conditioning. Phys. Sportsmed. 15:92–101, 1987.

Goldberg, B., A. Saraniti, P. Witman, M. Gavin, and J.A. Nicholas: Preparticipation sports assessment: An objective evaluation. Pediatrics 66:736–745, 1980.

Gomolak, C.: Problems in matching young athletes: Baby fat, peach fuzz, muscle and mustache. Phys. Sportsmed. 3:96–98, 1975.

Graham, T.P., J.T. Bricker, F.W. James, and W.B. Strong: Congenital heart disease. Med. Sci. Sports Exerc. 26:S246–S253, 1994.

Hutter, A.M.: Cardiovascular abnormalities in the athlete: The role of the physician. Med. Sci. Sports Exerc. 26:S227–S229, 1994

Lin, L.Y.: Scuba divers with disabilities, challenges, medical protocols, and ethics. Phys. Sportsmed. 15:224–235, 1987.

Linder, C.W., R.H. DuRant, R.M. Seklecki, and W.B. Strong: Preparticipation health screening of young athletes: Results of 1268 examinations. Am. J. Sports Med. 9:187–193, 1981.

Maron, B.J., J.M. Isner, and W.J. McKenna: Hypertrophic cardiomyelopathy myocarditis and other myopericardial diseases and mitral valve prolapse. Med. Sci. Sports Exerc. 26:S261–S267, 1994.

Minkoff, J.: Evaluating parameters of a professional hockey team. Am. J. Sports Med. 10:285–292, 1982.

Mitchell, J.H., G. Blomquist, W.L. Haskell, et al.: Classification of sports. J. Am. Coll. Cardiol. 6:1198–1199, 1985.

Mitten, M.J.: Athletic participation with a contagious blood-borne disease. Clin. J. Sports Med. 5:153–154, 1995.

Moore, M.: Preparticipation exams: Just "a lick and a promise"? Phys. Sportsmed. 10:113–116, 1982.

Round Table: The office examination of the athlete. Phys. Sportsmed. 4:86–105, 1976.

Savastano, A.A.: Physical basis for restriction of participation in sports. J. Maine Med. Assoc. 55:146–148, 1964.

Shephard, R.J., S. Thomas, and I. Weller: The Canadian home fitness test: 1991 update. Sports Med. 11:358–366, 1991.

Sterner, T.G., and E.J. Burke: Body fat assessment: A comparison of visual estimation and skinfold techniques. Phys. Sportsmed. 14:101–107, 1986.

Taunton, J.E., and D.B. Clement: The medical care of the elite athlete. Medicine North Am. Fall:84–90, 1987.

Thompson, P.D., F.J. Klocke, B.D. Levine, and S.P. Van Camp: Coronary artery disease. Med. Sci. Sports Exerc. 26:S271–S275, 1994.

Weidenbener, E.J., M.D. Krauss, B.F. Waller, and C.P. Taliercio: Incorporation of screening echocardiography in the preparticipation exam. Clin. J. Sports Med. 5:86–89, 1995.

Weistart, J.C.: Legal consequences of standard setting for competitive athletes with cardiovascular abnormalities. J. Am. College Cardiol. 6:1191–1197, 1985.

Zipes, D.P., and A. Garson: Arrhythmias. Med. Sci. Sports Exerc. 26:S276–S283, 1994.

Index